D0470765

POLICY & POLITICS

in Nursing and Health Care

Sixth Edition

Diana J. Mason, RN, PhD, FAAN
Rudin Professor of Nursing
Co-Director, Center for Health, Media, & Policy
Hunter College
City University of New York
New York, New York

Judith K. Leavitt, RN, MEd, FAAN
Health Policy Consultant
Barnardsville, North Carolina

Mary W. Chaffee, RN, PhD, FAAN
Captain, Nurse Corps, U.S. Navy (Retired)
Brewster, Massachusetts

ELSEVIER
SAUNDERS

SAUNDERS

3251 Riverport Lane
St. Louis, Missouri 63043

POLICY & POLITICS IN NURSING AND HEALTH CARE   ISBN: 978-0-323-24241-7

Copyright © 2014, 2012, 2007, 2002, 1998, 1993, 1985 by Saunders, an imprint of Elsevier Inc.

All rights reserved. No part of this publication may be reproduced or transmitted in any form or by any means, electronic or mechanical, including photocopy, recording, or any information storage and retrieval system, without permission in writing from the publisher. Details on how to seek permission, further information about the Publisher's permissions policies, and our arrangements with organizations such as the Copyright Clearance Center and the Copyright Licensing Agency can be found at our website: *www.elsevier.com/premissions.*

This book and the individual contributions contained in it are protected under copyright by the Publisher (other than as may be noted herein).

Notices

Knowledge and best practice in this field are constantly changing. As new research and experience broaden our understanding, changes in research methods, professional practices, or medical treatment may become necessary.

Practitioners and researchers must always rely on their own experience and knowledge in evaluating and using any information, methods, compounds, or experiments described herein. In using such information or methods they should be mindful of their own safety and the safety of others, including parties for whom they have a professional responsibility.

With respect to any drug or pharmaceutical products identified, readers are advised to check the most current information provided (i) on procedures featured or (ii) by the manufacturer of each product to be administered, to verify the recommended dose or formula, the method and duration of administration, and contraindications. It is the responsibility of practitioners, relying on their own experience and knowledge of their patients, to make diagnoses, to determine dosages and the best treatment for each individual patient, and to take all appropriate safety precautions.

To the fullest extent of the law, neither the Publisher nor the authors, contributors, or editors, assume any liability for any injury and/or damage to persons or property as a matter of products liability, negligence or otherwise, or from any use or operation of any methods, products, instructions, or ideas contained in the material herein.

The views expressed in this book are those of the authors and do not reflect the official policy or position of the Department of Defense, Department of Health and Human Services, Department of Veterans Affairs, any other government agency, or the U.S. Government.

Library of Congress Cataloging-in-Publication Data
Policy and politics in nursing and health care / [editors] Diana J. Mason, Judith K. Leavitt, Mary W. Chaffee. —6th ed.
    p. ; cm.
  Rev. ed. of: Policy & politics in nursing and health care. 5th ed. c2007.
  Includes bibliographical references and index.
  ISBN 978-0-323-24241-7 (pbk.)
  1. Nurses—Political activity—United States.   2. Nursing—Political aspects—United States.   3. Medical policy—United States.   4. Medical care—Political aspects—United States.   I. Mason, Diana J., 1948- II. Leavitt, Judith K. (Judith Kline)   III. Chaffee, Mary W.   IV. Policy & politics in nursing and health care.
  [DNLM: 1. Nursing—United States.   2. Delivery of Health Care—United States.   3. Politics—United States. 4. Public Policy—United States.   WY 16 AA1]
  RT86.5.P58 2012
  362.17'3—dc22

                                                        2011006309

Editor: Maureen Iannuzzi
Associate Developmental Editor: Julia Curcio
Publishing Services Manager: Jeff Patterson
Senior Project Manager: Clay S. Broeker
Designer: Paula Catalano

Printed in the United States of America

Last digit is the print number: 9   8   7   6   5   4   3   2   1

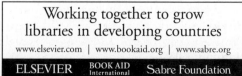

Working together to grow
libraries in developing countries

www.elsevier.com | www.bookaid.org | www.sabre.org

ELSEVIER   BOOK AID International   Sabre Foundation

About the Editors

Diana J. Mason, RN, PhD, FAAN, is the Rudin Professor of Nursing at the Hunter College-Bellevue School of Nursing of the City University of New York, where she directs the Hunter College Center for Health, Media, & Policy. For over 10 years, she served as Editor-in-Chief of the *American Journal of Nursing,* and she continues in an emeritus capacity. Under her leadership, the journal received numerous awards for editorial excellence and dissemination, culminating in the journal being selected by the Specialized Libraries Association in 2009 as one of the 100 most influential journals of the century in biology and medicine—the only nursing journal to be selected for this distinction.

In 2009, she was appointed to the National Advisory Committee for Kaiser Health News. Since 1986, she has been one of the producers and moderators of "Healthstyles," an award-winning, live radio program in New York City. She was project director for the WBAI-Global Kids' Sound Partners for Community Health Initiative (funded by the Benton and Robert Wood Johnson Foundations) to train New York City youth in producing radio programs on preventing teen substance abuse.

As a researcher, she published a series of studies on managed care arrangements with nurse practitioners. From 2006 to 2010, she served as Secretary for the American Academy of Nursing, and she continues to chair its "Raise The Voice" campaign, an initiative funded in part by the Robert Wood Johnson Foundation and the Independence Foundation for identifying and making visible to policymakers and journalists the innovative models of care developed by nurses and the public and private policies that are needed to sustain and support them.

Dr. Mason is the recipient of numerous awards and honors, including an Honorary Doctorate of Humane Letters from Long Island University; an Honorary Doctorate of Science from West Virginia University; fellowship in the American Academy of Nursing, the New York Academy of Medicine, and the West Virginia University Academy of Distinguished Alumni; and the Pioneering Spirit Award from the American Association of Critical Care Nurses. She is a graduate of West Virginia University School of Nursing (BSN, 1970), St. Louis University (MSN, 1977), and New York University (PhD, 1987).

Judith K. Leavitt, RN, MEd, FAAN, is a health policy consultant. She retired as Associate Professor from the University of Mississippi Medical Center, School of Nursing in 2005. She was formerly Executive Director of Generations United, a national organization dedicated to intergenerational policies and programs. She served on the National Advisory Council on Education and Practice for the Division of Nursing, U.S. Department of Health and Human Services. Ms. Leavitt was selected by President Clinton to serve on the Health Professional Advisory Group to the White House Task Force on Health Care Reform. She served as the upstate coordinator for Geraldine Ferraro's 1992 New York campaign for the United States Senate and was chairperson of the American Nurses Association Political Action Committee. She was chair of the New York State Nurses for Political Action and was instrumental in the founding of the New York State Nurses Association's Political Action Committee.

Ms. Leavitt is a noted speaker and author of extensive writings on policy and politics. Her many awards include the University of Mississippi Medical Center Nelson Award for Teaching Excellence, the Chancellor's Award for Teaching Excellence from the State of New York, the Health Policy Award from the Division of Nursing at New York University, the Legislative Award from the New York State Nurses Association, and the Mississippi Nurses Association Nurse of the Year, and she is a Fellow of the American Academy of Nursing. Ms. Leavitt earned her BSN from the University of Pennsylvania and her MEd from Teacher's College, Columbia University.

Mary W. Chaffee, RN, PhD, FAAN, served in the U.S. Navy Nurse Corps for 25 years. In her final assignment on active duty, she was the Disaster Research Coordinator in the Disaster Information Management Research Center, National Library of Medicine, National Institutes of Health in Bethesda, Maryland. Previously, she served as Director of the Navy Medicine Office of Homeland Security, Bureau of Medicine and Surgery, in Washington, DC and as a Senior Health Policy Analyst in support of the Office of the Assistant Secretary of Defense for Health Affairs. Following the events of September 11, 2001, she served on temporary assignment in the Federal Emergency Management Agency's Emergency Operations Center in Washington, DC.

Dr. Chaffee served as Vice President of the Federal Nurses Association, was elected to the American Nurses Association Congress on Nursing Practice and Economics, and was an intern in the Office of Senator Daniel K. Inouye. She was the founding managing editor of the journal *Policy, Politics & Nursing Practice.* A Fellow of the American Academy of Nursing, she was awarded an honorary doctor of science degree by the University of Massachusetts at Amherst in 2003. Her contributions to Navy Medicine and the Department of Defense have been recognized with multiple individual awards including the Legion of Merit. Dr. Chaffee led a Navy Medicine project to improve hospital preparedness that was recognized as a finalist in the Harvard University/Kennedy School of Government "Innovations in American Government" awards program in homeland security in 2004. She is a Distinguished Alumna of the University of Massachusetts at Amherst and received the Excellence in Caring Practices award from the American Association of Critical-Care Nurses. Dr. Chaffee is an honors graduate of the University of Massachusetts at Amherst where she received bachelor's degrees in nursing and public health and completed an internship at the Welsh National School of Medicine in Cardiff, Wales. She received her doctorate and master's degrees in nursing health policy and nursing administration from the University of Maryland at Baltimore.

Contributors

Charles Alexandre, MS, RN
Doctoral Candidate
College of Nursing and Health Sciences
University of Massachusetts Boston
Boston, Massachusetts
Chief, Health Professions Regulation
Division of Environmental & Health Services
    Regulation
Rhode Island Department of Health
Providence, Rhode Island

Norma Alicea-Alvarez, DNP, CRNP
Pediatric Nurse Practitioner
Pediatric Associates, Private Practice
New Castle, Pennsylvania

Susan Apold, PhD, RN, ANP-BC
Dean and Professor
Division of Nursing
Concordia College of New York
Bronxville, New York

Jane H. Barnsteiner, PhD, RN, FAAN
Professor of Pediatric Nursing
School of Nursing
University of Pennsylvania
Philadelphia, Pennsylvania

Mary L. Behrens, RN. MSN. FNP-BC
Family Nurse Practitioner,
Westside Woman's Clinic
Casper, Wyoming

Katherine N. Bent, RN, PhD, CNS
Chief
Healthcare Delivery and Methodologies Integrated
    Review Group
National Institutes of Health
Bethesda, Maryland

Jonathan Bentley, BS, RN
Governing Board Member
The Canary Coalition
Sylva, North Carolina

Bobbie Berkowitz, PhD, RN, FAAN
Dean
Columbia University School of Nursing
New York, New York

Sandra Bishop-Josef, PhD
Assistant Director and Associate Research
    Scientist
Edward Zigler Center in Child Development &
    Social Policy, Child Study Center
School of Medicine
Yale University
New Haven, Connecticut

Linda Burnes Bolton, DrPH, RN, FAAN
Associate Clinical Professor
University of California San Francisco
San Francisco, California
Vice President, Nursing
Cedars-Sinai Medical Center
Los Angeles, California
Associate Clinical Professor
University of California Los Angeles
Los Angeles, California

Rebecca (Rice) Bowers-Lanier, EdD, MS, MPH
Legislative Consultant
Macaulay & Burtch, PC
Richmond, Virginia

Patricia K. Bradley, PhD, RN
Associate Professor
College of Nursing
Villanova University
Villanova, Pennsylvania

Charlotte Brody, RN
National Field Director
Safer Chemicals, Healthy Families
Esmont, Virginia

Edie Brous, RN, BSN, MS, MPH, JD
Nurse Attorney
New York, New York

Mary Lou Brunell, RN, MSN
Executive Director
Florida Center for Nursing
Orlando, Florida

Kelly Buettner-Schmidt, RN, BSN, MS
Department of Nursing Chair
Minot State University
Minot, North Dakota

Laura Caramanica, RN, PhD
Westchester Medical Center
Executive Director
Nursing Institute of Excellence
Vahalla, New York

John T. Carlsen, PhD
Director
The Professional Development Institute
Chicago, Illinois

Cynthia Caroselli, RN, PhD
Associate HealthCare System Director for Patient
    Services & Chief Nurse Executive
VA New York Harbor HealthCare System
New York, New York

Christine Ceccarelli, RN, MBA
Adjunct Faculty Member
Division of Nursing
Elms College
Chicopee, Massachusetts

Pamela F. Cipriano, PhD, RN, NEA-BC, FAAN
University of Virginia Health System
Charlottesville, Virginia
Editor-in-Chief
American Nurse Today
HealthcomMedia
Doylestown, Pennsylvania

Dame June Clark, DBE, PhD, RN, FRCN
Professor
Swansea University
Swansea, Wales
United Kingdom

Sean P. Clarke, RN, PhD, FAAN
RBC Chair in Cardiovascular Nursing Research
Lawrence S. Bloomberg Faculty of Nursing
University of Toronto
Toronto, Ontario
Canada

Brenda Cleary, PhD, RN, FAAN
Director
Center to Champion Nursing in America
Washington, DC

Elaine Cohen, EdD, RN, FAAN
Associate Chief, Nursing Quality Improvement
The James A. Haley Veteran's Hospital
Tampa, Florida

Sally S. Cohen, PhD, RN, FAAN
Associate Professor and Director
Robert Wood Johnson Foundation
Nursing and Health Policy Collaborative
University of New Mexico
Albuquerque, New Mexico

Judith B. Collins, RN, MS, WHNP-BC, FAAN
Associate Professor Emeritus,
School of Nursing and Medicine
Virginia Commonwealth University
Medical College of Virginia
Richmond, Virginia

Johnnie Sue Cooper, RN, PhD, BC-FNP
Nursing Instructor
Graduate Nursing Department
Mississippi University for Women
Columbus, Mississippi

Leah L. Curtin, RN, ScD(h), FAAN
Clinical Professor
Nursing
University of Cincinnati
Cincinnati, Ohio
Executive Editor
American Nurse Today
Healthcom Media
Doylestown, Pennsylvania

Jessie Daniels, MA, PhD
Associate Professor
School of Public Health
Hunter College
City University of New York
New York, New York

Catherine R. Davis, PhD, RN
Director
Global Research and Test Administration
CGFNS International, Inc.
Philadelphia, Pennsylvania

Marie Davis-Williams, MSSW, LCSW
Assistant Commissioner, Recovery Services
  and Planning
Mental Health and Developmental Disabilities
Nashville, Tennessee

Betty R. Dickson
Lobbyist
Barnardsville, North Carolina

Joanne Disch, PhD, RN, FAAN
Clinical Professor and Director
School of Nursing
University of Minnesota
Minneapolis, Minnesota

Catherine Dodd, RN, PhD
Director
San Francisco Health Service System
City and County of San Francisco, California

Karen Drenkard, PhD, RN, NEA-BC, FAAN
Executive Director
American Nurses Credentialing Center
Fairfax, Virginia

Amanda L. Ebner, MA, MEd
PhD Candidate
University of California, Irvine
Los Angeles, California

Holly Edwards, RN, MEd
Registered Nurse
Health Services
Jefferson Board for Aging
Charlottesville, Virginia

Carroll L. Estes, PhD, FAAN
Professor & Founding Director,
Institute for Health & Aging University
San Francisco, California

William M. Enlow, DNP, CRNA
Assistant Professor of Clinical Nursing
Program in Nursing Anesthesia
School of Nursing
Columbia University
New York, New York

Nancy L. Falk, RN, PhD, MBA
Assistant Professor
School of Nursing
The George Washington University
Washington, DC

Stephanie L. Ferguson, PhD, RN, FAAN
Consulting Associate Professor
Stanford University
Amherst, Virginia

Loretta C. Ford, EdD, RN, PNP, FAAN, FAANP
Professor and Dean Emeritus
School of Nursing
University of Rochester
Rochester, New York
Director of Nursing
Strong Memorial Hospital, University of Rochester
  Medical Center
Rochester, New York

Rebecca Fox
Executive Director
National Coalition for LGBT Health
Washington, DC

Deborah B. Gardner, PhD, RN
Senior Advisor
Bureau of Health Professions
Health Resources and Services Administration
Rockville, Maryland

Carole Gassert, RN, PhD, FACMI, FAAN
Associate Professor Emeritus (Retired)
College of Nursing
University of Utah
Salt Lake City, Utah

Kristine M. Gebbie, DrPH, RN
Joan Hansen Grabe Dean
Hunter-Bellevue School of Nursing
Hunter College
City University of New York
New York, New York

Greer Glazer, RN, PhD, CNP, FAAN
Dean and Professor
University of Massachusetts Boston
College of Nursing and Health Sciences
Boston, Massachusetts

Barbara Glickstein, RN, MSN, MPH
New York, New York

Irma Goertzen, RN, MSN
Retired CEO and President
Magee Womens Hospital and Research Institute
Pittsburgh, Pennsylvania
Board Chair
Society of Women's Health Research
Washington, DC

Bethany Hall-Long, PhD, RNC, FAAN
State Senator
State of Delaware
Professor
University of Delaware and State of Delaware
Newark, Delaware

David Haltiwanger, PhD
Director of Clinical Programs and Public Policy
Chase Brexton Health Services
Baltimore, Maryland

Tine Hansen-Turton, MGA, JD
Executive Director
National Nursing Centers Consortium
Philadelphia, Pennsylvania

Alfreda Harper-Harrison, EdD, MSN, RN, CLNC
Assistant Professor
Winston Salem State University
Winston-Salem, North Carolina

Charlene Harrington, PhD, RN, FAAN
Professor Emeritus
Social and Behavioral Sciences
University of California
Oakland, California

Wylecia Wiggs Harris, MM, CAE
Doctoral Student
Capella University
Minneapolis, Minnesota
Executive Director
Center for American Nurses
Silver Spring, Maryland

Mary Ann Hart, SN, RN, NP-C
Assistant Clinical Professor of Nursing
Regis College
Weston, Massachusetts

Susan Hassmiller, PhD, RN, FAAN
Senior Advisor for Nursing
Director
RWJF Initiative on the Future of Nursing
  at the IOM
Robert Wood Johnson Foundation
Princeton, New Jersey

Barbara B. Hatfield, RN
Delegate
West Virginia House of Delegates
Charleston, West Virginia

Donna L. Haugland, MSN, CNP
Chief Nursing Officer
MinuteClinic
St. Paul, Minnesota

Pamela J. Haylock
Medina, Texas

Susan D. Hellier, DNP, CRNP
Women's Health Nurse Practitioner
Lawrence County OB/GYN Associates
New Castle, Pennsylvania

Karrie Cummings Hendrickson, PhD, RN
Postdoctoral Fellow
Yale University School of Nursing
New Haven, Connecticut

Catherine Hoffman, ScD, RN
Senior Researcher, Associate Director
Kaiser Commission on Medicaid and the Uninsured
Washington, DC

Anne Hudson, RN, BSN
Public Health Nurse
Coos County Public Health Department
North Bend, Oregon
Founder
Work Injured Nurses' Group USA (WING USA)
Coos Bay, Oregon

Patricia J. Hughes, EdD, MBA, CRNP
Campus Dean
Chamberlain College of Nursing
Arlington, Virginia

Brenda C. Isaac, RN, BSN, MA, NCSN
Lead School Nurse
School Health Services
Kanawha County Schools
Charleston, West Virginia

Jean E. Johnson, RN-C, PhD, FAAN
Senior Associate Dean,
Health Sciences
The George Washington University
School of Medicine and Health Sciences
Washington, DC

Pamela J. Johnson, RN, BSN
Clinical Team Leader
Advocate Health Care
Oakbrook, Illinois

Louise Kahn, MSN, MA, PNP
Clinical Educator
College of Nursing
University of New Mexico
Albuquerque, New Mexico

David M. Keepnews, PhD, JD, RN, FAAN
Associate Professor
Hunter-Bellevue School of Nursing
Hunter College
City University of New York
New York, New York

Mary Jo Kreitzer, PhD, RN, FAAN
Professor
School of Nursing
Director
Center for Spirituality & Healing
University of Minnesota
Minneapolis, Minnesota

Phyllis Beck Kritek, RN, PhD, FAAN
Professor, Tenured
School of Nursing
Director
Center for Spirituality & Healing
University of Minnesota
Minneapolis, Minnesota

Ellen T. Kurtzman, MPH, RN, FAAN
Assistant Research Professor
Department of Nursing Education
Washington, DC

Sandra B. Lewenson, EdD, RN, FAAN
Professor
Lienhard School of Nursing
Pace University
Pleasantville, New York

Elena Lopez-Bowlan, RN, MSN, APN
Family Nurse Practitioner
Reno, Nevada

Robert J. Lucero, PhD, MPH, RN
Post-Doctoral Research Fellow
School of Nursing
Center for Evidence-Based Practice in
    the Underserved
Columbia University
New York, New York

John Lumpkin, MD, MPH, FACEP, FACMI
Senior Vice President
Director Health Care Group
Robert Wood Johnson Foundation
Princeton, New Jersey

Beverly L. Malone, PhD, RN, FAAN
Chief Executive Officer
National League for Nursing
New York, New York

Ruth E. Malone, RN, PhD, FAAN
Professor and Director
Doctoral Specialty in Health Policy
San Francisco School of Nursing
University of California
San Francisco, California

Tracy A. Malone, RN, MSN
Executive Director
US Family Health Plan Alliance, LLC
Arlington, Virginia

Jeannee Parker Martin, RN, MPH
Associate Clinical Professor
School of Nursing
University of California San Francisco
President/Owner
The Corridor Group Inc.
San Francisco, California

Mary Lynn Mathre, RN, MSN, CARN, CLNC
Legal Nurse Consultant
Howardsville, Virginia
President
Patients Out of Time
Howardsville, Virginia

Margaret L. McClure, EdD, RN, FAAN
Professor
New York University
New York, New York

Janice M. McCoy, MSN, MSHSA, RN, CNAA, BC
Former Chief Nursing Officer
Cape Canaveral Hospital
Cocoa Beach, Florida

Ruth Merkatz, PhD, RN, FAAN
Director, Clinical Development, Reproductive
    Health
Center for Biomedical Research
Population Council
New York, New York

DeAnne K. Hilfinger Messias, PhD, RN, FAAN
Associate Professor
College of Nursing and Women's and
    Gender Studies
University of South Carolina
Columbia, South Carolina

Alfredo Mireles, RN, BSN
Staff Nurse, Psychiatry
San Francisco General Hospital
San Francisco, California
Jessie Marvin Unruh Assembly Fellow
Office of Assembly Member Anthony Portantino
California State Assembly
Sacramento, California

Alan Morgan, MPA
Chief Executive Officer
National Rural Health Association
Washington, DC

Ellen S. Murray, MS
Research Associate
The Roosevelt House Public Policy Institute
Hunter College, City University of New York
New York, New York

John S. Murray, PhD, RN, CPNP, CS, FAAN
Colonel, Air Force Nurse Corps (Retired)
Director, Nurse Scientist
Children's Hospital
Boston, Massachusetts

Mary V. Muse, MSN, RN
Correctional Health Care Consultant
Chicago, Illinois

Vanessa D. Newsome, MSEd
Program Coordinator
Will County Health Department
Dolton, Illinois

Barbara L. Nichols, DHL, MS, RN, FAAN
Chief Executive Officer
CGFNS International
Philadelphia, Pennsylvania

Karen O'Connor, JD, PhD
Jonathan N. Helfat Distinguished Professor of
    Political Science
American University
Washington, DC

Eileen T. O'Grady PhD, RN, NP
Lienhard School of Nursing
Pace University
New York, New York
Policy Editor
American Journal for Nurse Practitioners and
    NP World News
Cranbury, New Jersey

Doug Olsen, PhD, RN
Washington, DC

Judith A. Oulton, RN, BN, MEd, DSc(hon)
Partner
Oulton, Oulton & Associates
Geneva, Switzerland

Freida Hopkins Outlaw, PhD, RN, FAAN
Five Regional Mental Health Institutions
State Hospitals
Knoxville, Bolivar, Nashville, Memphis, and
    Chattanooga, Tennessee
Assistant Commissioner
Division of Special Populations
Tennessee Department of Mental Health and
    Developmental Disabilities
Nashville, Tennessee

Elizabeth Parry, MPP
Alexandria, Virginia

Patricia Reid Ponte, RN, DNSc, FAAN, NEA-BC
Adjunct Assistant Professor
School of Nursing
University of Massachusetts, Amherst
Amherst, Massachusetts
Associate Professor
College of Nursing and Health Sciences
University of Massachusetts, Boston
Boston, Massachusetts
Senior Vice President for Patient Care Services,
    Chief Nurse
Nursing and Patient Care Services
Dana-Farber Cancer Institute
Boston, Massachusetts
Director of Oncology Nursing and Clinical
    Services
Nursing and Patient Care Services
Brigham and Women's Hospital
Boston, Massachusetts

Lynn Price, JD, MSN, MPH
Associate Professor
Quinnipiac University
New Haven, Connecticut

Chad Priest, RN, JD
Chief Executive Officer
Managed Emergency Surge for Healthcare
Indianapolis, Indiana

Joyce A. Pulcini, PhD, RN, PNP-BC, FAAN
Associate Professor
William F. Connell School of Nursing
Boston College
Chestnut Hill, Massachusetts

Frank Purcell, BS
Senior Director
Federal Government Affairs
American Association of Nurse Anesthetists
Washington, DC

Joanne Rains Warner, DNS, RN
Dean and Professor
University of Portland
Portland, Oregon

Susan C. Reinhard, RN, PhD, FAAN
Public Policy Institute
AARP
Washington, DC

Donna R. Richardson, JD, RN
Director of Governmental Affairs and Professional
    Standards
CGFNS International
Philadelphia, Pennsylvania

Nancy Ridenour, PhD, APRN, BC, FAAN
Dean and Professor
University of New Mexico College of Nursing
Albuquerque, New Mexico

Ann Ritter, JD
Director, Health Center Development & Policy
National Nursing Centers Consortium
Philadelphia, Pennsylvania

Karen M. Robinson DNS, CNS, PMH-BC, FAAN
Professor
School of Nursing
University of Louisville
Louisville, Kentucky

Angela Ross, EdM
Assistant Director, Workforce Programs
Florida Center for Nursing
Orlando, Florida

Gail E. Russell, EdD, RN, NEA-BC
Professor and Graduate Program Director
College of Nursing
University of Massachusetts Dartmouth
North Dartmouth, Massachusetts

Yvonne Santa Anna, BSN, RN, MSG
Vice President, Congressional Relations
Fresenius Medical Care North America
Rockville, Maryland

Alice Sardell, PhD
Professor
Queens College
City University of New York
Flushing, New York

Rose Sherman, EdD, RN, NEA-BC
Director Nursing Leadership Institute & Associate
    Professor
Florida Atlantic University
Boca Raton, Florida

Dennis Sherrod, EdD, RN
Professor and Forsyth Medical Center Endowed
    Chair of Recruitment & Retention
Winston-Salem State University
Winston-Salem, North Carolina
President
Center for American Nurses
Silver Springs, Maryland

Judith Shindul-Rothschild, PhD, RNPC, DPNAP
Associate Professor
Nursing
William F. Connell School of Nursing
Boston College
Chestnut Hill, Massachusetts
Past President
Massachusetts Nurses Association
Canton, Massachusetts

Linda J. Shinn, MBA, RN, CAE
Principal
Consensus Management Group
Indianapolis, Indiana

James Mark Simmerman, PhD, RN
Epidemiologist
Bangkok, Thailand

Arlene M. Smaldone, DNSc, RN
Assistant Professor
School of Nursing
Columbia University
New York, New York

Andréa Sonenberg, DNSc, WHNP, CNM
Associate Professor
Lienhard School of Nursing
College of Health Professions
Pace University
Pleasantville, New York

Diane L. Spatz, PhD, RN-BC, FAAN
Helen M. Shearer Associate Professor of Nutrition &
    Associate Professor of Healthcare of Women and
    Childbearing Nursing
University of Pennsylvania
Philadelphia, Pennsylvania

Joanne Spetz, PhD
Professor
Community Health Systems
Senior Research Faculty
Center for the Health Professions
University of California San Francisco
San Francisco, California

Susan McDonough Stackpoole, MSN, RN
Former Director Nursing Operations
Cape Canaveral Hospital
Cocoa Beach, Florida

Patricia W. Stone, PhD, FAAN
Director of the Center for Health Policy
Professor
School of Nursing
Columbia University
New York, New York

Suzanne Stone, JD
Vice President
Finance and Administration
National Abortion Federation
Washington, DC

Elyse I. Summers, JD
Director
Division of Education and Development
Office for Human Research Protections
United States Department of Health and
    Human Services
Rockville, Maryland

Elaine Tagliareni, EdD, RN, CNE, FAAN
Chief Program Officer
National League for Nursing
New York, New York

Pamela Thompson, MS, RN, FAAN
Chief Executive Officer
American Organization of Nurse Executives
Washington, DC

Patricia E. Tobal
Hopwood, Pennsylvania

Corazon Tomalinas, RN, BSN, PHN
Santa Teresa Hospital (Former)
Kaiser Permanente
San Jose, California
Commissioner
FIRST 5
Santa Clara County, California

Virginia Trotter Betts, MSN, JD, RN, FAAN
Commissioner
Tennessee Department of Mental Health and
    Developmental Disabilities
Nashville, Tennessee

Lauren A. Underwood, MSN, MPH, RN
Johns Hopkins University
Baltimore, Maryland

Lynn Unruh, PhD, RN, LHRM
Associate Professor,
University of Central Florida
Orlando, Florida

Connie Vance, RN, EdD, FAAN
Professor,
College of New Rochelle, New York
New Rochelle, New York

Antonia M. Villaruel, PhD, FAAN
Associate Dean for Research and Scholarship
University of Michigan
Ann Arbor, Michigan

Catherine M. Waters, RN, PhD
Professor
Department of Community Health Systems
San Francisco School of Nursing
University of California
San Francisco, California
Health Commissioner
San Francisco Department of Public Health
City & County of San Francisco Department of
    Public Health
San Francisco, California

Jon L. Weakley
American University
Washington, DC

Scott Weber, EdD, PhD-c, MSN, RN
Assistant Professor
University of Pittsburgh School of Nursing
Pittsburgh, Pennsylvania

Ellen-Marie Whelan, RN, NP, PhD
Senior Health Policy Analyst and Associate Director
    of Health Policy
Center for American Progress
Washington, DC

Kathleen M. White, PhD, RN, NEA-BC, FAAN
Director, Doctor of Nursing Practice Program
Johns Hopkins University School of Nursing
Baltimore, Maryland

Eva Williams, MA, CPG
Staff Research Analyst II
Institute for Health & Aging
University of California
San Francisco, California

Michael P. Woody
Partner
East End Group
Washington, DC

Lynda Woolbert, MSN, RN, PNP
Executive Director
Coalition for Nurses in Advanced Practice
West Columbia, Texas

Reviewers

Michael D. Aldridge, MSN, RN, CCRN, CNS
Concordia University Texas
Austin, Texas

Margaret E. Barnes, RN, MSN
Indiana Wesleyan University, School of Nursing
Marion, Indiana

Deborah Becker, PhD, ACNP, BC, CCNS
School of Nursing
University of Pennsylvania
Philadelphia, Pennsylvania

Marylee Bressie, MSN, RN, CCRN, CCNS, CEN
Providence Hospital
Mobile, Alabama
Samford University
Birmingham, Alabama

Barbara Camune, RNC, CNM, WHNP-BC,
    DrPH, FACNM
Clinical Associate Professor Coordinator
Director
Nurse-Midwifery & Women's Health Nurse
    Practitioner Programs
Department of Women, Children & Family Health
    Science
College of Nursing
University of Illinois at Chicago
Chicago, Illinois

Karen Clark, PhD, MSN, BSN, RN, CCRN
University of Maryland School of Nursing
Rockville, Maryland

Rose E. Constantino, PhD, JD, RN, FAAN, FACFE
Department of Health and Community Systems
School of Nursing
University of Pittsburgh
Pittsburgh, Pennsylvania

Margaret Dean, RN, CS-BC, GNP-BC, MSN, APN
Associate Faculty
Nursing and Medical School
Texas Tech University Health Sciences Center
Amarillo, Texas

Deborah Dumphy, APRN, BSN, MS, IBCLC,
    RLC, NP-C
Family Nurse Practitioner and International Board
    Certified Lactation Consultant
Dawson Pediatrics
Dawsonville, Georgia
Assistant Professor of Nursing
North Georgia College & State University
Dahlonega, Georgia

Maurice Espinoza, RN, CNS, RN, BSN, MSN,
    WCC, CCRN
University of California Irvine Medical Center
Orange, California

Barbara L. Ferguson, RN, MSN, MHA, MBA
University of North Carolina Charlotte
Charlotte, North Carolina

Cris Finn, PhD, RN, FNP, MS, MA, FNE
Assistant Professor
Loretto Heights School of Nursing
Regis University
Denver, Colorado

Joyce Foresman-Capuzzi, BSN, RN,CEN, CTRN,
    CCRN, CPN, CPEN, SANE-A, EMT-P
Lankenau Hospital
Wynnewood, Pennsylvania

Mary Anne Hanley, RN, PhD
Perry School of Nursing
Texas Tech University Health Sciences Center
Lubbock, Texas

Joellen W. Hawkins, RN, PhD, WHNP-BC, FAAN, FAANP
Professor Emerita
William F. Connell School of Nursing
Boston College
Chestnut Hill, Massachusetts
Nursing Department
Writer in Residence Simmons College
Boston, Massachusetts

Leslie C. Hussey, PhD, RN
Associate Director of Doctoral Education
Wolford College
Naples, Florida

Karen Kelly, EdD, RN, NEA-BC
Associate Professor and Coordinator
Continuing Education
School of Nursing
Southern Illinois University Edwardsville
Edwardsville, Illinois

Linda U. Krebs, RN, PhD, AOCN, FAAN
College of Nursing
University of Colorado Denver
Aurora, Colorado

Jean Logan, RN, PhD
Professor of Nursing
Grand View University
Des Moines, Iowa

Jacqueline R. Meyer, RN, MSN
Associate Professor
Assistant Dean
Graduate Program
School of Nursing
Allen College
Waterloo, Iowa

Chad Rittle, DNP, MPH, BSN, RN
Adjunct Faculty
Waynesburg, University
Waynesburg, Pennsylvania

Mitchell J. Seal, EdD, Med-IT, BSN, RN-BC
Head
Ancillary Services Department
Medical Education & Training Campus
Fort Sam Houston, Texas
Adjunct Faculty
Health Careers & Nursing Department
Cerro Coso College
Ridgecrest, California

Nashat Zuraikat, PhD, RN
Indiana University of Pennsylvania
Indiana, Pennsylvania

To the contributors to this book
and
all nurses who influence the health of the public
through policy and politics.

Contents

UNIT 3   Policy and Politics in Research and Nursing Science

UNIT 4   Policy and Politics in the Workplace and Workforce

UNIT 6   Policy and Politics in Associations and Interest Groups

UNIT 7   Policy and Politics in the Community

Foreword

Donna E. Shalala

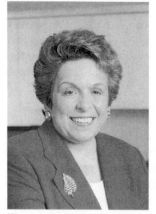

(Photo: University of Miami)

I have had the privilege of leading three institutions of higher learning with outstanding nursing education programs and have worked closely with many leaders in nursing. Nurses are key to the nation's health future. As Secretary of Health and Human Services during the administration of President Clinton, I nominated numerous nurses to leadership positions, including in Social Security. In addition, three nurses served as regional directors—an historic first. All were excellent leaders. They understood the health needs of people in their regions, built strategic relationships and partnerships, and developed public and private responses to regional health and welfare concerns.

My role as chairperson of the Initiative on the Future of Nursing at the Institute of Medicine (*www.iom.edu/nursing*) has made me even more knowledgeable of the challenges of producing and retaining an adequate supply of well-prepared nurses to serve in all sectors of our health care system. The barriers nurses face in sustaining and spreading their innovative models of care are on display in the American Academy of Nursing's "Raise the Voice Campaign" (*www.aannet.org*). As a predominantly female profession, nurses have long faced a daunting task to move their important patient-centered perspectives on health care to the conference rooms where important decisions are made about health policy. Health reform will only be achieved if nurses are unrelenting in pursuing their rightful place in policy leadership in partnership with others who are also committed to accessible, safe, effective, and equitable health care.

Some people may question whether nurses will be able to do this. According to a 2010 Gallup survey of over 1500 opinion leaders in health care, nurses are seen as influential in ensuring the quality and safety of health care but not in shaping health care policy reform. Some of those surveyed noted that many nurses shy away from leadership opportunities; they called for nurses to be more vocal and unified on important health care issues and more accountable for providing leadership in health care. Most leaders in health care will not wait for nurses to find their voices nor hand them the mantle of leadership. There is no better opportunity for nurses to lead health system change than now. We must and can shift the emphasis of care to health promotion, disease prevention, and chronic illness management with a patient- and family-centered focus. This is what nurses know and do so well.

The Initiative on the Future of Nursing's recommendations will hopefully put nurses in the forefront of transforming health care.

Policy & Politics in Nursing and Health Care provides information, perspectives, and strategies that nurses need to develop the capacity and skills to influence reform. We must rise to the challenges that lay before us as we continue to develop the policies and systems that are needed to make sure everyone has access to affordable quality care that promotes health.

Donna E. Shalala is president and professor of political science at the University of Miami. She was the longest-serving secretary of the U.S. Department of Health and Human Services, holding the position throughout the presidency of President Bill Clinton. She previously served as president of Hunter College, City University of New York, and Chancellor of the University of Wisconsin at Madison. Dr. Shalala is chair of the Initiative on the Future of Nursing at the Institute of Medicine and is a member of the National Advisory Committee of the American Academy of Nursing's Raise the Voice Campaign, serving as its first chairperson.

Foreword

Richard H. Carmona

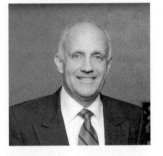

While many people recognize me as the 17th Surgeon General of the United States, and as a physician and public health leader, I am also a registered nurse.

Nurses have nearly unlimited opportunities to be catalysts for change in the today's health system—and change is clearly needed. To be effective in bringing about meaningful change in organizations and for populations, it is vital to understand political dynamics and policy processes. There is likely no better source for nurses to learn how to be influential than this book, the sixth edition of *Policy & Politics in Nursing and Health Care*.

Nurses have been successful advocates for improvement in the health of individuals, communities and, indeed, the Nation. However, much more work must be done to reduce health disparities, improve quality and safety in the health system as well as improve access to care, and formulate policies in organizations that focus on the needs of patients.

I challenge all nurses to take pride in the remarkable legacy of nursing's achievements in influencing health policy—and to build on that legacy by taking part in tackling the major health issues that face us. The problems are significant, but there are 2.7 million nurses who understand how the health system works and where change is needed. Advocacy, activism, and leadership in policy and politics will reduce the chronic problems that beleaguer the system that provides care and will open the doors to care for many who currently have no access. By working together, learning the ropes of policy and politics, and mentoring others, we can change the future of the nation's health.

Dr. Richard H. Carmona is the Distinguished Professor of Public Health at the Mel & Enid Zuckerman College of Public Health, University of Arizona and Vice Chairman of Canyon Ranch, a company that aims to inspire people to make a commitment to healthy living. He also serves as Chief Executive Officer of its Health Division and oversees Health Strategy and Policy for all Canyon Ranch businesses. He served as the 17th Surgeon General of the U.S., a position in which he advocated for strategies to address the Nation's major public health problems—chronic disease, tobacco use, obesity, and health disparities as well as global health and health diplomacy. A combat-decorated Army Special Forces veteran, Dr. Carmona trained as a general and vascular surgeon and started and directed Arizona's first regional trauma care system. As a physician, he recognized that most of his patient's clinical problems were preventable, and he changed course to establish a career in public health. Dr. Carmona also served for over 20 years as a deputy sheriff, detective, SWAT team leader, and department surgeon in Arizona. He has published extensively; is a nationally recognized expert in emergency management, trauma care, SWAT tactics, and tactical emergency medical support; and has received many awards for his contributions in health care, public health and law enforcement.

Preface

Diana J. Mason, Judith K. Leavitt, and Mary W. Chaffee

Welcome to the sixth edition of *Policy & Politics in Nursing and Health Care*. This book has been designed to meet the needs of nurses at all educational levels—from undergraduate students to masters and doctorally prepared professionals. We are excited to share with our readers the contributions of many nurses and others who have made a difference in the health of the public through shaping policy and political activism and are willing to share their expertise, experience, and analysis. While many of our contributors are well-known nursing leaders, others are first-time authors whose stories demonstrate how much can be accomplished by motivated nurses.

Since the last edition, Americans have witnessed the effects of a United States health system with worsening problems: limited consumer access to care, inconsistent quality, uncontrolled costs, and higher rates of morbidity and mortality than most other developed nations (Sultz & Young, 2009). Issues with health care quality and safety have sparked significant policy and political activity, including the passage of the most extensive health reform law since Medicare was enacted, the Affordable Care Act (ACA) of 2010. Some provisions of the law were enacted immediately, and others will continue to be enacted through 2018. More legislation will be needed in the coming years to make improvements in the original law. Until then, nurses will continue to be confronted with burgeoning problems that include:

- Unsustainable high cost of care
- Far too many health errors
- Inadequate access to care
- An unresolved shortage of nursing faculty to prepare the projected number of nurses needed to care for the population
- An insufficient primary care and public health workforce
- Significant disparities in access to care
- Inadequate focus on prevention of disease
- An economy in recession.

The health reform law will not resolve all these issues; our hope is it will initiate substantial progress in moving the U.S. to a universal system of health care for all.

WHAT'S THE REMEDY?

The remedy for many health system problems is a course correction directed by a new or revised policy. However, for a policy solution to effectively address a problem, the problem itself must be well understood—and that's where the need for nurses to actively participate in the policy process becomes apparent. Nurses understand how the health system really works and that perspective is critical in designing effective policy solutions. That's where this book comes in; it can support and guide nurses to be effective in advancing policy solutions and working in all environments.

WHAT'S NEW IN THE SIXTH EDITION?

An emphasis on evidence-based policy. Just as practice is expected to be evidence-based, so is policy. The book includes stronger attention to the research undergirding policy, the use of science to inform policy, and the problems that arise when ideology trumps evidence.

More focus on community activism. Recognizing that many nurses take their first political steps at the local level, we have expanded the unit on Policy and Politics in the Community. We added a chapter on community activism and have included powerful stories of nurses who took on problems in their local communities.

Exploration of health care reform. This book was in production during the debates on how to reform the U.S. health system. Many chapters include analysis and discussion of the changes resulting from implementation of the Affordable Care Act (ACA)—the most significant recent change in U.S. health policy. The revised reprint of this book includes a discussion of the ACA, its implementation as of summer 2013, and the implications for nursing. All printings include perspectives on the ACA at its inception.

Other new content. Because the world and the health care environment are continuously changing, we've added chapters to address critical issues for nurses. These include:

- Advocacy in nursing
- The uninsured and underinsured
- Rural health care
- Policy approaches to address health disparities
- Medical homes and primary care
- Science, policy, and politics
- Evidence-based practice and policy
- Workplace abuse policy
- Home health and hospice
- Quality and safety in health care
- Retail health care
- Global nurse migration
- Nursing education policy
- Showcasing nursing's leadership
- Policy problems like human trafficking, nurse staffing, and workplace injuries

WHAT'S CARRIED OVER FROM THE PREVIOUS EDITIONS?

We listen to our readers and faculty who use the book. You've told us about parts of the book that have been most valuable to you. We've updated every chapter from the previous edition of the book, including how nurses learn the ropes of policy and politics, the policy process, ethics in policymaking, the power of the media, and financing health care in the U.S. We've revised some chapters to reflect current policy issues in major health programs, including Medicare, Medicaid, TRICARE, the Veteran's Health System, and CHIP. We've updated the book's Appendix that acquaints readers with educational opportunities in policy and politics. We've highlighted inspiring stories by and about nurses who have taken action to address problems in health and health care; these are identified as Taking Action chapters.

USING THE SIXTH EDITION

Using the book as a course text. Faculty will find there is content in this book that will enhance learning experiences in policy, leadership, community, administration, research, and issues and trends courses at every educational level. Many of the chapters will help students in clinical courses understand the dynamics of the health system. Students will find chapters that assist them in developing new skills, building a broader understanding of nursing leadership and influence, and making sense of the complex business and financial forces that drive many actions in the health system.

Using the book in the workplace. Policy problems and political issues abound in nursing workplaces. This book offers critical insights into how to effectively resolve problems and influence workplace policy as well as to develop politically astute approaches to making changes in the workplace.

Using the book in professional organizations. Organizations use the power of numbers. The unit on associations and interest groups will help groups determine strategies for success and how to capitalize on working with other groups through coalitions.

Using the book in government activities. The unit on policy and politics in the government includes content that will benefit nurses considering running for elective office, seeking a political appointment, and learning to lobby elected officials about health care issues.

Using the book in community activism. With an expanded focus on community advocacy and activism, readers will find information they need to effectively influence remedies to policy problems in their local communities.

EXAMPLES OF PROMINENT NURSE LEADERS

Many nurses have addressed chronic and acute health and social problems in the past and are continuing their remarkable leadership today:

- **Dr. Mary Wakefield:** As the presidentially appointed Administrator of the Health Resources and Services Administration, she shapes federal policy to fill in the health care gaps for people who live outside the economic and medical mainstream.

- **Dr. Karen Daley:** Infected with HIV from a needle-stick while working as an emergency nurse, she became an advocate for needlestick safety measures, providing testimony at hearings and lobbying members of Congress. She was invited to witness President Clinton sign the Needlestick Safety and Prevention Act of 2000 into law at the White House, and she was elected president of the American Nurses Association in 2010.
- **Greg Mortenson:** Author of the award-winning best-seller *Three Cups of Tea: One Man's Mission to Promote Peace...One School At A Time,* he has established 131 schools in volatile areas of Pakistan and Afghanistan that provide education for 58,000 children, including 44,000 girls who generally have few educational opportunities. A former emergency nurse, he was nominated for the 2009 Nobel Peace Prize.
- **Virginia Trotter Betts:** She has served as the Commissioner of the Tennessee Department of Mental Health and Developmental Disabilities. Betts was president of the American Nurses Association from 1992-1996 during the national debate on health care reform from 1991-1994. She commissioned the development of professional nursing's "White Papers" on health reform.
- **Jennie Chin Hansen:** She served as AARP President in 2008-2010, representing the interests of 39 million older Americans. She began her career as a public health nurse in Idaho.
- **Dr. Linda Schwartz:** A retired Air Force Colonel, she serves as the Commissioner of the Connecticut Department of Veteran's Affairs, has given testimony to both house of Congress on veteran's issues, and has advocated throughout her career for America's military veterans.
- **Anneli Eriksson:** She is president of Médecins Sans Frontières (Doctors Without Borders) in Sweden. She received the 2007 International Achievement Award from the International Council of Nurse's Florence Nightingale International Foundation for her advocacy for endangered communities and humanitarian effort.
- **Dr. Stephanie Ferguson:** She has served as the Director of the International Council of Nurses' Leadership for Change Program and Consultant for Nursing and Health Policy. A former White House Fellow and the first chair for legislation and policy for the Association of Women's Health, Obstetrics, and Neonatal Nursing, she has worked throughout her career as an advocate for improving the health of children, families, and vulnerable populations.
- **Dr. David Keepnews:** He has served as director of policy development for the New York Academy of Medicine and director of policy for the American Nurses Association, and he was a regulatory policy specialist for the California Nurses Association. He is the Editor of the journal, *Policy and Politics in Nursing Practice.*
- **Marilyn Tavenner:** She was appointed as principal deputy administrator of the Centers for Medicare and Medicaid (CMS) as the Affordable Care Act was passed, making her the second highest ranking official at CMS. She came to the attention of the Obama administration after serving as secretary of Health and Human Services for the state of Virginia.
- **Dr. Catherine Dodd:** Now serving as Director of the San Francisco Health Service System, she served in San Francisco Mayor Gavin Newsom's Office as Deputy Chief of Staff overseeing Health, Human Services, Aging Services, and Children, Youth, and Family Services. Prior to this, she was District Chief of Staff to House Speaker Nancy Pelosi (D) and she served as Region IX Director of Health and Human Services as an appointee of President Bill Clinton.

The work of these nurses, and thousands of others in governments, communities, workplaces, and organizations across the U.S., demonstrates how nurses can influence critical changes in the health system and society through policymaking and political action. This book has been a resource for many of these activist nurses. However, there is much work remaining to be done and we hope this book will serve all nurses well who are not satisfied with the status quo.

REFERENCE

Sultz, H., & Young, K. (2009). *Health care USA—Understanding Its organization and delivery.* Sudbury, MA: Jones and Bartlett Publishers.

Acknowledgments

Each time we prepare a new edition of this book, we are impressed by and extremely grateful to the nurses who contribute their remarkable stories, knowledge, and experience. More than 150 nurses and others took part in writing the sixth edition. We think our readers will appreciate their contributions as much as we do. We remain grateful to Susan Talbott, the co-editor of the first two editions of the book, as well as the contributors to previous editions who helped establish this book's preeminence in its field.

We owe a huge thank you to Elizabeth (Beth) Lehr, our phenomenal editorial manager. Beth tracked and managed more than 100 manuscripts with great attention to detail. In the midst of her work, she had a baby, parented a toddler, and survived the "Snowmaggedon" blizzard of 2009. Beth, you are amazing and a delight to work with. This book would not have made it to press without your efforts.

We are quite grateful to the editors and staff at Elsevier. We appreciate the expert support and guidance we received from Maureen Iannuzzi, Editor, and Julia Curcio, Associate Developmental Editor. We also thank Yvonne Alexopoulos, Lisa Newton, and Mary Ann Zimmerman, who shepherded this text at the beginning of its journey. We are delighted to have worked for a third time with Clay Broeker, Senior Project Manager.

Developing an edition of this book takes about 2 years, produces thousands of email, consumes hundreds of hours on the phone and at the keyboard, and is fueled by many cups of coffee. Our families and friends sustain us while the book grows, and we each have some additional acknowledgments to add.

Life, as in politics, is about relationships. They sustain and help you through the tough times. Producing this book is always a nightmare (so much to do, so little time), but this edition was particularly challenging for me, as it occurred as I was changing jobs and took on more than I ended up feeling competent to manage well. So I'm grateful to my new colleagues at Hunter College of the City University of New York for their patience with my attempts to juggle too many commitments during my first year at the school of nursing.

I'm particularly appreciative of Judy and Mary for their willingness to pitch in when I faltered and their unwavering commitment to ensuring that this edition continued to reflect the prior editions' standard of excellence in thinking and writing. Even when we passionately disagreed about something, we always seemed to be able to support each other and build consensus. I am deeply indebted to these two fine colleagues.

Hard work is always made easier by friends and colleagues who are soul mates who bring creativity, passion, and joy to our lives. My dear friend, radio buddy, and trusted colleague Barbara Glickstein is always there for me. Working with her is a blast, though often overwhelming with too many ideas and riotous laughter. I adore her and value her continued support through the birthing of this book.

As I write this acknowledgement, I look up and see my husband, James Ware, washing the dishes after making dinner and saying to me, "I've got the dishes. You go ahead and finish what you're working on." It's a rerun of so many nights during the past 2 years. He's been steadfast in his support—whether walking our beloved dog Bling when I'm too tired or on deadline, or telling me I need to take a break from 12-hour days. Thank you.

Diana J. Mason
New York, New York

During the writing of this edition, my mentor and inspiration died—my 96-year-old Dad. He not only was my greatest champion as an activist nurse, but his words of wisdom and his example of political involvement guided my life. During the same time, my first grandson, Aryeh, was born. Through his great grandfather, his grandparents, and his parents, I know he will take up the mantle and work to improve our planet.

For me, writing this book provides an opportunity to work with two of the finest colleagues to create a work that is the result of our synergy, respect, gratitude, and caring for each other.

As always my sons, Noah and David, and their wives, Helen and Marnie, have supported me and the work of the book as health professionals and social activists who practice the lessons in these pages. Particular acknowledgment goes to my best buddy Betty Dickson, one of the finest lobbyists for nursing anywhere. There are too many friends and close family to acknowledge separately but without exception they have been patient and caring and will be glad that the book is published.

Judith K. Leavitt
Barnardsville, North Carolina

It was an honor and privilege to work with Diana and Judy as we created something we hope will make a difference in the lives of nurses and patients. Though it's a challenging journey, it is incredibly exciting when we are generating creative new ideas for content, learning about the achievements of remarkable nurses, and melding our individual visions into one. I am so grateful for the opportunity to work with these two tremendously accomplished nursing leaders.

Throughout the development of this book, my children, Thomas, Sandra, and Christopher, always put a smile on my face. Sandra deserves special recognition for enduring my doctoral journey, which was followed promptly by the launch of work on the book. Don't feel too sorry for her though; I'm sure she'll wangle some new shoes out of my gratitude. I'm appreciative of all my Dad and Ronnie do for me—and I enjoy their political analyses at the dining room table.

My car on the roller coaster of life is filled with great friends who make everything better. Thank you to George, Peggy, John, Kay, Connie, and Cherri' for being my personal "Morale, Welfare, and Recreation" committee. While the book was in progress, I was happy to get to know Karen, Rose, Lindsey, and Robin better. My special thanks and endless gratitude go to Don for all the reasons he knows.

Mary W. Chaffee
Brewster, Massachusetts

CHAPTER 1

A Framework for Action in Policy and Politics

Mary W. Chaffee, Diana J. Mason, and Judith K. Leavitt

"The true test of the American ideal is whether we're able to recognize our failings and then rise together to meet the challenges of our time. Whether we allow ourselves to be shaped by events and history, or whether we act to shape them."

—Barack Obama

On March 23, 2010, President Barack Obama signed the Patient Protection and Affordable Care Act (PPACA)—now known simply as the Affordable Care Act (ACA)—into law and 10 days later signed a reconciliation bill to fine-tune it. This law is arguably the most significant piece of social legislation passed in the United States since Medicare was implemented in 1965. For more than a century, there have been organized efforts to provide universal health coverage in the U.S. While ACA does not guarantee coverage for all, by 2019 it will cover up to 32 million of the 45 million who were uninsured when the bill was signed (94% of the population). It ends the ability of insurance companies to deny coverage to people with pre-existing conditions, to drop people once they acquire a costly illness, or to apply annual and lifetime caps on coverage.

But this landmark legislation promises to do more than reform the health insurance industry. It includes provisions for beginning to reform how care is delivered. The nation has realized that it can no longer afford a health care system centered on providing technology-intensive, acute care to individuals once they become sick or injured. Despite spending more on health care than most developed countries, the U.S. ranked last or next-to-last in 2004, 2006, and 2007 on five indicators of high-performing health systems (access, quality, equity, efficiency, and health lives) compared with five other nations (Australia,

Canada, Germany, New Zealand, and the United Kingdom) (Davis et al., 2007). To improve the health of the public and reduce health care costs, the foundation of the health system must be remade into one that focuses on health promotion and wellness, disease prevention, and chronic care management (Katz, 2009; Woolf, 2009; Wagner, 1998). Acute care must use fewer resources, be safer, and produce better outcomes (Conway & Clancy, 2009).

Nurses know how to do all of this and, in fact, do so every day. After decades marked by nurses' fighting to make their perspectives on health care count, the nation is realizing that they are key to making this shift a reality. The ACA contains a number of measures that reflect this (ACA, 2010). These include the following:

- The ACA is replete with opportunities to test models of care that already hold promise for improving health outcomes and lowering health care costs. A new Center for Medicare and Medicaid Innovations and other pilot programs and demonstration projects will test and develop ideas ranging from transitional care to nurse managed centers, both of which have been innovations led by and using nurses *(www.aannet.org/raisethevoice)*.
- One area identified in the law for testing is the patient-centered "medical" or "health homes."[1] Medical homes are single provider or health teams

---

[1] The ACA refers to refers to both "medical" and "health" homes; approval of such homes by the National Commission on Quality Assurance refers to a "medical home" designation, so this book will use that language, while recognizing that "health home" is more consistent with a health promotion model.

that take responsibility for coordinating all of the care for the patients it serves, whether this entails educating and coaching patients to better manage their chronic illnesses or ensuring that specialty care is provided and consistent with the patients' needs or providing transitional care from hospital to home. Nurses and social workers are the people who are and will be doing most of this care coordination.

- Community-based health centers will be expanded in areas where there are health care provider shortages. Expansion of the National Health Service Corps is expected to ensure that providers, including registered nurses (RNs) and advanced practice registered nurses (APRNs) will be available to staff these centers. An emphasis on primary care will increase the demand for nurse practitioners, and the law authorizes additional support for primary care workforce development (loans, scholarships, new educational program development, and expansion of existing programs).

- Payment reforms include piloting bundled payments and care coordination through "accountable care organizations" (ACO). ACOs are similar to integrated delivery systems that combine services across health care settings and are able to focus on ways to improve care delivery and health outcomes under a bundled payment scheme. Bundled payments will provide financial incentives to providers and health systems to keep patients healthy, rather than doing unnecessary tests and procedures that are currently covered on a fee-for-service basis. Again, nurses are key to preventing complications in hospitalized patients, ensuring smooth transitions to home, and coaching the patient and family caregivers in self-care management and health-promoting behavioral changes.

- The ACA authorizes demonstrations of "Independence At Home" models of care to keep older adults healthy and functioning in their own homes. The models' aim is improving the quality of life and health outcomes while reducing costly nursing home, hospital, and emergency department usage. Nurses are already leading such programs and are essential care providers, often as APRNs.

- Public health will get a boost from investments in prevention research, health screenings, health education campaigns, and other programs aimed at promoting health. Public health nurses are already providing such services and will be increasingly sought after as these programs expand. Nurse researchers study ways to promote health and prevent illness; their work will be highly relevant to the nation's understanding of how to improve health.

- A Center for Innovation will support research that focuses on how to improve the safety and quality of care. Nurses are key to quality and safety in health care; they are leading quality departments in hospitals and health systems. The new Center provides such nurse leaders and nurse researchers with opportunities to demonstrate new methods for improving care in cost-effective ways.

- Various measures authorize funding for nurse-managed centers, improved payment for advanced practice nurses including nurse midwives, and workforce development, including the nursing workforce.

This ACA demonstrates that nursing's time has come, but it doesn't mean complacency can now be acceptable. First, the law is only a first step in reforming health care delivery in the U.S. The Social Security Act, when first passed by Congress in 1935, excluded most minorities and women through exemption of specific job categories such as domestic workers. But over the subsequent years, the law was amended to extend coverage to all Americans. This perspective can alert nurses and others to the need to continue to develop statutes that improve upon the ACA. At the same time, some people who opposed the ACA will seek to dismantle it. Others will examine the ACA's impact on local and state health systems and policies and look for ways to use its mandates and provisions to improve care on a local level. Nurses can and must identify opportunities to implement and improve the law and shape local responses to it.

Second, the implementation of the law is dependent upon the regulations developed by the Department of Health and Human Services (HHS) and state responses including expansion of Medicaid (www.healthreformgps.org). For example, the ACA provides the HHS Secretary with wide authority to expand pilot programs once tested. The staff of the Center for Medicare and Medicaid (CMS) will write regulations that could remove barriers to APRN practice, such as the restriction that a physician must order hospice and home health services to be eligible for Medicare coverage. This requirement initially was intended to limit federal costs but now is viewed as (1) impeding efficient care delivery, (2) costing more because of duplication of providers and continuation of more expensive acute care services, and (3) presenting unnecessary barriers to access to care.

Another example is the law's call for an expansion of home visitation programs for high risk mothers and infants. The Nurse-Family Partnership is the model for this measure, but the law does not specify that the services be provided by nurses despite evidence that nurses produce significantly better outcomes than non-nurses as home visitors (Karoly, Killburn, & Cannon, 2005). States will be responsible for developing health insurance exchanges to provide options for coverage for those who are not covered by employers.

Third, while there are some measures in the law that bypass the Congressional appropriations process, most of the public health and workforce initiatives must have funding appropriated by Congress every year. As the nation's deficit increases, Congress is unlikely to appropriate funding for programs that do not have strong, vocal advocates. This became more evident after the 2010 elections. The election outcomes shifted the political landscape and will influence the implementation of the ACA and the future of health care reform. Control of the House of Representatives and eight governorships shifted to the Republican Party, whose platform included fiscal restraint and repealing the ACA. States are expected to play a more significant role in the implementation of the ACA, with some expected to fight its state mandates.

So while nursing is well positioned to contribute to a reformed health care system, we cannot assume that those making the decisions about how to reform it will automatically seek nurses' input. A 2010 Gallup poll of over 1500 non-nurse, health-care opinion leaders revealed that these leaders viewed nurses as essential for quality and safety in health care, but only 14% believed that nurses would be influential in reforming health care (Gallup, 2010). Whether developing new models of care, sharing ideas for regulations with policymakers, working with health care organizations to develop demonstration projects that the new law seeks to test, or advocating new legislation to amend and improve upon the law (or preventing it from being dismantled), nurses must assume

the mantle of politically savvy leaders who are shaping health policy at the local, state, and national levels within government, workplaces, health-related organizations, and communities. In fact, this mandate for nurses' leadership is one of the recommendations of the 2010 Institute of Medicine's report on *The Future of Nursing: Leading Change, Advancing Health*. This report, available at *www.iom.edu/nursing*, consists of four key messages, one of which is "Nurses should be full partners, with physicians and other health professionals, in redesigning health care in the U.S." This document provides an important blueprint for action by nurses and others concerned with improving access to affordable, quality health care and promoting the health of the nation.

POLICY AND THE POLICY PROCESS

Policy is the deliberate course of action chosen by an individual or group to deal with a problem (Anderson, 2006). *Public policies* are the choices made by public or government officials to deal with public problems (Kraft & Furlong, 2010). Public policies are authoritative decisions made in the legislative, executive, or judicial branches of government intended to influence the actions, behaviors, or decisions of others (Longest, 2005). When the intent of a public policy is to influence health or health care, it is a *health policy*. *Social policies* identify courses of action to deal with social problems. All are made within a dynamic environment and a complex policymaking process.

Policies are crafted everywhere from small towns to Capitol Hill. Federal health policy takes many forms including bills passed by Congress such as the Medicare Modernization Act of 2003 and workplace safety regulations enforced by the Occupational Safety and Health Administration. President Bill Clinton banned smoking in federal buildings by executive order, another type of policy (Cook & Bero, 2009). States use policies to specify requirements for licensure in the health professions, to set criteria for eligibility for Medicaid, and to mandate immunization requirements for public university students, for example. Hospitals use policies to direct when visitors may visit patients, to manage staffing, and to respond to disaster. Public schools employ policies to specify who may administer medications to schoolchildren.

Towns, cities, and other municipalities use policies to manage public water supplies, to define who may run for office, and whether or not residents may keep exotic pets.

In a capitalist economy such as the U.S., private markets are permitted to control the production and consumption of goods and services, including health services. The government "intrudes" with policies only when the private markets fail to achieve desired public objectives. When it is necessary for the government to intercede, two types of policy are used:

• *Allocative policies* are used to provide benefits to a distinct group of individuals or organizations, at the expense of others, to achieve a public objective (this is also referred to as the *redistribution of wealth*). The implementation of Medicare in 1966 was an allocative policy that provided health benefits to older adults and others using federal funds (largely from middle- and higher-income taxpayers).

• *Regulatory policies* are used to influence the actions, behavior, and decisions of individuals or groups to ensure that a public objective is met (Longest, 2005). The Health Insurance Portability and Accountability Act of 1996 is a regulatory policy. It regulates how individually identifiable health information is managed by users as well as other aspects of health records.

FORCES THAT SHAPE HEALTH POLICY

Many forces shape health policy. Some of the most prominent forces appear in Figure 1-1.

VALUES

Values influence all political and policymaking activities. Public policies reflect a society's values—and also conflicts between values. A policy reflects which value (or values) is given priority in a specific decision (Kraft

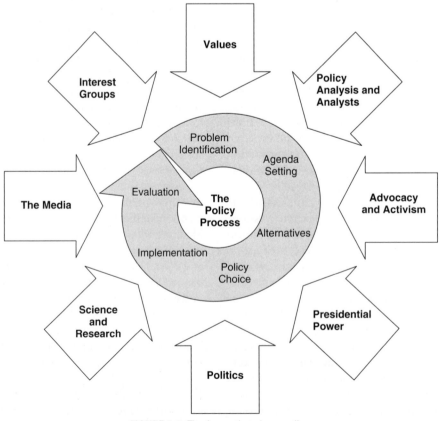

FIGURE 1-1 The forces that shape policy.

& Furlong, 2010). Once framed, a policy reveals the underlying values that shaped it. This is usually apparent in health policies; these often affect those who are unable to protect themselves like the young, poor, sick, old, and disabled. Different people value different things, and when resources are finite, policy choices ultimately bring a disadvantage to some groups; some will gain something from the policy, and some will lose (Bankowski, 1996). To support or oppose a policy requires value judgments (Majone, 1989). Conflicts between values were apparent throughout the debate on health care reform; for example, despite a strong contingent of advocates for a government-run, non-profit insurance option that would compete with private insurers, it was not included in the law after opposition from the insurance industry and from people who believed that it represented an increase in the government's control of health care.

POLITICS

Politics is frequently associated with a negative connotation, yet it is actually a neutral term. Politics is the process of influencing the allocation of scarce resources. Policymaking involves the distribution of resources; so politics or political action can be viewed as the efforts and strategies used to shape a policy choice. The definition of politics contains several important concepts. *Influencing* indicates that there are opportunities to shape the outcome of a process. *Allocation* means that decisions are being made about how to distribute resources. *Scarce* implies that there are limits to the amount of resources available—and that all parties likely cannot have all they want. Finally, *resources* are usually considered to be financial, but could also include human resources (personnel), time, or physical space such as offices (Mason, Leavitt, & Chaffee, 2007). Politics can also be considered to be how conflicts in a society are expressed and resolved in favor of one set of values or interests over another (Kraft & Furlong, 2010).

Political skill has a bad reputation; for some it conjures up thoughts of manipulation, self-interested behavior, and favoritism (Ferris, Davidson, & Perrewe, 2005). "She plays politics" is not generally considered to be a compliment, but true political skill is critical in health care leadership, advocating for others, and shaping policy. Ferris et al. (2005) consider political skill to be the ability to understand others and to use that knowledge to influence others

to act in a way that supports one's objectives. They believe political skill has four components:
1. *Social astuteness:* Skill at being attuned to others and social situations; ability to interpret one's own behaviors and the behavior of others.
2. *Interpersonal influence:* Convincing personal style that influences others featuring the ability to adapt behavior to situations and be pleasant and productive to work with.
3. *Networking ability:* The ability to develop and use diverse networks of people and the ability to position oneself to create and take advantage of opportunities.
4. *Apparent sincerity:* The display of high levels of integrity, authenticity, sincerity, and genuineness (p. 11).

POLICY ANALYSIS AND POLICY ANALYSTS

Analysis is the process of examining an object and breaking it down to understand it better. Policy analysis uses different methods to assess a problem and determine alternative ways to resolve it. This encourages deliberate critical thinking about the causes of problems, identifies the various ways a government or other group could act, evaluates the alternatives, and determines the policy choice that is most desirable. Policy analysts are individuals who, with professional training and experience, analyze problems and weigh potential solutions. Citizens can also use policy analysis to better understand a problem, alternatives, and potential implications of policy choices (Kraft & Furlong, 2010).

ADVOCACY AND ACTIVISM

Advocacy for one patient at a time has long been considered a core nursing role. Advocating for change through policy and politics permits nurses to advocate on a larger scale and is endorsed in *Nursing's Social Policy Statement* (American Nurses Association [ANA], 2003), a document that defines nursing and its social context. Political activism may be associated with protests and "sit-ins" but has grown to include diverse and effective strategies such as blogging, using evidence to support policy choices, and garnering media attention in sophisticated ways.

INTEREST GROUPS AND LOBBYISTS

Interest groups advocate for policies that are advantageous to their membership. Groups often employ lobbyists to advocate on their behalf, and their power cannot be underestimated. In the U.S. in 2009, about 1750 businesses and organizations spent at least $1.2 billion on lobbyists to advocate for their interests in the health care reform debate and on many other issues (Center for Public Integrity, 2010).

THE MEDIA

In 2009 and 2010, Pulitzer-prize winning journalist Charles Ornstein and his colleague Tracy Weber published a series of investigative reports on the California Board of Registered Nursing's excessive delays in acting on reports of professional misconduct by RNs for whom evidence of wrongdoing was well documented (Weber & Ornstein, 2010). The board took an average of 3 years to take disciplinary action, including against nurses who were charged with physically and sexually abusing patients or were in prison but still getting their licenses renewed. The journalists' initial reports resulted in more staff being hired by the board, but when it was not clear that they had successfully improved processing times and more reports were published by Ornstein and Weber, the governor dismissed the board's members and replaced them with new ones. The executive director of the board—a nurse—subsequently resigned. The governor advocated new legislation to require employers to notify the board whenever they fire or suspend a nurse for serious wrongdoing and permit a state official to suspend the license of any nurse who is deemed to represent a threat to the public. In 2010, the legislation was opposed by leading nurses' unions in the state (Weber & Ornstein, 2010).

Ornstein and Weber work for ProPublica, one of a growing number of non-profit investigative news organizations. They used traditional newspapers (the *Los Angeles Times*) to help disseminate their stories, but also created an interactive website *(www. propublica.org/series/nurses)* that profiled individual nurses and provided comparative data on disciplinary actions by other state boards for nursing. They also used new media, or social media, to further push their work out to other audiences. But new media have also introduced easily accessible tools for activists and advocates to use to become citizen journalists and influence policy.

SCIENCE AND RESEARCH

Scientific findings can play a powerful role in the first step of the policy process—getting attention for particular problems and moving them to the policy agenda. Research can also be valuable in defining the size and scope of a problem (Diers & Price, 2007). This can help to obtain support for a particular policy option and in lobbying for support for it. Evidence should be used to inform policy debates and shape policy choices to help ensure that the solution will be effective.

PRESIDENTIAL POWER

The president embodies the power of the executive branch of government and is the only person elected to represent the entire nation. As the most visible government official, the president is able to propel issues to the top of the nation's policy agenda. Though the president cannot introduce legislation, he can provide draft legislation and legislative guidance (Weissert & Weissert, 2006).

THE FRAMEWORK FOR ACTION

The first edition of this book, *Political Action Handbook for Nurses: Changing the Workplace, Government, Organizations and Community,* introduced readers to a model of political action for nurses (Mason & Talbott, 1985) named the Framework for Action. The model used "spheres of influence" to conceptualize the places where nurses use politics to shape policy and to work for change in the health system. The original Framework for Action's four spheres of influence were labeled: (1) the workplace, (2) the government, (3) organizations, and (4) the community. The original "workplace" sphere has been broadened now to include the workplace and the workforce. This addresses the policy work that is done in a variety of places to influence the size, educational preparation, and competence of the nursing workforce. The original "organizations" sphere was defined as professional nursing associations (Mason & Talbott, 1985, p. 444). Recognizing that nurses work to influence policy through other types of associations, such as interdisciplinary groups and unions, this sphere has now been reconceptualized as "associations and interest groups" (Figure 1-2).

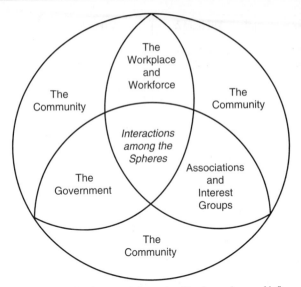

FIGURE 1-2 The framework for action. The four spheres of influence where nurses shape policy. The spheres overlap; activity in one can affect the others.

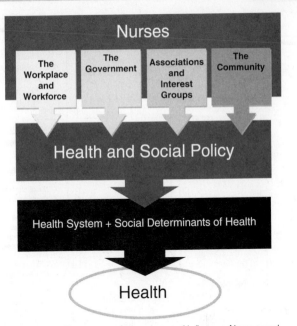

FIGURE 1-3 The targets of the spheres of influence. Nurses work in four spheres of influence to shape health and social policy. Policies are designed to remedy problems in the health system and to address social determinants of health to improve health.

The Framework for Action has been updated to reflect current knowledge about health care and the impact of social determinants on health (Figure 1-3). It more thoroughly explains nursing's role in improving health through influencing policy. Action in the spheres of influence can shape policy that can then influence the health system and social determinants of health.

The spheres of influence are not discrete silos. Each is a part of a broader, more complex system where change in one sphere often influences changes in others. Policy can be shaped in more than one sphere at one time, and action in one sphere can influence others. To achieve greater access to care for the uninsured, for example, nurses may work in their own organization to alter policy to increase access to services. They may also use political strategies in the media, such as blogging or being interviewed on television, to express their support for better access to care. They may work with their professional association, or an interest group, to communicate their views to policymakers. Additional context (the who, what, where, when, and why of nursing's policy influence) is provided in Figure 1-4.

SPHERE OF INFLUENCE 1: THE COMMUNITY

While a limited number of nurses will have the opportunity to influence policy at the highest levels of government, there are more extensive opportunities for nurses to influence health and social policy in communities. Nursing has a rich history of community activism with remarkable examples provided by leaders such as Lillian Wald, Harriet Tubman, and Dorothea Dix. This legacy continues today with the community advocacy efforts of nurses like Cora Tomalinas, Mary Behrens, Ruth Lubic, Patricia Tobal, Ellie Lopez-Bowlan, the Nightingales who took on big tobacco, and the nurses who are a part of the Canary Coalition for Clean Air (all of their stories appear in this book).

A community is a group of people who share something in common and interact with one another, who may exhibit a commitment with one another, and may share a geographic boundary (Lundy & Janes, 2001). A community may be a neighborhood, a city, an online group with a common interest, or a faith-based network. Nurses can be influential in communities by identifying problems, strategizing

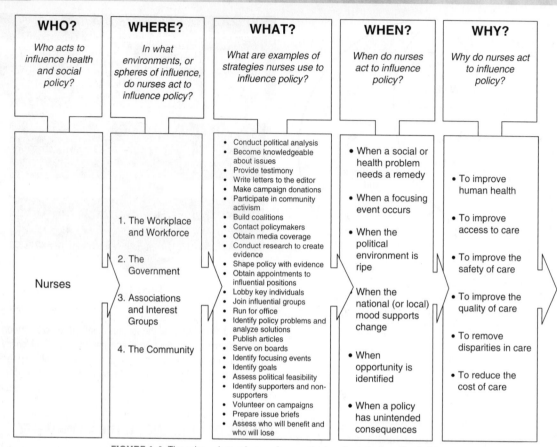

FIGURE 1-4 The who, what, where, when, and why of nursing's policy influence.

with others, mobilizing support, and advocating for change. In residential communities (such as towns, villages, and urban districts), there are opportunities to serve in elected and volunteer positions that influence policy. Many groups, such as planning boards, civic organizations, and parent-teacher associations, offer opportunities for involvement.

SPHERE OF INFLUENCE 2: THE WORKFORCE AND WORKPLACE

Nurses work in a variety of settings: hospitals, clinics, schools, private sector firms, government agencies, military services, research centers, nursing homes, and home health agencies. All of these environments are political ones—resources are finite, and nurses must work in each to influence the allocation of organizational resources. Policies guide many activities in the health care workplaces where nurses are employed. Many that affect nursing and patient care are internal

organizational policies such as staffing policies, clinical procedures, and patient care guidelines. External policies are operative in the health care workplace also, for example, state laws regulating nursing licensure and immunization requirements of clinical practitioners. Federal laws and regulations are evident in the nursing workplace such as Occupational Health and Safety Administration regulations regarding worker protection from bloodborne pathogens.

Outside of the workplace, policy is made that influences the size and composition of the nursing workforce. The ACA authorizes increased funding for scholarships and loans for nursing education—potentially augmenting existing workforce programs funded under Title VII and VIII of the Public Health Act. The non-governmental Commission on Graduates of Foreign Nursing Schools is authorized by the federal government to protect the public by ensuring that nurses and other health care professionals educated in countries other than the U.S. are eligible and qualified to meet licensure, immigration, and other practice requirements in the U.S. (Commission on Graduates of Foreign Nursing Schools, 2009). The National Council of State Boards of Nursing is a not-for-profit organization that brings together state boards of nursing to act on matters of common interest affecting the public's health, safety, and welfare, including the development of licensing examinations in nursing (National Council of State Boards of Nursing, 2009).

SPHERE OF INFLUENCE 3: THE GOVERNMENT

Government action and policy affects lives from birth until death. It funds prenatal care, inspects food, bans unsafe toys and cars, operates schools, builds highways, and regulates what is transmitted on airwaves. It provides for the common defense; supplies fire and police protection; and gives financial assistance to the poor, aged, and others who cannot maintain a minimal standard of living. The government responds to disaster, subsidizes agriculture, and licenses funeral homes (Heineman, Peterson, & Rasmussen, 1995).

Though most health care in the U.S. is provided in the private sector, much is paid for and regulated by the government. So, how the government crafts health policy is extremely important (Weissert & Weissert, 2006). Government plays a significant role in influencing nursing and nursing practice. States determine the scope of professional activities considered to be nursing, with notable exceptions of the military, veterans' administration, and Indian health service. Federal and state governments determine who is eligible for care under specific benefit programs and who can be reimbursed for providing care. Sometimes government provides leadership in defining problems for both the public and private sectors to address (Mason et al., 2007). At least eight House and Senate committees and subcommittees shape policy on health, and many more committees address social problems that affect health. In the House of Representatives, the House Nursing Caucus, an informal, bipartisan group of legislators who have declared their interest in helping nurses, lobbies for federal funding for nursing education (Walker, 2009).

Abraham Lincoln's description of a "government of the people, by the people and for the people" (1863) captures the intricate nature of the relationship of government and its people. There are many ways nurses can influence policymaking in the government sphere—at all levels of government (local, state, and federal). Examples include the following:

- Obtaining appointment or assignment to influential government positions
- Serving in federal, state, and local agencies
- Serving as elected officials
- Working as paid lobbyists
- Communicating to policymakers their support or opposition to a policy
- Providing testimony at government hearings or open meetings
- Participating in grassroots efforts, such as rallies, to draw attention to problems.

SPHERE OF INFLUENCE 4: ASSOCIATIONS AND INTEREST GROUPS

Professional nursing associations have played a significant role in influencing the practice of nursing. Many professional nursing associations have legislative or policy committees that advocate for policies that support their members' practice. For example, the American Nephrology Nurses Association identifies advocacy as a core value in their strategic plan. One of their goals is to be the leading advocate for nephrology nursing and to advocate for individuals, families, and communities affected by real or potential kidney disease (American Nephrology Nurses Association, 2009). Many nursing specialty groups provide training and workshops for nurses interested in learning the ropes of political involvement as well as online resources to assist members in their advocacy efforts. Working with a group increases the chances for advocacy to be effective, provides an environment where resources can be shared, and enhances networking and learning. Nurses can be effective in association policy activities by serving on public policy or legislative work groups, providing testimony, and preparing position statements.

When nursing organizations join forces through coalitions, their influence can be multiplied. For example, the American Nurses Association (ANA) is a member of the Safer Chemicals, Healthy Families coalition, a coalition whose members are united by a common concern about toxic chemicals in homes, workplaces, and products used every day. The Coalition for Patients' Rights is a group of 35 national organizations representing health care professionals who are working to fight the American Medical

Association's attempts to limit patients' access to non-physician providers (www.patientsrightscoalition.org). Twenty-six of the members are nursing organizations.

Nurses can be influential, not just in nursing associations, but through working with other interest groups such as the American Public Health Association and the Sierra Club. Some interest groups have a broad portfolio of policy interests, while others focus on one disease (e.g., breast cancer) or one issue (e.g., driving while intoxicated). Interest groups have become powerful players in policy debates; those with large funding streams are able to shape public opinion with television and radio advertisements.

HEALTH

The Framework for Action now includes health as an element of the model to represent that optimal health is viewed as the goal of nursing's policy efforts. Optimal health (either the individual patient's or a population's) is the central focus of the political and policy activity described in this book. This focus makes it clear that the ultimate goal for advancing nursing's interests must be to promote the public's health (see Figure 1-3).

HEALTH AND SOCIAL POLICY

Health and social policy now appear as elements in the Framework for Action. Many factors that affect health status are social factors such as income, education, and housing. Thus it was important to identify the important role that social policies play in influencing health (see Figure 1-3).

SOCIAL DETERMINANTS OF HEALTH

An important update to the framework is the inclusion of the concept of social determinants of health (see Figure 1-3). Even in the most affluent nations, people who are poor have substantially shorter life expectancies and experience more illness than the rich (Wilkinson & Marmot, 2003). While health can be improved with changes to the health system, an agenda for health improvement should be based on understanding the social determinants (Wilensky & Satcher, 2009). Policies are needed to address the social and economic conditions that make people ill. Universal access to care is one social determinant of health (Wilkinson & Marmot, 2003). Political aspects of the social determinants of health appear in Box 1-1.

> **BOX 1-1** **Political Aspects of the Social Determinants of Health**
>
> - The health of individuals and populations is determined significantly by social factors.
> - The social determinants of health produce great inequities in health within and between societies.
> - The poor and disadvantaged experience worse health than the rich, have less access to care, and die younger in all societies.
> - The social determinants of health can be measured and described.
> - The measurement of the social determinants provides evidence that can serve as the basis for political action.
> - Evidence is generated and used in a continuous cycle of evidence production, policy development, implementation, and evaluation.
> - Evidence of the effects of policies and programs on inequities can be measured and can provide data on the effectiveness of interventions.
> - Evidence about the social determinants of health is insufficient to bring about change on its own; political will combined with evidence offers the most powerful strategy to address the negative effects of the social determinants.
>
> Adapted from: National Institute for Health and Clinical Excellence. (2007). The Social Determinants of Health: Developing an Evidence Base for Political Action. Final report to the World Health Organization Commission on the Social Determinants of Health. Lead authors: J. Mackenbach, M. Exworthy, J. Popay, P. Tugwell, V. Robinson, S. Simpson, T. Narayan, L. Myer, T. Houweling, L. Jadue, and F. Florenza.

SUMMARY

Nurses are well-positioned for reforming health care in ways that promote a healthier public and reduce health care costs. But we must be strategic in our leadership, whether in clinical settings to improve the safety and quality of care or advocating for nurse-managed health centers that provide comprehensive primary care and community services to vulnerable and underserved populations. The health care opinion leaders in the 2010 Gallup poll discussed in the opening of this chapter identified two reasons why nurses would fall short of influencing health care reform: too many nurses didn't want to lead, and the myriad nursing organizations rarely presented a united front. We must not fall short. This book can help nurses to overcome barriers. It is time.

For a list of related websites, please refer to your Evolve Resources at http://evolve.elsevier.com/Mason/policypolitics/

REFERENCES

American Nephrology Nurses Association. (2009). Health policy overview. Retrieved from www.annanurse.org.

American Nurses Association. (2003). *Nursing's social policy statement.* Washington, DC: The Author.

Anderson, J. (2006). *Public policymaking: An introduction* (6th ed.). Boston: Houghton Mifflin.

Bankowski, Z. (1996). Ethics and human values in health policy. *World Health Forum, 17,* 146-149.

Center for Public Integrity. (2010). Washington lobbying giants cash in on health reform debate. Retrieved from www.publicintegrity.org/articles/entry/2010.

Commission on Graduates of Foreign Nursing Schools. (2009). Commission on Graduates of Foreign Nursing Schools—Mission and history. Retrieved from www.cgfns.org.

Conway, P. H., & Clancy, C. (2009). Transformation of health care at the front line. *JAMA, 301*(7), 763-765.

Cook, D., & Bero, L. (2009). The politics of smoking in federal buildings: An executive order case study. *American Journal of Public Health, 99*(9), 1588-1595.

Davis, K., Schoen, C., Schoenbaum, S., Doty, M., Holmgren, A., Kriss, J., & Shea, K. (2007). *Mirror, mirror on the wall: An international update on the comparative performance of American health care.* New York: The Commonwealth Fund.

Diers, D., & Price, L. (2007). Research as a political and policy tool. In D. Mason, J. Leavitt & M. Chaffee (Eds.), *Policy and politics in nursing and health care* (pp. 195-207). St. Louis: Elsevier.

Ferris, G., Davidson, S., & Perrewe, P. (2005). *Political skill at work—Impact on work effectiveness.* Mountain View, CA: Davies-Black Publishing.

Gallup. (2010). Nursing leadership from bedside to boardroom: Opinion leaders' perception. Retrieved from http://newcareersinnursing.org/sites/default/files/file-attachments/Top%20Line%20Report.pdf.

Heineman, R., Peterson, S., & Rasmussen, T. (1995). *American government.* New York: McGraw-Hill.

Karoly, L., Killburn, M. R., & Cannon, J. (2005). Early childhood interventions: Proven results, future promise. Arlington, VA: RAND Corporation. Retrieved from www.rand.org/pubs/monographs/2005/RAND_MG341.pdf.

Katz, M. H. (2009). Structural interventions for addressing chronic health problems. *JAMA, 302*(6), 683-685.

Kraft, M., & Furlong, S. (2010). *Public policy—politics, analysis, and alternatives* (3rd ed.): CQ Press.

Lincoln, A. (1863). Gettysburg Address. Retrieved from www.ourdocuments.gov/doc.php?flash=old&doc=36.

Longest, B. (2005). *Health policymaking in the United States* (4th ed.). Chicago: Health Administration Press.

Lundy, K., & Janes, S. (2001). *Community health nursing: Caring for the public's health.* Sudbury, MA: Jones and Bartlett.

Majone, G. (1989). *Evidence, argument, and persuasion in the policy process.* New Haven: Yale University Press.

Mason, D., Leavitt, J., & Chaffee, M. (2007). Policy and politics: A framework for action. In D. Mason, J. Leavitt, & M. Chaffee (Eds.), *Policy and Politics in Nursing and Health Care.* St. Louis: Elsevier.

Mason, D., & Talbott, S. (1985). Introduction: A framework for political action. In D. Mason & S. Talbott (Eds.), *Political action handbook for nurses—Changing the workplace, government, organizations, and community.* Menlo Park, CA: Addison Wesley.

National Council of State Boards of Nursing. (2009). National Council of State Boards of Nursing—About us. Retrieved from www.ncsbn.org/index.htm.

Patient Protection and Affordable Care Act and the Health Care and Education Reconciliation Act. (2010). Retrieved from http://dpc.senate.gov/dpcdoc-sen_health_care_bill.cfm.

Wagner, E. H., (1998). Chronic disease management: What will it take to improve care for chronic illness? *Effective Clinical Practice, 1*(1), 2-4.

Walker, I. (2009). Caucusing for a cause. *American Journal of Nursing, 109*(9), 26-27.

Weber, T., & Ornstein, C. (2010). When caregivers harm: California's unwatched nurses. *ProPublica.* Retrieved from www.propublica.org/series/nurses.

Weissert, C., & Weissert, W. (2006). *Governing health—The politics of health policy* (3rd ed.). Baltimore: The Johns Hopkins University Press.

Wilensky, G., & Satcher, D. (2009). Don't forget about the social determinants of health. *Health Affairs, 28*(2), w194-w198.

Wilkinson, R., & Marmot, M. (2003). *Social determinants of health—The solid facts* (2nd ed.). Denmark: World Health Organization.

Woolf, S. H. (2009). A closer look at the economic argument for disease prevention. *JAMA, 301*(5), 536-538.

CHAPTER 2

A Historical Perspective on Policy, Politics, and Nursing

Sandra B. Lewenson

"Organization is the power of the age."
—Sophia Palmer, founding editor of the
American Journal of Nursing

The history of the modern nursing movement, which began in 1873, tells the story of a pioneering group of women who responded to the changing role of women in society. They advocated a new profession for women and better health care for the public. In forging the nursing profession in this modern period, nurses had to enter the political arena to gain legitimate authority over their education and practice.

Over time, however, the history has blurred and often obscured from view the rich tapestry of nursing's political past. This can be explained in part by the fact that women are perceived by society to have historically played a small role in the political arena. Nursing, long considered "women's work," shares with the overall women's movement the many negative, devalued perceptions of the worth of its role (Reverby, 1987). The assumption that women's work is somehow free and expected perpetuates the negative aspects of "nursism"—"a form of sexism that specifically maligns the caring role in society" (Lewenson, 1996, p. 226).

The history of nursing is replete with stories of nurses' activism to advance the profession and health care, and this chapter provides some examples.

POLITICAL AWAKENING AND THE MODERN NURSING MOVEMENT

The modern nursing movement began when Florence Nightingale opened the nurse-training program at St. Thomas Hospital in England in 1860. This landmark event signaled to the world that nurses required schooling for the work they did and provided one of the first opportunities for women to work outside the home and be self-supportive. In turn, the rise of modern nursing catalyzed the political activism of nurses.

Nightingale's writing supports a feminist stance on who should control the education and work of nurses. Nightingale believed that nursing should be controlled by nurses. A 1908 editorial comment published in the *American Journal of Nursing* (*AJN*) acknowledged that her "brilliant essence lay in her taking from men's hands a power which did not logically or rightly belong to them, but which they had usurped, and seizing it firmly in her own, from whence she passed it on to her pupils and disciples" (Progress and reaction, 1908, pp. 333-334). Like women's education, education for nurses was considered unnecessary. Women were considered natural-born nurses and therefore did not require an education. After the extraordinary success of Nightingale's ideas about sanitation and nurses' education, nurses were educated to reform the deplorable conditions found in hospitals throughout the United States.

Nightingale, the reformer, emerges as a complex individual who often achieved her goals "by behind-the-scenes management of the committees and doctors" (Vicinus & Nergaard, 1989, p. 159). It was her letter-writing to influential people that helped Nightingale revolutionize health care and nursing education. Moreover, it was the acceptance, around the world, of her ideas about sanitation, education, and separation of nursing and medicine that contributed to her ability to facilitate change.

PROFESSIONAL EDUCATION AND NURSE-TRAINING SCHOOLS

Political activism of the early nursing pioneers took the form of creating the models for professional education. The year 1873 heralded the opening of Nightingale-influenced nurse-training schools and the beginning of the modern nursing movement in the United States. Early nursing leaders implemented many of Nightingale's ideas about nursing. They skillfully demonstrated to hospital administrators that using nursing students improved sanitary conditions on wards and led to better patient outcomes, creating great financial incentives for hospitals to open such schools (Dock & Stewart, 1931). Between 1873 and 1893, nurse-training schools proliferated, and by 1910 the number of schools had risen to more than 1129 (Burgess, 1928). But these early schools were not regulated by any professional group. Hospital administrators wanted these schools because it was cheaper to use student labor than to employ the graduates—education was secondary to work expected of the students.

Once a nurse's training was over, the school provided no support. Graduate nurses found themselves working in the only jobs they could find, such as private duty nursing or public health nursing. Physicians or pharmacists, as opposed to nurses, often controlled the private duty nursing directories, which distributed private duty work. This meant that the fee schedule rested outside the nurses' control, which often led to further exploitation of an already exploited group. The misuse of both the students and the graduate nurses contributed greatly to the strong political stance that early nursing leaders took when they formed professional nursing organizations.

POLITICAL ACTION AND THE RISE OF PROFESSIONAL ORGANIZATIONS

Professional nursing organizations began to form between 1893 and 1912. Their interests first revolved around the issues confronting the profession but later expanded to include social and political reforms affecting society.

NATIONAL LEAGUE FOR NURSING

The first national nursing organization to form was the American Society of Superintendents for Training Schools, founded in 1893 and renamed the National League of Nursing Education in 1912 and the National League for Nurses (NLN) in 1952. This organization originated at the nurses' congress that convened at the World's Columbian Exposition in Chicago in 1893. Superintendents, chief administrators, and hospital nursing staff sought uniformity in nursing curricula and standards of nursing practice. Alone in their work, they felt isolated and powerless to go before the entrenched powers, such as the hospital boards and medical groups, that sought to control the developing profession. The early speeches of leaders such as Isabel Hampton Robb, Lavinia Dock, and Sophia Palmer spoke out in favor of collective action and reflected the progressive nature of the newly founded organization (Birnbach & Lewenson, 1993).

AMERICAN NURSES ASSOCIATION

Training schools soon formed alumnae associations that would provide the basic structure for a second national nursing organization—the Nurses' Associated Alumnae of the United States and Canada in 1896 (renamed the American Nurses Association [ANA] in 1911). Isabel Hampton Robb was one of the founders and first president of the organization. She advocated nursing reforms that supported the ideas of the emerging nursing profession, such as moving toward an 8-hour workday versus a 12-hour workday and efforts to obtain nursing registration.

Considering "journalism … to be a necessary part of the trend of nursing progress" (The Editor, 1900, p. 65) the organization founded the *American Journal of Nursing (AJN)*, one of the first professional journals in nursing. Sophia Palmer, the first editor-in-chief of the *AJN* used the journal to call for a grassroots movement that would unite alumnae associations around the country for the purpose of political action and social reform (Figure 2-1). She urged small and large schools to organize alumnae associations "for the definite and separate purpose of promoting legislation for state registration of nurses" (Palmer, 1909, p. 956). She recognized the inherent power that nurses would wield, if they were united in a national organization. Palmer (1897) said, "Organization is the power of the age. Without it nothing great is accomplished. All questions having ultimate advancement of the profession are dependent upon united action for success" (p. 55).

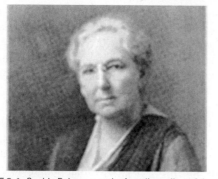

FIGURE 2-1 Sophia Palmer was the founding editor of the *American Journal of Nursing* and used the journal to stimulate discussion among nurses about the important policy and political issues of the day, such as nurse registration. She challenged nurses' alumnae associations to use their collective power to influence legislation of importance to the profession and to public health. (From *American Journal of Nursing*, June, 1920 [v.XX], No. 9, p. 677.)

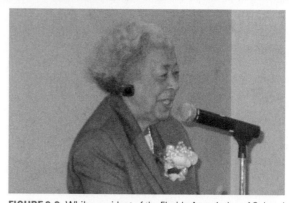

FIGURE 2-2 While president of the Florida Association of Colored Graduate Nurses, Dr. Mary Elizabeth Carnegie, noted nurse educator, historian, and civil rights activist, actively sought the integration of African-American nurses in the American Nurses Association and the dissolution of the National Association of Colored Graduate Nurses in 1951. The National Black Nurses Association was founded after this integration was accomplished and has provided African-American nurses with a venue for deeper explorations and actions regarding the issues confronting nurses of color and their communities.

The state alumnae associations organized around the highly political issue of state registration. Until 1903, anyone could call herself a nurse. It was not until 1903 that the first state nurse registration acts were passed and the title nurse was protected by law. Although the early registration acts varied in their protection of the public from inadequately prepared nurses, they signified the political efforts of organized nursing. Since nursing leaders did not yet have the vote, support for this legislation was gained through letter-writing campaigns, personal visits to the legislatures, use of the professional journals, and support of the public press.

NATIONAL ASSOCIATION OF COLORED GRADUATE NURSES

Discriminatory practices in parts of the United States barred many African-American nurses from membership in their state associations. This practice in turn prevented them from belonging to the ANA. Moreover, segregation and discriminatory practices throughout the country banned African-American nurses from attending most nurse-training schools and, in some states, prohibited them from taking state nurse registration examinations. In keeping with other women's organizations and the need for political activism, African-American nurses organized the National Association of Colored Graduate Nurses (NACGN) in 1908. Along with issues of blatant racial discrimination, the NACGN focused on education, standards of practice, and the passage of state nurse registration acts (Figure 2-2) (Staupers, 1937).

To determine the need for such an organization, Martha Franklin, nursing leader and founder of the NACGN, had undertaken a study on African-American nurses in 1906 and 1907. Franklin sent more than 1500 surveys to African-American graduates of nurse-training schools, most of which had opened in historically African-American hospital settings (Thoms, 1929), and found that African-American nurses needed an organization to address issues pertaining to their particular needs. Franklin also recognized that only in the collective would they gain enough power to change discriminatory practices and influence nursing and health care (Lewenson, 1996).

Members of the NACGN constantly faced the double-edged sword of sexism and racism, which led to their political activism. A primary concern for the NACGN was the nurse registration acts that the profession as a whole sought. Not only did the organization support the passage of such acts, but its members also fought to ensure that nurses of color could sit for the state examination and be given the same examination as their white counterparts.

The collective action of the NACGN around the issue of racial discrimination toward African-American nurses in the military during World War II serves as another example of political activism in nursing. Not until after the armistice in World War I were African-American nurses accepted into the Army Nurse Corps. It wasn't until after a great political campaign waged by the NACGN during World War II that they were integrated into the armed services, albeit in limited numbers. Mabel Staupers, considered one of the people instrumental in the integration of African-American nurses into the military, prepared the NACGN to engage in the political effort needed to effect change (Hine, 1993). Staupers not only mobilized the NACGN but also sought the "allegiance of sympathetic white nurses within the profession" (Hine, 1989, p. 170). The NACGN used letter-writing campaigns, alliances with the other professional nursing organizations, membership in the newly established National Nursing Council for War Service, meetings with politically significant people, and collective action to integrate nursing in the military.

NATIONAL ORGANIZATION FOR PUBLIC HEALTH NURSING

At the beginning of the twentieth century, the need for public health nurses increased as the U.S. experienced the effects of urbanization, industrialization, and immigration. Cities filled with people who wanted to find jobs in these growing industrialized centers. This change in demographics contributed to severely overcrowded housing, unsafe work conditions, inadequate sanitation, epidemics, and poor access to health care, causing progressive reformers to respond. The public health movement used trained nurses in public health departments and visiting nurse service agencies to bring their ideas about sanitation, immunization, and health care to the public. In 1902, there were fewer than 200 public health nurses; by 1912, there were more than 3000 (Gardner, 1933). With this steady proliferation of visiting nurse associations came unscrupulous home health care agencies that offered substandard visiting nurse services. To overcome poor and inferior nursing practices, the ANA and the NLN exerted their political expertise and in 1912 formed the National Organization for Public Health Nursing (NOPHN). This organization's members joined with other civic-minded citizens to improve the health of the American public.

To create the NOPHN, in 1911 nursing leaders of the ANA and the NLN developed a plan to organize public health nurses. Letters sent to organizations that employed public health nurses requested that they send a representative to the annual nursing convention of the ANA and the NLN who could vote on the issue of starting a new organization. Most of the agencies responded favorably, and one year later, in 1912, the NOPHN organized. The NOPHN objectives were to "stimulate responsibility for the health of the community by the establishment and the extension of public health nursing" and "to develop standards and techniques in public health nursing service" (Gardner, 1933, p. 27). From the outset, the NOPHN recognized the political expediency of forming coalitions with other health professionals and laypeople and included these other individuals as members.

ORGANIZED NURSING AND SUFFRAGE

While the four nursing organizations were forming, the campaign for suffrage was under way. Suffrage meant personal and political freedom and the means to control the laws that governed women. For nurses, suffrage meant gaining a political voice in the laws that regulated practice, education, and health. Professional nursing organizations provided the medium for nurses to share common experiences and thus find a collective voice. Once these organizations established themselves as viable associations, nurses expanded their horizons to include broader women's issues, including suffrage, in their political agenda (Lewenson, 1996). This period of political activism in nursing fits the description by Cohen and colleagues (1996) of the early stages of political development. Nursing, through the four organizations, had developed its identity, formed coalitions, built on its political base, and used the language needed for changing legislation. By advocating for patient rights, nurses began to shape policy. As nursing struggled to come to consensus over the issue of woman suffrage, they published a journal, formed coalitions among themselves and with non-nursing groups, and discussed the political ramifications of both sides of the suffrage question. Within the pages of the *AJN*, nurses had the opportunity to express their views on nursing's

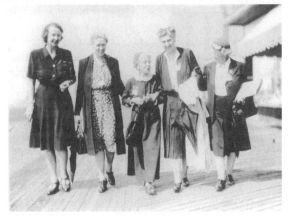

FIGURE 2-3 The international council of nurses (ICN) provided a venue for nurse activists throughout the world to develop a collective voice and policies on nursing and important health care issues. Lavinia Lloyd Dock *(center)*, and other nurses are shown on the Atlantic City boardwalk during the 1947 ICN meeting. (From the Gottesman Libraries, Special Collections, Teachers College, Columbia University, New York.)

support of woman suffrage. Although many nurses wanted to maintain the status quo and sought to avoid confrontational political battles, a sufficient number of nurses ardently believed that the survival of the profession rested on gaining suffrage.

Organized nursing's efforts to support the political agenda of the international nursing community led to the formation of the American Federation of Nurses (AFN) between 1901 and 1912. This newly created federation, a coalition forged between the ANA and the NLN, enabled organized nurses in the U.S. to join the National Council of Women and thus become members of the International Council of Women and later the International Council of Nurses (ICN) (Lewenson, 1996). It is significant to note that by 1901, nursing in the U.S. was ready to form strong coalitions with other nursing groups both domestically and abroad. Nurse organizations gained a political voice in international health issues affecting women and were specifically interested in supporting suffrage (Figure 2-3).

Proponents of nurses' support of woman suffrage linked health issues with the right to vote. Nurses could easily see the relationship between gaining the vote and improving the lives of their patients, families, and communities. Nursing's staunchest suffragist, Lavinia Dock (1907), argued for nursing's involvement in the suffrage movement and wrote that the national associations would fall short of their mission if they did not get politically involved. She warned against following "the narrow path of purely professional questions" (p. 895), and strongly advocated nursing's understanding and support of this movement. She urged nurses to examine how the franchise would improve social conditions that led to illness. Using tuberculosis as an example, Dock (1908) said, "… take the present question of the underfed school children in New York. How many of them will have tuberculosis? If mothers and nurses had votes there might be school lunches for all those children" (p. 926).

The argument that nurses used to oppose participation in the political suffrage campaign centered on fear that it would harm political efforts to obtain state nursing registration legislation. In 1908, at the ANA's eleventh annual convention held in San Francisco, the membership opposed a resolution in support of woman suffrage. Although often used as an example of nursing's conservatism and lack of political activism, this very defeat served as a catalyst for organized nursing to join forces with other women suffragists. Within 4 years, nursing had responded to the efforts of nursing leaders to support the political franchise. By 1912, nursing organizations had voted to support women's right to vote (Lewenson, 1996).

The NACGN, although not invited to participate in the ANA and NLN resolution to support woman suffrage, did express grave concern for social issues that affected health. The NACGN became an invited member of the international nursing community through its membership in the International Council of Women. This affiliation reflects the NACGN's involvement in woman suffrage. Active discussions about woman suffrage, membership in the international women and nursing councils, and support for the ICN resolution to attain suffrage by 1912 indicated strong political activism among African-American nurses (Lewenson, 1996).

SHAPING HEALTH AND PUBLIC POLICY

Several visionary leaders emerged during this initial period of organization. Some worked with the support of organized nursing, and others did not. Each leader who championed ideas about health care, equal rights, and professional opportunity had to be politically astute to attain the goals. They spoke to a large audience, served on national boards and commissions, and built strong coalitions around broad health concerns that went well beyond nursing. Lillian Wald typifies these visionary nurses.

Before the formation of the NOPHN, trained nurses such as Lillian Wald and her friend from training school, Mary Brewster, understood the ramifications of economic, political, social, and cultural factors in regard to health. In 1893, Wald and Brewster opened the Henry Street Nurses' Settlement in New York City, providing nursing care, health education, social services, and cultural experiences to the residents of the Lower East Side. Wald and the nurses at Henry Street lived within the community they served and became internationally noted for their success at addressing public health issues (Buhler-Wilkerson, 2001).

The work of the nurses at Henry Street reflected their ability to provide care in the home and to lobby for change in the body politic. Backer (1993) noted that Wald "connected her caring with activism by initiating practice and policy changes via administrative and organizational skills, persuasiveness, coalitions, delivering testimony and political power" (p. 128). Wald promoted public health nursing education and the formation of the NOPHN. Moreover, Wald's astute political awareness led to many social changes affecting the health and well-being of the Lower East Side residents.

Children's health and well-being struck a chord with Wald. Concerned for the welfare of children, Wald turned the backyard at Henry Street into a playground (Buhler-Wilkerson, 2001). Recognizing that too many children played in the overcrowded streets of the Lower East Side, Wald argued for the opening of city parks and in 1898 successfully formed the Outdoor Recreation League. This group obtained land in New York City and turned it into municipal parks (Siegel, 1983).

Wald's nursing knowledge, social concern, and political savvy joined forces when she maneuvered the board of health into hiring a school nurse in 1902. Wald writes her account in her 1915 book, *The House on Henry Street*, about how she and Brewster recognized a community health problem and kept records on those children excluded from school because of medical problems. After collecting these data, Wald convinced the president of the department of health of the need for nursing services in the public schools. Although the department of health decided to use physicians to inspect the children at schools, when the time was right, Wald encouraged the president to hire a public health nurse as well:

> *The time had come when it seemed right to urge the addition of the nurse's service to that of the doctor. My colleagues and I offered to show that with her assistance few children would lose their valuable school time and that it would be possible to bring under treatment those who needed it. Reluctant lest the democracy of the school should be invaded by even the most socially minded philanthropy, I exacted a promise from several of the city officials that if the experiment were successful they would use their influence to have the nurse, like the doctor, paid from public funds. (Wald, 1915, p. 51)*

To Wald's credit, the experiment was successful, and in October 1902 the city of New York paid for the services of a school nurse. The board of estimates had allotted more than $30,000 for the employment of trained nurses who were, in Wald's words, the "first municipalized school nurses in the world" (Wald, 1915, p. 53). New York City's Bureau of Child Hygiene was an outgrowth of this service (Wald, 1915).

ALLIANCES WITH THE WOMEN'S MOVEMENT: THE 1960s TO THE PRESENT

The political action of early nurse leaders set the stage for nurses' activism half a century later. In the 1960s, another women's movement spread throughout the U.S. This second wave of activists could conceivably harness the vote and gain equal status for women in the law, at work, and in the home. In the early 1960s, nursing's presence in the women's movement was "obscure" or "notably absent" (Chinn & Wheeler, 1985, p. 74). The political activism frequently associated with feminist groups was not reported to have carried over into nursing. An "uneasy" relationship existed between those in the traditional female profession of nursing and those engaged in feminist activities (Allen, 1985).

By the 1970s, some nursing leaders had enumerated the value of developing ties with the women's movement. Wilma Scott Heide (1973), a nurse and leader in the feminist movement who served as president of the National Organization for Women (NOW) between 1970 and 1974, called for nurses to embrace the ideas of the feminist movement. Heide (1973) believed that nurses and all women shared the similar dilemma of being characterized as caring, nurturing, compassionate, tender, submissive, passive, subjective, and emotional. Whereas some of the traits enhanced the professional role, others served to suppress proactive, empowering behaviors. Heide believed that nursing needed to join with the feminist movement in addressing the inequalities that women faced in society.

Another nurse and feminist, JoAnn Ashley (1976), argued that nurses could no longer be pacifists if they were to lead the health care changes that consumers needed. Ashley (1976, p. 133) recognized that "powerful, male-dominated groups, economically motivated, will not be reasonable with their interests and status threatened." Ashley challenged nurses to reflect on who they were and what their role was as nurses.

In the 1980s, nursing became a metaphor for the "struggle of women for equality" (Diers, 1984, p. 23). Personal and professional empowerment served as essential qualities for gaining political power, and nurse leaders recognized that public policy would not change without advocates who could successfully use persuasive, political strategies. Feminism gave nurses "a world view that values women and that confronts systematic injustices based on gender" (Chinn & Wheeler, 1985, p. 74). Nursing's acceptance of this definition of feminism has assisted nursing's struggle for equality and can be traced to the early 1970s with the ANA's support of the Equal Rights Amendment; the formation of a group called Nurses-NOW; and the establishment of the Nurses Coalition for Action in Politics, nursing's first political action committee.

Changes in women's roles mirror society's perceptions of nursing roles. As women in the second half of the twentieth century challenged inequality and sought political power, nurses did so as well. Yet the political savvy of early pioneer leaders was lost to later generations of nurses. Too often nurses are not included in policy decisions, not involved in policymaking, or just not recognized at all (Gordon, 1997). The nursism that exists within the broader society and at times within the women's movement has lessened, but nursing needs to be vigilant.

For a list of related websites, please refer to your Evolve Resources at http://evolve.elsevier.com/Mason/policypolitics/

REFERENCES

Allen, M. (1985). Women, nursing and feminism: An interview with Alice J. Baumgart, RN, PhD. *Canadian Nurse, 81*(1), 20-22.

Ashley, J. (1976). *Hospitals, paternalism and the role of the nurse.* New York: Teachers College Press.

Backer, B. (1993). Lillian Wald: Connecting caring with actions. *Nursing and Health Care, 14*(3), 122-129.

Birnbach, N., & Lewenson, S. B. (1993). *Legacy of leadership: Presidential addresses from the Superintendents' Society and the National League of Nursing Education, 1894-1952.* New York: NLN Press.

Buhler-Wilkerson, K. (2001). *No place like home: A history of nursing and home care in the United States.* Baltimore: Johns Hopkins.

Burgess, M. A. (1928). *Nurses, patients, and pocketbooks.* New York: Committee on the Grading of Nursing Schools.

Chinn, P. L., & Wheeler, C. E. (1985). Feminism and nursing: Can nursing afford to remain aloof from the women's movement? *Nursing Outlook, 33*(2), 74-76.

Cohen, S. S., Mason, J. M., Kovner, C., Leavitt, J. K., Pulcini, J., & Sochalski, J. (1996). Stages of nursing's political development: Where we've been and where we ought to go. *Nursing Outlook, 44*(6), 259-266.

Diers, D. (1984). To profess—To be a professional. *Journal of the New York State Nurses Association, 15*(4), 23.

Dock, L. (1907). Some urgent social claims. *American Journal of Nursing, 7*(10), 895-901.

Dock, L. (1908). The suffrage question. *American Journal of Nursing, 8*(11), 925-927.

Dock, L., & Stewart, I. (1931). *A short history of nursing.* (3rd ed., revised). New York: Putnam's Sons.

Gardner, M. S. (1933). *Public health nursing.* (2nd ed., revised). New York: Macmillan.

Gordon, S. (1997). *Life support: Three nurses on the front lines.* Boston: Little, Brown.

Heide, W. S. (1973). Nursing and women's liberation a parallel. *American Journal of Nursing, 73*(5), 824-827.

Hine, D. C. (1989). *Black women in white: Racial conflict and cooperation in the nursing profession. 1890-1950.* Bloomington, IN: Indiana University Press.

Hine, D. C. (1993). Staupers, Mabel Keaton (1890-1989). In D. C. Hine (Ed.), *Black women in America: An historical encyclopedia: Vol. 2.* Brooklyn, NY: Carlson.

Lewenson, S. B. (1996). *Taking charge: Nursing, suffrage and feminism in America, 1873-1920.* New York: NLN Press.

Palmer, S. (1897). First and second annual conventions of the American Society of Superintendents of Training Schools for Nurses, Harrisburg, PA.

Palmer, S. (1909). State societies: Their organization and place in nursing education. *American Journal of Nursing, 9*(12), 956-957.

Progress and reaction. (1908). *American Journal of Nursing, 8*(5), 334-335.

Reverby, S. (1987). *Ordered to care: The dilemma of American nursing, 1850-1945.* New York: Cambridge University Press.

Siegel, B. (1983). *Lillian Wald of Henry Street.* New York: Macmillan.

Staupers, M. (1937). The Negro nurse in America. Opportunity. *Journal of Negro Life, 15,* 339-341. (Also reprinted in Hine, D. C. [1985]. *Black women in the nursing profession: A documentary history.* New York: Garland.)

The Editor. (1900). *American Journal of Nursing, 1*(1), 64-66.

Thoms, A. (1929). *Pathfinders: A history of progress of the colored graduate nurses.* New York: Kay Printing House.

Vicinus, M., & Nergaard, B. (Eds.). (1989). *Ever yours, Florence Nightingale: Selected letters.* London: Virago.

Wald, L. (1915). The house on Henry Street. New York: Henry Holt.

CHAPTER 3

Learning the Ropes of Policy, Politics, and Advocacy

Judith K. Leavitt, Mary W. Chaffee, and Connie Vance

"I am not afraid of storms for I am learning how to sail my ship."

—Louisa May Alcott

Every politically active person, from United States presidents to chief executive officers, *learned* the political and policy skills that catapulted them into positions of power and responsibility. Nurses are no different. Though one can learn about the policy process and political analysis through formal education, it is only through experience and practice that one can apply what has been learned. A most important catalyst in becoming involved is to find mentors—colleagues and friends who are politically savvy—to teach us, to believe in and support us and to celebrate our success and learn from our failures.

This chapter explores how to become involved through mentoring, education, and experience. Students new to politics as well as experienced nurses have unlimited ways to expand their knowledge and involvement. Whatever our experience, we improve our skills as we engage in the process. There are infinite causes and issues in health care to stimulate our interest if we want to become engaged. We need only decide how much energy and time we are willing to devote. Success in the world of policy and politics demands the strengths and skills that nurses possess. Working in the policy arena will open doors to opportunities where nurses can become significant participants and leaders. This book includes many stories about nurses who have done this. These stories can be inspirational and motivate others to become active in policy and politics.

POLITICAL CONSCIOUSNESS-RAISING AND AWARENESS: THE "AHA" MOMENT

How does one get started? Many find that there is a defining moment when the old ways of reacting to issues of injustice, inequality, or powerlessness no longer work. It is the moment when a person realizes that an issue or problem is due to failures in the system. For instance, lack of support staff on an acute care unit may be related to decreased reimbursement rates rather than an uncaring hospital administration. Denial of care for a patient eligible to receive Medicaid or Medicare could be related to cuts in federal funding, rather than the patient's need for care. Realizing that a problem may be due to a policy failure is a critical first step toward becoming part of the policy solution. This is political consciousness-raising and an "aha" moment. It is the adrenaline rush that urges, "Something must be done—and I need to become involved."

Until that defining moment, nurses may feel frustrated, angry, or hopeless. When the "aha" hits, we begin to understand that we can and must influence those who make the laws and regulations that create the inequities. We recognize the personal nature of policy issues ("the political is personal") Many health care problems require policy solutions, and advancing a solution requires skills that can be learned. When nurses accept that they are not at fault for the inadequacies of the health care system and instead believe that nursing can shape solutions, the profession itself becomes political. Nurses then become proactive rather than reactive. The result is that the individual nurse, as well as the profession, become empowered to act. Feeling empowered is essential to true advocacy.

GETTING STARTED

Through interviews with 27 American nurses involved in health policy at the national, state, and local levels, Gebbie, Wakefield, and Kerfoot (2000) set out to discover how and why these activist nurses became involved. Their results corroborated what we knew anecdotally:

- The majority of respondents had parents, most often fathers, who were active in policy and politics and who created a mentoring, supportive environment.
- Many were raised to be independent and to believe in their capacity to accomplish what they wanted.
- High school provided a training ground in political socialization.
- Nursing education provided role modeling and mentoring by faculty, deans, and alumni as well as the opportunity to increase political awareness through courses in policy, political science, and economics.
- Clinical practice often provided strong role models, and experiences in public health and community health provided opportunities for political insights.
- Graduate education opened doors for many, through such avenues as the study of law, health economics, and health policy.
- Some had their consciousness raised gradually through work experiences that exposed them to public policy and the need to understand how to influence the process.

The nurses who were interviewed confirmed that there are multiple points of entry into the policy arena. Whether this chapter, this book, a course in policy and politics, or a conversation with a colleague is your first exposure, you have already started.

Political skills, such as how to be persuasive, how to identify and use power effectively, how to analyze barriers to goals, and how to mobilize people to work collectively, are all skills that can be learned. Nurses bring many skills to the political arena that are learned through education and further refined in clinical practice. Politics requires the kind of communication skills that nurses use to persuade an unwilling patient to get out of bed after abdominal surgery or a child to swallow an unpleasant-tasting medication. In addition, nurses, whether they realize it or not, are health care experts. Nurses can speak knowledgeably about what patients and communities need because they experience it firsthand.

ADVOCACY AND ACTIVISM

Nurses are considered to be powerful advocates—but what exactly does this mean? Florence Nightingale saw nursing in all of its forms as advocacy—a "calling" that required nurses to look for and act in ways to be world citizens for the sake of human health (Dossey, Slanders, Beck, & Attewell, 2005). Advocacy is increasingly recognized as a component of professional nursing practice. Nursing education at the baccalaureate level is expected to produce nurses who "advocate for health care that is sensitive to the needs of patients" and who "advocate for professional standards of practice using organizational and political processes" (American Association of Colleges of Nursing, 1998, pp. 15-17). Nurses who have been educated at the master's degree level are charged with assuming the role of advocate for consumers and the nursing profession as well as assuming the role of change agent in the health care system (American Association of Colleges of Nursing, 1996).

In the workplace, nurses work with patients to achieve mutual goals by advocating for the patient or for resources the patient needs. Outside the health system, nurses can be equally influential advocates. In the government, in professional associations, and in the community, nurses can use political skills to advocate for policies and change that will improve the health of populations (see Chapter 5).

THE ROLE OF MENTORING

At every stage of a nursing career—from student to novice to expert—mentor relationships are an essential element for professional success, socialization, and leadership development. In the traditional world of politics, the "old boys' network" consisted of strong mentoring components. Gaining entry into the inner circle required the mentorship of political party leaders who served as sponsors, role models, and door openers to aspiring "politicians." Nurses are discovering the necessity of receiving mentoring from a variety of leaders and peers at every career stage, particularly as they expand their influence from a clinical setting to policy and political involvement. For example, a nurse who has participated in lobbying elected representatives around an issue may need help learning the myriad rules of legislation particular to different legislative bodies. For instance, the two houses of Congress have different rules from most state legislatures. Knowing how to get bills passed requires understanding how to read legislative language and who can move legislation forward (see Chapters 64, 65, and 69). Mentors can guide others to learn about the processes and relationships.

A mentor or role model provides inspiration and encouragement to get involved, as well as coaching and tutoring in the nuts and bolts of political involvement. As explained by Kram (1983, 1985), mentoring has been compared to a dance relationship. The mentor is the dance teacher; the mentee is the pupil. The teacher supports, role models, guides, and critiques; the student/dancer seeks feedback, advice, and guidance and stays motivated to learn (Zauszniewski, 2009). It can be a long-term relationship as the dancer moves from acquiring knowledge and skills to refining and expanding learning. As with any other nursing skill, learning the political or policy process requires both theoretic and experiential knowledge.

In the nursing profession, the mentor model consists of both expert-novice and peer-peer partnerships. One example of developmental mentoring is the modeling of political behavior at lobby days in Congress or in state legislatures that are sponsored by nursing associations. At these events, nurse lobbyists and activists serve as mentor-guides and role models to nurses and students. They provide information and strategies and model effective behaviors while lobbying policymakers on specific legislation. These activists also provide the inspiration and vision for what can be done if nurses work together toward shared goals. This is real-life learning and it is a highly effective and practical way of developing political awareness and know-how. Check your state nurses association for lobby days.

FINDING A MENTOR

You can find a mentor, even if you don't know someone personally. Begin with an idea of what you would like to learn or in what area of politics and policy you would like to be involved. Then identify people whom you have noticed, heard, or read about who are activists in your area of interest. Good sources for finding mentors are nursing associations, schools of nursing, clinical organizations, and local political organizations and campaigns. You may contact the person directly, via e-mail, by phone, or with a note, or you can ask someone who knows the individual to provide an introduction. Tell them what you want to learn and why you would like them to assist you. For instance, nurses can get involved in local political campaigns, where they are warmly welcomed, particularly if one identifies himself or herself as a nurse. The mentor may or may not be a nurse. The important criteria for a mentor are knowledge and an interest in you. Sometimes the mentor need only get you started; in other situations, a mentor becomes a lifelong friend and role model.

COLLECTIVE MENTORING

Because the majority of nurses are newcomers to political and policy activism, every nurse should possess the mentality of being both a mentor and a protégé in the political process. Learning politics is not a solitary activity. This means that nurses should be on the lookout for mentors who can serve as their teachers and guides as they hone political and policy skills. Likewise, every nurse should assume responsibility for actively mentoring others as they refine their repertoire of skills and deepen their involvement. This reciprocal collective mentoring is extremely effective in expanding the political and power base of the profession and its members. Collective mentoring can occur in schools, clinical agencies, and professional associations. This means that wherever we practice, we can each refine our skills by seeking mentors and serving as mentors to others.

Inherent in this form of mentoring is the development of networks of persons who are active in policy and who take responsibility for expanding these networks. The nurses in these networks should develop strategies for mentoring political neophytes and for "claiming" nurses who may not be in traditional career paths (Gebbie et al., 2000). Organizational networks, including those in academic, clinical, and association settings, are a natural place to establish developmental mentoring activities. For example, politically active faculty members can network with political leaders in professional associations to provide undergraduate and graduate students with lobbying and leadership opportunities. Many state nursing associations are successfully reaching out to collectively mentor hundreds of nursing students through lobby days in national and state capitols. Nursing students and practicing nurses also have many opportunities to experience collective mentoring in learning the political ropes through relationships with leaders and peers in organizations such as the National Student Nurses Association, ANA, specialty and state nursing associations, and volunteer health-related organizations. In addition, local political parties, community organizations, and the offices of elected officials offer nurses opportunities to learn through mentored experiences. These organizations can offer numerous mentoring opportunities for involvement in lobbying, policy development, media contacts, fund-raising, and the political process in various venues.

Mentoring in policy development in any of the spheres also requires connections to knowledgeable leaders. In the workplace, one can learn from health professionals who serve as leaders on influential committees. For example, if you want to work on improving staffing systems, you would need to learn about the cost of staffing, the cost of bringing in temporary staff, and the budget allocation for staffing on the unit. A clinical unit manager should have that information and can help guide your learning. In addition, one would need to know how much Medicare and Medicaid allocates to particular types of patients (outside the control of the institution) and the acuity level of patients. By working with experienced and knowledgeable staff, one can learn how to put this information together, how to influence colleagues to support a proposed policy, and how to gain access to and support from organizational leaders.

EDUCATIONAL OPPORTUNITIES

There are many ways to learn how to influence health policy; some will depend on your own learning style, where you live, and your interests. Whatever your educational and political goals, there is something for everyone—from continuing education programs to graduate programs in political science and policy, from workshops run by campaign organizations to fellowships and conferences. With a little effort and some help getting started, an exciting world of educational possibilities is available.

Is it really worth putting the time and energy into learning new skills? Can nurses make a difference? Absolutely—many nurses and professional nursing associations have profoundly influenced health policy through their political efforts. Nursing's successful work is now being recognized by other professions as an example of how to be politically effective (see Chapter 85). The great success of nurse practitioners has been described as a model for how pharmacists can move their practices forward (O'Brien, 2003).

PROGRAMS IN SCHOOLS OF NURSING

A few degree programs in policy have been established in schools of nursing. More commonly, nursing programs offer courses, either as core requirements or electives, related to health policy or with health policy content embedded. Many of these can be taken as continuing education credits even if you are not enrolled as a part-time or full-time student. Examples include the following:

- The University of California, San Francisco, offers both master's and doctoral programs in Health Policy Nursing *(nurseweb.ucsf.edu/www/ps-dc-hp.htm)*
- The University of Pennsylvania School of Nursing collaborates with the Leonard Davis Institute of Health Economics to offer both a master and doctoral concentration in policy, health services research, and economics. *(www.upenn.edu/ldi/about.html)*
- Yale University in New Haven, Connecticut, offers both master's and doctoral programs through their Center for Health Policy in the School of Nursing *(nursing.yale.edu/Centers/HPE/)*

DEGREE PROGRAMS AND COURSES IN PUBLIC HEALTH, PUBLIC ADMINISTRATION, AND PUBLIC POLICY

College and university departments of public health, political science, policy science, political administration, and others are a rich source of policy content in academic programs. Programs in these areas take a little more effort to find because they reside under many different names. Programs leading to degrees that include health policy content are widely available at the baccalaureate, master, and doctoral levels. Numerous programs exist at all academic levels (associates, baccalaureate, masters, and doctorate). For courses in your area, examine the online listings for local colleges.

CONTINUING EDUCATION

Annual conferences on health policy topics are conducted by academic institutions and professional associations. Specialty nursing associations and state nursing associations often offer legislative workshops. Check websites and publications for the most current offerings, and monitor your state nursing association's meeting announcements. Search the Internet using health policy meeting, health policy conference, or health care meeting as search terms.

WORKSHOPS

A quick, intensive and participatory approach to learning is to take a one- or two-day workshop in politics, campaigning, or policy often from political or educational institutions. The following are examples:

- Rutgers University has a Center for American Women and Politics that offers ongoing workshops on a vast variety of topics *(www.cawp. rutgers.edu/education_training/index.php)*.
- The Women and Politics Institute at American University is the only training in the country that offers women how to run for student government *(www.american.edu/spa/wpi/campaign_college. cfm)*.
- Yale University has a series of workshops through their Center for the Study of American Politics *(www.yale.edu/csap/seminars)*.
- Both the two major political parties as well as third parties hold campaign workshops at state and national levels. Other political groups, from all political perspectives, do as well.
- Wellstone Action! Offers training programs in campaign management, community activism, and related topics *(www.wellstone.org)*.

LEARNING BY DOING

There are many ways to obtain valuable practical experience, from internships to self-study programs.
   Internships and Fellowships. Internships and fellowships provide great learning opportunities. In addition to teaching nurses the ropes, these practical experiences offer valuable mentoring and networking opportunities and may lead to employment opportunities. Internships may be arranged for credit in academic programs. Summer or year-long internships are

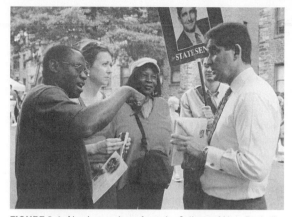

FIGURE 3-1 Nursing students from the College of New Rochelle, New York, with New York State Senator Jeff Klein.

available on Capitol Hill, in some federal agencies, and through professional associations. The Nurse in Washington Internship (NIWI) sponsored by The Nursing Organizations Alliance (The Alliance) is one of the most popular (see Chapter 4). See the Health Policy Internships and Fellowships list available in Appendix B and also on Evolve at *http://evolve.elsevier.com/ Mason/policypolitics/*.
   Volunteer Service. A great way to learn politics is to volunteer to work on a political campaign (Figure 3-1). Volunteer time and energy are welcomed by candidates for elective office at all levels of government—local, state, and federal. First-time candidates with tight budgets are especially appreciative of volunteer assistance. Building relationships through volunteer service is a critical part of learning the ropes. Also consider contacting Democratic or Republican national party headquarters for training and information about volunteer activities (see Chapter 74).
   Professional Association Activities. Many professional nursing associations offer opportunities for volunteer service that lead to rich educational, mentoring, and networking experiences (Figure 3-2). ANA members may participate on the Nurses Strategic Action Team (N-STAT), a national grassroots political activity program. N-STAT members are alerted about critical health care issues, are encouraged to contact their members of Congress, and are provided examples of how to write effective letters to legislators. Some N-STAT members who serve as statewide leaders interview and evaluate candidates for Congress and make endorsement recommendations to ANA's Political Action Committee (ANA-PAC).

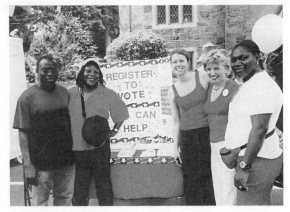

FIGURE 3-2 Nursing students with faculty member Dr. Connie Vance *(second from right)* participating in voter registration.

The American Association of Critical Care Nurses (AACN) and the Oncology Nursing Society (ONS), along with many specialty organizations, offer tool kits, training materials, legislative briefs, and mentoring around policy issues of concern to their practice. Other health professional associations such as the American Public Health Association, the American Cancer Society, and the American Heart Association have strong advocacy and legislative programs. Check their websites for learning and volunteer opportunities.

SELF-STUDY

The value of reading and self-directed learning cannot be underestimated in learning about policy and politics. Many types of literature exist for diverse interests:

Professional Journals. Many professional nursing, health care, and social sciences journals include updates on current political issues. Some are wholly focused on policy and politics; others publish regular political content (Box 3-1).

Books. Browse through the political science, government, or current events sections of your favorite bookstore and you are likely to find a goldmine (Box 3-2). You can also browse an online bookseller such as *www.amazon.com* or *www.barnesandnoble.com*. Search for the words *politics*, *policy*, or *health policy*, and see what piques your interest. (Many booksellers sell used books at discounted prices.)

Newspapers. Major metropolitan newspapers offer political analysis of national, regional, and local politics. Those recognized for in-depth political reporting on health issues include the *Washington Post* (www.washingtonpost.com), the *New York Times* (www.nytimes.com), the *Los Angeles Times*

> ### BOX 3-1 Professional Journals with Policy and Political Focus
>
> - *American Journal of Nursing,* a monthly publication that includes commentary on current political issues that affect nursing
> - *Health Affairs,* a bimonthly journal published by Project HOPE that is known for thought-provoking articles that inform and influence discussion of health policy issues
> - *Journal of the American Medical Association (JAMA),* a weekly publication of the American Medical Association, which covers health policy issues of interest to physicians
> - *Journal of Health Politics, Policy and Law,* a bimonthly peer-reviewed publication of Duke University Press
> - *New England Journal of Medicine,* published weekly by the Massachusetts Medical Society; a journal that publishes innovative perspectives and background on health policy issues
> - *Nursing Economic,* a bimonthly publication that includes "Capitol Commentary," a regular feature that examines health care policy issues
> - *Policy, Politics, & Nursing Practice,* a peer-reviewed quarterly journal that publishes articles on legislation that affects nursing practice, case studies in policy and political action, interviews with policymakers and policy experts, and articles on trends and issues
> - *Yale Journal of Health Policy, Law, and Ethics,* a biannual publication that provides a forum for interdisciplinary discussion of topics in health policy, health law, and biomedical ethics

(www.latimes.com), and the *Wall Street Journal* (www.wsj.com).

Television. Network and cable news programs and television news-magazines address political issues and government activities. The ultimate viewing experience for true political voyeurs is C-SPAN. This channel is available as a public service created by the U.S. cable television industry to provide access to the live gavel-to-gavel proceedings of the U.S. House of Representatives and the U.S. Senate and to other forums in which public policy is discussed, debated, and decided. C-SPAN provides a wealth of information about the democratic process, without editing, commentary, or analysis. Television programs have become interactive by integrating social media such as Twitter so viewers can participate in televised stories and discussions.

Radio. Radio continues to be a rich source of political information and debate—on AM, FM, and

---

BOX 3-2 Policy and Politics Books

- *Politics for Dummies* (2nd ed.) by Ann DeLaney (For Dummies, 2002). This is a great book for anyone who slept through civics class in high school. Related reading: *Congress for Dummies* and *The Complete Idiot's Guide to American Government.*
- *What You Should Know About Politics ... But Don't: A Nonpartisan Guide to the Issues* (2008) by Jessamyn Conrad. She explores both sides of major issues in an unbiased and witty way.
- *The One-Hour Activist: The 15 Most Powerful Actions You Can Take to Fight for the Issues and Candidates You Care About* by Christopher Kush (Jossey-Bass, 2004). Practical guidance on how to influence policymakers.
- *The Politics of Health Legislation: An Economic Perspective* (3rd ed.) by Paul Feldstein (Health Administration Press, 2006). An economist explores how individuals, groups, and legislators act in their own self-interest.
- *Governing Health: The Politics of Health Policy* (3rd ed.) by Carol Weissert and William Weissert (Johns Hopkins University Press, 2006). Excellent overview of health policy and how politics shapes policy.
- *Don't Think of an Elephant! Know Your Values and Frame the Debate* by George Lakoff (Chelsea Green Publishing Company, 2004). An examination of how conservatives and liberals think differently.
- *Agendas, Alternatives, and Public Policies* by John Kingdon (Longman, 2002). Kingdon is highly revered and constantly quoted by policy experts.

---

satellite radio stations. Policy-focused stations include the following:

- National Public Radio. (NPR) via public radio stations and the Internet *(www.npr.org)*. NPR provides carefully researched in-depth reporting.
- C-SPAN Radio. C-SPAN Radio offers public affairs commercial-free programming 24 hours a day. Listeners may listen through the radio or Internet. The broadcast schedule is available at *www.c-span.org*.
- Liberal and conservative political talkfests. Many political "talking heads" have radio programs that serve as forums to debate hot political topics. Check your local radio program website for air time and station.

Internet. An all-you-can-eat political buffet exists on the Internet. All major news organizations, activism groups, political parties, issue advocates, and many others have a presence on the Internet. A diverse universe of political discussion exists, from well-substantiated journalism to blogs with absolutely no quality control. Unlike print sources, the Internet provides an interactive medium.

APPLYING YOUR POLITICAL, POLICY, ADVOCACY, AND ACTIVISM SKILLS

The purpose of learning the ropes of policy, politics, and advocacy is to influence health care or broader social agendas that influence human health. The process of learning to be an effective activist, advocate, or leader often involves ongoing experiential learning as well as self-directed activities like reading. There are diverse opportunities to apply what is learned—and there are opportunities to make a difference regardless of experience or expertise.

Individuals can exert influence on decisions made by governments, communities, organizations, and associations. Much political activity (though not all) occurs in the sphere of the government. The U.S. government is a complicated system that determines the direction of a complex nation. Citizens are permitted, but not compelled, to participate in the process of governing (Kush, 2004). Activism has made a difference in many communities and has been recognized as a powerful counterbalance in a political system often dominated by cash and corporations (Shaw, 1996). Kush (2004) described the grassroots efforts of Maryland citizens in fending off the powerful and rich gambling lobby. Maryland's neighbors (Delaware, West Virginia, and New Jersey) reap the benefits of slot machines, and Maryland residents were urged to support slot machine legislation to increase funding for public schools. The gambling industry spent $1.5 million in 2003 to support legislation in the Maryland legislature that would have legalized slot machines. An effective grassroots campaign proved more effective than the gambling lobby and was able to convince Maryland voters not to support the slot machine legislation.

Nurses, individually, collectively, and in working with others, can influence the political and policy decisions made by organizations, communities, and governments. The Spectrum of Political Competencies (Figure 3-3) portrays the range of activities that nurses may choose to use to influence health and health care. It demonstrates the breadth and variety of competencies ranging from novice level to more

LEARNING THE ROPES	PARTICIPATING IN DEMOCRACY	INFLUENCING AND ADVOCATING	USING ADVANCED POLITICAL SKILLS

- Get a mentor
- Educate self about policy and politics
- Read and consider health care and social issues
- Get an internship
- Read, listen to and discuss the news and current issues
- Network with other nurses
- Participate in nursing legislative events
- Learn about advocacy and activism
- Study policy
- Obtain a degree in policy, political science, or related field
- Strengthen communication skills (written and verbal)
- Attend educational programs or 'camps'
- Learn the structure of governments
- Identify your elected representatives
- Learn the scope of influence of groups with authority (e.g., local board of health, organizational leadership groups, commissions, congressional committees)

- Volunteer on a political campaign
- Vote
- Explain political views to others
- Learn about political candidates and their views
- Participate in voter registration activities
- Sign petitions
- Post candidates' signs on your property or vehicle
- Weigh pros and cons of political positions
- Join a political party
- Research the status of a bill
- Serve as a volunteer poll worker on election day

- Post opinions on blogs
- Host a blog
- Participate in professional organization's legislative activities
- Write an op-ed piece for a newspaper
- Write letters to the editors of magazines and journals
- Express opinions via social media (e.g., Twitter)
- Create an address book of important contact information
- Identify all stakeholders with an interest in your issue
- Speak at public hearings
- Cultivate a relationship with elected representatives
- Work on the solution to a policy problem
- Use data and evidence to support your efforts
- Respond to 'action alerts' sent out by professional organizations
- Participate in rallies and protests
- Network with opinion-leaders (local organizers, business owners, health professionals and others)
- Use your life, your professional expertise and your experience in your advocacy efforts
- Support a political candidate (go door-to-door, attend meetings, make calls)
- Develop strategies for political action
- Express opinions to elected officials via letter, e-mail, call or visit
- Make financial contributions to political action committees and candidates who share your views
- Hold a house party fundraiser for a candidate
- Volunteer to work on a phone bank for a candidate
- Participate in community meetings
- Participate in grassroots community organizing
- Launch a petition
- Mobilize others around an issue

- Run for elective office
- Obtain a political appointment
- Serve as a paid political staff member
- Provide expert testimony
- Hold a media event
- Host television, radio or other media broadcasts
- Write a newspaper column
- Serve as a policy analyst
- Obtain an appointment to a board or committee
- Serve as a speechwriter
- Participate in political surveys and polling
- Manage a political campaign
- Become a lobbyist
- Publish articles on health care issues and solutions
- Provide an interview with the media

FIGURE 3-3 The spectrum of political competencies.

sophisticated ones including running for elective office.

The Spectrum of Political Competencies includes skills that can be learned and applied in a wide variety of activities aimed at improving health and health care. There are many environments where nurses may test out new skills. Some nurses have their initial experience using new activism and advocacy skills in school. For example, students in the RN-to-BSN program at Valdosta State University in Georgia learned to address community health problems through political strategies aimed at fluoridating a community water system (Wold, Brown, Chastain, Griffis, & Wingate, 2008). Senior nursing students at New York Institute of Technology attended New York State Nurses Association's Lobby Day to develop skills in civic engagement (Zauderer, Ballesas, Cardoza, Hood, & Neville, 2008-2009). New political and advocacy skills can be exercised in the workplace and in communities to advocate for nursing issues and health improvement. For example, Pennsylvania nurses established the Lehigh Valley Hospital and Health Network Professional Excellence Council to foster professional nursing advocacy (Hartman, 2008). In the community, nurses can participate in a variety of activities aimed at influencing decisions, including working on campaigns, serving in volunteer positions, speaking at hearings, and participating in rallies (Figure 3-4).

More sophisticated political skills are required for effective organizational leadership, obtaining political appointments, and in seeking elective office. Many skills that nurses learn in clinical roles are directly transferrable to influential leadership roles and paid political positions. Ohio State Senator Sue Morano, RN, identified skills that nurses can bring to elective office that help them become effective advocates. These include skill in setting priorities, leadership, conflict resolution, collaboration, communication, and having conversations about difficult issues (Iacono, 2008). Regardless of education, background, and experience, there are limitless opportunities for nurses to learn new skills and use them to improve health for individuals and populations.

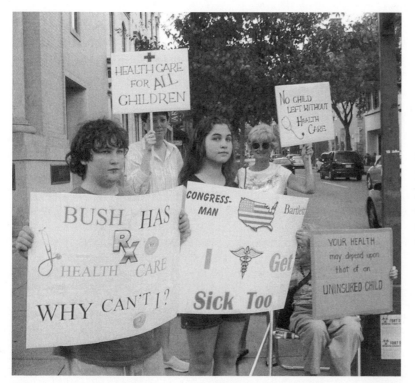

FIGURE 3-4 Nurses Peggy McNeill and Mary Chaffee participate in a rally in Frederick, Maryland, to draw attention to the need for ongoing funding for the State Children's Health Insurance Program (S-CHIP) in 2008. Photo used with permission of author.

For a list of related websites, please refer to your Evolve Resources at http://evolve.elsevier.com/Mason/policypolitics/

REFERENCES

American Association of Colleges of Nursing. (1996). *The essentials of master's education for advanced practice nursing.* Washington, DC: AACN.

American Association of Colleges of Nursing. (1998). *The essentials of baccalaureate education for professional nursing practice.* Washington, DC: AACN.

Dossey, B., Slanders, L., Beck, D. M., & Attewell, A. (2005). *Florence Nightingale today: Healing, leadership, global action.* Silver Spring, MD: ANA.

Gebbie, K. M., Wakefield, M., & Kerfoot, K. (2000). Nursing and health policy. *Journal of Nursing Scholarship, 32*(3), 307-315.

Hartman, N. (2008). An advocacy work group: Impacting legislative, regulatory, and professional practice issues. *Pennsylvania Nurse, 63*(3), 8.

Iacono, M. (2008). Senator Sue Morano, RN: Nursing advocacy in the Ohio Senate. *Journal of PeriAnesthesia Nursing, 23*(3), 204-206.

Kram, K. E. (1983). Phases of the mentoring relationship. *Academy of Management Journal, 26,* 608-625.

Kram, K. E. (1985). *Mentoring at work: Developmental relationships in organizational life.* Glenview, IL: Scott Foresman.

Kush, C. (2004). *The one-hour activist.* San Francisco: Jossey-Bass.

O'Brien, J. M. (2003). How nurse practitioners obtained provider status: Lessons for pharmacists. *American Journal of Health System Pharmacy, 60*(22), 2301-2307.

Shaw, R. (1996). *The activist's handbook.* Berkeley, CA: University of California Press.

Wold, S., Brown, C., Chastain, C., Griffis, M., & Wingate, J. (2008). Going the extra mile: Beyond health teaching to political involvement. *Nursing Forum, 43*(4), 171-176.

Zauderer, C., Ballesas, H., Cardoza, M., Hood, P., & Neville, S. (2008-2009). United we stand: Preparing nursing students for political activism. *Journal of the New York State Nurses Association,* Fall/Winter, 4-7.

Zauszniewski, J. (2009). Mentoring our next generation: Time to dance. *Journal of Child and Adolescent Psychiatric Nursing, 22*(3), 14.

CHAPTER 4

TAKING ACTION
How I Learned the Ropes of Policy and Politics

Alfredo Mireles

"Learning is a treasure that will follow its owner everywhere."

—Chinese proverb

I stood at the podium facing the San Francisco Board of Supervisors and took a deep breath. I worked for a county-funded hospital, and the board was debating whether or not to stop funding my psychiatric unit. I thought of my patients' challenges and told the board, "Inpatient psychiatry treats the most vulnerable people in our community. Our patients struggle with mental illness, homelessness, substance abuse and many other co-morbidities. There are few places equipped to deal with all of these issues simultaneously, and by cutting this funding you are placing some of the most vulnerable people in our community in serious risk." I was nervous, but my patients needed somebody to stand up for them. Although it did not come naturally, I felt it was my responsibility as a nurse.

I believe nurses need to advocate for patients with equal vigor at the bedside and at city hall. However, after my first foray into political advocacy with the Board of Supervisors, I knew I needed to learn more about how to be an effective policy and political advocate. So, I sought out more experiences and training. First, I enrolled in a graduate program in health policy at the University of California at San Francisco. In the first year, I learned about policy theory, health economics, and current issues in health care. I became involved in student government and was part of a team that negotiated the student health insurance policy. I had a phenomenal time in graduate school

and learned a tremendous amount, but I still needed more practical experiences.

I was overjoyed when I won a scholarship to attend the Nurse in Washington Internship (NIWI). The NIWI conference equips nurses with the knowledge, strategy, and courage to advocate for patients in legislative arenas. The NIWI program is a great opportunity to network with other nurse leaders from all over the country and to gain valuable insight from their experiences. I benefited greatly from the Nurse in Washington Internship and can apply the knowledge I gained to advocate more effectively for my patients.

Next, I got to participate in another wonderful opportunity called the Paul Ambrose Scholars Program. I traveled to Washington D.C. and met other graduate health science student leaders from all disciplines and dozens of different schools. The three-day program included discussions with national public health officials. Scholarships were granted to students who proposed community projects that were focused on prevention. My project was focused on showing how public health programs save money for the California state government. I felt that because of the recent budget cuts to health programs it was important to show how many public health programs actually reduce state spending. I left the conference inspired by the passion of the other students and public health officials.

My interest in California politics led me to apply to the Jessie Marvin Unruh Assembly Fellow program, a one-year paid fellowship. It includes graduate seminars on California state government, mentorship, and

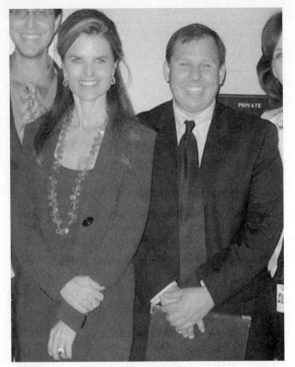

FIGURE 4-1 Governor Schwarzenegger's State of the State Address on January 6, 2010, First Lady Maria Shriver, and Alfredo Mireles.

direct policy experience in a California State Assembly member's office. I was fortunate to be selected and was assigned to Assembly member Anthony Portantino's office. I worked on health, human services, and aging and long-term care issues. I attended policy briefings, proposed bill ideas, researched bills, and met many interesting and influential people. It has been an incredible experience, and it has helped me to become an even more effective patient advocate (Figure 4-1).

Nurses are perceived as people who care about others. This is a tremendous advantage in the political environment. Nurses are practical and natural problem solvers. We have all "made things work" in challenging clinical situations, and the same skills can be applied to challenging policy situations. Influencing policy requires patience and unconventional thinking—two things nurses also possess.

For a list of related websites, please refer to your Evolve Resources at http://evolve.elsevier.com/Mason/policypolitics/

CHAPTER 5

Advocacy in Nursing and Health Care

Chad Priest

*"I come to present the strong claims of suffering human-
ity. I come to place before the Legislature of Massachusetts the condition of the miserable, the desolate, the
outcast. I come as the advocate of helpless, forgotten,
insane men and women; of beings sunk to a condition
from which the unconcerned world would start with real
horror."*

—Dorothea Dix

Nurses have a long history of advocating on behalf of
and alongside patients, families, and communities to
promote health, equality, and justice. Nursing is
widely respected for effective professional advocacy
that has expanded the professional role of the registered nurse and created safer working conditions for
nurses. Florence Nightingale's revolutionary advocacy around the environment of care and Margaret
Sanger's pursuit of reproductive freedom for women
exemplify nursing advocacy.

Despite a history rooted in speaking for and
working on behalf of the most vulnerable among us,
nursing's relationship with advocacy is complicated.
Perhaps this is because the profession was for many
years defined by loyalty to others—namely to physicians and hospitals—and not to patients. Echoes of
this tension reverberate today, as nurses are routinely
challenged as they navigate between loyalty to physicians and hospitals, and advocacy on behalf of
patients, families, and communities. Complicating
matters, nursing schools and institutions do not necessarily prepare students to serve as advocates. Many
nurses find the idea of advocacy on behalf of patients
(and even themselves) to be daunting. The nursing
profession has also sent mixed signals about the value
of advocacy, and there has been scant research into
what exactly nursing advocacy looks like.

This is a chapter about advocacy at the individual,
community, and system levels—and advocacy's
relationship to policy. Because this is a chapter
about advocacy, this is also a chapter about nursing.
Although nursing's relationship with advocacy
deserves refinement, nursing practice is rooted in
advocacy on behalf of and alongside those who are
sick, vulnerable, and in need of care.

THE DEFINITION OF ADVOCACY

The word *advocacy* is derived from the Latin word
advocatus, meaning to plead the cause of another
(Advocate, n.d.). While the word *advocacy* is most
frequently associated with legal and political settings,
the definition has expanded to encompass a wide
range of activities undertaken in support of individuals, families, systems, communities, and issues. Nurses
are widely viewed as advocates for patients and their
families. Some have suggested that patient advocacy
is an integral part of nursing practice (Vaartio, Leino-
Kilpi, Salantera, & Suominen, 2006). In modern
nursing practice, nurses serve as advocates when they
ensure that patients understand the treatments they
are receiving while in the hospital, or serve as a trans-
lator between the patient and members of the health
care team. Many nurses work to coordinate care and
help patients navigate the complexities of the health
system.

In the community setting, nurses frequently work
with residents and community leaders to advocate
for healthier neighborhoods. Working alongside
members of the community, community health
nurses seek to mitigate the social determinants of
illness through advocacy at the individual, system,
and policy levels. As experts in the delivery of health

care and the promotion of health, nurses are also frequently engaged in issue advocacy, addressing such issues as access to care and disease prevention.

Through professional organizations such as the American Nurses Association (ANA) and the American Association of Nurse Anesthetists (AANA) (see Chapter 35), nurses serve as advocates for the nursing profession itself by educating and appealing to state and federal legislators and policymakers to promote safe workspaces for nurses and to safeguard the nursing scope of practice.

THE NURSE AS PATIENT ADVOCATE

Patient advocacy is a frequently described, but poorly understood, concept in nursing. It is viewed as a central tenet of nursing practice, both in the U.S. and around the world (Allcock, 1989; Altun & Ersoy, 2003; Bu & Jezewski, 2007; Foley, Minick, & Kee, 2000; Gale, 1989; Hanks, 2005; Kohnke 1978; Mathes, 2005; McSteen & Peden-McAlpine, 2006; Morra, 2000; Vaartio, et al., 2006). Despite widespread acceptance of the role of patient advocate by nurses in the published literature, there is little understanding of what nursing advocacy is, how (and whether or not) it is performed by nurses, and what results from nursing advocacy (Baldwin, 2003; Grace, 2001; Mallik, 1998).

Winslow (1984) identified two major metaphors— loyalty and advocacy—espoused by nursing leaders and educators from the profession's birth through the mid 1980s. Loyalty as a metaphor for practice was rooted in the "battle against disease" and featured rigid hierarchies that were prevalent in military practice settings through the 1940s (Winslow, 1984). Instructional books from the early period of the profession characterized the nurse as a warrior in the battle against disease and illness, glamorizing a life of "toil and discipline" in which nurses pledged loyalty to their physician leaders (Winslow, 1984). The primary goal of loyalty by nurses was to project and reinforce confidence in the health care enterprise. Nurses were explicitly taught that loyalty to the physician equated with faithfulness to the patient (Winslow, 1984). This was particularly important prior to the advent of penicillin and other modern therapies, when many infectious diseases could not be effectively treated and seeking medical care often made

little difference in whether the patient's condition improved or deteriorated.

The primacy of loyalty as a nursing ethic came under attack in 1929 in a most unusual place. In a hospital in Manila, The Philippines, a physician ordered a new graduate nurse, Lorenza Somera, to administer cocaine injections, instead of *procaine* injections, to a tonsillectomy patient (Winslow, 1984). Somera loyally carried out the physician's order, resulting in the death of the patient. Although it was clear that the physician had erred in ordering the wrong medication, he was acquitted of all charges while Somera was found guilty of manslaughter for failing to question the orders of the physician (Winslow, 1984). The Somera case sparked worldwide protests from nurses and served to push nursing toward independent practice and accountability. It was also one of many events that led to a reconceptualization of the dominant nursing metaphor from loyalty to physicians to advocacy for patients (Winslow, 1984).

CONSUMERISM, FEMINISM, AND PROFESSIONALIZATION OF NURSING: THE EMERGENCE OF PATIENTS' RIGHTS ADVOCACY

During the 1960s and 1970s, influenced by feminist and consumer-rights ideologies, nursing advocacy became the dominant metaphor for nursing (Hewitt, 2002; Mallik, 1998; Winslow, 1984). The concept of "nurse as advocate for the patient" recognized the inherently oppressive nature of patienthood, wherein the patient is vulnerable as a result of his or her illness and unable to care for himself or herself (Bu & Jezewski, 2007). Advocacy for the patient was thus framed as rejection of loyalty to the physician, freeing nurses to develop their own professional identity. Indeed, adoption of the patient advocate role occurred simultaneously with the professionalization of nursing (Porter, 1992; Shirley, 2007). As a construct for nursing practice, advocacy had the advantage of being seen as morally good for patients, as well as providing an opportunity for nursing to promote professional autonomy (Kosik, 1972; Winslow, 1984). Typical of the literature produced during this period, Kosik (1972) asserted that "nurses must serve as advocates," arguing that:

[N]ursing cannot afford not to allow nurses to become patient advocates. Advocacy is where the action is. Through patient advocacy we can all begin to address ourselves to the real issues of the day. Patient advocacy is our hope for the future. (Kosik, 1972, p. 698)

Early forms of nursing advocacy borrowed heavily from legal models of advocacy and centered on consumerism and patients' rights. Through this lens, the nurse acted as a guardian and intervened when these rights were threatened by the medical establishment (Bramlett, Gueldner, & Sowell, 1990; Mallik, 1997a; Mallik & Rafferty, 2000; Winslow, 1984). This form of advocacy was eventually codified in the ANA Code of Ethics in 1978, which proclaimed that:

[I]n the role of client advocate, the nurse must be alert to and take appropriate action regarding any instances of incompetent, unethical, or illegal practice(s) by any member of the health care team or the health care system itself, or any action on the part of others that is prejudicial to the client's best interests. (Bernal, 1992, p. 18)

The Canadian Nurses Code of Ethics also identifies areas where nurses must advocate on behalf of their patients. The Code provides in part that "nurses must intervene if others fail to respect the dignity of persons in care" and that "nurses must advocate for appropriate use of interventions in order to minimize unnecessary and unwanted procedures that may increase suffering" (Code of Ethics for Registered Nurses, 2002). The Canadian code also commands that nurses should "advocate for health and social conditions that allow persons to live and die with dignity" as well as "intervene if other participants in the health care delivery system fail to maintain their duty of confidentiality" (Code of Ethics for Registered Nurses, 2002).

Some U.S. state boards of nursing have codified, and thus mandated, nursing advocacy by including language in nurse practice acts that either explicitly or implicitly define an advocacy role. For example, the Indiana Nursing Practice Act defines Registered Nursing to include "advocating the provision of health care services through collaboration with or referral to other health professionals" (Indiana Nursing Practice Act, 2008).

PHILOSOPHICAL MODELS OF NURSING ADVOCACY

GADOW

While patients' rights advocacy formed the basis of nursing advocacy and remains the dominant conception of nursing advocacy, nursing theorists have advanced competing conceptualizations of advocacy that seek to define a unique nursing advocacy. Sally Gadow advanced an "existential advocacy" whereby the nurse's role is to help patients clarify their values and the illness experience, and exercise their right to self-determination (Gadow, 1983). The premise underlying existential advocacy was that nurses are uniquely situated to advocate for patients, because they frequently spend the most time with patients and have an intimate connection with patients and their families. She also viewed advocacy as a moral imperative, with the ultimate goal being to increase patient autonomy (Hanks, 2005).

CURTIN

Writing during the same period as Gadow, Curtin (1979) sought to situate nursing advocacy as "human advocacy." Curtin invited nurses to help patients identify meaning and purpose in their illness with the ultimate goal of enhancing patient autonomy (Curtin, 1979; Mallik, 1997a).

KOHNKE

Occupying something of a middle ground between patients' rights advocacy and the philosophical advocacies of Gadow and Curtin (1979), Kohnke developed a model of functional advocacy that called nurses to serve as brokers of information and supporters of patient decision making (Kohnke, 1978, 1980). Like the other models, Kohnke assumed that patients were in need of advocacy so they could be freed of oppression by the medical structure. More than any other theorist of the time, Kohnke expressly suggested that physicians persecuted patients (whom she calls victims) through their "we know best" attitude (Kohnke, 1980). An illustration appearing with her work in the *American Journal of Nursing (AJN)* depicts the physician as a puppet-master manipulating a helpless patient, with the nurse as a "rescuer," attacking the physician with the banner of health (Kohnke, 1980).

While nursing advocacy has been widely internalized as a core professional value by many nurses, critics have questioned the utility of nursing advocacy as a framework for practice and have argued that few nurses are actually engaged in advocacy activities. Several critics have questioned whether or not nurses have the capacity to serve as advocates, noting that many nurses lack the institutional and personal power required to advocate for patients' rights (Bernal, 1992; Grace, 2001; Hanks, 2007; Hewitt, 2002; Mackereth, 1995; G. W. Martin, 1998). Hewitt (2002) points out that "for the nurse to be in a position to empower patients, it is necessary for the nurse to be first empowered" (p. 444).

While it is well understood that the oppressive nature of the medical establishment impairs patient autonomy, it is less clear why nurses view themselves as well suited to act as patient advocates (Mallik, 1997b; G. W. Martin, 1998; Negarandeh, Oskouie, Ahmadi, & Nikravesh, 2008; O'Connor & Kelly, 2005). One central theme in the nursing advocacy literature is that nurses are uniquely situated to serve as patient advocates because they spend the most time with patients and have the most influence over the patient's experience while the patient is hospitalized or ill (Bu & Jezewski, 2007; Curtin, 1979; Hanks, 2007; G. W. Martin, 1998; Schroeter, 2002, 2007). The intimacy of nursing care has been suggested as the mechanism by which nurses are able to engage in existential advocacy behaviors (i.e., empowerment advocacy) (Curtin, 1979). In a study of nursing elite in the United Kingdom, Mallik (1998) found that nursing leaders viewed the intimate nursing relationship with suspicion. One subject in her study stated:

> [T]his complete "under the skin oneness" is a piece of impertinence really. I mean somebody who has 55 years of history behind them walks through the door and suddenly you are their best friend and you know everything there is to know about them, it's a bit beyond the pale. (Mallik, 1998, p. 1005)

Others have argued that when nurses assume the role of advocate, they unfairly and inappropriately stake an exclusive claim to the role, alienating other health care team members that arguably engage in advocacy behaviors in the course of their professional duties (Hewitt, 2002; Mallik, 1997a).

Perhaps the most devastating critique of nursing advocacy, especially considering the high value nurses place on evidence-based practice, is that the phenomenon is poorly understood (Hewitt, 2002). Despite substantial attention to nursing advocacy since the early 1970s, there is a dearth of scientific research exploring the phenomenon. Only a handful of researchers have undertaken any scientific exploration of nursing advocacy. Most of these are qualitative researchers who have focused on understanding the concept of nursing advocacy and how nurses internalize and enact the nursing advocacy role. Despite their inability to fully explain nursing advocacy, these studies have resulted in remarkable consistency with respect to identifying advocacy functions and personal traits and characteristics of nurses that appear to promote or inhibit advocacy behaviors. A flaw in these analyses is that they operate within the constructs of existing nursing advocacy frameworks, leading to a repetition of existing constructs and ideas.

ADVOCACY OUTSIDE THE CLINICAL SETTING

Nursing advocacy isn't limited to clinical settings. Nurses are expert health care providers who are well positioned to advocate for policies and practices that promote and encourage health. Three types of nursing advocacy influence policy, population health, and the profession of nursing: issue advocacy, community and public health advocacy, and professional advocacy.

ISSUE ADVOCACY

The nursing care of patients necessarily extends beyond the hospital or clinic. Consider that symptom management for many patients requires interventions that are not purely medical. For example, mental health nurses frequently set goals with their patients to integrate patients into the community. The reality is that patients with mental illness cannot be expected to integrate into the community without the existence of health care services and programs that support such integration. Mental health nurses are frequent advocates for these programs and services. This issue advocacy directly promotes improved patient outcomes, although it does not involve advocacy on behalf of any one individual.

Importantly, issue advocacy is almost always best accomplished through the formation of coalitions. Nurses are excellent coalition partners, bringing evidence-based expertise and professional credibility to any debate. Muckian (2007) describes a successful grassroots coalition of nurses, patients, families, and other advocates that organized to reverse budget cuts to a Wisconsin in-home Medicaid program for children with autism. The in-home service program provided one-on-one behavioral care to children with autism (Muckian, 2007). Despite the fact that research had demonstrated the effectiveness of the program in promoting learning and improving integration of autistic children into traditional education classrooms, Wisconsin eliminated the program in the face of a substantial budget shortfall (Muckian, 2007). A coalition of advocacy organizations, parents, and health care professionals, including nurses, quickly mobilized to save the program (Muckian, 2007). The coalition lobbied members of the legislature and officials at the Wisconsin Department of Health and Family Services to restore the program (Muckian, 2007). Although the coalition became fragmented, as different interests emerged in the development of an ultimate policy solution, the program was eventually restored and services resumed (Muckian, 2007). Nurses were instrumental in the effort as they provided evidenced-based expertise that was used to help craft policies directly impacting children. Nurses have been active in influencing health reform legislation. Organizations such as the ANA have called for universal health care, and nurses have testified about the importance of health reform (Olshansky, 2009).

COMMUNITY AND PUBLIC HEALTH ADVOCACY

While reforming the health care system is important, and nurses' input into reform is critical, advocacy in support of health extends beyond issue advocacy. There is wide agreement among researchers, policymakers, and providers that social structures and behaviors have a significant impact on health. The quality of the environment, the nature of human relationships, the durability of the social infrastructure, and the justice inherent in the social order are all, in isolation and in combination, powerful determinants of health status. These social determinants of health and illness are complex, multifactorial, and almost entirely unresponsive to the biomedical interventions that are the core of the current health system.

Nurses, however, are well positioned to work with communities to mitigate social determinants of illness and promote health. Community health nurses routinely interact with community leaders to improve community conditions that impact health. For example, Longo and colleagues (2010) describe a nursing-led indoor air quality assessment for persons exposed to volcanic air pollution from the ongoing eruption of the Kilauea volcano in Hawaii. Previous research identified that toxic emissions from the volcano resulted in an increase in cardiopulmonary symptoms among the residents of the Ka'u District of Hawaii (Longo, et al., 2010). Nurse-researchers evaluated the penetration of toxic volcanic emissions at hospitals, schools, and libraries in the District and found elevated levels of toxins (Longo, et al., 2010). This research added evidence that supported ongoing and new prevention programs to reduce the impact of toxic air pollution. It serves as an example of how community health nursing research and interventions serve to advocate for health at the population level.

PROFESSIONAL ADVOCACY

Nursing, and nurses, matter. Consider the following:
- Nurses compose the largest segment of the health care workforce;
- Patients are in frequent contact with nurses who deliver almost all of the care to patients in the hospital setting (Needleman, 2008); and
- Research has demonstrated that the amount and quality of nursing care that patients receive is directly related to a number of health outcomes (Needleman, 2008).

Because nurses have a direct relationship to the health of patients, advocacy on behalf of the nursing profession is a powerful form of patient advocacy. Advocacy on behalf of the profession frequently involves examining issues such as workplace safety, nurse/patient ratios, expanded scope of practice, and limitations on malpractice liability. At the national level, organizations such as the ANA attempt to provide broad representation of nursing interests to members of congress, policymakers, and thought leaders. Advanced practice nurses (APRNs) and their representative organizations are known to be highly effective advocates at the state and federal level. Through advocacy of advanced practice nursing, these nurses also advocate for improved access to care and the reduction of health disparities in communities. Major policy issues impacting APRNs and frequent areas of advocacy include: reimbursement for services at the same level as physicians when delivering similar services; advocacy of neutral terms to describe health care providers (e.g., "provider" instead of "physician"); and obtaining and securing prescriptive authority for appropriately qualified APRNs (Ray, 2008).

BARRIERS TO SUCCESSFUL ADVOCACY

Like any political activity, advocacy is time-consuming and requires a significant commitment on the part of the nurse. Whether it is direct patient advocacy requiring the nurse to stay late after a shift to work with a family, or issue advocacy involving research around an issue and meetings with members of the legislature, some nurses are unwilling or unable to devote the time needed for successful advocacy.

For those who make the commitment of time and energy to become advocates, other barriers may exist, including lack of education and training about advocacy skills or outright fear of retribution from employers or governmental organizations as a result of advocacy activities (Galer-Unti, Tappe & Lachenmayr, 2004). Each of these barriers is discussed in the following paragraphs.

EDUCATION AND TRAINING

One of the major barriers to successful nursing advocacy is a lack of education and training in advocacy during formal nursing education. While some schools of nursing offer programs or units to expose students to political processes, typically limited to visits to state board of nursing meetings or legislative committees, few educational programs are designed to promote advocacy skills in nurses. Faculty may not model effective advocacy behaviors. Since nursing remains a heavily female-populated profession, this has resulted in oppressed group behaviors that have inhibited faculty in schools of nursing from effectively training students in advocacy (Hewitt, 2002).

In one of the few examples of research into how nurses learn and engage in advocacy, Foley, Minick, & Kee (2002) discovered that some nurses reported feeling as though advocacy was "deeply rooted in who they were" so that advocacy skills were essentially ingrained in their personhood (Foley, Minick, & Kee, 2002, p. 184). Other nurses reported learning advocacy skills by watching their colleagues or mentors engage in advocacy behaviors (Foley, Minick, & Kee, 2002). Still others reported that it wasn't until they gained confidence as a nurse that they felt comfortable engaging in advocacy (Foley, Minick, & Kee, 2002). These findings are problematic for those interested in teaching advocacy skills, as they suggest that advocacy skills are primarily a part of individual personality or are learned in practice, and not during formal education.

Zauderer and colleagues (2008) outlined a political-organizing educational program for nursing students that focused on empowering students to be aware of, and to participate in, the political process. This program focused on political activism and included a trip to the state capital to lobby legislators (Zauderer, Ballestas, Cardoza, Hood, & Neville, 2008). While this training approach is likely useful to build skills in advance of a specific legislative encounter and is certainly valuable, it is not clear if a political-organizing framework is sufficient to prepare students to act as advocates in their practice upon graduation.

McDermott-Levy (2009) described a unique opportunity to train students in advocacy for environmental health. During a clinical experience, one of McDermott's students cared for a patient with laryngeal cancer (McDermott-Levy, 2009). In the course of caring for the patient, the student discovered a history of laryngeal cancer in the patient's immediate family. Further investigation revealed that the family may have been exposed to carcinogens while living in a coal-mining community (the patient's father worked in a coal mine as well). McDermott suggests that nurses trained in environmental health would be well positioned to advocate for patients and communities in these situations. Considering the work of Foley and colleagues (2002) described earlier in the chapter, organic clinical encounters are likely to be extraordinary opportunities to introduce students to advocacy skills. Consider that these students could have engaged in any number of advocacy activities related to the environmental exposure—all from an encounter with one patient. In their groundbreaking study of nursing education, Benner and colleagues (2010) call for greater attention to nursing advocacy in the schooling, learning, and teaching process. They accurately point out that "[e]nthusiasm for nursing as a social good is a motivation for both students and teachers, and a 'moral source' against frustration and fatigue" (p. 206).

INSTITUTIONAL BARRIERS AND FEAR OF RETRIBUTION

Advocacy, whether on behalf of patients or in support or opposition to issues, is typically associated with some degree of "rocking the boat." After all, if the status quo were effective, there would be no need for advocacy (unless, of course, you were advocating for the preservation of the status quo). Speaking up for what you believe can be a risky endeavor. Consider that many nurses fear advocating for better workplace conditions, or for patient safety, for fear that their employers will retaliate against them. While many health care institutions respect the contribution of nursing and promote nursing autonomy, nurses who fear retaliation for doing the right thing have plenty of examples to substantiate their concerns. And it isn't just health care organizations that have retaliated against nurses who were strong advocates: governmental organizations such as state boards of nursing also send mixed signals about nursing advocacy.

Consider the interesting, and perhaps troubling, case of Ellen Finnerty, a Registered Nurse from California who was terminated from her job and had her Registered Nursing license revoked by the California Board of Registered Nursing based on her advocacy for a patient under her care. Finnerty had worked as a Registered Nurse for 20 years and was serving as a charge nurse on a medical-surgical floor when one of her patients developed respiratory problems (*Finnerty v. Board of Registered Nursing*, 2008). According to the court records, the patient was exhibiting labored breathing, but had stable vital signs. The treating physician ordered that the patient be intubated immediately while on the medical-surgical unit. Finnerty disagreed with the physician's order, claiming that the patient should be taken to the ICU for the intubation because the medical-surgical unit lacked the appropriate equipment to perform the procedure and nurses were distracted handling many patients during the change of shift. Despite Finnerty's objection, the physician reaffirmed the order for the intubation. Finnerty then countermanded the order directly, unplugged the patient's bed, and transferred the patient directly to the ICU where the patient arrived in stable condition and was successfully intubated.

Unfortunately, the patient experienced respiratory arrest a few minutes later and died. Although the patient's demise was not related to any delay in intubation that may have taken place due to the transfer to the ICU, Finnerty's employer terminated her employment (although the termination was later changed to a resignation) as a result of her "gross negligence—failure to follow direction from [the] treating physician." Shortly thereafter, the California Board of Registered Nursing filed a complaint against Finnerty alleging unprofessional conduct and gross negligence and incompetence and seeking the revocation or suspension of her license (*Finnerty v. Board of Registered Nursing*, 2008). The Board determined that Finnerty had inappropriately substituted her clinical judgment for the physician's and that her actions violated the nurse practice act, and they issued a revocation of her license.

Finnerty appealed the decision up to the California Court of Appeals, claiming that "she was required by the Board's standards of competent performance 'to act as Mr. C.'s advocate by taking him to the ICU for intubation, rather than permitting intubation to take place in an environment that was not equipped for intubation.'" The case of Ellen Finnerty calls into question whether and how nurses can act as advocates for patients in the face of questionable decision making by other members of the health care team. What would happen if the nurse didn't question the intubation in the medical-surgical environment and the patient had an adverse outcome?

SUMMARY

Advocacy is widely viewed as a fundamental nursing role—whether on behalf of patients, communities, or the profession, and in crafting policy solutions. While many nurses are engaged in advocacy behaviors, there are significant barriers to advocacy by nurses. First, while some boards of nursing require that nurses engage in advocacy, others appear to punish nurses who stand up for what is right. Second, there is tension between nurses' loyalty to patients (or communities, the profession, or policies) and nurses' obligations to institutions (e.g., hospitals). Finally, advocacy education and training is not a routine component of most formal nursing education programs, leaving nurses to rely on their colleagues to learn effective advocacy behaviors. Despite these barriers, advocacy on behalf of health can be extremely rewarding, and nurses are in a unique position to advance the cause of patient's interests in our complex health care system.

For a list of related websites, please refer to your Evolve Resources at http://evolve.elsevier.com/Mason/policypolitics/

REFERENCES

Advocate. (n.d.). Dictionary.com unabridged. Retrieved from http://dictionary.reference.com/browse/advocate.

Allcock, D. (1989). The psychiatric nurse as advocate. *Nursing Standard, 3*(37), 29-30.

Altun, I., & Ersoy, N. (2003). Undertaking the role of patient advocate: A longitudinal study of nursing students. *Nursing Ethics, 10*(5), 462-471.

Baldwin, M. A. (2003). Patient advocacy: A concept analysis. *Nursing Standard, 17*(21), 33-39.

Benner, P., Sutphen, M., Leonard, V., & Day, L. (2010). *Educating nurses: A call for radical transformation.* San Francisco, CA: Jossey-Bass.

Bernal, E. W. (1992). The nurse as patient advocate. *Hastings Center Report, 22*(4), 18-23.

Bramlett, M. H., Gueldner, S. H., & Sowell, R. L. (1990). Consumer-centric advocacy: Its connection to nursing frameworks. *Nursing Science Quarterly, 3*(4), 156-161.

Bu, X., & Jezewski, M. A. (2007). Developing a mid-range theory of patient advocacy through concept analysis. *Journal of Advanced Nursing, 57*(1), 101-110.

Code of ethics for registered nurses. (2002). Canadian Nurses Association/Association des Infirmières et Infirmiers du Canada.

Curtin, L. L. (1979). The nurse as advocate: A philosophical foundation for nursing. *Advances in Nursing Science, 1*(3), 1-10.

Finnerty v. Board of Registered Nursing, Cal.App. 4th 219, 2008.

Foley, B. J., Minick, P., & Kee, C. (2000). Nursing advocacy during a military operation. *Western Journal of Nursing Research, 22*(4), 492-507.

Foley, B. J., Minick, P., & Kee, C. (2002). How nurses learn advocacy. *Journal of Nursing Scholarship, 34*(2), 181-186.

Gadow, S. (1983). Existential advocacy: Philosophical foundations of nursing. In C. P. Murphy & H. Hunter (Eds.), *Ethical problems in the nurse-patient relationship.* Boston, MA: Allyn and Bacon.

Gale, B. J. (1989). Advocacy for elderly autonomy: A challenge for community health nurses. *Journal of Community Health Nursing, 6*(4), 191-197.

Galer-Unti, R. A., Tappe, M. K., & Lachenmayr, S. (2004). Advocacy 101: Getting started in health education advocacy. *Health Promot Pract, 5*(3), 280-288.

Grace, P. J. (2001). Professional advocacy: Widening the scope of accountability. *Nursing Philosophy: An International Journal for Healthcare Professionals, 2*(2), 151-162.

Hanks, R. G. (2005). Sphere of Nursing Advocacy Model. *Nursing Forum, 40*(3), 75-78.

Hanks, R. G. (2007). Barriers to nursing advocacy: A concept analysis. *Nursing Forum, 42*(4), 171-177.

Hewitt, J. (2002). A critical review of the arguments debating the role of the nurse advocate. *Journal of Advanced Nursing, 37*(5), 439-445.

Indiana Nursing Practice Act. Ind. Code §23-25-1-1.1(b)(4) (2008).

Kohnke, M. F. (1978). The nurse's responsibility to the consumer. *American Journal of Nursing, 78*(3), 440-442.

Kohnke, M. F. (1980). The nurse as advocate. *American Journal of Nursing, 80*(11), 2038-2040.

Kosik, S. H. (1972). Patient advocacy or fighting the system. *American Journal of Nursing, 72*(4), 694-698.

Longo, B. M., Yang, W., Green, J. B., Longo, A. A., Harris, M., & Bibilone, R. (2010). An indoor air quality assessment for vulnerable populations exposed to volcanic vog from Kilauea Volcano. *Fam Community Health, 33*(1), 21-31.

Mackereth, P. A. (1995). HIV and homophobia: Nurses as advocates. *Journal of Advanced Nursing, 22*(4), 670-676.

Mallik, M. (1997a). Advocacy in nursing—A review of the literature. *Journal of Advanced Nursing, 25*(1), 130-138.

Mallik, M. (1997b). Advocacy in nursing—Perceptions of practising nurses. *Journal of Clinical Nursing, 6*(4), 303-313.

Mallik, M. (1998). Advocacy in nursing: Perceptions and attitudes of the nursing elite in the United Kingdom. *Journal of Advanced Nursing, 28*(5), 1001-1011.

Mallik, M., & Rafferty, A. M. (2000). Diffusion of the concept of patient advocacy. *Journal of Nursing Scholarship, 32*(4), 399-404.

Martin, G. W. (1998). Communication breakdown or ideal speech situation: The problem of nurse advocacy. *Nursing Ethics, 5*(2), 147-157.

Mathes, M. (2005). On nursing, moral autonomy, and moral responsibility. *Medsurg Nursing, 14*(6), 395-398.

McDermott-Levy, R. (2009). Education: Nurses' tool for advocacy in environmental health. *The Pennsylvania Nurse, 64*(2), 10-13.

McSteen, K., & Peden-McAlpine, C. (2006). The role of the nurse as advocate in ethically difficult care situations with dying patients. *Journal of Hospice and Palliative Nursing, 8*(5), 259-269.

Morra, M. E. (2000). New opportunities for nurses as patient advocates. *Seminars in Oncology Nursing, 16*(1), 57-64.

Muckian, J. (2007). Influencing policy development: The whirling dervish of the autism in-home program. *Journal of Pediatric Nursing, 22*(3), 223-230.

Needleman, J. (2008). Is what's good for the patient good for the hospital? Aligning incentives and the business case for nursing. *Policy, Politics & Nursing Practice, 9*(2), 80-87.

Negarandeh, R., Oskouie, F., Ahmadi, F., & Nikravesh, M. (2008). The meaning of patient advocacy for Iranian nurses. *Nursing Ethics, 15*(4), 457-467.

O'Connor, T., & Kelly, B. (2005). Bridging the gap: A study of general nurses' perceptions of patient advocacy in Ireland. *Nursing Ethics, 12*(5), 453-467.

Olshansky, E. (2009). Nursing's role in health care reform. *Journal of Professional Nursing, 25*(4), 193-194.

Porter, S. (1992). The poverty of professionalization: A critical analysis of strategies for the occupational advancement of nursing. *Journal of Advanced Nursing, 17*(6), 720-726.

Ray, M. M. (2008). Advanced practice registered nurse policy issues in today's health care climate. *Journal of Emergency Nursing, 34*(6), 555-557.

Schroeter, K. (2002). Ethics in perioperative practice—Patient advocacy. *AORN Journal, 75*(5), 941-944, 949.

Schroeter, K. (2007). Advocacy: The tool of a hero. *Journal of Trauma Nursing, 14*(1), 5-6.

Shirley, J. L. (2007). Limits of autonomy in nursing's moral discourse. *Advances in Nursing Science, 30*(1), 14-25.

Vaartio, H., Leino-Kilpi, H., Salantera, S., & Suominen, T. (2006). Nursing advocacy: How is it defined by patients and nurses, what does it involve and how is it experienced? *Scandinavian Journal of Caring Sciences, 20*(3), 282-292.

Winslow, G. R. (1984). From loyalty to advocacy: A new metaphor for nursing. *Hastings Center Report, 14,* 32-40.

Zauderer, C. R., Ballestas, H. C., Cardoza, M. P., Hood, P., & Neville, S. M. (2008). United we stand: Preparing nursing students for political activism. *J N Y State Nurses Assoc, 39*(2), 4-7.

CHAPTER 6

A Primer on Political Philosophy

Sally S. Cohen

"If I were to attempt to put my political philosophy tonight into a single phrase, it would be this: Trust the people."

—Adlai Stevenson

All of the politics and policies discussed in this book have underlying issues that are infused with some basic understanding of political philosophy. Although most people engaged in health policymaking focus primarily on the strategies used in advocating for a particular issue, it is also important to understand the fundamental themes that structure debates, limit options, and motivate many of those in positions of power. Most of these themes are derived from political philosophy and have historical roots that have evolved over time and assume slightly different meaning in contemporary health policy deliberations.

In this chapter, we present major concepts from political philosophy so that nurses will be mindful of the ideologic, philosophical, and political themes that structure contemporary health policy debates. Such knowledge can enhance the ability of nurses to develop strategies that take into account political and ideologic perspectives, many of which are not always evident but nonetheless often drive political deliberations and outcomes. After an introduction to political philosophy, we present an overview of the state and its relationship with individuals. Next, major political ideologies and their evolution are explained. This leads to a discussion of what policy analysts often refer to as the "welfare state" and its differences across nations in terms of public and private roles and

This chapter provides a cursory overview of political philosophy, but in no means is meant to be a comprehensive discussion. Readers interested in more detail are encouraged to pursue items on the reference list or consult the Internet Encyclopedia of Philosophy, available online at *www.iep.utm.edu*.

responsibilities. We conclude with a discussion of the implications of political philosophy for nurses involved in health politics and policy.

POLITICAL PHILOSOPHY

Political philosophy examines, analyzes, and searches for answers to fundamental questions about the state (discussed later) and its moral and ethical responsibilities. It asks questions such as, "What constitutes the state?" "What rights and privileges should the state protect?" "What laws and regulations should be implemented?" "To what extent should government control people's lives?" Political philosophy encompasses the goals, rules, or behaviors that citizens, states, and societies ought to pursue. It provides generalizations about proper conduct in political life and the legitimate uses of power (Hacker, 1960). Political philosophers take into account the capabilities of people and societies. Therefore philosophers' moral assumptions and the realities of their times shape their perceptions and writings. Today's political philosophers build on the classic works of the past and apply them to contemporary issues, including health policy. From another perspective, political philosophy addresses two issues. The first is about the distribution of material goods, rights, and liberties. It encompasses the rights and responsibilities of residents of a specific geographic locale and how people can exercise those privileges and duties to meet their personal and social needs. The second issue pertains to the possession and determination of political power. It includes questions such as, "Why do others have rights over me?" "Why do I have to obey laws that other people developed and with which I disagree?" "Why do the wealthy often have more power than the majority?" (Wolff, 1996).

Political philosophy is a normative discipline, meaning that it tries to establish how people ought to be, as expressed through rules or laws. It involves making judgments about the world, rather than simply describing or observing people and society. Political philosophers attempt to explain what is right, just, or morally correct. It is a constantly evolving discipline, prompting us to think about how the concerns and questions just described, although as ancient as society, affect us today.

For nurses, political philosophy offers ways of analyzing and handling situations that arise in practice, policy, organizational, and community settings. For example, it helps determine how far government authorities may go in regulating nursing practice. It offers ways of understanding complex ethical situations—such as end-of-life care, the use of technology in clinical settings, and reproductive health—when there is no clear answer regarding what constitutes the rights of individuals, clinicians, government officials, or society at large. Political philosophy offers normative ways of addressing such situations by focusing on the relationships among individuals, government, and society. Finally, political philosophy enables nurses to think about their roles as members of society, organizations, and health care delivery facilities in attempting to attain important health policy goals, such as reducing the number of people without health care coverage and eliminating disparities among ethnic groups. To achieve these goals, nurses also need to address larger issues of poverty, income distribution, and allocation of resources, all of which entail the balance among the rights and responsibilities of individuals, health care professionals, and the state.

THE STATE

The "state" in political philosophy (and political science) does not pertain to the 50 states of the United States. Rather, it is a "particular kind of social group" (Shively, 2005, p. 13). Centuries ago government as we know it today did not exist. Rather, kings and their soldiers held power. Over time, states developed control over war, peace, governance, and industry. The nineteenth century Industrial Revolution greatly contributed to the growth of the modern state. Commerce and industry relied on states to support the expansion of transportation and communication through laws and other policy venues. Conversely, commerce and industry enhanced the development of the state as

the latter sought ways to levy taxes, build their defense apparatuses, and develop internal operations.

The state arose from the notion that people cannot rule at their will. As Andrew Levine (2002) explained, "Few, if any, human groupings have persisted for very long without authority relations of some kind" (p. 6). Concentration of power in a "single, centrally controlled mechanism of administration and coercion" characterizes the origins of the modern state (Levine, 2002, p. 6). This coercion or, more precisely, the ability to influence people's compliance with rules, is necessary for sustaining peace and orderly conduct and for advancing the good of individuals and society as a whole. Political ideologies, described later, provide ways of discerning the best way to achieve those ends.

Today's modern state is a highly organized government entity that influences many aspects of our lives (Shively, 2005). It typically refers to the "governing apparatus that makes and enforces rules" (Shively, 2005, p. 56). Therefore the terms *state* and *government* may be interchangeable. It is the role of the state (or government) in health policy issues—such as licensure of health professionals and institutions, financing care, ensuring adequate environmental quality, protecting against bioterrorist attacks, and subsiding care—that affects nurses in their professional practice and personal lives. Usually people think of national governments as the modern state. However, local and state governments also assume important roles in protecting individuals, regulating trade, and ensuring individual rights and well-being. In distinguishing between a nation and a state, note that a state is a political entity "with sovereignty," meaning it has responsibility for the conduct of its own affairs. In contrast, a nation is "a large group of people who are bound together, and recognize a similarity among themselves, because of a common culture" (Shively, 2005, p. 51).

Despite these distinctions, the terms *state* and *nation* often overlap in common parlance because government leaders often appeal to the "emotional attachment of people in their nation" in building support for the more legal entity, a state (Shively, 2005, p. 52). Furthermore, our global society, with the cultural diversity of most countries, makes claims of common cultural ties as the distinguishing feature of any nation increasingly difficult to uphold. That said, few would dispute that the political culture of the

U.S. is different from that of other countries. We pride ourselves on individualism, a laissez-faire approach to government and economics, and a strong belief in the rights of individuals. Policy analysts often point to our unique political culture as an explanation for why U.S. social policy deviates from that of other countries. Two examples are our difficulty in establishing any type of national health insurance program, despite historical progress in the 110th congressional session (2009-1010) and our being one of the last nations to ratify the United Nations Convention on the Rights of the Child. [As of Jan. 20, 2010, the U.S. had yet to ratify the Convention, despite promises from the Obama administration (Carrera, 2009). These policies follow a strong American tradition of a carefully delineated relationship between individuals and the state.

INDIVIDUALS AND THE STATE

Thomas Hobbes. One of the major political philosophers to describe the relationship between individuals and the state was Thomas Hobbes (1588-1679). (See Table 6-1 for a summary of the contributions of Hobbes and other major philosophers discussed in this chapter.) Hobbes developed the concept of the "social contract," which basically claims that "individuals in a hypothetical state of nature would choose to organize their political affairs" (Levine, 2002,

TABLE 6-1 Major Political Philosophers*

Political Philosopher	Major Contributions
Thomas Hobbes (1588-1679)	Social contract; individuals will voluntarily form governments to provide for common good
Thomas Locke (1632-1704)	Individual inalienable rights; different from legal rights
Jeremy Bentham (1748-1832)	Utilitarianism—individuals are utility maximizers; government exists to maximize happiness for greater good
John Stuart Mill (1806-1873)	Liberalism, but not to the extent that it might harm others
Karl Marx (1818-1883)	Socialism—reliance on state policies to protect working class and ensure equity; common ownership of resources

*An excellent resource for reading about these and other major philosophers is the Internet Encyclopedia of Philosophy (www.iep.utm.edu).

p. 18). As Shively succinctly explained, "Of their free will, by a cooperative decision, the people set up a power to dominate them for the common good" (Shively, 2005, p. 38). Hobbes's theory was intended to defend the rights of kings, but one can use it to justify other forms of government and authority. His thinking was important in establishing governance and authority, without which people would live in a natural state of chaos. To avoid such situations, according to Hobbes, people living in communities voluntarily establish rules by which they abide.

Nurses can view the social contract as a rationale for government intervention in aspects of practice, public health, and delivery of care. We turn to government to protect us from situations such as unregulated care and unlicensed practice, which might cause harm to patients if professionals and administrators were left to their own devices. We voluntarily adhere to these rules to prevent danger and minimize the consequences of unmonitored care.

John Locke. Despite its advantages, the social contract doesn't adequately address the importance of individual rights. British political philosopher John Locke (1632-1704) greatly influenced liberal thinkers, including the writers of the U.S. Constitution, by emphasizing the importance of individual rights in relationship to the state. His defense of individual rights was fundamental to liberalism (discussed later) and the development of democracies around the world. For Locke, individual rights were more important than state power. States exist to protect the "inalienable" rights afforded mankind. One of the premises of Locke's theories is that people should be free from coercive state institutions. Moreover, the rights inherent in such freedom are different from the legal rights established by governmental authority under a Hobbesian contract. They are basic to the nature of humanity.

Jeremy Bentham. Jeremy Bentham (1748-1832), heralded as the father of classic utilitarianism, rejected the natural law tradition. His utilitarianism theory basically asserted that individuals and governments strive to attain pleasure over pain. When applying this "happiness principle" to governments, "it requires us to maximize the greatest happiness of the greatest number in the community" (Shapiro, 2003, p. 19). Instead of relying on natural law, Bentham favored the establishment of legal systems "enforced by the sovereign" (Shapiro, 2003, p. 19). Acknowledging that people are "individual utility-maximizers who care nothing for the overall good of society," Bentham called for a "robust role for government in computing people's utilitarian interests and enacting policies to further them" (Shapiro, 2003, pp. 22-23). Therefore quantitative reasoning and cost-benefit calculations to "determine the best course for society" were central to his thinking (Shapiro, 2003, p. 24). Bentham's utilitarianism has become foundational to many contemporary theories in economics, political science, bioethics, and other disciplines.

The tension between individual rights and the role of the state is inherent in many health policy discussions. Consider, for example, substance abuse. On one hand, individuals have the right to smoke tobacco and drink alcohol. One might even argue that the state should protect individuals' rights to do so. On the other hand, such freedoms may interfere with others' rights to fresh air and freedom from harm (e.g., from second-hand smoke inhalation or from incidents related to alcohol use). In such cases, the state has a legitimate role to intervene and protect the rights of others—the greater good. The challenge lies in finding the right balance between the rights of individuals on both sides of the issue and balancing them with the rights of the state.

Hobbes, Locke, and Bentham are among the classic philosophers whose work set the stage for subsequent moral, political, and ethical discourse. Locke's concepts of liberty, in particular, are basic to other versions of liberalism, a description of which is beyond the scope of this chapter. Liberalism has also been the underlying premise of many contemporary political ideologies.

POLITICAL IDEOLOGIES

A political ideology is a "set of ideas about politics, all of which are related to one another and that modify and support each other" (Shively, 2005, p. 19). Political ideologies are characterized by distinctive views on the organization and functioning of the state. Ideologies give people a way of analyzing and making decisions about complex issues on the political agenda. They also provide a way for policymakers to convince others that their position on an issue will advance the public good. Three major political ideologies—liberalism, socialism, and conservatism—originated with eighteenth and nineteenth century European philosophers and are the basis of political

deliberations and policies throughout the world (Shively, 2005). Each is described in the following sections, followed by an overview of contemporary American ideologies, which are variations of traditional liberalism and conservatism. It is important to remember that terms and definitions of *liberalism* and *conservatism* as they have evolved over time are not necessarily consistent with these two ideologies as they exist today. Nonetheless, without appreciating their origins, the nuances in their rhetoric and their role in health policy cannot be fully understood.

LIBERALISM

American political thought was greatly influenced by eighteenth century European liberalism and the political thinking of Hobbes, Locke, and others. To fully grasp the impetus for such intellectual revival, one must recall that medieval Europe was a repressive agricultural society with wealthy nobility, monarchs, and clergy (especially the Roman Catholic Church) holding power. The seventeenth and eighteenth centuries brought industrialists, who sought to move goods across land and sea; scientists, who sparked innovation in work and family life; and artists, whose creativity freed the mind from parochialism. Thus, eighteenth century liberalism meshed well with political, economic, scientific, and cultural trends of the time—all of which sought to free people from confining and parochial values. Liberalism relies on the notion that members of a society should be able to "develop their individual capacities to the fullest extent" (emphasis in original) (Shively, 2005, p. 24). People also must be responsible for their actions and must not be dependent on others.

John Stuart Mill. John Stuart Mill (1806-1873), a British political philosopher, is considered a major force behind contemporary liberalism. His essay On Liberty (1859) is foundational to modern liberal thinking. Mill was committed to individual rights and freedom of thought and expression, but not unconditionally. He based his work on Locke's philosophies, tempered by Bentham's utilitarian philosophy.

Mill contended that individuals were sovereign over their own bodies and minds but could not exert such sovereignty if it harmed others. In a sense, Mill provides a way of reconciling Locke's emphasis on individual rights with Hobbes' focus on the importance of an authoritarian state. A leading contemporary political philosopher and political scientist, Ian Shapiro, applied Mill's balancing of individual rights with his "harm principle" as follows:

> … *although sanitary regulations, workplace safety rules, and the prevention of fraud coerce people and interfere with their liberty, such policies are acceptable because the legitimacy of the ends they serve is "undeniable." (Shapiro, 2003, p. 60)*

The best form of government under liberal ideology is a democracy, in which individuals participate in political decision-making and express their views freely. The right to vote confers an important privilege to members of a democracy in that it is a form of political expression free from domination by others.

In sum, liberal ideology is based on the importance of democracy; intellectual freedom (e.g., freedom of speech and religion); limited government involvement in economic activities and personal life; government protections against abuse of power by one person or group; and placing as many choices as possible in the private realm (Shively, 2005). In many ways, liberalism lies at the center of American political thought. Our early settlers came here seeking a new life, free from the old, more-rigid order in Europe. Centuries later the liberal tenets that motivated our founders and those who followed endure.

CONSERVATISM

In response to liberals' calls for changing the existing social and political order, conservatives countered with a preference for stability and structure. They preferred patterns of domination and power that had the benefit of being predictable and gave people familiar political terrain. Under conservative thought, those in power had the "awesome responsibility" to "help the weak." In contrast, liberals preferred to give such individuals "responsibility for their own affairs" (Shively, 2005, p. 26). Liberals wanted people to be free of government intrusion in their lives; conservatives favored a strong government role in helping those in need of assistance.

Guided by the notion that government had a responsibility to provide structured assistance to others, nineteenth century European conservatives, especially in Great Britain and Germany, developed many programs that featured government support to the disadvantaged (e.g., unemployment assistance and income subsidies). They accepted welfare policies (discussed later) that were foundational to the revival of Europe after World War II. Despite the upheavals of the war, which destroyed the status quo, conservatives have found their place in European politics today. They have been major players in contemporary European politics, especially in Great Britain, offering a synergy with American conservatism (discussed later).

SOCIALISM

Socialism grew out of dissatisfaction with liberalism from many in the working class. Unable to prosper under liberalism, which relied on individual capacities, socialists looked to the state for policies to protect workers from sickness, unemployment, unsafe working conditions, and other situations.

Karl Marx. Karl Marx (1818-1883), a German philosopher, is widely considered the father of socialism. For Marx, individuals could improve their situation only by identifying with their economic class. The nineteenth century Industrial Revolution had created a new class—the working class—which, according to Marx, was oppressed by capitalists who used workers for their profits. According to Marx, only revolution could relieve workers of their oppression.

As a political ideology, socialism encompasses many ideas. Among them are equality regardless of professional and/or private roles; the importance of a classless society; an economy that contributes equally to the welfare of a majority of citizens; the concept of a common good; lack of individual ownership; and lack of any type of privatization. Therefore socialism is also an economic concept under which "the production and distribution of goods is owned collectively or by a centralized government that often plans and controls the economy" (Socialism, 2005). The collective nature of socialism is in contrast to the primacy of private property that characterizes capitalism.

Socialism originated and proliferated in Europe toward the end of the nineteenth and in the early twentieth centuries. Then it split into two parties: Communist and Democratic Socialist. In 1917, Communists, under the leadership of V. I. Lenin, took over the Russian Empire and formed a socialist state, the

Union of Soviet Socialist Republics (USSR). Lenin and his Communist followers believed in revolution as the only way to advance socialism and achieve total improvement in workers' conditions. Democratic Socialists, in contrast, were more willing to work with government institutions, participate in democracies, and "settle for partial improvements for workers, rather than holding out for total change" (Shively, 2005, p. 33). Communism prevailed in most Eastern European countries until the late 1980s. Between 1989 and 1991, communist regimes in Eastern Germany, in the USSR, and throughout Eastern Europe collapsed. In their quest for economic and political change, the new Eastern European governments have turned to democracy, democratic socialism, capitalism, and other economic and political models.

Today, only a handful of countries (e.g., Cuba, China, North Korea, and Vietnam) are under communist rule. Socialists, especially Democratic Socialists, have prevailed in Scandinavia and Western Europe. They have been instrumental in advancing the modern welfare state in those countries and elsewhere around the world (Shively, 2005).

CONTEMPORARY CONSERVATISM AND LIBERALISM

Contemporary political conservatism, which grew in popularity in the late twentieth century, is similar to classic conservatism (described previously) but differs from it in several ways. In particular, conservatives oppose a strong government role in assisting the disadvantaged. Recall that the conservative political philosophers of the eighteenth and nineteenth centuries supported the state's role in helping individuals through social policies. Now, liberals are the ones who generally favor a strong government role in social policies such as health, welfare, education, and labor, whereas conservatives prefer minimal government intervention and reliance on privatization and individual choice.

As proponents of earlier models of conservatism did, contemporary conservatives oppose rapid and fundamental change. They call for devolution of federal responsibility for health and other social issues to state governments, a diminished presence of government in all aspects of policy, reduced tax burden, and the importance of traditional social values. Many political observers point to the 1980 election of President Ronald Reagan as a turning point for the rise of

American conservatism. Reagan had a strong conservative constituency, and once in office he promoted policies that were in keeping with its views. For health care this meant a decrease in federal spending on public health initiatives such as maternal and child health, mental health, and reproductive health services, especially abortions. The 1980s and the rise of conservatism diminished the influence of liberal voices on the American political and health care scene.

In contrast to conservatives' calls for a decreased federal presence in health care policy, liberals today support an expanded government role to help people who need income support, health care coverage, child care assistance, vocational guidance, tuition, and other aspects of social policy. They follow their liberal predecessors, who in the 1930s and 1940s supported President Franklin D. Roosevelt's New Deal policies, which aimed to help the disadvantaged in the wake of the Great Depression. The Great Society programs of President John F. Kennedy and Lyndon B. Johnson in the 1960s and early 1970s further boosted American liberal policies. Among the highlights of the Great Society initiatives were the enactment of Medicare, Medicaid, and Head Start. These federal government programs are founded on the importance of the state helping the disadvantaged through government-sponsored programs. They are in line with traditional liberal philosophies, described previously, which support the notion that individuals should be given equal opportunities to pursue their inalienable rights. Such rights include their health and welfare, broadly defined, even though the right to health care is not a legal one under our Constitution.

Since the mid 1990s, conservatives and liberals have found themselves in a somewhat ironic situation. Conservatives have deviated from their preference for the status quo by favoring rampant changes in certain aspects of social policy. Among them are privatizing Social Security and inserting the federal government into the public education domain under the No Child Left Behind (NCLB) law. Liberals, on the other hand, often find themselves as the defenders of the status quo as they fight to sustain public programs, such as Medicaid. Each of these stances also reflects ideologies of their respective camps. In calling for the privatization of Social Security, for example, conservatives are staking their claim for a diminished federal role and for a stronger market orientation. In wanting to preserve and increase funding for

Medicaid and other social policy programs, liberals retain their position that the federal government has an important role in helping the disadvantaged.

George Lakoff, a well-known linguist and political scientist, has developed an interesting way of explaining the differences between contemporary liberals and conservatives by designating each as a particular type of parent. For Lakoff, conservatism revolves around the so-called "Strict Father" model. It is an authoritarian structure that emphasizes the traditional nuclear family in which the father plays the essential role in supporting and protecting the family as well as in establishing rules for the behavior of children and strictly reinforcing these policies. Parental authority is expressed through "tough love" (Lakoff, 2002, p. 33).

According to Lakoff, liberalism favors an entirely different approach to family life, the so-called "Nurturant Parent." "Love, empathy, and nurturance are primary" (Lakoff, 2002, p. 33). "Children become responsible and self-reliant through being cared for, respected, and caring for others, both in their family and in their community" (Lakoff, 2002, p. 34). This metaphor of caring for children applies to liberals who support policies for other dependents, such as welfare recipients and the disabled. These liberals want to make sure that basic needs such as food, shelter, health care, and education of members of society are met. They focus on investing in social programs as a form of social support. Conservatives oppose this approach because it fails to sustain self-discipline and reinforces moral weakness.

These differences between conservatives and liberals can be seen with many issues, such as health care. Conservatives think that government regulation interferes with individual choice and "the pursuit of self-interest" (Lakoff, 2002). They prefer policies that increase coverage of the uninsured through tax credits. The latter would give money to individuals and families in the form of a credit on taxes owed. The recipients could then use the money to purchase health care of their choice.

Liberals regard governmental regulation of issues as protection against the flaws of relying solely on the free market. Citizens must be protected against those who pollute the natural environment, jeopardize workers' safety and health, deceive customers, and manufacture dangerous products. Their approach to covering the uninsured is typically to extend existing

government entitlement programs, such as Medicaid and Medicare, and the Children's Insurance Program (CHIP), to those who are ineligible under existing law.

This description places liberals and conservatives at two extremes of an ideologic continuum. Most people's views, however, lie between these two extremes. Moreover, although conservatives are usually Republicans and liberals are usually Democrats, this is not always the case. Moderate Republicans often side with Democrats on issues such as covering the uninsured, abortion, and women's rights. Similarly, conservative Democrats might side with Republicans on those and other issues. Many organizations are aligned with a liberal or conservative ideology (Table 6-2). They often take policy positions on health care and other issues that are in concert with a certain ideologic perspective. However, similar to elected officials, they may deviate from these positions on any given issue. Nursing organizations welcome members of all political persuasions and strive to foster tolerance among different ideologic and partisan points of view.

TABLE 6-2 Organizations and Think Tanks That Are Aligned with a Political Ideology on Health Policy Issues

Organization	Website
Conservative	
American Enterprise Institute	www.aei.org
American Family Association Foundation	www.afa.net
Concerned Women of America	www.cwfa.org/main.asp
Family Research Council	www.frc.org
Heritage Foundation	www.heritage.org
Hudson Institute	www.hudson.org
National Center for Public Policy Research	www.nationalcenter.org
Liberal	
Americans for Democratic Action	www.adaction.org
Center for Public Policy Priorities	www.cppp.org
Center for Law and Social Policy	www.clasp.org
Center for the Study of Social Policy	www.cssp.org
Center for American Progress	www.americanprogress.org
Choice USA	www.choiceusa.org
Families USA	www.familiesusa.org
People for the American Way	www.pfaw.org/pfaw/general

THE WELFARE STATE

The welfare state refers to the "share of the economy devoted to government social expenditures" (Hacker, 2002, pp. 12-13). Health policy analysts often compare aspects of the welfare state among developed countries. In such comparisons, the United States typically ranks lowest for public social expenditures as a percentage of the gross domestic product (GDP). Explanations for this "American exceptionalism" include the philosophical traditions inherent in American culture, as discussed previously. However, if one adjusts for tax burdens, such as income taxes, and other public subsidies, then the United States ranks closer to the middle (Hacker, 2002).

Social policies have many different components. When health care expenditures alone are considered, the United States ranks highest among industrialized nations for health care spending as a percentage of GDP. Another unique aspect of the American welfare state is that most health care spending comes from the private sector. Nonetheless, escalating public expenditures, primarily for Medicare and Medicaid, are a main cause of concern to federal and state policymakers and are an important aspect of the American welfare state.

The origins for much of the modern welfare state in Europe and the United States can be traced to the post–World War II period, when, after the war's devastation, government leaders wanted to provide health and other social services to rebuild their economies and their people. One of the best examples of such activities was the establishment of the British National Health Service (NHS), a government-administered and government-financed health insurance and delivery system to which all United Kingdom residents are entitled (see Chapter 38). In the late 1930s, the U.S. also expanded its welfare state to ameliorate the devastation of the Depression. The 1935 Social Security Act, which established the Social Security program, welfare, federal maternal and child health programs, and other important initiatives, is the cornerstone of our welfare state. As described earlier in the chapter, it was expanded in the 1960s and early 1970s, when activist government again prevailed.

Since the 1980s, the welfare state has been in a state of flux in the U.S. and across Europe. Government budgetary constraints and a wave of conservatism put a brake on the expansion of the welfare state and made policy analysts question its future direction. One response to the constraints on the welfare state in countries such as the U.S. and Canada, the United Kingdom, and Germany has been the infusion of competition, accountability, and requirements for increasing private sector responsibility in the provision of health care. This was exemplified by the growth of managed care in the U.S., the increased accountability of physicians and the infusion of market-oriented practices in the United Kingdom, and tightening of rules regarding physician income in Canada. Shifts in political mood, as with the 2008 election of President Barack Obama and the Democratic gains in both the House of Representatives (256 Democrats, 178 Republicans, 1 vacant) and the Senate (56 Democrats, 42 Republicans, 2 other), demonstrate how the ideologic pendulum can swing from one side to another in a relatively short time.

TYPES OF WELFARE STATES

There are many different types of welfare states, based on the division of responsibilities for social services between public and private sectors and the role of a central government authority. The most well-known categorization is Esping-Andersen's (1990) description of three types of welfare states: social-democratic, corporatist, and liberal. Remember that this categorization encompasses all aspects of social policy. Health care as a specific component of welfare policy is discussed later.

Social-democratic welfare states refer to the Scandinavian countries, where most social programs are publicly administered and relatively few privately sponsored social benefits are offered. In these countries, social democratic regimes, as described previously, "were the dominant force behind social reform." These countries have "pursued a welfare state that would promote an equality of the highest standards." This means that services are generally all on a par with those provided to the "new middle classes" and that workers are guaranteed "equality of rights enjoyed by the better-off" (Esping-Andersen, 1990, p. 27).

Corporatist welfare states are typically the Western European nations (e.g., France, Italy, Germany), where social rights and status differentials have endured and affected social policies. These countries grant social rights to many but primarily provide state interventions when family capacities fail. They lack the universal tendencies of social-democratic states. Because of the strong influence of the church, especially the Catholic Church, in these nations, they tend to preserve traditional values.

Liberal welfare states stand apart from the more socially stratified corporatist welfare states and include the U.S., Canada, and Australia, where privately sponsored benefits dominate. Among liberal welfare states, the U.S. is distinctive for its large percentage of social spending in the form of privately sponsored benefits (Hacker, 2002). In liberal welfare states, the "traditional, liberal, work ethic norms" prevail. Welfare and other social benefits are highly stigmatized, and the state encourages market involvement as much as possible (Esping-Andersen, 1990, p. 26).

HEALTH CARE AND THE WELFARE STATE

Moran distinguishes between the "welfare state" and the "health care state." The latter is part of the welfare state but needs to be analyzed separately. "Health care institutions are influenced by, and of course influence, the wider welfare state; but they are also shaped by dynamics of their own—some of which are internal to, and some of which are external to, the health care system" (Moran, 2000, p. 139). The concept of "health care state" is important because states and health care institutions are joined symbiotically" (Moran, 2000, p. 147). As Moran explained:

> [H]ealth care is the biggest single consumer of resources in the modern welfare states and states are either directly the dominant financiers of health care or are central to the regulation of institutions that provide the money. Health care looms large in the modern welfare state, and states loom large in modern health-care systems. (Moran, 2000, pp. 138-139)

Moran proposed three "governing areas" of the health care state: health care consumption, provision of care, and the development and use of technology. Each involves a particular role for the state and its own "system of politics" (Moran, 2000, p. 146).

Consumption. Regarding consumption, many schemes exist for a package of services to the whole population or a subgroup, each involving a key role for the state. They may be the "only third-party payer who matters (United Kingdom and Scandinavia); the biggest single third-party payer (United States); they

may be centrally involved in struggling with the inadequacies of existing systems of third-party payment (United States, again)"; or they may "provide a public law framework for the institutions that dominate third-party payment" as in Germany and other countries (Moran, 2000, p. 142).

Provision of Care. Moran identifies two major aspects of the provision of care: hospital government and professional government. Arrangements for hospital government vary from the NHS, where the "central state" owns and controls hospital care, to the United States, where most hospitals are privately operated with large public subsidies. As for professional government, analyses typically focus on physicians, whom most politicians think are the most important and perhaps only health care providers. This provides an excellent opportunity for nurse researchers to examine how nursing care varies in its governance and arrangements across countries as part of welfare and health care policy analysis. Nonetheless, regarding physicians, variations across nations persist—for example, in Scandinavian nations, physicians are salaried state employees and in the United Kingdom, physicians are "self-employed contractor[s] with little freedom to generate discretionary income" (Moran, 2000, p. 143).

Development and Use of Technology. States have been crucial for the development of technology, especially regarding its funding. States also regulate technology by "promoting drug safety" or "classifying medical devices" (Moran, 2000, p. 145). It is also important to recognize that much technology is produced by private corporations. Even though the state regulates their commerce and development, entrepreneurs from the private sector own the technology and have a huge deal of discretion over property rights, marketing strategies, and other aspects of technology production (Moran, 2000, p. 146).

POLITICAL PHILOSOPHY AND THE WELFARE STATE: IMPLICATIONS FOR NURSES

How might nurses apply these concepts of political philosophy to their involvement in health politics and policy? Rather than sitting on the sidelines, nurses—regardless of partisan preference—can participate in the ideologic and political debates that shape health policies. Each of us has perspectives on the role of government and the rights of individuals with regard to certain health policies. They form our own ideology and political positions. Figure out where you stand on an issue and the underlying ideology that informs your views. Then use that knowledge as the basis for advocating for policies that have the potential to improve health policy and patient outcomes. In so doing, be mindful of the philosophical traditions that shape your views.

When engaging in political deliberations, listen to the rhetoric that others use and identify the underlying political and philosophical threads. Use similar language, as long as it is based on sound knowledge, when you meet with policymakers, or use written texts to advance your positions. Two cases, covering the uninsured and motorcycle helmet use, make these points more clearly.

First, consider the issue of reducing the number of uninsured Americans. If one believes that the government's role should be minimal and individuals should largely be accountable for health care purchasing and costs, then tax credits and other types of individual health care accounts would be the policy of choice. If, on the other hand, one believes that the state is largely responsible for ensuring a basic minimum of health care, then one would prefer the expansion of government-sponsored programs, such as Medicare, Medicaid, and CHIP, to cover those presently lacking insurance. People in this camp might also lean toward a single-payer option, with the state or federal government being the designated payer. The same model can be used for the issue of health care quality—that is, one would rest responsibility with the private sector or the state, depending on one's ideology.

Similar issues arise when considering issues of public health, such as motorcyclists' use of helmets. For example, one view, taken predominantly by traditional liberals, might be that motorcyclists have the right to decide for themselves whether or not they wear helmets. Others, using a Hobbesian or social contract framework, might argue that it is in the best interest of society at large for riders to wear helmets and abide by laws requiring them to do so. This is partly because of the cost to society, but mostly because the state has a responsibility to protect individuals, which in turn promotes a peaceful and orderly society. Individuals, in turn, have a responsibility to yield to the state in its attempts to maintain order. There are some cases in which the state may

need to limit individual freedoms in order to protect the state at large. Variations among the American states in helmet laws depict the different approaches to the balance of power among individuals, the state, and the community at large. The relationship between nursing and the state has yet to be carefully explored. Connolly (2004) states, "Undertaking political history requires an understanding of how government works, in both theory and practice" (p. 16). Yet, there are many aspects of nursing's political history that remain untapped and that warrant a close examination of how the profession has interacted with state structures in the policy process. Recent examples that come to mind are the 2002 Nursing Reinvestment Act and the role of nursing under health care reform.

Whether working with public officials, strategizing to create links between policy and practice, or studying the role of the state in public policies that pertain to nursing, political philosophy is the foundation of thought and action. It can be a lively aspect of nurses' strategic thinking in linking policy, politics, and practice.

For a list of related websites, please refer to your Evolve Resources at http://evolve.elsevier.com/Mason/policypolitics/

REFERENCES

Carrera, J. M. (2009, May 6). Why fear U.S. ratification of UN convention? Retrieved from http://theunitednations.suite101.com/article.cfm/why_fear_us_ratification_of_un_convention.

Connolly, C. A. (2004). Beyond social history: New approaches to understanding the state of and the state in nursing history. *Nursing History Review, 12,* 5-24.

Esping-Andersen, G. (1990). *The three worlds of welfare capitalism.* Princeton, NJ: Princeton University Press.

Hacker, A. (1960). *Political theory: Philosophy, ideology, science.* New York: MacMillan.

Hacker, J. S. (2002). *The divided welfare state: The battle over public and private social benefits in the United States.* New York: Cambridge University Press.

Lakoff, G. (2002). *Moral politics: How liberals and conservatives think.* Chicago: University of Chicago Press.

Levine, A. (2002). *Engaging political philosophy from Hobbes to Rawls.* Malden, MA: Blackwell Publishers.

Moran, M. (2000). Understanding the welfare state: The case of health care. *British Journal of Politics & International Relations, 2*(2), 135-160.

Shapiro, I. (2003). *The moral foundations of politics.* New Haven: Yale University Press.

Shively, W. P. (2005). *Power and choice: An introduction to political science* (9th ed.). Boston: McGraw-Hill.

Socialism. (2005). Online encyclopedia, thesaurus, dictionary definitions and more. Retrieved from www.answers.com/topic/socialism.

Wolff, J. (1996). An introduction to political philosophy. Oxford, UK: Oxford University Press.

CHAPTER 7

The Policy Process

Bobbie Berkowitz

"A problem clearly stated is a problem half solved."
—Dorothea Brande

The purpose of this chapter is to provide a conceptual basis and framework for understanding policymaking. When pursued with a clear understanding of the issue, the data, the interests, and the options, the policy process can be highly effective in resolving problems. This chapter includes boxes titled "Think Like a Policymaker." They are designed to help the reader consider policy options and to begin thinking like a policymaker. While the emphasis of this chapter is on public policy and its process, four spheres of policy development are discussed along with their context, conceptual basis, and research and practice implications. Policy terms used in the chapter are defined in Box 7-1.

CREATING POLICY: SEEKING SOLUTIONS TO SOCIETAL, WORKPLACE, AND ORGANIZATIONAL CHALLENGES

How does a problem require a policy solution? Key factors to consider include the generation of public interest, the potential of developing an effective and efficient policy solution, the likelihood that the policy will serve most of the people at risk in a fair and equitable fashion, and a judgment about the organizational, community, societal, and political viability of the policy solution. The first step is to get the problem on the agenda of those who have the power to implement a solution.

Public interest is a fascinating dynamic related to the development of public policy. How does the public become interested in a health-related problem that impacts society at large?

Taft and Nanna (2008) have classified the sources of health policy within three domains. The first is professional, such as the need for standards and guidelines for practice. The second is organizational consistent with the needs of health care purchasers (employers), payers (insurers), and suppliers (health systems and providers). The third rests with community stakeholders (patients and consumers) and public sources, including the needs of special interest groups and government entities.

Whatever the source, public awareness and concern are often necessary for political action to get the policy process moving. For example, trends associated with health behaviors, such as the increased rates of childhood obesity, smoking prevalence, or youth violence must be seen as unacceptable and generate enough interest that people will organize to find a solution. When the costs associated with accessing health care become prohibitive for not just the poor, but middle class families as well, interest and concern are generated and public policy solutions become more viable. Unsafe products such as toys, appliances, or flammable clothing; outbreaks of disease such as influenza; or environmental threats such as air, food, or water borne toxins may raise concern about exposure of large numbers of people to the risk of disease and injury.

Moving from interest in a policy solution to action can be stimulated by interest groups where people can collectively share their concerns and work together to find solutions. Unions, trade associations, and political action committees are examples. For example, professional nursing organizations have served as a place where nurses not only explore issues about the advancement of nursing but also focus on societal issues, such as the need for health reform; exposure of the public to emerging diseases; the consequences of health disparities; and other health-related problems that affect individuals, families, and communities.

BOX 7-1 Policy Definitions

Policy is authoritative decision making (Stimpson & Hanley, 1991) related to choices about goals and priorities of the policymaking body. Generally, policies are constructed as a set of regulations (public policy), practice standards (workplace), governance mandates (organizations), ethical behavior (research), and ordinances (communities) that direct individuals, groups, organizations, and systems toward behaviors and goals.

Health policy, as defined by Longest (2006), consists of the decisions (laws, rules, judicial decisions) made within government structures (executive, legislative, judicial branches) that direct or influence the actions, behaviors, and decisions pertaining to health and its determinants.

Policy analysis is the process leading to a study of the background, purpose, content, and effects of various options within a policy and their relevant social, economic, and political factors (Dye, 1992).

Stakeholders are those directly impacted by specific policy decisions and tend to be highly involved in the policymaking process.

Advocacy is a role, often performed by nurses, that works to protect rights, values, access to support, interests, and equality. Much of the policy process involves advocating for policy that if enacted, will provide protection and support.

Think Like a Policymaker: Nurse Staffing Ratios

Staffing ratios have been mandated in some states through legislative action as a solution to inadequate nurse staffing and concerns about the quality and safety of patient care. Opinions vary widely about whether the implementation of mandatory staff ratios in hospitals will have the desired effect. Some would say that these mandatory ratios will remove the ability of hospitals to effectively manage their costs resulting in higher costs for taxpayers and patients. Others argue that voluntary methods to improve safe staffing have not worked and nurses are placed in high risk care environments. Buerhaus (2009) has proposed several non-regulatory solutions to safe staffing including improving hospital work environments, incentives to hospitals for high quality care, and a focused effort on reducing the nursing shortage. Do you think this health related issue is amenable to a public policy solution or, could safe staffing standards be managed as a policy within the workplace? As a policymaker, what information would you need to decide whether this problem would benefit from a policy solution?

Recommended Reading: Buerhaus, P. (2009) Avoiding mandatory hospital nurse staffing ratios: An economic commentary. *Nursing Outlook, 57*(2), 107-112. (Also see Chapters 53 and 61.)

The opportunity to create *effective and efficient policy solutions* answers the "so what do we do?" question. Identifying a problem is the first step, but it is necessary to identify potential solutions that might be used. For example, concerns were raised in Washington State about the ability of insured workers to access health care in rural areas. This resulted in delay of workers in returning to work as well as insufficient reporting of injuries. Because nurse practitioners had been restricted from performing some of the functions related to certifying worker disability compensation, workers access to these providers was underutilized. The Washington State legislature enacted a pilot program to allow nurse practitioners (NPs) to expand their scope of practice to include serving as attending providers for injured workers. Despite some stakeholder concerns, the evidence concerning NP competency in serving this population was compelling. To assure that the pilot program resulted in a more permanent solution, a study was done to evaluate the effectiveness of this approach. The study concluded that this was not only an effective role for NPs, it was also efficient in terms of utilization (Sears & Hogg-Johnson, 2009). A policy intervention that will solve the problem is dependent on a thorough understanding of the problem itself as well as viable policy options and an examination of the underlying evidence that the option will work in an effective and efficient manner.

Fairness and equity are important aspects of policy development. Fawcett and Russell (2001) consider the equity of a policy as the extent to which it allows the benefits and burdens of nursing practice to be equally distributed to all; in particular equal access to health services. This may be one of the primary drivers that inspire nurses to participate in the policy process. For many nurses, advocating for fairness and equity is an application of patient advocacy, in particular when human rights and health disparities are at stake.

Political viability is essential for a policy solution to a societal problem. Policy that is considered desirable to politicians and stakeholders will have the best chance of passage by a policymaking body. In addition, a policy that furthers the interests of multiple constituents will have a better chance of success. For example, public concerns about health effects from exposure to second hand smoke have been communicated to policymakers many times. While policymakers may want to take action to protect the public from tobacco smoke in public places, the pressure from tobacco companies not to act has been equally powerful. As a result, public policy related to second hand smoke languished for years in many states. However, when local communities changed their ordinances to restrict smoking in public, there was increased pressure on state legislators to take action.

CONCEPTUAL BASIS FOR POLICYMAKING

The policy process consists of a series of actions, each critical to resolving a problem through analysis and formulation of solutions. The process can involve many organizations and individuals and requires multiple steps; it is seldom logical or unidirectional. Frameworks are helpful in understanding the process. We will discuss several: the concept of incrementalism, the policy streams model, the stage-sequential model, rational decision making, and the advocacy coalition framework.

INCREMENTALISM

Lindblom (1979) first described the concept of incrementalism in the early 1950s. Most health policy change in the United States has been incremental. When policymakers face a highly complex, theoretical, or resource-intensive decision and lack the time, capacity, or understanding to analyze all of the various policy options, they may limit themselves to a set of strategies instead of tackling the whole problem. An incremental approach is often restricted to familiar policy options related to the status quo, and the analysis may focus more on the problems than on the solutions (Lindblom, 1979). Because the development of the strategies and the analysis of options may be fragmented, the process may produce limited results.

Weiss and Woodhouse (1992) stated that the concept had become associated with a process that is neither proactive, goal-oriented, nor ambitious and tends to be conservative, with limited usefulness.

POLICY STREAMS MODEL

Kingdon (1995) proposed a "policy streams" model to reflect the issue of "policy looking for a problem." He described three streams of policy activity: the problem stream, the policy stream and the political stream. The problem stream describes the complexities in getting policymakers to focus on one problem out of many facing constituents. For example, early in the process of developing the language for health reform legislation, policymakers engaged in a long process to define exactly which problems associated with our health care system should be included in a legislative package. Part of the challenge was the lack of agreement about which problems were the most urgent and which required legislation. Some felt that cost was the biggest problem, others wanted to limit health reform to tort reform, and others wanted to improve access. Until the problem is adequately defined, an appropriate policy solution cannot be effective.

The second stream is the policy stream. This describes policy goals and ideas of those in policy subsystems, such as researchers, congressional committee members and staff, agency officials, and interest groups. Ideas in the policy stream float around policy circles in search of problems. The third stream, the political stream, describes factors in the political environment that influence the policy agenda, such as an economic recession, special interest media, or pivotal political power shifts.

Kingdon sees these streams as moving constantly and waiting for a "window of opportunity" to open through "couplings" of any two streams (particularly in the political stream), creating new opportunities for policy change. However, such opportunities are time-limited: if change does not occur while the window is open, the problems and options return to the soup and continue floating. For example, while health reform was a high priority for the newly elected President Obama, the economic crisis and recession became a powerful political "stream" bringing to bear a major debate about the short-term costs of health care reform as opposed to a discussion about long-term savings.

THE STAGE-SEQUENTIAL MODEL

The stage-sequential model is a dynamic process that includes four stages: agenda setting, policy formulation, program implementation, and policy evaluation (Ripley, 1996). Each stage contains a set of actions and activities that produce outcomes or products that influence the next stage. Theoretically, the stages flow in a circular pattern, each informing the next with the process beginning again at the evaluation stage. While simple in design, this model and the rational decision-making model are deceptively complex. Defining the policy problem with adequate clarity so that it gains the attention of policymakers and stakeholders is challenging; each policy problem has many competitors seeking a place on the policy agenda. Though policy formulation is dependent on good data and evidence about what works, data and evidence may not be enough to outweigh the influence of special interests. Program implementation is carried out by the executive branch of government through guidelines and regulations. It is not unusual for the intent of a policy to get lost in the translation to program. Policy evaluation is the opportunity to evaluate whether or not a policy solved the problem either through a program, regulation, or law. However, if the intent of the policy was vague or if it was misinterpreted on its way to program design, the evaluation may highlight a policy solution that failed to solve the problem.

RATIONAL DECISION MAKING

Longest (1998, 2006) described an approach to public policymaking that features a series of actions that are highly dependent on relationships among individuals, organizations, and policymakers. It assumes that policymaking is a rational decision-making process that combines influence from interest groups, data, political negotiations, and ideology. The process holds promise for major policy change because it reflects a broad view of the problem to be solved, the many options through which the problem could be solved, and a clear focus on intent and outcomes. While the model is circular rather than linear, it is described in stages that closely resemble the stage-sequential model.

THE ADVOCACY COALITION FRAMEWORK

The advocacy coalition framework may be most familiar to nurses as an activist approach to working on problems related to health inequity and disparities. The role of the advocate is to empower others to make informed decisions (Spenceley, Reutter, & Allen, 2006). The authors define policy advocacy as the knowledge-based action that is intended to improve health through the influence of system-level decisions. The advocacy coalition framework is primarily concerned about how interest groups are organized within policy domains. It is a powerful tool used to develop an understanding of the various policy disputes among stakeholders (Birkland, 2005). Sabatier (2007) stated that beliefs matter a great deal in policymaking. The preferences that individuals hold are deeply engrained and drive their thinking about policy options. Therefore, public opinion matters and the use of public opinion through the mobilization of coalitions to support or change legislation or regulations or to shift resources in favor of different programs is the strategy of the advocacy coalition framework (Weible, 2006). (See Chapter 86 on coalitions.)

STEPS IN THE POLICY PROCESS

The following steps are most closely related to the rational approach and the stage-sequential model. They combine the four primary stages of the stage-sequential model, but focus on the importance and value of explicit analysis of various policy alternatives. Examples are used to provide a picture of how policymakers, advocates, analysts, and citizens can engage in the policy process.

DEFINE THE PROBLEM AND GET IT ON THE AGENDA

This occurs through a series of actions to define the real issue. Policymakers need to understand what the problem is, what the concerns of interest groups are, why it requires a policy solution, what trends are supporting the growth and criticality of the problem, and what if any relationship this problem has to other issues of concern. Anderson (1997) describes identifying the policy problem as a "situation that produces needs or dissatisfaction among people for which relief is sought through governmental action" (p. 94). It requires getting the attention of policymakers.

RESEARCH THE PROBLEM

Learning as much as possible about the problem is critical to understanding it and formulating possible solutions. Evidence may range from empirical research to expert opinion and come from all sectors such as economics, sociology, health services research, and biological sciences. An important source for utilizing data to transform health practices are the outcomes from translational research. Woolf (2008) described translational research as taking knowledge gained from research and using it in the clinical environment. In relation to the policy process, translational research that provides new knowledge on incentives within health care to improve quality can help policymakers evaluate options about different incentive models. In nursing practice, for example, translational research can provide evidence that a model of care such as the transitional care model (Naylor, et al., 2004) can reduce hospital readmission rates (see Chapter 85).

The idea is to make the case that the problem is significant from both an evidence-based perspective as well as a public or political perspective. Public policy generated through political and public discourse may not always use data in a strictly empirical way. For example, new guidelines on mammography were developed by the U.S. Preventive Services Task Force (USPSTF) and released in 2009. The committee's guidance, based on the best available evidence on the risks and benefits for screening mammography, concluded that women should access biennial screening between ages 50 and 74. The recommendation was an update from their 2002 statement that recommended screening start at age 40 (USPSTF, 2009). The ensuing debate was over whether or not the data on risks and benefits should outweigh the opportunity to save even a limited number of lives. The American Cancer Society released a statement that said, "The American Cancer Society strongly believes that screening saves lives and continues to recommend that women start regular screening through mammography starting at age 40" (AScribe Newswire, 2009). Health care organizations and providers must decide how these changes in the recommendations will impact their own practice standards and policies. Group Health Cooperative, a large integrated health plan in the Northwest, released a statement on their website on November 17, 2009, that stated "Group Health will make no immediate changes to its guideline for breast cancer screening. Our clinical experts will review the new USPSTF recommendations in early 2010 and determine if we need to make changes"

(Group Health, 2009). The intent is to study the issue in more depth and decide whether or not to change practice policy within the organization.

DEVELOP POLICY OPTION

This step relies on evidence and opinion. For example, if we were developing alternative options for improving access to health care for uninsured or underinsured individuals, we might look at three issues related to access. Access is often characterized by its structure (supply and distribution of services), its process (financial ability to pay for services), and its outcomes (health disparities among those who seek care) (McLaughlin & McLaughlin, 2008). Any of these three factors may lead to alternative options for seeking to improve access to care. Solutions are also influenced by whether policymakers believe that one or more options are likely to solve the problem. Confidence in the ability to solve a problem is improved when the solution has a track record, the support of evidence, political and public support, and a method to communicate and carry out the solution.

The process of selecting alternative options for consideration requires considerable analysis of the various options. For example, the National Quality Forum (NQF) is a nonprofit organization that sets national priorities and goals for performance improvement; endorses national consensus standards for measuring and publicly reporting on performance; and promotes the attainment of national goals through education and outreach programs. They use a formal consensus development process to select standards and performance measures from many options submitted for review and possible selection. The process of selecting from among the many options includes: a call for nominations of candidate standards, a review of each standard, public and NQF member comment, voting process, decision, ratification, and appeal. The process is designed to ensure that each measure received a robust review and is adopted through a rigorous consensus process.

INVOLVE INTEREST GROUPS AND STAKEHOLDERS

There are many ways to think about stakeholders and interest groups. For example, some interests may be considered "public interest" rather than "self interest." Policy development that is dominated by public interest generally follows a course of action that is based on data, information, and community values and addresses a solution to an actual or potential problem. It tends to be practical decision making. Policy generated by self interest often follows a course of action with a predominantly special interest focus connected to the concerns of individual preferences or group interests over public interest. Both are important in generating dialogue and debate during the policy process so that all sides of an issue are considered. For example, professional nursing organizations (e.g., the American Academy of Nursing, the American Nurses Association, and many nursing specialty groups) are concerned not only with public policy that impacts the health of all people, but also with policy that impacts nurses and the practice of nursing. These organizations, individually and collectively, support policies that are in the best interest of their members.

IMPLEMENT THE SELECTED POLICY

How the policy is implemented will depend on the type of policy. If it is federal legislation, a series of steps will occur including the development of regulations. If it is an organizational policy, affected parties will need to be informed and educated about the decision and the issues around implementation.

EVALUATE THE IMPACT OF THE POLICY

Once implemented, it is critical to determine if the policy worked and resolved the problem it was designed to address. It is also important to determine if any unintended consequences occurred. These may require additional policy development if they are significant.

MODIFY, REPEAL, OR LEAVE THE POLICY ALONE

A policy is an attempt to solve a problem at a particular point in time. Policymakers and stakeholders always have the option of bringing a policy back through the policy process for modification if it does not achieve the desired outcome. In the public arena, repeal may be an option, if the political will changes and the policy is no longer desirable.

COMMUNICATE POLICY OPTIONS

Policy options can be summarized through either a short policy issue or decision brief (generally a one-page summary with a recommended course of action; see Box 7-2) or an issue analysis paper (an in-depth analysis and comparison of options; see Box 7-3).

ENGAGING IN ANALYSIS

Issue analysis is similar to the nursing process: One must clearly identify the problem (including context of the problem, alternatives for resolution and consequences of each, and specific criteria for evaluating alternatives) and, finally, recommend the optimal solution. (See Figure 7-1 for a useful model for decision making.)

Issue papers provide the mechanism to do this. It is a process that identifies the underlying issue, the stakeholders, and specifies alternatives with their positive and negative consequences. Issue papers help to clarify arguments in support of a cause, to recognize the arguments of the opposition, and to develop strategies to advance the issue through the policy cycle.

FIGURE 7-1 Policy analysis scorecard example: comparison of policy alternatives for federal financing of nursing education. (Authored by Nancy L. Falk and Barbara Hanley in the 5th edition.)

		Alternatives		
		Title VIII, Public Health Service Act	Capitation Funding PLUS Title VIII	Medicare Funding of Nursing Education
Criteria				
	Substantive Funding Stream	+	+	++
	Likelihood of Ongoing Funding	+	+	++
	Ability to Meet Current/Future Demands	–	+	++
	Political Feasibility	++	+	– –
		4+/1–	4+/0–	6+/2–
Score for Each Alternative		3	4	4

BOX 7-2 Example of a Policy Decision Brief

To: Chief of Staff, Senator Wynne

From: Helen Luce, Health Policy Analyst

Re: **Health Care Fraud in the Military Health System**

ISSUE SUMMARY: Health care fraud burdens the Department of Defense (DOD) with enormous financial losses while threatening the quality of health care. Assuming that between 10% and 20% of paid claims are fraudulent, the annual loss to DOD is $600 million to $1.2 billion.

Background

- The U.S. Attorney General has identified health care fraud as the second priority for law enforcement, following only violent crime.
- Because health care fraud perpetrators target DOD, Medicare, Medicaid, and private health insurers simultaneously, the Defense Criminal Investigative Service (DCIS) cooperates extensively with many federal agencies in joint health care fraud investigations.
- Federal agencies fighting health care fraud, except DOD, have received additional resources to enhance their efforts.
- The TRICARE Program Integrity Office currently has a staff of 10, and a caseload of 1000 active cases.
- The 1996 Kennedy-Kassebaum legislation provided for 80 additional U.S. Attorneys to be hired specifically to prosecute health care fraud and abuse.

Alternatives

1. **Enhance prosecution.** Provide state attorneys general with an incentive to participate in the prosecution of DOD health care fraud by offering a portion of recovered funds from successfully prosecuted cases.

   Advantages: Could increase the total number and speed with which DOD health care fraud cases are prosecuted.

   Disadvantages: Does not address the problem of inadequate resources dedicated to detecting and investigating DOD health care fraud cases.

2. **Enhance detection and investigation.** Provide a portion of recovered funds (5% to a maximum cap of $15 million annually) to the federal agencies charged with detection and investigation of DOD health care fraud to enhance their efforts.

   Advantages: The bottleneck in government efforts to control military health care fraud is at the first two steps: detection and investigation. Returning a portion of recovered funds would serve both as an incentive for superior performance, as well as permit increased efforts in the anti-fraud fight. Current budget restrictions have precluded significant deterrent efforts; additional resources would be used to develop computer applications that detect and deter health care fraud more effectively.

   Disadvantages: Funds previously recovered and returned to the DOD would be returned specifically to detection/investigation agencies.

3. **Continue current efforts.** No change in current detection, investigation, and prosecution efforts.

   Advantages: Current efforts will uncover a certain level of health care fraud and will continue to recover a portion of fraudulent claims to the government.

   Disadvantages: Fraud perpetrators will become increasingly sophisticated in their activities and will be able to outwit overburdened government investigators.

4. **Develop additional data about the problem.** Direct the Government Accountability Office to conduct a study on the feasibility of alternatives.

Recommendation: Direct the Controller General of the U.S. to undertake a study and provide a report to Senator Smith on the feasibility of above alternatives. Because of the magnitude of federal expenditures on health care, and the loss from health care fraud, it is essential to determine the best alternative based on data.

It is helpful to compare alternatives by creating a scorecard. This is a two-dimensional grid, with the evaluation criteria on the vertical axis and the alternative policies on the horizontal axis. A summarizing notation is made for each alternative on the criteria, facilitating comparison of their strengths and weaknesses.

An easily usable mechanism for understanding an issue is a policy decision brief. This briefing paper, often referred to as a "one pager" is helpful if you are meeting with a policymaker or staff. It provides an easy document for the policymaker to read quickly and get a grasp of the issue. On the other hand, the issue paper is helpful to policy analysts to provide more depth understanding of an issue. A standard format for a policy brief includes: summary of the issue, background information, analysis of alternatives, your recommendation for action, and your contact information.

THE EVIDENCE BASE FOR HEALTH POLICY

The role of data and research is highly valuable in understanding a health policy issue and in developing a solution to the problem. It is assumed that health policy driven by an evidence base will link the evidence, policy solution, and the significance of the situation. However, evidence may support opposing views of a policy solution. For example, the public health insurance plan offered as one component of health reform is based in part on the experience of Medicare. Medicare has saved money through reduced administrative expenses as compared to private insurance providers. Others argue that the funding of a public plan, based on data from the Medicare Hospital Insurance Trust Fund, may not be sustainable (Jaffe, 2009). Here we have evidence that supports both sides of the policy debate.

Another barrier to the use of evidence in crafting policy is that it may be unclear about the kind of evidence that is needed. Nurses generally understand that evidence-based practice is based on science. However, there is a hierarchy of what constitutes evidence that ranges from systematic review, randomized controlled trials, cohort studies, case control studies, cross-sectional surveys, case reports, expert opinion, and anecdotal information (Glasby & Beresford, 2006). This hierarchy can make it difficult to reach an agreement among stakeholders, policymakers, and the public about what evidence is appropriate for health policy. As noted by Hewison (2008), the experience of practitioners and consumers may be at odds over which type of evidence is more valuable.

Despite the debate over what constitutes evidence and which evidence is relevant for health policy, health services research can be most effective in developing policy options. These include issues such as the restructuring of health services, human resource use in health care settings, primary care design, patient safety and quality, and patient outcomes (Reutter & Duncan, 2002). For example, Linda Aiken's work on safe staffing (Aiken, 2007a; Aiken, et al., 2002), Mary Naylor's work on transitions in care for older adults (Naylor, et al., 2004), and Mary Mundinger's work on the utilization of nurse practitioners (Mundinger, et al., 2000) are widely cited in policy literature as supporting specific policy action.

Think Like a Policymaker: Utilization of Advanced Practice Nurses

High on the health reform agenda in 2009 was the development of more cost-effective models for delivering high-quality care. One model in particular that gained a great deal of support from the health sector was the "Medical Home." The model was consistent with earlier patient-centered primary care models that were intended to integrate the team concept of providing care with features such as care coordination, transitions across care settings, accountability for total care of patients, innovation in improving effectiveness and efficiency, utilization of advanced technology, and assuring that patients have access to both primary and specialty care. As this model gained prominence and demonstration sites for the medical home were developed, the utilization of nurse practitioners was not made explicit. The medical home model continued to evolve as promoting a relationship between the patient and physician without a clear role for the nurse practitioner. While evidence supports the role of nurse practitioners as providers of both primary and specialty care (Ingersoll, 2009), support for the role remained controversial among the national physician organizations.

As a policymaker, how would you use this evidence to advance the full utilization of advanced practice nurses? How could the political and societal viability of such a policy be strengthened?

Recommended Reading: Ingersoll, G. (2009) Outcomes evaluation and performance improvement: An integrative review of research on advanced practice nursing. In Hamric, A., Spross, J., & Hanson, C. (Eds.), *Advanced practice nursing: An integrative approach* (4th ed.), St. Louis: Saunders.

POLICYMAKING AS PRACTICE

Many opportunities exist for nurses to become involved in the policy process. Involvement in health policy is a natural extension of the role as advocate. Nurses who seek elective office have chosen to take on the role of policymaker as their primary practice. In this case, the public policy process is the tool that a professional nurse uses to advance the public's health (Hall-Long, 2009). In addition to elective office, nurses serve in policy research roles; as policy analysts within professional nursing organizations and health care institutions and within state or federal agencies; and as staff to policymakers. Nursing leaders have had considerable impact on policy from their leadership positions in organizations such as the AARP, the Institute of Medicine (IOM), the Health Services and Resources Administration (HRSA), and the Centers for Disease Control and Prevention (CDC). At the end of the day, as Atul Gawande (2009) noted in his New Yorker article, it is the leaders within the health care sector that will implement policies on health reform. Nurses should be active in all policy arenas to assure that solutions improve the health of people.

For a list of related websites, please refer to your Evolve Resources at http://evolve.elsevier.com/Mason/policypolitics/

REFERENCES

Aiken, L. (2007a). Supplemental nurse staffing in hospitals and quality of care. *Journal of Nursing Administration, 37*, 335-342.

Aiken, L. (2007b). U.S. nurse labor market dynamics are key to global nurse sufficiency. *Health Services Research, 42*(3P2), 1299-1320.

Aiken, L., Clarke, S., Sloane, D., Sochalski, J., & Silber, J. (2002). Hospital nurse staffing and patient mortality, nurse burnout, and job dissatisfaction. *JAMA, 288*(16), 1987-1993.

Aiken, L. H., Cheung, R. B., & Olds, D. M. (2009). Education policy initiatives to address the nurse shortage in the United States. *Health Affairs (Project Hope), 28*(4), w646-w656.

Aiken, L. H., & Gwyther, M. E. (1995). Medicare funding of nursing education: The case for policy change. *JAMA, 273*(19), 1528-1532.

American Association of Colleges of Nursing. (2001). *Expand the reach of the Nurse Education Act with new initiatives—AACN recommendations to address the nursing shortage.* Washington, D.C.: Author.

American Association of Colleges of Nursing. (2010a). *2010 Federal policy agenda.* Washington, D.C.: Author.

American Association of Colleges of Nursing. (2010b). *Addressing the nursing shortage: A focus on nurse faculty.* Washington, D.C.: Author.

Anderson, J. E. (1997). *Public policymaking* (3rd ed.). Boston: Houghton Mifflin.

AScribe Newswire. (2009), American Cancer Society joins call for more information about changes to breast cancer screening program. Retrieved from www.ascribe.org

Birkland, T. (2005). *An introduction to the policy process: Theories, concepts, and models of public policy making.* London: M.E. Sharpe.

Buerhaus, P. (2009). Avoiding mandatory hospital nurse staffing ratios: An economic commentary. *Nursing Outlook, 57*(2), 107-112.

Buerhaus, P. I. (2008). Current and future state of the US nursing workforce. *JAMA, 300*(20), 2422-2424.

Buerhaus, P. I., Auerbach, D. I., & Staiger, D. (2009). *The future of the nursing workforce in the United States: Data, trends, and implications.* Sudbury, MA: Jones & Bartlett.

Bureau of Labor Statistics. (2010). *Occupational outlook handbook, 2010-2011 edition.* Washington, DC: U.S. Department of Labor.

Coffman, J., Mertz, B., & O'Neil, E. (1999). *Medicare funding of nursing education: Policy options.* San Francisco: UCSF, Center for Health Professions.

Dye, R. R. (1992). *Understanding public policy* (7th ed.). Englewood Cliffs, NJ: Prentice Hall.

Fawcett, J., & Russell, G. (2001). A conceptual model of nursing and health policy. *Policy, Politics, & Nursing Practice, 2*(2), 108-116.

Federal Interagency Forum on Aging-Related Statistics. (2008). *Older Americans 2008: Key indicators of well-being.* Washington, D.C.: U.S. Government Printing Office.

Gawande, A. (2009). The cost conundrum. *The New Yorker*, June 1, 2009, 36-44.

Glasby, J., & Beresford, P. (2006). Who knows best? Evidence-based practice and the service user contribution. *Critical Social Policy, 26*, 268-284.

Greene, D. L., Allan, J. D., & Henderson, T. (2003). *The role of states in financing of nursing education.* Washington, D.C.: National Conference of State Legislatures, The Nursing Workforce, Institute for Primary Care and Workforce Analysis.

Group Health. (2009). Group Health Mammogram recommendation remains unchanged. Retrieved from www.ghc.org/news/20091117-mammography.jhtml.

Hall-Long, B. (2009). Nursing and public policy: A tool for excellence in education, practice, and research. *Nursing Outlook, 57*(2), 78-83.

Hewison, A. (2008). Evidence-based policy: Implications for nursing and policy involvement. *Policy, Politics & Nursing Practice, 9*(4), 288-298.

H.R. 3185, 111th Congress Sess. (2009).

Ingersoll, G. (2009). Outcomes evaluation and performance improvement: An integrative review of research on advanced practice nursing. In A. Hamric, J. Spross, & C. Hanson (Eds.), *Advanced practice nursing: An integrative approach* (4th ed.). St. Louis: Saunders.

Jaffe, S. (2009). A public health insurance plan. Health Policy Brief, Health Affairs. Retrieved from www.healthaffairs.org/healthpolicybriefs/brief.php?brief_id=4.

Kalisch, P. A., & Kalisch, B. J. (1986). *Advance of American nursing.* Boston: Little, Brown.

Kingdon, J. W. (1995). *Agendas, alternatives, and public policies.* Boston: Little, Brown.

Kline, D. S. (2003). Push and pull factors in international nurse migration. *Journal of Nursing Scholarship, 35*(2), 107-111.

Lindblom, C. (1979). Still muddling, not yet through. *Public Administration Review, 39*, 517-526.

Longest, B. (1998). *Health policymaking in the United States* (2nd ed.). Chicago: Health Administration Press.

Longest, B. (2006). *Health policymaking in the United States* (4th ed.). Chicago: Health Administration Press.

McLaughlin, C., & McLaughlin, C. (2008). *Health policy analysis: An interdisciplinary approach.* Sudbury, MA: Jones & Bartlett.

Medicare Graduate Nursing Education Act, S. 1569, 111th Congress Sess. (2009).

Mundinger, M., Kane, R., Lenz, E., Totten, A., Tsai, W., Cleary, P., et al. (2000). Primary care outcomes in patients treated by nurse practitioners or physicians: A randomized trial. *JAMA, 283*, 59-68.

National League for Nursing. (2008). Graduations from basic RN programs by program type. *NLN DataView.* From www.nln.org/research/slides/images/full_size/AS0708_F10.jpg

National Quality Forum. (2009). Consensus Development Process. Retrieved from www.qualityforum.org/Measuring_Performance/Consensus_Development_Process.aspx.

Naylor, M., Brooten, D., Campbell, R., Maislin, G., McCauley, K., & Schwartz, J. (2004). Transitional care of older adults hospitalized with heart failure: A randomized, controlled trial. *Journal of the American Geriatric Society, 52*, 675-684.

Nurse Education, Expansion, and Development Act, H.R. 2043, 111th Congress Sess. (2009).

Nurse Education, Expansion, and Development Act, H.R. 5324, 108th Congress Sess. (2004).

Nurse Education, Expansion, and Development Act, S. 497, 111th Congress Sess. (2009).

Patient Protection and Affordable Care Act, Public Law 111-148, 111th Congress Sess. (2010).

Reutter, L., & Duncan, S. (2002). Preparing nurses to promote health-enhancing public policies. *Policy, Politics, & Nursing Practice, 3*(4), 294-305.

Reyes-Akinbileje, B., & Coleman, S. K. (2005). *Nursing workforce programs in Title VIII of the Public Health Services Act.* Washington, D.C.: Congressional Research Service.

Ripley, R. B. (1996). Public policy theories, models and concepts: An anthology. In D. C. McCool (Ed.), *Stages of the policy process.* Englewood Cliffs, NJ: Prentice-Hall.

Rollet, J. (2010). 2009 National Salary & Workplace Survey: Good news in troubled economy. *Advance for Nurse Practitioners, 18*(1), 24-26, 29-30.

Rother, J., & Lavizzo-Mourey, R. (2009). Addressing the nursing workforce: A critical element for health reform. *Health Affairs, 28*(4), w620-w624.

Sabatier, P. (Ed.), (2007). *Theories of the policy process* (2nd ed.). Boulder, CO: Westview Press.

Sears, J., & Hogg-Johnson, S. (2009). Enhancing the policy impact of evaluation research: A case study of nurse practitioner role expansion in a state workers' compensation system. *Nursing Outlook, 57*(2), 99-106.

Spenceley, S., Reutter, L., & Allen, M. (2006). The road less traveled: Nursing advocacy at the policy level. *Policy, Politics, & Nursing Practice, 7*(3), 180-194.

Stimpson, M., & Hanley, B. (1991). Nurse policy analyst. Advanced practice role. *Nursing and Health Care, 12*(1), 10-15.

Taft, S. H., & Nanna, K. M. (2008). What are the sources of health policy that influence nursing practice? *Policy, Politics, & Nursing Practice, 9*(4), 274-287.

Thies, K. M., & Harper, D. (2004). Medicare funding for nursing education: Proposal for a coherent policy agenda. *Nursing Outlook, 52*(6), 297-303.

U.S. Preventive Services Task Force. (2009). Screening for breast cancer. Retrieved from www.ahrq.gov/clinic/USpstf/uspsbrca.htm#summary.

Weible, C. (2006). An advocacy coalition framework approach to stakeholder analysis: Understanding the political context of California marine protected area policy. *Journal of Public Administration Research and Theory, 17,* 95-117.

Weiss, A., & Woodhouse, E. (1992). Reframing incrementalism: A constructive response to the critics. *Policy Sciences, 25,* 255-273.

Woolf, S. (2008). The meaning of translational research and why it matters. *JAMA, 299*(2) 211-213.

BOX 7-3 **Policy Issue Paper Example: Federal Funding of Nursing Education (by Nancy L. Falk)**

Policy Problem

The U.S. currently faces a number of highly significant challenges posed by an aging nurse workforce, a shortage of nurses and nurse educators, and an increasing demand for nursing services due to the health issues that accompany an aging population. To ensure that the U.S. has an RN workforce prepared to meet societal demands, federal policymakers should aim to implement solutions that would address current and future nursing education funding challenges. Health care and policy professionals view federal support of nursing school programs as "inconsistent and insufficient" (Rother & Lavizzo-Mourey, 2009). Despite current, critical shortages and a growing demand for nurses and nurse educators, federal funding falls far short of addressing these serious health care workforce challenges. Workforce projections suggest that the U.S. will face a shortage of 285,000 nurses by 2015 and 500,000 by 2025 (Buerhaus, 2008). Because nursing shortages jeopardize health care quality and access, it is essential that we examine options that will foster healthy growth and development of nursing education programs.

A Brief History of Funding of Nursing Education

Historically, the federal government has played a major role in funding and supporting nursing education. Federal funding for nursing education began in 1935 with provisions established by the Social Security Act whereby nurses pursuing education in public health received financial assistance. Similarly, the government supported psychiatric nursing, another nursing shortage practice area, with scholarship assistance from 1947 to 1955 (Kalisch & Kalisch, 1986). Additional measures were taken to

curb the nursing shortage when Congress enacted provisions in Title II of the Health Amendment Act of 1956 to provide traineeships for RNs to embark on full-time study in administration and education. These funds covered travel, tuition, fees, and allowances (Kalisch & Kalisch, 1986).

In 1963, the U.S. Surgeon General's Consultant Group on Nursing identified nursing shortage concerns that closely mirror those of today. Their recommendations led to the 1964 enactment of the Nurse Training Act in the Public Health Service Act (Public Law [PL] 88-581), the first comprehensive federal legislation to consolidate a number of nurse education and training programs. The act provided funds for construction grants to nursing schools, student loans, education grants, and traineeships (Reyes-Akinbileje & Coleman, 2005). This program was a major stimulus to enhancing the quality of nursing education, encouraging a shift from student-labor training to a professional model.

Nurse Education Funding on a Capitation Basis

PL 92-158 provided capitation funding (a set sum per student) to schools of nursing, enabling them to increase enrollment. Enacted in 1971, this legislation provided capitation until 1978 (American Association of Colleges of Nursing, 2001). Capitation was repealed in PL 99-92, the Nurse Education Amendments of 1985 (Reyes-Akinbileje & Coleman, 2005). In 2004, the Nurse Education, Expansion, and Development (NEED) Act was introduced in Congress with the goal of reinstating capitation funding (Nurse Education, Expansion, and Development Act, H.R. 5324, 2004).

BOX 7-3 Policy Issue Paper Example: Federal Funding of Nursing Education (by Nancy L. Falk)—cont'd

In February 2009, U.S. Senate Bill 497 was introduced by Senator Richard Durbin (D-IL), and in April 2009, a companion bill (House of Representatives Bill 2043) was introduced by Representative Nita Lowey (D-NY) (Nurse Education, Expansion, and Development Act, H.R. 2043, 2009). Like the Nurse Training Act of 1971, the NEED bills were written and introduced in an attempt to ease the nursing shortage by assisting nursing education programs. They seek to provide nursing school funding on a per-student basis with assistance ranging from $966 for each associate degree student to $1405 per bachelor's degree nursing student and $1800 for each master's degree or doctoral student. The funds could be used to hire and retain faculty, enhance clinical laboratories, purchase educational equipment, repair and expand infrastructure, or recruit students. The bill would amount to costs projected at $75 million in fiscal year (FY) 2010, $85 million in FY 2011, and $95 million in FY 2012 (Nurse Education, Expansion, and Development Act, S. 497, 2009).

Funding Through Title VIII of the Public Health Service Act

Since 1964, Title VIII of the Public Health Service Act has been the key federal initiative that provides funds in support of nursing education. Title VIII has been amended or reauthorized at least 14 times (Reyes-Akinbileje & Coleman, 2005), most recently in the 2010 Patient Protection and Affordable Care Act (2010). Earlier names include the Nurse Training Act, the Nursing Education Act, and the Nurse Reinvestment Act. Title VIII programs are administered by the Division of Nursing within the Bureau of Health Professions of the Health Resources and Services Administration (HRSA) of the Department of Health and Human Services (HHS). The breadth and scope of Title VIII is significant, with provisions for programs in health disparities, advanced education nursing, nursing workforce diversity, nursing education, practice and retention, loan repayment and scholarships, nursing faculty loans, and geriatric education (Reyes-Akinbileje & Coleman, 2005). In the American Recovery and Reinvestment Act (ARRA) of 2009, funding was also available for simulation laboratories for the purpose of updating nursing education and applying new solutions that maximize faculty time and resources (Aiken, Cheung, & Olds, 2009).

Funding takes the form of grants, loans, and scholarships. In 2008, Title VIII of the Public Health Service Act provided about $156 million for nursing workforce development programs. Fiscal year 2009 funding increased by an additional 9.6% (American Association of Colleges of Nursing [AACN], 2010a). Also, in 2009, $42.2 million was provided for Title VIII programs through the American Recovery and Reinvestment Act. In the Consolidated Appropriations Act of 2010, close to $243.9 million was allocated to the Title VIII programs. President Obama's FY 2011 budget proposal requests level funding for nursing workforce development programs (AACN, 2010a).

Funding Nursing Education through Medicare

Since 1965, Medicare has reimbursed hospitals for a portion of the educational costs of training nurses, physicians, and other health personnel. The intent of PL 89-97, the Social Security Amendments of 1965, was to promote high-quality inpatient care for beneficiaries of Medicare (Aiken & Gwyther, 1995). In medicine, Medicare funds are used to pay salaries of interns and residents who in turn teach medical students and provide patient care (Thies & Harper, 2004), whereas in nursing, these funds have been used to support hospital-based diploma nursing education programs. Yet, the nursing education model has shifted in such a way that it is now based primarily in associate, bachelor's, and higher-degree programs. In the 1960s, about 80% of nurses were prepared in hospital diploma programs' (Coffman, Mertz, & O'Neil, 1999). Conversely, in 2007-2008, approximately 3% of the prelicensure basic RNs graduated from diploma programs (National League for Nursing, 2008). Advanced practice registered nurses (APRNs) (e.g., nurse practitioners, certified nurse-midwives, certified registered nurse anesthetists, and clinical nurse specialists) with graduate degrees represent a growing segment of the clinical nursing workforce and must be considered within the scope of Medicare funding. Historically, advanced practice registered nurse programs have not been well funded, receiving a small percentage of the over $9 billion focused on expanding the overall health care workforce via federal initiatives (AACN, 2010b).

Therefore, Congress must review and revise Medicare funding provisions to ensure that the laws are consistent with current nursing education models and nursing workforce supply and demand. There is a growing realization that change is needed with respect to Medicare funding of nursing education. In July 2009, House of Representatives Bill 3185, the Medicare Graduate Nursing Education program, was introduced into the House of Representatives by nurse and Representative Lois Capps (D-CA) (H.R. 3185, 2009). Senator Debbie Stabenow (D-MI) introduced Senate companion Bill 1569 seeking a full-scale funding program focused on providing additional support for graduate nursing education (GNE) for historically underfunded clinical education of APRNs (Medicare Graduate Nursing Education Act, S. 1569, 2009). Going one step further—the Patient Protection and Affordable Care Act, Public Law 111-148 (2010) includes a provision for a $200 million 4-year demonstration project that would amend Title XVIII of the Social Security Act to expand programs for the clinical education of APRNs. If funded, project evidence and outcomes will need to be examined closely by the Medicare Payment Advisory

Continued

BOX 7-3 **Policy Issue Paper Example: Federal Funding of Nursing Education (by Nancy L. Falk)—cont'd**

Commission (MEDPAC) and others to determine the feasibility of providing additional Medicare payments for educating and training nonphysician health professionals. The role of the federal government in the funding of nursing education must be examined in light of history as noted above, but also within the context of current and future social, economic, ethical, political, and legal factors.

Background
Social Factors

Examination of the broad array of social factors reveals multi-faceted circumstances and challenges. The population of the United States is aging. Projections indicate that the 85-years-and-older age group could potentially grow from 5.3 million in 2006 to 21 million in 2050 (Federal Interagency Forum on Aging-Related Statistics, 2008). The population aged 65 years and older is projected to be two times larger in the year 2030 than it was in the year 2000, composing about 20% of the population (Federal Interagency Forum on Aging-Related Statistics, 2008). An increase in demand for health care services accompanies population aging.

In addition to an aging population, the United States has an aging clinical and academic nursing workforce. With the many career options available to women today, nursing is attracting fewer young women than in the past. Nurses seeking advanced practice degrees often opt for higher-paying clinical job opportunities over lower-paying academic roles. Moreover, the average age of nurses and nurse educators continues to rise. In 2006, the average age of working RNs was 43.7 years; expectations are that this figure will increase to 44.5 years by 2012 (Buerhaus, 2008). It is estimated that by 2025, 12% of the RN workforce will be over 60 years of age (Buerhaus, Auerbach, & Staiger, 2009) with potential retirement close at hand.

Concurrently, workforce projections suggest that the demand for nurses will increase by 2% to 3% over the next two decades with no expected increase in the overall supply of nurses. Between 2015 and 2025, the deficit of full-time equivalent (FTE) RNs is anticipated to grow from 285,000 to 500,000. At the 2025 level, the deficit would be three times larger than any the U.S. has ever faced (Buerhaus, 2008).

Economic Factors

Hospitals, health care systems, and students alike face mounting economic challenges. Historically, hospitals have received graduate medical education (GME) funding, which has included support for diploma nursing education. In this way, they gained a ready source of staff through hospital diploma programs. In addition to the continuing shift in nursing education away from diploma programs toward associate-, baccalaureate-, and graduate-degree level programs, hospitals and health care

systems face new economic pressures and staffing challenges. Increasing staff shortages have forced hospitals to close units, thereby decreasing the services available to some communities. In other cases, hospital systems that have had to hire temporary nurses are coping with the financial burden of increased operating costs. Workforce shortages have temporarily eased as aging nurses have reentered the workforce to meet personal and family financial challenges. In short, the magnitude of the future supply of nurses will be impacted by the overall state of the economy.

Economic challenges also impact the situation at the student level. A shorter education pathway via a diploma or community college program reduces the need for student loans and expedites entry into the workforce. Advanced education options, such as bachelor's degree or master's-level advanced practice, provide valuable skills that are much needed in the nursing and health care world. Clinical nurses are qualified to practice with a minimum of a diploma, associate, or baccalaureate degree. Nurse educator roles typically require graduate education. The requisite time commitment and graduate school education costs can serve as barriers to pursuing nursing education as a career option.

Clinical nurses who are interested in assuming educational roles also grapple with the reality of compensation differences between clinical practice and academia. Earning potential can be significantly higher in clinical practice. For example, in 2009, the average annual salary for nurse practitioners across various settings was $89,579 (Rollet, 2010) versus approximately $69,000 for master's prepared faculty (American Association of Colleges of Nursing, 2010b). Such salary differentials impact the ability of nursing education programs to attract and retain faculty. Nursing education shortages at the institutional level contribute to the nationwide nurse faculty deficit. Because of the recent adoption of the Doctor of Nursing Practice degree and the small number of graduates to date, it is difficult to assess its potential impact on human resources issues over the long haul.

An assortment of other economic factors must be considered. The aging of both faculty and facilities, the need for a sizeable qualified faculty to meet the required faculty-to-student ratios, and the overall economic challenges of operating a nursing program are problematic (Greene, Allan, & Henderson, 2003). Furthermore, tighter state budgets have led to cuts in funds for higher education. States, educators, and employers are therefore looking at a variety of financing options that include state and local workforce investment boards and employer-matched state funding. Medicaid funding has historically been available for nursing education in some states (Greene et al., 2003).

BOX 7-3 Policy Issue Paper Example: Federal Funding of Nursing Education (by Nancy L. Falk)—cont'd

Ethical Factors

Two ethical factors are of primary concern. As the nursing shortage increases, there is a growing dependence on foreign-trained nurses. Opportunities for higher pay, better working and living conditions, political and economic stability, and travel pull foreign nurses to the U.S. Although dependence on foreign nurses may alleviate workforce challenges in the U.S., it also contributes to a resource drain in poor, underdeveloped countries with a limited number of trained health care professionals (Aiken, 2007b; Kline, 2003).

Legal and Political Factors

The belief that nursing education should be financed by Medicare dollars has existed for many years. Although institutions currently receiving little to no funding have a strong incentive to support policy change, the current federal political and fiscal climate will be problematic for changing Medicare law related to GNE funding. With the U.S. government facing fiscal deficits and curtailed domestic spending, costly programs face strong scrutiny. Medicare costs have been trending upward, due in part to an aging and needy population. Other legal and political issues serve as drivers. Immigration laws, for example, are already under review; the loosening or tightening of such laws will have a direct bearing on the supply of available nurses.

Political factors internal to nursing have affected and continue to impact the development and enactment of legislation. Historically, the nursing community's weak lobbying presence, internal divisions, and inconsistent message have resulted in weak support on Capitol Hill, thereby limiting its ability to contribute to substantive policy changes impacting federal funding for nursing education. However, with time comes change. The Robert Wood Johnson funded Center to Champion Nursing in America has added a new dimension to the workforce landscape, making great strides in raising awareness and exploring solutions for nursing workforce issues nationally. Likewise, the shortage of primary care providers and the ability of nurse practitioners to help address current and future primary caregiving challenges have drawn increasing attention to the nursing community. Conversely, physician and hospital lobbies are very strong and may oppose some changes, particularly changes to GME funding and provider scope of practice, if the perception is that such changes may diminish anticipated or actual benefits to the medical community.

Issue Statement

How should the federal government fund nursing education to ensure the necessary supply of entry-level and advanced practice nurses to meet future health care demands?

Stakeholders

There is a broad range of stakeholders, each with vested interests, including hospitals, academic programs, patients, families, and both domestic and foreign-trained nurses. Staff shortages hinder both access to care and the quality of care. New streams of funding have the potential to enhance education and staffing, and thereby enhance patient access to high-quality care. As history has demonstrated, however, hospitals and health systems have much at stake. In the 1960s, approximately 80% of RNs were trained in hospital-based diploma programs strongly supported by Medicare funding (Coffman et al., 1999), Today, a mere 3% of basic RN preprofessionals graduate from diploma programs (National League for Nursing, 2008) and Medicare funding, while significant, is less than ideal for hospitals in regard to nursing education.

Available data tracking Medicare funding of Graduate Medical Education and nursing education are limited. However, existing data from 2006 indicate that Medicare direct graduate medical education payments exceeded $2 billion in 2006 with only about 6% paid to hospitals for nursing education—a sum equal to or greater than the funds available through Title VIII (Aiken et al., 2009). Medicare funding of nursing education thus has significant upside potential for the nursing community and patient care—a potential far exceeding funding levels historically provided through Title VIII. In addition, academic programs and related institutions could benefit from a funding increase to nursing education through Medicare dollars. Depending on program specifics, nurses and other employees would directly benefit. These changes, coupled with other institutional policy improvements, would likely create a more positive work environment and encourage nurse retention. Ultimately, positive changes to nursing education and training can only serve to enhance patient care. Finally, if more students from the United States enrolled in nursing programs and dependence on foreign nurses declined, this would have a mixed impact on other countries. While fewer nurses would be sending earnings to their homelands to help support families, more nurses would remain in their homelands to provide valuable health care human resources.

Policy Goals and Objectives

The goal of federal nursing education legislation is to ensure adequate recruiting, education, and retention of RNs and nursing faculty in order to meet patient care and health care service demands. Policy objectives include the following:

Continued

BOX 7-3   Policy Issue Paper Example: Federal Funding of Nursing Education (by Nancy L. Falk)—cont'd

1. Establish funding policies consistent with the demands of the existing and future health care systems.
2. Acknowledge that the structure of nursing education has changed and that policies must be updated to reflect current and future demand.
3. Develop policies, legislation, and regulations that provide steady funding to establish and support a solid foundation for nursing education at all levels.
4. Establish and develop programs that address both short-term and long-term attraction, education, and retention of high-quality students from traditional and nontraditional backgrounds.
5. Build funding and recruitment policies based on sound ethics, and strive to ensure positive national and international outcomes.

Policy Options and Alternatives

Policy alternatives for resolving the issue of federal funding of nursing education include the following:

1. Do Nothing Option: Title VIII of the Public Health Service Act. Continue primary federal support of nursing education as in current practice.
2. Incremental Change Option: Capitation payments in addition to Title VIII. Enact legislation to increase financial support for nursing education institutions based on enrollment.
3. Major Change Option: Medicare funding of nursing education. Although the GME program has traditionally supported hospital-based nursing programs, this is only one avenue for funding through Medicare.

Note: For the purposes of this analysis, we have assumed that, as in the past, the government will continue to support funding of nurse education. One could make the case that other alternatives should be considered. For instance, one might take a position that the federal government should not be supporting education for nursing or any of the health professions. Or, one could assert that other policy alternatives are feasible, such as funding of programs focused on workforce diversity, nurse practitioner residencies, and new career ladders (American Association of Colleges of Nursing, 2010a).

Criteria for Evaluation

1. Likelihood of ongoing funding
2. Size and availability of funding stream
3. Ability to meet current and future demand
4. Political feasibility

Analysis of Option 3

Because this is a sample paper, only the third option, Medicare funding, will be analyzed using the four criteria listed above. In an actual analysis, the process that follows would be repeated for each option.

Criterion 1: Likelihood of Ongoing Funding
Pro

Whereas other options, such as Title VIII, are funded through discretionary spending and are made available through Congressional appropriations, Medicare is an entitlement program funded through mandatory spending. If a law is passed to authorize spending for nurse education through the Medicare entitlement program, the federal government is obligated to make payments to those persons, institutions, or governments that meet the legal criteria delineated in the law. Therefore, the funding stream will be ongoing, unless the law is changed. Discretionary funds are made available through the Congressional appropriations process and may fluctuate significantly depending on politics and the priorities of the country at any given point in time.

Con

The cost of health care continues to rise each year. Changing demographics, increased health care needs, and enhanced health care coverage in the Patient Protection and Affordable Care Act may lead to higher health care costs. If costs increase and prove unsustainable over time, provisions in the new law may come under increasing scrutiny. Major policy changes that raise costs will have a lower likelihood of acceptance. Trends toward pay-for-performance, quality outcomes, evidence-based medicine, and development of a high-value workforce will have an impact on decision-making and federal expenditures.

Criterion 2: Size and Availability of Funding Stream

This criterion looks at the total dollars available through the major change option.

Pro

Precise information on current payments to nursing education via Medicare is difficult to obtain. Yet, the total funds available to support education through Medicare have been significantly higher than discretionary funds through Title VIII as noted above. Overall, the potential dollars at stake are substantially higher through Medicare than through Title VIII.

BOX 7-3 Policy Issue Paper Example: Federal Funding of Nursing Education (by Nancy L. Falk)—cont'd

Con

It is difficult to fully analyze the funding availability and use of GME support for diploma nursing education because data are incomplete. However, we do know that with the decline in the number of diploma programs, few nursing programs are benefiting from Medicare GME funds. With the shift away from diploma programs and toward associate and baccalaureate programs, it is critical to revisit federal, state, and local funding policies, now and on an ongoing basis, to ensure that nursing programs remain adequately funded as shifts take place.

Criterion 3: Ability to Meet Current and Future Demand

Pro

Hospitals with diploma nursing education programs are currently benefiting from GME funding. Physicians and hospitals currently reaping benefits from GME funding will continue to lobby to ensure that GME funding is not cut.

Con

Although nursing has received some benefit from GME funding, the benefit continues to trend downward as diploma programs close. Medicare funding for nursing education has supported primarily preprofessional education (Aiken & Gwyther, 1995). Current federal law has not kept pace with the nursing education models in place today. To be most effective, laws need to be updated to account for changes in nurse education and practice models, as well as current and future nurse and nurse educator supply and demand.

Criterion 4: Political Feasibility

Pro

An aging nursing workforce and a shortage of new nurses will grow increasingly visible as the baby boomers age and our overall population faces increased health care needs. As the shortage heightens, legislators, health care systems, regulatory agencies, academic institutions, and both public and private health care institutions will be open to new and creative solutions to meet society's nursing needs. There are 2.6 million RN jobs in the U.S., making nursing the largest health care occupation (Bureau of Labor Statistics, 2010). A feasible strategy is for the RN community to develop a consistent message and exercise a concerted lobbying effort to educate legislative and regulatory bodies regarding Medicare funding in support of nursing education to help alleviate the nursing shortage.

Con

Medicare funding is sizeable. Significant funds flow from Medicare to physician education in GME. In addition, a small number of diploma programs receive critical funds to support nursing education. Those who benefit from GME funds, such as hospitals and physicians, will use their formidable power to protect their turf by lobbying and influencing legislators to maintain the status quo.

Comparison of Alternatives and Results of Analysis

Analysis and comparison of the three policy alternatives on the criteria and alternatives matrix as outlined on the scorecard (Figure 7-1) reveal a tie score between alternative 2 (the capitation and Title VIII combination for federal nurse education funding) and alternative 3 (expansion of Medicare funding for nursing education, similar to the program for medicine). The capitation and Title VIII alternative scores positively on each of the four criteria, but not strongly on any one individual criterion. Alternative 3, Medicare funding, strongly meets three of the criteria (substantive funding, likelihood of ongoing funding, meeting current and future demand for nursing education), but demonstrates a major weakness in the area of political feasibility. Amendment of the Medicare professional education components are likely to stimulate strong opposition from the medical, professional, and hospital lobbies, as they fear competition for scarce dollars.

Option 1, continuation of Title VIII funding, fails on the criterion of meeting current and future demand. However, it is politically the most feasible, as it would produce the least direct political opposition.

When using an alternatives and criteria matrix, a "tie score" is not unusual. On the matrix, as in life, alternatives and decisions are not always black and white. There are shades of gray. The key is to look beyond the tie to complete the analysis.

In our example, the tie represents two potentially viable alternatives, each presenting different challenges. Given the current political climate and fiscal challenges, particularly with regard to Medicare, a two-pronged approach would be feasible. Capitation funding could be pursued through legislation immediately. This is a solution that fits well, given the current political climate and concern for improving the nursing supply through federal support of education.

Concurrently, the nursing community could continue to ramp up educational efforts, develop the political base, and mobilize for broad professional, congressional, and agency support. This effort would raise the visibility of the Medicare funding

Continued

BOX 7-3 **Policy Issue Paper Example: Federal Funding of Nursing Education (by Nancy L. Falk)—cont'd**

opportunity. Likewise, it would push policymakers to examine the potential for increased Medicare funding of nurse education as a solution that goes well beyond Title VIII and capitation to provide funding that is of greater magnitude and less tied to the appropriations process. The graduate nursing education provisions in the Patient Protection and Affordable Care Act provide hope that the voices of nurses are being heard as they seek to secure funds that could go a long way toward alleviating the nurse and nurse faculty shortages, thereby promoting quality care to patients and families.

This example was revised from the 5th edition of this book and was initially authored by Nancy L. Falk and Barbara Hanley.

CHAPTER 8

Political Analysis and Strategies

Judith K. Leavitt, Diana J. Mason, and Ellen-Marie Whelan

"You campaign in poetry and you govern in prose."
—Mario Cuomo

Nursing and politics are a good match. First, nurses understand people. Success in any political situation depends on one's ability to establish and sustain strong interpersonal relationships. Second, nurses appreciate the importance of systematic assessments. Nurses engaged in the politics of the policy process will find that their efforts are most effective when they systematically analyze their issues and develop strategies for advancing their agendas. Finally, nurses bring to the deliberations of any health policy issue an appreciation of how such policies affect clinical care and patient well-being and can foresee possible unintended consequences. Few policymakers have such an ability. Thus nurses have much to offer public and private sector discussions and actions around health policy issues.

COMPONENTS OF POLITICAL ANALYSIS

The best approach to accomplish change must include a thoughtful analysis of the politics of the problem and proposed solutions. This must be done simultaneously with policy analysis, as explored in Chapter 7 (Box 8-1).

THE PROBLEM

The first step in conducting a political analysis is to identify the problem. Answering several questions is useful for framing the problem:

- What are the scope, duration, and history, and whom does it affect?
- What data are available to describe the issue and its ramifications?
- What are the gaps in existing data?
- What types of additional research might be useful?

Not all serious conditions are problems that warrant government attention. The challenge for those seeking to get public policymakers to address particular problems (e.g., poverty, the underinsured, or unacceptable working conditions) is to define the problem in ways that will prompt lawmakers to take action. This requires careful crafting of messages so that calls for public, as opposed to private sector, solutions are clearly justified. This is known as "framing" the issue. In the workplace, framing may entail linking the problem to one of the institution's priorities or to a potential threat to its reputation, public safety and wellbeing, or financial standing. For example, inadequate nurse staffing could be linked to increases in rates of infection, morbidity, and morality—outcomes that can increase institutional costs and jeopardize an institution's reputation and future business.

Sometimes what appears to be a problem is not. For example, proposed mandatory continuing education for nurses is not a problem. Rather, it is a possible solution to the challenge of ensuring competency of nurses. After an analysis of the issue of clinician competence, one might review the policy outcomes and establish a goal that includes legislating mandatory continuing education. The danger of framing solutions as problems is the possibility that it can limit creative thinking about the underlying issue and leave the best solutions uncovered.

Proposed Solutions. Typically, there is more than one solution to an identified problem, and each option differs with regard to cost, practicality, and duration. These are the policy options. The political analysis revolves around what is politically feasible. By identifying and analyzing possible solutions, nurses will acquire further understanding of the issue and what is possible for an organization, workplace, government agency, or professional organization to undertake. There needs to be a full understanding of

---

BOX 8-1 Steps of a Political Analysis

1. Identifying and analyzing the problem
2. Outlining and analyzing proposed solutions
3. Understanding the background of the issue: its history and previous attempts to address the problem
4. Locating the political setting and structures involved
5. Evaluating the stakeholders
6. Conducting a values assessment
7. Recognizing the resources (both financial and human) needed to reach the intended goals
8. Analyzing power bases

---

the big picture and where the issue fits into that vision. For example, if nurses want the federal government to provide substantial support for nursing education, they need to understand the constraints of federal budgets and the demands to invest in other programs, including those that benefit nurses. Moreover, support for nursing education can take the form of scholarships, loans, tax credits, aid to nursing schools, or incentives for building partnerships between nursing schools and health care delivery systems. Each option presents different types of support, and nurses would need to understand the implications of the alternatives before asking for federal intervention.

The amount of money and time needed to address a particular problem also needs to be taken into account. Are there short-term and long-term alternatives that nurses want to pursue simultaneously? Is there a way to start off with a pilot or demonstration program with clear paths to expansion? How might one prioritize various solutions? What are the tradeoffs that nurses are willing to make to obtain stated political goals? Such questions need to be considered in developing the political strategy.

BACKGROUND

When striving to affect policy formation, one must know about previous attempts to move an issue. This will provide insight into the feasibility of a particular approach and provide lessons on what worked and what did not. Knowledge of past history will also provide insight into the position of key public officials so that communications with those individuals and strategies for advancing an issue can be developed

accordingly. For example, if one knows that a particular legislator has always questioned the ability of advanced practice nurses (APNs) to practice independently, then that individual would need special coaxing and perhaps a stronger emphasis on the evidence about the quality and value of APNs to support legislation allowing direct billing of APNs under Medicare.

Historical precedent for one issue can affect the politics of another. For example, in the United States today, one would not expect to be successful in moving social welfare legislation that was associated with high taxes because of the predominant value of "get government out of our lives"—as was evident during the debate preceding the passage of health care reform. This was not always the case. Social Security, Medicare, and Medicaid were all passed because at that time the public understood the need for government support to help those lacking adequate resources. In a classic work, Fox-Piven and Cloward (1993) documented that societies go through cycles of expanding and contracting social policies and programs aimed at supporting vulnerable citizens. As the size and need of the vulnerable population increases, social policies for safety nets are more likely to be put into place as a response to escalating social unrest and upheaval. This work reminds us that historical precedent does not mean that what happened in the past will remain the same. In fact, it suggests that we should be cognizant of cycles of change, seek to support a shift in political climate that will support our agendas, and be prepared to act when the time is right. The Affordable Care Act (ACA) is a good example of how lessons learned from the health care reform debate under President Clinton was instrumental in final passage under President Obama (Table 8-1).

POLITICAL SETTING

Once the problems and solutions have been clearly identified and described, the appropriate political arenas for influencing the issue need to be analyzed. Usually this begins by identifying the entities with jurisdiction over the problem. Is the issue primarily within the public domain, or does it also entail the private sector? Many issues require a mix of public and private sector players, but responsibility for decision-making will ultimately rest with one sector more than the other. For example, nurses interested

TABLE 8-1 Historical Precedent: Lessons That Helped Pass the Patient Protection and Affordable Care Act

	President Clinton	President Obama
Strike while the iron is hot	Clinton hoped to send legislation to Congress within the first 100 days of his new Administration, but it took nearly a year. By that time, fear had escalated and momentum had waned.	Like Clinton, Obama made health care reform a top priority. Although it took longer than expected, Obama worked on health care after his election and kept working until he signed the bill into law.
It's not what you say, it's how you say it	Clinton spoke about health care reform more as a moral imperative: "It's the right thing to do for the nation."	Obama learned that the message didn't resonate with the public. Instead he reiterated that under his plan: "If you like what you have (health insurance) you can keep it."
Proposed solutions	Clinton worked out all the details of a plan within the administration and presented the completed plan to Congress. The members of Congress were unhappy about not having input.	Obama learned that Congress needed to be involved—from the very beginning. Instead of working out the details, he presented Congress with a set of seven principles for health reform and instructed them to write the legislation.
Stakeholders	Clinton did not negotiate with key stakeholders in the development of the plan. As a result, the insurance industry launched the now infamous "Harry and Louise" commercials that some credit with successfully killing the legislation.	From the beginning, Obama met with key stakeholders including health professional groups, hospitals, insurance companies, and drug companies. He told them he was moving forward and wanted them at the table from the very beginning to help map out a health reform plan. In the end, most of the major stakeholders supported the final product.
United we stand, divided we fall	Clinton was forceful in telling Congress that if they sent him a health care proposal that "did not guarantee every American private health insurance that can never be taken away," he would veto the legislation.	Obama's team declared early on they would try to get bipartisan agreement on the legislation and be willing to negotiate to accomplish this. The Senate Finance Committee deliberated for months trying to get bipartisan support in their committee and succeeded, though with only one Republican vote. In the end, despite a bipartisan summit held by Obama and the inclusion of many GOP ideas, the bills were passed with only Democratic support.

in improving workplace conditions would first turn to their employers and other local stakeholders. It is seldom prudent to turn to public officials until other efforts in the private sector have failed. Additionally, making a change in one arena, such as Medicare in the public arena, affects other sectors such as private payers.

With regard to public policy, nurses need to clarify which level of government (federal, state, or local) is responsible for a particular issue. When one communicates with legislators and develops strategies, it is critical to understand the level of government responsible for a particular issue and how the levels interrelate. Scope of practice is a good example.

Although typically defined by the states, there are examples where the federal government has superseded the state's authority—such as in the Veteran's Administration and the Indian Health Service. (See Chapter 64 for a full discussion of how government works.)

In addition to the level of government, nurses need to know which branch of government (legislative, executive, or judicial) has primary jurisdiction over the issue at a given time. Although there is often overlap among these branches, nurses will find that a particular issue falls predominantly within one branch (see Chapter 65 on the legislative and regulatory processes).

If the issue is in the problem definition and policy formation stage, then nurses will focus on the legislative branch. If an issue entails the implementation of a program, including promulgating regulations, then nurses will focus on the executive branch while maintaining an eye toward the legislative role in oversight. Issues that are within the courts call for knowledge of the judicial system.

Nurses can also apply a political analysis to the workplace or community organization. Regardless of the setting, nurses will want to identify who has responsibility for decision-making for a particular issue; which committees, boards, or panels have addressed the issue in the past; the organizational structure; and the chain of command.

At an institutional level, once the relevant political arenas are identified, the formal and informal structures and functioning of that arena need to be analyzed. The formal dimensions of the entity can often be assessed through documents related to the organization's mission, goals, objectives, organizational structure, constitution and bylaws, annual report (including financial statement), long-range plans, governing body, committees, departments, and individuals with jurisdiction.

Does the entity use parliamentary procedure? Parliamentary procedure provides a democratic process that carefully balances the rights of individuals, subgroups within an organization, and the membership of an assembly. The basic rules are outlined in Robert's Rules of Order (*www.rulesonline.com*). Whether in a legislative session or the policymaking body of large organizations, such as the American Nurses Association (ANA) House of Delegates, one must know parliamentary procedure as a political strategy to get an issue passed or rejected. Countless issues have failed or passed because of insufficient knowledge of rule making.

It is also vital to know the informal processes and methods of communication. A well-known example of the power of informal processes and communication is the case of the business lunch or the golf game that in the past excluded women.

STAKEHOLDERS

Stakeholders are those parties who have influence over the issue, who are directly influenced by it, or who could be mobilized to care. In some cases, stakeholders are obvious. For example, nurses are

stakeholders in issues such as staffing ratios. In other situations, one can develop potential stakeholders by helping them to see the connections between the issue and their interests. Many individuals and organizations can be considered stakeholders when it comes to staffing ratios. Among them are employers (i.e., hospitals, nursing homes) payers (i.e., insurance companies), legislators, other professionals, and, of course, consumers. The role of consumers cannot be underestimated. In the political arena, these are the constituents and therefore the voters.

In many cases, nurses are working on behalf of stakeholders, the patients, who are affected by the care they receive. Nursing has increasingly realized the potential of consumer power in moving nursing and health care issues. For example, nurses have worked with the National Alliance for Mental Illness on mental health parity and with the American Cancer Society on tobacco and breast cancer issues. A consumer advocacy organization such as AARP represents significant lobbying power. When nursing wanted to advance the idea of a Medicare Graduate Nursing Education benefit, similar to the Medicare Graduate Medical Education funding to hospitals for the clinical training of interns and residents, AARP championed the proposal and it was included in the ACA as a pilot project. AARP advocated this benefit because it views the nursing shortage as a threat to its members' ability to access health care.

What kind of relationships do you or others have with key stakeholders? Look at your connections with possible stakeholders through your schools, places of worship, or business. Which of these stakeholders are potential supporters or opponents? Can any of the opponents be converted to supporters? What are the values, priorities, and concerns of the stakeholders? How can these be tapped in planning political strategy? Do the supportive stakeholders reflect the constituency that will be affected by the issue? For example, as states expand coverage of health services through each state's Medicaid, it is vital to have parents of enrolled children let their policymakers know how important the issue is for them. These parents can share their personal stories of how the program has made a difference for their children. Yet stakeholders who are recipients of the services are too often not identified as vital for moving an issue. Nurses as direct caregivers have an important role in ensuring that recipients of services are included as stakeholders—especially when bringing issues to elected officials.

VALUES ASSESSMENT

Every political issue, especially those issues that entail "morality policies," could prompt discussions about values. Morality policies are those that primarily revolve around ideology and values, rather than costs and distribution of resources. Among well-publicized morality issues are abortion, stem cell research, immigration, and the death penalty. But even issues that are not classified as morality policies require that stakeholders assess their values and those of their opponents.

Values underlie the responsibility of public policymakers to be involved in the regulation of health care. In particular, calls for extending the reach of government in the regulation of health care facilities implies that one accepts this as a proper role for public officials, rather than as a role of market forces and the private sector. Thus, electoral politics affect the policies that may be implemented. An analysis that acknowledges how congruent nurses' values are with those of individuals in power can affect the success of advancing an issue.

Although nurses may value a range of health and social programs, legislators will hear their calls for increased funding for nursing research and education within the context of demands from other constituencies. Here timing is critical. When a request is made, it is critical to link it to the "problem" it may solve. It is also important to make sure issues are framed to show how they will help the public at large and not just the nursing profession. Any call for government support of health care programs implies a certain prioritization of values: Is health more important than education, or jobs, or the war in Afghanistan? Elected officials must always make choices among competing demands. And their choices reflect their values, the needs and interests of their constituents, and their financial supporters such as large corporations. Similarly, nurses' choice of issues on the political agenda reflects the profession's values, political priorities, and ways to improve health care.

RESOURCES

An effective political strategy must take into account the resources that will be needed to move an issue successfully. Resources include money, time, connec-

tions, and intangible resources, such as creative ideas. Analyzing resources requires both short-term and long-term needs.

The most obvious resource is money, which must be considered in relation to both the proposed policy solution and the campaign to champion it. The proposed solution needs to include an analysis of the resources needed for the solution to be successful. Thus, before launching a campaign for a particular bill or program, campaign leaders must know how much the proposed solution will cost, who will be bearing those costs, and the source of the money. It is also critical to fully examine—despite the initial financial outlay—the potential for cost savings it may produce. In addition, it is helpful to know how budgets are formulated for a given government agency or institution. What is the budget process? How much money is allocated to a particular cost center or budget line? Who decides how the funds will be used? How is the use of funds evaluated? How might an individual or group influence the budget process?

Money is not the only resource. Sharing available resources, such as space, people, expertise, and in-kind services, may be best accomplished through a coalition (see Chapter 86). It may require a mechanism for each entity to contribute a specific amount or to tally their in-kind contributions such as office space for meetings; use of a photocopier, telephone, or other equipment; or use of staff to assist with production of brochures and other communications. Other cost considerations include accessing the media or other publicity efforts; printing brochures and other educational materials; paying for postage; and establishing access to electronic communications.

Nurses can also provide in-kind contributions. When nurses and other volunteers are recruited for a political issue, project, or campaign, a common response is lack of time for involvement. Nurses need to figure how to get volunteers while simultaneously protecting one of their most precious commodities, time. One must find creative ways to use available resources. For instance, an option for limited volunteer time might be contracting for specific services; such as writing testimony or other communications, or producing white papers or other scholarly activities to help elucidate complicated policy details around an issue.

Creativity is a precious resource that enables nurses and others to develop strategies that will be inspiring and captivating to one's audience. How much creativity is evident among the stakeholders? How can one stimulate and channel creativity? Allocating enough time for brainstorming and strategic planning, especially among a diversified coalition, will pay off in the end if well-designed and creative approaches result.

POWER

In the workplace, government, professional organizations, and community, effective political strategy requires an analysis of the power of proponents and opponents of a particular solution. Power is one of the most complex political and sociologic concepts to define and measure. It is also a term that politicians and policy analysts use freely, without necessarily giving thought to what it means.

Power can be a means to an end, or an end in itself. Power also can be actual or potential. The latter implies power as undeveloped but a "force to be reckoned with" (Joel & Kelly, 2002). Many in political circles depict the nursing profession as a potential political force, given the millions of nurses in this country and the power we could wield if most nurses participated in politics and policy formation—and if nurses could identify issues on which they could speak with a single voice.

Any discussion of power and nursing must acknowledge the inherent issues of hierarchy and power imbalance that arise from the long-standing relationships between nurses and physicians. Some of nurses' discomfort with the concept of power may arise from the inherent nature of "gender politics" within the profession. Male or female, gender affects every political scenario that involves nurses. Working in a predominantly female profession means that nurses are accustomed to certain norms of social interactions (Tanner, 2001). In contrast to nursing, the power and politics of public policy-making typically are male dominated, although women are steadily increasing their ranks as elected and appointed government officials. Moreover, many male and female public officials have stereotypic images of nurses as women who lack political savvy. This may limit officials' ability to view nurses as potential political partners. Therefore nurses need to be sensitive to gender issues that may

affect, but certainly not prevent, their political success.

Many nurses find political work unsavory because of the inevitability of conflict this power struggle sometimes causes. Conflicts between political parties, between those with different ideologic values, and between nurses and other stakeholders are inherent to the political process. Conflict is unavoidable, and it is also necessary for identifying the different viewpoints that will structure subsequent negotiations. Conflict presents opportunity. Especially when there is disagreement, it is important to find a way to move forward. In this case, nurses as natural problem solvers, can excel. Unlike other situations in which conflict may be unwelcome, in politics it is necessary for establishing the parameters of discourse and the terms of compromise. This holds true for any setting, whether in the workplace, the community, organizations, or governmental arenas (see Chapter 12 for a discussion of conflict management).

Although individuals develop political skill and expertise, it is the influence of large organizations, coalitions, or like-minded groups that wield power most effectively. Too often nurses become concerned about a particular issue and try to change it without help from others. Although the individual may hold expert power, it will be limited if one attempts to "go it alone." In the public arena particularly, an individual is rarely able to exert adequate influence to create long-term policy change. For instance, many APNs have tried to change state Nurse Practice Acts to expand their authority. As well intentioned and knowledgeable as the policy solutions may be, they will likely fail unless nurses can garner the support of other powerful stakeholders such as members of the state board of nursing, the state nurses association, and physicians, either through the medical association or the state Board of Medicine. Such stakeholders often hold the power to either support or oppose the policy change.

Any power analysis must include reflection on one's own power base. Power can be obtained through a variety of sources (Ferguson, 1993; French & Raven, 1959; Joel & Kelly, 2002; Mason, Backer, & Georges, 1991):

1. *Coercive power* is rooted in real or perceived fear of one person by another. For example, the supervisor who threatens to fire those nurses who speak out is relying on coercive power, as is a state commissioner of health who threatens to develop

regulations requiring physician supervision of nurse practitioners.

2. *Reward power* is based on the perception of the potential for rewards or favors as a result of honoring the wishes of a powerful person. A clear example is the supervisor who has the power to determine promotions and pay increases.

3. *Legitimate (or positional) power* is derived from an organizational position rather than personal qualities, whether from a person's role as the chief nurse officer or the state's governor.

4. *Expert power* is based on knowledge, special talents, or skills, in contrast to positional power. Benner (1984) argues that nurses can tap this power source as they move from novice to expert practitioner. It is a power source that nurses must recognize is available to them and tap. Policymakers are seldom experts in health care; nurses are.

5. *Referent power* emanates from associating with a powerful person or organization. This power source is used when a nurse selects a mentor who is a powerful person, such as the chief nurse officer of the organization or the head of the state's dominant political party. It can also emerge when a nursing organization enlists a highly regarded public personality as an advocate for an issue it is championing.

6. *Information power* results when one individual has (or is perceived to have) special information that another individual desires. This power source underscores the need for nurses to stay abreast of information on a variety of levels: in one's personal and professional networks, immediate work situation, employing institution, community, and the public sector, as well as in society and the world. Use of information power requires strategic consideration of how and with whom to share the information.

7. *Connection power* is granted to those perceived to have important and sometimes extensive connections with individuals or organizations. For example, the nurse who attends the same church or synagogue as the president of the home health care agency, knows the appointments secretary for the mayor, or is a member of the hospital credentialing committee will be accorded power by those who want access to these individuals or groups.

8. *Empowerment* arises from shared power. This power source requires those who have power to recognize that they can build the power of colleagues or others by sharing authority and decision-making. Empowerment can happen when the nurse manager on a unit uses consensus building when possible instead of issuing authoritative directives to staff or when a coalition is formed and adopts consensus building and shared decision-making to guide its process.

An analysis of the extent of one's power using these sources can also provide direction on how to enhance that power. This analysis can be done both for short-term and long-term purposes. For example, consider the nursing organization that finds itself unable to secure legislative support for a key piece of legislation. It can develop a short-term plan for enhancing its power by finding a highly regarded, high-profile individual to be its spokesperson with the media (referent power), by making it known to legislators that their vote on this issue will be a major consideration in the next election's endorsement decisions (reward or coercive power), or by getting nurses to tell the media their stories that highlight the problem the legislation addresses (expert power). Its long-term plan might include extending its connections with other organizations by signing onto coalitions that address broader health care issues and expanding connections with policymakers by attending fundraisers for key legislators (connection power); getting nurses into policy-making positions (legitimate power); hiring a government affairs director to help inform the group about the nuances of the legislature (information power); and using consensus building within the organization to enhance nurses' participation and activities (empowerment).

CREATING A PLAN OF ACTION

Once a political analysis is completed, it is necessary to develop a plan that identifies strategies for action. Political strategies are the methods and guidelines used in the formulation of a plan to achieve desired goals, including policy goals. They are the means to the goal. Well-planned and practiced strategies can make the difference between success and failure.

INCREMENTAL VERSUS REVOLUTIONARY CHANGE

Policy implementation almost always happens through incremental change. Incremental changes or actions may have a better chance of success than a change of major proportions. Resistance to change can often be overcome if a pilot or demonstration project is created to test an idea on a small scale.

Many times we are confronted with situations in which we may not get all we want. One must be clear about what are acceptable solutions or alternatives and what are not. Identification of alternatives represents a good way to test one's convictions and to consider what the long-term and short-term goals are. For example, the ACA fell short of covering all uninsured and of reforming health care delivery. But it was viewed as creating a foundation for universal coverage and improving the nation's health care system that could be strengthened through future amendments.

The "Pilot" Approach. Change is difficult for people, particularly major policy change. Proposing even modest changes in an organization or to a public policy can be met with skepticism and outright opposition by key decision-makers and those who will be affected by the change. Even when the change is dictated at the highest administrative level, it can be sabotaged or dismissed at the local or unit level. Demonstration or pilot projects can make the change more palatable by suggesting that it be tested before being implemented on a full scale, whether in one hospital or in society, particularly when the idea is seen as radical or risky (Roberts, 1998).

Demonstration projects are planned implementation and evaluation of models or ideas to determine their merits, problems, and costs before adopting them for a larger population. They test the effects of new ideas, develop solutions to barriers that arise, explore costs, and provide justification for future policies. They are time-limited. Pilot projects are initiatives that can be scaled up if successful. This strategy has been applied to making changes in the workplace, as demonstrated with Transforming Care At the Bedside (TCAB), an initiative sponsored by the Institute for Healthcare Improvement and the Robert Wood Johnson Foundation (see Chapter 54). TCAB targets change on medical-surgical nursing units in participating hospitals to identify ways to improve care, increase patient and family satisfaction, empower multidisciplinary teams, and position staff nurses as the key change agents on these units.

Pilot and demonstration projects can also advance major public policy initiatives. The ACA includes a variety of both. The pilot projects can be scaled up, if shown to be effective, without Congressional action. For example, the Act includes a provision for pilot projects for transitional care that can be institutionalized under Medicare if the Secretary of Health and Human Services deems them to be cost-effective. Getting a full-fledged Medicare transitional care benefit into the Act was not possible, despite data demonstrating the cost-effectiveness of this service.

When the innovation requires cooperation from other departments or key decision-makers, the pilot or demonstration project can provide them with first-hand experience with the change and turn them into supporters. Consulting key stakeholders early on during a pilot project can be instrumental in reducing the risk of opposition because of "wounded egos." In public policy, this translates into building the political support for the demonstration project from legislators (if legislation is needed to authorize it), executive branch support (for signing such legislation), and public employees (who will be responsible for government oversight of the project).

It is important to plan well for the evaluation of the demonstration project. What are the expected outcomes of the project? What data are needed to demonstrate the efficacy and cost impact of the idea? Who will design and who will conduct the evaluation of the demonstration project? What biases does the evaluator bring to the evaluation? What are the potential problems expected during the demonstration project? Is there sufficient time for achieving the stated aims in utilization rates, clinical outcomes, or costs? Is there enough funding for undertaking a well-designed evaluation of the project?

STRATEGIES FOR SUCCESS

LOOK AT THE BIG PICTURE

It is human nature to view the world from a personal standpoint, focusing on the people and events that influence one's daily life. However, this strategy requires that one step back and take stock of the larger environment. It can provide a more objective perspective and increase nurses' credibility as broad-minded visionaries, looking beyond personal needs. It also means that one should not get bogged down in details that may seem important at the time but that in the larger schema may not be critical to the success of the issue. For example, legislation to address "patients' rights" under managed care plans was sidetracked by issues around medical liability and the high cost of malpractice insurance for physicians. The intent of the legislation was to give patients more choices for care under managed care plans. The original intent of the legislation became lost because certain stakeholders were more concerned with liability than with patients' rights.

In the heat of legislative battles and negotiations, it is easy to get distracted. However, the successful advocate is the one who does not lose sight of the big picture and is willing to compromise for the larger goal. It is critical for nurses to look beyond successes for the profession and focus on how nursing innovations improve the health of patients and the broader health delivery system.

DO YOUR HOMEWORK

We can never have all the information about an issue, but we need to be sufficiently prepared before we advocate. Usually one does not know beforehand when a particular policy will be acted on. It is not sufficient to claim ignorance when confronted with questions that should be answered. However, if one has done everything possible to prepare and is asked to supply information that is not anticipated, it is reasonable and preferable to indicate that one does not know the answer. It does mean that one must get the information as soon as possible and distribute it to the policymaker who requested it. Remember not to let perfection be the enemy of good; gather the requested information, and present it as clearly and simply as possible.

There are numerous ways to be adequately prepared:

- Clarify your position on the problem and possible solutions.
- Gather data, and search the clinical and policy literature.
- Prepare documents to describe and support the issue.
- Assess the power dynamics of the players.
- Assess your own power base and ability to maneuver in the political arena.
- Plan a strategy, and assess its strengths and weaknesses.
- Prepare for the conflict.

- Line up support.
- Know the opposition and their rationale.

IT'S NOT WHAT YOU SAY, IT'S HOW YOU SAY IT

The content of an issue is important, but it may be secondary to the way the message is framed and conveyed to stakeholders. Know the context of the issue (as described earlier). Learn to use strong, affirmative language to describe nursing practice. Use the rhetoric that incorporates lawmakers' lingo and the "buzz words" of key proponents. This requires having a sense of the values of the target audiences, be they policymakers, the public, hospital administrators, or community leaders.

Appealing to a variety of stakeholders often requires developing rhetoric or a message to frame your issue that is succinct and appealing to the values and concerns of those you want to mobilize or defeat. For example, "Cut Medicare" was an ineffective political message that the Republicans used in 1997 to try to gain public support for decreasing spending on Medicare. When the message was changed to "Preserve and Protect Medicare," the public was more supportive, even though the policy goals were the same. During health reform discussions, APNs framed their issue in terms of quality of care and cost savings. Since the nation continues to be concerned about the amount of money spent on health care, the message of reducing costs without compromising quality resonated with the Administration, Members of Congress, insurers, employers, and the public alike. How you convey your message involves developing rhetoric or catchy phrases that the media might pick up and perpetuate. Nurses need to develop their effectiveness in accessing and using the media, an essential component of getting the issue on the public's agenda.

READ BETWEEN THE LINES

Often issues are not what they seem. It is just as important to be aware of the way one conveys information as it is to provide the facts. Communication theory notes that the overt message is not always the real message (Gerston, 1997). Some people say a lot by what they choose not to disclose. When legislators say they think your issue is important, it does not necessarily mean that they will vote to support it. The real question that needs to be asked is, "Will you vote in support of our bill?" What are the hidden agendas of the stakeholders concerned with the issue? What is not being said? When framing an issue, be aware of the covert messages. Be careful to make the issue as clear as possible and test it on others to be certain that reading between the lines conveys the same message as the overt rhetoric.

IT'S NOT JUST WHAT YOU KNOW, IT'S WHO YOU KNOW

Using the power that results from personal connections is often the most important strategy in moving a critical issue. Sometimes it comes down to one important personal connection. In the example of APRN reimbursement, the original legislation that gave some APNs Medicare reimbursement was greatly facilitated because the chief of staff for the Senate Majority Leader was a nurse. Or consider the nurse who is the neighbor and friend of the secretary to the chief executive officer (CEO) in the medical center. This nurse is more likely to gain access to the CEO than will someone who is unknown to either the secretary or the CEO. Networking is an important long-term strategy for building influence; however, it can be a deliberate short-term strategy as well.

QUID PRO QUO

Developing networks involves keeping track of what one has done for you and not being afraid to ask a favor in return. Often known as *quid pro quo* (literally, "something for something"), it is the way political arenas work in both public and private sectors. Networking is an important skill for achieving personal and political goals. Leaders expect to be asked for help and know the favor will be returned. It makes the one doing the favor feel good to be asked. Because nurses interface with the public all the time, they are in excellent positions to assist, facilitate, or otherwise do favors for people. Too often, nurses forget to ask for help from those whom they have helped and who would be more than willing to return a favor. Consider the lobbyist for a state nurses association who knew that the chair of the Senate public health and welfare committee had a grandson who was critically injured in a car accident. She visited the child several times in the hospital, spoke with the nurses on the unit, and kept the legislator informed about his grandson's progress and assured him that the boy was well cared for. When the boy recovered, the legislator was grateful and asked the lobbyist what he could do

to move her issue. Interchanges like this occur every day and create the basis for quid pro quo.

STRIKE WHILE THE IRON IS HOT

The timing of an issue is often the strategy that makes the difference in a successful outcome. A well-planned strategy may fail because the timing is off. An issue may languish for some period because of a mismatch in values, concerns, or resources. Yet suddenly, something can change to make an issue ripe for consideration. Before September 11, 2001, the issue of bioterrorism was of limited concern to the public and a low priority for most health care professionals. Yet warnings and preparations had actually begun. In response to the first bombing of the World Trade Center in 1993, President Clinton had convened a group of experts to develop a national strategy for responding to a bioterrorist attack. However, the effort received limited resources. After the attacks of September 11 on the World Trade Center and the Pentagon, the issue moved to the top of the congressional and presidential agenda. President Bush asked for and got billions of dollars to prevent and respond to bioterrorism.

The recent passage of the ACA is another good example. Candidate Obama knew from history that the best chance of passing sweeping legislation was in the early years of a president's term. Once elected, with both the U.S. House of Representatives and the U.S. Senate under the control of the Democratic Party, President Obama knew that the only hope of passing comprehensive health care reform would be if it became his priority within his first year (see Box 8-2).

UNITED WE STAND, DIVIDED WE FALL

The successful achievement of policy goals can be accomplished only if supporters demonstrate a united front. Collective action is almost always more effective than individual action. Collaboration through coalitions demonstrates broad support for the issue. Besides having your own group organized and ready to be mobilized, what other networks do you have or can you develop?

Sometimes diverse groups can work together on an issue of mutual support, even though they are opponents on other issues. Public and private interest groups that identify with nursing's issues can be invaluable resources for nurses. They often have influential supporters or may have research information that can help nurses move an issue. Rallies, letter-writing campaigns, and grassroots efforts by such groups can turn up the volume on nursing's issues and create the necessary groundswell of support to overcome opposition.

This is especially true within nursing itself. It is in nursing's best political interest to end the divisiveness among nurses and professional nursing organizations and to foster ways for nurses to become flexible and politically responsive. When one specialty organization can support another—even if not their issue—they should expect the same when the other encounters an issue to be addressed. For example, when the issue of increasing faculty salaries in public institutions came up in the Mississippi legislature, other nursing groups, including specialty organizations, lobbied legislators in support of nursing faculty. The expectation was that faculty would help the other groups as issues arose.

Of course nurses cannot be expected to agree on everything. A 2010 Gallup poll of health care leaders found that the lack of a united front by national nursing organizations was viewed as a major reason why nursing's influence on health care reform would not be significant. To maximize nursing's political potential, we must look for opportunities to reach consensus or remain silent in the public arena on an issue that is not of paramount concern.

NOTHING VENTURED, NOTHING GAINED

Nurses have always been risk takers. Margaret Sanger fled to England after she was sentenced to jail for providing women with information about birth control (Chesler, 1992). Harriet Tubman risked her life to transport and care for more than 300 slaves who sought freedom in the North before and during the Civil War (Carnegie, 1986). Such thoughtful risk takers weigh the costs and benefits of their actions. They consider possible outcomes in relation to the expenditure of available resources. For example, a nurse may decide to run for Congress, knowing that she has little chance of winning. She risks losing, but running will give her the opportunity to bring important health issues to the public's attention and will help her gain name recognition for her next race.

Risk taking requires analyzing both the risks and the benefits of an action. This can be much easier for an individual than for an organization, but nonethe-less it warrants open and thoughtful discussion by those taking the risk. The strongest case for risk taking comes when the core values of an individual or organization are at stake.

THE BEST DEFENSE IS A GOOD OFFENSE

A successful political strategy is one that tries to accommodate the concerns of the opposition. It requires disassociating the emotional context of working with opponents—the first step in principled negotiating. The person who is skillful at managing conflict will be successful in politics. The saying that "politics makes strange bedfellows" arose out of the recognition that long-standing opponents can sometimes come together around issues of mutual concern, but it often requires creative thinking and a commitment to fairness to develop an acceptable approach to resolving an issue.

One must also anticipate problems and areas for disagreement and be prepared to counter them: When the opposition is gaining momentum and support, it can be helpful to develop a strategy that can distract attention from the opposition's issue or that can delay action. For example, one state nurses' association continually battled the state medical society's efforts to amend the Nurse Practice Act in ways that would restrict nurses' practice and provide for physician supervision. Nurses became particularly concerned about the possibility of passage during a year when the medical society's influence with the legislature was high. Working with other health provider organizations engaged in similar battles (e.g., optometrists, pharmacists), the nurses proposed a bill that would go after the medical practice act by removing all oversight authority. The physicians knew that there would be a large coalition supporting such a bill. As a result they agreed to drop efforts to amend the Nurse Practice Act.

The other dimension of this axiom is creating opportunities for your opposition and power holders to gain firsthand experience with your issue. The many "walk a mile with a nurse" campaigns, when legislators or others spend time trailing a nurse, have provided hospital executives and public officials with the opportunity to understand the complexities of a nurse's daily work and the barriers that nurses confront. Once they have seen issues through the nurse's lens, they may be more willing to find satisfactory policy solutions. Media coverage of your issue can also help to accomplish this end, particularly when personal stories are used to illustrate the conflicts or concerns raised by an issue.

SUMMARY

The future of nursing and health care may well depend on nurses' skills in moving a vision. Without a vision, politics becomes an end in itself—a game that is often corrupt and empty. Instead, nurses can use the vision to define the goals.

For a list of related websites, please refer to your Evolve Resources at http://evolve.elsevier.com/Mason/policypolitics/

REFERENCES

Benner, P. (1984). *From novice to expert.* Menlo Park, CA: Addison-Wesley.

Carnegie, M. E. (1986). *The path we tread: Blacks in nursing, 1854-1984.* Philadelphia: Lippincott.

Chesler, E. (1992). *Woman of valor: Margaret Sanger and the birth control movement in America.* New York: Anchor Books.

Ferguson, V. D. (1993). Perspectives on power. In D. J. Mason, S. W. Talbott, & J. K. Leavitt (Eds.), *Policy and politics for nurses: Action and change in the workplace, government, organizations, and community* (2nd ed.). Philadelphia: Saunders.

Fox-Piven, F., & Cloward, R. (1993). *Regulating the poor: The functions of public welfare.* New York: Vintage Press.

French, J. R. P., & Raven, B. (1959). The basis of social power. In D. Cartwright (Ed.), *Studies in social power.* Ann Arbor, MI: University of Michigan Press.

Gallup. (2010). Nursing leadership from bedside to boardroom: Opinion leaders' perception. Retrieved from http://newcareersinnursing.org/sites/default/files/file-attachments/Top%20Line%20Report.pdf.

Gerston, L. N. (1997). *Public policy making: Process and principles.* Armonk, NY: M.E. Sharper.

Joel, L., & Kelly, L. (2002). *The nursing experience: Trends, challenges, and transitions* (4th ed.). New York: McGraw-Hill.

Mason, D. J., Backer, B. A., & Georges, C. A. (1991). Towards a feminist model for the political empowerment of nurses. *Image: Journal of Nursing Scholarship, 23*(2), 72-77.

Roberts, N. (1998). Radical change by entrepreneurial design. *Acquisitions Review Quarterly.* Retrieved from www.au.af.mil/au/awc/awcgate/dau/roberts.pdf.

Tanner, D. (2001). *Talking from 9 to 5: Women and men in the workplace—Language, sex, power.* New York: Quill.

CHAPTER 9

Health Policy, Politics, and Professional Ethics

Leah L. Curtin

"To see what is right and not do it is want of courage."
—Confucius

To frame a discussion of policy, politics and ethics, I will present some actual situations: a "no-admit" list, dying with dignity, and the passage of the Patient Protection and Affordable Care Act of 2010.

CASE STUDY I: A "NO-ADMIT" LIST

A graduate student asked about the use of a no-admit list and described the following situation. A 29-year-old male patient with diagnoses of bipolar disorder, substance use disorder, and antisocial personality disorder comes to the emergency department (ED) one midnight shift under the law enforcement Baker Act. This law permits a 72-hour involuntary placement for psychiatric assessment. The law says the patient is to be admitted to the nearest Baker Act receiving facility. The ED staff provided me with the following unsolicited information: "Get rid of this guy fast; he's trouble"; the patient is an "abuser of the system," they say, and he has assaulted several health care workers. He is a drain on overextended resources because his behavior requires constant intervention to maintain safety.

I find in our assessment office that the patient is on a "do not admit" list. The unit nursing staff on duty that night provides me with the information that this patient assaulted a nurse on one of the adult psychiatric units and was jailed and charged for this offense. The nurse sustained permanent damage to her knee and currently has a restraining order against this patient. At this time, the patient is calm and cooperative during my assessment—other than making continuous, aggressive requests to smoke and

several attempts to leave the ED without an escort to do so. The psychiatrist on call was new to this facility, as was I at the time, so we were unaware of the patient's history and past treatment record. In addition, the psychiatrist and I had a previous positive professional relationship at another facility, and I knew that he respected my recommendations. Before calling him, I make inquiries at area psychiatric units and find out that earlier in the day this patient left treatment at a facility 70 miles away and is not welcome back because of his aggressive behavior. The local community mental health facility also is not amenable to a referral because this patient assaulted personnel there in the past. My colleague at the community center says that this patient has "burned all his bridges in a hundred mile radius."

I now have a great deal of information from various sources about this patient. To pose this question realistically and succinctly, do I say, "Doc, this guy is bad news and the unit will have your head and mine if we admit him" or "Doc, this patient is suicidal with a plan and we have the closest bed"? What about the law*? How legal is a "do not admit" list, and what are my ethical obligations particularly when administration is aware of this patient's situation and has

---

*Section 1867 of the Social Security Act imposes specific obligations on Medicare-participating hospitals that offer emergency services to provide a medical screening examination (MSE) when a request is made for examination or treatment for an emergency medical condition (EMC), including active labor, regardless of an individual's ability to pay. Hospitals are then required to provide stabilizing treatment for patients with EMCs. If a hospital is unable to stabilize a patient within its capability, or if the patient requests, an appropriate transfer should be implemented.

opted not to address options that might break the cycle of continued abuse of acute services and the abuse of resources this facilitates?

CASE STUDY II: DEATH WITH DIGNITY

The Oregon Health Department published an accounting of Oregon's experience with the first Death with Dignity Act in the nation, excerpts from which follow:

Physician-assisted suicide (PAS) has been legal in Oregon since November 1997, when Oregon voters approved the Death with Dignity Act (DWDA) for the second time ... In response to a lawsuit filed by the State of Oregon on November 20, 2001, a U.S. district court issued a temporary restraining order against Attorney General Ashcroft's ruling pending a new hearing. On April 17, 2002, U.S. District Court Judge Robert Jones upheld the Death with Dignity Act. On September 23, 2002, Attorney General Ashcroft filed an appeal, asking the Ninth U.S. Circuit Court of Appeals to overturn the District Court's ruling, which was subsequently denied on May 26, 2004 by a three-judge panel. On July 13, 2004, Ashcroft filed an appeal requesting that the Court rehear his previous motion with an 11-judge panel; on August 13, 2004, the request was denied. On November 9, 2004, Ashcroft asked the U.S. Supreme Court to review the Ninth Circuit Court's decision and on February 22, 2005, the court agreed to hear the appeal. Arguments were held during the Supreme Court's term beginning in October of 2005, and in a stunning blow to the Bush Administration, the Supreme Court upheld the Oregon law in January of 2006; thus Oregon's law remains in effect.

As a result of this ground-breaking legislation as well as the court decisions, three states have abolished the common law of crimes and do not have statutes criminalizing assisted suicide (North Carolina, Utah, and Wyoming). However, 9 states criminalize assisted suicide through common law, and 34 states have statutes explicitly criminalizing assisted suicide. Only the states of Oregon and Washington permit physician-assisted suicide under carefully controlled situations (*www.euthanasia.com/bystate.html*).

CASE STUDY III: HEALTH REFORM LEGISLATION

Any discussion of health reform must include a review of human rights and a discussion of whether or not there is such a thing as a human right to health care services, and whether or not a just society would provide a legal right to such services. A human right is a just claim to an essential, universal human need. The justice of the claim is affected by (1) the universality of the need, (2) the extent to which a person can meet his or her own needs, and (3) the extent to which others can help meet these needs without compromising their own fundamental needs.[1] Some argue that health care services—or at least illness care services—is not a human right; however a far larger number think that such needs can easily meet each of these criteria, at least under a variety of circumstances.[2]

For almost a century, presidents and members of Congress have tried and failed to provide universal health benefits to Americans. There are a few simple facts that are important: (1) the U.S. is the only industrialized country in the world that does not offer some type of universal health care; (2) each year tens of thousands of Americans lose their health care coverage due to circumstances beyond their control; and (3) the main reason that Americans file bankruptcy is outstanding medical bills.

In 2010, Congress passed, and the president signed into law, the Patient Protection and Affordable Care Act of 2010. The core of the massive law is the extension of health care coverage to 32 million Americans who now lack it, a goal to be achieved through a complex mixture of new mandates for individuals and employers, subsidies for people who can't afford to buy coverage, consumer-friendly rules required of insurers, tax breaks, and "exchanges" to shop for health plans.

---

[1]Nickel, J. (2009). Human rights. In Zalta, E. N. The Stanford encyclopedia of philosophy. Retrieved from http://plato.stanford.edu/archives/spr2009/entries/rights-human/. First published February 7, 2003; substantive revision July 29, 2006.
[2]Universaruary Declaration of Human Rights, Article 25 in 1948. The article says that "Everyone has the right to a standard of living adequate for the health and wellbeing of himself and his family...." The Preamble to the WHO constitution also declares that it is one of the fundamental rights of every human being to enjoy "the highest attainable standard of health." Inherent in the right to health is the right to the underlying conditions of health as well as medical care.

The law's most far-reaching changes will not start until 2014, including a requirement that most Americans have health insurance—whether through an employer, a government program, or their own purchase—or pay a fine. To make that a reality, tax credits to help pay for the premiums will be provided to middle-class families, and Medicaid will be expanded to cover more people with low incomes. This law will prohibit insurance companies from putting lifetime dollar limits on policies, denying coverage for pre-existing conditions, and cancelling a policy when someone gets sick. Insurers also will have to allow parents to keep children on their plans up to age 26. For seniors, the plan will gradually close the prescription coverage gap and improve preventive care. But it also will cut funding for popular private insurance plans offered through Medicare Advantage.

The changes are to be paid for with cuts in projected government payment increases to hospitals, insurance companies, and others under Medicare and other health programs; an increase in the Medicare payroll tax for some; fees on insurance companies, drug makers, and medical device manufacturers; a new excise tax on high-value insurance plans; and a tax on indoor tanning services.

So much for substance. Now, on to process. There has been much controversy about the various proposals to reform the health care system, perhaps more about the process than the content of the legislation. A Center for Public Integrity analysis of Senate lobbying disclosure forms shows that more than 1750 companies and organizations hired about 4525 lobbyists—eight for each member of Congress—to influence health reform bills in 2009.[3] Whether the reasons can be attributed to lobbying or to partisan politics, the tactics used on both sides (Republicans used lies, scare tactics, and obstructionism to block health reform,[4] and Democrats were accused of abuse of power for using several parliamentary maneuvers[5]) raise questions about the ethics of the processes used.

[3]Retrieved from http://www.publicintegrity.org/articles/entry/1953/.
[4]Pearlstein, S. Republicans propagating falsehoods in attacks on health-care reform. Retrieved from www.washingtonpost.com/wp-dyn/content/article/2009/08/06/AR2009080603854.html.
[5]Gallup: Majority says Dem health reform tactics were "abuse of power." Retrieved from http://theplumline.whorunsgov.com/senate-republicans/gallup-majority-says-dem-health-reform-tactics-were-abuse-of-power.

THE ENDS AND THE MEANS

Why bring these particular situations to your attention? Principally this: Each involves a variation of the same question—that is, what means can be legitimately used to achieve an end that someone (or a political party, or even the electorate) believes to be good? We have laws that require screening, stabilizing, and treating all people who come to an ED (a good) even though it may enable abuse of the system (an evil), as in Case Study I. In Case Study III, proponents of health insurance reform are accused of "abuse of power" to provide access to care for millions of people (a good) even though it may create partisan divisions (an evil). In Case Study II, the situation is far more ambiguous and controversial because it is a generally accepted principle of both law and ethics that killing a person is wrong—and therefore encouraging suicide is wrong. Others believe that enabling medically assisted suicide is a good because it promotes personal autonomy and therefore respects the dignity of individuals facing inevitable and painful deaths. The difference is this: In Cases I and III, the law provides for a good (equity of access in both), which may occasionally produce an evil (abuse of the system); in Case II, the law enables what is generally considered an evil (killing, or suicide) in order to produce a good (autonomy and relief of suffering). This inevitably leads to a discussion of whether or not the ends can ever justify the means.

The ends-and-means argument often is explained as follows. We can cut a man open (an evil means) to save his life (a good end). We can remove a perfectly healthy kidney from one person (an evil means) to transplant it to save the life and health of another (a good end). And we admire the person who sacrifices his life (an evil means) to save the life of his friend (a good end). If our intention (to produce a good) can justify the means (doing an evil), then why can't we torture one man (an evil means) to gain information that might save another person's life or even the lives of many people (a good end)? Should we assure the passage of health care insurance reform (a good end) by strong-arm tactics (an evil means)?

A FEW THINGS THAT MUST BE SAID

Before we get into more ticklish problems, it is important to note that cutting a person open, even to save his life, is not a good thing unless the person consents to it. Similarly one cannot "steal" one person's kidney even to save another; rather, the consent of both donor and recipient is required. The prisoner does not choose to be tortured, although it is very tempting to justify "beating the facts out" to protect innocent lives. But hard as it is to say, if a man can be tortured on the suspicion that he may know something subversive, who is safe from governmental oppression? For we, just as they, are members of society. The price we pay for freedom and human rights is to grant them to all people, not just a favored few. And yes, it is risky, and yes, it may reduce our "efficiency" and in some cases even lead to loss of life. But the alternative is that no one has rights (i.e., just claims); rights become the privilege of a favored group, while all other individuals are utterly helpless before the power of the state.

Certainly the electorate does not consent to the corruption of the legislative process—and even if a majority did approve of bending the rules of fair engagement to ensure that a particular piece of legislation is passed, would that make it right? Would it not end up threatening the very foundations of a free society (because the foundation of a republic lies in the honesty of its processes)? What are the differences between normal legislative "wrangling" and abuse of power? What does it mean when political parties refuse to participate in the legislative process and/or use blatant scare tactics? What is legitimate dissent, and what is a refusal to accept democratic outcomes unless you happen to agree with them? Without civil disobedience, we would still have the "Jim Crow" laws. And without respect for the law, a society degenerates into either despotism or anarchy.

As for the children used in medical research, the consequence of these and other cases that came to light in the 1970s was the establishment of institutional review boards and stringent guidelines that were put in place to curtail medical research. Why? Because our laws require us to protect the well-being of the vulnerable, even though sacrificing the vulnerable may end up benefiting large numbers of the general population. Put another way, if the human rights of patients, organ donors, and children can be sacrificed to expediency, so can your rights and mine. Therefore, it is in the public's best interest to protect children (and prisoners and other vulnerable people), even at the cost of slower development of medical treatments. Gandhi, one of the twentieth century's most principled political leaders, taught and demonstrated through his life and political actions that there

is no difference between ends and means—that, in fact, what we choose to do (the means) is what actually is manifest in the world, regardless of what we intend to produce (the ends) (Gandhi, 1958). In short, the means are the ends, because the means are what we have chosen to bring into existence. Another author puts it this way:

> One man in the twentieth century led us back into morality as a practical thing and that was Mohandas Gandhi. His greatest contribution to the discussion of politics and morality was his insistence that 'the distinction that the Cartesians and the Marxists had made between ends and means was a false distinction'. Gandhi demonstrated that the means were the end; that how you did things determined the end, that violence as a means to solving a problem was in fact the nature of the solution. He was able to destroy the mightiest empire in history without the use of a single gun. So the proof he gave was that morality was not impractical, and what is practical and worth practicing is only morality. (Kidder, 1994, p. 222)

ETHICS, RIGHT AND WRONG

Ethics has to do with right and wrong in this world, and politics has everything to do with what happens to people in this world. Moreover, both ethics and politics have to do with making life better for oneself and others. Surely both deal with power and powerlessness, with human rights and balancing their claims, with justice and fairness—and, yes, with good and evil. And good and evil are not the same as right and wrong. Right and wrong have to do with adherence to principles; good and evil have to do with the intent of the doer and the impact the deed has on other people. Surely politics involves justice in the distribution of social goods; fairness and equity in relationships among and between people of different races, genders, and creeds; and access to education and assistance when one is in need. And, yes, it has to do with intent and social impact (good and evil). According to a contemporary philosopher, the discipline of ethics proposes to identify, organize, examine, and justify human acts by applying certain principles to determine the right thing to do in specific situations (Wellman, 1975). Although the goodness of an action lies in the intent and integrity of the human being who performs it, the rightness or wrongness of an action is judged by the difference it makes in the world. Therefore the principles applied in ethical analysis generally derive from a consideration of the duties one person owes another by virtue of commitments made and roles assumed, and/or a consideration of the effects that a choice of action could have on one's own life and the lives of others.

PROFESSIONAL ETHICS

A professional ethic is built around three essential components:

1. Its purpose. All professions develop in response to a social need—one that the members of the profession promise to meet. Put in legalistic terms, this need (along with the power and privileges society grants to the profession to help the professionals meet the need) and the profession's promised response to it constitute the profession's contract with society.
2. The conduct expected of the professional. The ethical code developed and promulgated by the profession—its code of ethics—describes the conduct society has a right to expect from professionals as they go about the business of the profession. However, it is not a list of prescribed do's and don'ts but rather an articulation of those values that, in fact, outline the scope of the profession's practice and the relationships that ought to pertain between its members and the lay public, among the practitioners of this profession, between the practitioner and the profession itself, and between the professional and the community within which he or she practices.
3. The skills and outcomes expected in professional practice. Nursing's standards of practice state with some precision the obligations of nurses in specific areas of practice. Clearly, each of these components is dynamic—that is, subject to change and reevaluation as the profession grows, as knowledge increases, and as social mores and expectations develop. This is not to claim that there are no constants (e.g., a general imperative to respect persons), but rather to say that the meaning and application of the imperatives change.

Professional ethics is the study of how personal moral norms apply or conflict with the promises and duties of one's profession. Society demands that professionals be held to a separate moral standard of conduct because the choices professionals make affect other people's lives more than their own. Generally speaking, the kinds of choices that fall within this context encompass: (1) the human rights of the patient and the degree to which he or she is capable of exercising them; (2) choices about the technical options available and their appropriate application to the human being as well as the "value options" open to patients—whether or not and to what extent they want or reject the technical options; (3) choices about research and learning on human beings; (4) choices about resource allocation in situations of scarcity; (5) choices about futile care and patient autonomy; (6) choices about the preeminence of one's own self-interest—ranging from exposure to biologic and other workplace hazards, to recompense for services rendered, to weighing an institution's interests into the equations; and (7) questions of law and regulation—what laws are needed to assure the public's well-being, and to assure some equity in the distribution of resources. It is unbelievably easy to justify—for the sake of financial security, for the sake of research, for the sake of the "greater good," even for the sake of our own intellectual curiosity—sacrificing the comfort, well-being, or even the very lives of other people—even, or most particularly, because they are in our power. Therefore to an increasing extent there is public oversight of health care practice and health care research.

As members of the profession face specific ethical quandaries, they are obliged morally and sometimes even legally to keep in mind the promises their professions both infer and imply. Once the profession as a whole adopts a code of ethics, the professional views the occupation and all of its requirements as an enduring set of normative and behavioral expectations. Thus, the ethics of a profession not only delimit the role and scope of its activities and prescribe the nature of the relationship that should exist between its members and the public but also establish duties that professionals owe to one another and to the profession itself. Codes of professional ethics also usually include a pledge to exert one's best efforts to maintain the honor of the profession and to uphold its public standing. The reason for this is that a profession's members cannot practice effectively without the public's trust—and although this is true for all professions, it is especially so for the politician, whose reputation is undercut as intense media scrutiny lays every infraction of every politician before the entire public. Thus it is that the *U.S. House Ethics Manual* prescribes as a member's first duty: "to conduct himself at all times in a manner which shall reflect creditably on the House of Representatives" *(www.house.gov/ethics)*.

Unfortunately, professions develop unevenly because the professionals who comprise them are in diverse states of awareness, intellectual attainment, and commitment. Member's perceptions of their roles and their character traits affect the problems they see, the personal presence they bring to them, the manner in which they address them, and the reservoir of personal resources they can call on to serve another day. At the same time, their moral commitments (or lack of them), as repeated in hundreds of their colleagues, create or destroy the credibility of the profession. In no profession is this truer than in politics because the stakes are so high, the power so great, and the temptations so insistent.

Just as the license to practice nursing does not include a permission to practice it poorly but rather presupposes an obligation to practice it well, election to office carries with it a compelling obligation to serve all of the people well all of the time *(www.house.gov/ethics)*. If election to office entails an obligation to work for the good of all, then the power to govern entails an obligation to judge and to monitor well one's own conduct and the conduct of one's colleagues. Therefore each member of a profession shares the obligation of assuring that every member follows established standards and codes.

Although the practice of medicine has existed since ancient times, it is important to realize that the practice of curative or clinical medicine had virtually zero impact on human survival until about 1950, when antibiotics became available to the general population (McKeown, 1976). This observation, although thoroughly documented, runs counter to the common impression that improvements in our health and life expectancy are a result of medical progress. This is not true. We have long known that the dramatic improvement in health and life expectancy from 1900 to 1950 (from 49 years in 1900 to 74 by 1950) is due almost entirely to an improved standard of living, a sufficient and clean food supply, social justice, public sanitation, vaccination, personal hygiene, and other such

public health measures (Canadian Institute for Advanced Research, 1994).

The obvious result of these largely social and environmental improvements is that most people began living long enough to age—and with age comes an increased risk for chronic illnesses and their acute manifestations. However, modern medicine as practiced in the United States has little to do with treating anything other than the acute manifestations of chronic illness.

When one explores the field of public health research, one begins to realize that the nature of the factors that cause disease can be better understood in light of what produces healthy people, and that social rather than medical interventions make a far greater contribution to the health of any community. Thus, a good case could be made that to advance the health of the population, nurses should be advocating for social and environmental change, not funding for more research and treatment for the ill and that far from advocating for their own advantage, or even the best interests of the ill, nurses and physicians should be lobbying for better environmental conditions, nutrition, education, and social supports for young families.

However, the principles of distributive justice, indeed the personal security of every member of society, are affected by whether or not someone will care for them if they are injured or ill or when they become older adults. Therefore what is in the profession's best interests and the patients' (those who are ill) best interests does indeed promote society's best interests—as long as this concern does not undermine the economic viability of that society. So, it is possible to reconcile competing interests; in fact, that's what politics is all about, on every level. To frame this discussion, a review of the principles of distributive justice is in order.

PRINCIPLES OF DISTRIBUTIVE JUSTICE

Health care professionals, who are ideally situated to make micro-distributive decisions and whose social role enables them to speak with authority to the general population about the impact of resource allocation decisions on the health and welfare of various segments of the population, must not allow social decisions to influence their clinical decisions. For one thing, their ethical codes require—and for good reason—that health care professionals act in the best interests of the person on whom they are laying hands (Frankl, 1959). For another thing, the will of the citizenry, as expressed through the votes of their elected representatives, should determine the distribution of the resources they have so diligently (if unwillingly) supplied to their governments. In general, the principles of distributive justice ought to be used to guide decision-making at the sociopolitical levels. They are as follows:

1. To each the same thing. One of the simplest principles of distributive justice is that of strict or radical equality. The principle says that every person should have the same level of material goods and services. Even with this ostensibly simple principle, some of the difficult specification problems of distributive principles can be seen, specifically, construction of appropriate indexes for measurement, and the specification of time frames. Because there are numerous proposed solutions to these problems, the "principle of strict equality" is not a single principle but a name for a group of closely related principles.

2. To each according to his need. The most widely discussed theory of distributive justice in the past three decades has been that proposed by John Rawls in *A Theory of Justice* (Rawls, 1971) and Political Liberalism (Rawls, 1993). Rawls proposes the following two principles of justice: (1) Each person has an equal claim to a fully adequate scheme of equal basic rights and liberties, and (2) social and economic inequalities are "to be to the greatest benefit of the least advantaged members of society" (Rawls, 1993, pp. 5-6). These principles give fairly clear guidance on what type of arguments will count as justifications for inequality.

3. To each according to his ability to compete in the open market place. Aristotle argued that virtue should be a basis for distributing rewards, but most contemporary principles owe a larger debt to John Locke. Locke argued that people deserve to have those items produced by their toil and industry, the products (or the value thereof) being a fitting reward for their effort. His underlying idea was to guarantee to individuals the fruits of their own labor and abstinence. According to some contemporary theorists (Feinberg, 1970), people freely apply their abilities and talents, in varying degrees, to socially productive work. People come to deserve varying levels of income by providing goods and services desired by others (Feinberg, 1970). Distributive systems are just insofar as they distribute incomes according to the different levels earned or deserved by the individuals in the society for their productive labors, efforts, or contributions.

4. To each according to his merits (desserts). Merit-based principles of distribution differ primarily according to what they identify as the basis for deserving. Most contemporary proposals regarding merit fit into one of three broad categories (Miller, 1976, 1989):
   - Contribution: People should be rewarded for their work activity according to the value of their contribution to the social product.
   - Effort: People should be rewarded according to the effort they expend in their work activity.
   - Compensation: People should be rewarded according to the costs they incur in their work activity.

THE NITTY GRITTY

Ethical theory is relatively unambiguous and rational. Unfortunately, the real world—whether it be the world of organizational politics or the world of national health policy development—is, generally speaking, murky at best. It operates on opinion, emotion, and, as often as not, relationships. Therefore to a great extent one could say that what is wrong in relationships is also wrong in politics—so that, for example, lying to further a political aim is as wrong as lying to a friend, a loved one, an employer, or a patient.

When people ask whether it is right to lie about something (e.g., the number of people affected by a particular disease) to get funding for research and/or treatment of patients with a particular disease, in a word the answer is yes. It is wrong. Why is lying wrong? It's wrong because it undermines the foundation of any relationship: trust. In like manner, lying to further a political agenda is wrong—not only because it undermines trust, but also because it fosters further dishonesty. Judging by the amount of political dishonesty reported in the media, one is led to the conclusion that there is a lot of lying going on! Adding to it—telling more lies to further our own agenda—will only make matters worse.

Is it right for nurses to endorse health reform legislation even if the legislation is not perfect? The answer is yes, it may indeed be the right thing to do. Remember, politics is about relationships, and relationships cannot prosper when one party insists that the other party must agree with them on every (or even any) issue. "In the end, to thrive—even to exist—invariably means to tolerate in oneself a certain degree of inconsistency, but that is a far cry from deserting one's sense of right and wrong. It means, rather, that this is a world chock-full of small mindedness and inequity, a world in which greed and vanity are encouraged—promoted—at every turn. Each of us should know which lines she will not cross—would not even consider crossing—both in one's professional life and in the world at large, and those principles must remain inviolate" (Stein, 1982, p. 149). It is not wrong to compromise; compromise is part of the give and take of relationships, and it is part of the give and take of politics.

Well, one might ask, if it's acceptable to compromise, can it be acceptable to distort an issue to manipulate public opinion or to win the support of a particular piece of legislation? Here one must be very careful, because deliberate distortion is lying by intent if not by actual fact. One can frame a discussion in a manner that is more acceptable to a certain constituency without lying. For example, in the health care arena, one can use words that appeal to known values; words such as *tradition, legitimate authority,* and the like tend to appeal to conservatives, whereas words such as *autonomous* and *experimental* tend to appeal to liberals. Knowing the target audience and framing the issue in words that will help them listen (or at least not harden their opposition) is smart, not unethical.

Now we will return to the issue of nurses' (and others') lobbying activities: Here compromise is in order. Any professional group has a duty, imposed on it by both its social role and its code of ethics, to push forward laws and policies that protect or advance the best interests of those whom they serve. And finally, any citizen, particularly a knowledgeable one, has a civic duty to speak out for the common good.

The issues are not easy, nor are their proposed solutions. But ignoring them not only may lead to social disaster, it will also place the onus of decision-making on nurses and physicians. The real irony of the situation is that health policy questions are resolved everyday on our clinical units. Why? The health care system as it is currently structured and financed leaves access and decision-making up to insurers and to individuals who work at the "point of care." Resources to provide care are shrinking, as government and third-party purchasers (employers who represent small and large businesses, alike) pressure the system to control, if not shrink, spending.

How much is too much to spend on medical care? This question is not easily answered at either the micro-level or the macro-level. On the micro-level, it is handled a bit more easily, as individuals decide whether to spend their money on food or drugs or to see a physician because they or their children are suffering a certain symptom. As we move incrementally from the individual to the social level, matters become more complex.

THE CASE OF BARBARA HOWE

An example is the case of Barbara Howe. On March 11, 2004, the *Boston Globe* ran an article about a 79-year-old woman who is now completely paralyzed from Lou Gehrig's disease (Kowalczyk, 2004). When Barbara Howe was diagnosed with Lou Gehrig's disease, she knew that it would cripple her before killing her. Therefore she repeatedly told her daughters and doctors and nurses to do whatever it took to keep her alive as long as she could appreciate her family. Howe also discussed end-of-life care with her family and physicians. Nonetheless, she ended up in a situation that neither she nor her family foresaw: long before her death, she was unable to make the slightest gesture while her doctors and her family argued in court about whether she still wanted everything done to keep her alive, given the advanced stage of her disease and the fact that she had been unable to communicate anything for more than 3 years.

Mrs. Howe did not leave the hospital from the time of her admission on November 15, 1999, until the time of her death in 2004. Blue Cross and Blue Shield of Massachusetts stopped covering her hospital stay in 2002. Her physicians and nurses believed that she was in pain and that keeping her alive was tantamount to torture. However, the patient's oldest daughter, who was her mother's health care proxy, disagreed, stating that it was her belief that her mother still recognized family members when they entered the room and would not have wanted to die at that point. The daughter also said that when she sensed that her mother no longer appreciated her family, she would have the ventilator turned off.

Howe's case epitomizes a shift in American medicine, one outcome of patients and families who are more educated and opinionated about health care—and more suspicious that physicians may deny care because of soaring costs. As late as August 2000, Mrs. Howe told her physicians that being alert was more important to her than being pain free—even though she suffered from constant headaches and facial pain. She also indicated that she wanted to continue receiving aggressive care, even though her ability to interact was fading fast. At the beginning of 2001, she could follow people with her eyes and move one finger. By the end of the year, even these tiny gestures had disappeared.

In July 2001 the hospital's end-of-life committee reviewed the case. During this meeting, the patient's daughter insisted that her mother wanted aggressive treatment as long as she was able to enjoy and respond to her family. The ethics committee agreed to honor the request. However, shortly thereafter, Howe lost the ability to blink and to lubricate her eyes. Subsequently the dry tissue of her right cornea tore, and the end-of-life committee met immediately to reconsider her situation. As quoted by the journalist, the chairman of the ethics committee, Dr. Edwin Cassem (a psychiatrist and Jesuit priest), wrote in the minutes of the ethics committee, "There is now 100 percent unanimous agreement that this inhumane travesty has gone far enough. This is the Massachusetts General Hospital, not Auschwitz" (Kowalczyk, 2004, p. 7F).

The next day, surgeons removed Howe's right eye. Later that month, the hospital's lawyers asked the Probate and Family Court to intervene, but they ruled that there was not sufficient cause to remove the patient's daughter as her health care proxy. However, the judge did urge the daughter to refocus her assessment from the patient's wishes to the patient's best interests. On January 13, 2004, physicians and nurses again asked Massachusetts General's end-of-life committee to order withdrawal of life support, saying the patient was now in danger of losing her left eye, which was taped shut except when her daughters visited. The daughter returned to court, saying her mother's left eye had improved; she said that when the patient was in danger of losing it, she would allow the hospital to turn off the ventilator. On February 22, 2004, the parties met with the probate judge for $2\frac{1}{2}$ hours but failed to agree on a course of action (Kowalczyk, 2004). Barbara Howe died at the age of 80, 26 days before a court settlement would have allowed the hospital to turn off her ventilator (Kowalczyk, 2005).

The Howe case, so far at least, has not progressed beyond the local level—and that is difficult enough. The next case, though, went to state supreme courts and to federal courts, as well as to local, state, and national legislatures. What follows is a summary of testimony given in the Terri Schiavo case in the Pinellas County Circuit Court.

THE CASE OF TERRI SCHIAVO

Terri Schiavo, 25, was found unconscious by her husband in the early morning of February 25, 1990. She had suffered a full cardiac arrest. Defibrillation was performed seven times during initial resuscitative efforts, with eventual restoration of a normal cardiac rhythm. The initial serum potassium level was 2.0, undoubtedly the cause of her cardiac arrest. Terri had a history of erratic eating habits, including probable bulimia, with a major weight loss several years before this event. In November 1992, Michael Schiavo won a malpractice suit against Terri's physicians for failing to diagnose her health problems leading up to the cardiac arrest resulting directly from her eating disorder (George W. Greer, Circuit Court, Pinellas County, Florida, File No. 90-2908-GD-003).

Terri was in a coma for approximately one month, and then her condition evolved into a persistent vegetative state (PVS). Four board-certified neurologists in Florida consulting on her care diagnosed PVS. The initial computed tomography (CT) scan on the day of admission, February 25, 1990, had normal findings, but further CT scans documented a progression of widespread cerebral hemisphere atrophy, eventually resulting in CT scans in 1996 and 2002 that showed extreme atrophy, specifically, "diffuse encephalomalacia and infarction consistent with anoxia, hydrocephalus ex vacuo, neural stimulator present." Clinical examinations over the years were entirely consistent with the diagnosis of permanent vegetative state secondary to hypoxic-ischemic encephalopathy (George W. Greer, Circuit Court, Pinellas County, Florida, File No. 90-2908-GD-003).

For purposes of discussion, it helps to make some important distinctions, such as the distinction between a coma and a PVS. "A coma is a profound or deep state of unconsciousness. An individual in a state of coma is alive but unable to move or respond to his or her environment. Coma may occur as a complication of an underlying illness, or as a result of injuries, such as head trauma. A persistent vegetative state (commonly, but incorrectly, referred to as "brain-death") sometimes follows a coma. Individuals in such a state have lost their thinking abilities and awareness of their surroundings, but retain noncognitive function and normal sleep patterns. Even though those in a persistent vegetative state lose their higher brain functions, other key functions such as breathing and circulation remain relatively intact. Spontaneous movements may occur, and the eyes may open in response to external stimuli. They may even occasionally grimace, cry, or laugh. Although individuals in a persistent vegetative state may appear somewhat normal, they do not speak and they are unable to respond to commands" *(www.ninds.nih.gov/disorders/coma/coma.htm)*.

Another problem that needs to be addressed is whether or not feeding is a medical intervention, especially whether or not a permanent feeding tube could be considered a "futile medical intervention," and therefore could be legitimately withdrawn. Although feeding per se is not a medical intervention, tube feedings may indeed be considered one. At any rate, the courts in the Schiavo case held this to be so (George W. Greer, Circuit Court, Pinellas County, Florida, File No. 90-2908-GD-003). If Schiavo could have been fed by mouth and swallow her food, the courts may have taken a different position. However, whether Terri was fed via a PEG tube or orally, she was still in a permanent vegetative state, and feeding her would not have resulted in any change in her clinical condition, except she would probably die much sooner were attempts made to feed her orally—that is, the feeding tube could not improve her medical condition. If feeding is not a medical treatment, can medical personnel refuse to provide it, or remove a feeding tube if it already is in place? The answer is unclear and may depend on the patient's wishes and values, or those of a legal guardian. In the Schiavo case, despite her parents' monumental efforts, Schiavo's husband repeatedly was recognized by the courts as her legal guardian.

Although numerous court cases have irrefutably established a patient's right to refuse medical treatment, few have dealt with a patient's right (if there is one) to undergo medical treatment when all medical authorities agree that the treatment is useless. Although a case can be made that a right to refuse treatment isn't worth much if there is no right to treatment, one must ask if there is a right "to treatment that can in no way benefit one." Surely not even the most zealous advocates for universal access to health care would insist that patients have a right to medical treatments that do not benefit them and that may, indeed, harm them.

How much can any citizen or family demand from society? This is, indeed, a political question that, according to the best information available to us, should not be answered in a manner that undermines support for policies that improve living and working conditions; provide support for young families; reduce domestic and social violence; and assure fair wages, educational benefits, and a clean environment, for these are the elements of a health-producing society (Black, Morris, Smith, & Townsend, 1982). And the questions do not stop at difficult cases, or even with a determination of futility. In fact, these questions must be asked about all socially funded care.

For a list of related websites, please refer to your Evolve Resources at http://evolve.elsevier.com/Mason/policypolitics/

REFERENCES

Black, D., Morris, J. N., Smith, C., & Townsend, P. (1982). *Inequalities in health: The Black report.* Harmondsworth, Middlesex, England; New York: Penguin Books.

Canadian Institute for Advanced Research. (1994). *The determinants of health.* CIAR publication #5. Toronto: CIAR.

Ethics manual for members, officers, and employees of the U.S. House of Representatives. Retrieved from www.house.gov/ethics/Ethicforward.html.

Feinberg, J. (1970). *Justice and personal desert, doing and deserving.* Princeton, NJ: Princeton University Press.

Frankl, V. (1959). *Man's search for meaning.* Boston: Beacon Press.

Gandhi, M. (1958). *The collected works of Mahatma Gandhi.* Publications Division, Ministry of Information and Broadcasting, Government of India, New Delhi.

George W. Greer, Circuit Court, Pinellas County, Florida, File No. 90-2908-GD-003.

Kidder, R. M. (1994). *Shared values for a troubled world: Conversations with men and women of conscience.* San Francisco: Jossey-Bass.

Kowalczyk, L. (2004, March 11). Hospital, family spar over end-of-life care. *Boston Globe,* 2F-8F.

Kowalczyk, L. (2005, June 8). Woman dies after battle over care. *Boston Globe,* 2F.

McKeown, T. (1976). *The role of medicine: Dream, mirage or nemesis?* Oxford: Basil Blackford.

Miller, D. (1976). *Social justice*. Oxford: Clarendon Press.
Miller, D. (1989). *Market, state, and community*. Oxford: Clarendon Press.
Rawls, J. (1971). *A theory of justice*. Harvard, MA: Harvard University Press.
Rawls, J. (1993). *Political liberalism*. New York: Columbia University Press.
Stein, H. (1982). *Ethics and other liabilities*. London: St Martin's Press.
Wellman, C. (1975). *Morals and ethics*. Glenview, IL: Scott, Foresman.

CHAPTER 10

Using the Power of Media to Influence Health Policy and Politics

Jessie Daniels, Barbara Glickstein, and Diana J. Mason

"Whoever controls the media—the images—controls the culture."

—Allen Ginsberg

In February 2007, then United States Senator Barack Obama (D-IL) had a conversation with Marc Andreessen, a founder of Netscape (one of the original browsers, pre-dating Google) and member of the board of directors of Facebook. The conversation was about using social media to build a political campaign that could upset frontrunner Hillary Rodham Clinton in the Democratic primary election for the U.S. presidency. In 2004, presidential candidate Howard Dean had used a viral Web strategy to build a campaign war chest through small donations from large numbers of people. Obama had a vision for building upon Dean's success, and he hired Chris Hughes, another founder of Facebook, to manage his presidential campaign's social media effort. David Axelrod, Obama's top adviser, was formerly a partner in ASK Public Strategies, a public relations firm. Together, Hughes and Axelrod built a team that marshaled every tool in the social media and marketing tool box to create and sustain the Obama campaign and brand.

They launched an expert viral marketing campaign including: Obama ringtones, product placement (Obama ads in sports video games), and a 30-minute infomercial that was played on YouTube. The campaign's effort spawned additional digital videos as well, including the "I Got a Crush…On Obama," video and the celebrity-filled video called "Yes We Can," featuring Black-Eyed Peas front man Wil.I.Am, both of which went viral, spreading to millions of viewers in just days of being posted online. The Obama campaign led competitors in using social media to connect with a growing audience of

followers on Facebook, Twitter, MySpace, and blogs. In the general election, he had 118,107 followers on Twitter, outpacing his opponent John McCain's 2865 followers by a factor of 40 to 1 (Lardinois, 2008). Obama used social media to build a grassroots movement that resulted in his historic election (Talbot, 2008).

But he knew that the use of social media is not simply a campaign technique—it's a way of interacting, building an activist community, and engaging people in ways that matter to them. As president, he quickly launched *www.change.gov* for people to share their ideas for reforming the country, sending the message that he had no intention of regressing to a traditional media operation as president. Rather, he was going to continue to engage people in supporting his agenda for the nation. When health care reform was teetering from a growing army of discontents blocking its passage, he continued using social media to mobilize supporters to pressure Congress to act before the April 2010 recess. President Obama also took to the road and held town meetings in key communities because he knew that these town meetings would garner reports on primetime television, radio coverage, and front page position in newspapers. He could count on the primetime news including a sound bite and visual image of him speaking before a crowd of enthusiastic Ohioans, cheering for passing some form of health care reform legislation. The personal appearances were a way to get his message to those who were not yet social media mavens and to reinforce it with those who were already his followers on Twitter and Facebook.

The Web has dramatically changed how we think about communicating with others, whether to connect with family or build a grassroots political movement to push policymakers to pass new laws. Even traditional media outlets are now augmenting their work with all sorts of social media to extend their reach and impact. Legislators are launching blogs, using Facebook, and "Tweeting" to make their voices heard and connect with their constituents. In fact, engaging citizens in government is reshaping the way government works. This chapter looks at the integration of traditional and social media as powerful tools for nurses to harness in shaping health policy and politics.

SEISMIC SHIFT IN MEDIA: ONE-TO-MANY AND MANY-TO-MANY

There has been a seismic shift in the way media is created and distributed. For many years, the dominant paradigm in media was a model in which one broadcaster sent a message out to a mass audience. This broadcast model is referred to as "one-to-many." Today, this model is being challenged by the advent of the Internet and user-generated-content in which many people create media and distribute it to their networks. This new model is sometimes referred to as "many-to-many."

MASS MEDIA: THE ONE-TO-MANY MODEL

Traditional media in radio, television, film, and newspapers was based on the idea that one broadcaster would try to reach as many audience members as possible. But for those interested in influencing health policy and politics through the media, there were many advantages and some significant disadvantages to the one-to-many model of broadcast media (Abramson, 2003).

Radio, film, and television have all been used to communicate messages about health to consumers and policymakers alike. What all these media share is the ability to broadcast a message to a mass audience, sometimes in the millions or tens of millions. When there were very few media outlets, it was possible to broadcast a consistent message to a wide audience. The use of mass media has been a major tool in health promotion campaigns because it reaches a large audience. Media is a powerful tool that is capable of promoting healthy social change (Whitney & Viswanath, 2004).

There are also disadvantages to mass media communications. Large corporations own media outlets and control what goes out through their channels. The expense of buying time or space in major media outlets can be prohibitive, especially for non-profit organizations. Mass media campaigns, by definition, are intended to reach a wide audience but are not as effective at reaching specific, target populations. For example, a mass media campaign about HIV prevention may reach a wide audience but may fail to reach the specific population that is most vulnerable to infection. However, political operatives have developed increasingly sophisticated approaches to segmenting and targeting specific electoral districts with mass media when they want to pressure a policymaker who may hold a deciding vote on an important bill. They buy commercial time on the dominant television station in that policymaker's district. But what no form of mass media does very well (or, at all) is to allow users to create and distribute their own content with messages they find most important.

MANY-TO-MANY: USER-GENERATED CONTENT AND THE RISE OF THE "PROSUMER"

The rise of the Internet, and specifically websites that rely on users to generate content, are part of a new landscape of media creation and distribution. The early Internet featured "brochure" websites that were one-way flows of information. The paradigm-shifting quality of the Internet began to emerge with the rise of Web 2.0 (pronounced: "web two point oh"), a term coined by Tim O'Reilly (2005) at a conference in 2004. Web 2.0 refers to a range of web-based Internet practices based on information sharing, social networks, and collaboration rather than the one-way communication style of the early era of the Internet. The key idea with the concept of Web 2.0 is that people are using the Internet to connect with other people, through their old face-to-face networks and through newly formed online networks.

"Prosumption" is another way that some people talk about this shift. Prosumption is the idea that "producing" and "consuming" are combined in this new many-to-many paradigm. Rather than an elite few who "produce" media for a mass audience to "consume," now we are all both "producers" and "consumers," or *prosumers* of media. The many-to-many paradigm does not refer to a new form of technology but rather a new way that everyday people make use of that technology (Ritzer & Jurgenson, 2010).

The collaborative, information-sharing Internet practices have broad implications for health media, policy, and politics, but they do not mean the end of mass media.

THE POWER OF MEDIA

A classic example of the power of media in shaping health policy arose during the first months of William Jefferson Clinton's presidency, when he tried but failed to enact health care reform legislation despite campaigning on a policy platform that sought to guarantee comprehensive health care coverage for every American. In September 1993, he proposed the Health Security Act to Congress and the public with the hope and anticipation that this would become landmark legislation. Clinton's proposal initially had substantial public support, because many believed the country had a moral imperative to extend health care coverage to all who live here. However, according to an analysis by the Annenberg Public Policy Center of the University of Pennsylvania (1995), one of the top factors that unraveled the legislation's progress was the "Harry and Louise" campaign (a series of television advertisements about two curious characters, Harry and Louise), which was sponsored by the Health Insurance Association of America (HIAA), an ardent opponent to the president's plan.

Actors portrayed this couple voicing grave concerns about the bill. They said, "Under the President's bill, we'll lose our right to choose our own physician," and "What happens if the plan runs out of money?" Although the advertisements were not the only reason for the demise of the Health Security Act, the Harry and Louise television spots effectively planted fear and negativity in the hearts and minds of many citizens within the span of 60 seconds. Suddenly, many of the Americans who had been concerned about the growing numbers of uninsured became more concerned about how the bill would affect their own health care options and withdrew their support from the Act.

What many do not realize about the Harry and Louise ads is that the target audience was not the public, directly. Rather, it was policymakers and those who could influence how the public perceived the issue: journalists. The ads originally aired in the country's major media centers: Washington, DC; Los Angeles; New York City; and Atlanta. They were seen and reported on by journalists. In fact, the ads got more airtime by becoming part of the journalists' news stories. Many people who saw the ads did so through viewing them as part of the evening news, not as a paid advertisement.

The Harry and Louise commercials are an example of a deliberate media strategy to reframe a public policy issue and mobilize a public constituency around it. It is one illustration of the power of the media in policy and politics. The media saturate this nation and much of the world with images that change people's opinions, shape their attitudes and beliefs, and transform their behavior (McAlister, 1991). In today's media landscape, the Harry and Louise television ads would also be posted on YouTube for millions more to view. Bloggers would include links to the video, as would people who write about it on their Facebook or Twitter pages. Yet, the current media landscape would also spawn critical analyses of the ads by bloggers and unmasking the HIAA and their motives, potentially limiting the impact of the ads.

Media campaigns such as these often rely on cloaked websites to enhance the effectiveness of their deception. Cloaked websites are published by individuals or groups who conceal authorship in order to deliberately disguise a hidden political agenda (Daniels, 2009). Consider an ad from the more recent, successful effort to pass the Affordable Care Act of 2010. During this political battle, an unknown political group with no clear affiliation to a political party created a video opposing the reform. In the ad, a variety of attractive-looking people declare, "I guess I'm racist" because they oppose health care reform. The central message of the video, although not immediately obvious, was a signal that a growing number of people opposed Obama's policy on health care reform but that opposition was not rooted in any individual racism. The video had fairly high-quality production values, meaning it looked professionally produced and good enough to appear on broadcast television; yet, it was released exclusively on YouTube. The provocative video quickly went viral (meaning it was very popular and links to it spread via e-mail and blogs from person to person, much like a biological virus). Within 24 hours, it was one of the most viewed videos on YouTube—no small accomplishment among the millions of videos on the site. Once again, the political operatives behind this video did not have to buy airtime on television to get their message out. After the video became the top video on YouTube, several mainstream broadcast news media outlets re-aired it on television. Some of these were critical of the video, such as the Rachel Maddow Show on MSNBC, but the fact is that what started as a YouTube video was featured on several broadcast television shows within 24 hours. Health care reform legislation did eventually pass despite these types of campaigns. Yet, this instance of converging media[1] illustrates just how sophisticated the use of multiple forms of media has become.

WHO CONTROLS THE MEDIA?

The traditional media industry has been owned by six major corporations that, prior to the growth of social media, controlled 90% of the news Americans read, saw, or heard (Harris, 2005). In 2003, the Federal Communications Commission (made up of political appointees reflecting the then-dominant Republican party's values) voted to ease the restrictions on cross-ownership between different news entities, permitting one corporation to own the primary television, radio, and newspaper outlets in a community, thus enabling one corporation to control messages and put forth a particular perspective. CNN founder Ted Turner objected to this consolidation of corporate media power, arguing that allowing this cross-ownership "will extend the market dominance of the media corporations that control most of what Americans read, see, or hear" and "give them more power to cut important ideas out of the public debate" (Harris, 2005, p. 83).

Today, social media can actually drive traditional media to cover issues that major newsrooms may not deem worthy of their limited space and time. On June 12, 2009, Iran held its presidential elections between incumbent Mahmoud Ahmadinejad and rival Hossein Mousavi. The result was a landslide victory for Ahmadinejad; yet there was strong suspicion of voting fraud. This led to violent riots across Iran and protests worldwide. As protests erupted in the streets of numerous cities in Iran and in some cases turned

violent, major broadcast media in the U.S. had almost no news on these events at all. Americans and others around the world and in Iran used the Twitter hashtag (e.g., a # symbol used to group messages on a specific topic) "#CNNfail" to track and share updates on what was happening in Iran that were pouring in from around the world. Twitter was the best source of information for second-by-second updates and breaking news on what was happening in Iran. People on-the-ground and across the globe chatted about the news out of Iran fed by social media more than mainstream news divisions. YouTube was a central distribution medium for the Iran riots with videos shot by people on the ground using their cell phones and small handheld cameras. The blogosphere was far quicker with news and multimedia from Iran then traditional news, illustrated by the spectacle of highly paid cable news anchors reading Twitter and blog updates on the air as part of their "reporting" a story. The social media photo site Flickr was quickly filled with gut-wrenching imagery from the ground showing photos of beatings, protests, and military action. This groundswell of news from and about Iran spread globally and nearly instantly through social media turned into a news item itself and was reported on by all traditional media outlets. Eventually, the focus shifted and CNN and other news outlets started covering stories about Iran.

This example illustrates the power of social media to offset the corporate takeover of traditional media. This bodes well for nurses who have not always been able to garner media attention for their issues. Two studies during the 1990s documented nursing's invisibility in the media (Buresh et al., 1991; Sigma Theta Tau International, 1998). Commissioned by The Honor Society of Nursing, *Sigma Theta Tau* International, the *Woodhull Study on Nursing and the Media* found that nurses were included in health stories in major print media (newspapers and news magazines published in September 1997) less than 4% of the time, even when they would have been germane to the story. An even more disturbing finding was the fact that nurses were represented in health care industry publications (such as *Modern Healthcare*) less than 1% of the time.

Buresh and Gordon (2006) suggest that findings such as these could be a systematic journalistic bias against nursing. But they also note that nurses have not been proactive in accessing traditional media.

---

[1]"Converging media" refers to the interweaving of traditional and new social media, rather than these platforms remaining separate.

Social media provides an opportunity for nurses to not wait for traditional media to value their perspectives. Instead, nurses can use social media to create and distribute messages and to engage others to care about an issue and discuss it from various vantage points.

But will nurses seize this opportunity? On March 15, 2010, *Medical, Marketing & Media*, a monthly business publication for health care marketers, published the results of an online survey on nurses' and physicians' use of social media (Arnold, 2010). The survey found that only 11% of nurses said they used Twitter and 77% had visited Facebook. The authors noted that this was about one year behind the general population. If nurses want visibility, they must become cyberactivists,[2] fusing the old and new media methods to allow for the widest range of engagement of the public.

Nursing organizations are particularly well-positioned to mount focused social media campaigns because they already have a list of people who can begin the viral spreading of messages. But the social network lines are getting crowded; and establishing a reputation for reliable, important information that others want to regularly take note of requires a thoughtful strategy. Distributed campaigns are increasingly a part of a political strategy, whether for winning an election, getting an issue on policymakers' or the public's agenda, or garnering support for a new policy initiative.

DISTRIBUTED CAMPAIGNS

Obama's social media campaign strategy is called a *distributed campaign*—a bottom-up rather than a top-down approach to political campaigns that depends upon viral spreading from the grassroots rather than message broadcasting and control by the campaign staff (Ozimek, 2005). These campaigns are designed to involve more than core supporters. They seek to engage swing voters, provide opportunities for core supporters to craft messages that may appeal to these swing voters more effectively than messages created by central campaign staff, and thereby strengthen the commitment of core supporters to the campaign. E-mail, blogs, and various other social media venues are used by campaign staff to begin a dialogue that is subsequently taken over and developed by a broad community of supporters.

Whether people are reached by e-mails, Facebook or Twitter updates, or other means, distributed campaigns provide people with tools for activism, such as petitions to sign, e-mail scripts to send, or letters to sign and send to legislators. Organizations such as Democracy In Action *(http://salsalabs.com/democracyinaction)* are available to help build the capacity of groups that want to develop action tools that reach diverse audiences in distributive campaigns. Living in a media-saturated world can sometimes feel like being in a cacophony of conflicting voices. The challenge is how to use these powerful tools most effectively as the media model changes.

GETTING ON THE PUBLIC'S AGENDA

One of the most important roles that media plays is getting issues on the agendas of the public and policymakers. What the mainstream media do or do not cover is equally powerful in determining what issues are considered by policymakers.

The news media are instrumental in getting issues onto the agenda of policymakers, but non-news entertainment television programs can mobilize public constituencies around an issue. Television continues to be the dominant form of media in most people's lives, despite the rise of new forms of media online. The television is on more than 8 hours a day in the average American household (Nielsen Reports, 2007). Teenagers still spend more time watching TV than they do online (Generation M2, 2010). The Internet may be where people go to find out about a health issue, but they often first become aware of the issue through television.

Turow (1996) points out that non-news television entertainment is particularly loaded with rhetoric that often stereotypes power relationships and may be more successful than the news in shaping people's images of the world. Highly viewed TV presentations of health care hold political significance that should be assessed alongside news. Medical and nursing dramas on broadcast and cable television, such as *Grey's Anatomy, ER*, and *Nurse Jackie,* are often important sources of information about health and health policy for a wide audience. Researchers Turow

---

[2]Cyberactivists are people who want to create change involving a variety of issues and have taken up the use of new media technologies and strategies that characterize Web 2.0 (McCaughey & Ayers, 2003).

and Gans (2002) systematically evaluated one television season of four hour-long medical dramas and found that health care policy issues appeared regularly in the programs. Evidence from a national telephone survey indicates that the percentage of regular viewers of the show *ER* who were aware that HPV is a sexually transmitted disease was higher (28%) one week after viewing an episode of the show about HPV than before seeing the show (9%). Even 6 weeks after viewing the episode, 16% had retained this knowledge. This capacity to quickly get a message out to millions of people through an hour-long drama is part of the reason that many health advocates work to get their particular issue included in a storyline of a major network drama. For many working in public health, storyline placement is considered the "gold standard" for achieving advocacy goals.

Perhaps not surprisingly then, when National Institutes of Health (NIH) wanted to get out a message that "drug addiction is a brain disease," they turned to HBO. In a landmark collaboration between HBO, the NIH, and the Robert Wood Johnson Foundation, the cable network launched *The Addiction Series* (2007), an award-winning collection of documentary films about substance use, each by a leading director. Of course, *The Addiction Series* also included a website with more information about treatment options and a lively discussion board (Bauder, 2007).

Documentary films, in conjunction with online campaigns, are influencing health policy and politics, while achieving mainstream commercial success. For example, Morgan Spurlock's *Super Size Me* (2004) explored the health impact of fast food on childhood obesity, fueling changes in local school and community policies requiring posting of calories in fast food stores, changing the foods and beverages available in schools, and ramping up exercise options in schools. Michael Moore's documentary *SiCKO* (2005) examined health care policy in the U.S., helping to raise the public's awareness of how bad the U.S. health care system had become at a time when health care reform was on the nation's agenda. Many of those who were uncertain about whether or not health care reform was needed became converts after watching *SiCKO*.

For some media activists concerned with health policy, Internet technologies have transformed documentary films into just one element in a multimodal social action campaign. Perhaps the archetypal example of how media is converging across multiple platforms and creating change in awareness about

health and galvanizing movement for policy change around an important health issue is the development of *Food, Inc.* (2008). In 2001, journalist and filmmaker Robert Kenner read *Fast Food Nation*, a book by Eric Schlosser about the rise of agribusiness, and Kenner was appalled. He wanted to do something about the industrialization of the food supply, so he started work on the documentary that would eventually become *Food, Inc.* Kenner collaborated with Schlosser on the film (Schlosser is listed as co-producer). The online presence for *Food, Inc.* (*http://www.foodincthemovie.com*) is a vast repository of further information about the issues surrounding the industrialization of food. It includes opportunities to participate in activism, such as signing the online petition to reauthorize the Child Nutrition Act, which would support healthy food choices in schools. The film also inspired another book (*Food, Inc.*), an e-version that can be downloaded at the website, or a hard copy can be ordered from online booksellers. The social action campaign around *Food, Inc.* started with a heavily researched book and became a documentary film, a website, another book, and links for people to take action. This exemplifies how people are converging media to shape health and health policy.

MEDIA AS A HEALTH PROMOTION TOOL

Media can promote health in three ways: public education, social marketing, and media advocacy. The first two are often used to help people change their health behaviors by acquiring important information that they lacked (public education) or through visual or verbal messaging that can shift the individual's thinking, attitudes, and values (social marketing). Both of these can also be used to shape public policy and in political campaigns, but media advocacy specifically targets public policy.

MEDIA ADVOCACY

Media advocacy is the strategic use of media to apply pressure to advance a social or public policy initiative (Dorfman, Wallack, & Woodruff, 2005; Jernigan & Wright, 1996; Wallack & Dorfman, 1996). It is a tool for policy change—a way of mobilizing constituencies and stakeholders to support or oppose specific policy changes. It is a means of political action (DeJong, 1996). It differs from social marketing and

TABLE 10-1 Media Advocacy Versus Social Marketing and Public Education Approaches to Public Health

Media Advocacy	Social Marketing and Public Education
Individual as advocate	Individual as audience
Advances healthy public policies	Develops health messages
Changes the environment	Changes the individual
Target is person with power to make change	Target is person with problem or at risk
Addresses the power gap	Addresses the information gap

Adapted from Wallack, L., & Dorfman, L. (1996). Media advocacy: A strategy for advancing policy and promoting health. *Health Education Quarterly, 23*(3), 297. Copyright 1996 by Sage Publications. Reprinted by permission of Sage Publications.

public education approaches to public health, as noted in Table 10-1. Media advocacy defines the primary problem as a power gap, as opposed to an information gap, so mobilization of stakeholders is needed to influence the development of public policies.

The success of Mothers Against Drunk Driving (MADD) is illustrative of the power of media advocacy. MADD was formed in 1980 at a time when a drunk driver could kill a child and it would not be treated as a crime. MADD developed a policy agenda aimed at preventing drunk driving. It developed a "Rating the States" program to bring public attention to what state governments were and were not doing to fight alcohol-impaired driving. Then, just after Thanksgiving (the beginning of a period of high numbers of alcohol-related traffic accidents), MADD representatives held local press conferences with their state's officials and members of other advocacy groups to announce the state's rating. Local and national broadcast and print press brought the story to an estimated 62.5 million people. Subsequently, lawmakers in at least eight states took action to address drunken driving (Russell, Voas, DeJong, & Chaloupka, 1995).

Today, MADD's website *(www.madd.org)* advocates a number of policy changes that people can sign onto, a walk to raise funds to support the organization's work, a link to its Twitter page, and news about drunk driving initiatives. Getting on the news media's agenda is one of the functions of media advocacy

(Wallack, 1994). With numerous competing potential stories, media advocacy employs strategies to frame an issue in a way that will attract media coverage. For example, MADD often created media events by putting a wrecked car in front of a local high school a few days prior to a prom. Journalists flocked to these events. The visual of the wrecked car got people's attention, particularly from reporters. The news accounts and parental outrage that resulted from these media events eventually led to wide social support for the concept of "designated driver" and harsher penalties for "driving under the influence."

How a message is presented is as important as simply getting the attention of the news media. The demise of Clinton's Health Security Act demonstrates this point. It got on the media's agenda, but the important messages were lost in the strategic use of the Harry and Louise commercials.

FRAMING

Getting an issue on the agenda of the public and policymakers and shaping the message require framing (Dorfman et al., 2005). *Framing* "defines the boundaries of public discussion about an issue" (Wallack & Dorfman, 1996, p. 299). *Reframing* involves breaking out of the dominant perspective (or frame) on an issue to define a new way of thinking about it that can lead to very different ideas about potentially effective policy responses. Reframing requires working hard to understand the dominant frame, the values that undergird it, and its limitations, and then exploring new frames.

Framing applies to all messaging and policy work, whether changing staffing policies in a hospital or promoting legislation that will remove soft drinks from school vending machines. From a media perspective, *framing for access* entails shaping the issue in a way that will attract media attention. It helps to attach the issue to a local concern or event, anniversaries, or celebrities or to "make news" by holding events that will attract the press, such as releasing new research at a press conference (Jernigan & Wright, 1996). Most importantly, it requires some element of controversy (albeit not over the accuracy of advocates' facts), conflict, injustice, or irony. The targeted medium or media will shape how the story is presented. For example, television requires compelling visual images. If a broad audience is to be reached, a powerful, brief message on television can provide a quick frame for an issue and narrow how people will view it. But the interactive nature of social media provides the opportunity for others to continue to reframe a message, helping people to break out of a dominant frame.

Framing for content is more difficult than for access. A compelling individual story may gain visibility in some media, but there is no guarantee that the reporter or social media activists will focus on the public policy changes that you want. Wallack and Dorfman (1996) suggest that this reframing can be accomplished by the following:

- Emphasizing the social dimensions of the problem and translating an individual's personal story into a public issue
- Shifting the responsibility for the problem from the individual to the corporate executive or public official whose decisions can address the problem
- Presenting solutions as policy alternatives
- Making a practical appeal to support the solution
- Using compelling images
- Using authentic voices—people who have experience with the problem
- Using symbols that "resonate with the basic values of the audience" (Wallack & Dorfman, 1996, p. 300)
- Anticipating the opposition and knowing all sides of the issue

Framing is not just about verbal messages. Jacob Riis was a social reformer who used visual imagery and the latest technology to frame issues in ways that would influence policymakers. Riis emigrated to the U.S. from Copenhagen in 1871 and found work as a reporter in New York City. As a reporter, his beat was writing about the Lower East Side of New York where, in the 1880s, 334,000 people were crammed into a single square mile, making it the most densely populated place on earth. The people there were living in disease-ridden tenements, often with 10 or 15 to a room (Burrows & Wallace, 2000). Riis wrote often about their plight for his newspaper; he identified with the people on the Lower East Side, mostly immigrants like himself. Moved as he was, he grew frustrated by the lack of response from his readers. Riis had considered using photography to tell the stories of these New Yorkers, but the photographic technology of the day required a lot of light—which was scarce in a dark, airless tenement. Then, Riis read about a new technology from Germany called "flash photography." Riis started using flash technology to photograph some of the poorest New Yorkers and the deplorable conditions in which they lived and worked. In 1899, *Scribner's Magazine* published an 18-page article by Riis that included 19 of his photographs. Based on that article, a publisher invited Riis to publish an entire book, and his *How the Other Half Lives* became influential in shaping the early progressive movement working on behalf of immigrants' rights. Riis' photographs also influenced a young New York politician by the name of Theodore Roosevelt to implement public health laws that improved the city's health and are still in place today.

Many bloggers now include a photo or image with each post to draw attention to an entry. The images help to convey the frame that the bloggers want.

FOCUS ON REPORTING

One can argue that individual journalists are equally responsible for their choice of issues to cover and how they cover them. Journalists rarely have the same depth of knowledge about a topic as insiders. In fact, prior to the rise of social media, journalists and traditional media contributed to a public cynicism of politics and policymakers that resulted in a largely uninvolved citizenry (Fallows, 1996). This is due partially to journalists' having limited expertise on particular issues; as a result, they often cover only the political dimensions of an issue rather than the details of the policy options. This, in combination with the growth in polarized television "news" programs and politicized talk radio shows, requires careful analysis of "news." But social media also provides myriad opportunities for false, biased, and inflammatory messaging.

Getting to know the nature and quality of a particular journalists' or cyberactivist's work can help you to decide how much trust to place in it. Ask the following questions:

- Do they frequently misrepresent issues?
- Are their stories sensationalized, overplayed, or exaggerated?
- Do they present all sides of an issue with accuracy, fairness, and depth?
- Can you substantiate wild claims through sites such as *www.snopes.com*, *www.urbanlegends.about.com*, and *www.truthorfiction.com*?

In reality, few journalists have the time and the editorial support or the breadth and depth of knowledge about science to provide thorough reporting on health issues that have policy implications. This often results in less-than-adequate reporting on important issues, such as the reporting on how communities should respond to the West Nile virus. Roche (2002) examined print media coverage of the approaches to reducing the mosquito population to reduce the incidence of and mortality from West Nile encephalitis. None of the newspapers or magazines examined gave any information about risk of mortality from pesticide exposure or a cost analysis of this approach. Roche concluded that the public is "operating 'in the dark' in evaluating the question of whether pesticides should be deployed."

Nurses can assist journalists and cyberactivists by both reframing health policy issues and providing the depth of detail that others may lack. For example, a journalist covering a story on the nursing shortage has focused on the faculty shortage and producing more nurses. You could help the journalist to see that framing the story as purely one of a supply issue—getting more people into the pipeline—misses the important issues of retention of existing nurses and ways to reduce the demands on their time. While talking with this journalist does not ensure that your frame will be incorporated into the journalist's story, you can push out the frame you believe is important through your blog, Facebook page, or Twitter account.

One strategy is to facilitate information exchange in the public arena by becoming news makers, aggregators, or curators of health news. Posting links to news articles and research on critical policy issues on social media sites such as Facebook makes the news easy to find. Nurses are positioned to explain complex health policy issues by breaking them down, not just for information sharing but for civil engagement, so people will act, whether by having a conversation with a co-worker about the issue or contacting government representatives. Facebook friends, including other nurse colleagues, can click "share" on Facebook, which reposts these articles to their personal networks to widen the community in infinite ways. Social networking can generate a buzz and create conversations about an issue or policy. It is "digital activism" and has enormous potential to build networks, propagate power, and frame issues.

EFFECTIVE USE OF MEDIA

Nurses are seldom educated about using media to promote health or for media advocacy purposes. The following recommendations provide readers with a starting point for effectively using traditional and social media.

POSITIONING YOURSELF AS AN EXPERT

Whereas health policy was once the domain of a limited field of experts setting the agenda for the rest of us, the rise of user-generated content signals a radical departure from this approach. The emergence of user-generated content means a profound transformation in what it means to be an expert and opens the possibility of a wider range of types of expertise. New media provides nurses with platforms to reach the public as media makers and aggregators of reliable health research information.

Gain Credentials. There are many types of credentials, although they are typically thought of as degrees from educational institutions, work titles, and affiliations. Some institutions require that their employees notify them of any interaction with media; but this may be unnecessary if you don't name the institution in your interview or other communication. For example, you could be a "nurse practitioner in women's health at a community hospital."

Become an Expert in Your Field. Becoming the "go to" person who is *the* expert on a topic or particular field is another way to establish yourself as an expert. You can establish this by launching your own professional website, blog, and Twitter and Facebook pages, as well as by meeting with local journalists who cover health.

Use Personal Experience. Part of why this MADD's campaign has been compelling is their strategic use of stories from women whose children have been killed as a result of drunk driving. These bereaved mothers involved with MADD have transformed themselves into experts on the policy of driving while intoxicated and used their experience to make this point with policymakers. Similarly, people who were infected with HIV/AIDS in the 1980s and believed that the federal government was acting too slowly to move treatment through clinical trials made themselves experts on the science of the disease and, using a variety of tactics, forced policymakers to speed up the time for drugs to market. The Internet facilitates the rise of this kind of expertise.

Create Your Own Brand of Expertise. You can also become an expert in your field through some unique-to-you combination of all these. Individual policymakers weigh these differently. For example, after the death of her 2½-year-old son from *E. coli*, Barbara Kowalcyk became an expert in food-borne illness. Eventually, she started a non-profit organization called Center for Foodborne Illness & Prevention (CFI) *(www.foodborneillness.org)* and lobbied Congress to adopt laws for better food safety.

GETTING YOUR MESSAGE ACROSS

Getting your message to the appropriate target audience requires careful analysis and planning. For example, you might want to target a message to local homeowners, many of whom watch a particular TV station's evening news. To get television coverage, you must have a visual story. California nurses staged a media event on a senior health issue by staging a "rock around the clock" marathon, with seniors in rocking chairs outside an insurance company. They received press coverage of the event, which elicited some supportive letters to the editor as well as some negative press from seniors who said that they were stereotyping older adults. See Box 10-1 for guidelines for getting your message across in traditional media, and Box 10-2 for ways to use social media tools to reach an audience.

BLOGGING AND MICROBLOGGING

A 2006 random sample telephone survey conducted by the Pew Internet and American Life Project found that the American blogosphere was dominated by those who use their blogs as personal journals. When asked to choose just one topic that they blog about, 37% of bloggers responded that "my life and experiences" are their primary focus. Politics and government ran a very distant second with 11% of bloggers citing issues of public life as the main subject of their blog. Entertainment-themed topics were the next most popular category of blog (7%), followed by sports (6%); general news and current events (5%); business technology (4%); religion, spirituality, or faith (2%); and a specific health problem or illness (2%). Of interest here is the 2% that blog about a specific health problem or illness. While this is a comparatively small percentage of the total blogosphere, this 2% still constitutes a vast universe of health blogs. A conservative estimate would place the number of health blogs in the hundreds of thousands, and a less conservative estimate would be upwards of five million; and these blogs are consulted by an estimated 60 million users in the U.S., according to research conducted in 2008 (Manhattan Research, 2008). While most blogs are maintained by individuals who are affected by a particular health condition, some health-related blogs are sponsored by traditional newspapers or by community activist organizations.

Theresa Brown is an oncology nurse living and working in Pittsburgh. Her first career was as a doctorally-prepared English professor before deciding that she wanted to work more closely with people. She wrote a narrative about a dying patient that was published on the first page of the *New York Times* Science section, which until then had been dominated by physicians' narratives. She was then invited to contribute to the *Times'* health blog, *Well,* and now does so on a regular basis. As a result, issues of concern to practicing nurses get regular visibility through her posts. Her expertise as a nurse in cancer care is clearly valued by those who post responses to her blog entries.

Twitter, an example of microblogging, is a great way for nurses to listen as well as talk to others on a very direct level. Twitter allows users to post short, 140-character, messages. For longer conversations, people use hashtags (# symbols) to track topics. People are very creative in the way they use Twitter, and it holds a great deal of potential for nurses. For example, you can use it to convey your position on legislation that is up for a vote on the local, state, or national level to inform public debate on how this policy will impact the health and well being of individuals and communities. You can also use Twitter— and other social media such as Facebook—to link to relevant data supporting your position and to see what others are saying about this policy: Is it positive? Negative? Misinformed? Journalists frequently use Twitter to find sources and information on stories they're covering, or to simply uncover new stories. Following key health journalists can provide opportunities for recommending yourself or other nurses as experts on specific topics or to help them to reframe their stories.

BOX 10-1 Guidelines for Getting Your Message Across

The following guidelines will help you shape your message and get it delivered to the right media:

The Issue

- What is the nature of the issue?
- What is the context of the issue (e.g., timing, history, and current political environment)?
- Who is or could be interested in this issue?

The Message

- What's the angle or "so what"? Why should anyone care? What is news?
- Is there a sound bite that represents the issue in a catchy, memorable way?
- Can you craft rhetoric that will represent core values of the target audience?
- How can you frame nursing's interests as the public's interests (e.g., as consumers, mothers, fathers, women, taxpayers, and health professionals)?

The Target Audience

- Who is the target audience? Is it the public, policymakers, or journalists?
- If the public is the target audience, which segments of the public?
- What medium is appropriate for the target audience? Does this audience watch television? If so, are the members of this audience likely to watch a talk show or a news magazine show? Or do they read newspapers, listen to radio, or surf the Internet? Or are they likely to do all of these?

Access to the Media

- What relationships do you have with reporters and producers? Have you called or written letters or thank-you notes to particular journalists? Have you requested a meeting with the editorial board of the local community newspaper to discuss your issue and how the members of the board might think about reporting on it?
- How can you get the media's attention? Is there a "hot" issue you can connect your issue to? Is there a compelling human interest story? Do you have a press release that describes your issue in a succinct, compelling way? Do you have other printed materials that will attract journalists' attention within the first 3 seconds of viewing it? Are there photographs you can take in advance and then send out with your press release? Can you digitalize the images and make them available on a website for downloading onto a newspaper?
- Whom should you contact in the medium or media of choice?

- Have you been getting prepared all along? Are you news conscious? Do you watch, listen, clip, and track who covers what and how they cover it? What is the format of the program, and who is the journalist? What is the style of the program or journalist?
- Who are your spokespersons? Do they have the requisite expertise on the issue? Do they have a visual or voice presence appropriate for the medium? What is their personal connection to the issue, and do they have stories to tell? Have they been trained or rehearsed for the interview?

The Interviews

- Prepare for the interview. Get information on your interviewer and the program by reviewing the interviewer's work or talking with public relations experts in your area. Select the one, two, or three major points that you want to get across in the interview. Identify potential controversies and how you would respond to them. And rehearse the interview with a colleague.
- During the interview, listen attentively to the interviewer. Recognize opportunities to control the interview and get your primary point across more than once. What is your sound bite? Even if the interviewer asks a question that does not address your agenda, return the focus of the interview to your agenda and to your sound bite with finesse and persistence.
- Try to be an interesting guest. Come ready with rich, illustrative stories. Avoid yes or no answers to questions.
- Know that you do not have to answer all questions and should avoid providing comments that would embarrass you if they were headlines. If you don't know the answer to a question, say so and offer to get back to the interviewer with the information.
- Avoid being disrespectful or arguing with the interviewer.
- Remember that being interviewed can be an anxiety-producing experience for many people. It's a normal reaction. Do some slow deep-breathing or relaxation exercises before the interview, but know that some nervousness can be energizing.

Follow-Up

- Write a letter of thanks to the producer or journalist afterward.
- Provide feedback to the producer or journalist on the response that you have received to the interview or the program or coverage.

BOX 10-2 Using Social Media

MobileText Messaging

Mobile, and particularly text, messaging is the ideal medium for communicating with everyone equally, regardless of their age, gender, or economic status. To get started, do the following:

- Create a subscriber base with zip codes so text alerts can be targeted to subscribers; you can then ask people in a specific Congressional district to contact their representative about an important issue.
- Send alerts about a news item, an action, or a "meet-up"— the calling of a gathering of people for a shared interest.
- Send a link to a website or local news item.
- Feature a text-alert campaign on your website homepage.

Blogging

Blogs are great ways for you to share your opinions and ideas on health and social topics, and to bring attention to important issues. The following are some tips for blogging:

- Be creative.
- Engage your audience and invite readers to get involved.
- Tell important stories.
- Share your process (how your organization works).
- Share successes and challenges.
- Write short, action-oriented posts.
- Link to interesting local news.
- Find your niche.
- Be a subject matter expert.
- Be conversational.
- Write like you'd talk to your neighbor.
  One website that provides easy tools for starting a blog is www.wordpress.com.

Facebook (www.facebook.com)

Facebook provides a vehicle for building and growing a community. Lots of people are on Facebook to stay connected with friends and family. You can also create a Facebook page for your professional life, since mixing the two can be dicey if you're a clinician.

- Create a page for your organization or specific causes or issues; you can always have a new cause up that includes a new action item and a new goal.
- Upload relevant videos, photos, and articles.
- Turn your cause into a campaign.
- Set an achievable goal, and find a creative way to engage people to invite their friends.
- Host short-term causes.
- Use the announcements feature to keep cause members informed.
- Always send new info.
- Keep it short.
- If one idea doesn't work too well, don't be afraid to shut it down and try a new idea!

Twitter (www.twitter.com)

Twitter asks one question, "What are you doing?" Answers must be under 140 characters in length and can be sent via mobile texting, instant message, or the Internet.
TWITTER IS NOT DUMB IF YOU FOLLOW SMART PEOPLE.

Photo and Video Sharing Sites: YouTube (www.youtube.com) and Flickr (www.flickr.com)

Photos and videos can provide important visual messages, enabling issues to get on the public's agenda, providing an important frame to an issue, or simply drawing attention to a cause. YouTube has created an online video community. Flickr is a way to manage and access photos.

FACEBOOK AND MYSPACE: USING SOCIAL NETWORKING SITES (SNS)

The development of Web 2.0 has meant increased participation and media attention on virtual communities, most frequently in social networking sites (SNS) such as Facebook and MySpace. The impact that SNS will have on health policy is still emerging, but there are some intriguing early examples of the advantage they may hold for advocacy. For instance, Facebook is emerging as an important venue for debate about health policy, and not just among people typically thought of as policymakers. The health care reform battle sparked a huge number of for- and against-themed pages, such as Ohio Against Health Care Reform (81 fans), Wyoming For Health Care Reform (247 fans), and the perennial Facebook meme, "I bet we can find 1,000,000 people who support/oppose" health care reform. While measuring the effectiveness of such Facebook campaigns remains elusive, we should expect to see more of this type of activity as health care reform gets implemented over the coming years.

The promise of online communities and SNS for community health advocacy has captured the attention of major funders in health policy, including the Robert Wood Johnson Foundation *(www.rwjf.org)* and the Benton Foundation *(www.benton.org)*. In a unique joint venture between Robert Wood Johnson and Benton, in 2007 the two foundations launched New Routes to Community Health *(www.newroutes.org/)*. New Routes, a Madison, Wisconsin-based initiative, is an attempt to bring the power of a social networking site to bear on improving the health of immigrants. It does this through immigrant-created media and by funding other immigrant-led collaborations across the U.S. In each of these efforts, immigrants have worked to create locally focused media and outreach campaigns that speak directly to immigrants' health concerns in their area.

BUILDING COMMUNITY AND WORKING WITH PARTNERS

In the pre-Internet era, activists made use of existing technology to mobilize supporters through the use of "phone trees." One person would call ten others, and each of those ten would call ten others, and so on. In the digital era, cyberactivists use Web 2.0 to accomplish a number of different goals, including public representation of their cause through an online presence, information distribution to and solidarity with other cyberactivists, outreach to potential new supporters, fund-raising, and direct action (Costanza-Chock, 2003). With Web 2.0 technologies, social networks can be built, accessed, and amplified, particularly with features such as always-on connectivity. Taken together, these features allow tremendous potential to leverage Web 2.0 to advocate for change with cybertools that are constantly evolving.

ANALYZING MEDIA

The first obligation that all nurses have is to be knowledgeable consumers of media. Nurses must seek out factual unbiased information from many sources before taking positions on policy issues and be able to critically evaluate media messages, assess who controls the media, and identify whose vested interests are being protected or promoted. Nurses should add *www.mediachannel.org* and *www.mediareform.net* to their Internet favorites and evaluate their sources.

When nurses assess patients and families, they get information from many sources; assessing the media is no different.

WHAT IS THE MEDIUM?

The first step is to ask yourself where you get your information and news.

- What TV and radio news programming do you regularly tune in to? Do you read a daily newspaper or go online to a trusted news website every morning?
- What is the station's, program's, paper's, or website's reputation? Is it known for balanced coverage of health-related issues? Is it partisan?
- Does it cover national as well as state and local issues?
- Is it a credible source of information about health issues and policies?

These questions provide a basis for you to judge whether or not the information and news you are getting are credible and representative of a broad sector of public opinion. For any particular issue of concern, you will want to sample various media presentations of the issue and evaluate their messages and effectiveness.

WHO IS SENDING THE MESSAGE?

Part of understanding what the real message is about comes from knowing who is behind the message and why. You could interpret the real message behind the Harry and Louise commercials against President Clinton's health care reform legislation once you knew they were sponsored by the HIAA. If the legislation had passed, the majority of insurance companies would have been locked out of the health care market. Instead, their media success left them in control of health care in the U.S. until 2010.

For news media, ask the following questions: Who owns this medium? Who sponsors the website? What are the owner's biases? In addition, more and more newspapers and online venues are using the Associated Press (AP), or other major national papers, as their source for stories. The AP does not investigate; they attend events, accept news releases, and file reports. If newspapers are using abridged stories from other papers, the news slant or bias of the other paper reflects the bias or slant of the paper you are analyzing. As newspaper and television newsroom budgets get slashed, few news outlets are able to afford investigative journalism. To preserve this important aspect of journalism, non-profit investigative news organizations have arisen to fill the void, such as the online Kaiser Health News *(www.kaiserhealthnews.org)* founded and supported by Kaiser Family Foundation, and ProPublica, supported by a major multiyear commitment of funding by the Sandler Foundation. While Kaiser Health News is specific to health, Pro-Publica is not. Nonetheless, the latter does cover health issues. For example, in collaboration with the *Los Angeles Times,* it published a series of reports on the excessive delays in the California State Board of Registered Nursing's actions on complaints against nurses who were found guilty of drug abuse, sexual assaults on patients, and homicides *(www.propublica.org/series/nurses).* The reporting by Pulitzer Prize-winning journalist Charles Orstein and his colleague Tracy Weber resulted in the firing of the board members and resignation of its head.

WHAT IS THE MESSAGE, AND WHAT RHETORIC IS USED?

What is the ostensible message that is being delivered, and what is the real message? What rhetoric is used to get the real message across? In a protracted debate on Social Security during the administration of George W. Bush, his administration attempted to create a "crisis" of solvency that needed immediate reform. Economists and organizations such as the AARP were successful in pointing out that the government's own actuaries demonstrate that the Social Security Trust is solvent through 2042 and that the fund will begin to spend more than it is receiving only in 2018, so there is no immediate crisis. But Bush's messages also appealed to individual self-interest in talking about an "ownership society" and "private accounts," which are contrary to the purpose of the Social Security system, which was set up in 1935 to protect all of society—especially older adults, the widowed, and the disabled. Bush's message avoided talking about the Trust's solvency because his proposals actually contributed to insolvency earlier than what had been projected without any changes.

In 2005, pollster Frank Luntz of the Luntz Research Companies provided an analysis of the rhetoric used in the 2004 presidential campaign and outlined rhetoric that Republicans would use to win legislative battles and political campaigns in 2006. Luntz's analysis also provides insight into the language used to frame some of the major issues that would confront the federal Republican policymakers. For example:

> *Sometimes it is not what you say that matters but what you don't say. Other times a single word or phrase can undermine or destroy the credibility of a paragraph or entire presentation … [E]ffectively communicating the New American Lexicon requires you to stop saying words and phrases that undermine your ability to educate the American people. So from today forward YOU are the language police. From today forward these are the words never to say again. (Luntz, 2005, Appendix, p. 1)*

One of the words "never to say" was "privatization/private accounts." Rather, the document advocated the phrase "personalization/personal accounts." The report noted that "Many more Americans would "personalize" Social Security than "privatize" it. Personalizing Social Security suggests ownership and control over your retirement savings, while privatizing it suggests a profit motive and winners and losers. "BANISH PRIVATIZATION FROM YOUR LEXICON" (Luntz, Appendix, p. 1). Democrats were well aware of this difference in language and consistently framed the issue as "privatization." On health care, the document admonished never to say "healthcare choice" but rather to say "the right to choose," noting:

> *This is an important nuance so often lost on political officials. Almost all Americans want "the right to choose the healthcare plan, hospital, doctor and prescription drug plan that is best for them," but far fewer Americans actually want to make that choice. In fact, the older you get, the less eager you are to have a wide range of choices. One reason why the [Medicare] prescription drug card earned only qualified public support was that it offered too many choices and therefore created too much confusion for too many senior citizens. (Luntz, 2005, Appendix, p. 4)*

Every issue has "spin doctors" who develop believable messages based on focus groups and polling. As messages are repeated in the media, they become normalized and believable. It is essential to be attentive to the language used in media messages—whether delivered directly by policymakers, pundits, or advocates—and evaluate the credibility, bias, and intentions of sources. What and whom should we believe?

Images also convey important messages. As the Luntz document notes, "Language is your base. Symbols knock it out of the park. The American people cannot always be expected to directly grasp the connection between your policies and your principles. Symbols bridge this gap, so use them" (Section 2, p. 2). The document promotes the obvious symbols of the American flag and Statue of Liberty. But consider the symbols used by health insurance companies to advertise to employed individuals and families. These ads use pictures of healthy active adults and bright-eyed children. Health insurers have never used images of obese individuals or people disabled by arthritis to attract new members to their insurance products. These are examples of targeted media messages in which images are symbols to augment carefully crafted rhetoric to sway a target audience to believe or act in a particular way.

IS THE MESSAGE EFFECTIVE?

Does the message attract your attention? Does it appeal to your logic and to your emotions? Does it undermine the opposition's position?

IS THE MESSAGE ACCURATE?

Who is the reporter or cyberactivist, and what reputation do they have? Are they credible, with a reputation for accuracy and balanced coverage of an issue? What viewpoints are missing? Whose voice is represented in the message or article?

Box 10-3 provides an exercise for critically analyzing print and online news reporting.

RESPONDING TO THE MEDIA

One of the most important ways to influence public opinion is to respond to what is read, seen, or heard in the media. Letters to the editor or call-ins to talk radio programs can be powerful ways to reframe an issue or put it on the public's agenda.

Opinion editorials ("op eds") allow more in-depth response to current issues and provide a way to get an issue on the public's agenda. Although they are often solicited by a newspaper or magazine, particularly in large cities, local community papers are often eager to receive editorials that describe an important

---

BOX 10-3 How to Analyze Newspaper Reporting

- Get a recent copy of two or more national newspapers or review them online. Find an issue of concern, and compare the papers on their coverage of the issue.
- First, note where the article is placed. Is it on the front page of print and the mail page of the online version? Is it buried in a small portion of one column in the last section of the paper? Why do you think it received front or last, top or bottom page coverage?
- Second, note who wrote the article. The reputation of journalists can give you a sense of what bias might appear in the reporting, whether or not the coverage is likely to be balanced, and whether or not this journalist is known for in-depth investigative reporting.
- Third, what are the sources of information that are reported in the article? Every time a government official (e.g., president, other administration official, congressional representative, or staff) says something, highlight the passage with a yellow marker. This includes "anonymous high-placed public officials" whose names and formal titles are not included. Every time the source is nongovernmental, highlight the passage with a pink marker. With a blue marker, note every time a woman or a person of color is mentioned or quoted. Now compare these passages. The ratio of yellow to pink to blue suggests what and who are routinely considered most important.
- For health reporting, note how often journalists quote or refer to nurses as opposed to physicians. How might the article be different if nurses were a primary source of information on the topic?
- What is the focus of the story? Does it present all sides of an issue? Is the coverage confined to the politics of an issue, rather than the content of the issue itself? (Fallows, 1996)
- Do any photographs included in the article reflect the issue and the people involved in it? If it is a story on some aspect of patient care, for example, does the photograph include and name nurses who are providing the care? Or are only the physicians shown and named?
- Who sits on the board of directors of the newspaper or sponsors the website, and what interests do they represent? What is or is not being said in the editorials that might be directly or indirectly critical of these interests?

---

issue or problem, include a story that illustrates the local impact of the problem, and suggest possible solutions.

Tips for successful Op Eds include the following:

- Keep it short and within the word limit specified by the publication.
- Hook it to a national event if the publication or website has a national focus, or to a local event for local publications.
- Have a timely topic, concisely and clearly written in a conversational style, and with an unexpected or provocative slant.
- Include details or examples to bring the commentary alive.
- Define the problem and the solution(s).

Similarly, letters to the editor should be written immediately after the original story is published and follow the publication's guidelines for letters. They should be concise and make a specific point relevant to the article.

Calling in to talk radio provides another opportunity for sharing your perspectives. Remember to identify yourself as a registered nurse and to stay on the line while the host or program guest responds to your point or question. You may need to correct a misunderstanding or offer additional clarifying information.

Finally, it's always a good idea to contact a journalist to thank him or her for a good story. If you have a blog, be sure to link to the story in a post. If you see a Tweet you like, you can "re-Tweet" it to others who follow you. If you're on Facebook and like someone's posting, you can click on the "Like" phrase to register your approval and continue the viral spread of the posting.

CONCLUSION

Nurses have not always been taught how to use the media as a health promotion tool. But sometimes we have to teach ourselves how to navigate in this rapidly changing world. Certainly, harnessing the new social media will provide myriad opportunities for nurses to shape healthy public policies and engage in political activism. But use of traditional media can also help to spread a message.

This should come naturally to nurses since we're educated to interact in therapeutic ways and are often quite skilled in communicating with the public. In this new cyberworld, it's up to nurses to ensure that their voices are heard.

For a list of related websites, please refer to your Evolve Resources at http://evolve.elsevier.com/Mason/policypolitics/

REFERENCES

Abramson, A. (2003). *The history of television, 1942 to 2000*. New York: McFarland.

Annenberg Public Policy Center of the University of Pennsylvania. (1995). *Media in the middle: Fairness and accuracy in the 1994 health care reform debate*. Philadelphia: Annenberg Public Policy Center.

Arnold, M. (2010). Docs, nurses use social media for work. Medical, Marketing & Media. Retrieved from www.mmm-online.com/docs-nurses-use-social-media-for-work/article/166982/.

Bauder, D. (2007). For HBO executive, series on "Addiction" is personal. *Boston Globe*, March 14. Retrieved from www.boston.com/ae/tv/articles/2007/03/14/for_hbo_executive_series_on_addiction_is_personal.

Buresh, B., & Gordon, S. (2006). *From silence to voice: What nurses know and must communicate to the public*. Ithaca, NY: ILR Press, Cornell University.

Buresh, B., Gordon, S., & Bell, N. (1991). Who counts in news coverage of health care? *Nursing Outlook, 39*(5), 204-208.

Burrows, E., & Wallace, M. (2000). *Gotham: A history of New York City to 1898*. New York: Oxford University Press.

Costanza-Chock, S. (2003). Mapping the repertoire of electronic contention. In A. Opel & D. Pompper (Eds), *Representing resistance: Media, civil disobedience and the global justice movement* (pp. 173-191). New York: Greenwood Press.

Daniels, J. (2009). Cloaked websites: Propaganda, cyber-racism and epistemology in the digital era. *New Media & Society, 11*(5), 659-683.

DeJong, W. (1996). MADD Massachusetts versus Senator Burke: A media advocacy case study. *Health Education Quarterly, 23*(3), 318-329.

Dorfman, L., Wallack, L., & Woodruff, K. (2005). More than a message: Framing public health advocacy to change corporate practices. *Health Education and Behavior, 323*, 320-336.

Fallows, J. (1996). *Breaking the news: How the media undermine American society*. New York: Vintage Books.

Generation M2: Media in the lives of 8- to 18-year-olds. (2010). Menlo Park, CA: Kaiser Family Foundation.

Harris, J. (2005). To be our own governors: The independent press and the battle for "popular information." In Cohen E. D. (Ed.), *News incorporated* (pp. 79-95). Amherst: Prometheus Books.

Jernigan, D. H., & Wright, P. A. (1996). Media advocacy: Lessons from community experiences. *Journal of Public Health Policy, 18*, 306-329.

Lardinois, R. (2008). Obama's social media advantage. ReadWriteWeb, November 5, 2008. Retrieved from www.readwriteweb.com/archives/social_media_obama_mccain_comparison.php.

Luntz, F. (2005). *The new American lexicon*. Alexandria, VA: The Luntz Research Companies. Retrieved from www.dailykos.com/story/2005/2/23/3244/72156.

Manhattan Research. (2008). Cybercitizen Health™, v 8.0. Retrieved from www.manhattanresearch.com/cch.

McAlister, A. L. (1991). Population behavior change: A theory-based approach. *Journal of Public Health Policy, 12*(3), 345-361.

McCaughey, M., & Ayers, M. (Eds.). (2003). Cyberactivism: Online activism in theory and practice. New York: Routledge.

Nielsen reports television tuning remains at record levels. (October 17, 2007). Retrieved from http://en-us.nielsen.com/content/nielsen/en_us/news/news_releases/2007/october/Nielsen_Reports_Television_Tuning_Remains_at_Record_Levels.html.

O'Reilly, T. (2005). What is Web 2.0: Design patterns and business models for the next generation of software. O'Reilly, September 30. Retrieved from www.oreillynet.com/pub/a/oreilly/tim/news/2005/09/30/what-is-web-20.html?page=1.

Ozimek, T. (2005). Distributed campaigns: Using the Internet to empower action. In D. Mason, J. Leavitt, & M. Chaffee (Eds.). *Policy and politics in nursing and health care* (5th ed.) (pp. 171-176). St. Louis: WB Saunders/Elsevier.

Ritzer, G., & Jurgenson, N. (2010). Production, consumption, prosumption: The nature of capitalism in the age of the digital "prosumer." *Journal of Consumer Culture, 10*(1), 13-36.

Roche, J. P. (2002). Print media coverage of risk-risk tradeoffs associated with West Nile encephalitis and pesticide spraying. *Journal of Urban Health, 79*(4), 482-490.

Russell, A., Voas, R. B., DeJong, W., & Chaloupka, M. (1995). MADD rates the states: Advocacy event to advance the agenda against alcohol-impaired driving. *Public Health Reports, 110*(3), 240-245.

Sigma Theta Tau International. (1998). *The Woodhull study on nursing and the media: Health care's invisible partner.* Indianapolis: Sigma Theta Tau Center Nursing Press.

Talbot, D. (2008). How Obama really did it: The social-networking strategy that took an obscure senator to the doors of the White House. Technology Review (September/October). Retrieved from www.technologyreview.com/web/21222.

Turow, J., & Gans, R. (2002). *As seen on TV: Health policy issues in TV's medical dramas.* Menlo Park, CA: The Henry J. Kaiser Family Foundation.

Turow, J. (1996). Television entertainment and the U.S. health-care debate. *Lancet, 347*(9010), 1240-1243.

Wallack, L. (1994). Media advocacy: A strategy for empowering people and communities. *Journal of Public Health Policy, 15,* 420-436.

Wallack, L., & Dorfman, L. (1996). Media advocacy: A strategy for advancing policy and promoting health. *Health Education Quarterly, 23*(3), 293-317.

Whitney, R., & Viswanath, K. (2004). Lessons learned from public health mass media campaigns: Marketing health in a crowded media world. *Annual Review of Public Health, 25,* 419-437.

CHAPTER 11

Communication Skills for Success in Policy and Politics

Mary W. Chaffee

"You don't have to be a person of influence to be influential."

—Scott Adams

Effective communication skills are essential to advance policy initiatives and advocate for solutions to problems. Politics is the process of influencing the allocation of scarce resources. The act of influencing others occurs through communication. The process of influencing or persuading can occur in many ways, for example, in conversation at social events, through testimony, by e-mail, through social networking websites such as Facebook, and in meetings. This chapter will explore how you can communicate effectively—in person and in electronic formats— so your political efforts are more likely to be successful.

COMMUNICATION BASICS

Communication is simply the transfer of information. We communicate for specific reasons: to gather information, to direct, to educate, to provide feedback, to question, and to understand. The tools we use are spoken words and written symbols as well as nonverbal movements including eye contact and body movement. An important aspect of communicating is that we can learn to do it better and we can learn new communication skills.

PERSUASION

Being able to influence others, to orchestrate support, and to inspire trust and confidence are the hallmarks of political skill (Ferris, Davidson, & Perrewe, 2005). Communicating effectively is how those activities are accomplished. People's attitudes can be changed when they come in contact with information that alters their beliefs. This provides us with the opportunity to design the messages we write and speak in ways that can influence how people think. According to Perkins (2008), there are three ways to persuade someone about an issue:

1. Facts and reasoning (logic)
2. Credibility of the speaker (ethics)
3. Appealing to a basic emotion, need, or desire (emotions) (p. 145).

Speaking or writing to persuade is different from communicating to only share information. The goal of informational communications is to have your audience remember specific facts. The goal of persuasive speaking or writing is to have your audience draw a conclusion about information to get them to believe something or take action (Young & Travis, 2008). Persuasion happens over time, but you may only have an e-mail, a short meeting with a policymaker, or a chance encounter in an elevator to convince someone to take action. This means your spoken and written words should be clear, concise, logical, and, ideally, rooted in evidence. When you advocate for solutions to problems by attempting to persuade others to support you or join you, don't expect success each time. Rejection will occur no matter how effectively you make your case. Rejection can be difficult to deal with, but it demonstrates that you are working to solve problems and can provide you with guidance toward an alternative solution (Kush, 2004).

LISTENING: A CRITICAL COMMUNICATION SKILL

The listening skills that permit nurses to gather and process information from patients can be successfully applied in policy and politics. Effective communication depends on effective listening. Effective listeners exercise conscious control over listening and maintain awareness of the message, voice tone, and nonverbal messages. Effective listeners remain objective until the entire message has been communicated (Chambers, 2001). Effective listening includes being patient, being curious, and paraphrasing what has been heard to ensure that it was received accurately. Asking questions indicates the listener is engaged and interested (Patterson, Grenny, McMillan, & Switzler, 2002).

EFFECTIVE COMMUNICATION "IN PERSON"

FIRST IMPRESSIONS

When we meet another person, we instinctively assess, appraise, and form opinions within about 30 seconds (Boothman, 2000). It is important to recognize this instinct, especially if you are greeting someone with whom you want to obtain support from or assist you in your advocacy efforts. To make a good first impression, do the following:

- Make your first words count, and introduce yourself clearly. Repeat the name of the person you are meeting (this will help you remember the name, and people like to hear their own names).
- Smile and make eye contact. Let your smile reflect that you are glad to be meeting the other person.
- Face the person you are meeting. If you are seated, stand up for the introduction.
- If you're asked to make a name tag, write your name clearly.

ATTIRE

Are you any less knowledgeable or committed if you wear comfortable old jeans and sandals to a meeting with a policymaker? No. Will you be taken as seriously as if you had on a business suit? Probably not. When it is important for you to be perceived as a credible professional, a professional image is important. Take care with your attire and how you present yourself, just as you do with your language and nonverbal communication. Whether we like it or not, opinions are formed about us initially based on our appearance.

MINGLING AT SOCIAL EVENTS

Many people are uncomfortable attending social events where they know few people (or none). But social events that accompany business meetings, political events, or conferences offer many opportunities for networking. One way to consider these events, rather than with dread or fear, is to approach them with a plan to "work the room." RoAne (2000) defines working a room as the ability to circulate comfortably and graciously through a gathering of people; meeting, greeting, and talking with as many of them as you wish; creating communication that is warm and sincere; establishing an honest rapport on which you can build a professional or personal relationship; and knowing how to start, how to continue, and how to end lively and interesting conversations (p. xxviii). Working a room isn't a cold, calculated process, but it does involve some thought and care. Before attending an event, think about what it is you'd like to accomplish. Do you want to learn about a Medicare funding proposal? Do you want to meet people in your professional association? Do you need to find colleagues to work on a grassroots campaign? As you make connections that turn into ongoing professional relationships, or even friendships, you'll feel better about tackling the next event or meeting on your schedule. Working a room is a new skill for many professionals. Learn from others who are experienced. Watch what they do to move effortlessly between conversations and what they do to make people feel comfortable.

MAKING CONVERSATION ("SMALL TALK")

Your mother may have taught you that silence is golden and not to talk to strangers, but those rules are problems at social events (Fine, 2005). "Small talk" lays the groundwork for more substantial conversation and for building relationships. One of the most effective ways to communicate is to assume the burden of introducing yourself to others and initiating a conversation. Many people find it easier to attend social events with a friend; this allays anxiety. If you are alone at an event, consider that there are likely others like you who don't know other attendees. Take responsibility and initiate conversations with a greeting and an introduction. You may approach an individual or group, introduce yourself, and start chatting about a general topic (the weather, the meeting topic, the food). Some conversations will

BOX 11-1 Behaviors and Attitudes That Draw People into a Conversation

- Sense of humor
- Good manners
- Confidence
- Nonthreatening appearance
- Smiling and eye contact
- Starting a conversation rather than waiting for someone else to do it
- Knowledge of the subjects at hand
- Not taking oneself too seriously
- Fearlessness
- Respect for cultural differences

Adapted from Mandell, T. (1996). *Power schmoozing: The new etiquette for social and business success.* New York: McGraw-Hill.

become interesting, and others won't. Some groups will welcome you and include you in the conversations, and others won't. The more you try, the more comfortable you'll be and you'll know what works best for you. Box 11-1 demonstrates behaviors that draw people into a conversation.

ETIQUETTE

Etiquette is the set of expected behaviors in social situations that help make the situation go smoothly. Pagana (2008) describes in a book written for nurses how to make introductions and remember names, handle compliments and gossip, and deal with many other social issues. These are all situations where knowledge and comfort with the rules of etiquette make social interactions easier to manage. Being comfortable and competent with etiquette at meetings, when dining, and at work will enhance your communication skills.

NETWORKING IN PERSON

Networking can be defined as making contacts that may be valuable to you in some aspect of your professional activities. Networking is critical for nurses involved in policy and politics because most issues are advanced with the support and power of allies, colleagues, and those interested in attaining the same goal. Networking can occur in many places—at a social event or meeting, in a hallway, even when traveling or shopping. Sharing information is seen as a valuable benefit derived from developing a healthy network of professional contacts. Everyone

needs information—to learn about employment opportunities, to track the status of a legislative issue, to identify colleagues who share a common interest, or to influence a policy. Effective networking is based on developing relationships with "contacts," or individuals from whom you may obtain information, advice, or business. Always carry business cards, and keep the ones you collect organized and accessible. Jot down notes about conversations on the back of a card to jog your memory. The social role of networking cannot be minimized. It is much more enjoyable to tackle a problem, write a press release, or plan a campaign when working with a team of friends and colleagues than to do it alone.

BUSINESS CARDS

Your card is a vital networking tool—both the paper and electronic versions. Carrying business cards is important in fostering new connections; you won't impress new acquaintances by tearing a napkin in half and writing your name and number on it. As you collect business cards from colleagues, you may want to jot notes about the acquaintance on the card so you don't forget an important connection. Keep the cards you collect in a file so you can access a needed card quickly. E-mail systems permit the creation of an electronic business card that can be attached to your outgoing e-mail traffic and saved in an electronic file.

BRIEF BIOGRAPHY

Your brief biography can be an important tool to introduce you, and it can be an important networking tool. You may be asked for a brief biography if you are going to be introduced at a meeting or other events. It should be a concise (less than one page) overview of who you are and what you do. Be concise, write in the third person, and briefly highlight your major achievements (Sundquist, 2010). Templates can be found on the Internet. Read the biographies of others when you have the opportunity to locate people who may have similar interests as you.

SKILLS TO IMPROVE COMMUNICATION EFFECTIVENESS IN PERSON

ASK FOR WHAT YOU WANT

To make things happen—whether you are at a reception, a congressional hearing, or a meeting with your boss—you often have to ask for things. Whether you are asking for a budget increase for your unit or the support of a policymaker, there are several key points to keep in mind. Your chances of success will increase if you do the following:

- Say exactly what you want.
- Say exactly when you want it.
- Say exactly whom you want it from (Krisco, 1997).

A key word is *exactly.* The less precise you are in your request, the more chance there is for a less-than-desirable response. Make it as easy as possible for the person you are making a request of to help you. If you are asking someone to provide a letter of reference, bring a draft that you have prepared and offer to e-mail an electronic version. If you are asking someone to be the keynote speaker at a meeting, explain what you need and discuss how you'll make the appearance as easy as possible for them.

After you've made a request, there are several potential outcomes. The person you approached may do one of the following:

- Accept. Your request is accepted as is.
- Decline. Your request is turned down; a reason may or may not be provided.
- Make a counteroffer. Some aspect of your request is modified.
- Promise to reply later. The response is on hold. If you are met with this delaying tactic, agree on when you can expect a decision.
- Make a referral. You may be referred to another individual for assistance.

Even when you make a clear request, you may receive a non-response. Non-responses include "I'll think about it," "That's a great idea," "I'll see what my boss thinks," and "I'll look into it." These are all dodges or avoidance techniques. If you find yourself dealing with one, be respectfully persistent. "Does that mean you will do it?" or "I'd like to call you tomorrow to follow up on this issue." These comments send a message that you desire an answer.

SHAKE HANDS

A handshake is the expected business greeting in the United States. Greet a stranger with an extended hand, and shake hands with a firm, but not crushing, grip. At social events and meetings where introductions are likely, keep your right hand free in order to greet others quickly. Make sure to stand up or come out from behind a desk when greeting someone.

BE CULTURALLY SENSITIVE

Recognizing cultural differences is vital in communicating effectively. When you interact with others from cultural backgrounds different from your own, whether you are in the United States or traveling internationally, the key to success is respecting differences. Physical gestures and language that are acceptable in one culture may be vague or even offensive in another. Not recognizing or respecting cultural differences can lead to disaster in business and social communications. The following paragraphs describe general caveats that may be helpful in navigating the slippery slope of intercultural communication.

Gestures. Recognize that gestures and other nonverbal language mean different things in different cultures. For example, the traditional North American thumb and forefinger symbol for "okay" may be offensive to someone from Denmark, the Chinese do not like to be touched by people they don't know, and the Irish consider winking inappropriate (Morrison & Conaway, 2006). Take time to learn about the etiquette and behavior codes of other cultures if you will be working with or socializing with people from a background unfamiliar to you.

Handshakes. In some cultures, touching is a sensitive issue. In Europe and North America, the handshake is a welcome gesture, but this may not be the case in the Middle East, especially if you are a woman greeting a man. If you are traveling in unfamiliar territory, find out in advance what is acceptable and what is considered rude.

Personal Space. The British and North Americans tend to require more personal space and are more likely to move away from others if their space is "invaded."

Jokes. Be careful in using jokes to communicate with people from other cultures, especially if you are dealing with a language barrier. Jokes may not translate well and could be embarrassing.

EXPRESS YOUR GRATITUDE

One simple act can set you apart from others and demonstrate your exceptional social expertise: saying thank you. As you advocate for action on issues, request help from others, and lead others, it is vital to recognize the contributions and support you receive. Never pass up an opportunity to show your appreciation. When people extend themselves, they appreciate knowing that their efforts were recognized, whether the person is a U.S. Senator or one of your neighbors who helped stuff envelopes for a candidate. When you receive any type of significant assistance, send a brief thank-you note. A phone call or e-mail note will suffice for other efforts to assist you or help you advance a project. When you are writing a note to express gratitude, describe in some detail exactly what you are grateful for. Comment on why you are appreciative, and close with one or two sentences unrelated to the thank you. Try to avoid general remarks such as "Thanks for your help."

SPEAK EFFECTIVELY IN PUBLIC

Polls suggest that some people are more frightened of public speaking than of dying. Speaking publicly may be frightening (at first), but it can be a powerful tool in advocating for a specific issue or moving a project forward. You may not recall the first steps you took as a toddler, but odds are, you fell down. After some practice, walking becomes effortless. Public speaking may never be effortless, but with practice you can become comfortable and effective. You may not recognize it, but you have been speaking publicly all your life—from reading a paragraph aloud in your sixth grade class to talking about the work schedule at a staff meeting. To develop comfort and skill in speaking to audiences, start with some "low-risk" situations, such as speaking at your place of worship, presenting to a small group of colleagues in your workplace, teaching a class in your community, or even practicing in front of family or friends. Hone your skills every chance you get, then take advantage of speaking to more-challenging groups. Some suggestions for success include the following:

Practice. Plan your comments to fit the allotted time, and practice, whether it's in front of your mirror or with a tape recorder. Ask for feedback from a trusted friend. Consider learning the ropes with a group like Toastmasters International.

Keep Focused. Be clear about your objective and why you are speaking to a specific group.

Know Your Audience. What is the background of the people in the audience, and what do they expect from you? How many will be present? If you are speaking to an organized group, do your homework. Learn about them through their website or by talking to members.

Meet and Greet Your Audience. If you have the chance to speak with members of your audience in advance, it will be less frightening to merely continue your conversation with them from the podium.

Observe the Experts. Watch expert public speakers, and note what they do that works.

Watch the Clock. Do not go beyond your allotted time period.

PROVIDE AN EFFECTIVE BRIEFING

Providing a briefing can be a powerful method of influencing how someone views an issue or a course of action. You may have the opportunity to brief a leader in your organization, a policymaker, or a community leader about a health care topic. The following factors will contribute to successful briefings:

Know Your Topic. Really know your topic.

Present the Topic in a Concise and Logical Manner. It is called a "briefing" for a reason.

Be Prepared for Questions. But be able to say "I don't know."

Make Yourself Available for Follow-up. It will be helpful to prepare a one-page summary as a handout for your audience. It might be referred to as a *position paper,* a *decision brief,* or simply a *"one-pager"* (a one-page summary). It will reinforce your verbal comments and leave your listeners with a document to refer to. And writing the paper will force you to carefully think about the issue, consider alternatives, and make a case for a solution. A standard briefing paper usually includes the following:

- A summary of the issue
- Background information
- Analysis of alternatives
- Your recommendation for action
- Your contact information

DON'T FORGET YOUR NON-VERBAL COMMUNICATION

When you're speaking, don't forget the physical messages you communicate along with your spoken ones. Body language—the wide range of conscious and unconscious physical movements we make—can either strengthen your verbal messages or sabotage you. Because of the range of movements and subtlety, body language can sometimes be tough to interpret—and to control (Heller, 1998). However, in a business or social situation it's extremely important to monitor your body language and to monitor the nonverbal cues you receive from those who are speaking with you.

YOUR SIGNALS

You signal interest in others by maintaining eye contact, by holding a comfortable body position, and by not doing anything that signals your mind is wandering. If you want to continue a conversation, try to avoid fidgeting with jewelry, checking your watch, scanning the room, or constantly shifting position—these all indicate you are trying to break contact.

READING BODY LANGUAGE IN OTHERS

Be alert to physical cues that are being sent to you while you are engaged in conversation. If the person you are speaking with is maintaining eye contact and remains facing you, she is probably comfortably engaged and interested in continuing to speak with you. If you are speaking with someone who is looking behind you, checking the food table, picking lint off his sleeve, or backing up, you're being told that he is ready to move on and speak with someone else.

SEXUAL MESSAGES

Sexual body language excludes others from conversation. Nonsexual body language keeps conversation open and keeps you a part of the group rather than in a private, exclusive huddle. In business and professional situations, sexual body language is inappropriate. It can include leaning in closely to the person with whom you're speaking (which excludes others from the conversation); speaking in soft, intimate tones that discourage others from joining the conversation; and touching the other person or touching your own body, hair, or clothes (Mandell, 1996).

TOOLS FOR EFFECTIVE COMMUNICATION IN THE DIGITAL WORLD

Technology has transformed how, when, and where we communicate with one another. Just as with face-to-face communication, there are steps you can take that will help you communicate your position, recommendation, or request effectively. Having a professional "electronic" face will lend to your credibility and make it easier for others to communicate with you. While phone and e-mail use are common, using professionalism and courtesy when using them will set you apart from others. Newer means of communication, including social media, can be helpful in influencing others when used appropriately.

THE PHONE

Answer your phone with a professional greeting and your full name ("Good morning. This is Salvatore Shireman."). If you answer calls directly (without first being referred by another person), greet callers with both your name and organization ("Good afternoon, Frederick Research Center, this is Max Zangaro.").

- When you place a call, identify yourself and the purpose for your call ("Hello, Ms. Chanel, this is Riley Murray. I'm calling about the animal protection legislation you are sponsoring.")
- Return every phone call—quickly. Returning calls promptly demonstrates your respect for the caller and is always appreciated.
- If you must put a caller on hold, ask permission ("May I put you on hold for a moment?"). Use this feature only when it is absolutely essential. Don't leave a caller on hold for more than 30 to 60 seconds. When you return, thank your caller.
- If you are speaking with someone and are using your phone's speaker feature or your car's Bluetooth system, alert the caller if others are present that can hear what they say. This is a courtesy and will be appreciated by the caller.

Mobile phones can be problematic as well as useful. Despite widespread use over many years, mobile phone users should attend to some specific etiquette. It's easy to be rude with a cell phone (and this will not be helpful in your efforts to influence others). Annoyingly loud ringtones, loud conversations about personal issues, taking calls or texting when in the midst of a conversation, and texting while driving are some of the ways mobile phones cannot just be a problem, but can even be dangerous (Elgan, 2010). Many situations call for turning off a cell phone (or setting it to silently vibrate) so that it does not disturb others.

VOICEMAIL

If you use voicemail to greet callers and record messages when you are not available, record a clear and coherent outgoing message that lets callers know when they can expect to hear from you. The words you use and your inflection project an image to

To:	SenatorWashington@Senate.us.gov
From:	marydyre@email.com
Subject:	Support for Increased Funding for NIH Cancer Research

Senator Washington,

My name is Mary Dyre. I'm a constituent who lives at 100 North Street in Boston, MA.

I'm writing as a cancer survivor, and as a nurse, to encourage you to vote for increasing the NIH budget for cancer research. Research breakthroughs are changing the lives of people like me. I work on a pediatric oncology (cancer) unit and see how new drugs are giving children the chance to grow up.

I also directly benefitted from scientific advances when I was treated for cancer. Five years later, I live a healthy, productive life.

I hope you will support increasing the NIH research budget so their remarkable research can continue to benefit others. Please co-sponsor Senator Lincoln's bill, SB 1234, that aims to increase NIH funding for cancer research. It will make a difference in many lives.

Thank you,
Mary Dyre, RN

Subject line clearly identifies the topic

Writer indicates clearly they are a constituent

Writer indicates their credibility and knowledge related to the issue

Writer clearly defines what they would like the recipient to do

FIGURE 11-1 An example of an effective e-mail to a policymaker.

callers. Your outgoing message should include your name, title, and location, as well as a brief message to inform the caller when he or she may receive a call back from you: "Hello, you've reached Morgan Turcketta, Legislative Director for Congressman Hill. I'll be out of the office on August 12 but will return calls on August 13. Please leave a message and I'll contact you when I return." Change your outgoing message whenever your circumstances change.

When you leave a voicemail message for someone, summarize the reason for your call in a few sentences and be brief. A lengthy message can be tedious, and the recipient may hit the delete button before getting to the most important part. Make it easy for someone to return your call by speaking clearly when you leave your name and phone number. If you are a first-time caller, consider repeating your name and number.

USING THE FAX

The key to success with sending a fax is to ensure it arrives where you send it—and that the receiver knows where it came from. Use a cover sheet that provides your contact information so the recipient may contact you. When you send faxes, check the transmission record to determine if the fax was sent successfully. If you misdial a phone number and reach the wrong number, you know immediately, but the same is not so with a fax. Make sure you send your fax to the correct number. If you are faxing to an individual who shares a fax machine in a workplace, you may want to send a courtesy e-mail to let the person know that a fax has been sent.

E-MAIL

The Internet is a major thoroughfare for communications carrying millions of messages a day. Use an e-mail "signature" that contains your name and contact information. If your e-mail system offers an automatic response feature, use it to send an automatic reply to e-mail you receive when you will not be responding to messages. Figure 11-1 is an example of an effective e-mail. Crafting effective e-mail messages can be critical to your ability to influence others. When writing to a policymaker, government official,

Dear Secretary Salazar,

I love Cape Cod and I support Cape Wind.

I am a Cape Cod resident and a nurse - and I have great concern about our Nation's dependence on oil. The Cape is one of the most beautiful places on earth and is at risk from the effects of continued climate change. The Cape Wind project offers Massachusetts an opportunity to become a pioneer in clean energy. If approved, Cape Wind will not just provide a smart, efficient and renewable source of energy but will provide jobs at a critical time for our economy.

I've traveled through Europe and marveled at the beauty of wind farms - and at their ability to harness a completely renewable resource. Developing wind power technology is a smart choice for the U.S. The Cape Wind developers have demonstrated their willingness to adapt their plan, their sensitivity to the environment, and the cost savings for cash-strapped Cape communities.

Please permit Cape Wind to begin establishing their pioneering offshore windfarm in Nantucket Sound. This project can be a shining example of America's commitment to a clean environment and our ability to use sophisticated technology for the public good.

Sincerely,

Mary Chaffee, PhD, RN, FAAN

FIGURE 11-2 An example of an effective comment submitted at *www.regulations.gov.*

or someone in your workplace, use the following tips to create effective e-mail:

1. Be brief and clear about what you want.
2. Personalize your message; include your contact information and explain why this issue is important.
3. Proofread your message for errors and clarity.
4. Avoid anger, emotional pleas, and threats (Kush, 2004).

There are opportunities to submit electronic messages to influence legislation and federal decision-making at *www.regulations.gov*. In these electronic messages you have an opportunity to comment on legislation or offer your opinion on an issue being considered by a cabinet department. Figure 11-2 is an example of an effective message posted at *www.regulations.gov*.

SOCIAL MEDIA

In the beginning, the Internet (and its user interface the World Wide Web) was a pipeline that delivered information in the form of bytes between senders and receivers. Explosive use and sophisticated technology led to the development of Web 2.0—a much more social and interactive electronic world. Populating the Internet now is an array of social media that permits users to network, communicate, share, and interact in diverse ways. Social media can be used in advocacy efforts and to influence others about your point of view. Examples of social media and their uses appear in Table 11-1.

The growth of social media permits users to post their opinions, views, and responses to others in an environment where many others may read and react. When you post your opinions or write a blog, craft your posting with care, use evidence to support your opinions, and carefully proofread before you dispatch your posting for the world to read. Social media are being used widely in government and politics. CNN and YouTube partnered, as did ABC News and Facebook, to sponsor debates leading up to the General Election in 2008. Facebook has a full-time employee working on Capitol Hill to coach members of Congress and key staffers in how to use Facebook (Shapira, 2009).

Website. If you maintain a website, accuracy and currency of information is critical. Before launching a site, make sure all the content has been carefully reviewed as it will represent you to the world. Review content carefully or have a colleague with a sharp eye review it for you to catch mistakes. Frequent updates are important to bring readers back to your site.

TABLE 11-1 Social Media Examples and Their Uses

Type of Social Media	Examples	What It Is and What It's Used For
Blog	The Huffington Post *(Huffingtonpost.com)* Townhall *(Townhall.com)* Political Junkie *(www.npr.org/blogs/politicaljunkie)*	Publish opinions Respond to other's posts
Micro-blog	Twitter *(www.twitter.com)*	Social network that uses brief messages between users
Social bookmarking	Delicious *(www.delicious.com)* StumbleUpon *(www.stumbleupon.com)*	Permits users to save favorite websites so others can visit them and search websites tagged by other people
Social network	Facebook *(www.facebook.com)* MySpace *(www.myspace.com)* LinkedIn *(www.linkedin.com)* aSmallWorld *(www.asmallworld.net)* BigTent *(www.bigtent.com)*	Users interact with others via their profile (personal information page), communicate in groups, post photos, and use website widgets
Social photo and video sharing	YouTube *(www.youtube.com)* Flickr *(www.flickr.com)* Photobucket *(www.photobucket.com)*	Users post and share video and photos
Social news	Digg *(http://digg.com)* Reddit *(www.reddit.com)* Propellor *(www.propeller.com)*	Readers vote on the value of news stories
Wiki	Wikipedia *(http://en.wikipedia.org)* Wikia *(www.wikia.com)*	Interactive linked webpages; users edit posted articles

For a list of related websites, please refer to your Evolve Resources at http://evolve.elsevier.com/Mason/policypolitics/

REFERENCES

Boothman, N. (2000). *How to make people like you in 90 seconds or less.* New York: Workman.

Chambers, H. (2001). *Effective communication skills for scientific and technical professionals.* New York: Basic Books.

Elgan, M. (2010, January 22). Here comes the new cell phone etiquette. *ComputerWorld—Mobile and Wireless.*

Ferris, G., Davidson, S., & Perrewe, P. (2005). *Political skill at work.* Mountain View, CA Davies-Black.

Fine, D. (2005). *The fine art of small talk.* New York: Hyperion.

Heller, R. (1998). *Communicate clearly.* New York: DK Publishing.

Krisco, K. (1997). *Leadership and the art of conversation.* Rocklin, CA: Prima.

Kush, C. (2004). *The one-hour activist.* San Francisco: Jossey-Bass.

Mandell, T. (1996). *Power schmoozing: The new etiquette for social and business success.* New York: McGraw-Hill.

Morrison, T., & Conaway, W. (2006). *Kiss, bow, or shake hands* (2nd ed.). Avon, MA: Adams Media.

Pagana, K. (2008). *The nurse's etiquette advantage.* Indianapolis, IN: Sigma Theta Tau International.

Patterson, K., Grenny, J., McMillan, R., & Switzler, A. (2002). *Crucial conversations—Tools for talking when stakes are high.* New York: McGraw-Hill.

Perkins, P. (2008). *The art and science of communication—Tools for effective communication in the workplace.* Hoboken, NJ: John Wiley and Sons.

RoAne, S. (2000). *How to work a room.* New York: HarperCollins.

Shapira, I. (2009, December 30). Can Facebook, Capitol Hill be friends? Lawmakers learn social networking. The Washington Post, p. C01. Retrieved from www.washingtonpost.com/wp-dyn/content/article/2009/12/29/AR2009122901436.

Sundquist, B. (2010). How to write a brief bio. Retrieved from www.howtowritebio.com.

Young, K., & Travis, H. (2008). *Oral communication—Skills, choices, and consequences.* Long Grove, IL: Waveland Press.

CHAPTER 12

Conflict Management in Health Care: The Tipping Point Arrives

Phyllis Beck Kritek

"There is no power for change greater than a community discovering what it cares about."

—Margaret Wheatley

All human endeavors eventually find the participants differing, becoming oppositional about incompatible needs, drives, wishes, or demands. Conflict is intrinsic to human interaction, and health care environments are not exempt. This propensity to differ with an antagonistic response is familiar, dynamic, emergent, often surprising, and always contextual. The overriding context in the United States is germane: The emergence of conflict is often experienced as a threat.

In part, this can be traced to the central metaphor of our culture—one of competition, argument, and indeed war (Lakoff & Johnson, 1980). Within this metaphor is the unstated assumption that the person with the power "wins." The primary meaning of power—self-agency—has been culturally supplanted by the secondary meaning of power—dominance over another (Kritek, 2002). So, difference and disagreement can trigger a predictable sequence of threat, strife, discord, and defeat. We are habituated to conflict as adversarial, evoking both fear and defensiveness, often reactive.

Management also has a variety of meanings; it can mean both "directing with skill" and "keeping others compliant." Confronted with interpersonal volatility, we often try to do both, while concurrently managing our own responses. Managing conflict is always a challenge.

MANAGING CONFLICT THROUGH ALTERNATIVE DISPUTE RESOLUTION

It is within this context that the field of conflict resolution, usually referred to as Alternative Dispute Resolution (ADR), emerged in the U.S. ADR refers to a rich array of processes used by individuals and groups to resolve disputes, make decisions, or improve relationship outcomes. It is rooted in international diplomacy practices, the historic relationships between employers and employees (particularly through the union movement), and a variety of social technologies emergent from social sciences. ADR as a distinct practice and discipline began to flourish in the 1990s. In the first decade of the 21st century, it became "normalized" in government structures and corporations, often viewed not so much as an attractive alternative but more as a cost-saving option. It was cheaper than litigation. ADR educational programs multiplied and flourished. The U.S. health care delivery system, though, was unique in its resistance to this ADR expansion. That has changed.

I have worked for almost 25 years to build a bridge between my colleagues in health care and my colleagues in the burgeoning field of ADR. My motivation stemmed from experiential and anecdotal data: The conflict aversive and avoidant behaviors of health care professionals put patients at risk. Databased evidence was slowly building (e.g., Shortell et al., 1994), substantiating my concern. Our failure to manage conflict effectively was a threat to patient safety.

In the previous edition of this book, I briefly traced the history of ADR in the U.S., mapping the policies, executive orders, and legislative initiatives that have embedded ADR in governmental structures (Kritek, 2005). I also discussed the most high-profile approach to conflict resolution, the use of principled negotiation as the tool of choice. Principled negotiation is an interest-based approach that focuses primarily on conflict resolution. It is considered an "integrative" approach, one in which negotiations aim to create outcomes that meet all parties' essential needs and maximize benefits for everyone (Mayer, 2000, p. 151). The concept of principled negotiation was introduced in the landmark, now classic book, *Getting to Yes* by Fisher and Ury (1981; 1994). They also introduced the concept of "win-win" negotiations, drawing on game theory, the theoretical roots of much of the early conflict resolution research. These two authors and their colleagues were responsible for much of my early training in ADR, and hence this focus on "interest-based" negotiation shaped my worldview as it has many, if not most ADR practitioners. Newer models are now emerging.

ADR has increasingly been adopted as an essential resource in a variety of conflict arenas including labor and industrial disputes but also consumer, community, family, environmental, organizational, federal and state governmental, and international disputes. The primary focus of these initiatives was to create mediation options for disputants. These options could reduce obstacles to communication, explore alternatives, transcend adversarial behaviors, and address the needs of all parties. The assistance of a "third party," who was described as "neutral"—a mediator—helped participants through this process (Folberg & Taylor, 1984).

HEALTH CARE: THE LAST FRONTIER IN ADR

As ADR intensified its impact on all aspects of the U.S. culture, the health care community was generally disengaged and reactive. We gave lip service to the importance of collaboration while concurrently avoiding or suppressing conflict. Robson and Morrison (2003) posited that health care was the last big ADR frontier. They listed four health care characteristics that explain why it may be less likely to use ADR approaches in solving its problems. Specifically, health care:

1. is a complex adaptive system, which makes it harder to understand;
2. has widespread inequalities and imbalances of power, knowledge, and control;
3. has widely divergent "cultures" and value systems among the various professional and nonprofessional groups working within the system; and
4. struggles with the difficulty inherent in identifying the parties who should sit at the table.

There were additional germane forces in play. Reliance on litigation as a problem-solving device is a difficult behavior to overcome. Conflict avoidance was a normalized cultural norm. Leadership practices grounded in the exercise of power over others were equally normalized, though often denied. Health professionals did not welcome ADR professionals as helpful or valued consultants but as potential threats, requiring unwelcome behavior changes, manifesting a propensity for "naming elephants in the room" (Hammond & Mayfield, 2004).

In lieu of investing in ADR, the health care community invested in other related or contrasting services and programs. Ombudspersons addressed some of the concerns of patients and their families about care or experiences that they viewed as troublesome. The human resources division of many health care systems and hospitals integrated some cursory brief training on conflict management into their educational programs. Ethics committees attempted to address the moral dilemmas that confront health care providers today and provided reasoned reflection on options and opportunities. And, finally, the legal representatives of health care communities often viewed disputes as their terrain, where the use of the justice system was accessed embracing traditional approaches and models. All of these factors shed some light on the reluctance of health care communities to become active participants in ADR.

THE TIPPING POINT ARRIVES

The past is always prologue. "The Tipping Point" refers to the moment when an idea, trend, or social pattern meets a threshold that leads to rapid change. It was popularized as a concept through Malcolm Gladwell's book of the same name where he posited that "Ideas and products and messages and behaviors spread just like viruses do" (Gladwell, 2000, p 7). Gladwell suggests that three principles create the conditions for a tipping point to occur: contagiousness, the fact that little causes can have big effects, and that change happens not gradually but at one dramatic moment (p. 9). The U.S. health care community, historically resistant to ADR policies and practices, has reached this threshold of change. Health care communities are now actively exploring the possibilities presented by ADR practices due to the convergence of a cornucopia of forces and factors. Some of the most salient forces are described in the following paragraphs and provide context.

THE INSTITUTE OF MEDICINE FOCUSES ON SAFETY, CREATES A MOVEMENT

The Institute of Medicine (IOM), established in 1970, is an independent, nonprofit organization that works outside of government to provide unbiased and authoritative advice to decision makers and the public. In 1999, at the conclusion of a fractious decade in health care awash with downsizing, re-engineering, and hostile takeovers called mergers, the IOM captured the attention of the nation by publishing a report, "To Err is Human: Building a Safer Health Care System" (Institute of Medicine, 1999). This report documented the magnitude and severity of preventable medical errors, which they called "adverse events," and called for a shift from a blame response to one of finding causes and fixing problems. They provided an array of proactive recommendations to that end. And they catalyzed the patient safety movement.

Two subsequent reports by the IOM added to the impact of this report. "Crossing the Quality Chasm: A New Health System for the 21st Century" (2001) called for an overhaul of the U.S. health care system and further energized the focus on health care quality and safety. "Keeping Patients Safe: Transforming the Work Environment of Nurses" (2004) amplified the focus on patient safety by identifying the problems in health care environments that threaten patient safety and impact nursing care. The push for improved patient safety created a tipping point.

The Patient Safety and Quality Improvement Act of 2005 (Patient Safety Act) authorized the creation of Patient Safety Organizations (PSOs) to improve quality and safety by reducing the incidence of events that adversely affect patients. The Patient Safety Act authorized the Agency for Healthcare Research and Quality (AHRQ) to facilitate the development of a network of patient safety databases (NPSD) to which PSOs, health care providers, and others could voluntarily contribute nonidentifiable patient safety work products. The Patient Safety Act directs AHRQ to incorporate the nonidentifiable trend data from NPSD in its annual National Health Care Quality Report (NHQR), available at *www.ahrq.gov/qual/qrdr07.htm*.

These data swiftly revealed that one of the most consistent findings in emergent research focused on the inability of health care providers, individually and collectively, to collaborate and constructively engage in conflict. This inability became an underlying theme in these and related studies that could no longer be denied or ignored. Abruptly, the need to craft a new relationship model became apparent. After decades of purportedly supporting collaboration, health care professionals were confronted with a new meaning to their central ethos: "Do No Harm." Authentic collaboration and constructive relationships were not optional; they had become a moral imperative. The refusal to take action could now be viewed as a form of negligence and harm. A tentative bridge between health care and ADR communities began to emerge.

THE JOINT COMMISSION

The Joint Commission (TJC), previously called The Joint Commission for the Accreditation of Health Care Organizations, is an independent, not-for-profit accrediting body founded in 1951. TJC conducts on-site evaluations of over 17,000 health care organizations in the U.S. every 3 years to ensure that they provide "safe and effective care of the highest quality and value" (TJC Mission Statement, 2010).

Accreditation surveys are organized through established standards that health care organizations must demonstrate they have met; TJC standards thus carry disproportionate impact on health care organizations' policies and practices. Risking accreditation is risking a viable future.

TJC introduced new standards, effective January 2009, which focused on two new areas of concern: disruptive behavior on the part of health care professionals and the need for conflict resolution competencies as a component of health care leadership. Box 12-1 provides the actual language of the new

---

BOX 12-1 Joint Commission Leadership Standards—Effective January 2009 (Components Referring to Conflict Management and Disruptive Behavior)

Leadership Standard (LD 2.40)

Standard: "The organization *manages conflict* between leadership groups to protect the quality and safety of care."

Elements of Performance

1. Senior managers and leaders of the organized medical staff work with the governing body to develop an ongoing process for *managing conflict* among leadership groups.
2. The governing body approves the process.
3. The process is implemented when needed.
4. Individuals who implement the process are *skilled in conflict management.*

Leadership Standard (LD 01.03.01)

Standard: "The governing body is ultimately accountable for the safety and quality of care, treatment, and services."

Elements of Performance

- The governing body *provides a system for resolving conflicts* among individuals working in the hospital.

Leadership Standard LD.3.01.01

Standard: "Leaders create and maintain a culture of safety and quality throughout the hospital."

Rationale for LD.3.01.01

- Safety and quality thrive in a work environment that supports team work and respect for other people, regardless of their position in the organization.
- *Disruptive behavior* that intimidates staff and affects morale or staff turnover can also harm care. Leaders must address disruptive behavior of individuals working at all levels of the organization, including management, clinical and administrative staff, licensed independent practitioners, and governing body members.

Elements of Performance

- The hospital has a code of conduct that defines acceptable and disruptive and inappropriate behaviors.
- Leaders create and implement a process for managing disruptive and inappropriate behaviors.
- Relevant language is italicized.

Joint Commission Leadership Standards—Effective January 2009 (Components Referring to Conflict Management and Disruptive Behavior). Copyright © 2009 by The Joint Commission.

---

standards and/or performance measures now embedded in the accreditation process. These changes accelerated the engagement of the health care community in the possibilities of ADR in health care.

FRONT RUNNERS ADVOCATING FOR ADR IN HEALTH CARE

A less visible factor creating this tipping point was the efforts of a community of frontrunners who built bridges between the health care and ADR communities. Composed largely of health care providers concerned about the impact of conflict among providers and established ADR professionals eager to bring their competency to the health care community, this group has worked to integrate the expertise generated by the ADR community into health care environments. Scholars augmented this effort with useful documentation of the problem. Examples that had a significant impact on nursing included the seminal work of Alan Rosenstein, who documented the severity and dangers of disruptive physicians and nurses (Rosenstein, 2002; Rosenstein & O'Daniel, 2005), and Gerardi (2004, 2005, 2007), who has provided both the ADR and health care communities with thoughtful guidance in bridge building.

The frontrunners, of which I am a member, created ADR services relevant to health care communities. These included organizational and group conflict assessments, facilitation of groups, training of health care professionals in basic ADR, assistance with conflict change initiatives, mediation services, individual and group conflict coaching, and conflict systems design. Useful social technologies such as World Café and Mind Mapping were integrated into the services and adapted to the challenges of conflict and collaboration. World Café is a conversational process that uses structured principles designed to reveal a deeper living network pattern within a group. Mind Mapping is the use of a visual diagram to represent words,

TABLE 12-1 A Map of Levels of Discourse in Potential Responses to Conflict

If the Conflict Focuses On:	The Response Focus Is:
POWER: authority and competition	⇒War
RIGHTS: entitlement and adjudication	⇒Policy and Legislation
INTERESTS: needs/desires/hopes of all involved parties	⇒Negotiation
RELATIONSHIPS: inclusive, fair, respectful, and transparent	⇒Collaboration

Copyright Phyllis Beck Kritek, RN, PhD, FAAN.

ideas, tasks, or other items linked to and arranged around a central key word or idea.

Using these and other ADR resources, this group has also been instrumental in shifting the emphasis in health care ADR from interest-based negotiation to relationship-based collaboration, which is more congruent with the traditions and values of health care and essential to crafting long-term, systemwide collaborative practices and policies. Table 12-1 provides a visual mapping of the levels of discourse that emerge from the point of a conflict. Only ADR, which is grounded in relationship building and maintaining, can ensure collaboration as an outcome.

The international community of frontrunners has been loosely affiliated since their first gathering in Vancouver, British Columbia, in 2002. Since that time, we have continued to meet and work with Etienne Wenger to build our "community of practice … groups of people who share a concern, a set of problems, or a passion about a topic, and who deepen their knowledge and expertise in this area by interacting on an ongoing basis" (Wenger, et al., 2002). This model ensures that our efforts will be congruent with health care values.

This 2002 gathering and the subsequent interactions were organized under the sponsorship of Emerging Health Care Communities, Inc. (EHCCO), a community of practice led by Debra Gerardi, RN, JD. EHCCO's website (www.ehcco.com/) provides access to "Conflict Engagement Training for Health Professionals: Recommendations for Creating Conflict Competent Organizations—A White Paper for Healthcare and Dispute Resolution Professionals" (Emerging Health Care Communities, 2010). This paper provides a comprehensive overview of best practices to date in incorporating ADR training into health care environments and provides principles to guide decision-making.

NURSE LEADERS IN CONFLICT ENGAGEMENT

Nurses have provided critical leadership in advocating for focused attention on conflict among health care professionals. The American Association of Critical Care Nurses spearheaded the landmark study "Silence Kills" that identified the seven topics of crucial conversations that are especially difficult for health care professionals (AACN, 2005) and developed "Standards for Establishing and Sustaining Healthy Work Environments" in collaboration with some other national nursing organizations (Fontaine & Gerardi, 2005).

Nurses have created a robust body of literature focused on the nurse-to-nurse conflict characterized as "bullying" or "lateral violence" (Griffin, 2004; Woelfle & McCaffrey, 2007; Martin, et al., 2008; Johnston, et al., 2009). The Center for American Nurses conducted a national online survey of nurses (n = 858) to better understand how nurses experience conflict (Dewitty, et al., 2009). Fifty-three percent of the respondents reported that conflict while on the job was "common," the most prevalent being nurse-to-nurse conflict either with managers or peers. Following the study, the center initiated a well-developed program on preventing and managing bullying with useful resources about conflict engagement (www.centerforamericannurses.com).

Nurses are seeking basic and advanced preparation in conflict engagement skills. Nursing faculty are including conflict resolution content in course work. More hospitals are providing conflict engagement training for their nurses, particularly those in leadership roles. Nursing leadership programs have integrated such training (e.g., the American Organization of Nurse Executives [AONE] Nurse Manager Fellowship Program [2010]). The American Nurses Credentialing Center's (ANCC) program "Pathways to Excellence" requires that its participants have "non-adversarial, non-retaliatory, and alternative dispute resolution mechanisms in place to address concerns about the professional practice of healthcare professionals" (ANCC, 2009).

AND THERE IS STILL MUCH TO BE DONE

The most frequently used conflict research tool, the Thomas-Kilmann Conflict Mode Instrument (TKI), is designed to understand how we respond to conflicts. The TKI identifies five potential responses: avoidance, compromise, accommodation, competition, and collaboration. All are appropriate given specific situational factors (Thomas & Kilmann, 2002) The five responses parse degrees of cooperativeness and assertiveness, each offering both costs and benefits. All modes except collaboration lead to short-term solutions; thus their use creates the conditions for a repeat of the same conflict in the near or distant future. Collaboration is also the only mode that effectively merges cooperativeness with assertiveness.

Valentine (2001) analyzed studies conducted on nurses using the TKI. Nurses' preferred response to conflict was avoidance, followed by compromise and accommodation. The least likely response was collaboration. The three modes preferred by nurses are all either unassertive or only moderately assertive. Accommodation, the most cooperative of the three, involves neglecting one's own concerns to satisfy the concerns of others. More recently, Sportsman and Hamilton (2007) further highlighted the disconnect between nurses' commitment to collaboration and their likely responses to the conflict—ones that deter collaboration. This dissonance is heightened by the repeated assertion in the ANA Code of Ethics (ANA, 2001) that nurses will engage in conflict resolution.

While there is still work to be done, nurses have a distinct advantage because their educational preparation emphasizes the importance of relationships in health care. Historically this emphasis has focused on patients and families. Nurses are faced daily with conflicts surrounding care that involve the patient or family members. The same skills that are needed to respond to this challenge are needed to deal with our conflicts with our colleagues. After nearly 25 years of training what is now thousands of nurses in conflict engagement skills, I have learned to respect the "starter set" of skills nurses bring to ADR. But advanced skills are needed and can be acquired. The skill sets most critical to expanding our competencies are listed in Box 12-2 and provide a useful guide for planning systematic skill acquisition.

BOX 12-2 Expanding Conflict Engagement Competencies: Necessary Skills in Negotiation, Mediation, Facilitation, and Conflict Coaching

Expanding personal self-awareness
Being present and engaged in the process
Manifesting empathy
Unveiling and integrating your shadow dimensions
Monitoring for projection, inflation, and deflation
Owning your "stuff"; owning only your "stuff"
Acknowledging the other
Conducting a conflict assessment and analysis
Asking nonjudgmental questions
Actually listening to the answers
Reframing
Mirroring
Managing the process and timing
Option generation
Offering help
Agreement management
Managing closure
Disciplined self-assessment
Integrating humor

Copyright Phyllis Beck Kritek, PhD, RN, FAAN.

EMERGING INSIGHTS

The "tipping point" reported here intensified and accelerated the work of bringing ADR into health care environments. Our community of practice has refined insights into its collective work, identifying research needs and programmatic possibilities. Some of the most salient of these insights are listed here as a roadmap to the future.

1. In 2004, Bernard Mayer, one of ADR's iconic figures, introduced the concept of conflict engagement, which involves "accepting the challenges of a conflict, whatever its type or stage of development may be, with courage and wisdom and without automatically assuming that resolution is an appropriate goal" (Mayer, 2004, p. 184). This deemphasizes the expectation of resolution while supporting engagement in the conflict to do whatever is possible. Changing our language to capture this insight is an important shift that ensures ADR adapts to the world of health care, e.g., the competitive relationships between two service areas

may never be eliminated, but their relationships can be managed with civility and professionalism and collaborative initiatives can be initiated.

2. Conflict is very costly, and preparing staff to be competent in conflict engagement can have a dramatic impact on the bottom line. Analyses of the costs and potential cost savings related to conflict are needed to guide decision-making.

3. Conflict prevention is a burgeoning field that could be invaluable in health care. Training programs that include this emphasis will also generate real cost savings.

4. Although interest-based negotiation dominates the ADR literature, an emerging emphasis on relationship-based conflict engagement better fits the ethos and traditions of health care. Developing clear parameters for this style of conflict management is essential in ensuring collaborative relationships and teams. Shifting from "conflict management" to the language of "conflict engagement" is equally important as we blend the worlds of health care and ADR. By way of example, if a nurse manager merely "manages" a persistent conflict between two staff members, unconsciously using avoidance and accommodation, the high cost of the conflict will persist and most likely will spread and infect the entire unit.

5. Patient safety and quality care concerns catalyzed the shared initiatives of health care and ADR professionals. Safety and quality are system issues. Relationship-based conflict engagement competency is therefore not only an individual goal but an organizational goal. Collaboration can only occur in a conflict engagement–competent organization.

I would like to give Mohandas Gandhi, a model of nonviolent conflict management, the last word: "We must be the change we hope to see in the world."

Using Relationship-Based Conflict Engagement in Daily Nursing Practice: An Example

Margaret is a nurse with 22 years of OR experience. She has been appointed the Perioperative Quality Director and asked to implement the World Health Organization (WHO) Surgical Safety Checklist. She has initiated the process in collaboration with the Chief of Surgery and the Chief of Anesthesiology. Representatives of each of these disciplines have specific roles and tasks designated in using the checklist during a surgical case. The new policy includes a requirement that failure to participate in the procedure must be acted upon immediately by the responsible discipline's leader.

Jane has worked in the OR for 13 years, feels she is quite careful about safety, and thinks the new policy simply adds to her workload and is just "nonsense." The checklist policy requires that the circulating nurse function as the checklist coordinator, and must confirm that there are no particular problems with the equipment required for the procedure (instrument table, aspiration equipment, medical devices). Jane, serving as the circulating nurse, jokes about the expectation and does not provide the required verbal assurance before a scheduled case. Shortly after the case was completed, Margaret is told about Jane's behavior by the surgeon who witnessed it. Margaret realizes she must take prompt action and asks Jane if she could speak with her privately in her office. Jane agrees and walks with Margaret to the office while joking about how silly the WHO checklist procedure really seems to her.

This is an invitation to a conflict. Margaret can practice her recently expanded conflict engagement skills in a variety of ways. She can first notice her anger at this comment, and accept that her anger is her issue. She can decide that rather than ignoring the comment or overreacting, she can take a moment to focus, manage her own emotions, and then choose to engage Jane and stay present to her as she starts their conversation. She can recall that she is trying to honor a collegial relationship that can have an impact on what happens to patients in the future. She can try to see Jane's comment from her perspective (try for a moment to understand what might have evoked Jane's attitude). She can acknowledge to Jane that she knows that many times new policies just seem like more work when they are first introduced.

She can then try to reframe the situation, perhaps offering Jane more extensive information on the policy, including copies of some of the studies that demonstrated the positive impact of the checklist. She can ask Jane to tell her a bit more about what she is trying to communicate (why she thinks that the checklist is silly). She can then work very hard to listen to what Jane says and try to understand it, asking more questions not from a place of judgment but from a place of curiosity. She can watch for opportunities to ask Jane if she would ever imagine herself changing her viewpoint about the policy and what would change her viewpoint. She can even begin to imagine ways to make that possible and share them with Jane.

In the past, Margaret would have tried to ignore Jane's behavior and distance herself from Jane, or simply mandated that Jane comply. She would have spent part of her day ruminating on the behavior, increasing her anger and frustration. She might have told others about the comment, engaged in criticism with her peers, and increased the anger in the Perioperative Service.

She is now practicing conflict engagement. It is not easy, but it is creative, constructive, and will not only improve relationships, it will also improve patient safety and quality of the care. It actually takes less time and energy than her old practice of fretting and spreading discontent. She knows that she is not only practicing new skills; she knows she is functioning in a more responsible and professional manner. She has learned a new way to manage conflicts.

For a list of related websites, please refer to your Evolve Resources at http://evolve.elsevier.com/Mason/policypolitics/

REFERENCES

American Association of Critical-Care Nurses (AACN). (2005). *Silence kills: The seven crucial conversations for healthcare.* Final report cosponsored by Vitalsmarts. Retrieved from www.aacn.org/WD/Practice/Docs/PublicPolicy/SilenceKillsExecSum.pdf.

American Nurses Credentialing Center (ANCC). (2009). *Pathway to excellence organizational self-assessment tool.* Retrieved from www.nursecredentialing.org.

American Nurses Association (ANA). (2001). *Code of ethics for nurses with interpretive statements.* Washington, DC: American Nurses Association.

American Organization of Nurse Executives (AONE). (2010). *Nurse Manager Fellowship Program.* Retrieved from www.aone.org.

Dewitty, V. P., Osborne, J. W., Friesen, M. A., & Rosenkranz, A. (2009). Workforce conflict: What's the problem? *Nursing Management, 40*(5), 31-33, 37.

Emerging Health Care Communities. (2010). Conflict engagement training for health professionals: Recommendations for creating conflict competent organizations—A white paper for healthcare and dispute resolution professionals. Retrieved from www.ehcco.com.

Fisher, R. & Ury, W. (1981; 1994). *Getting to yes.* Boston: Houghton Mifflin.

Folberg, J., & Taylor, A. (1984). *Mediation: A comprehensive guide to resolving conflicts without litigation.* San Francisco: Jossey-Bass.

Fontaine, D. K. & Gerardi, D. (2005). Healthier hospitals? *Nursing Management, 36*(10), 34-44.

Gerardi, D. (2004). Using mediation techniques to manage conflict and create healthy work environments. *AACN Clinical Issues, 15*(2), 182-195.

Gerardi, D. (2005). The culture of health care: How professional and organizational cultures impact conflict management. *Georgia Law Review, 21*(4), 857-890.

Gerardi, D. (2007). The emerging culture of health care: Improving end-of-life care through collaboration and conflict engagement among health care professionals. *Ohio State Journal on Dispute Resolution, 23*(1), 105-142.

Gladwell, M. (2000). *The tipping point: How little things can make a big difference.* Boston: Little, Brown.

Griffin, M. (2004). Teaching cognitive rehearsal as a shield for lateral violence: An intervention for newly licensed nurses. *The Journal of Continuing Education in Nursing, 35*(6), 257-263.

Hammond, S. A. & Mayfield, A. B. (2004). *The thin book of naming elephants: How to surface undiscussables for greater organizational success.* Bend, OR: Thin Book.

Institute of Medicine. (1999). *To err is human: Building a safer health care system.* Washington, DC: National Academies Press.

Institute of Medicine. (2001). *Crossing the quality chasm: A new health system for the 21st century.* Washington, DC: National Academies Press.

Institute of Medicine. (2004). *Keeping patients safe: Transforming the work environment of nurses.* Washington, DC: National Academies Press.

Johnston, M., Phanhtharath, P., & Jackson, B. (2009). The bullying aspect of workplace violence in nursing. *Critical Care Nursing Quarterly, 32*(4), 287-295.

Kritek, P. B. (2002). *Negotiating at an uneven table: Developing moral courage in resolving our conflicts.* (2nd ed.). San Francisco: Jossey-Bass.

Kritek, P. B. (2005). Alternative dispute resolution: A tool for managing conflict. In D. Mason, J. K. Leavitt, & M. W. Chaffee (Eds.). *Policy and politics in nursing and health care.* St Louis: Saunders Elsevier.

Lakoff, G. & Johnson, M. (1980). *Metaphors we live by.* Chicago: University Press.

Martin, M. M., Stanley, K. M., Dulaney, P., & Pehrson, K. M. (2008). The role of the psychiatric liaison nurse in evidence-based approaches to lateral violence in nursing. *Perspectives in Psychiatric Care, 44*(1), 58-60.

Mayer, B. (2000). *The dynamics of conflict resolution: A practitioner's guide.* San Francisco: Jossey-Bass.

Mayer, B. (2004). *Beyond neutrality: Confronting the crisis in conflict resolution.* San Francisco: Jossey-Bass.

National Health Care Quality Report. Retrieved from www.ahrq.gov/qual/qrdr07.htm.

Robson, R., & Morrison, G. (2003). ADR in healthcare: The last big frontier. *ACResolution,* Spring, 1-6. Retrieved from http://mediate.com/articles/robmorr1.cfm.

Rosenstein, A. H. (2002). Original research. Nurse-physician relationships: Impact on nurse satisfaction and retention. *American Journal of Nursing, 102*(6), 2634.

Rosenstein, A. H., & O'Daniel, M. (2005). Disruptive behavior and clinical outcomes: Perceptions of nurses and physicians. *American Journal of Nursing, 105*(1), 54-64.

Shortell, S., Zimmerman, J. E., Rousseau, D. M., Gillies, R. R., Wagner, D. P., et al. (1994). The performance of intensive care units: Does good management make a difference? *Medical Care, 32*(5), 508-525.

Sportsman, S., & Hamilton, P. (2007). Conflict management styles in the health professions. *Journal of Professional Nursing, 23*(3), 157-166.

The Joint Commission Mission Statement. (2010). Retrieved from www.jointcommission.org.

Thomas, K. W., & Kilmann, R. H. (2002). *Thomas-Kilmann Conflict Mode Index.* Palo Alto, CA: CPP.

Valentine, P. E. B. (2001). Gender perspective on conflict management strategies of nurses. *Journal of Nursing Scholarship, 30*(2), 69-74.

Wenger, E., McDermott, R., & Snyder, W. M. (2002). *Cultivating communities of practice: A guide to managing knowledge.* Boston: Harvard Business School Press.

Woelfle, C. Y. & McCaffrey, R. (2007). Nurse on nurse. *Nursing Forum, 42*(3), 123-131.

CHAPTER 13

The United States Health Care System

Gail E. Russell

"No reform is ever complete. We must constantly keep moving forward."

—Senator Edward Kennedy

The U.S. health care system is complex and pluralistic. It is a mix of private and public initiatives and institutions that employ millions of workers in a myriad of settings to provide a wide range of health-related goods and services to the diverse U.S. population across geo-political environments that range from sophisticated cities to stretches of wilderness. The purpose of this chapter is to provide a description of this system and a framework for evaluation of the system for current and future reforms.

CHARACTERISTICS OF SYSTEMS

A system is a group of interacting people and processes that are organized for the purpose of producing goods and services and delivering them to the people who need or want them. A system openly interacts with its environment to procure raw materials and identify consumers of its goods and services and to respond to changes in need and demand, technology and innovation, demographic and economic trends, political realities, and natural and man-made disasters. Organizational and systems theories indicate that the effectiveness and survival of systems require continuous adaptation to internal and external factors. Systems must self-adjust to remain relevant and viable. If systems become too complex to function efficiently and effectively, adaptations falter, resulting in poor outcomes for the system and the population it serves.

Health care in the U.S. is an example of a very complex system. Its basic elements are patients, providers, and payers. However, the patients are diverse in age, education, social and economic status, and cultural/ethnic roots and include people who are: well but need routine examinations, screenings, health education/promotion, and guidance; experiencing critical illnesses or injuries and need extensive diagnostics and technology intensive care; experiencing common illnesses or life events that respond to routine interventions; experiencing chronic diseases or disabilities that vary in intensity and number and require monitoring and care over time; or experiencing terminal illnesses that require symptom management and supportive care. The health care providers are also diverse and include: institutions with a wide range of mission and capacity from high-technology diagnostics and interventions to homemaker services; clinicians drawn from multiple professional disciplines with different training and competencies; support services that range from the simple (e.g., greeters who welcome patients) to the sophisticated (e.g., diagnostic testing or information systems); and suppliers that provide goods and services that range from tissue paper to genetic material, from spiritual support to computer support, from paper clips to titanium replacement parts. Finally, health care payers vary widely and include: insurance companies that are regulated differently by each of the 50 states; various federal and state programs for special populations and the uninsured; individuals who pay out of pocket for premiums, services not covered by insurance, and philanthropy. Even these basic building blocks of the health care system are complicated.

Patients, providers, and payers interact at different times and with different motivations. Insurance companies seek to make money by designing benefit packages to market to individuals and employers and by managing benefits to enrollees to maximize patient outcomes and patient satisfaction. Employers purchase insurance packages for their employees to attract and retain workers. Individuals with insufficient knowledge of their future health care needs choose health insurance plans based on cost of premiums, co-payments, and deductibles. Individuals then use their health insurance to pay to visit an array of providers depending on the specific need for health care, the availability of providers, the nature and urgency of the problem, and even the time of day. Each provider has patients covered by many insurance plans, all with different benefits and administrative process for approving and paying for services. In the ideal world, there is synergy among patient, provider, and payer. In the real world, the variety and complexity of patient needs and health providers can lead to very disjointed service. Another real world fact is that up to one third of people under age 65 do not have health insurance and another 25 million are underinsured (Whelan & Feder, 2009). Uninsured people often delay treatment, become more seriously ill, and need more extensive and expensive treatments in more complex settings when they do present for care. And their care is financed by shifting the cost to insured patients, the insurance plans, and the taxpayer in a way that makes tracking the true cost of this care almost impossible.

EVALUATION OF THE HEALTH CARE SYSTEM

It is common to evaluate the health care system on three dimensions—how well it does in providing safe and effective patient care to the people who need it at a cost that is reasonable and equitably distributed; quality, access and cost. Several respected organizations use closely related concepts to define and monitor health systems performance. The World Health Organization (WHO) (2000) and the Institute of Medicine (IOM) (2001) use equity, efficiency, and healthy life years (Box 13-1). The Commission on a High Performance Health System (Commonwealth Fund, 2007) identifies six drivers of high-performance health care systems—again very related concepts (Box 13-2). These dimensions or concepts or drivers are interrelated and interconnected; changes in one dimension creates changes in other dimensions.

How does the U.S. health care system compare with industrialized counties on these dimensions of health care? In 2000, the WHO survey ranked the U.S. health system 37th in the world. The U.S. was 24th in terms of health attainment; 32nd in terms of equity of health outcomes across its population; and 54th in terms of

BOX 13-1	The Dimensions of Health Care Systems

Safety: Avoiding injury and harm from care that is meant to aid patients.

Effectiveness: Assuring that "evidence-based" care is actually delivered by avoiding overuse of medically unproven care and underuse of medically sound care.

Patient-centeredness: Involving patients thoroughly in their care decision-making process, thereby respecting their culture, social circumstances, and needs.

Timeliness: Avoiding unwanted delays in treatment.

Efficiency: Seeking to reduce waste—low-value-added processes and products—in all its forms, including supplies, equipment, capital, and space.

Equity: Closing racial, ethnic, gender, and socioeconomic gaps in care and outcomes.

Timeliness: Avoiding unwanted delays in treatment.

Efficiency: Seeking to reduce waste—low-value-added processes and products—in all its forms, including supplies, equipment, capital, and space.

Equity: Closing racial, ethnic, gender, and socioeconomic gaps in care and outcomes.

Adapted from Institute of Medicine. (2001). *Crossing the quality chasm: A new health system for the 21st century.* Washington, DC: National Academies Press; and World Health Organization. (2000). *World health report, 2000.* Geneva, Switzerland: Author.

fairness of financial contributions toward health care. There has been no progress on these issues.

According to the Commission on a High Performance Health System (2008), the U.S. health system gets Cs, Ds, and Fs on these dimensions and ranks last among Australia, Canada, Germany, New Zealand, and the United Kingdom (Table 13-1). These data propel the continuing health reform debate.

QUALITY

Quality of care is the degree to which health services for individuals and populations increase the likelihood of desired outcomes and are consistent with current knowledge. Quality care is collaborating with patients to perform appropriate assessments; make the most accurate diagnoses; implement appropriate treatments in the most convenient and efficient setting in a timely manner to maximize patients' outcome and minimize any pain, disability, and down time for patients; monitor the treatment and its effectiveness; and make any needed adjustments or changes.

BOX 13-2 Six Drivers of High Performance Health Care Systems

- Clinically relevant patient information is available to all providers at the point of care and to patients through electronic health record systems.
- Patient care is coordinated among multiple providers, and transitions across care settings are actively managed.
- All providers both within and across settings have accountability to each other, review each other's work, and collaborate to reliably deliver high-quality, high-value care.
- Patients have easy access to appropriate care and information, including after hours with multiple points of entry to the system; and providers are culturally competent and responsive to patients' needs.
- There is clear accountability for the total care of patients.
- The system is continuously innovating and learning in order to improve the quality, value, and patients' experiences of health care delivery.

Adapted from Commonwealth Fund Commission on a High Performance Health System. (2006, August). *Framework for a high performance health system for the United States.* New York: The Commonwealth Fund.

TABLE 13-1 Scores for the U.S. on Dimensions of High Performance Health Systems, 2006

Equity	71%
Efficiency	51%
Access	67%
Quality	71%
Long, healthy, productive lives	69%
Overall score	66%

Adapted from Commonwealth Fund. (2006, September). National scorecard on U.S. health systems performance; Complete chartbook. Retrieved from *www.commonwealthfund.org/publications.htm?doc_d=403925.*

Patient Safety. Patient safety is the freedom from accidental or preventable injury while receiving health care. Because health care interventions are complex, can be high risk, and are rendered to people when they are most vulnerable, extra effort must be directed to preventing injury or harm. Preventing avoidable harm or injury is the first level of quality. While the focus of patient safety is on adverse events and comparing rates to benchmarks, the need is for more innovation on effective measures for early detection and prevention.

Healthy Life Years. The goal of any health care system is to ensure that people lead healthy lives. Common indicators deal with aggregate data and include deaths that could have been prevented with timely and effective care; infant mortality; and healthy life expectancy. U.S. health indicators lag behind other industrialized nations in several areas (Anderson, Frogner & Reinhardt, 2007). In a comparison of the U.S. health care system to the United Kingdom, Germany, Australia, New Zealand, and Canada, the U.S. was last in delivering safe care, and next to last in delivering the right care, coordinated care, and patient-centered care (Commonwealth Fund, 2007). Half of chronic care patients in the U.S. do not fill prescriptions, get the recommended care, or see a doctor due to cost. In seven other industrialized countries, the rate is only 7% to 36% (Commonwealth Fund, 2008). Recognizing the interconnectedness of reimbursement policy to quality, experts recommend a shift in resources and priorities to primary care, care coordination, prevention, and wellness and a change in how providers are paid by rewarding care management and coordination, not expensive and unnecessary tests, images, and procedures—by rewarding the quality not the quantity of care services (Kaiser Family Foundation, 2009).

ACCESS

Access is the ability to obtain needed, affordable, convenient, acceptable, and effective health care in a timely fashion. Over the years, many federal initiatives have focused on access to health care. Some examples include: Hill Burton funds that brought hospitals to rural and new suburban settings in the post–World War II era; education and training for the health professions that not only provide access to professional work and status for financially disadvantaged students but also brings newly minted providers to medically underserved areas of the country; and Medicare and Medicaid legislation that provides health insurance to elderly and disabled persons and poor children.

Despite many initiatives, access to health care remains a serious problem. Although access has many dimensions in the current health care debate (e.g., geographic availability of qualified providers and well-equipped facilities, convenient hours of operation, and culturally sensitive providers), access is a euphemism for adequate health insurance coverage. Over 46 million Americans lacked health coverage for all of 2008, up from 45.7 million in 2007 (U.S. Census Bureau, 2009). In addition, the number of individuals insured by the government rose from 83.0 million to 87.4 million, while the number insured by employer-sponsored insurance declined from 177.4 million in 2007 to 176.3 million in 2008 (U.S. Census Bureau, 2009). Another 25 million American adults are considered to be underinsured with high out-of-pocket health care expenditures (Fronstin, 2008). Nearly 83% of the uninsured live in families headed by workers (Fronstin, 2008). Almost two-thirds of uninsured workers have an employer who doesn't offer coverage (Keehan, et al., 2008). Although the importance of health insurance cannot be underestimated, the Massachusetts experience with universal health coverage highlights other access issues, especially the critical shortage of primary care providers and urgent care and emergency services (Kaiser Commission on Medicaid and the Uninsured, 2009). (See Chapter 21.)

Equity. Equity bridges the dimensions of quality and access. The IOM (2001) defines equity as health care that does not vary in quality because of gender, ethnicity, geographic location, or socioeconomic status. In the U.S., persistent health disparities in segments of our population underscore this as a problem area. The U.S. Department of Health and Human Services (2008) defines health disparities as differences in the occurrence, frequency, death, and burden of diseases and other unfavorable health conditions that exist among specific population groups, including racial and ethnic minority groups. In 2002, the IOM reported that minorities are in poorer health, experience more substantial obstacles to receiving care, are more likely to be uninsured, and are at greater risk of receiving care of poor quality than other Americans. A recent National Healthcare Disparities Report (U.S. Department of Health & Human Services Agency for Healthcare Research and Quality, 2007) finds that limited progress is being made to eliminate health care disparities and that many significant gaps in quality and access have not been addressed. An increasingly diverse population demands that the U.S. address these disparities.

Another dimension of equity is highlighted by Wennberg's work on practice variations in health care (Mullan, 2004). Different practices are based on things other than patient need and standards of care. So how do patients know that what they get is actually good for them? Equity demands that patients have access to the right care.

COST

The cost of health care must be considered from several perspectives. For patients or consumers, cost is the price of purchasing needed health care goods and services and includes insurance premiums, co-pays and deductibles; out-of-pocket health expenditures not covered by insurance; taxes (social security, federal, and state) that support health programs; in-kind services such as caring for aging parents or sick children; and voluntary contributions to health-related charities. For health care providers, the cost of health care is the cost of producing health care products and services and delivering them to patients in a timely and relatively convenient manner. From a broader perspective, the cost of health care is how much the state or nation spends on health care; the percent of the total domestic production that health care consumes. Incentives and policy initiatives that address the "cost" of health may be beneficial to one, some, or none of these perspectives. When discussing cost, it is important to clarify what perspectives are or are not being addressed.

Because health care costs are high, different methods of financing health care have evolved. In the U.S., most health care is provided by privately owned organizations and is financed by private health insurance purchased by individuals or in many cases by employers for groups of employees and their families. This is supplemented by government supported or operated programs for special populations, such as people who are on active duty military service, veterans, Native American, disabled, mentally ill, elderly, or poor women and children. However, the government support of these programs varies widely and the budget drives how fully they are implemented.

Efficiency. An efficient health care system maximizes quality of care and outcomes within the resources available and ensures that investments in new programs and services yield net value over time (Commonwealth Fund, 2006). Efficiency is usually measured by the total national expenditures on health as a percent of GDP and the percent of those expenditures that go to administration or overhead rather than health care goods and services. Rapid growth in health care costs is a major problem facing the U.S. economy (Table 13-2). In 2008, the U.S. spent nearly

TABLE 13-2 **Actual and Projected National Health Expenditures, Selected Years**

	Expenditure in Dollars	Expenditure as % of DNP
1993	0.91 trillion	13.7
2005	1.97 trillion	15.9
2006	2.11 trillion	16
2007*	2.25 trillion	16.3
2008*	2.40 trillion	17.6
2012*	3.00 trillion	17.7
2017*	4.28 trillion	19.5

*Projected.
Adapted from Keehan, S., Sisko, A., Truffer, C., Smith, S., Cowan, C., Poisal, J., & Clemens, M.K., the National Health Expenditure Accounts Projections Team. (2008, February 26). Health spending projections through 2017: The baby-boomer generation is coming to Medicare. *Health Affairs Web Exclusive*, w145-w155.

17% of its gross domestic product (GDP) on health care. If health care costs continue to grow at the current rate, health care will be 25% of the U.S. GDP in 2025 (Whelan & Feder, 2009). This is not sustainable because more diversity in our economy is essential. In addition, because the government pays for half of all health services, health care usurps public funds from other important programs such as education, housing, and infrastructure.

The U.S. health care delivery system has issues in all dimensions. The current and future reform of the U.S. health care system must consider all these dimensions to be effective.

FRAGMENTATION IN CARE DELIVERY

One of the key factors behind these issues of quality, access, and cost in the U.S. health care system is fragmentation at the national, state, community, and practice levels (Commonwealth Fund Commission on a High Performance Health System, 2007, 2008; Shih et al. 2008; Cantor et al., 2007). There is no systematic assessment of aggregate health care need; no systematic design or development of needed services at the local, regional, or national level; no systematic evaluation of effectiveness of the current services against national norms or targets; and no systematic feedback to improve the quality of health care and assure both patients and payers that they are getting good value for their money. Nor are there local,

regional, or national entities to set policies or guidelines for the global health system. Rather multiple governmental agencies and health organizations manage segments of the health system without consideration for unintended consequences.

In addition, there is little patient focus to the system. Providers caring for the same patient work independently of each other. The patient moves among different providers for services that should be coordinated along a continuum but instead are disjointed causing frustration and many dangerous patient experiences. Poor communication and lack of clear accountability for the patient among multiple providers lead to medical errors, waste, and duplication. The absence of peer accountability, quality improvement infrastructure, and clinical information systems across providers and settings fosters poor quality of care.

Perhaps, the most fragmented part of U.S. health care is how it is financed with high insurance premiums, co-payments, and deductibles; high out-of-pocket spending for needed services that are not covered by health insurance; and high taxes for programs to care for the uninsured or special populations such as our veterans. Health insurance rates and benefits are regulated by each state, and there is wide variation across the 50 states. People who qualify for public programs like Medicaid—predominantly children and individuals who are disabled—receive health care services at modest cost sharing, but benefits vary by state. Health plans offered by large employers have comprehensive benefits, but premiums, deductibles, and co-pays vary across employers and have risen in recent years. Small employers, if they offer health benefits, do so at higher cost to the employee than large employer plans. People who are self-employed buy insurance from the non-group market generally at a substantially higher cost and with fewer benefits. In many states, non-group purchasers with pre-existing conditions can be excluded from coverage, charged higher premiums, or have benefits restricted (Kaiser Family Foundation, Health Research & Educational Trust, 2008). Finally, the employer-based health insurance model has created problems for workers and their families when changing jobs, during times of economic downturn, and when businesses make decisions to change health insurance benefits or plans or to close or move their operations.

These problems in health care are obviously complex and interconnected with business and government and multiple stakeholder groups with competing interests. For many years, the U.S. health system has changed incrementally through local market initiatives for health care services and legislation or regulation to address the most egregious problems for populations or groups. But this incremental reform has created a patchwork of programs with conflicting rules or regulations, eligibility requirements, incentives, and benefits and has increased the administrative burden for payers, providers, and patients.

THE TECHNOLOGY IMPERATIVE

Another key factor influencing quality, access, and cost in the U.S. health care system is the fascination of Americans with science and technology. What U.S. health care does well, it does very well. Patient and provider choice and the incentives in the U.S. health care system have promoted the use of innovation and high technology services. High-cost intensive intervention is rewarded over primary care, such as preventive medicine and the management of chronic illness. While specialty-based interventions are financially rewarded, both primary care practices and safety net providers such as emergency rooms are stressed beyond endurance (Commonwealth Fund Commission on a High Performance Health System, 2008).

HEALTH INFORMATION TECHNOLOGY

The expansion of health care information technology (HIT) is now driving many changes in health care. Health information systems include computer hardware, software, and communication devices that assimilate data, understand medical terminology, store data, and transmit clear communication. This technology creates greater operating efficiencies in three basic functions of health care: clinical, administrative, and financial. Used across health care environments (including homes, primary care and specialty care practices, hospitals, rehabilitation, and long-term care), HIT can facilitate timely and effective communication and promote patient safety and quality. Health care informatics is pivotal in the movement to cut costs and enhance patient care by implementing a standardized system for electronic health records, developing expedited systems for billing, clinical research, client scheduling, and the exchange of other health care information. With HIT,

valid and reliable aggregate data replaces anecdotal cases as the basis for decisions. Although relatively new health information technology is rapidly being disseminated, especially with the award of federal stimulus money and the requirements of Medicare regulations. However, there are problems. There is the lack of interoperability of the various information systems and the expense of purchase, migrating data to electronic formats, training personnel, and updating hardware and software. In addition, it creates divisions among providers with many older clinicians feeling challenged and uncomfortable with this new technology and with some well-funded facilities having more and better information technology.

SOCIO-ECONOMIC AND POLITICAL TRENDS

A range of socio-economic and political trends are also factors influencing quality, access, and cost in the U.S. health care system. There are dramatic changes occurring in the U.S. and the larger world that impact the need for health care and the capacity to meet this need. Perhaps the most significant is the *aging population*. For the next 50 years, this aging cohort brings increased incidence of chronic disease and disability; a smaller portion of the population who work and pay taxes; a smaller segment of the population who work to provide health-related (and other) services; and older adults in the workplace who may require more workplace accommodations. For health care workers, these may include job sharing to reduce fatigue, the use of new equipment such as bariatric beds and lifts to prevent injuries, and the redesign of work so that the accumulated knowledge of older workers can be shared with newer generations with accommodation for any physical limitation.

Another significant demographic is population shift with countries like China and India growing in both population and influence. As evolving industrialized nations assume a larger role in the world's economy, the prominence of the U.S. and its way of doing things is diminished. *Globalization* means increasing diversity in the production and distribution of health related goods and services. While the U.S. still attracts large numbers of immigrants and workers and students from other countries, it also outsources much of its production. Variations in products and services are likely and must be monitored. Increasing workforce and patient diversity, lower-cost drugs from Canada, and the distribution of health information (both good and bad) on the Internet are examples that have significant impact on health care.

Certainly, the *economic downturn* with banks and large and small corporations failing, unemployment rising, home mortgage foreclosures, government bailouts, and the U.S. debt and debt service rising threatens the status quo for the health care system. There is increased need for services but lower tax base to support programs to address this need. There is a limit to wealth and resources in the U.S., and health care and other programs are confronted with that reality.

Environmental issues influence health care need, including access to clean air and water; exposure to health hazards and toxic chemicals; natural disasters and their aftermath; and the easy spread of infectious disease because of the interconnectedness of our world. Other community resources (e.g., schools, transportation, recreational facilities, safe neighborhoods, and sidewalks) influence the quality of life in our communities and the health of individuals and aggregate health outcomes. How can a resource-constrained health care system maintain the flexibility to respond to infrequent but catastrophic disasters? With tax-supported public health programs and advocacy initiatives challenged by economic realities, how do we promote and maintain healthy communities?

Consumerism empowers people to make good choices about how to spend their limited resources on goods and services. Patients have assumed increasing responsibility for the management of their health and health-related problems. Access to good information on the Internet and patient education activities has fostered this movement. Building on this trend will be a key in the future health care system.

Despite Americans' desire for small government, there has been an expansion of the role of state and federal governments as provider and payer for health care services. Currently, the government pays for just under 50% of all health care. It is projected that the private share of national health spending will fall to 49% by 2018 and that public spending will rise to 51% as the oldest baby boomers enroll in Medicare (U.S. Department of Health and Human Services, 2006).

Health care is a significant component of state and federal spending and is a driving force in rising taxes.

CHALLENGES FOR THE U.S. HEALTH CARE SYSTEM

Some unique issues in the U.S. health care systems present special challenges at this time. Changing care models, the issue of waste, fraud and abuse, high administrative overhead, and malpractice in the health system are such issues and impact health care cost and quality.

CHANGING MODELS OF CARE DELIVERY

The U.S. health care system is rooted in an acute care model and does not meet the health care or economic needs of a nation that has as its biggest health challenge chronic disease among an aging population (National Center for Chronic Disease Prevention and Health Promotion, 2008). Almost 44% of the U.S. population has one or more chronic conditions; 20% report living with one chronic condition; 10.7% report two conditions; and 13.3% have three or more chronic conditions. The prevalence of chronic disease has risen by 32% among young adults age 20 to 44 and by 63% among midlife adults age 45 to 64 (Paez, Zhao, & Hwang, 2009).

The reimbursement system for health care in the U.S. does not support coordinated care and the establishment of a delivery system with appropriate capacity and utilization, especially for people with chronic illness. Several proposals for the design of new models of care to address this situation have been proposed including the Accountable Care Organization (ACO) (Devers & Berenson, 2009) and the Medical Home. An ACO is a local organization of related health care providers (primary care, specialists, and hospitals at a minimum) that agree to be accountable for the cost and quality of care delivered to a defined population. The goal of the ACO is to deliver coordinated and efficient care. ACOs that achieve quality and cost targets receive a financial bonus from the insurance company; those that fail are subject to a financial penalty. An ACO is able to do the following:
- Care for patients across the continuum of care, in different institutional settings.
- Plan, prospectively, for its budgets and resource needs.

- Support comprehensive, valid, and reliable measurement of its performance.

It is providers, not insurers, who are best able to make the changes that address cost and quality problems such as fragmented care, variation in practice patterns, and volume-based payment systems. Current proposals for ACOs allow flexibility in both the organizational design of the ACO and the methods by which providers would be paid so that local markets can address their known strengths and weaknesses.

Medical home was a term coined by the American Academy of Pediatrics in 1967. Now also called *health home,* it is an approach in which a primary care provider heads a team of professionals to provide round-the-clock access to care. Unlike managed care, in which primary care providers act as gatekeepers and the overriding goal is managing costs, in a medical home the primary care provider helps patients get specialty care when they need it and, through electronic records, keeps careful track of treatments and informs specialists of the patients' progress. The connections between the professionals who work on each case are seamless and convenient. Providers and patients have easy access to medical information, and patients with chronic ailments are called regularly to reinforce treatment regimens and see how they are doing. In whatever revised model of care is adopted, the emphasis will be on prevention and management of disease and disability with more patient involvement and more collaboration across practice settings.

CONTROLLING FRAUD AND ABUSE

Many identify waste and high administrative overhead in the current health care system as key factors in low quality and high cost. The U.S. Department of Health and Human Services and Department of Justice (2008) report annually on coordinated federal, state, and local law enforcement activities focused on *health care fraud and abuse* in the Medicare and Medicaid programs. In 2007, the federal government won or negotiated approximately $1.8 billion in health care fraud judgments and settlements. In addition, U.S. Attorneys' Offices opened 878 new criminal health care fraud investigations, and 1612 health care fraud criminal investigations are in process. A total of 560 defendants were convicted for health care fraud–related crimes during the year. Finally, the Department of Justice opened 776 new civil health care fraud investigations and had 743 civil health care fraud investigations pending at the end of the fiscal year. The health care system consumes vast amounts of public and private resources for the care of people when they are sick and vulnerable. Because patients are often unaware of the full costs of service and the health system is so complex, this scrutiny is necessary.

ADMINISTRATIVE OVERHEAD

Costs for marketing, billing, mortgage payments, executive compensation, maintaining buildings and grounds, and records management are higher in the U.S. than in most industrialized countries. The use of electronic medical records, standardization of benefits and claims processes across insurance companies, and other efficiencies are needed.

MALPRACTICE

The tort system in the U.S. enables patients to seek redress for alleged injury. Health providers owe a duty of care to their patients. Patients may attempt to recover from providers losses that result from breaches of such duty. This places the court in a position to deter negligent behavior on the part of providers and compensate claimants for losses they incur (including medical costs, lost wages, and pain and suffering) as the result of an injury that occurs because of negligence.

Critics argue that the threat of malpractice claims drives clinicians to order unnecessary and expensive tests and treatments and that unrealistic malpractice settlements drive up the cost of health care. The concern is that the tort system for claims of medical malpractice is too subjective. Many states have implemented restrictions on tort claims for medical malpractice, and Congress has considered nationwide tort limits. Limits on tort claims for medical malpractice could reduce both malpractice awards and malpractice insurance premiums (Congressional Budget Office, 2009). Lower malpractice premiums, in turn, reduce providers' costs and result in somewhat lower private health insurance premiums and costs for federal health programs.

HEALTH CARE REFORM

The current reform initiatives are broad-based system changes to address issues of quality, access, and cost.

This legislation, the Patient Protection and Affordable Care Act and the Health Care and Education Reconciliation Act of 2010 are focused on the pragmatic issues of health insurance coverage and how to pay for it. Long-standing ideologic differences made passing this legislation difficult and are likely to continue to influence its scheduled implementation over the next few years (see Chapter 63 and Appendix A).

The legislation makes a set of health benefits available and affordable to most people (Merlis, Dentzer, Haislmaier & Turnbull, 2010). Under reform, insurers must accept all applicants; can place no limits on benefits on the basis of pre-existing conditions; cannot use enrollee's health status to vary premium rates; and can use age to vary premiums only by a specified amount. As compensation for these concessions, health insurance companies have access to new markets—uninsured Americans. An *individual mandate* requires all individuals to purchase health insurance (Box 13-3). Employers are required to offer health insurance, so called *play-or-pay*. The cost of extending coverage to many of the 47 million uninsured is paid by subsidizing low-income individuals and small employers so they can purchase health insurance; imposing penalties on individuals and employers who do not purchase insurance; changing incentives in the health care systems to promote primary and preventative services while constraining

---

BOX 13-3 What Is an Individual Mandate?

The individual mandate requires everyone to have or to contribute toward health insurance. For an individual mandate to be effective, the insurance coverage has to be defined and must be available to everyone who is included in the mandate. Since some people cannot afford the full costs of coverage, financial or other assistance must be available. People who fail to obtain coverage pay a penalty.

Economic/Market Reasons for the Individual Mandate

Individual mandate is key to improving how the U.S. public-private system of health insurance works. Health insurance markets work best when everyone is insured because the risk of high medical expenses for a relative few is spread among a large and diverse group of people in the insurance pool.

Ethical/Moral Reasons for the Individual Mandate

If there is no mandate to buy health coverage, some healthy people will not buy it because they believe they will not need it. These people become free riders if they become ill and use health services. The cost of their care is shifted to the insured populations in the form of higher charges by providers that in turn lead to higher insurance premiums. When only sick people buy coverage because they know they will incur large medical expenses and use insurance extensively (adverse selection), premiums rise to cover costs. These premium increases cause healthier people to drop coverage or go to cheaper insurance

plans, leaving a shrinking pool of very high-cost enrollees in the plan. This is economically not viable.

With everybody in the health insurance pool, insurers eliminate such practices as medical underwriting that denies coverage or leads to dramatically higher premiums for sicker individuals; cancellation of coverage after enrollees submit claims for previously undisclosed illness; or coverage exclusions for treatment of pre-existing medical conditions.

Those opposed to the individual mandate argue that it infringes on personal freedom. Other opponents say it is unreasonable to compel people to buy insurance that they consider unnecessary or less important than other things they want.

Another objection is that the individual mandate won't make health coverage affordable. The benefit package will be too generous and the cost too high. Even if the mandate were initially linked to a basic, low-cost plan, constant pressure will expand the benefits. Since health care costs vary widely across the country, it is not fair to require the same amount of insurance nationwide.

Others argue that if insurance under health reform is a good buy for people, a mandate will not be necessary, because most people will elect to buy coverage. Whether health insurance charges are reasonable and its benefits are good depends on other factors in health reform. Reform health insurance first and see if people enroll before an individual mandate is imposed.

Finally, some opponents of a mandate are skeptical that it could be enforced.

Adapted from Merlis, M., Dentzer, S., Haislmaier, E., & Turnbull, N. (2010, January 13). Health policy brief: Individual mandate. *Health Affairs*. Retrieved from *www.healthaffairs.org/healthpolicybriefs/brief.php?brief_id=14*.

access to low-value but high-cost services; promoting coordination and collaboration across practice settings; implementing information technology to improve and monitor patient care safety and quality; and rewarding quality care and penalizing poor care and service.

BENEFITS

Defining the minimum level of coverage involves difficult tradeoffs between the level of protection offered to people; the cost to individuals, the government, and employers; and the degree of disruption relative to the insurance people have today (Emanuel & Fuchs, 2006; Lambrew, Podesta, & Shaw, 2006). The covered services for the minimum health plan must be specified. To expand Medicaid to those with low incomes, there is a need for clear policies on states supplementing federal matching funds to create coverage and specific cost sharing policies. A health insurance exchange—an organized, competitive market for health insurance offering a choice of plans—must establish common rules regarding the offering and pricing of insurance, providing information to help consumers better understand the options available to them as well as defining minimum covered benefits and structuring tiers of benefits (Box 13-4).

Play-or-pay requires employers to offer coverage to workers or pay a fee to the government to offset the cost of insurance subsidies. Minimum standards must be developed for plans to be offered by employers to include defined benefits and cost sharing and defined benefits and contributions toward the premium for workers and their families.

COST OF REFORM

President Obama and Congressional leaders demand that health reform be budget neutral. Any additional spending on health reform must be offset by new revenues or savings in existing government spending. The largest costs for health reform are subsidies to the uninsured of whom 65% are below 200% of the poverty level (U.S. Census Bureau, 2009). These subsidies can take the form of expanded public programs like Medicaid, direct financial assistance for the purchase of private insurance, or tax credits to offset the cost of health insurance. While adding costs to the federal budget, theses subsidies reduce the cost of health care for families. Other costs in the health reform initiative include: investments in

---

BOX 13-4 Functions of Health Insurance Exchanges

1. Focus competition on the price of coverage, and minimize benefit variation to attract enrollees
2. Organize covered services and cost sharing to make comparisons across plans easier for consumers
3. Provide consumers with information about plan provisions such as premium costs and covered benefits, as well as a plan's performance in encouraging wellness, managing chronic illnesses, and improving consumer satisfaction
4. Facilitate enrollment in a plan and payment of the premium for individuals and small businesses
5. Provide customer assistance around billing or access problems
6. Determine eligibility for and administer income-related subsidies
7. Make health insurance more portable for people moving from job to job
8. Coordinate enrollment shifts between Medicaid and subsidized private coverage for people with very low and potentially changing incomes
9. Facilitate changes in the rules governing how insurers sell coverage
10. Monitor market practices and administer uniform system for enrolling in a health insurance plan

Adapted from Kaiser Family Foundation (2009, May) Explaining health care reform: What are health insurance exchanges? Retrieved from *www.kff.org/healthreform/7908.cfm*.

---

infrastructure such as information technology; administrative expenses; and other subsidies such as assistance for small businesses to meet new requirements. The Congressional Budget Office (2009) estimates that health reform will cost $100 billion per year or $1 trillion or more over 10 years.

The financing approaches to cover the costs will fall into three broad categories that are bound to generate contentious debate:

Savings from Existing Programs Such as Medicare and Medicaid. Some of the saving proposals include: reducing payments to the private Medicare Advantage plans by moving to a system of competitive bidding; incorporating increases in productivity into Medicare payments to providers (pay for performance); reducing subsidies to hospitals for treating the uninsured as coverage expands; negotiating lower prices for drugs under Medicare; reducing readmissions to hospitals under Medicare; and higher Medicaid rebates from drug manufacturers.

New Revenues from Sources within the Health Care System. Reform will restructure the health system to raise new federal revenues. The play-or-pay requirement on employers will build employer-based coverage and increase revenue. Changing the tax treatment of employer-sponsored health insurance will yield substantive new revenue. Now contributions for health insurance are not taxed; in effect the government is subsidizing a portion of the cost of health insurance (Kleinbard, 2008). Capping the tax exemption at the level of the standard option plan will be an incentive to change health behaviors, encouraging employers and employees to move to less generous plans. Workers and their families will use less health care and pay more out of pocket for their care (Joint Committee on Taxation, 2009).

New Revenues from Sources Outside of the Health Care System. The proposals are many and varied. The Obama Administration proposes to cap itemized deductions for higher-income people and to dedicate these new revenues to a health care reform reserve fund. A House Tri-Committee proposal includes a graduated tax surcharge on income in excess of $280,000 for single taxpayers and $350,000 for families. There are also proposals for a values added tax and taxes related to lifestyle that could encourage healthier behaviors and decrease health costs (Emanuel & Fuchs, 2006; Lambrew et al., 2006). The Senate Finance Committee proposes a uniform tax on beverages based on alcohol content and a new excise tax on sugar-sweetened drinks.

Any assessment of impact of health reform will depend on who benefits and who loses, driven in large part by how it is financed—whether by additional taxes that people or employers must pay or savings from public programs that affect beneficiaries, providers of health care, and insurers. Researchers from the Urban Institute (Holahan, Garrett, Headen, & Lucas, 2009) used a simulation model to estimate coverage and cost trends between now and 2019 in the absence of health reform. Under the worst-case scenario, within 10 years the following would have occurred:

- Increased numbers of people without insurance—by more than 30% in 29 states; and in *every* state by at least 10%.
- Increased premiums for health insurance, more than doubling in 27 states. Even in the best-case scenario, employers in 46 states would have seen premiums increase by more than 60%.
- Less employer-sponsored health coverage. In half the states, the number of people with employer-sponsored health insurance would have fallen by more than 10%.
- A greater than 75% increase in spending for the Medicaid/Children's Health Insurance Program (CHIP).
- A doubling of uncompensated care in the health system in 45 states.

Given these predictions, failure to reform the health care system was not an option. In addition, reform will continue to evolve. Whether it is national or state by state innovations or driven by regional market-based initiatives, more health reform is in our future.

OPPORTUNITIES AND CHALLENGES FOR NURSING

Nurses are positioned to play a significant role in the changing health care system. They know the many forces that have come together to create poor health outcomes and rising health care costs. Nurses are patient-focused and have a unique perspective that can inform health system change. Educating themselves and their patients about important health system issues and engaging in reform processes are vital nursing responsibilities.

The reform initiative affords nurses a prime opportunity to collaborate with professional colleagues to redesign our health care processes to provide high-quality, efficient, and cost-effective care to all people in the U.S. Because nurses are often the last line of defense against poor care and costly errors, they have the best opportunity to improve systems of care (Lavizzo-Mourey & Berwick, 2009). The health care system needs highly qualified nurses in all practice settings to involve patients in their care management, to coordinate care across practice environments, to communicate effectively with patients and other providers, and to assess and monitor systems change.

Commitment to continuous learning, evidence-based innovation, and flexibility are the personal characteristics of the nurse of the future. The challenges and the potential benefits are great.

For a list of related websites, please refer to your Evolve Resources at http://evolve.elsevier.com/Mason/policypolitics/

REFERENCES

Anderson, G., Frogner, B., Reinhardt, U. (2007). Health care spending in OECD countries in 2004: An update. *Health Affairs, 26*(5), 1481-1488. Retrieved from http://content.healthaffairs.org/cgi/reprint/26/5/1481.

Cantor, J., Schoen, C., Belloff, D., How, S., & McCarthy, D. (2007, June). *Aiming higher: Results from a state scorecard on health system performance.* New York: The Commonwealth Fund Commission on a High Performance Health System.

Commonwealth Fund. (2006, September). National scorecard on U.S. health systems performance: Complete chartbook. Retrieved from www.commonwealthfund.org/publications.htm?doc_id=403925.

Commonwealth Fund. (2007, May 16). Mirror, mirror on the wall: An international update on the comparative performance of American health care. Retrieved from www.commonwealthfund.org/publications/publications_show.htm?doc_id=482678.

Commonwealth Fund. (2008). In Chronic condition: Experiences of patients with complex health care needs in eight countries, 2008. Retrieved from www.commonwealthfund.org/publications/publications_show.htm?doc_id=726492.

Commonwealth Fund Commission on a High Performance Health System. (2006, August). *Framework for a high performance health system for the United States.* New York: The Commonwealth Fund.

Commonwealth Fund Commission on a High Performance Health System. (2007, November), *A high performance health system for the United States: An ambitious agenda for the next president.* New York: The Commonwealth Fund Commission on a High Performance Health System.

Commonwealth Fund Commission on a High Performance Health System. (2008, July). *Why not the best? Results from a national scorecard on U.S. health system.* New York: The Commonwealth Fund Commission on a High Performance Health System.

Congressional Budget Office. (2009, June 16). Letter to the Honorable Kent Conrad, Chairman, Senate Committee on Budget. Retrieved from www.cbo.gov/ftpdocs/103xx/doc10311/06-16-HealthReformAndFederalBudget.pdf.

Devers, K. & Berenson, R. (2009, October). Can accountable care organizations improve the value of health care by solving the cost and quality quandaries: Timely analysis of immediate health policy issues. Retrieved from www.rwjf.org/files/research/acobrieffinal.pdf.

Emanuel, E., & Fuchs, V. (2006). *Comprehensive Cure: Universal Health Care Vouchers.* Washington DC: Brookings Institution. Retrieved from www.brookings.edu/~/media/Files/rc/papers/2007/07useconomics_emanuel/200707emanuel_fuchs.pdf.

Fronstin, P. (2008). *Sources of coverage and characteristics of the uninsured: Analysis of the March 2008 Current Population Survey. EBRI Issue Brief no. 321.* Washington, DC: Employee Benefit Research Institute. Retrieved from www.ebri.org/pdf/briefspdf/EBRI_IB_09a-2008.pdf.

Holahan, J., Garrett, B., Headen, I., & Lucas A. (2009, May 21). *Health reform: The cost of failure.* Princeton, NJ: Robert Wood Johnson Foundation and the Urban Institute.

Institute of Medicine. (2001). *Crossing the quality chasm: A new health system for the 21st century.* Washington, DC: National Academies Press.

Joint Committee on Taxation. (2009, June 2). Letter to Senate Finance Committee Chair Max Baucus and ranking member Charles Grassley. Retrieved from www.newamerica.net/blog/files/Exclusion%20revenue%20estimates.pdf.

Kaiser Commission on Medicaid and the Uninsured. (2009). Massachusetts health care reform: Three years later. Retrieved from www.kff.org/uninsured/upload/7777-02.pdf.

Kaiser Family Foundation. (2008). 2008 Presidential candidate health care proposals: Side-by-side summary. Retrieved from www.health08.org/sidebyside_results.cfm?c=5&c=16.

Kaiser Family Foundation. (2009, May). Explaining health care reform: What are health insurance exchanges? Retrieved from www.kff.org/healthreform/7908.cfm.

Kaiser Family Foundation, Health Research & Educational Trust. (2008). Employer Health Benefits Survey, 2008. Retrieved from www.kff.org/insurance/7790.

Keehan, S., Sisko, A., Truffer, C., Smith, S., Cowan, C., Poisal, J., & Clemens, M. K., the National Health Expenditure Accounts Projections Team. (2008, February 26). Health spending projections through 2017: The baby-boomer generation is coming to Medicare. Health Affairs Web Exclusive, w145-w155.

Kleinbard, E. (2008, July 31). Testimony for Senate Finance Committee Hearing: Health benefits in the tax code: The right incentives. Retrieved from www.jct.gov/publications.html?func=startdown&id=1194.

Lambrew, J. M., Podesta, J. D., & Shaw, T. L. (2006). Change in challenging times: A plan for extending and improving health coverage. Health Affairs Web Exclusive, w5-119–w5-132.

Lavizzo-Mourey, R., & Berwick, D. (2009). Nurses transforming care. *American Journal of Nursing, 109*(11 Supplement), 3.

Merlis, M., Dentzer, S., Haislmaier, E., & Turnbull, N. (2010, January 13). Health policy brief: Individual mandate, Health Affairs. Retrieved from www.healthaffairs.org/healthpolicybriefs/brief.php?brief_id=14.

Mullan, F. (2004, October 7). Wrestling with variation: An interview with Jack Wennberg. Health Affairs. Retrieved from http://content.healthaffairs.org/cgi/content/full/hthaff.var.73/DC2.

National Center for Chronic Disease Prevention and Health Promotion. (2008, March 20). *Chronic disease overview.* Atlanta, GA: Centers for Disease Control and Prevention. Retrieved from www.cdc.gov/nccdphp/overview.htm#related.

Paez, K., Zhao, L. & Hwang, W. (2009). Rising out-of-pocket spending for chronic conditions: A ten-year trend. *Health Affairs, 28*(1), 15-25.

Schoen, C. et al. (2008). How many are underinsured? Trends among U.S. adults, 2003 and 2007. The Commonwealth Fund, 102. Retrieved from www.commonwealthfund.org/Content/Publications/In-the-Literature/2008/Jun/How-Many-Are-Underinsured--Trends-Among-U-S–Adults–2003-and-2007.aspx.

Shih, A., Davis, K., Schoenbaum, S., Gauthier, A., Nuzum, R., & McCarthy, D. (2008, August). *Organizing the U.S. health care delivery system for high performance.* New York: Commonwealth Fund Commission on a High Performance Health System.

U.S. Census Bureau. (2008, August). Income, poverty, and health insurance coverage in the United States: 2007. Current population survey. Retrieved from http://factfinder.census.gov/home/saff/aff_acs2008_quickguide.pdf.

U.S. Census Bureau. (2009). Table HIA-1. Health insurance coverage status and type of coverage by sex, race and hispanic origin: 1999 to 2008. Retrieved from www.census.gov/hhes/www/hlthins/historic/hihistt1.xls.

U.S. Department of Health and Human Services, Agency for Healthcare Research and Quality. (2006). Medical Expenditure Panel Survey (MEPS). Retrieved from www.meps.ahrq.gov/mepsweb/survey_comp/household.jsp.

U.S. Department of Health & Human Services, Agency for Healthcare Research and Quality. (2007). National healthcare disparities report. Retrieved from www.ahrq.gov/qual/qrdr07.htm.

U.S. Department of Health and Human Services and Department of Justice. (2008, November). *Health Care Fraud and Abuse Control Program annual* report for FY 2007. Washington DC: Author. Retrieved from http://oig.hhs.gov/publications/docs/hcfac/hcfacreport2007.pdf.

Whelan, E., & Feder, J. (2009, June). *Payment reform to improve health care: Ways to move forward.* Washington DC: Center for American Progress. Retrieved from www.americanprogress.org.

World Health Organization. (2000). *World health report, 2000.* Geneva, Switzerland: Author.

CHAPTER 14

Financing Health Care in the United States

Joyce A. Pulcini and Mary Ann Hart

"When any human being is denied a life of dignity and respect, no matter whether they live in Anacostia or Appalachia or a village in Africa; when people are trapped in extreme poverty or are suffering from diseases we know how to prevent; when they're going without the medicines that they so desperately need—we have more work to do."

—Barack Obama speech at 99th
NAACP Convention, July 12, 2008

Health care financing is a central issue in every discussion on problems in the health system—and was a primary driver in the 2010 health care reform legislation. The cost of health care continues to rise with poorer outcomes over the past 30 years. An aging population and the demands for chronic care are having a major impact on increasing costs. This chapter will provide a historical perspective focusing on how and why our current system has evolved to this point. The new model for health care reform will be discussed and summarized in light of evolving trends in health care financing and system design.

HISTORICAL PERSPECTIVES

Some dominant values underpin the U.S. political and economic systems. The U.S. has a long history of individualism, an emphasis on freedom to choose alternatives, and an aversion to large-scale government intervention into the private realm . Compared to other developed nations with capitalist economies, social programs have been the exception rather than the rule and have been adopted primarily during times of great need or social and political upheaval, such as in the 1930s and 1960s. Because health care in the U.S. had its origins in the private sector, partly because of the power of physicians, hospitals, and

insurance companies, the degree to which government should be involved in health care remains controversial. Unlike other developed capitalist countries, such as Canada, the United Kingdom, France, Germany, and Switzerland, where health care is viewed as a right and considered a social good that should be available to all, the U.S. has viewed health care as a market-based commodity, readily available to those who can pay for it.

The debate over the role of government in social programs was heightened in the decades after the great depression. While the Social Security Act of 1935 brought sweeping social welfare legislation, which provided for social security payments; workman's compensation; welfare assistance for the poor; and certain public health, maternal, and child health services, it did not provide for health care coverage for all Americans. Also, during the decade following the Great Depression in the 1930s, Blue Cross and Blue Shield (BC/BS) were developed as private insurance plans to cover hospital and physician care. The rationale that persons should pay for their medical care before they actually got sick ensured some level of security for both providers and consumers of medical services. The creation of these insurance plans effectively defused a strong political movement toward legislating a broader, compulsory government-run health insurance plan at the time (Starr, 1982). After a failed attempt by President Truman in the late 1940s to provide Americans with a national health plan, no movement occurred on this issue until the 1960s, when Medicare and Medicaid were developed.

BC/BS dominated the health insurance industry until the 1950s, when commercial insurance companies entered the market and were able to compete with BC/BS by holding down costs through excluding sicker people from insurance coverage. Over time, the distinction between BC/BS and commercial insurance companies became increasingly blurred as BC/BS offered competitive for-profit plans (Jonas & Kovner, 2005). In the 1960s, the U.S. enjoyed relative prosperity, along with a burgeoning social conscience, an appetite for change that led to a heightened concern for the poor and elderly and the impact of catastrophic illness. In response, Medicaid and Medicare, two separate but related programs, were created in 1965 by amendments to the Social Security Act. Medicare is a federal government–administered health insurance program for the disabled and those over 65, and Medicaid is a state and federal government administered health insurance program for low-income people within certain categories.

THE PROBLEM OF CONTINUAL RISING COSTS

Since the 1970s, continually rising health care costs and insurance premiums have strained government budgets, become a costly expense to businesses that offer health insurance to their employees, and put health care increasingly out of reach for individuals and families. Figure 14-1 depicts the costs of health care from 1960 to 2008 (Kaiser Family Foundation [KFF], 2010d). Stakeholders in small and large businesses, government, organized labor, health care providers, and consumer groups have convened over the years to tackle the problem of rising health care costs, with little lasting success. Appendix A provides a more thorough discussion of the Affordable Care Act, its implementation as of mid-2013, and the implications for nursing.

A range of strategies have been used to curb rising health care costs over the last 40 years. Health care expenditures as a percentage of the gross domestic product (GDP) have been increasing steadily. National health care spending reached $2.5 trillion in 2009, accounting for 17.6% of the GDP. By 2018, national health spending is expected to reach $4.4 trillion if costs are not controlled, and national health expenditures are projected to rise 6.2 percent per year as compared to a general GDP increase of 4.1% (Siska et al., 2009). Another example of increased costs is the fact that all other industrialized countries spend significantly less on health care. For example, in 2009, health care costs per capita in the U.S. were $7290 or 16% of GDP, compared to the next highest, Norway, whose comparable costs are $4763 or 11% of GDP continuing our country's rank as number one for cost per person among industrialized nations (KFF, 2009; OECD, 2009).

Economic factors also impact health care costs and services. During the Clinton administration, universal health care legislation was introduced and failed. From 1995 to 2001, the U.S. experienced a booming economy and an unprecedented budget surplus after years of budget deficits under previous Republican administrations. In 2001, Congress approved a $1.35 trillion tax cut for higher-income Americans as recommended by President George W. Bush. This tax

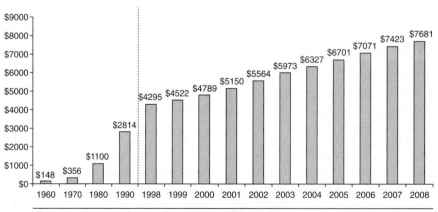

FIGURE 14-1 National health expenditures per capita and their share of gross domestic product, 1960-2008. (Source: Centers for Medicare and Medicaid Services, Office of the Actuary, National Health Statistics Group. From Kaiser Family Foundation. [2010]. National health expenditures per capita and their share of gross domestic product, 1960-2008. Retrieved from *http://facts.kff.org/chart.aspx?ch=854.*)

cut, along with a weakening economy made worse by the impact of the terrorist attacks of September 11, 2001, plunged the U.S. into another recession. Concerns rose regarding the solvency of Medicare, the Social Security system, and an inability to contain rising health care costs.

Only about 60% of firms offered health benefits in 2009 compared to 63% in 2008. While 98% of large firms offered health insurance to employees, only 59% of small firms offered it in 2009 (KFF, HRET, 2009). Only 52% of people in the U.S. were covered by employer-based health insurance compared to 66% in 1999, with over 90% of these enrolled in a managed care organization (MCO) (KFF & HRET, 2009, p. 5; KFF, 2010b). The recession of 2008 only exacerbated the replacement of full-time jobs with health benefits to part-time jobs without health benefits, leaving more Americans uninsured. Massachusetts, in its 2006 state health reform law, has reaffirmed the responsibility of employers to provide health insurance to employees or pay a penalty fee. Establishing the concept of "shared responsibility," it also was the first state to institute an individual mandate requiring individuals to have health insurance or pay a tax penalty.

Another option for health care reform that is being debated is employer mandates. Rising health care costs continue to impact both citizens and employers who provide health insurance for their employees. From 1999 to 2009, average health insurance premiums increased 131% and average worker contributions increased 128% over that time period, an amount much higher than inflation, which was 31.44% (KFF, 2009). The burden of higher premiums falls most heavily on those with lower incomes and on small businesses. Disproportionate shares of health care costs also fall on lower-income people further exacerbating the problem of inequities.

WHY ARE COSTS RISING?

Multiple factors are responsible for rising health care costs as a percentage of GDP. These include financial incentives for providers to increase services created by fee-for-service payment systems, the rising cost of pharmaceuticals and health care technology, high administrative costs, fears of malpractice litigation and the practice of defensive medicine, and a disproportionate number of expensive medical specialists. Other factors include a lack of consumer knowledge

of actual costs for care received, leading to inability of the market to accurately respond to cost and differential health care prices by region, type of hospital, or health care facility. For example, patients usually do not receive an itemized bill for costs incurred that are paid by insurance companies, nor do they receive information on differential costs for care by hospital or region. Future costs will also be largely determined by the aging of the population and subsequent higher health care cost utilization.

Another important factor in the rising cost of health care is the disproportionate impact of a small percentage of the population on costs. For example, from 1977 to 2007, a very stable 5% of the population, who had complex chronic illness, accounted for nearly half of the health care expenditures (Stanton, 2006; KFF, 2010d), in spite of efforts to control costs among this population. This trend continues with those in the top 1% of the population, who are most ill, spending 22.9% of health care dollars in 2007, while those in the bottom 50% spent 3% of health care dollars as shown in Figure 14-2 (KFF, 2010a). Interestingly, the majority of those in the high-expenditure group were not older adults but instead had complex chronic illnesses (Stanton, 2006). Health services research is being conducted in the area of high-cost care, but more studies are needed to explore nursing models of care delivery and their effect on cost outcomes.

Finally, as the number of uninsured has increased to more than 52 million persons in 2010 and as the population ages, the number of Medicaid enrollees, which was relatively stable for 30 years, has greatly increased (Gilmer & Kronick, 2009).

Health care costs are projected to continue to rise as the average life expectancy is extended and the "baby boomers" age and need more health services. Another factor in cost increases was the addition of coverage of prescription drugs by Medicare in 2006, as a result of the Medicare Prescription Drug Improvement and Modernization Act of 2003. Cost shifting is another problem that continues to plague the health care industry. For example, while Medicare spending for inpatient hospital services has been declining, outpatient costs and administrative costs have been increasing (National Coalition on Health Care, 2009).

Long-term care costs promise to be a major factor in the future, and some of these costs may be tied to the general economic trends in health care. Costs for skilled nursing facilities (SNFs) and home care

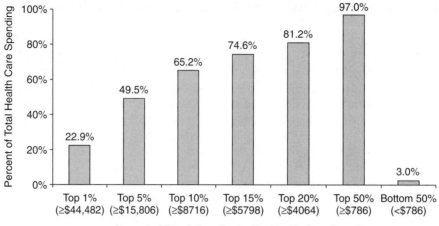

FIGURE 14-2 Concentration of health care spending in the U.S. population, 2007. Note: Dollar amounts in parentheses are the annual expenses per person in each percentile. Population is the noninstitutionalized population, including those without any health care spending. Health care spending is total payments from all sources (including direct payments from individuals, private insurance, Medicare, Medicaid, and miscellaneous other sources) to hospitals, physicians, other providers (including dental care), and pharmacies; health insurance premiums are not included. (Source: Kaiser Family Foundation calculations using data from U.S. Department of Health and Human Services, Agency for Healthcare Research and Quality, Medical Expenditure Panel Survey [MEPS], 2007. From Kaiser Family Foundation. [2010]. Concentration of health care spending in the U.S. population, 2007. Retrieved from *http://facts.kff.org/chart.aspx?ch=1344.*)

increased rapidly, especially for the most elderly until 2007. After record-setting prices in 2007, the average price paid for skilled nursing facilities fell 17% in 2008 to $45,500 per bed, according to Levin's report, The Senior Care Acquisition Report, (14th Edition), (2009). Along with the housing market declines, the average price for assisted living fell by 21% in 2008 to $124,900 per unit as the volume of transactions declined with the recession. The average price per unit in independent living units also fell in 2008 more than 32% to $118,100 from the 2007 high (Senior Living Business, 2009).

COST-CONTAINMENT EFFORTS

Over time, several approaches have been used to contain costs. None have adequately changed the trajectory of increasing costs and higher insurance premiums.

REGULATION VERSUS COMPETITION

During the 1970s, modest government regulation attempted to contain health care costs through health planning mechanisms such as Certificate of Need (CON) programs and regional Health Systems

Agencies (HSAs), which evaluated and approved applications for the construction of new facilities, beds, and new technology. During the 1980s, when proponents of competition and free market health care became politically more powerful, CON programs were weakened and HSAs were eliminated. While the free-market system has few similarities to a fully competitive market in economic terms , competition among health plans as they marketed themselves to employers in the 1980s may have slowed growth in health costs for short periods of time before they began to rise again. Co-payments, deductibles, and coinsurance are economic incentives to discourage care, putting the onus of cost-containment on the consumer/patient. However, ample research shows that low-income people may avoid necessary care when there are co-payments and deductibles. Chapter 16 focuses on economics and more fully describes the mechanisms underlying the market system in health care.

PROSPECTIVE PAYMENT VERSUS FEE-FOR-SERVICE FINANCING

Until the 1980s, Medicare paid providers through fee-for-service (FFS) reimbursement. In FFS, providers charge a fee for each service, and then patients submit claims to their insurance company, with potentially relatively high co-payments and deductibles. According to this payment methodology, hospitals reported on their total costs for the previous year, and the federal government paid these hospitals according to their percentage of Medicare recipients, which was inherently inflationary. The federal government replaced the old system with a prospective payment system (PPS) for hospital care, establishing payment based on as diagnosis-related groups (DRGs). DRGs set a payment level for each of approximately 500 diagnostic groups typically used in inpatient care. Prospective payment measures helped to slow the rate of growth of hospital expenditures and had a major impact on length of stay and increased patient acuity in hospitals (Heffler, et al., 2001). In March 1992, physician payment reform was initiated by means of the resource-based relative value scale (RBRVS). Its goal was not only cost savings but also a redistribution of physician services to increase primary care services and decrease the use of highly specialized physicians. The Medicare program also limits the amount physicians can charge for care. In 1997, Congress instituted a prospective payment system for skilled nursing facilities and home health agencies.

MANAGED CARE

The origins of the current managed care plans were in early prepaid health plans of the 1920s. A managed care system shifts health care delivery and payment from open-ended access to providers, paid for through fee-for-service reimbursement, toward one in which the provider is a "gatekeeper" or manager of the client's health care and assumes some degree of financial responsibility for the care that is given. Managed care implies not only that spending will be controlled, but other aspects of care will be managed, such as price, quality, and accessibility. In managed care, the primary care provider has traditionally been the gatekeeper, deciding what specialty services are appropriate and where these services can be obtained at the lowest cost. During the 1990s, negative media regarding the restriction of services in managed care for cost savings fueled a political backlash against restrictive managed care policies. Consumer and provider demand for greater "choice" for services and access to providers have led managed care plans to become less

restrictive, and also less effective in holding down the growth in health care expenditures.

Government health insurance programs such as Medicaid and Medicare also have incorporated managed care into their plans to cut costs. All fifty states offer some type of Medicaid managed care plans, and states can decide if participation is voluntary or mandatory. Some states have created state-run Medicaid-only plans, but others enroll Medicaid recipients in private managed care organizations (MCOs). By 2010, 70% of the Medicaid population received some or all of their services through Medicaid managed plans (Kaiser Health News, 2010).

During the 1990s, media attention to the concerns of consumers and providers who questioned the quality of care provided by managed care organizations (MCOs) resulted in state and federal health plan accountability laws to further regulate managed care plans (Kongstvedt, 2001). These laws included provisions for grievance procedures, confidentiality of health information, requirements that patients are fully informed of the benefits they will receive under a managed care plan, antidiscrimination clauses, and assurances that various quality mechanisms are in place so that patient satisfaction is measured and efforts to control costs do not curtail needed care. In addition, most states adopted policies giving health plan enrollees a right to appeal plan determinations involving a denial of coverage to an independent medical review entity, which is often a private organization approved by the state (American Association of Health Plans, 2001). Efforts to pass into law the federal Patient's Bill of Rights, which contains many consumer protections related to managed care, have not been successful.

PUBLIC/FEDERAL FUNDING FOR HEALTH CARE IN THE UNITED STATES

In the U.S, no single public entity oversees or controls the entire health care system, making the payment for and delivery of health care complex, inefficient, and expensive. Instead, the system is composed of many public and private programs that form interrelated parts at the federal, state, and local levels. The public funding systems, which include Medicare, Medicaid, the Child Health Insurance Plan, (CHIP), the Veterans Administration (VA), and the Defense Health

Program (TRICARE) for military personnel, their families, military retirees, and some others, continue to represent a larger and larger portion of health care spending. Other examples of federal programs are the Indian Health Service, which covers American Indians and Alaskan Natives, and the Federal Employees Health Benefits (FEHB) Program, which covers all federal employees unless excluded by law or regulation. In 2010, federal health expenditures totaled $829 billion, or 22% of all federal expenditures in that year (U.S. Government Spending, 2010). This number is expected to grow as the baby boomer population ages and becomes eligible for Medicare. Medicare outlays are projected to be $504 billion in 2010 with 46 million enrollees (KFF, 2010c). Medicaid outlays in 2009 were $378.3 billion with 60 million or one in five individuals receiving care through this program (KFF, 2010b).

MEDICARE

Before enactment of Medicare in 1965, older adults were more likely to be uninsured and more likely to be impoverished by excessive health care costs. Half of older Americans had no health insurance; but by 2000, 96% of seniors had health care coverage through Medicare (Federal Interagency Forum on Age-Related Statistics, 2000). Medicare and Medicaid legislation were controversial when they were debated in Congress because they were government insurance programs, but groups like the American Medical Association, who originally opposed the legislation, later benefited from these programs because older and low-income patients became insured.

Medicare had a beneficial effect on the health of older adults by facilitating access to care and medical technology, and, in 2006, prescription drug coverage helped improve the economic status of older adults. The percentage of persons over age 65 living below the poverty line decreased from 35% in 1959 (when older adults had the highest poverty rate of the population) to 9.7% in 2008 (U.S. Census Bureau, 2010).

Americans are eligible for Medicare Part A at age 65, the age for Social Security eligibility or sooner, if they are determined to be disabled. Medicare Part A accounted for 35% of benefit spending in 2010 and covers 46 million Americans. Medicare Part A covers hospital and related costs and is financed through payroll deduction to the Hospital Insurance Trust Fund at the payroll tax rate of 2.9% of earnings paid by employers and employees (1.45% each) (KFF, 2010c). Medicare Part B, which accounted for 27% of benefit spending in 2010, covers 80% of the fees for physician services, outpatient medical services and supplies, home care, durable medical equipment, laboratory services, physical and occupational therapy, and outpatient mental health services (KFF, 2010c). Part B is financed through subscriber premiums and general revenue funding.

Medicare Part C or the Medicare Advantage Program, through which beneficiaries can enroll in a private health plan and also receive some extra services such as vision or hearing services, accounts for 24% of benefit spending and has more than 10 million beneficiaries (KFF, 2010c). Medicare Part D is a voluntary, subsidized outpatient drug plan with additional subsidies for low and modest income individuals. It accounts for 11% of benefit spending and enrolls more than 27 million beneficiaries (KFF, 2010c). Figure 14-3 presents Medicare benefit payments by payment type (KFF, 2010c).

FEE-FOR-SERVICE VERSUS MANAGED CARE MEDICARE

At its inception in 1965, Medicare was modeled after private employer-provided fee-for-service insurance plans (Atherly, 2001). In 1982, Medicare beneficiaries were given the choice of remaining in traditional fee-for-service Medicare or enrolling in an MCO. Many older adults took advantage for the choice of this option through Medicare + Choice (now Medicare Part C). But with the passage of the 1997 Balanced Budget Act, Medicare enrollees were given a choice of three types of Medicare plans, including the original fee-for-service coverage plan, Medicare managed care, and the privately insured fee-for-service (Medicare Advantage). The original Medicare fee-for-service plan, which covered 83% of Medicare beneficiaries in 2000 (Oberlander, 2000), offers the beneficiary a choice of hospital and provider, but requires an annual deductible and, unless prohibited by state law, the beneficiary may have to pay the difference between what Medicare will pay and what the provider charges. Under Medicare, this practice, called "balance billing", occurs when certain providers may opt to bill patients a portion of what Medicare does not cover for medical services. Medicare Part B will also pay for the difference between the physician charges and the cost of care, but not all older adults

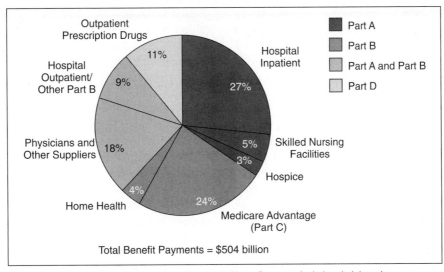

FIGURE 14-3 Medicare benefit payments by type of service, 2010. Note: Does not include administrative expenses such as spending to administer the Medicare drug benefit and the Medicare Advantage program. (Source: CBO Medicare Baseline, March 2009. From Kaiser Family Foundation. [2010]. Medicare at a glance: Fact sheet. Retrieved from *www.kff.org/medicare/upload/1066-12.pdf*.)

have Part B "Medigap" insurance because it involves an additional premium. Medigap health insurance is sold by private insurance companies to fill the "gaps" in Medicare Plan coverage. Over the past 20 years, out-of-pocket expenses for health care have increased for older adults across all income groups, with lower-income Americans paying a larger portion of their income for health care.

Between 1996 and 2009, Medicare enrollment in managed care plans increased to 22% (KFF, 2009), but still the majority of older adults continue to be enrolled in fee-for-service plans. In another option, Medicare will pay fixed monthly payments to certain plans, from which beneficiaries purchase private indemnity health insurance policies. The consumer maintains choice of provider and health care setting and receives extra services such as partial prescription drug coverage, but the individual must pay deductibles and premium fees that may exceed those charged by the original Medicare. The plan, not the provider, determines the rate of provider reimbursement, and providers may be allowed to balance-bill Medicare patients 15% above the payment level set by the plan. Medicare fee-for-service is not available in all areas. Patients with end-stage renal disease who are covered under Medicare Parts A and B are not covered with the private fee-for-service option (USDHHS, CMS, 2010).

Although the majority of Medicare recipients remain in traditional fee-for-service plans, Medicare managed care has received increased attention as part of a strategy to control escalating health care costs. In 1983, under the Tax Equity and Fiscal Responsibility Act (TEFRA), Congress authorized Medicare payments to qualified "risk-contract" HMOs (Social Security Administration, 2000). In risk plans or "coordinated care plans," the beneficiary is required to receive all services from within the organization's network of providers. Medicare beneficiaries can also enroll in "cost plans." Under cost plans, care may be received outside of the provider network or service area. Costs not covered under fee-for-service Medicare, including preventive care and prescription drugs, may be covered under Medicare managed care plans. Participation in a managed care plan may offer additional consumer savings by negating the need for supplemental Medigap insurance.

MEDICARE REFORM

Because the shift by some beneficiaries to Medicare managed care in the 1990s did not produce intended savings, there have been numerous other proposals for insuring the solvency of Medicare. Proposals for Medicare reform have included delaying the age of retirement; increasing payroll taxes for higher income taxpayers; offering so-called premium support (where

Medicare pre-funds premiums for individuals) to Medicare enrollees to encourage them to join HMOs; and improved risk-sharing between Medicare and HMOs (Etheredge, 2000; Oberlander, 2000).

MEDICARE MEDICAL SAVINGS ACCOUNTS (MSAS)

In the late 1990s, demonstration projects were funded with federal dollars to test the hypothesis that the application of market principles could cut Medicare costs (Nichols & Reischauer, 2000). As a result, the Medicare Medical Savings Account Plan was touted as a way to cut costs to consumers and Medicare by establishing a tax-sheltered Medicare-funded savings account for health care expenses and a private catastrophic health insurance plan with a high deductible (Kendix & Lubitz, 1999; Hall & Havighurst; 2005; IRS, 2010).

Recipients receive a capitated (capped) amount as part of the Medicare Advantage program, equal to 95% of the traditional costs of fee-for-service Medicare. From the capitated amount, Medicare pays the premium for the catastrophic insurance and deposits money into the individual's MSA. Money in the savings account is used to pay the deductible on the insurance policy, if needed. Beneficiaries who have insufficient money in the savings account must pay the balance of the deductible out of private funds. If the beneficiary does not use the money in the savings account in a given year, the money accumulates in the savings account for use in another year. These high deductible Medicare Advantage plans could potentially cut Medicare costs, because Medicare saves 5% on the capitated amount. The intent here is for consumers to save health care dollars, because they would be responsible for costs incurred over the amount in the MSA up to the deductible. MSAs are intended to eliminate the need for supplemental, or Medigap, coverage, again resulting in consumer savings particularly if the person is not chronically ill nor a user of high-cost care (Kendix & Lubitz, 1999). These plans will not work well for people with chronic illness or with high-cost care.

Another option, outside of the Medicare program, is the High Deductible Health Plan (HDHP)/Health Reimbursement Arrangement (HRA), which is "a consumer-driven health plan in which the plan member is reimbursed for covered health expenses by his/her employer up to a predetermined amount.

Unused funds may be carried over to the next year, subject to limits set by the employer" (CIGNA, 2010). In 2009, at least 12% of companies providing health insurance offered high-deductible plans, covering about 8 million workers (KFF/HRET, 2009; Yoo, 2009).

MSAs and other attempts at premium support or high-deductible plans have been criticized for moving the healthiest and wealthiest persons from traditional fee-for-service Medicare to the private insurance sector. This results in overall increased costs for those left in the Medicare system (Baker & Weisbrot, 1999; Kendix & Lubitz, 1999; Oberlander, 2000). According to Oberlander (2000), premium-support plans actually reduce choice for many Medicare recipients, who are already overwhelmed by the options available under Medicare. These older adults, many who will be chronically ill, frail, and financially challenged, may choose a plan according to what they can afford, rather than according to what they need.

FEDERAL/STATE/LOCAL FINANCING PROGRAMS

MEDICAID

Medicaid is the main public program jointly funded and administered by states and the federal government, available to low-income people within certain categories. Medicaid eligible people include low-income persons receiving Temporary Assistance to Needy Families (TANF) blind and totally disabled persons who received cash assistance under the Supplemental Security Income (SSI) program; pregnant women; and children born after September 1983 in families with incomes at or below the poverty line. To qualify for federal Medicaid matching grants, a state must provide a minimum set of benefits, including hospitalization, physician care, laboratory services, radiology studies, prenatal care, and preventive services; nursing home and home health care; and medically necessary transportation. Medicaid programs are also required to pay the Medicare premiums, deductibles, and co-payments for certain low-income persons. Medicaid is increasingly becoming a long-term care financing program of last resort for older adults in nursing homes. Many older adults have to "spend down" their life savings to become eligible for Medicaid. Figure 14-4 indicates the current numbers

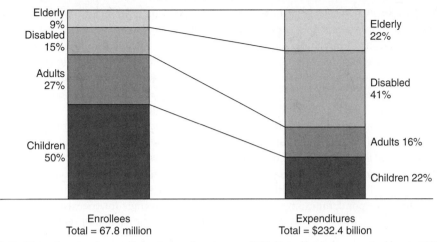

FIGURE 14-4 Medicaid enrollment and expenditures by enrollment group, 2009. Note: Numbers may not add up to 100% due to round-ing. (Source: Center for Children and Families analysis of March 2009 CBO Medicaid baseline. Retrieved from *ccf.georgetown.edu/pix/Graphs/Medicaid%20Expenditures%20and%20Enrollment.jpg.*)

served by category and amounts of money attributed to each group, (CBO, 2009). Family nurse practitio-ners (NPs), pediatric NPs, geriatric NPs, and certified nurse midwives must also be reimbursed under Medicaid if, in accordance with state regulations, they are legally authorized to provide Medicaid-covered services.

CURRENT FINANCING FOR MEDICAID

Medicaid is funded partially through general funds in the federal budget and through general funds in the state budget. The federal match makes Medicaid an attractive payer for state governments which are com-mitted to covering as many of their residents as pos-sible with comprehensive health insurance. States may be given permission to expand their Medicaid programs to cover certain otherwise uninsured people, and many have taken advantage of this oppor-tunity through obtaining a Medicaid waiver from the federal government. In Massachusetts, where 97% of residents now are covered by health insurance through the state's health reform initiative, federal Medicaid funds have been used to help subsidize insurance pre-miums for people not eligible for traditional Medic-aid, but who cannot afford to pay full premiums for private health insurance. Lawmakers have found expanding coverage to uninsured people, through an existing program such as Medicaid, is more palatable because of the cost-sharing between the federal and

state governments and because Medicaid already has a built-in administrative structure.

The Child Health Insurance Program (CHIP) is also funded through state federal matching funds and has had much controversy since its passage particu-larly as to the number of children covered according to income level. This program will be discussed in Chapter 18.

STATE HEALTH CARE FINANCING

State governments not only administer some federally funded insurance programs such as Medicaid and CHIP, but also may administer specific state public health programs. The definition of public health as compared to other types of health programs is not always well understood. The mission of public health as defined by the Institute of Medicine (IOM) is to ensure conditions in which people can be healthy (IOM, 1988). While medicine focuses on the patient, public health focuses on populations. Public health programs are often funded by states or localities, which also may combine state funding with grants from the federal government in areas such as maternal and child health, smoking cessation, obesity prevention, HIV/AIDS, substance abuse, and envi-ronmental health. Many of these population-based prevention programs are not reimbursable by private or government insurance programs, and the burden will fall on the state public health department. States have a major responsibility in determining how access to care, health care quality, and cost-containment programs will be carried out on behalf of their own residents. States also have a major responsibility for oversight of health insurance, health care providers, and public health activities.

Reduction of public budgets for public health during times of fiscal constraint have resulted in the resurgence of infectious diseases such as tuberculosis and sexually transmitted diseases. The tragedy of September 11, 2001, and a series of natural disasters also brought to light gaps in our public health system, especially our ability to respond, for example, to mass casualty events.

LOCAL/COUNTY LEVEL

Like state governments, local and county governments in many states also have the responsibility for protecting the public health. Some provide indigent care by funding and running public hospitals and clinics, like New York City's Health and Hospitals Corporation and Chicago's Cook County Hospital. While receiving a subsidy from their local government, these hospitals (which serve primarily poor patients and older adults) get a large amount of operating money from Medicaid and Medicare. Because public hospitals and clinics are so dependent on public funds, their budgets are frequently squeezed during times of fiscal restraint by local, state, and federal governments, making them vulnerable to long-term sustainability.

PRIVATE HEALTH CARE SYSTEM

The U.S. health care system historically has been predominantly a private one that operates more like a business and according to free market principles. Yet the latest data indicate that by 2012, the government will pay more than 50% of the costs for health. Most care has been delivered through privately run for-profit or nonprofit corporations such as hospitals and health care systems and private insurance plans (Truffer et al., 2010). Pharmaceutical companies, suppliers of health care technology, and the various service industries that support the health care system in the U.S. are part of what has been called the "medical industrial complex" (Meyers, 1970). While the private delivery system is dependent on payment from private insurers as well as government insurers,

it has usually been resistant to government-directed efforts to expand access to care or cost-containment measures. Private insurance companies have likewise been successful in defeating regulations proposed to make private insurance more available and more affordable. For example, employers can decide to offer health insurance or not, except in Massachusetts, which has required employers to provide insurance or pay a penalty fee. Insurers can reject an application for insurance, if the applicant has a preexisting medical condition, although this practice has been outlawed in Massachusetts. The issue of mandating coverage for preexisting conditions is a major tenet of national health reform.

NURSING AND NATIONAL HEALTH REFORM

With the inauguration of Barack Obama and a Democratic Congress in January 2010, expanding access to care through significant national health reform became an immediate top domestic priority agenda of the new president and majority party. In March 2010, a landmark national health reform law, The Patient Protection and Affordable Care Act, was finally signed by the President with no Republican support. This legislation, which was modeled after the highly successful reform model Massachusetts implemented in 2006, projects it will enable 94% of all Americans to obtain health insurance, reduce the growth in health care costs, and decrease the federal budget deficit by $143 billion over the next 10 years (Congressional Budget Office, 2010). It accomplishes this through some of the provisions outlined in Table 14-1.

The new law is projected to cost $940 billion over 10 years, and is paid for through reductions in projected payment increases to providers; taxes levied on expensive "cadillac" insurance plans, medical device manufacturers, tanning salons, and certain cosmetic treatments; reductions in extra payments for Medicare Advantage Plans; and an increase in the Medicare payroll tax for the top 5% of American income earners.

The debate over national health reform consumed Congress for all of 2009 and early 2010, proving once again, that just like the debate on Medicare and Medicaid in the 1960s, major health reform legislation is difficult to pass in the U.S.

TABLE 14-1 Summary of the Patient Protection and Affordable Care Act of 2010

Insurance Reform to Improve Access to Coverage	Prohibits insurance exclusion based on pre-existing conditions and bars insurance premiums from being based on health status. Lifetime limits on coverage are prohibited. Allows children to stay on their parents' plan up to age 26. Requires all plans to cover essential benefits.
Shared responsibility between individuals and employers	By 2014, most people will be required to have health insurance or pay a penalty, unless health insurance is deemed unaffordable for them. Employers with 50 or more employees will be required to offer employees health insurance and pay a penalty if any employee would otherwise be receiving public assistance to pay for insurance.
Affordable health insurance for low- and moderate-income Americans	Low- and moderate-income families up to 400% of the Federal Poverty Level ($88,000 for a family of 4) will be given tax credits to help them afford insurance. Health Benefit Exchanges in each state will help individuals and small businesses obtain affordable health insurance coverage.
Medicaid coverage for more Americans	Medicaid will be expanded to include all non-elderly Americans with incomes below 133% of the federal poverty level ($30,000 for a family of 4).
Investments in primary care and prevention programs	Co-pays and deductibles are eliminated for recommended preventative care. Reimbursement to primary care providers is increased. Provider neutral language is adopted to recognize the important role of advanced practice nurses in primary care delivery and management.
Payment for Medicare Part D prescription drugs	Helps seniors pay for prescription drugs and will eventually eliminate the Medicare Part D "donut hole," which has left older adults without coverage for their medications.
Investments in innovative models of health care delivery	Makes investments in new delivery models such as Nurse Managed Clinics, Accountable Care Organizations, Medical Homes, and chronic disease management programs; enables non-physician providers, such as advanced practice nurses, to play a greater role in managing patient care in these new entities.
Health care workforce development	Invests in initiatives to increase access by expanding the number of primary care providers, including advanced practice nurses, through loan repayment programs and scholarships and support for higher educational programs

SUMMARY

Since 1970, the U.S. health care system has grown to almost unmanageable proportions and complexity. The medical-industrial complex pervades all sectors of the economic system and employs a vast number of citizens. It consumes more than 15% of the GDP and is continuing to rise after a short leveling-off period. The projected large-scale retirement of the baby boomers beginning in 2010 and growing health care costs present challenges to a fragmented private delivery system and to public and private sector budgets.

The primary purpose of national health reform law was to increase access to health care through regulating the health care insurance industry, providing tax credits to low- and moderate-income families for health insurance, and implementing innovative financing and delivery models. The new law also embraces a greater and more significant role for advanced practice nurses and invests in nursing education.

For a list of related websites, please refer to your Evolve Resources at http://evolve.elsevier.com/Mason/policypolitics/

REFERENCES

American Association of Health Plans. (2001). *Independent medical review of health plan coverage decisions: Empowering consumers with solutions.* Washington, DC: Author.

Atherly, A. (2001). Supplemental insurance: Medicare's accidental stepchild. *Medical Care Research and Review, 58*(2), 131-161.

Baker, D. & Weisbrot, M. (1999). *Social Security: The phony crisis.* Chicago: The University of Chicago Press.

Congressional Budget Office (CBO). (2009). Medicaid enrollees and expenditures by enrollment group: 2009. Retrieved from http://ccf.georgetown.edu/pix/Graphs/Medicaid%20Expenditures%20and%20Enrollment.jpg.

Congressional Budget Office. (2010, March 20). Retrieved from www.cbo.gov/ftpdocs/113xx/doc11379/Manager'sAmendmenttoReconciliationProposal.pdf.

CIGNA. (2010). CIGNA medical plans. Retrieved from www.cigna.com/our_plans/medical/hra/for_you.html.

Etheredge, L. (2000). Medicare's governance and structure: A proposal. *Health Affairs, 19*(5), 60-71.

Federal Interagency Forum on Age-Related Statistics. (2000). *Older Americans 2000: Key indicators of well-being.* Hyattsville, MD: Author.

Gilmer, T. P. & Kronick, R. G. (2009). Hard times and health insurance: How many Americans will be uninsured by 2010? *Health Affairs, 28*(4), w573-w577.

Hall, M. A., & Havighurst, C. C. (2005). Reviving managed care with Health Savings Accounts: HSAs with active benefit management by high-deductible plans could lessen patients' resistance to managed care. *Health Affairs, 24*(6), 1490-1500.

Heffler, S., Levit, K., Smith, S., Smith, C., Cowan, C., Lazenby H., & Freeland, M. (2001). Health care spending growth up in 1999: Faster growth expected in the future. *Health Affairs, 20*(2), 193-203.

Inflationdata.com. (2010). Retrieved from www.inflationdata.com.

Institute of Medicine, National Academy of Sciences. (1988). *The future of public health*. Washington, DC: National Academy Press.

Internal Revenue Service. (2010). Medical savings accounts. Retrieved from www.irs.gov/publications/p969/ar02.html.

Jonas, S. & Kovner, A. (2005). *Jonas and Kovner's health care delivery in the United States* (7th ed.). New York: Springer.

Kaiser Family Foundation (KFF). (2009). Medicare spending and financing, May 2009. Retrieved from www.kff.org/medicare/upload/7305-04-2.pdf.

Kaiser Family Foundation. (2010a). Concentration of health care spending in the U.S. population, 2007. Retrieved from http://facts.kff.org/chart.aspx?ch=1344.

Kaiser Family Foundation. (2010b). Medicaid and managed care: Key data, trends, and issues. Retrieved from www.kff.org/medicaid/8046.cfm.

Kaiser Family Foundation. (2010c). Medicare at a glance: Fact sheet. Retrieved from www.kff.org/medicare/upload/1066-12.pdf.

Kaiser Family Foundation. (2010d). National health expenditures per capita and their share of gross domestic product, 1960-2008. Retrieved from http://facts.kff.org/chart.aspx?ch=1344.

Kaiser Family Foundation and Health Research Educational Trust (KFF/HRET). (2009). Employer health benefits: 2009 summary of findings. Retrieved from http://ehbs.kff.org/pdf/2009/7937.pdf.

Kaiser Health News. (2010). Research Roundup: Medicare spending, community health centers, children's dental services. Retrieved from www.kaiserhealthnews.org/Daily-Reports/2010/February/05/Research-Roundup.aspx.

Kendix, M. & Lubitz, J. D. (1999). The impact of medical savings accounts on Medicare program costs. *Inquiry, 36*(3), 280-290.

Kongstvedt, P. (2001). *The managed health care handbook* (4th ed.). Gaithersburg, MD: Aspen.

Levin, Irving and Associates. (2009). *The senior care acquisition report*. (14th ed.). Norwalk, CT: Author.

Meyers, H. (1970, January). The medical-industrial complex. *Fortune, 90-91*, 126.

National Coalition on Health Care. (2009, Sept). Health care facts costs. Retrieved from http://nchc.org.

Nichols, L. M. & Reischauer, R. D. (2000). Who really wants price competition in Medicare managed care? *Health Affairs, 19*(5), 30-43.

Oberlander, J. (2000). Is premium support the right medicine for Medicare? A challenge to the emergent conventional wisdom. *Health Affairs, 19*(5), 84-99.

Organization for Economic Co-operation and Development. (OECD). (2009). Health data 2009. Retrieved from www.oecd.org/health/healthdata.

Senior Living Business. (2009). The acquisition market. *Senior Living Business, 3*(3), 12.

Siska, A., et al. (2009, March/April). Health care spending projections through 2018: Recession effects add uncertainty to the Outlook. *Health Affairs, 28*(2), w346-w357.

Social Security Administration. (2000). *Annual statistical supplement, 2000*. Washington, DC: Author. Retrieved from www.socialsecurity.gov/policy/docs/statcomps/supplement/2000.

Stanton, M. (2006). *The High Concentration of U.S. Health Care Expenditures. Research in Action, Issue 19*. Washington, D.C.: Agency for Health Care Research and Quality (AHRQ).

Starr, P. (1982). *The social transformation of American medicine*. New York: Basic Books.

Truffer, C., Keehan, S., Smith, S., Cylus, J., Sisko, A., Poisal, J., Lizonitz, J., & Clemens, M. K. (2010, February). Health spending projections through 2019: The recession's impact continues. *Health Affairs, 29*(3), 522-529.

U.S. Census Bureau. (2010). Poverty rates by age. Retrieved from www.census.gov/hhes/www/poverty/poverty08/pov08fig04.pdf.

U.S. D.H.H.S., CMS. (2010). Medicare coverage of kidney dialysis and kidney transplant services. Retrieved from www.medicare.gov/Publications/Pubs/pdf/10128.pdf.

U.S. Government Spending.com. (2010). Retrieved from www.usgovernmentspending.com/.

Yoo, H. (2009). Census shows 8 million people covered by HSA/high-deductible health plans, America's health insurance plans. Retrieved from www.ahipresearch.org/pdfs/2009hsacensus.pdf.

CHAPTER 15

Could a National Health System Work in the United States?

Kristine M. Gebbie

"There are always alternatives."

—Mr. Spock, Star Trek

"Don't we have one? Didn't the president sign health reform on March 23, 2010?" Maybe the best answer is "No, Virginia, he wasn't Santa Claus." The reform bill signed in March does make an enormous difference in the flow of money for illness care, and prevention, in the United States. And it does widen the number of individuals who have access to an affordable way to pay. The majority of provisions are financial (Kaiser Family Foundation, 2010):

- Most U.S. citizens and legal residents must purchase health insurance.
- State-based exchanges allow individuals to purchase coverage, with premium and cost-sharing credits available to individuals/families with income between 133% and 400% of the federal poverty level ($18,310 for a family of three in 2009)
- The exchanges allow small businesses to purchase coverage.
- Large employers pay penalties for employees who receive tax credits for health insurance through an exchange, with exceptions for small employers.
- Exclusion of pre-existing conditions has been eliminated.
- Medicaid is expanded to 133% of the federal poverty level.

However, better ways to pay do not create a national system. The use of evidence to push expenditures toward prevention and the least costly alternatives is not required, and the current unconnected array of individually driven professionals, hospitals, clinics, and other components is largely left untouched. While there is some attention to making sure that there are caregivers to respond to the newly insured (e.g., more primary care providers, more funding for community health centers), it is not clear that this new law will do much to assure that care is centered on support of the well to allow them to stay well, rather than centered on reaction to emergencies and crises.

The significant but limited change embodied in the 2010 health reform means that the U.S. has not quite yet ended its isolation as the only economically developed country on the globe that does not assure universal access to health services for its population. It also leaves the U.S. as the country that spends more in both total dollars and per capita dollars than any other nation. For example, between 1970 and 2005, the U.S. had the largest increase (8.3%) of all economically developed countries, reaching 15.3%. The cost per capita ($6401) is more than double the $2922 median for 30 industrialized countries routinely compared by the Organization for Economic Cooperation and Development. Unlike many of these other countries, the U.S. uses public insurance for only 26.2% of the population and is in the top half for only 8 of 16 quality measures used for comparison. For example, the U.S. is second in controlling tobacco use, but next to the bottom (16th of 17 countries reporting) in adult hospital admissions for asthma. The U.S. is 12th of 23 countries in screening women over 50 for breast cancer, though 5th in survival rate in women treated for the same. One translation: we may not find breast cancer, but if we do, we treat it well. We are also at the bottom (23rd of 24 countries reporting) in vaccinating children against pertussis. The U.S. has fewer hospital beds (2.7 per 1000 people compared with France's 3.7 per 1000). In an economic analysis of purchasing power, the U.S. is the most isolated outlier with far more than expected spending and far less than expected successful outcomes (Anderson & Frogner, 2008).

Near universality of access is achieved in other countries through a variety of arrangements, including government-operated care systems, government-managed finance systems, and government-mandated financing. The U.S. has experience with most of these: the Veteran's Administration system is fully government-operated, as is the care provided our military forces (and their dependents) by the Department of Defense. Medicare is fully government-managed, and one state (Hawaii) has long-mandated insurance coverage of all employees. Massachusetts has recently made a move to require insurance, either through employers or individually purchased. We leave insurance regulation to 50 differing state systems, patch together care for the very poor with Medicaid, managed individually in each state, require many tests of newborns, and forbid use of some money for some purposes (e.g., the ban on federal funding of abortion). Moves toward a universal financing system and universal access to care have been made at several points during the twentieth century, most recently in the 1993-1994 proposal by President Clinton that died without ever coming to a vote in Congress. Advocates were revitalized by the fact that President Obama put this on his priority agenda despite the competing issues of economic disaster and wars and held out hopes that this time would be the time for true health reform. Given the worldwide economic depression that preoccupied his administration, it was not surprising that negotiations narrowed the promise to changes that bring more individuals into the finance system without any serious impacts on the actual delivery of care. The election of a Republican to the seat vacated by the death of Ted Kennedy made passage more complicated, as it ended the 60-vote (filibuster-proof) majority the Democrats had held in the Senate, and it took extremely careful parliamentary and political maneuvering to get the law now in place. Since a fully national system is not yet in law, exploring the potential for such an approach can reveal strengths and weaknesses and begin to answer whether it is possible in the U.S.

POSSIBLE APPROACHES TO A NATIONAL SYSTEM

The two major approaches to a national system that have been successfully used elsewhere are some form of financing that is universal or a service system that is universally available. For each of these there are at least two structural options.

UNIVERSAL PAYMENT

Universal payment as a route to a national health system assumes that the lack of access to services is primarily associated with lack of ability to pay and therefore that if funds were available, the services would follow. This discussion of payment will not take up the problematic reality of such an assumption. It is notable, however, that even some people who have financing for care are unable to get access because practitioners are not available for reasons such as geographic maldistribution, professional workforce shortages, or some form of social discrimination (e.g., denial of Medicaid to some immigrants, or provider prejudice regarding sexual orientation).

National Tax. The simplest form of universal payment would be a national program in which tax funds are used to pay providers for care rendered as needed. The tax could be a special one (such as that currently used to support Medicare for those over 65 or disabled) or some portion of general revenues. The payment from this single national payer could go directly to those providing care (as in the province-based single-payer system of Canada) or could be managed through contracts with fiscal intermediaries (as is now the case for Medicare). If truly universal, there would be little or no administrative burden for enrollment, as everyone would automatically be eligible. There would be a need to negotiate with providers of care for fee levels and methods of reimbursement; a single payer controlling all health dollars would be a formidable bargaining agent for hospitals and clinicians to confront. The fear of such a single agent clearly affects policy decisions, such as the prohibitions on national contracts for lower-cost drugs under the Medicare drug benefit legislated in 2003. This program is to be managed through the usual range of nongovernmental providers, each of which may negotiate with manufacturers for lower prices. However, the most powerful negotiator, the nationwide Medicare program as a whole, is prohibited from negotiating for a single lowest price for all seniors across the country.

Multiple Payers. Alternately, a universal payment system could be constructed with multiple payers, and this is the model that the new health reform law comes close to. For example, all employers, no matter how small or large, could be required to provide a certain level of health insurance for all employees and their families, with Medicare continuing for those over 65 or disabled and a form of Medicaid used for the unemployed and their families. This less-monolithic system is the heart of the rejected Clinton plan and shares features with that in place, as in Germany. It allows for a range of payment mechanisms, with more room for bargaining and less sense of the government as the overwhelming controller of the purse strings. For a system such as this to work successfully, there would have to be rules governing the components of coverage and dual coverage in families with more than one worker. The employment-based coverage would be financed as it is now, with funds that would otherwise be available for wages or other benefits; coverage for those not in working families would require tax support, as it does now to the extent that they are available. Although this might be more palatable to practitioners or institutions, many employers, especially those with few employees, would find the mandate objectionable.

UNIVERSAL CARE

A more radical approach to a national health system would be to make the actual provision of care universal.

National Health System. This is the approach begun after World War II in Great Britain when it established the National Health Service. National tax dollars (general or special taxes) are used to pay primary care providers throughout the country for basic health services and to pay specialists and hospitals for their share of needed services. This essentially makes the provision of care a government service, whether the caregivers and hospital staff are put directly on a government payroll or are employed by contract. The managers of the system are obligated to find sources of care for everyone throughout the country; to do so, they might need to make differential fees available to recruit providers—for example, to serve remote areas. This approach also lends itself to careful investment in only as many hospital beds and specialized services as population size and health statistics suggest are needed, with a clear disincentive for continuing the expensive practice of having large numbers of excess beds or competing diagnostic services. It is for this reason that Britain, as most other countries, invests far less in multiple, identical pieces

of diagnostic equipment. For example, the United Kingdom has only 5.5 magnetic resonance imaging (MRI) units for each million in the population, compared with the U.S. at 8.2 per million (Anderson & Frogner, 2008). There are many fears, however, that such a system has too many incentives to control cost and not enough incentives to be user-friendly or of high quality.

State-Based System. Universality could be achieved with similar results but greater flexibility by placing the requirement for access on the states through some combination of funding incentives and penalties. Expecting each state to use its tax authority and funds provided through national tax resources to assure access for everyone would allow each state to employ and deploy its own preferred mix of generalists and specialists, and community-based and hospital-based services. Within a national minimum expectation, states with more income could choose a richer mix of services, but no one would be without access to care. This approach to national minimums and state options on organization and final mix of services is the overall structure for our present Medicaid system. There are risks here, as even states with a relatively high income level could adopt a more miserly approach to access for health and illness services.

For providers of care, either form of a universal care system presents a far more radical change from current realities than a move to assure payment for care for everyone. It is the approach that most surely would push us toward truly evidence-based care and a serious dialogue about the limits of technological intervention in human life span. Such centralized control of purse strings makes it far less likely that individual entrepreneurs or entrepreneurial systems would survive. And it is not clear that the current infusion of private capital into development of pharmaceuticals or equipment would continue, or whether a leveling of incomes across types of providers might prove discouraging to those considering entering a health profession.

THE PARTICIPANTS

Understanding the debate about universal coverage in the U.S. is almost impossible without at least some awareness of the groups that have participated in the arguments that have kept the system as it is now. These include the following myriad groups that maintain political and economic power through the present nonstructure:

- For-profit insurance companies, which might not be allowed to sell competing products at whatever price they can command
- Pharmaceutical and technology manufacturers, which might experience limits in the volume of what can be sold or have to face monopsonistic buying power
- Medium-sized and small businesses that believe that they would be forced to pay either taxes or premiums beyond what is affordable
- Health professionals, particularly those in small group, fee-for-service practices, who perceive that their degree of freedom may become limited.

From other perspectives, there are also groups whose focus is more on what is currently missing and therefore that speak out on behalf of change:

- Labor unions, aware of the vulnerability of their members to arbitrary changes in work-related and retiree coverage
- Advocates for population groups with decreased access in the current system
- Health professionals in salaried positions, particularly those in system-oriented organizations such as public health agencies and community-based health centers
- Businesses that have grasped the potential economic benefit of leveling the cost playing field by bringing everyone to the table.

Although neither of these perspectives is absolutely the purview of one political party or the other, the Republican party and those identified as farther to the right on the political spectrum are more identified with opposition to any form of mandated universality or any changes in care that can be labeled as big government having the power of life and death over individuals. The Democratic Party and those identified as farther to the left on the political spectrum have been traditionally more identified with the campaigns for comprehensive approaches and have led the current debate for such major changes as a single payer system, or a public insurance option.

BARRIERS TO RESOLVING THE LACK OF UNIVERSALITY

Describing ways that true universality of a system driven to support health could be achieved does not

deal with the reality that universality of access to care or funding for care has not been popular in the U.S. The history of care and payment has been a blend of entrepreneurship, private charity, and public charity.

AMERICAN ENTERPRISE

Entrepreneurs have been free to develop care or care products and sell them freely, subject for just over 100 years to the strictures of federal and state safety regulation and professional licensing laws. Private groups, particularly religious ones, have offered hospitals, clinics, and home care and other services to those unable to purchase such services, although this charity role has diminished in the face of rising costs and a greater number of reimbursement programs. Governments have offered public hospitals, various clinics, and a few finance systems, to assure that the neediest citizens have had access to at least the rudiments of care. There is a personal cost to these "free" services, paid in such currency as extended waiting time for care or loss of personal dignity.

INCREMENTALISM

Over the latter half of the twentieth century, the U.S. edged closer toward universality with the convergence of specialized programs such as Medicare, community and migrant health centers, expanded Medicaid, state insurance purchasing initiatives, and the Child Health Insurance Program. However, these positive moves on the part of governments have been offset by the growing number of jobs that do not offer a health insurance benefit either for workers or for worker families or do so at a cost that is not affordable. Furthermore, these incremental moves are open to the fluctuations in year-to-year budgets and changing political philosophies. There is no indication that this trend will be reversed any time soon.

POLITICAL HISTORY

It is also important to remember that the political history of the U.S. is one of suspicion about government and a reluctance to use government as the solution to a problem.[1] The election of 2004 returned to

---

[1]For a more complete discussion of the modern political history of this debate, see Blumenthal, D., & Morone, J. A. (2009). *The heart of power: Health and politics in the oval office.* Berkeley: University of California Press.

office a party that has consistently run against government, proposes tax cuts in part so that the funds will not be there to tempt Congress to spend, and touts private solutions to social concerns. The 2005 Bush administration proposals to make major changes in the Social Security Administration died with little attention, but the mere suggestion illustrates that even this most basic of social contracts among citizens and their government cannot be assumed sacrosanct.

Recollecting multiple panel discussions and academic presentations during the 1993-1994 health reform debate, the overall impression was that, while people were willing to agree that lack of access to care is a problem, they were divided about whether or not this improvement should be publicly financed and were reluctant to support either spending more money or giving up some of their own current services to make it possible. If this is accurate, it means that decision-makers were receiving sufficiently mixed messages that any action they took would please only a few. There is a history of abrupt reversal of public policy on catastrophic coverage for older adult in the 1980s (Congress enacted in one session and repealed in the next a system of higher Medicare taxes that assured a limit on personal expenditures for extremely high medical expenses, in large part because of anger by older adults claiming they were misled regarding the increased premiums they would have to pay for this protection) and the disastrous 1993-1994 health reform debate (when President Clinton attempted to keep his campaign promise of health care for all by sending to Congress a complex proposal developed largely behind closed doors by a panel headed by his spouse; the idea died an agonizing death through attacks by every established interest that stood to lose control or funding). Those events, coupled with the conflicting views of the public, have been read by many as making it highly unlikely that any major effort to achieve universality of care will be attempted in the near future. Even the most popular of changes, creating a Medicare prescription drug benefit, was accomplished by crafting a benefit that is incomplete, complex, and extremely confusing to many participants. For example, the period of full implementation in January 2006 led to many individuals being denied access to medication essential to the management of chronic mental illness, with an echo effect of increased hospitalization costs.

POTENTIAL POSITIVE FORCES

Despite the negatives, there are some forces that might push the country in the direction of universality.

A BALANCING ACT

The major force is the conundrum of balancing cost and quality without leaving an even larger number of individuals without care. A number of states attempting health reform and universal coverage in the 1980s and 1990s dealt with this problem extensively. The problem can be described as similar to trying to get complete control of a large, slightly underfilled balloon: when you grab on one place, it simply bulges out in another. The expectation that the care system will achieve a higher quality of error-free care may require additional staff, different staff, or new information systems, all of which entail cost. Under the existing system, adding any staff or capital equipment without jeopardizing quality or raising cost can be accomplished by reducing the number of individuals cared for. If, however, it is very clear that no one can be moved outside—that is, left without care—we will be forced to have the dialogue needed to make a collective agreement on all three points: how much care, of what quality, and at what cost. However, no state has the legal authority to require participation in any state-specific universal plan on the part of Medicare or companies choosing to self-insure and thereby be exempted from state regulation by ERISA,[2] so state efforts have at best had only partial success and for limited periods of time.

ECONOMICS MATTER

The sense that there is a problem has dissipated since the wave of support for health reform in 1992 and 1993, when President Bill Clinton tried to live up to his campaign promise of providing universal access

---

[2]The employee retirement income security act (ERISA) exempts self-insured health benefits plans from regulation by the states, meaning that self-insured companies may limit benefits, arbitrarily change coverage, or exempt certain conditions in ways that would otherwise be limited by state law if coverage were offered through ordinary insurance companies. When the law was enacted in 1974, the focus was primarily on eliminating duplicate oversight of pension plans for companies operating in many states. Hawaii had a mandate for universal employment-based insurance that predated ERISA and is the only exemption to the law.

to care. Because those who are uninsured are disproportionately from often-disenfranchised groups, their concerns have not been heard. Emergence of a larger group more representative of the economic and ethnic mix of the nation would make the problem real. Many hope that awareness of the problem would be rekindled if the economy were to take a serious downturn, bringing home to many more individuals the reality that under the present nonsystem they are only one paycheck or one layoff away from being unable to finance needed health care for themselves and their families. There is a resurgence of reports from large employers that they are experiencing crippling increases in costs for health insurance for employees (even if they ignore families and retirees). The most well-known of these complaints is from General Motors: When the cost of materials and labor is broken out per vehicle manufactured, the attributable cost of health insurance exceeds the cost of raw metals used. Public awareness of such stories can stimulate the political will to make the needed changes.

THE PUBLIC'S ROLE

Public awareness and concern may be, in the end, what makes the change possible. The public voted overwhelmingly for change in national leadership by selecting Barack Obama as president and a Congress with a Democratic Party in both houses. As often happens, the euphoria of the election and inauguration have become tempered by the realities of governing in the face of a global economic depression and armed conflicts in Iraq and Afghanistan. It did take the president's personal intervention and expenditure of political capital to achieve the change that is now being put into place. The further policy change needed to develop a fully comprehensive and inclusive national health policy can happen only when there is a confluence of a perceived problem, a potential solution, and the political will to act. These may be driven by documentation of the continuing gaps in service and excessive expenditures that continue under the new law. The potential solutions are many and have been in circulation for many years. The

exact combination of funding and organization that would achieve universality in the U.S. may not be known, but its component parts are most likely already within the policy menu. The widespread awareness that there really is a problem has strengthened the political will of those currently in power.

However, the use of an awakened public can cut both ways. From the far right, the use of demagoguery to arouse fears of "death panels killing grandma" and "big government in your examining room" made it impossible for Republican members of the House or Senate to vote for health reform without risk of losing the next election. Advocates at the far left of the political spectrum remain unhappy that the new law focuses primarily on financing issues and did not incorporate what are seen as radical solutions, such as a single national payer. The memorial message of enacting change in memory and honor of the life and work of the late Senator Ted Kennedy was a definite push. Even an endorsement by the long-time opponent of change, the American Medical Association, did not produce a well-spring of confidence. There does not appear to be a sustained lobbying effort that will last longer than one election cycle and is loud enough to be heard over the voices of the currently enfranchised nonsystem. The fears of clinicians, hospitals, suppliers, employers, and insurance companies that they will lose autonomy and face tough regulation and even tougher price negotiations continues to mean that they will argue loud and long against any single national voice about health, even if benefiting from the new financial arrangements. And there is no way to achieve true universality, or a truly national system, without that single national voice.

For a list of related websites, please refer to your Evolve Resources at http://evolve.elsevier.com/Mason/policypolitics/

REFERENCES

Anderson, G. F., & Frogner, B. K. (2008). Health spending in OECD countries: Obtaining value per dollar. *Health Affairs, 27*(6), 1718-1727.
Kaiser Family Foundation. (2010). Focus on health reform: Summary of new health reform law (publication #8061). Retrieved from www.kff.org/healthreform/upload/8061.pdf.

CHAPTER 16

A Primer on Health Economics

Lynn Unruh and Joanne Spetz

"All models are wrong, but some are useful."
—George Box

It would be great if we could provide all the health care we wanted to anyone needing it at any time. It is becoming clearer and clearer, however, that health care resources are limited, and that choices must be made—and *are* being made—as to *what* health care is provided, *who* receives health care, and *how much* health care is received.

The choices that must be made among scarce resources can be seen from the following: The United States (U.S.) spends more than any other nation on health care, around $2.5 trillion per year. This translates to 17.6% of the Gross Domestic Product, or $8160 per person (Kaiser Family Foundation [KFF], 2009a). Yet around 17% of our population goes without regular care due to lack of health insurance (KFF, 2008), primary care is often difficult to obtain (Schoen, et al., 2004), and many of our health outcomes are worse than those of other countries (The Commonwealth Fund [CWF], 2007).

These realities of our health care system are important to *consumers* of health care, yet they equally affect nurses as *providers* of health care. First, they impact the health of nurses' patients. When someone goes without preventative care because she cannot pay for the services, she may enter the health care system sicker and use more nursing resources. Second, they impact the *types of nursing services* that are provided. Over the past decades, health care services have moved away from inpatient hospital care toward outpatient care such as home care, same-day surgery, and urgent care centers. Care also has shifted to nursing homes, rehabilitation centers, or other subacute care centers. As a result, demand for nurses has shifted away from inpatient hospital care. Third, they affect the *quantity and quality of resources* that are available to provide health care, including physical, technological, and human resources. In turn, these resources (such as nurse-to-patient ratios and nursing skills) affect the quality of health care, nurses' work environments, and nurses' physical and mental health (Unruh, 2008).

Health economics helps us make decisions about what and how much health care to produce, how to provide it, and to whom to provide it. Health economics strives to provide insight into how our health care system operates, and ways to make it operate better. It assists in quantifying and evaluating the pros and cons of the multiple potential uses of limited resources. While it is useful as an input in decision-making, it should not be seen as the "last word." Many other considerations are involved, such as cultural, social, and political concerns.

This chapter begins with a discussion about the application of economic theory to health care. Following that, the chapter addresses the following specific topics: the demand for health care, of which insurance and managed care play big roles: the supply of health care, including the roles of hospitals, physicians, and nurses; the markets for hospitals and nurses; the evaluation of costs and benefits of specific health care policies; and the future health care system.

ECONOMIC THEORY AND REALITY IN HEALTH CARE

Economic theory addresses the question of how communities allocate scarce resources. Individuals have different preferences for goods, services, time, and other things of value. Moreover, individuals have different abilities to produce things that people need, such as food, equipment, and services. As a result of these two types of differences, opportunities for trade abound. A highly-productive farmer can trade food she will not eat for a doctor's services, and a carpenter can trade her construction work for clothing.

In a freely competitive economy, prices can adjust as needed to ensure that the supply and demand for goods and services are balanced. When the demand for a product is greater than its supply, purchasers bid up the price of the scarce product. As the price rises, fewer purchasers are interested in the product, because its cost becomes greater than its value to some buyers. Thus, the demand drops. At the same time, the higher price that can be received for the product causes suppliers to increase their supply, because they can receive greater profit for each item sold. The combined effect of the decrease in demand and increase in supply, caused by the free-market change in price, is that the market will reach an equilibrium point at which supply and demand are equal. When supply exceeds demand, a similar story can be told, with the price falling so that more buyers are interested in the product and sellers want to offer less of it.

A freely competitive market, often called a "perfectly competitive" market, never faces a shortage or surplus of a product. Several conditions must be met for a market to be perfectly competitive, the most important of which are that there must be many buyers and sellers, there is no cost to becoming a seller or buyer, the products must be uniform ("homogenous"), and buyers and sellers must have perfect information about the qualities of products. Some markets exhibit many of these characteristics. For example, the low-wage labor market has many buyers (employers) and sellers (workers), job attributes are generally well-known, employers can assess that workers have few skills, and employers and workers can enter the labor market easily.

It requires little analysis to recognize that health care markets violate all the basic requirements of perfectly competitive markets. For many types of health care markets, there are not many, but instead few sellers. Hospital or nursing home markets, for example, are closer to "monopolies" or "oligopolies" (characterized by one or only a few sellers in the market, respectively) than to competitive markets. Similarly, health care professionals such as physicians or nurses cannot enter the market freely; most professionals are licensed by state or professional organizations. The health care "product" is not uniform: each physician or hospital provides different care

compared to another. Given these characteristics, these health care providers have some degree of market power over the *sale* of their product. This can lead to shortages and higher prices for care than would exist in a competitive environment. Market power can also extend to the *buying* of inputs such as labor ("monopsony" or "oligopsony") and lead to shortages in the labor force because wages and benefits stay below equilibrium levels.

Perhaps more importantly, buyers and sellers do not have perfect information about patients' need for health care or the quality of health care products. Patients do not know whether or when they will need health care in the future. They may not even be sure that they are ill, nor will they know how to treat their ailments. Providers often do not know what a patient's ailment is until further tests are conducted. Moreover, providers do not know how effective a course of treatment is for an individual patient.

Most economists agree that policy intervention can be used to address problems in markets that are not perfectly competitive. Some regulations are widely accepted, such as the licensure of health professionals and hospitals so patients have assurance of the quality of their providers. Government provision of health insurance for certain populations—older adults and the poor—is designed to address the fact that these populations cannot obtain insurance otherwise, and is generally accepted. But there is also much debate about the appropriate role of government. Should governments regulate health care prices? To what extent should governments invest in research that leads to new health care treatments? Should employers receive tax breaks for providing health insurance? Most debates about government intervention focus on the question of whether the health care market can be made sufficiently competitive to function with some regulation, or whether the health care market is so dysfunctional that a complete government takeover is needed.

THE DEMAND FOR HEALTH CARE

In recent years, health policy in the U.S. has focused on the needs of those who demand health care services. The demand for health care is often intermediated by the purchase of health insurance. In the U.S., people obtain health insurance in three general ways: their employers offer health insurance as a component of compensation for work; they purchase insurance individually from an insurance company; or they are enrolled in a government-funded program.

Once a person has insurance, she is insulated from the costs of each health care service. Apart from small payments that might be required for each service, the insurance enrollee pays only the fixed cost of the insurance, and in fact might not even pay this if insurance is provided by an employer or government entity. As a result, the enrollee tends to demand more health care than would be demanded without insurance. This is called *moral hazard*. Moral hazard leads to greater health care demand, and thus greater health care expenditures, than would occur in a perfectly competitive market. A fundamental issue faced by all health care systems is how to reach the socially optimal level of health care utilization given the presence of health insurance.

Insurance companies try to address moral hazard in a variety of ways. Most common is the requirement that the enrollee pay some part of the cost of each health service in the form of co-payment (a flat fee paid for each service) or co-insurance (a fixed percentage of the cost of each service). Many traditional insurance plans also require that the enrollee pay some amount of health care costs before the insurer pays any of the costs; this is called a *deductible*. Although the RAND Health Insurance Experiment of the 1980s found that increased out-of-pocket expenses were not associated with worse health, other studies indicate that needed health care might be neglected (Karter et al., 2003), which could lead to greater emergency department utilization (Wright et al., 2005) and poorer health outcomes.

Since the 1940s, insurance companies have provided "managed care," in which the insurance company plays a role in directing the overall care of enrollees. One of the first managed care insurance plans was the Kaiser Foundation Health Plan, which still operates today. In the Kaiser plan, a medical group exclusively contracts with the insurance company to provide health care, and Kaiser Permanente operates its own hospitals. Employees pay small co-payments for health services, and physicians receive extensive education and guidance about providing preventative care and evidence-based practice. A patient must be referred to a specialist by a primary care physician; self-referral is not allowed, and care

received outside the Kaiser network is not covered by the insurance.

There were few other insurance companies offering managed care insurance until the past three decades, during which time numerous variants of the managed care concept have evolved. Many new HMOs are not "closed panel," and allow the physicians with whom they contract to treat both HMO and non-HMO patients. These HMOs maintain control over care provided to patients either directly by placing restrictions on the services offered or indirectly by providing physicians and hospitals incentives to care for patients in certain ways. Enrollees are assigned to primary health care providers, called "gatekeepers," who manage the overall care of enrollees.

Preferred provider organizations (PPOs) encourage enrollees to select certain care providers by providing lower co-insurance rates if preferred providers are chosen. They allow members to go to specialists without having to use a gatekeeper first. A point-of-service plan (POS) is a hybrid of an HMO and a PPO. Patients are assigned a primary health care provider, as in an HMO, but they can seek care from other providers, albeit at a higher out-of-pocket cost.

The goal of these benefit conscriptions, in-network requirements, gatekeeper requirements, and other enrollee incentives is to control costs by better managing the care of enrollees, and reducing "moral hazard." In theory, managed care insurance plans focus on preventative health care services and try to eliminate unneeded medical care.

Because people have little information with which to judge the quality of care offered by health care providers and thus by insurance companies, they often select insurance based on price rather than quality. Moreover, a hospital that provides excellent quality care is usually reimbursed at the same rate as a hospital that provides mediocre quality care. When managed care pressures cause providers to focus on reducing costs, they often do so at the expense of quality. At a minimum, amenities are eliminated, and in some cases registered nurse (RN) staff.

These problems arise due to the difficulty of obtaining information about health care products, and are a reason for intervention by governmental regulatory or private credentialing organizations such as The Joint Commission (TJC). Through regulation or certification, quality can be monitored, standardized, and improved, and information about quality can be conveyed to consumers.

This discussion on the demand for health care in the U.S. omits one important issue: the high share of Americans who lack adequate health insurance. About 28% of non-elderly adults did not have health insurance at some time in 2007, while another 20% were underinsured, with a high economic burden of health care relative to income (Schoen et al., 2008). The uninsured tend to be poor or near poor adults in families with at least one wage earner. Most have gone without coverage for at least two years. Rates of uninsurance are higher among minorities. For these people, the primary issue is that they do not use primary and preventative health services as much as they should because they cannot afford the out-of-pocket costs. As a result, health problems that could be treated effectively grow into acute problems that must be treated aggressively, are more costly, and have poorer outcomes. A universal health insurance program continues to be a controversial policy for Americans. The health reform legislation passed in 2010, though not completely universal, will reduce the number of uninsured by about 32 million people.

THE SUPPLY OF HEALTH CARE

The supply of health care also has been a focus of health policy. Direct suppliers of health care are professionals (such as physicians and advanced practice nurses), and institutions of care (such as hospitals, nursing homes, home care, and doctor's offices). Institutions of care, in turn, employ a number of non-professional and professional staff, such as the nursing staff, who enter into employment through the "derived demand" of their institutional employers.

These suppliers, or providers, of health care offer services in exchange for payment from the various demanders of health care discussed earlier in the chapter. Providers have experienced drastic changes in the reimbursement for their services. In general, payers have moved away from paying providers what they charge after the service is provided (retrospective payment) to amounts set in advance of the service (prospective payment). Both public and private payers have been responsible for these changes, starting with the introduction of Diagnostic Related Groups (DRGs) and Resource Based Relative Value Scales (RBRVS) for payment under Medicare, and

continuing with various negotiated fees and charges under managed care. At this time, prospective payment systems (PPSs) exist for all types of health care: inpatient hospital, nursing home, home care, and ambulatory care.

PPSs have, in turn, prompted providers to find efficiencies in delivering care in order to provide care for the agreed-upon amount of money. The search for efficiencies can take the form of technology improvements that reduce the time needed to perform the services, or cost-cutting measures such as staff reductions and substitutions.

One practice that providers may engage in to compensate for reduced payment is "provider-induced demand." In this practice, providers instruct patients, who generally know less about their health problem and treatment than the providers, to consume more health care than would be demanded if the patient had perfect information. Demand inducement is not necessarily a malicious phenomenon; care providers might encourage patients to seek every medical intervention or test that could have any benefit, even if the benefit is so small that the costs exceed the benefits. Patients do not pay the full cost of health services in most cases, so they do not make cost-benefit comparisons. Demand inducement is a problem because it leads to greater overall health care spending and can lead to iatrogenic illnesses among the patients who receive "too much" or inappropriate health care.

One set of health care providers—physicians—play a central role in the provision of medical care services, and therefore make many of the demand decisions for their patients. They act as agents for their patients. When physicians are able to induce demand for health care, it is called "physician-induced demand." Whether physicians or other providers can actually induce demand for health care has been an area of research and debate in health care economics.

In the previous section, we discussed how managed care attempts to reduce "moral hazard." Managed care also attempts to reduce supplier-induced demand. One of the most drastic methods is through capitation, in which providers are paid a fixed amount per patient per year, regardless of how much care the person requires. Providers' incentives are to keep the utilization of resources down—for example, the number of office visits, or the use of tests and procedures. The use of capitation is currently in decline due to consumer and provider backlash.

Per diem and DRG-based reimbursements to hospitals limit the amount of reimbursement hospitals may receive for each patient's stay. Under these systems, greater utilization of resources by providers may lead to financial losses. Physicians may be paid bonuses to keep resource utilization down, and pay may be withheld for overutilization. Case management, utilization management, disease management, the use of second opinion, and the use of practice guidelines also are aimed at reducing unnecessary medical care. The research evidence tends to confirm that these managed care methods reduce health care utilization (Yelin, et al., 2004).

THE MARKET FOR HOSPITAL SERVICES

Hospitals are an important part of the U.S. health care system. They provide emergency care, surgeries, highly technical tests and treatments, and institutional care for those too sick to be cared for at home. Although hospitals in 2007 received 33% of all health care dollars, demand for their services fell during the 1990s, primarily due to managed care influence (AHA, 2009). The number of annual admissions fell 14% from 1980 to 1995, and has not yet returned to its 1980 level (CDC, 2008). Many health care services have moved to the hospital outpatient setting, as indicated by a 163% increase in emergency department, outpatient surgery, and other outpatient care from 1980 to 2006 (CDC, 2008).

Hospitals are classified according to length of stay, type of service, and type of ownership. Short-term hospitals are those with average lengths of stay less than 30 days. Community hospitals are short-stay hospitals that offer general services, and some also provide specialty care and rehabilitation. They may be owned by state or local governments, non-profit voluntary organizations, or for-profit organizations.

Hospital ownership can be private not-for-profit, private for-profit, and governmental. The most prominent form of ownership of hospitals is private not-for-profit (around 60% of all hospitals). However, for-profit ownership grew in the 1980s and 1990s. By 2006, 18% of community hospitals in the U.S. were for-profit (KFF, n.d.).

Some believe that the quality of care in non-profit hospitals must be better because they don't focus on the "bottom line." Actually, non-profit hospitals have to be just as conscious of costs and revenues as for-profits. Both for-profit and non-profit hospitals can generate surplus revenue. Where they differ is that for-profits can distribute the surplus in the form of profit to stockholders or owners, whereas non-profits must maintain the surplus within the institution or use it to provide some benefit to the community. The research record on whether non-profit hospitals provide better care is mixed (Eggleston et al., 2006).

Because of the reimbursement and managed care pressures described earlier, hospital organization, finances, services, and employment patterns underwent dramatic change in the past decades. At the beginning of the 1990s, hospitals found themselves negotiating unfavorable contracts with managed care companies because those companies had power on the buyer's side of the market. In response to this pressure, hospitals merged and formed multihospital systems in the 1990s. Some hospitals merged or expanded vertically by adding non-inpatient types of health care such as home care, nursing home care, rehabilitation, or ambulatory care. Some hospitals closed.

These changes provided integrated hospital systems with greater market power to counter that of managed care, greater economies of scale (efficiencies due to size), and greater economies of scope (efficiencies due to producing many different types of products). It also produced hospital markets that are classically "monopolistic" or "oligopolic" as sellers—that is, one or a handful of hospital systems have carved out the market for hospital care in each geographic area. Managed care plans must negotiate with these few sellers of hospital services. As a result, the cost savings that managed care achieved in the 1980s and early 1990s began to dissipate in the late 1990s as the hospital oligopolies arrived on the scene.

It is thought that hospitals respond to reduced public reimbursement by charging privately-insured patients higher prices. Those who believe that hospitals cost-shift point to the fact that the gap between payment-to-cost ratios of private to public payers widened during the 1980s and early 1990s. With the rise of managed care, the differential declined significantly but began widening again starting in 2000. By 2007, the payment-to-cost ratio of public payers was around 90%, while that of private payers was 130% (Avalere Health, 2009). Internally, in response to lower demand and reduced public and private payments in the 1990s, hospitals downsized and restructured. Both nursing and non-nursing staff were affected. We will discuss the changes and their impact on nursing staff in the next section. In addition, hospitals reorganized care so that patients complete their hospital stays in a shorter amount of time. Average lengths of stay in short-stay hospitals fell from 7.5 days in 1980 to 4.7 days in 2006, a drop of 37% (CDC, 2008). Because hospitals are often paid a fixed or maximum amount per patient stay, length of stay reductions allows them to provide care at costs lower than the fixed reimbursements, and keep the additional revenue.

THE MARKET FOR NURSES

The term *nurse* means different things to different people. By "nurse" we refer to both licensed nurses, such as RNs and licensed practical nurses (LPNs), and unlicensed nurses, such as nursing assistants. We focus primarily on the market for RNs.

Because most nurses are employees of health care institutions, the demand for their employment is derived from their employers, who employ nurses based on the demand and prices for their services, and the productivity and prices (wages, salaries, and benefits) of the nurses being hired. As reimbursement changed to prospective systems, and as managed care practices grew, the growth in demand for inpatient care slowed and the prices paid for care were constrained. As a consequence, hospital demand for licensed nurses fell in the 1990s, as reflected in lower staffing ratios (RNs or licensed nurses per acuity-adjusted patient day) and lower skill mix (RNs or licensed nurses as a proportion of total nurses) (Unruh & Fottler, 2006).

On the other hand, the demand for nurses in other areas such as ambulatory surgery centers and home care has grown. This growth slowed in home care after 1997, when the Balanced Budget Act (BBA) introduced a Prospective Payment System (PPS) for home care. With that, the demand for home care nurses plunged. In other areas, such as nursing homes and physicians' offices, demand has been more stable.

After reports of surpluses of nurses (demand lower than supply) in hospitals in the mid-1990s, a shortage of RNs in hospitals reemerged in the late 1990s. At that time, public reimbursement improved and managed care pressures lessened. Admissions increased, and length of stay stabilized. In addition, the typical hospitalized patient was acutely ill. Suddenly, demand for nurses, particularly RNs, rose. Hospital vacancy rates peaked at 12% to 15% in 2001 (AHA, 2002). In 2007, hospital vacancy rates still stood at 8.1% (AHA, 2007).

The RN shortage that began in the late 1990s is considered to be structural rather than temporary. It is expected that the gap between RN supply and demand will grow: by 2020 the gap between supply and demand is projected to climb to 16% (Buerhaus et al., 2008). This structural shortage has several causes. On the demand side, population growth and an aging population exerts growing health care consumption pressure. Other factors affecting demand include levels of access afforded by public and private insurance, and the efficiency of health care delivery. On the supply side, factors include a large population of older RNs who are expected to retire soon; educational bottlenecks that restrict the growth of nursing supply; and difficult work environments that discourage entry into, and encourage withdrawal from, the profession.

In 2008, the RN shortage took an unexpected turn. A general economic crisis in the U.S., with high unemployment levels and reduced hospital utilization, is thought to have contributed to an increase in RN supply and a drop in hospital demand for RNs. Given the fact that supply increased and demand fell, the gap between supply and demand in hospitals may have narrowed considerably. It is generally agreed, however, that this adjustment is temporary and that the overall forces leading to a severe shortage within 10 years have not changed.

It was mentioned earlier that in a competitive market shortages would not occur. Why do we see shortages in the market for nurses? One economic theory is that the primary employers of nurses—hospitals—enjoy a monopsony over the hiring of nursing labor; they have market power in the buying of nursing labor, which they use to keep wages, benefits, and working conditions at lower-than-equilibrium levels. Even though employers would like to employ more nurses, the wages, benefits, and working conditions they offer do not attract people to their jobs. Raising wages alone may not be the answer to this problem, however, as long as working conditions remain difficult (Di Tommaso et al., 2009; Spetz & Given, 2003).

It may be that wages, benefits, and working conditions for nurses are at suboptimal levels because nursing care is not appropriately valued and priced. At the societal level, market economies have tended to downplay the value of "caring" services, as well as "women's work," both of which are the cultural and historical legacy of nursing (Nelson & Folbre, 2006). At the payer level, specific nursing services have generally not been included in reimbursement systems. Studies of the DRG payment system have shown that DRG values are not strongly associated with the intensity of nursing care for that category (Welton & Halloran, 2005). At the organizational level, health care facilities typically treat nursing care only as "expense" items in their budget, not as revenue-generating items. The price of nursing is wrapped into the room rate.

To receive adequate wages, benefits, and working conditions, these societal, financial, and organizational impediments to properly valuing and pricing nursing services need to be overcome. Ways to accomplish this include conducting and disseminating research on the following:

- What nurses do, including their caring activities, but also their intellectual, technical, managerial, and other activities
- How what they do affects health outcomes
- What the costs of adequate nursing care are versus the costs of inadequate care

As the value of nursing care is understood, nursing advocates can work for societal, financial, and organizational change that will allow for valuing and pricing nursing services. The changes in reimbursement and the cost-consciousness of public and private payers have increased the demand for advance practice nurses. In acute care, nurse clinicians and nurse practitioners are needed to clinically manage a more acutely ill patient population. In ambulatory care, demand for nurse practitioners is on the rise. However, the expansion of advanced practice nursing continues to face opposition by the medical establishment, and many legal barriers remain.

CLINICAL ECONOMICS: EVALUATING HEALTH CARE PERFORMANCE

Given the limited resources in health care, methods to help us choose among them are welcome.

Economics offers the following six techniques for health care decision-making:

- Cost of illness
- Cost identification
- Cost minimization
- Cost-consequence analysis
- Cost-effectiveness analysis
- Cost-benefit analysis

When performing *cost-of-illness* analyses, investigators only look at the total costs of one or more *illnesses* in order to ascertain whether they should be a priority for treatment and/or public health measures. Often the entire economic burden of a disease is described, including not only the medical costs, but also days lost from work. A recent example is a study on the cost of prematurity (Cuevas et al., 2005). It finds that charges for initial hospitalization increased as birth weight and gestational weight decreased, and concludes that interventions to improve prenatal care targeted to high-risk pregnancies would reduce costs.

Cost identification looks at the costs of a health care *service*. This can be done for several different services for a given health care problem. Then, the cost of the different services can be compared, and the service with the lowest cost can be chosen. At this point, the analysis becomes a *cost-minimization* study.

Several strategies measure both the costs and effectiveness of health care interventions. In *cost-consequence* analysis, one creates a comprehensive listing of all the benefits of competing interventions, and lets decision-makers determine which benefits are most important. A *cost-effectiveness analysis* (CEA) measures the benefits of projects with a consistent unit of measure, such as "cost per life saved," cost per quality-adjusted life years (QALYs), or "cost per case of breast cancer detected." With CEA, the objective is to find the treatment that has the relatively best effectiveness for the relatively best costs. Treatments that have both higher costs and less effectiveness are eliminated. While CEA enables the investigator to relatively rank treatments, a judgment about the absolute effectiveness of the treatments is not possible. In other words, in CEA, even though one or some treatments are better, all the treatments could entail high costs for little benefits. Box 16-1 contains an example of a study concerning sleep apnea (Mar et al., 2003).

BOX 16-1 Example of Cost-Effectiveness Analysis

Objective: To compare the cost-effectiveness of nasal continuous positive airway pressure (nCPAP) with conventional null treatment for those with moderate to severe obstructive sleep apnea (OSAS).

   Methods: A Markov-type decision tree was used to diagram the possible progression of obstructive sleep apnea. The measure of effectiveness of treatments was quality adjusted life years (QALYs). Direct costs of diagnosis and treatment of OSAS as well as costs of not being treated were considered. The incremental cost-effectiveness ratio (ICER) was calculated for various scenarios.

   Results: The ICER was similar to that of other interventions, indicating that nCPAP is a cost-effective treatment modality.

Mar, J., Rueda, J. R., Duran-Cantolla, J., Schechter, C., & Chilcott, J. (2003). The cost-effectiveness of nCPAP treatment in patients with moderate-to-severe obstructive sleep apnoea. *European Respiratory Journal, 21*(3), 515-522.

Finally, sometimes the technique of *cost-benefit analysis* (CBA) is used. In CBA, both costs and benefits are in dollar amounts. The total costs are subtracted from the total benefits of each treatment to find the *net benefits*, which are then compared. CBA is not used nearly as much as CEA in health care because dollar amounts must be placed on human life and health.

REFORM OF THE U.S. HEALTH CARE SYSTEM AND THE FUTURE OF NURSING

The U.S. health care system presents three challenges: lowering costs, improving access, and improving quality. Being able to implement a reform that would do all three has been difficult. Some believe that market forces should be used, and the government's role is to ensure that health care markets are competitive. Market-oriented reforms include medical savings accounts, tax credits, and vouchers. Others believe a single national health care system should be established. There are many policy proposals that seek intermediate ground.

   Some policymakers have suggested that medical savings accounts would help reduce costs without worsening access or quality. Medical savings accounts would be created for every individual either through their employer, themselves, or public assistance. Individuals would use the money in their savings accounts for primary health care, such as routine physician visits, medications, and tests. For larger medical expenses, including hospitalization, individuals would buy a low-cost, high-deductible insurance plan. For low-income individuals, vouchers could be used to subsidize the costs of obtaining these plans. This type of health plan is favorable to healthy and wealthy families, and is generally more expensive for people with chronic illnesses. Moreover, poor families might avoid seeking primary health care services due to the out-of-pocket costs, and thus allow problems to reach a catastrophic level before seeking care.

   At the other extreme, advocates of a single-payer health care system believe that eliminating the multiple payers of the U.S. system and providing everyone with the same access to health care will both reduce costs and improve access. They cite that current administrative costs take away 31 cents of every health care dollar (Woolhandler et al., 2003). If the system could be streamlined by creating a single governmental payer, around half of these costs could disappear. The "single payer" system could use payroll taxes and the money saved from reduced administrative costs to provide health care to all. Issues with this system involve those having to do with moral hazard and supplier-induced demand. Unless the system also maintains a managed care approach to delivering care, the easy availability of health care could lead to a rise in health care expenditures and to waiting periods to receive health care.

   Other reform alternatives take a middle-of-the-road approach to these two. At the time of this writing, the Obama administration is exploring a middle approach that would keep in place the current employer-based private insurance system plus require individual mandates for those who are not covered by employers. It would provide support for individuals who can't afford health insurance by expanding Medicaid and SCHIP eligibility and providing subsidies to low-income individuals to purchase insurance (KFF, 2009b).

   Economists believe that the U.S. has not been able to enact a major health care reform plan because of a combination of interests and power (Feldstein, 2005). The constituents who are most affected by a reform must be able to influence policymakers, and multiple constituents need to agree on a plan. In health care, powerful interest groups (e.g., insurance companies, hospitals, pharmaceuticals, unions, and others) influence politicians to move in different directions rather than a unified one, and the group that would most benefit from reforms—the poor and uninsured—have little influence at all.

The future of nursing depends very much on the future of the U.S. health care system. Reforms that focus on cost-containment at the expense of access and/or quality could lead to continuing problems with staffing and working conditions as institutions attempt to tighten their belts even further. Reforms that do not constrain costs while providing greater access could lead to even greater shortages of nursing personnel. The best situation for nursing, as for health care consumers in general, will be finding a solution that has the fewest tradeoffs between costs, access, and quality yet improves all three.

For a list of related websites, please refer to your Evolve Resources at http://evolve.elsevier.com/Mason/policypolitics/

REFERENCES

AHA. (2002). Chartbook: Trends affecting hospitals and health systems. November, 2002. Retrieved from www.aha.org/aha/trendwatch/2002/cb2002chapter5.pdf.

AHA. (2007). The 2007 state of America's hospitals: Taking the pulse. Findings from the 2007 AHA Survey of Hospital Leaders, American Hospital Association, Retrieved from www.aha.org/aha/research-and-trends/health-and-hospital-trends/2007.html.

AHA. (2009). Chartbook: Trends affecting hospitals and health systems, Chart 1.5. Retrieved from www.aha.org/aha/research-and-trends/chartbook/index.html.

Avalere health analysis of American Hospital Association annual survey data, 2007, for community hospitals (from American Hospital Association Trend Watch Chartbook, 2009). Retrieved from www.aha.org/aha/trendwatch/chartbook/2009/chapter4.ppt.

Buerhaus, P. I., Staiger, D. O., & Auerbach, D. I., (2008). The future of the nursing workforce in the United States: Data, trends and implications. Sudbury, MA: Jones & Bartlett.

Centers for Disease Control and Prevention (CDC). (2008). Health United States, 2008, Tables 94, 102, 106. Retrieved from www.cdc.gov/nchs/hus.htm.

The Commonwealth Fund (CWF). (2007). Mirror, mirror on the wall: An international update on the comparative performance of American health care. May 15, 2007, The Commonwealth Fund. Retrieved from www.commonwealthfund.org/Content/Publications/Fund-Reports/2007/May/Mirror-Mirror-on-the-Wall-An-International-Update-on-the-Comparative-Performance-of-American-Healt.aspx.

Cuevas, K. D., Silver, D. R., Brooten, D., Youngblut, J. M., & Bobo, C. M. (2005). The cost of prematurity: Hospital charges at birth and frequency of rehospitalizations and acute care visits over the first year of life. American Journal of Nursing, 105(7), 56-64.

Di Tommaso, M. L., Strøm, S., & Saether, E. M. (2009). Nurses wanted: Is the job too harsh or is the wage too low? Journal of Health Economics, 28(3), 748-757.

Eggleston, K., Shen, Y., Lau, J., Schmid, C., & Chan, J. (2006). Hospital ownership and quality of care: What explains the different results? National Bureau of Economic Research, NBER Working Papers: 12241.

Feldstein, P. (2005). Health policy issues: An economic perspective (3rd ed.). Chicago: Health Administration Press.

Karter, A. J., Stevens, M. R., Herman, W. H., Ettner, S., Marrero, D. G., Safford, M. M., et al. Translating Research Into Action for Diabetes Study Group. (2003). Out-of-pocket costs and diabetes preventive services: The Translating Research Into Action for Diabetes (TRIAD) study. Diabetes Care, 26(8), 2294-2299.

Kaiser Family Foundation (KFF). (n.d.). Trends and indicators in the changing health care marketplace, Kaiser Family Foundation website. Retrieved from www.kff.org/insurance/7031/print-sec5.cfm.

Kaiser Family Foundation (KFF). (2008). The uninsured: A primer. Kaiser Family Foundation. Kaiser Commission on Medicaid and the Uninsured. Retrieved from www.kff.org/uninsured/upload/7451_04_Data_Tables.pdf.

Kaiser Family Foundation (KFF). (2009a). Trends in healthcare costs and spending. Kaiser Family Foundation. Retrieved from www.kff.org/insurance/upload/7692_02.pdf.

Kaiser Family Foundation (KFF). (2009b). Focus on health reform: A side-by-side comparison of major health care reform proposals, last modified July 24, 2009. Retrieved from www.kff.org/healthreform/upload/healthreform_sbs_full.pdf.

Mar, J., Rueda, J. R., Duran-Cantolla, J., Schechter, C., & Chilcott, J. (2003). The cost-effectiveness of nCPAP treatment in patients with moderate-to-severe obstructive sleep apnoea. European Respiratory Journal, 21(3), 515-522.

Nelson, J. A., Folbre, N. (2006). Why a well-paid nurse is a better nurse. Nursing Economics, 24(3), 127-130.

Schoen, C., Collins, S. R., Kriss, J. L., & Doty, M. (2008). How many are underinsured? Trends among U.S. adults, 2003 and 2007. Health Affairs Web Exclusive, June 10, 2008, W298-309, Retrieved from http://content.healthaffairs.org/cgi/reprint/27/4/w298.

Schoen, C., Osborn, R., Trang Huynh, P., Doty, M., Davis, K., Zapert, K., et al. (2004). Primary care and health system performance: Adults' experiences in five countries. Health Affairs, Web Exclusive, October 28, 2004, W4-487, 487-503. Retrieved from http://content.healthaffairs.org/cgi/reprint/hlthaff.w4.487v1.

Spetz, J., & Given, R. (2003). The future of the nurse shortage: Will wage increases close the gap? Health Affairs, 22(6), 199-206.

Unruh, L., & Fottler, M. (2006). Patient turnover and nursing staff adequacy. Health Services Research, 41(2), 599-612.

Unruh, L. (2008). Nurse staffing and patient, nurse, and financial outcomes. American Journal of Nursing, 108(1), 62-71.

Welton, J. M. & Halloran, E. J. (2005). Nursing diagnoses, diagnosis related group, and hospital outcomes. Journal of Nursing Administration, 35(12), 541-549.

Woolhandler S., Campbell T., Himmelstein, D. U. (2003). Costs of health care administration in the United States and Canada. New England Journal of Medicine, 349(8), 768-775.

Wright, B. J., Carlson, M. J., Edlund, T., Devoe, J., Gallia, C., & Smith, J. (2005). The impact of increased cost sharing on Medicaid enrollees. Health Affairs, 24(4), 1106-1116.

Yelin, E., Trupin, L., Earnest, G., Katz, P., Eisner, M., & Blane, P. (2004). The impact of managed care on health care utilization among adults with asthma. Journal of Asthma, 41(2), 229-242.

CHAPTER 17

Reforming Medicare

Susan C. Reinhard

"Only in growth, reform, and change, paradoxically enough, is true security to be found."

—Anne Morrow Lindbergh

THE ISSUE

The 2010 Affordable Care Act (ACA, P.L, 111-148) as amended by the Health Care and Education Reconciliation Act (HCERA, P.L. 111-152) opens up the 45-year old Medicare program to the biggest changes since its inception. The reforms are intended to protect older adults from financial hardships associated with illness, improve prevention and prescription coverage, and strengthen Medicare by increasing its solvency by about a decade. Most important, many provisions will drive innovation, changing care delivery for people of all ages. The nursing profession has the opportunity to reshape health care in ways we have long advocated but feared would never happen.

INITIAL INTENT AND EVOLUTION OF THE MEDICARE PROGRAM

Before 1965, over half of the United States population age 65 years and older had inadequate or no health insurance coverage. After years of debate, modification, and compromise, Medicare was established with the signing of HR 6675, the Social Security Amendments of 1965. The initial intent of the Medicare program was to improve the availability of health care for older adults (Gluck & Reno, 2001). Since its inception, this complex social program has gone through periodic reform. Addition of the outpatient drug benefit in 2003 was one of the most radical reforms, but it did not change the way care is provided, particularly for those with multiple chronic conditions.

In its initial form in the 1960s, Medicare offered compulsory hospital insurance for persons over the age of 65 and an optional program of government assistance in covering doctors' fees. Participants could opt not to participate in this latter part. These provisions established a substantive role for the private sector, because participants would purchase health care services in the open fee-for-service market and the federal government would pay the bills. Amendments to Medicare in 1972 extended benefits to certain individuals under the age of 65 with disabilities. These amendments also included provisions to review the quality of patient care and encourage the use of health maintenance organizations (Kaiser Family Foundation [KFF], 2005). In 1980, Congress expanded coverage of home health services and established major hospital reimbursement reform. The prospective payment system (PPS) and diagnostic-related groups (DRG) methodology for hospital payment radically altered the hospital industry by replacing the cost-based ("open checkbook") payment method and financially discouraging long hospital stays. In the latter half of the 1980s, the Medicare Catastrophic Coverage Act added a drug benefit to Medicare, but it was repealed almost immediately when older adults complained that their personal contribution to this program was too high (KFF, 2005).

The Balanced Budget Act (BBA) of 1997 again reformed Medicare payment policies by adding a prospective payment system (PPS) for five services: home health services; skilled nursing facilities (nursing homes); hospital outpatient services; outpatient rehabilitation services; and inpatient rehabilitation hospitals. It also created the Medicare + Choice program, which promised to increase Medicare enrollment in managed care by offering beneficiaries more private sector, managed care choices. Initially Medicare +

Choice enrollments in private plans increased, but as Medicare entered the new millennium, the number of plans participating in Medicare + Choice began dropping significantly. As plans dropped out, more than 2 million beneficiaries were left to find other options. Beneficiaries and providers became upset and confused, and their confidence in the managed care alternative eroded (Gold et al., 2004).

This upheaval helped to drive more changes to the Medicare program. After years of debate, in 2003 the Medicare Prescription Drug Improvement and Modernization Act (PL 108-173) established the Medicare Advantage program (previously called Medicare + Choice) and a voluntary prescription drug benefit. Known by its shorter name, the Medicare Modernization Act (MMA), this legislation launched the voluntary Medicare "Part D" Prescription Drug Benefit program with "extra help" (a subsidy) for low-income Medicare beneficiaries (KFF, 2005).

THE MEDICARE PROGRAM TODAY: THE BASICS

Medicare is a popular and trusted government-run health insurance program for America's older adults and certain people with disabilities. The original policy intent was to ensure that all older adults have access to medically necessary acute care services, regardless of where they live, their health status, or their income. Current Medicare policy continues this entitlement status for older adults, starting the first day of the month an individual turns 65. People with end-stage renal disease are also entitled to Medicare Part A, regardless of their age. Individuals who are under the age of 65 and become disabled receive Medicare benefits after having received Social Security benefits for two years. The number of Medicare beneficiaries has more than doubled since 1970. In 2010, Medicare covered 39 million older adults and 8 million younger persons with disabilities (KFF, 2010).

Contrary to popular belief, Medicare does not cover all of beneficiaries' health care costs. It covers about half of their total health care expenses. Beneficiaries spent an average of $4394 of their own money on health care in 2005—almost one third of their income (Nonnemaker & Sinclair, 2009). This is because Medicare does not cover all health care services and because it is not a free program. For example, it does not cover routine vision and hearing care,

dental care, or long-term care. Medicare beneficiaries pay 25% of the cost of the Part B program through premiums and co-payments; taxpayers pay the other 75%. As required by MMA, the Part B premium a beneficiary pays each month is now based on his or her annual income.

Over the past 45 years, the cost to Medicare beneficiaries has risen. For example, the Medicare Part B standard premium increased from $3 per month in 1965 to $110 per month in 2010, and $354 a month for those with incomes greater than $214,000 (CMS, 2009). Low-income Medicare beneficiaries can get help paying these costs through the Medicare Savings programs, which are administered by the states through Medicaid funding (Reinhard et al., 2004). Unfortunately, only about half of those who are entitled to receive this help actually apply for it.

MEDICARE PARTS A, B, C, AND D

Medicare pays for health care for older adults and some people with disabilities, although it does not pay for all acute and long-term care. As the program has evolved, it has become more complex. Currently, Medicare has four "parts" and is administered by the Center for Medicare & Medicaid Services (CMS).

PART A (THE HOSPITAL INSURANCE PROGRAM)

Part A helps to cover medically necessary costs for hospital stays, skilled nursing facility care, home health care, and hospice care.

PART B (SUPPLEMENTAL MEDICAL INSURANCE)

Part B assists in the coverage of outpatient care and services from physicians and advanced practice registered nurses. It also covers some services not included in Part A, such as physical and occupational therapists and home health care when medically necessary. Part B also covers some clinical laboratory services and preventive services, such as cardiovascular screening and blood tests. Participation is voluntary (95% of those enrolled in Part A also enroll in Part B), and the program has deductibles and premiums.

PART C (MEDICARE ADVANTAGE)

Originally called "Medicare + Choice," this part of Medicare allows beneficiaries to enroll in a variety of managed care plans, such as health maintenance organizations, preferred provider organizations, or private fee-for-service plans. Enrolled beneficiaries receive their Part A and B services through these plans, and sometimes their prescription drug benefits.

PART D (PRESCRIPTION DRUG BENEFIT PROGRAM)

Part D refers to the voluntary coverage of outpatient prescription drugs that was created under Medicare as part of the 2003 MMA. The government-sponsored prescription drug plans, which began to be offered in 2006, are offered by private companies and require payment of a premium, copayments, and deductibles. Plans can establish their own premiums, subject to CMS approval; therefore the cost of premiums varies from plan to plan. In 2010, beneficiaries who chose to enroll in Part D paid a monthly premium (average of $32), a $310 deductible, and 25% of total medication costs between $310 and $2830. Until health care reform was enacted, those who spent more than this fell into the coverage gap or "doughnut hole," paying 100% of their drug costs until they spent $4550 out of pocket (excluding premiums). After that, they paid 5% of cost of the prescription or a co-payment ($2.50/generic or $6.30/brand for each drug) for the rest of the year. These standard benefit amounts rise annually. In 2010, the size of the doughnut hole was $3610 (Purvis, 2010).

Medicare beneficiaries with low incomes and limited assets can get "extra help" that is intended to reduce or eliminate the out-of-pocket expenses associated with Part D, including premiums, deductibles, copayments, and costs in the coverage gap. In a major departure from traditional Medicare policy, the MMA imposed asset and income tests on people seeking a low-income subsidy to receive federal assistance with their Medicare Part D coverage. One in three Medicare beneficiaries is eligible for this extra help.

DRIVING FORCES FOR CHANGE IN MEDICARE

Medicare is part of America's social fabric. It has succeeded in its initial promise of lifting older adults out of the ranks of the uninsured. It has changed over the last 45 years, and the health care reform laws will change it further in the decades ahead. Various stakeholders push for change based on their differing perspectives. But in 2009, major stakeholders (nurses, physicians, hospitals, pharmaceutical manufacturers, providers, health insurers, and labor and consumer organizations) agreed that change was needed and that they had to share responsibility for change. Stakeholders' varying perspectives helped to shape the debate for changes to Medicare and health care in general, but escalating costs is the greatest driving force for change.

Over the last several years, two major arguments shaped the policy and political dialogue. First, health care costs are rising and age only accounts for a small part of that rise. We need to deal with underlying health care costs (Figure 17-1).

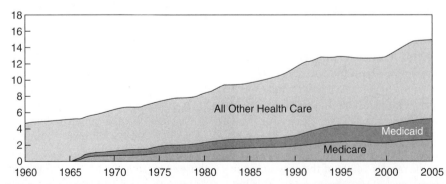

FIGURE 17-1 Spending on health care as a percentage of gross domestic product, 1960 to 2005. Note: Amounts for Medicare are gross federal spending on the program; amounts for Medicaid include spending by the federal government and the states. Source: Congressional Budget Office based on data on spending on health services and supplies, as defined in the national health expenditure accounts, maintained by the Centers for Medicare and Medicaid Services. (From Congressional Budget Office. [n.d.]. The long-term outlook for health care spending. Retrieved from *www.cbo.gov/ftpdocs/87xx/doc8758/MainText.3.1.shtml.*)

Second, there are stark regional variations in Medicare spending and service use. Service use in higher-use areas is greater than in lower-use areas, and the variation in spending is even greater (MedPAC, 2009). Research findings indicate that Medicare spending does not necessarily translate into better care or improved health (Fisher et al., 2003a, 2003b). People on Medicare who live in higher-spending regions of the country receive 60% more care than those who live in lower-spending regions. But that spending difference does not lead to better health outcomes. It might be possible to reduce Medicare spending by 30% without negatively affecting the health of Medicare beneficiaries.

As a new administration listened to experts in this field, the call for more "value" took hold. Instead of paying for services on a volume basis, more policymakers began to talk more about paying for value (price in relation to quality). Ideas such as "bundled payments" and Accountable Care Organizations (ACOs) took hold (discussed later in the chapter). So too did the focus on better chronic care management, and prevention of avoidable rehospitalizations. And to make all of this possible, there was greater attention to a workforce prepared to deliver evidence-based care, often in teams, across settings.

CHANGES IN THE MEDICARE PROGRAM UNDER HEALTH CARE REFORM

While most of the attention in health care reform has been on improving coverage for people under the age of 65, there are four important things nurses should know:

- The health care reform law provides coverage for people of all ages and is funded in large part by Medicare savings.
- People on Medicare do achieve some significant improvements in benefits.
- Because Medicare is the major payer of health care, innovations in serving people on Medicare will fuel innovations across the system for people of all ages; nurses need to help drive these innovations.
- Workforce provisions will support the preparation of nurses for the future and faculty to teach them.

MEDICARE SAVINGS AND FINANCING

The 2010 health care reform law was funded in part by $390 billion in savings from Medicare over 10 years (Congressional Research Service, 2010). The savings do not come from cuts in basic benefits; indeed beneficiaries will see improvements in coverage for prevention and prescription drugs. The savings come from reductions in future provider payment increases. Instead of the average annual growth in spending of 8% over the last two decades, the reforms could slow down spending to about 6% over the next two decades. This is known as "bending the curve."

Providers will feel the effects. For example, $196 billion in Medicare savings over the next 10 years comes from smaller increases in payments to hospitals, nursing homes, home health workers, and other health care providers (Congressional Budget Office, 2010). But some clinicians will see increases in payment. To ensure that Medicare beneficiaries have access to advanced practice nurses and primary care physicians, Medicare will give a 10% bonus to physicians and nurses providing primary care, and to general surgeons working in shortage areas. Community health centers will receive $11 billion starting in 2011, allowing them to serve some 20 million new patients. Hospitals that prevent readmissions or hospital-acquired infections will be paid more than those that do not.

About $136 billion in Medicare savings comes from reductions in subsidies paid to Medicare Advantage private health insurance plans, which in 2010 got an average of 14% more to care for a member than it would cost if that person remained in traditional Medicare. CMS will start lowering payments to Medicare Advantage plans, replacing the current payment system with one that rewards plans that meet certain quality standards for care (Dubow, 2010). Plans cannot reduce or eliminate essential guaranteed Medicare benefits. At least 85 cents of every dollar insurers receive must be spent on benefits.

Consumers will share in the responsibility to reform health care. In the next decade, more Medicare beneficiaries will pay higher-income premiums because the current income levels on which they are based will be frozen until 2020. And for the first time, Medicare beneficiaries with higher incomes will pay higher premiums for drug coverage.

The law also requires the government to spend Medicare dollars more wisely. A new Independent Payment Advisory Board is expected to make recommendations to reduce net Medicare program spending, saving Medicare $16 billion over 10 years. Cracking down on fraud and waste will save an estimated $7 billion (CBO, 2010).

MEDICARE IMPROVEMENTS

Despite the $390 billion in savings, Medicare spending will increase. In addition to the rising costs of health care for all people, there will be more Medicare beneficiaries. And existing basic benefits will not decline for Medicare beneficiaries; there will be important improvements. Two are highlighted in the following paragraphs.

Better Prescription Coverage. Those who enter the doughnut hole in 2010 will get a one-time rebate of $250. Starting in 2011, they will get a 50% discount on brand-name and biologic drugs and a 7% discount on generic drugs while they are in the coverage gap. These discounts will gradually increase until 2020, when Part D enrollees will only be responsible for 25% of their prescription drug costs in the doughnut hole (Purvis, 2010).

Better Coverage of Prevention Services. Starting in 2011, beneficiaries will get free annual physicals and many preventive services. Any Medicare-covered service that has a grade A or B by the United States Preventive Services Task Force (USPSTF) must be fully covered with no cost sharing (Flowers & Nonnemaker, 2010).

INNOVATIONS

There are many important provisions in the health care reform laws that can serve as platforms for improving quality and stimulating innovations. Several (but not all) that should interest nurses are highlighted here.

One of the most significant provisions is the establishment of the Center for Medicare and Medicaid Innovation (CMI). This Center will test innovative payment and service delivery models, with the focus on reducing Medicare spending while preserving or enhancing quality. The secretary of the U.S. Department of Health and Human Services (HHS) must select models for testing where there is evidence that the model addresses a population that is experiencing deficits in care that lead to poor clinical outcomes or potentially avoidable costs. Through the CMI, the potential for translating evidence-based nursing models is enormous. And if the model is shown to reduce spending without reducing quality, or improve patient care without increasing spending, the HHS secretary through rule-making can implement that model on a national basis without going back to Congress for another authorization. The speed to market of successful models will be significantly enhanced through this provision.

Beginning in 2012, ACOs will qualify for a new "Medicare shared savings program." Providers who meet certain criteria can be recognized as ACOs and enter into a 3-year agreement with the HHS secretary to be accountable for the quality, cost, and overall care of at least 5000 Medicare fee-for-service beneficiaries assigned to them. An ACO includes groups of providers and suppliers who have established shared governance, including partnerships or joint venture arrangements between hospitals and ACO professionals, defined as a physician, physician assistant, nurse practitioner, or clinical nurse specialist (Health Policy Alternatives [HPA], 2010). This is a "bottom up" innovation that offers opportunities for advanced practice registered nurses in their own communities.

Another locally-based innovation involves "bundling" pilots. The HHS secretary will develop, test, and evaluate alternative Medicare payment methodologies for "episodes of care" through a national, voluntary five-year pilot program. The pilot will focus on an episode that begins three days prior to a hospital admission and ends 30 days following hospital discharge, with the goal of integrating care across settings to improve the coordination, quality, and efficiency of health care services. Services include hospitalization, physician care inside and outside of the hospital setting, outpatient and emergency room care, postacute care home health, skilled nursing, inpatient rehabilitation, and other services that the secretary identifies. Eligible entities for this pilot include hospitals, physician groups, skilled nursing facilities, and home health agencies. The entity must furnish or direct all services and will receive the bundled payment, including payment for care coordination, medication reconciliation, discharge planning, transitional care services, and other patient-centered activities determined appropriate. Again, the secretary can expand the new methodology through rule-making if expansion would reduce spending while improving or not reducing the quality of care. The secretary will work with the Agency for Healthcare Research and Quality (AHRQ) and the National Quality Forum (NGF) to develop episode of care and other quality measures (HPA, 2010).

The Independence at Home demonstration program will test Medicare shared savings for physician and nurse practitioner–directed home-based primary care provided to chronically ill beneficiaries who require coordinated health care across all treatment settings. The demonstration will include no more than 10,000 beneficiaries who have two or more chronic illnesses, two or more functional dependencies, a non-elective hospital admission within the past 12 months, and previous acute or subacute rehabilitation services. Each participating group must serve at least 200 of these Medicare beneficiaries and use electronic health information systems, remote monitoring, and mobile diagnostic technology (HPA, 2010).

High hospital readmission rates have been identified as problematic. One in four Medicare beneficiaries who are discharged from hospitals is readmitted within 30 days (Jencks et al., 2009). This pattern is costly in both financial and human terms. The health care reform laws use both a stick and carrot approach to spurring innovation to solve this problem. The "stick" approach is known as the hospital readmissions reduction program that reduces payments to Medicare PPS hospitals with excess readmissions. Initially, the policy will apply to readmissions in three high-volume/high-expenditure conditions with NQF-endorsed measures (heart attack, heart failure, and pneumonia), but it will be expanded to other high-volume or high-expenditure conditions. Hospitals will also have to report readmission rates on the Hospital Compare Internet website, and some hospitals will be eligible to participate in a quality improvement program (HPA, 2010). Nurses who have expertise in caring for chronically ill persons and their families will find many opportunities to create programs that hospitals will need to avoid the penalties they face with excessive rehospitalizations.

Similar opportunities exist for nurses who can lead or participate in reducing unnecessary rehospitalizations. Known as the Community-Based Care Transitions Program, this 5-year program will fund hospital and community-based partnership organizations to provide patient-centered, evidence-based care transitional care services to individuals at the highest risk

of repeated, unnecessary hospitalizations (HPA, 2010). Applications to participate must include a detailed proposal with at least one evidence-based care transition intervention, such as those advanced by Naylor and colleagues (2004). The secretary can expand the program through rule-making to reduce spending while improving or not reducing the quality of care.

WORKFORCE

There are many workforce-related provisions in health care reform. For example, there are measures to attract more doctors, nurses, and physician assistants to primary care by forgiving student loans, especially for those who practice in areas that need health care professionals (Center to Champion Nursing in America [CCNA], 2010). But one of the most significant workforce provisions is a four-year demonstration to test a Medicare Graduate Nursing Education program. The goal is to modernize the way we spend Medicare dollars to prepare advanced practice RNs who can provide primary care, chronic care, and transitional care services to people on Medicare in a reformed system. Payments go to hospitals for the clinical training costs of preparing advanced practice nurses with the skills necessary to provide primary and preventive care, transitional care, chronic care management, and other nursing services appropriate for the Medicare population. This graduate nursing education would be provided through affiliations with accredited schools of nursing in partnership with two or more community-based care settings where at least half of all of the training occurs. Hospitals would reimburse the schools of nursing and community-based care settings for their portion of these training costs (CCNA, 2010).

IMPLICATIONS

The reforms enacted are numerous, interlocking, and ambitious. Nurses have an unprecedented opportunity to shape the future of the health care delivery system and their places in it. Since changes in Medicare drive system reforms more generally, all nurses should pay attention to what happens in the CMS Innovation Center and all the pilots and demonstrations that CMS will oversee. Some of those noted in the statute explicitly identify nurses as potential leaders, while others are silent but do not exclude that possibility. This is the time to step up and lead at the local and national levels. There are many boards and commissions that should count nurse leaders among their prestigious members (CCNA, 2010). Nurses need to be there because consumers need the expertise that nurses can bring to the urgent, historic deliberations that will ensue.

For a list of related websites, please refer to your Evolve Resources at http://evolve.elsevier.com/Mason/policypolitics/

REFERENCES

Center to Champion Nursing in America. (2010). Nursing Provisions P.L. 111-148, the Patient Protection and Affordability Care Act (PPACA). Retrieved from http://championnursing.org/sites/default/files/NursingandHealthReformLawTable_0.pdf.

Centers for Medicare & Medicaid Services. (2009). CMS announces Medicare premiums, deductibles for 2010. Retrieved from www.cms.gov/apps/media/press/factsheet.asp?Counter=3534.

Congressional Budget Office. (March March 20, 2010). H.R. 4872, Reconciliation Act of 2010 (Final Health Care Legislation). Retrieved from www.cbo.gov/doc.cfm?index=11379.

Congressional Research Service. (2010). Medicare: Changes made by the Reconciliation Act of 2010 to Senate-passed H.R. 3590. 7-5700 R41124. Retrieved from http://law.slu.edu/library/research/Reconciliation%20Act%20and%20Medicare.pdf.

Dubow, J. (2010). *How health reform adjusts Medicare Advantage (MA) payments, rewards quality of care.* Washington, D.C.: AARP Public Policy Institute. Retrieved from www.aarp.org/health/health-care-reform/info-07-2010/fs197-health.html.

Fisher, E. S., Wennberg, D. E., Stukel, T. A., Gottleib, D. J., Lucas, F. L., & Pinder, E. L. (2003a). The implications of regional variations in Medicare spending: Part 1: The content, quality, and accessibility of care. *Annals of Internal Medicine, 138*(4), 273-287.

Fisher, E. S., Wennberg, D. E., Stukel, T. A., Gottleib, D. J., Lucas, F. L., & Pinder, E. L. (2003b). The implications of regional variations in Medicare spending: Part 2: Health outcomes and satisfaction with care. *Annals of Internal Medicine, 138*(4), 288-299.

Flowers, L., & Nonnemaker, L. (2010). *Improvements to Medicare's preventive services under health reform.* Washington, D.C.: AARP Public Policy Institute. Retrieved from http://assets.aarp.org/rgcenter/ppi/health-care/fs180-preventive.pdf.

Gluck, M. G., & Reno, V., (Eds.), (2001). *Reflections on implementing Medicare.* Washington, D.C.: National Academy of Social Insurance.

Gold, M., Achmats, L., Mittler, J., & Stevens, B. (2004). *Monitoring Medicare + Choice: What have we learned?* Washington, D.C.: Mathematica Policy Research.

Health Policy Alternatives. (2010). *Summary of Patient Protection and Affordable Care Act.* Washington D.C.: Author.

Jencks, S. F., Williams, M. V. & Coleman, E. A. (2009). Rehospitalizations among patients in the Medicare fee-for-service program. *New England Journal of Medicine, 360*(14), 1418-1428.

Kaiser Family Foundation (KFF). (2005). Medicare: A timeline of key developments. Retrieved from www.kff.org/medicare/medicaretimeline.cfm.

Kaiser Family Foundation (KFF). (2010). Medicare: A primer 2010. Retrieved from www.kff.org.

Medicare Payment Advisory Commission (MedPAC). (2009). *Measuring regional variation in service use.* Washington, D.C.: MedPAC.

Naylor, M. D., Brooten, D. A., Campbell, R. L., Maislin, G. M., McCauley, K. M., & Schwartz, J. S. (2004). Transitional care of older adults hospitalized with heart failure: A randomized clinical trial. *Journal of the American Geriatrics Society, 52*(5), 675-684.

Nonnemaker, L. & Sinclair, S. (2009). *Medicare Beneficiaries' Out-of-Pocket Spending for Health Care Services.* Washington, D.C.: AARP Public Policy Institute. Retrieved from http://assets.aarp.org/rgcenter/health/i30_oop.pdf.

Purvis, L. (2010). *Health care reform legislation closes the Medicare Part D coverage gap.* Washington, D.C.: AARP Public Policy Institute. Retrieved from https://assets.aarp.org/rgcenter/ppi/health-care/fs182-doughnut-hole-reform.pdf.

Reinhard, S. C., Scala-Foley, M. A., Caruso, J. T., & Archer, D. (2004). Medicare savings programs. *American Journal of Nursing, 104*(6), 62-64.

CHAPTER 18

Children's Health Insurance Coverage: Medicaid and the State Children's Health Insurance Program

Kathleen M. White

"It was once said that the moral test of government is how that government treats those who are in the dawn of life, the children; those who are in the twilight of life, the elderly; and those who are in the shadows of life—the sick, the needy, and the handicapped."

—Hubert H. Humphrey

HEALTH INSURANCE COVERAGE FOR LOW-INCOME CHILDREN

Health insurance coverage for the children of the United States (U.S.) has improved over the last 30 years. In 2009, twenty-nine million children were enrolled in Medicaid and 7 million in the Children's Health Insurance Program (CHIP), yet many children remain uninsured and eligible for Medicaid or CHIP, but are not enrolled. Since 2008, the U.S. has experienced a severe economic recession with unemployment levels greater than 10% resulting in a decline in employer-sponsored health insurance; yet the numbers of uninsured children dropped from 9 million in 2005 to 8.1 million in 2009 due to increasing public insurance coverage for children. However, nearly 72% of the uninsured children live in families with household incomes below 200% of the federal poverty level (FPL) or about $44,000 for a family of four (Kaiser Commission on Medicaid and the Uninsured, 2010a). This trend began in the early 1980s as the country saw an increase in child poverty resulting from the stagnating economic situation and an increase in single-parent families. The uninsurance rates increased from 20.9% to a high of 30.8% between 1977 and 1987 (Cunningham & Kirby, 2004; Selden,

Hudson, & Banthin, 2004). During the same period, there was also a steady decline in the percentage of private insurance coverage for children. The Medicaid program was not able to address this worsening situation, as many of the children came from homes that did not meet Medicaid eligibility criteria. An expansion of public coverage was needed, and the State Children's Health Insurance Program (now referred to as CHIP, not SCHIP) was developed.

PUBLIC HEALTH INSURANCE COVERAGE FOR CHILDREN

MEDICAID

Medicaid is a federal entitlement program enacted in 1965 that guarantees eligible children access to a health care benefit package with little or no cost to them or their families. It is jointly financed and administered by the federal and state governments. The federal government has established minimum standards for the Medicaid program, including eligibility requirements and the minimum benefit package, and the states administer the program within those parameters. The states may vary their programs if they receive permission in the form of a "waiver" to depart from the federal standards, which has resulted in significant variation among the states.

Because of the increasing uninsurance rates between 1984 and 1990, which reached a high of 30%, the Medicaid program implemented several poverty-related expansions to include many poor and near-poor children who were not eligible for welfare, the traditional pathway to receive Medicaid coverage (Selden et al., 2004). States were required to cover children 6 years of age and under from families earning up to 133% of the FPL and were allowed to expand coverage to include families earning up to 185% of the FPL and still receive federal matching funds (Sasso & Buchmueller, 2004). "From 1988 to 1998, the proportion of children insured through Medicaid increased from 15.6% to 19.8%. At the same time, the percentage of children without health insurance increased from 13.1% to 15.4%, mostly as a result of fewer children being covered by employer-sponsored health insurance" (Centers for Medicare and Medicaid Services [CMS], 2005). However, many low-income children who were above the poverty level were still not eligible for these Medicaid expansion programs, and it was widely recognized that something else was needed to address the coverage gap for low-income children not eligible for Medicaid.

CHILDREN'S HEALTH INSURANCE PROGRAM

After the defeat of President Clinton's universal health insurance plan, many in Congress felt that it was time to expand health care coverage to the most vulnerable in the population; children became a likely choice. In 1997, the State Children's Health Insurance Program (SCHIP) was enacted as part of Title XXI of the Social Security Act (Balanced Budget Act of 1997, PL 105-33). This legislation provided health insurance coverage to children, up to age 19, in low-income families that were not eligible for Medicaid. This included families whose income was too high to qualify for Medicaid or that were not covered by private health insurance, often because the family income was too low for them to afford the private coverage. The original SCHIP legislation apportioned $40 billion in federal matching funds over a 10-year period to allow participating states to receive federal contributions to expand Medicaid eligibility, to create a new health care coverage program under the SCHIP legislation, or to develop a program that combined Medicaid with a new program. The SCHIP program provided the funds to the states, not to the individual as in Medicaid, and the states could design the program to meet their own needs. Under this program, the states could provide health care coverage to children in families earning up to 200% of the FPL.

The procedure for the development of the SCHIP programs was similar to that of Medicaid. The state had to develop a program plan and submit it to CMS for approval. CMS then had to approve or disapprove the plan within 90 days of submission. States were allowed to modify the state plan by again submitting it to CMS for approval. The amount of federal funding for each state participating in SCHIP is defined in the statute appropriation, with annual allotments determined by a statutory formula based on the number of children and the state cost factor. The state cost factor is a geographic factor based on the annual wages in the health care industry for that state. The state plan must address eligibility standards, enrollment caps, disenrollment policies, type of health benefits covered, basic delivery system approach, cost sharing, and screening and enrollment procedures.

The original SCHIP legislation had several important goals: to expand health insurance for children whose families earn too much money to be eligible for Medicaid but not enough money to purchase private health insurance; to provide access to quality medical care without dependence on cost; to develop a system that establishes a medical home for clients; to simplify the enrollment process for a public insurance program; and finally, to provide flexibility and innovation for the states to design a program that met the needs of their population, such as cost sharing different benefit packages in order to cover a wider segment of the population.

The states were allowed to develop different eligibility criteria and coverage. Eligibility in most states began for uninsured children whose family income was at 185% to 200% of the FPL. Generally, all plans were required to cover well-baby and well-child care, immunizations, hospitalization, and emergency room visits. For states that opted for a Medicaid expansion, the services provided under SCHIP needed to mirror the Medicaid services provided by that state. For states that opted for a separate child health program, there were four options for determining coverage:

1. Benchmark coverage: This coverage package is substantially equal to either the Federal Employee Health Benefits Program Blue Cross/Blue Shield Standard Option Service Benefit Plan; a health benefits plan that the state offers and makes generally available to its own employees; or a plan offered by a Health Maintenance Organization that has the largest insured commercial, non-Medicaid enrollment of any such organization in the state.

2. Benchmark equivalent coverage: In this instance, the state must provide coverage with an aggregate actuarial value at least equal to that of one of the benchmark plans. States must cover inpatient and outpatient hospital services, physicians' surgical and medical services, laboratory and x-ray services, and well-baby and well-child care, including age-appropriate immunizations.

3. Existing state-based comprehensive coverage: In the states where existing state-based comprehensive coverage existed before the enactment of SCHIP (i.e., New York, Pennsylvania, and Florida), the existing health benefits package was deemed to be meeting the coverage requirements of the SCHIP program.

4. Secretary of HHS approved coverage: This includes a provision for coverage that is the same as the state's Medicaid program; comprehensive coverage for children offered by the state under a Medicaid demonstration project approved by the Secretary; coverage that either includes full Early and Periodic Screening, Diagnosis, and Treatment (EPSDT) benefits or has been extended by the state to the entire Medicaid population in the state; coverage that includes benchmark coverage plus any additional coverage; coverage that is the same as the coverage provided by New York, Florida, or Pennsylvania; or coverage purchased by the state that is substantially equal to coverage under one of the benchmark plans through the use of benefit-by-benefit comparison.

By fall 1999, all states had adopted some type of SCHIP program. Initially, in all but 12 states the coverage was given to children in families with incomes of at least 200% of the FPL, allowing more near-poor families to meet the states' eligibility criteria. By 2001, 19 states had expanded Medicaid, 15 states had created a separate SCHIP program, and 17 states had implemented some type of combination program (Sasso & Buchmueller, 2004) (Box 18-1). The Kaiser Commission on Medicaid and the Uninsured (2004) found that between 1997 and 2003, the percentage of poor children who were uninsured declined from 22.4% to 15.4% and that uninsurance rates have declined even more dramatically for the group of slightly higher income children who were the main target of SCHIP: those with family incomes of 100% to 200% of the FPL. Uninsurance rates for that group fell from 22.8% to 14.7% in 2003, a decline of more than one third (36%). However, the number of children eligible for public coverage who remain uninsured was still estimated to be about 21%, and an estimated 5.6 million children were eligible but not enrolled.

"The SCHIP Dip". The original budget allocations for SCHIP included $40 billion over 10 years, with stable dollar allocations over the first 4 years. However, because of early projected budget shortfalls, the allocations for 2002 to 2004 were over $1 billion less annually to the SCHIP program than in the previous 4 years. States that had not spent their full allocations in previous years could use that unused portion to help during these lower-funded years because the legislation allowed them to carry over unspent funds to the next budget year in the early years of the program. However, the dip in available funds for SCHIP also came at a time when many states were beginning to experience budget constraints or shortfalls and led most states to make cuts in their Medicaid and SCHIP program budgets. Some of the cutbacks have included reduction in the eligibility requirements, enrollment caps or freezes on enrollment, increased premiums, increased cost-sharing amounts, and limited outreach and marketing efforts.

THE CHILDREN'S HEALTH INSURANCE PROGRAM REAUTHORIZED

In 2007 the 10-year SCHIP program was due to expire, and both houses of Congress passed SCHIP reauthorization. The House bill, the Children's Health and Medicare Protection Act (HR 3162), increased funding by $50 billion to increase coverage, provided incentives to enroll more children and grants for outreach, and provided for expanded coverage for children up to 21 years of age and legal immigrant children and pregnant women. The Senate bill, the Children's Health Insurance Program Reauthorization Act (S 1893), increased funding by only $35 billion to expand coverage and included the incentives for enrollment and grants for outreach, but limited matching funds for children below 300% of the poverty level and prohibited the submission of new SCHIP waivers to cover parents (Kaiser Commission on Medicaid and the Uninsured, 2009). Both bills included increased quality measurement and reporting.

BOX 18-1 Comparison of CHIP to Medicaid

Medicaid and CHIP are both joint federal- and state-funded programs. The Medicaid program is an open-ended entitlement program to the individual. Under CHIP, each state is funded by a capped grant to the state, with the amount of funding determined by a formula set by Congress. Federal matching money is about 30% higher under SCHIP than under Medicaid.

Medicaid provides a full range of health care services for children, including screening and treatment, preventive check-ups, physician and hospital services, and vision and dental care. At a minimum, state Medicaid eligibility is given to children under 6 years of age who live in families at or below 133% of the FPL ($29,327 for a family of 4 in 2009) and to children 6 to 18 years of age in families at or below 100% of the poverty level.

The original SCHIP legislation prevented children who were already enrolled in Medicaid from enrolling in the SCHIP program, preventing the states from shifting children from Medicaid to SCHIP and taking advantage of the more generous matching funds under SCHIP. The legislation set up a procedure that required all SCHIP applicants to be screened for Medicaid eligibility as part of the SCHIP application process. It has been noted that this screening requirement has had an indirect effect on increasing the numbers eligible for and enrolled in Medicaid (Government Accountability Office [GAO], 2000). The increased number of children covered by Medicaid because of SCHIP has been important in reducing the total number of uninsured children in the U.S. The innovation allowed in the application procedures for the SCHIP program has also been credited for better enrollment and reenrollment procedures for Medicaid. With the implementation of SCHIP in 1997, innovations in outreach and enrollment have been the hallmark of the program's success. SCHIP also offers states more flexibility in designing the program that meets their needs, including eligibility criteria and benefits. Income eligibility levels have remained relatively stable over recent years (Kaiser Commission on Medicaid and the Uninsured, 2005). Unlike Medicaid, SCHIP required states to include outreach efforts as part of their expansion program. The outreach campaigns were designed to get the word out to eligible families and have included mass media campaigns and community-based efforts. Many states created television, radio, and print media campaigns to educate the public and increase awareness of the new program. Toll-free numbers were used; the public could call in to get enrollment information.

The SCHIP programs have also included reforms to the application process, making it simpler. The most important enrollment innovation has been the adoption of an electronic submission application that is a short, joint application for both Medicaid and SCHIP, eliminating the face-to-face interviews that had previously been required of all Medicaid applications. In addition, the resource and asset tests were also eliminated, which allowed applicants to self-declare their income. The final innovation relies on passive renewal so that 12-month continuous eligibility for SCHIP has been established.

The CHIPRA legislation continues these program requirements and puts in place additional innovations to create "Express Lane Eligibility" through "Express Lane Agencies" that are used by both Medicaid and CHIP for enrollment and eases up on citizenship documentation procedures.

In fall 2007, Congress passed HR 976, the Children's Health Insurance Program Reauthorization Act (CHIPRA) with bipartisan support. CHIPRA was similar to the Senate bill passed in the summer. However, President Bush vetoed the legislation and the House was unable to override the veto. In the winter, Congress again attempted reauthorization and passed HR 3963, a revised version of the CHIPRA bill. The bill addressed issues raised by opponents about income eligibility and limits to crowd-out, and provided stricter requirements for verification of citizenship. The president once again vetoed the bill (Box 18-2).

In order to keep the program in operation, Congress passed the Medicare, Medicaid and SCHIP Extension Act of 2007, a temporary reauthorization through April 2009, and President Bush signed it. This extension maintained funding at current levels with slight increases for the next 2 years for state budget shortfalls, but did not address other important critical issues to the future of the program.

Finally, in January 2009, the 111th Congress passed one of its first pieces of legislation, the Children's Health Insurance Program Reauthorization Act of 2009 (CHIPRA), to reauthorize and expand the program and fund it through increased tobacco taxes. President Obama signed the bill on February 4, 2009. The reauthorization of the CHIP (no longer referred to as SCHIP) was for $4\frac{1}{2}$ years and provides $34 billion through fiscal year 2013. The CBO estimated that CHIPRA would provide coverage to an additional 6.5 million children in CHIP and Medicaid by

BOX 18-2 What Is Crowd Out?

The "crowd out" provision of the original SCHIP legislation and the rules that followed were developed to ensure that SCHIP did not "crowd out" or substitute for existing employer-sponsored coverage. However, this created inequities across the program. Some states permitted children to be enrolled if they met the eligibility criteria. Other states developed policies to exempt children from SCHIP if they had access to employer-sponsored coverage, even if the family met the income thresholds. This was especially difficult for families with children with special health care needs, who were often carrying a high-cost catastrophic insurance plan.

During the reauthorization process, CMS offered guidance to the states in August 2007 to require them to show that they have enrolled 95% of children who are 200% below the federal family poverty income levels before they could expand coverage to 250%. This guidance also included showing that employer-based health insurance coverage for these same children had not declined by more than 2% during the prior five years (Kaiser Commission on Medicaid and the Uninsured, 2009a, 2009b, 2009c). However, this was never enforced, and the guidance was withdrawn by President Obama after CHIPRA legislation was passed in 2009. "Crowd-out" will remain an important concern over the short term because of the economic recession and high unemployment rates with resultant loss of employer-based health insurance coverage.

2013. About two-thirds of those enrolled (4.1 million children) would have otherwise been uninsured.

In addition to the increased funding to expand coverage, CHIPRA provided $100 million in outreach funding and included new outreach and enrollment requirements to increase participation, provided additional monies for translation and interpretation services, proposed quality measures and reporting, promoted the use of health information technology, and realigned incentives to focus on quality and outcomes in the program (Simpson et al., 2009). The CHIPRA benefit package was basically the same but required states to include dental services and allowed states the option to provide dental-only coverage for a child who qualifies for CHIP but has other health insurance coverage without dental.

The legislation created the Medicaid and CHIP Payment and Access Commission (MACPAC) to review Medicaid and CHIP enrollment and payment policies and develop quality measures and electronic health records. The program also addressed four key areas of prior concern:

1. Pregnant Women and Adults—the legislation provided for options to cover pregnant women, but CHIPRA placed limits on current coverage for adults and prohibited the development of any new waivers for parental coverage. However, the legislation provided for a separate program for parental coverage available to states at the Medicaid rate who met performance benchmarks on the child program.

2. U.S. Citizenship requirements—CHPIRA allowed states to comply with citizenship documentation requirements by using the process created by the Social Security Administration data exchange for Medicaid eligibility. In addition, the legislation allowed the states to provide coverage to legal immigrants who had been in the U.S. under five years.

3. Express Lane Eligibility (ELE)—was created to increase the efficiency and effectiveness of the eligibility process. The ELE allowed both Medicaid and CHIP enrolling agencies to use eligibility findings from other needs-based programs, such as food stamps, the National School Lunch Program, and the Nutrition Program for Women, Infants and Children (WIC) to enroll or renew children and allowed states to decide if ELE would be used for enrollment, renewal, or both, and to streamline the process and create the entry point for eligibility determination. The legislation also provided for flexibility and discretion in selecting express lane agencies. It allowed states to decide whether to use ELE for just Medicaid or for both Medicaid and CHIP to reach more moderate-income children who are uninsured. It enabled states to use presumptive eligibility to grant temporary health coverage while final eligibility determination was made. Finally, CHIPRA stressed an increasing role for technology to automate the processes and recommended using available federal resources to upgrade technology systems.

4. Performance Bonus—CHIPRA provided for a federal bonus paid to the states for exceeding enrollment targets for children in Medicaid, thereby increasing a state's federal Medicaid match. In order to be eligible for the performance bonus, a state must implement five of eight policies:

a. Provide 12-month continuous coverage
b. Require no asset test or a simplified asset verification
c. Require no face-to-face interview
d. Use joint application and the same verification process for Medicaid and CHIP
e. Allow for administrative and ex parte renewals
f. Have presumptive eligibility
g. Express lane eligibility
h. Offer a premium assistance option

FEDERAL HEALTH CARE REFORM AND CHIP

The Patient Protection and Affordable Care Act (PL 111-148), major comprehensive health care reform legislation, was signed by President Obama into law on March 23, 2010. This law, as well as new provisions from the Health Care and Education Affordability Act of 2010 signed into law on March 30, 2010, created an individual requirement or mandate to obtain health insurance and significant provisions for Medicaid expansion and subsidies to help low-income individuals buy coverage through a newly established health insurance exchange. The Congressional Budget Office (CBO) estimates that the legislation will increase Medicaid/CHIP coverage by 16 million from 35 million by 2019. The bill will have a federal Medicaid/CHIP cost of $434 billion from 2010 to 2019 and an estimated increase in state spending of $20 billion during the same period (Kaiser Commission on Medicaid and the Uninsured, 2010b).

The new legislation creates a national floor for Medicaid eligibility of up to 133% of the FPL, or $14,404 for an individual or $29,326 for a family of 4 in 2009 (Kaiser Commission on Medicaid and the Uninsured, 2010b). This would begin to eliminate the state-to-state variations in eligibility for the Medicaid program. The law includes an immediate provision to cover childless adults through a Medicaid State Plan and provides the expansion of Medicaid coverage to all non-Medicare–eligible individuals under age 65 based on the 133% FPL guidelines by 2014. It also includes federal matching dollars for newly eligible individuals. The legislation also provides for subsidies for individuals to buy health care insurance coverage through Health Benefit Insurance Exchanges for those

who are above the 133% and up to 400% of the FPL by 2014.

The new law provides for continuation of CHIP through 2019 and funding for CHIP through 2015 (an additional two years). The law also includes a new immediate provision to allow states to offer CHIP coverage to children of state employees eligible for health benefits if state premium contributions for family coverage are less than 1997 levels or if the employee's premiums and cost sharing exceeds 5% of the family's income.

The legislation expands the role of the Medicaid and CHIP Payment and Access Commission (MACPAC), initially created for quality and outcomes monitoring for children. The MACPAC will now include monitoring for all enrollees and establishes the Center for Medicare and Medicaid Innovation to test demonstrations for innovative payment and service delivery models that improve quality and efficiency and pilot programs for patient-centered medical home and accountable care organizations.

SUMMARY AND THE FUTURE FOR CHILDREN'S COVERAGE

The CHIPRA legislation of 2009 provided the states, facing severe economic situations because of the recession, with additional funding and financial incentives to expand their child health insurance programs and enroll additional lower-income and uninsured children. The Patient Protection and Affordable Care Act of 2010, by requiring all individuals to obtain health insurance, poses a challenge for state and federal governments to work collaboratively to make these requirements successful. The Medicaid and CHIP program provisions, as defined in the new health reform law, will significantly reduce the number of uninsured children in the U.S., and as part of a comprehensive health care reform plan should impact the provision of health care for all U.S. citizens.

For a list of related websites, please refer to your Evolve Resources at http://evolve.elsevier.com/Mason/policypolitics/

REFERENCES

Centers for Medicare and Medicaid Services (CMS). (2005). State Children's Health Insurance Program. Retrieved from www.cms.hhs.gov/schip.

Cunningham, P., & Kirby, J. (2004). Children's health coverage: A quarter-century of change. *Health Affairs, 23*(5), 27-38.

Government Accountability Office (GAO). (2000). *Medicaid and SCHIP: Comparison of outreach, enrollment practices and benefits.* GAO/HEHO-00-86. Washington, D.C.: GAO.

Kaiser Commission on Medicaid and the Uninsured. (2004). *SCHIP program enrollment: December 2003 update.* Washington, D.C.: Kaiser Commission.

Kaiser Commission on Medicaid and the Uninsured. (2005). Enrolling uninsured low-income children in Medicaid and SCHIP. Washington, D.C.: Kaiser Commission.

Kaiser Commission on Medicaid and the Uninsured. (2009). *State children's health insurance program (CHIP): Reauthorization history.* Washington, D.C.: Kaiser Commission.

Kaiser Commission on Medicaid and the Uninsured. (2010a). *Health coverage of children: The role of Medicaid and CHIP.* Washington, D.C.: Kaiser Commission.

Kaiser Commission on Medicaid and the Uninsured. (2010b). *Focus on health reform: Medicaid and children's health insurance program provisions in the new health reform law.* Washington, D.C.: Kaiser Commission. Retrieved from www.kff.org/healthreform.

Sasso, A. T., & Buchmueller, T. C. (2004). The effect of the state children's health insurance program on health insurance coverage. *Journal of Health Economics, 23*(8), 1059-1082.

Selden, T. M., Hudson, J. L., & Banthin, J. S. (2004). Tracking changes in eligibility and coverage among children, 1996-2002. *Health Affairs, 23*(5), 39-50.

Simpson, L., Fairbrother, G., Touscher, J., & Guyer, J. (2009). Implementation choices for the children's health insurance reauthorization act of 2009. *The Commonwealth Fund*, September 2009.

CHAPTER 19

The United States Military Health System: Policy Challenges in Wartime and Peacetime

John S. Murray and Mary W. Chaffee

"Our team provides optimal health services in support of our nation's military mission—anytime, anywhere."

—Military Health System Mission

Members of the U.S. uniformed services have received Federal health benefits for more than 200 years since Congress first enacted legislation requiring that medical care be provided for ill soldiers and sailors. Over the years, Congress added provisions that care be provided for military families, military retirees and their family members, and others (Department of Defense [DOD], 2007).

The Military Health System (MHS) has dual missions (Figure 19-1):

- A *military readiness mission* focused on maintaining readiness and providing support during military operations.
- A *health care benefits mission* focused on providing care and support to members of the uniformed services, their family members, and others entitled to DOD health services (Hosek and Cecchine, 2001).

In 2009, the MHS cared for approximately 9.5 million eligible beneficiaries around the world (Table 19-1). It is staffed by about 133,000 personnel consisting of 86,000 military and 47,000 civilian personnel working at 59 military hospitals, 413 medical clinics, and 413 dental clinics worldwide (TRICARE Management Activity, 2009). Care in the MHS is provided in diverse settings including major medical centers, outpatient clinics, aircraft carriers, submarines, medical evacuation aircraft, combat medical units (tents), and other environments.

ORGANIZATION OF CARE

DIRECT CARE

Care for active duty personnel, and for others when space is available, is provided through military medical facilities known as the *direct care system.* Care for wounded military personnel begins in the direct care system. This entails providing care in theatre (the area of combat operations), and transport back to the U.S. Rehabilitation may continue in the hospitals and clinics operated by the U.S. Department of Veterans Affairs (VA). Collaboration between the DOD and VA is vital; significant coordination is required for continuity of care for military members.

TRICARE

Hospitals and clinics operated by the military services do not have adequate capacity to provide all the care required by eligible beneficiaries so a civilian network of care has been developed to augment the direct care system. TRICARE is the health benefit plan for military beneficiaries (those who are entitled by law to receive care in the DOD health system). TRICARE includes multiple program options to meet the medical and dental needs of beneficiaries. TRICARE Prime is similar to a Health Maintenance Organization (HMO) and uses military and civilian facilities. TRICARE Extra is structured like a Preferred Provider Organization (PPO), and TRICARE Standard is a fee-for-service option. TRICARE For Life is an option for military retirees enrolled in Medicare Part B (Burelli, 2003). The DOD also manages dental and pharmacy benefit programs.

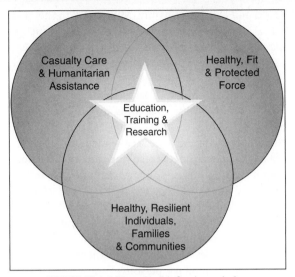

FIGURE 19-1 Military Health Services mission.

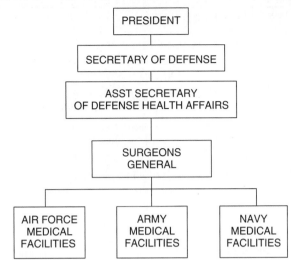

FIGURE 19-2 Military Health Services organizational structure.

TABLE 19-1 **Groups Eligible for Care in the U.S. Military Health System**

- Members of the Uniformed Services (active duty and retired members and their family members)
  - U.S. Army
  - U.S. Air Force
  - U.S. Navy
  - U.S. Marine Corps
  - U.S. Coast Guard
  - Commissioned Corps of the Public Health Service
  - Commissioned Corps of the National Oceanic and Atmospheric Association
- National Guard members and military reservists and their families as well as retired Guard and reserve
- Medal of Honor recipients
- Dependent parents and parents-in-law of uniformed service members who are eligible
- Certain foreign military service members and their families
- The president, vice president, and members of Congress
- Specially designated others

Sources: TRICARE.mil/mybenefit/home/overview/eligibility; Military Medicare care: Questions and answers, March 7, 2007, CRS Report for Congress (RL33537).

HUMANITARIAN EFFORTS AND MEDICAL DIPLOMACY

The MHS also provides disaster relief and humanitarian assistance around the world. Humanitarian assistance is an element of national diplomacy in the war on terrorism. It helps to build bridges to peace around the world (DOD MHS, 2008; 2009). The military's hospital ships, U.S. Naval Ship (USNS) COMFORT and USNS MERCY, have responded to numerous crises including the 2004 Asian tsunami. Military medical personnel have carried out humanitarian missions in Honduras, Afghanistan, Nicaragua, Bangladesh, and many other areas, bringing much-needed care to underserved areas and in response to disaster (Caring for America's Heroes, 2008).

LEADERSHIP AND VISION

MHS leadership consists of more than 36 senior military and civilian health care leaders including the Surgeons General of the Air Force, Army, and Navy (the chief executive officers of their respective organizations) (DOD MHS, 2008, 2009) (Figure 19-2). The MHS leadership structure includes career military and civilian political appointees. For example, the U.S. president is responsible for nominating senior leaders to become the Assistant Secretary of Defense for Health Affairs and the Surgeons General of the Air Force, Army, and Navy. Following a nomination, Congress is responsible for confirming the selection. Although the MHS is a military system, policy shifts occur when administrations change, as a result of the civilian political leadership.

THE MHS BUDGET

Each year, the National Defense Authorization Act is passed by Congress specifying the budget for DOD including the MHS through the Defense Health Program (DHP). The military medical departments, the MHS financial management staff along with the DOD comptroller and key members of Congressional oversight committees, work to develop an executable budget. Following preparation of the budget, each military Surgeon General, along with other leaders from the MHS, testifies before the Senate Armed Services Committee outlining accomplishments from the past year and their plan for the next year's budget execution. DHP funding provides for the delivery of health services and also funds the education and training of medical personnel, research, procurement of medical equipment for military hospitals and clinics, and other select health care activities.

The 2009 defense appropriations bill included increases for traumatic brain injury (TBI) and psychological health of military personnel returning from war. The $24.6 billion funding represents an approximate 9% increase from the previous year. This growth in the budget represents a commitment on the part of MHS and Congressional leadership to address this important issue (DOD, 2009).

MAJOR POLICY ISSUES IN THE MHS

COMBAT INJURIES CAUSING PTSD AND TBI

Following September 11, 2001, two major military campaigns were initiated in response to the terrorist attacks on the U.S. The first, Operation Enduring Freedom (OEF) in Afghanistan, began in October 2001. The second, Operation Iraqi Freedom (OIF) in Iraq, commenced in March 2003. Since 2001, military members have been deployed for long periods of time in extreme combat conditions with subsequent exposure to life-changing experiences. These events have placed them at great risk for developing a variety of mental health conditions including posttraumatic stress disorder (PTSD).

PTSD

Military personnel are exposed to numerous psychological and social stressors that can be immediate,

acute, and chronic in nature. Military personnel with PTSD often relive their stressful experiences such as exposure to combat, death of fellow comrades, devastated communities, and homeless refugees, through nightmares and flashbacks. Not only do they have concerns about their own safety in the war zone; they also worry about the well-being of family members at home (GAO, 2008a; Gahm & Lucenko, 2007; Romanoff, 2006). Affected service members often feel detached and estranged, resulting in family relationship disruptions. It is estimated that as many as 20% of service members who served in Iraq and Afghanistan have screened positive for PTSD or other behavioral health symptoms such as depression and anxiety (GAO, 2008a; Gahm & Lucenko, 2007).

The DOD developed and implemented standards for screening military personnel for mental health conditions related to deployment. However, policies requiring health care providers to review medical records to screen for conditions were inconsistent. To address this deficit, the DOD issued a policy establishing baseline mental health standards military personnel must meet in order to deploy to support the wartime mission. This policy recognized the predeployment mental health assessment as a mechanism for screening personnel within 60 days before an individual deploys (GAO, 2008a). To further improve care for military personnel serving in areas of conflict, a postdeployment health assessment was also developed to provide screening 90 to 180 days following return from combat. This tool affords the DOD the ability to obtain information on service members' health concerns that emerge over time after return from deployment (Gahm & Lucenko, 2007).

TBI

Military personnel serving in OEF and OIF are also at risk for exposure to physical injury related to combat. TBI is one of the most frequently reported injuries among service members in Iraq and Afghanistan and may account for as much as 20% to 30% of battlefield-related injuries (GAO, 2008a). Exposure to improvised explosive devices; motor vehicle accidents; gunshot injuries to the face, head, and neck; and falls are the mechanisms of injury responsible for the greatest number of cases of TBI (Martin et al., 2008; Meyer et al., 2008). Improved effectiveness of body armor in protecting military personnel from injuries that would have resulted in death in prior conflicts is likely the reason for the increasing numbers of TBI cases reported (Warden, 2006). With this high survival rate has come policy issues related to identifying and meeting the demand for care of patients with TBI including training and research as part of the policy solutions.

In 2007, the Defense and Veterans Brain Injury Center (DVBIC) was reorganized to work with the newly established Defense Centers of Excellence for Psychological Health and Traumatic Brain Injury. The purpose of this was to provide evaluation, treatment, and follow-up care for military personnel on active duty or retired from military service who have a brain injury. DVBIC's mission is accomplished through patient care, educational programs, and clinical research conducted to identify evidence-based care and treatment for patients with TBI (DVBIC, 2009).

Research is aimed at identifying the effectiveness of various medications in treating or eliminating the effects of TBI such as headaches, confusion, agitation, and alterations in memory and cognition. In collaboration with the Centers for Disease Control and Prevention (CDC), efforts are underway to follow TBI patients over time to identify long-term problems associated with TBI. Research initiatives are critical for providing data on the consequences of TBI injuries so MHS policymakers can base policy on evidence (DVBIC, 2009).

Another critical issue for policymakers, as with PTSD, is appropriate screening of OEF/OIF veterans for TBI. In collaboration with the DVBIC, the VA is refining a tool to screen all veterans for TBI. Training has been established for providers to ensure that screening protocols are used accurately and that veterans are properly evaluated and treated for TBI (GAO, 2008b). Beginning in 2008, the DOD required screening for TBI in all military personnel who were identified for combat duty (GAO, 2008a).

SUICIDE

Suicide rates among both active duty military members and veterans continue to rise despite efforts by the DOD to address the problem (Kuehn, 2009; Tanielian & Jaycox, 2008). It is estimated that approximately 37% of military personnel returning from Iraq and Afghanistan have challenges with their mental health (Seal et al., 2009). The military has grappled for years with the issue of stigma associated

with seeking mental health services. Service members may have reservations about disclosing symptoms because of the possible implications for their careers (Kuehn, 2009; Hill et al., 2006). Current policies need to be examined and new policies need to be created that encourage those who need help to seek mental health care without fear of risk to their professional livelihood and with certainty that they can seek treatment in a confidential manner (Tanielian & Jaycox, 2008).

BASE REALIGNMENT AND CLOSURE/INTEGRATION

Base Realignment and Closure (BRAC) is mandated by Congress and serves as a mechanism by which a major reorganization of military installations, including health services, occurs periodically. A major goal of BRAC for the MHS is planning for the effective and efficient delivery of health care services for all beneficiaries—especially the care for casualties returning from Iraq and Afghanistan (Murray, 2009). From a health care perspective, under BRAC law the Air Force, Army, and Navy are responsible for working jointly to ensure that health care resources are properly utilized to achieve the MHS mission. BRAC presents an opportunity for greater integration and coordination of health care assets. This more integrated health system is expected to improve effectiveness and efficiency (Murray, 2009).

Congress has directed the MHS to establish and maintain partnerships with other federal agencies such as the VA and Health and Human Services (HHS) as well as explore similar partnerships with the private health care sector (Murray, 2009). The MHS and VA are currently coordinating health care delivery services working through barriers that exist like different computer systems. In fact, in the fiscal year 2010 DOD budget, funding was specifically set aside for the DOD and the VA to work collaboratively to develop an interoperable electronic health care record.

PERSONNEL

Staff in military hospitals consists of military, civilian, and contracted civilian personnel. A major personnel policy issue is the congressional direction to shrink the size of military staff and convert their positions to civilian ones. Determining the appropriate mix of military and civilian personnel to support U.S. forces during a war or other conflict and to provide high-quality, cost-effective medical care during peace-time has not occurred without controversy. The conversion has begun, but each military department took a different approach. At the end of fiscal year 2007, the Air Force projected that 1216 military positions would be converted. During the same time period, the Navy planned to change 2675 positions and the Army approximately 1588 (DOD, 2007).

There are concerns with this personnel policy. Uniformed health care professionals are viewed as the foundation of the MHS because of their training for missions such as wartime and disaster response. Many MHS leaders worry that significant reductions in military medical personnel will decrease the agility needed to respond to wartime and disaster response missions. Military to civilian conversions have also contributed to unfilled vacancies. With the increasing shortage of health care personnel (e.g., nurses) and strong competition with the civilian sector for health care providers, the MHS is confronted with significant challenges in filling these vacancies. Recruiting and retaining highly qualified health care professionals is becoming more challenging for all of the military services, which have been challenged for years by chronic shortages in certain essential health care specialties (e.g., critical care, internal medicine, and orthopedic surgery) that are required for sustained operational readiness. Further complicating personnel shortages, military departments compete not only with the civilian health care sector for qualified medical personnel, but also with each other (DOD, 2007).

TOBACCO USE

Researchers are reporting that not only are military personnel who are deployed to Iraq and Afghanistan at increased risk for injury related to dangers inherent in war, they are also at risk for diseases associated with smoking (Smith & Malone, 2009). Use of tobacco products causes both short-term and long-term complications such as reducing overall general fitness; pulmonary diseases such as chronic obstructive pulmonary disease; oral, pancreatic, and lung cancers; and cardiovascular diseases such as heart attack and stroke (Institute of Medicine, 2009). Despite the DOD's attempts to curtail tobacco use in those serving in the military, use of tobacco products continues to remain high (Smith & Malone, 2009). DOD policies have focused on smoking-cessation programs,

smoke-free environments, and efforts to either prohibit the sale of tobacco products or restrict the sale of such products on military installations (Institute of Medicine, 2009; Smith & Malone, 2009). However, this issue remains a significant health concern that impedes the ability of military personnel to be medically ready to serve. In order to prevent illness of military personnel as a result of tobacco use, stronger policies addressing comprehensive tobacco-free environments and wide-ranging tobacco-control programs are needed (Institute of Medicine, 2009; Smith & Malone, 2009).

EMERGENCY CONTRACEPTION

Another policy issue being analyzed in the MHS is the availability of emergency contraception (EC) in military hospitals. Although approved by the FDA since 1997 as a safe and essential method for avoiding unplanned pregnancies following unprotected sexual intercourse, EC remains underutilized in both the military and civilian health care sectors (Chung-Park, 2008). Unintentional pregnancies have implications on the military readiness of women serving in uniform. The MHS is considering policy that will make EC readily available to all female service members at all locations where they serve as well as examining the impact such a policy might have on their health and medical readiness (DOD MHS, 2009).

For a list of related websites, please refer to your Evolve Resources at http://evolve.elsevier.com/Mason/policypolitics/

REFERENCES

Burelli, D. F. (2003). *Military health care: The issue of "promised" benefits.* Washington D.C.: Congressional Research Service/The Library of Congress.

Caring for America's heroes—2008 MHS stakeholders' report. (2008). Retrieved from www.health.mil.

Chung-Park, M. (2008). Emergency contraception knowledge, attitudes, practices, and barriers among providers at a military treatment facility. *Military Medicine, 173*(3), 305-312.

Defense and Veterans Brain Injury Center (DVBIC). (2009). Defense and veterans head injury program. Retrieved from www.dvbic.org.

Department of Defense. (2007). Future of military health care. Retrieved from www.health.mil/dhb/downloads/103-06-2-Home-Task_Force_FINAL_REPORT_122007.pdf.

Department of Defense. (2009). FY 2009 Defense health program. Retrieved from www.whitehouse.gov/omb/budget/fy2009/defense.html.

Department of Defense Military Health System (DOD MHS). (2008). The military health system strategic plan. Retrieved from www.health.mil/StrategicPlan/2008%20Strat%20Plan%20Final%20-lowres.pdf.

Department of Defense Military Health System (DOD MHS). (2009). Military health system mission. Retrieved from www.health.mil.

Gahm, G., & Lucenko, B. (2007). Screening soldiers in outpatient care for mental health concerns. *Military Medicine, 173*(1), 17-24.

Government Accountability Office (GAO). (2008a). Mental health and traumatic brain injury screening efforts implemented, but consistent pre-deployment medical record review policies needed. Retrieved from www.gao.gov/products/GAO-08-615.

Government Accountability Office (GAO). (2008b). Mild traumatic brain injury screening and evaluation implemented for OEF/OIF veterans, but challenges remain. Retrieved from www.gao.gov/new.items/d08276.pdf.

Hill, J., Johnson, R. & Barton, R. (2006). Suicidal and homicidal soldiers in deployment environments. *Military Medicine, 171*(3), 228-232.

Hosek, S. D., & Cecchine, G. (2001). Reorganizing the military health system—Should there be a joint command? (Rand Monograph). Retrieved from www.rand.org/pubs/monograph_reports/MR1350.

Institute of Medicine. (2009). Combating tobacco in military and veteran populations. Retrieved from www.health.mil/include/exitwarning.aspx?link=http://www.iom.edu/Object.File/Master/70/990/Combating%20Tobacco%20Military%20for%20web.pdf.

Kuehn, B. (2009). Soldier suicide rates continue to rise: Military, scientists work to stem the tide. *JAMA, 301*(11), 1111-1113.

Martin, E., Lu, W., Heimick, K., French, L., & Warden, D. (2008). Traumatic brain injuries sustained in the Afghanistan and Iraq wars. *Journal of Trauma Nursing, 15*(3), 94-101.

Meyer, K., Helmick, K., Doncevic, S., & Park, R. (2008). Severe and penetrating traumatic brain injury in the context of war. *Journal of Trauma Nursing, 15*(4), 185-191.

Murray, J. S. (2009). Joint task force national capital region medical: Integration of education, training & research. *Military Medicine, 174*(5), 448-454.

Romanoff, M. (2006). Assessing military veterans for posttraumatic stress disorder: A guide for primary care clinicians. *Journal of the American Academy of Nurse Practitioners, 18*(9), 409-413.

Seal, K., Metzler, T., Gima, K., Bertenthal, D., Maguen, S., & Marmar, C. (2009). Trends and risk factors for mental health diagnoses among Iraq and Afghanistan veterans using Department of Veterans Affairs health care, 2002-2008. *American Journal of Public Health, 99*(9), 1651-1658.

Smith, E., & Malone, R. (2009). Everywhere the soldier will be: Wartime tobacco promotion in the U.S. military. *American Journal of Public Health, 99*(9), 1595-1602.

Tanielian, T., & Jaycox, L. (2008). *Invisible wounds of war; Psychological and cognitive injuries, their consequences, and services to assist recovery.* Arlington: RAND Corporation.

TRICARE Management Activity. (2009). What is TRICARE? Retrieved from http://tricare.mil/mybenefit/home/overview/WhatIsTRICARE.

Warden, D. (2006). Military TBI during the Iraq and Afghanistan wars. *Journal of Head Trauma Rehabilitation, 21*(5), 398-402.

CHAPTER 20

The Veterans Administration Health System: An Overview of Major Policy Issues

Cynthia Caroselli

"Caring for our veterans is the duty of a grateful nation."
—Senator Patty Murray

The United States Department of Veterans Affairs (VA), the second largest of the 15 Cabinet departments of the executive branch of the federal government, was established in 1989, succeeding the Veterans Administration. It operates nationwide programs for health care, financial assistance, and burial benefits. As the most visible component, the Veterans Health Administration (VHA) is one of the largest integrated health systems in the world, providing a variety of services to veterans in every state and Puerto Rico. Funding for VA services is provided through congressional and presidential authorization and is managed via submissions to the Office of Management and Budget. As opposed to private sector organizations, VA budgets are disbursement models rather than expenditure budgets. Additionally, it serves as an important venue for training the next generation of health care professionals in a variety of disciplines, with approximately 90,000 health professionals receiving clinical education in VA facilities each year. The VHA provides clinical learning sites for the majority of nurses and physicians in the country. Advances in care and policy implementation at VA facilities have wide-ranging effects on health care throughout the nation, since so many patients are served by so many providers and learners from all of the health care professions.

MISSION AND ORGANIZATION

The VHA provides services to almost 8 million enrollees (Department of Veterans Administration Information Technology Center, 2008) in 153 medical centers and over 800 community-based outpatient centers (Department of Veterans Affairs, 2010). Staffed by almost 300,000 employees, services provided include outpatient primary care; social services; inpatient medical-surgical care; acute and chronic psychiatric care; specialty services such as audiology and dialysis; and tertiary care such as emergency services, transplant, neurosurgery, and the full range of cardiovascular services.

Veterans Administration Medical Centers (VAMCs) are categorized according to complexity and acuity of services. For instance, a level 1A facility will provide the full range of acute medical, surgical, psychiatric, specialty, critical care, long-term, and outpatient services, and generally includes tertiary/subspecialty care, as well as supporting community-based outpatient centers and affiliating "vet centers." At the other end of the complexity spectrum, a level 3 facility may provide only long-term or outpatient services.

Veterans must enroll to receive VA health care benefits. They are then placed in priority groups that determine which specific benefits they are eligible for, and which co-payments they are required to pay in relation to their income levels. Veterans who have a service-connected disability rating of 50% or greater are not required to enroll. Veterans who served in Operation Enduring Freedom and Operation Iraqi Freedom (OEF/OIF) are eligible to receive VA health care for five years following separation from the military, regardless of disability rating.

PATIENT POPULATION AND CHANGING DEMOGRAPHICS

A look at current VA patient demographics reveals a changing portrait. While the World War II veteran population is well advanced in age and close to 1000 die each day, less than 40% of the population of veterans is 65 years of age or older. Currently, the veteran population is composed of growing numbers of those who have served in the Persian Gulf War, Iraq, and Afghanistan, as well as those who have served in Korea and Viet Nam. As of 2008, the projected total veteran population was 24 million. It is expected that many of these veterans will choose to receive their care at VA facilities for the rest of their lives, thus the system has a lifelong relationship with these individuals.

Women veterans have been a numerical minority in VA settings for many years, reflective of the limited role that women were allowed to play in the military in the past (Yano, 2008). However, it is expected that the number of women seeking VA care over the next several years will double, with the greatest proportion from the influx of women recently deployed and discharged from service in OEF/OIF, where the active duty military is 14% female (Hayes, 2008). Further, more than 42% of all discharged women have utilized VA health care at least once, with over 45% having visited 2 to 10 times (Kang, 2008). It is expected that women will comprise a continuously growing component of both the military and the subsequent veteran population.

Given this significant increase in women in the eligible population, VA leadership has mandated that the needs of this unique population be addressed in a focused manner. In 2008, the Secretary of Veterans Affairs mandated that a full-time Women Veterans Program Manager be in place at every VA facility and that every woman veteran have access to a VA primary care provider who can meet all her primary care needs, including gender-specific care (Hayes, 2008). Additionally, since PTSD rates are higher in women than in men (Tolin & Foa, 2006), and since over 20% of women seen in VA outpatient care have reported military sexual trauma (Kimerling et al., 2007), the VHA has mandated that services specific to these needs are available to all veterans, with women veterans receiving gender-specific care. The VHA has made women's health services research a priority solicitation area for over a decade and mandates the inclusion of women in all VA studies (Yano, 2008).

QUALITY AND SAFETY: "THE BEST CARE ANYWHERE"

The VHA established a performance measure system that allows individual facilities to measure clinical care on a national, facility, and individual provider level. Thus, it is possible to determine success on such measures as diabetic control, immunization, heart failure readmission rates, and ventilator-acquired pneumonia, among others. The performance measure program has given rise to a number of clinical initiatives and has fostered the implementation of Institute for Healthcare Improvement bundles, MRSA prevention, and other safety programs. Nationally, the VA established the National Center for Patient Safety (NCPS) to develop and nurture a culture of patient safety, including the presence of patient safety managers in all VA hospitals. Notable for its emphasis on prevention rather than blame, the NCPS has fostered the use of root cause analysis to investigate how well patient care systems function and to create "hard fixes" for identified problems. These efforts have become widely emulated models for systems redesign in the private sector.

The performance measure system provides an important opportunity for internal and external benchmarking. The subsequent analysis and dissemination of data in lay and professional publications has significantly altered the public image of VHA. It is now possible to state that the VHA cares for an older, sicker, and poorer population and achieves clinical outcomes that match or surpass similar organizations in the private sector, and at a lower cost. This has led many to claim that the VHA provides "the best care anywhere" (Longman, 2007).

THE PATIENT-CENTERED MEDICAL HOME

A patient-centered "medical home" is now established for each patient. In this model, also known as

Advanced Primary Care, the primary care team takes responsibility for providing all of the patient's health care needs, either directly or by facilitating the involvement of the appropriate specialty service. The basic primary care team includes a provider (physician, nurse practitioner, or physician assistant), an RN care manager, a clinical associate (health technician or licensed practical nurse), and a clerical associate. The patient is expected to act as a full partner with shared decision making for all actions. Other clinicians such as pharmacists and nutritionists, as well as tertiary specialists, are involved as appropriate to the patient's needs. Electronic communication and secure messaging enhance communication between the patient and team members.

HEALTH CARE ISSUES OF THE NEWEST VETERANS

Traumatic brain injury (TBI) has emerged as the signature injury of the OEF/OIF conflicts. Screenings for TBI, depression, and substance use are carried out for all newly returned veterans on a regular basis. Ending homelessness among veterans has also become both a presidential and VHA priority, and social service programs are in place at every VHA facility to assist veterans with obtaining jobs and housing, on both a temporary and permanent basis.

Suicide among veterans is an issue that has assumed a prominent place in VA care. Rates of suicide among VA health care users are at least 66% higher than the age and gender–adjusted U.S. population (McCarthy et al., 2009). All VHA facilities employ suicide prevention coordinators. These clinicians provide direct service to those at risk for suicide as well as educate staff, assess clinical environments, develop prevention strategies, and coordinate with community agencies.

THE ELECTRONIC MEDICAL RECORD

The VA has long been recognized for the development and implementation of a world class electronic medical record (EMR). It has evolved into a completely paperless system that is not only a robust data repository for documenting care rendered; it is also a uniquely configured system that ensures continuity of care. The EMR can be accessed by an unlimited number of personnel simultaneously. Thus,

information is available as soon as it is entered by the clinician. Since the record is not stored in a remote location, clinicians do not need to "wait their turn" to access the record, and it is always available at the point of care. The ubiquitous nature of the data renders verbal orders obsolete because providers can enter orders from any location. Thus, an attending surgeon can monitor a postoperative patient from his or her home, enter orders, check on laboratory data, and change an intervention plan without requiring the nurse to receive and transcribe a verbal order.

The Bar Code Medication Administration (BCMA) system has revolutionized the way in which nurses administer, evaluate, and document medication regimens. As medication orders are entered into the EMR, they migrate to the BCMA data base. The prescription is automatically sent to the pharmacy, where it is verified for accuracy, allergy status, and interaction with other medications. It is also transmitted to the inventory control system, which monitors institutional use, pricing, reordering, and other actions. After verification, it generates a medication administration record. At the time of medication administration, the nurse brings the medication cart to the bedside, scans the patient's wristband with a handheld scanning device, and administers the medication to the patient.

The chief nursing informatics officer in the Office of Nursing Services directs a comprehensive program. This expert nursing role manages a vast nursing outcomes database; systems design, simulation training, terminology standardization. Nurse executives at the various medical centers are provided with various management reports, including executive-level dashboard reports, nursing hours per patient day, RN satisfaction, clinical indicators, and demographic databases. These initiatives have wide-ranging utility and are more than mere recordkeeping devices. They provide an opportunity to create knowledge, to refine nursing practice, and to deliver the basis for evidence-based care.

NURSING ISSUES

The VA employs more than 76,000 nursing staff (45,000 RNs, 13,000 LPN/LVNs, and 11,000 nursing assistants), making it one of the largest nursing staffs of any health system in the world. Approximately

80% of these individuals are in direct care positions, which demonstrates efficient staff utilization and a flat hierarchical structure. The variety of practice roles and specialty areas is vast. National mobility allows nurses to transfer from facility to facility without losing seniority or benefits; licensure is only required in one state. Educational benefits allow nurses to increase their knowledge in formal academic programs as well as enrichment programs. Additionally, unlicensed personnel can participate in mobility programs that advance them into technical and professional positions. All VHA employees have access to on-line programming that can be completed at the employee's convenience, including programmed instruction and on-demand video learning.

Most VHA facilities have formal affiliation agreements with academic nursing partners, as well as with other health professions schools. As such, VHA is a major educator of future nurses, providing sites for clinical practice from the undergraduate to postdoctoral level. The VHA Office of Nursing Services (ONS) seeks to bridge the gap between basic nursing education programs and the realities of professional nursing practice by piloting RN residency programs. Begun in 2009, eight sites have implemented year-long programs to assist new nursing graduates with refinement of clinical competencies and development of professional behaviors and leadership skills. It is anticipated that this program will result in improved practice and staff satisfaction, as well as decreased turnover (ONS Annual Report, 2009).

Nursing faculty find the VHA to be a hospitable and fruitful partner for research, with faculty conducting research at VHA facilities as well as mentoring VHA staff in the research process. VHA's ONS has formed liaison task forces with the American Association of Colleges of Nursing to explore issues of mutual interest such as nursing residencies, the clinical nurse leader role, and scope and development of the Doctor of Nursing Practice role.

A growing number of VHA facilities have achieved Magnet® status, with many facilities actively pursuing this achievement. As of March 2010, five sites achieved this distinction. In addition, at least one VHA facility has achieved the Beacon Award from the American Association of Critical Care Nurses for excellence in nursing practice.

THE CLINICAL LADDER

VA nurses participate in a clinical ladder that allows them to be recognized for expertise, experience, and excellence. The National Professional Standards Board has established criteria that allow nursing practice to be categorized from Nurse I, or entry level with no experience, through Nurse V, the chief nurse executive level. Progression is rewarded with salary increases. Each local facility has a peer review professional standards board composed of nurses at the various levels who review each nurse on a regular basis to determine progression through the clinical ladder and provide advice on ways in which the nurse can advance, such as serving on committees, publishing, assuming formal and informal leadership, and certification.

GROWTH OF ADVANCED PRACTICE ROLES

The VA utilizes many nurses in advanced practice roles including nurse practitioners, nurse anesthetists, and clinical nurse specialists. Many completed some or all of their clinical education at VA facilities, and many received educational benefits that allowed them to participate in these academic programs. Recently, the VA has partnered with the American Association of Colleges of Nursing to develop and implement the Clinical Nurse Leader role. This innovative role prepares nurses to act as clinical leaders while remaining at the bedside or point of care. A unique feature of these programs is the partnership developed between the academic institution and the VA facility in which both partners collaborate on curriculum development and shape clinical experiences around specific practice roles that the VA facility finds important to achieve excellent clinical outcomes. The Office of Nursing Services has set a goal of implementing the CNL role in every VA facility by 2016. As of 2009, 32 VAMCs employed 87 CNLs in various settings (ONS Annual Report, 2009).

THE VA NURSING ACADEMY

A national shortage of RNs is a constant challenge to the delivery of care and a serious policy issue as health care organizations confront current and future staffing needs. The shortage of nursing faculty forces colleges and universities to turn away thousands of qualified students each year. To address this serious and growing policy issue, the VA has established the

VA Nursing Academy (VANA). Established as a five-year pilot project, this program is centrally administered through the Office of Academic Affiliations in partnership with the Office of Nursing Services. Based upon partnerships between a VA facility and an academic institution, this competitive program has awarded $59 million in funding to 15 partnerships. The goals of the initiative are to expand the number of nursing faculty, enhance the professional and scholarly development of nurses, and increase student enrollment by approximately 1000 students. Students receive most of their clinical instruction at the VA and are mentored by VA professional nurses. As they near graduation, it is anticipated that these students will gravitate to VA employment. Similarly, since each VA has invested significant energy in these students and has had the opportunity to guide them in experiences that are unique to the needs of the veteran patient, the VA will be more likely to employ these students after graduation. Thus, the return on investment by the taxpayer is enormous.

SUMMARY

The VHA is one of the largest health care systems in the world, providing a full range of health care and social services. This federally funded system also acts as a training ground for the majority of the nation's health care professionals. The VA's excellent clinical outcomes can be documented by a robust performance measure program.

The opinions expressed herein are those of the author and do not represent the official position of the Department of Veterans Affairs.

For a list of related websites, please refer to your Evolve Resources at http://evolve.elsevier.com/Mason/policypolitics/

REFERENCES

Department of Veterans Administration Information Technology Center. (2008). Washington, D.C. Federal Computer, February 7, 2010.

Department of Veterans Affairs. (2010). United States Department of Veterans Affairs health care. Retrieved from www1.va.gov/health/MedicalCenters.asp.

Hayes, P. M. (2008). The evolution of women's health services in VA. *Forum*, November, 1-2.

Kang, H. (2008). OEF/OIF Utilization Data FY 2008, First Quarter. Office of Public Health and Environmental Hazards.

Kimerling, R., et al. (2007), The Veterans Health Administration and military sexual trauma. *American Journal of Public Health, 97*, 2160-2166.

Longman, P. (2007). *Best care anywhere: Why VA health care is better than yours.* Sausalito, CA: PoliPointPress.

McCarthy, J. F., Valenstein, M., Kim, H. M., et al. (2009). Suicide mortality among patients receiving care in the veterans health administration health system. *American Journal of Epidemiology, 169*, 1033-1038.

Office of Nursing Services. (2009). Annual report 2009, VA Nursing: Connecting all the pieces of the puzzle to transform care for veterans. Washington, D.C.

Tolin, D. F. & Foa, E. B. (2006). Sex differences in trauma and posttraumatic stress disorder: A quantitative review of 25 years of research. *Psychological Bulletin, 132*(6), 959-992.

Yano, E. M. (2008). Achieving high quality care for women veterans. *Forum*, November, *3*, 8.

CHAPTER 21

The Uninsured and Underinsured— On the Cusp of Health Reform

Catherine Hoffman

"Everybody should have some basic security when it comes to their health."
—President Barack Obama on signing health care reform legislation, 2010

While the large majority of Americans have either private or public health insurance, gaps in our pluralistic health insurance system leave many millions—15% of the population—without health insurance coverage of any kind. Just over one half of the total population is covered privately as a benefit of their job, and a small share (5%) purchase private health insurance plans for themselves in the non-group market (Figure 21-1). The public arms of the system cover nearly all older adults through Medicare (14% of the population), with Medicaid and other public programs covering many, but not all, of those with low incomes (13% of the population) (Kaiser Commission on Medicaid and the Uninsured and the Urban Institute, 2009).

The problem of the uninsured has challenged the country for decades, but universal coverage had eluded policymakers. The combination of unabated growth in the number of uninsured, the unchecked growth in health care costs, questionable health care quality, and a deep economic recession created a consensus that the health care system was truly in crisis at this point and in need of major national health reform. Historic legislation that will markedly decrease the majority of the uninsured in the years ahead was passed and signed by the president on March 23, 2010. The policy work to implement the new laws is critically shaped by what is known about those who do not have health insurance today.

There were 46 million uninsured under the age of 65 in the United States in 2008. The problem affects people of all ages, colors, and income and educational levels—and bears real consequences. Not having insurance makes a substantial difference in people's access to needed health care. In addition, millions of Americans who have health insurance do not have the financial security health insurance coverage should promise.

This chapter profiles the uninsured, who they are, why they do not have health coverage, and the difference not having health insurance makes in their lives. It also provides an overview of our health insurance system, describing the holes in the system, why they exist, and the funding of "charity care." The chapter concludes with key elements of the current national health reform legislation that attempt to address the many barriers to access to health insurance in the U.S..

HOLES IN THE HEALTH INSURANCE SYSTEM

Gaps in health insurance coverage, be they short or last for years, are primarily a problem only among the nonelderly because nearly all who are 65 years and older are covered by Medicare. More than one half of the nonelderly receive health coverage as an employer benefit. Those who do not have access to or cannot afford employer-sponsored or private non-group insurance go without health coverage unless they qualify for Medicaid, the Children's Health Insurance Program (CHIP), or other subsidized insurance programs.

The number of nonelderly uninsured has been growing steadily every year since 2000 by about 1 to 2 million, with the exception of a dip in 2007 when the otherwise steady decline in employer-sponsored coverage leveled off briefly (Figure 21-2). By 2008, however, the number of nonelderly uninsured Americans rose again and is expected to continue to climb

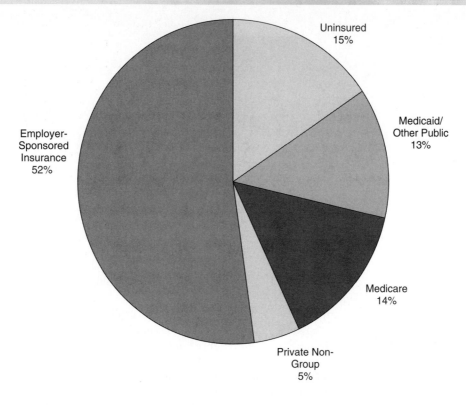

Total Population = 300.5 million

FIGURE 21-1 Health insurance coverage in the U.S., 2008. Note: Includes those over age 65. Medicaid/Other Public includes Medicaid, CHIP, other state programs, and military-related coverage. Those enrolled in both Medicare and Medicaid (1.9% of the population) are shown as Medicare beneficiaries. (From Kaiser Commission on Medicaid and the Uninsured/Urban Institute analysis of 2009 ASEC Supplement to the Current Population Survey.)

as a consequence of the country's recession and persistently high unemployment rate.

The holes in the health insurance system for the nonelderly left 1 in 6 (17%) of the nonelderly uninsured in 2008. And because being insured is largely a condition of being able to afford insurance, the chances of being uninsured are considerably higher for those who have low incomes (Figure 21-3). The nonelderly poor are seven times as likely to be uninsured compared to those with high family incomes (35% uninsured vs. 5% among those with incomes of four times the federal poverty level [FPL] and higher) (Kaiser Commission on Medicaid and the Uninsured and the Urban Institute, 2009).

EMPLOYER-SPONSORED HEALTH INSURANCE

About 60% of people in the U.S. under the age of 65 obtain their health insurance through an employer,

making it the most common form of health coverage. However, having a job does not guarantee a person will have access to employer-sponsored coverage; in fact, about 37 million of the uninsured are in families that have at least one working member (Kaiser Commission on Medicaid and the Uninsured and the Urban Institute, 2009). The share of the nonelderly population with employer-sponsored coverage has been declining since 2000—even during periods when the economy was stronger and growth in health insurance premiums was slowing—and has been exacerbated by two recessions.

Businesses are not required to offer job-based coverage to their workers, although 60% of businesses did in 2009. Almost all large firms with more than 200 workers offer a health insurance benefit. Smaller firms and those with more low-wage workers are much less likely to offer health benefits. Across

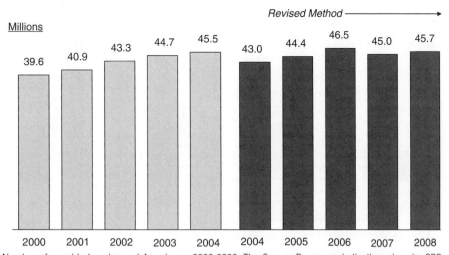

FIGURE 21-2 Number of nonelderly uninsured Americans, 2000-2008. The Census Bureau periodically revises its CPS methods, which means data before and after the revision are not comparable. Comparison across years can be made from 2000 through 2004, and revised estimates for 2004 through 2008. (From Kaiser Commission on Medicaid and the Uninsured/Urban Institute analysis of Current Population Survey Supplements for each year.)

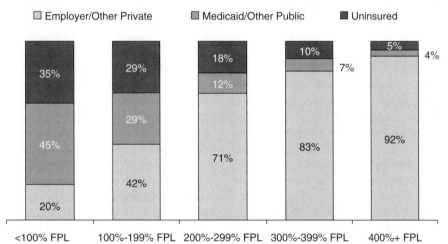

FIGURE 21-3 Health insurance coverage by poverty level, 2008. The federal poverty level (FPL) was $22,025 for a family of four in 2008. Data may not total 100% due to rounding. (From Kaiser Commission on Medicaid and the Uninsured/Urban Institute analysis of 2009 ASEC Supplement to the Current Population Survey.)

industries, uninsured rates for workers range from 35% in agriculture to just 5% in public administration. But even in industries where uninsured rates are lower, the gap in health coverage between blue-collar and white-collar workers is often two-fold or greater. More than 80% of uninsured workers are in blue-collar jobs. More than half of employees in poor families are not offered coverage either through their own employer or their spouse's employer, compared to just 4% of employees at or above 400% of the FPL (Clemans-Cope & Garrett, 2006).

Even when businesses offer health benefits, not all employees are eligible because they work part-time or have been recently hired. Among firms that offered health insurance benefits in 2009, an average of 79% of their workers were eligible for them (Kaiser Family Foundation and Health Research & Educational Trust, 2009). Other workers may not participate in their company's health benefits because they cannot afford the employee share of the premium.

The high cost of health insurance is the most common reason employers report for not offering

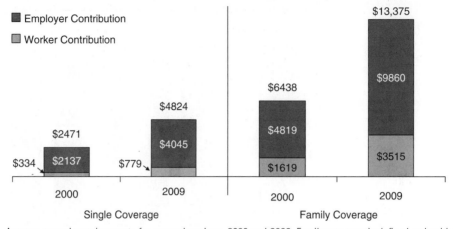

FIGURE 21-4 Average annual premium costs for covered workers, 2000 and 2009. Family coverage is defined as health coverage for a family of four. (From Kaiser Family Foundation/Health Research and Educational Trust Employer Health Benefits Survey, 2009.)

coverage and why individuals do not buy it for themselves. Health insurance premiums have been escalating, outpacing the growth in wages and general inflation by three-fold in the past decade. In 2009, annual employer-sponsored group premiums averaged $4824 for individual coverage and $13,375 for family coverage. Total family premiums and the employee's share of the premium have doubled since 2000 (Figure 21-4) (Kaiser Family Foundation and Health Research & Educational Trust, 2009). Despite the high cost, the majority of employees participate in their employer's health plan when they are offered coverage, even among those with very low incomes (Clemans-Cope & Garrett, 2006).

MEDICAID'S ROLE FOR THE NONELDERLY

Medicaid is the nation's major public health insurance program for low-income Americans, a partnership between each state and the federal government to provide a health insurance safety net. Unlike Medicare, which covers nearly all older adults, Medicaid is an entitlement for only certain categories of the nonelderly. Medicaid limits its reach to four main groups: children, their parents, pregnant women, and people with disabilities—with the program playing its broadest role among children.

Federal law requires states to cover school-age children up to 100% of the FPL and 133% of the FPL for preschool children. The Children's Health Insurance Program (CHIP), created in 1997 to expand coverage to more low-income children, complements Medicaid by covering low-income children with family incomes higher than Medicaid eligibility levels.

Through the combination of Medicaid and CHIP, most states cover children up to or above 200% of the FPL (see Chapter 18). Together these programs cover more than one half of all low-income children and have played a critical role in improving access to care for children.

In contrast to coverage for children, the role of Medicaid for nonelderly adults is more limited. While all poor children are eligible for Medicaid, many of their parents are not. States are only required to cover parents with incomes below their state's 1996 welfare eligibility levels, which is often below 50% of the FPL. In addition, although Medicaid covers some low-income individuals with disabilities, most adults without dependent children—regardless of how poor—are ineligible for Medicaid. As a result, over 40% of poor parents and adults without children are uninsured (Figure 21-5) (Kaiser Commission on Medicaid and the Uninsured and the Urban Institute, 2009).

Over the past decade, growth in Medicaid enrollment has helped buffer the loss of employer-sponsored coverage, containing the growth in the number of uninsured. As the health insurance safety net for the nonelderly, enrollment in Medicaid always increases during economic downturns when people lose their jobs. However, at the same time, recessions also decrease state revenues and they are less able to meet the increased need.

In recent years, states have used their Medicaid and CHIP programs as a foundation for broader health care coverage expansions, taking advantage of the existing delivery and administrative systems as

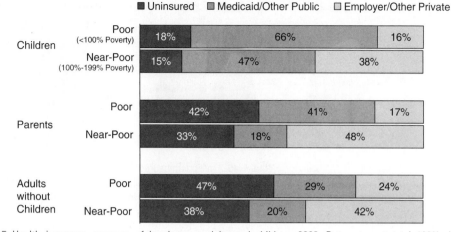

FIGURE 21-5 Health insurance coverage of low-income adults and children, 2008. Data may not total 100% due to rounding. (From Kaiser Commission on Medicaid and the Uninsured/Urban Institute analysis of 2009 ASEC Supplement to the Current Population Survey.)

well as federal matching funds to help finance the expansions. In addition, several states have obtained waivers of federal requirements to expand coverage to childless adults through their Medicaid programs (Artiga & Schwartz, 2009). These programs, along with coverage expansions for low-income children and families, have been a cornerstone of state strategies to address the problem of the uninsured.

PROFILE OF THE UNINSURED

In 2008, 45.7 million people in the U.S. under age 65 did not have health insurance (Kaiser Commission on Medicaid and the Uninsured and the Urban Institute, 2009). Most of them were adults, and were from working families earning low incomes. In fact, more than 8 in 10 of the uninsured are members of working families—about two thirds are from families with one or more full-time workers, and 14% are from families with part-time workers. Only 19% of the uninsured are from families that have no connection to the workforce (Figure 21-6). Even at lower income levels, the majority of the uninsured are in working families. Among the uninsured with incomes below the FPL ($22,025 for a family of four in 2008), 55% have at least one worker in the family (Kaiser Commission on Medicaid and the Uninsured and the Urban Institute, 2009).

About two-thirds of the uninsured are poor or near-poor (see Figure 21-6). These individuals are less likely to be offered employer-sponsored coverage or to be able to afford to purchase their own coverage.

Those who are poor (below 100% of the FPL, which was an income of $22,025 for a family of four in 2008) are about twice as likely to be uninsured as the entire nonelderly population (35% vs.17%). Were it not for the Medicaid program, many more of the poor would be uninsured. The near-poor (those with incomes between 100% and 199% of the FPL) also run a high risk of being uninsured (29%), in part because they are less likely to be eligible for Medicaid. Only 10% of the uninsured are from families at or above 400% of the FPL.

Adults make up more than their share of the uninsured (80%) because, as mentioned earlier, they are less likely than children to be eligible for Medicaid. Young adults, ages 19 to 29, compose a disproportionately large share of the uninsured, largely due to their low incomes. They have a higher uninsured rate (30%) because they are more likely to be earning low incomes, in new jobs and not yet eligible for benefits, and are less likely to be married so have no other connection to job-based coverage. While young adults are more likely to be uninsured, they do not compose the majority of the uninsured. More than one half (52%) of the uninsured are age 30 and older, and these older adults are at increased risk of serious health problems.

The uninsured tend to be in worse health than the privately insured. About 11% of the uninsured are in fair or poor health, compared to 5% of those with private coverage. Almost half of all uninsured nonelderly adults have a chronic condition (Davidoff and Kenney, 2005). Without employer-sponsored

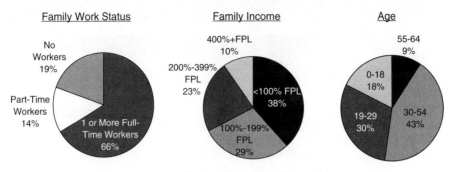

Total = 45.7 million uninsured

FIGURE 21-6 Characteristics of the uninsured, 2008. The federal poverty level (FPL) was $22,025 for a family of four in 2008. Data may not total 100% due to rounding. (From Kaiser Commission on Medicaid and the Uninsured/Urban Institute analysis of 2009 ASEC Supplement to the Current Population Survey.)

insurance, those with such conditions and others who are not in good health often find non-group coverage to be unavailable or unaffordable.

More than half (62%) of nonelderly uninsured adults have no education beyond high school, making them less able to get higher-skilled jobs where health benefits are provided. Those with less education are also more likely to be uninsured for longer periods of time (National Center for Health Statistics, 2008).

Minorities account for a disproportionate share of the uninsured (making up 37% of the nonelderly population but 54% of the uninsured) because they are much more likely to be uninsured than whites. About one third of Hispanics and one fifth of African Americans are uninsured compared to 13% of whites. Because racial and ethnic minority groups are more likely to come from low-income families, Medicaid is an important source of health insurance for them. However, its limited reach leaves large numbers of minorities uninsured.

Although non-citizens (legal and undocumented) are about three times more likely to be uninsured than citizens, the majority of the uninsured (80%) are native or naturalized U.S. citizens. Non-citizens have less access to employer coverage because they are more likely to have low-wage jobs and work for businesses that do not offer coverage. In addition, federal law bars undocumented immigrants from enrolling in Medicaid and CHIP.

Finally, insurance coverage varies by state depending on the share of families with low incomes, the nature of the state's employment, and the reach of state Medicaid programs (Marks, Schwartz, & Donaldson, 2009). The chances of being uninsured

are greater among those living in the southern and western regions of the U.S.. State uninsured rates range from less than 10% in Hawaii, Massachusetts, and Minnesota to over 25% in New Mexico and Texas (Kaiser Commission on Medicaid and the Uninsured, 2009a).

HEALTH INSURANCE AND ACCESS TO CARE

Health insurance makes a difference in whether and when people get necessary medical care, where they get their care, and ultimately, how healthy people are. The problems begin when they postpone or forgo health care they know they need because they cannot afford it.

Nearly 25% of uninsured adults say that they have forgone care in the past year because of its cost—compared to 4% of adults with private coverage (Figure 21-7) (Kaiser Commission on Medicaid and the Uninsured, 2009b). Anticipating high medical bills, many of the uninsured are not able to follow recommended treatments. Over one fourth of uninsured adults say they did not fill a drug prescription in the past year because they could not afford it (27% vs. 5% of those with private insurance). Regardless of a person's insurance coverage, those injured or newly diagnosed with a chronic condition receive similar follow-up care plans, however the uninsured are less likely than the insured to actually follow through and obtain all the services that are recommended (Hadley, 2007).

Another fundamental barrier is that more than one half of uninsured adults do not have a regular

Percentage of adults (age 18 – 64) reporting:

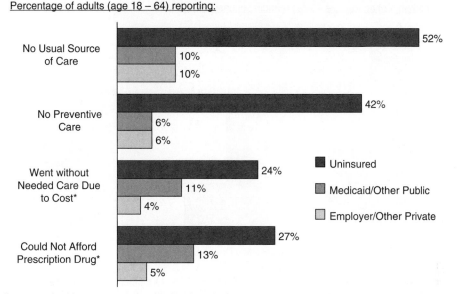

FIGURE 21-7 Barriers to health care among nonelderly adults, by insurance status, 2008. Respondents who said usual source of care was the emergency room were included among those not having a usual source of care. *In the past 12 months. (From Kaiser Commission on Medicaid and the Uninsured analysis of 2008 NHIS data.)

place to go when they are sick or need medical advice (see Figure 21-7). Silent health problems, such as hypertension and diabetes, often go undetected without routine checkups. Uninsured nonelderly adults compared to those with coverage are far less likely to have had regular preventive care, including cancer screenings (NewsHour with Jim Lehrer/Kaiser Family Foundation National Survey on the Uninsured, 2003). Consequently, uninsured patients are diagnosed in later stages of a disease, including cancer, and die earlier than those with insurance (Ayanian et al., 2000; Roetzheim et al., 2000).

Because the uninsured are less likely than the insured to have regular outpatient care, they are more likely to be hospitalized for avoidable health problems and experience declines in their overall health. When they are hospitalized, the uninsured receive fewer diagnostic and therapeutic services and also are more likely to die in the hospital than insured patients (Hadley, 2003; Canto et al., 2000). Even among those injured in severe automobile accidents who are unable to participate in the initial treatment decisions, the uninsured receive less hospital services and have a substantially higher mortality rate (Doyle, 2005).

Access to health care has eroded over time for many. Rising health care costs have made health care less affordable, particularly for the uninsured. Between

1997 and 2006, the differences in access to care between the uninsured and insured widened, even among those with chronic conditions. The insurance disparities in access to a usual source of care, annual checkups, and preventive health care are the greatest and grew the most over the decade (Hoffman & Schwartz, 2008a, 2008b).

Research has shown that gaining health insurance restores access to health care considerably and diminishes the adverse effects of having been uninsured. Middle-aged adults who are continuously uninsured vs. insured are much more likely to experience a decline in their health (Baker et al., 2001). However, among previously uninsured adults who acquire Medicare coverage at age 65, use of preventive care increases, their access to physician and hospital care increases, and they experience improved health and functional status. When uninsured children gain health coverage, they receive more timely diagnoses, have fewer preventable hospitalizations, and miss fewer days of school (Institute of Medicine, 2009).

HEALTH INSURANCE AND FINANCIAL SECURITY

In addition to improving access to health care, health insurance provides the security of knowing that when

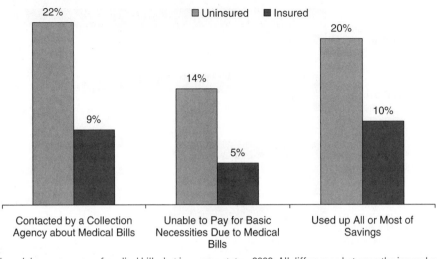

Percentage of adults (age 18-64) reporting in past 12 months:

FIGURE 21-8 Financial consequences of medical bills, but insurance status, 2009. All differences between the insured and the uninsured are statistically significant ($p < 0.05$). (From Kaiser Family Foundation's Health Tracking Poll, August 2009.)

needed, health services will be paid for in large part. The majority of the uninsured come from low-income families and have very limited savings and assets to fall back on when their health fails. One half of uninsured households in 2004 had total assets, other than their home and car, of $600 or less, leaving little to no financial reserve to pay unexpected medical bills (Jacobs & Claxton, 2008). One in five uninsured adults reported in 2009 that they used up all or most of their savings to pay for medical bills (Figure 21-8) (Kaiser Family Foundation's Health Tracking Poll, August 2009). This leaves the uninsured at high risk of being unable to pay off medical debt, and, like any unpaid bill, this debt is turned over to a collection agency, jeopardizing a person's credit profile for years.

FINANCING CARE FOR THE UNINSURED

Inadequate access to care means that the uninsured use less health care; in fact, they spend less than one half of what the insured do on health care. In 2008, the average person who was uninsured for a full year incurred $1686 in total health care costs compared to $4463 for the nonelderly with coverage. The uninsured pay for about one third of their care out of their own pocket; in 2008 this totaled to $30 billion (Hadley et al., 2008).

The remaining costs of their care, the uncompensated costs, amounted to about $57 billion in 2008 and was, in fact, paid to providers through a patchwork of federal, state, and private funds. Three fourths of this total ($42.9 billion) was paid by federal, state, and local government funds appropriated for care of the uninsured. Nearly one half of all funds for uncompensated care come from the federal government, with the majority of federal dollars flowing through Medicare and Medicaid. To put this in perspective—while this amount was substantial, government dollars for uncompensated care amounted to only a small slice (just 2%) of total health care spending in the U.S. in 2008.

Hospitals, community clinics, and physicians all provide care to the uninsured. While physicians and community clinics see more uninsured patients, 60% of uncompensated care costs are incurred in hospitals because medical needs requiring hospitalization are the most expensive. The cost of uncompensated care provided by physicians is not reimbursed by public dollars, either directly or indirectly (Hadley et al., 2008). Financial pressures and time constraints, coupled with changing physician practice patterns, have contributed to a decline in charity care provided by physicians. The percent of all doctors who provided charity care fell to 68% in 2004-2005 from 76% in 1996-1997 (Cunningham & May, 2006).

In contrast, uncompensated care costs in service programs, such as the Veterans Affairs health system and community health centers, are funded largely by public dollars. Community health centers and public hospitals also rely heavily on the Medicaid program as their largest source of third-party insurance payments. About one third of all revenues in Federally Qualified Health Centers and public hospitals are paid by Medicaid, evidence of the large share of low-income patients they serve (National Association of Public Hospitals and Health Systems, 2009; National Association of Community Health Centers, 2008).

THE UNDERINSURED

Health insurance alone is no longer a guarantee of financial protection from the costs of health care for many. What it means to have health insurance has changed considerably as premiums, cost-sharing requirements, and limits on benefits have increased the amounts that people pay out of pocket for health care, even with "good" health insurance plans. Consumers weigh how much they can afford in a health plan against their best guess of what their health needs may be in the upcoming year—all with little knowledge of the costs of services they most likely have never used. It is a difficult choice and one that leaves millions underinsured each year.

The problem has continued to grow over time (Schoen et al., 2008). Moreover, research has also found that the underinsured are significantly more likely than those with adequate insurance to have problems with access to care due to costs, including access to preventive care, prescription drugs, and recommended treatments.

In addition to the problem of accessing needed care, medical debt can accumulate quickly—whether a person is uninsured or underinsured. Survey research documents that over one half of bankruptcies were tied to medical debt and/or health problems in early 2007. The majority of those filing for bankruptcy related to medical problems actually had health insurance when they filed, but having a gap in coverage in the preceding two years was a predictor of a medically-caused bankruptcy (Himmelstein et al., 2009).

EXPANDING HEALTH INSURANCE COVERAGE THROUGH NATIONAL HEALTH REFORM

With the onset of a deep economic recession in 2008 and the number of uninsured growing as jobs and health benefits were lost, both Congress and newly elected President Obama made national health reform a top domestic priority in 2009. Increasing the availability and affordability of coverage were fundamental tenets of the major proposals put forth. The basic framework is similar in some respects to that used by the state of Massachusetts when it mandated universal health insurance for all of its residents in 2006 and shared the responsibility for financing the expanded coverage across consumers, businesses, and the government.

Congress enacted historic national health insurance reform which was signed by the president on March 23, 2010. The legislation was broad in scope and addressed many health system concerns in addition to health insurance coverage. It enacted new laws for Medicare, including an expanded drug benefit and improvements for safety net services; addressed the quality of health care delivery, including better preventive care and management of chronic conditions; improved long-term care and its financing; and addressed needs for the health care workforce (see Chapter 17).

The key elements that address the rising numbers of uninsured included the following:

- An individual mandate requiring that most individuals have health insurance beginning in 2014. Exceptions to the mandate exist, but those who do not have coverage will be required to pay a penalty.
- Medicaid expanded. Medicaid will be opened to all individuals with incomes under 133% of the FPL, thereby creating a uniform minimum income eligibility threshold across all states and eliminating the current restriction that prohibits most adults without dependent children from enrolling. The costs of those newly eligible for Medicaid will initially be fully paid for by the federal government, later transferring a share of the costs back to the states. Eligibility for Medicaid and the Children's Health Insurance Program for children will continue at their current eligibility levels until 2019. Undocumented immigrants, as under current law, will not be eligible for public programs or allowed

to purchase coverage in the newly created American Health Benefit Exchanges.

- American Health Benefit Exchanges created. People with incomes above 133% of the FPL who do not have access to employer-sponsored insurance will be able to obtain coverage through these new Exchanges—new marketplaces that will provide consumers with information to help them better choose among plans. Federal premium and cost-sharing assistance (applying a sliding scale) will be available for those with incomes between 133% and 400% of the FPL. Small businesses will be allowed to purchase coverage for their employees through separate Exchanges.
- Changes in employer participation. There is no employer mandate, but businesses with more than fifty employees will be charged a fee per employee if they do not offer health benefits and if at least one of their employees receives a premium credit through an Exchange. Employers who offer health benefits but have an employee receiving insurance subsidies through an Exchange will be required to pay fees as well.
- Private insurance market changes. Private health plans will no longer be able to deny coverage for any reason, including a person's health status, and will be prohibited from charging people more based on their health status and gender. Plans will no longer be allowed to have annual and lifetime limits on coverage, nor be able to rescind coverage. Preventive services will be covered without beneficiary cost-sharing. Young dependent adults will be allowed to remain on their parents' plan to age 26. Health plan premium increases will be subject to review.

The Congressional Budget Office estimated that the number of uninsured will be reduced by 32 million by 2019, leaving only those exempted from the mandate and undocumented immigrants without insurance of any kind.

As this chapter goes to publication, the nation's economy has begun to stir, but high unemployment levels and uncertainty about economic recovery persist. Employer-sponsored insurance, the primary source of coverage for the majority of Americans, has been steadily declining over the past decade. In this recession, as in the past, state budgets are inadequate to meet the greater demand for Medicaid coverage while state tax revenues plummet. The combination of these trends greatly heightens the challenge of making health insurance more available and affordable, but also underscores the urgency for implementing national reforms.

For a list of related websites, please refer to your Evolve Resources at http://evolve.elsevier.com/Mason/policypolitics/

REFERENCES

Artiga, S. & Schwartz, K. (2009). Expanding Health Coverage for Low-Income Adults: Filling the Gaps in Medicaid Eligibility. Kaiser Commission on Medicaid and the Uninsured Report #7900.

Ayanian, J., et al. (2000). Unmet health needs of uninsured adults in the United States. *Journal of the American Medical Association, 284*(16), 2061-2069.

Baker, D., Sudano, J. J., Albert, J. M., Borawski, E. A., & Dor, A. (2001). Lack of health insurance and decline in overall health in late middle age. *New England Journal of Medicine, 345*(15), 1106-1112.

Canto, J. G., Rogers, W. J., French W. J., Gore, J. M., Chandra, N. C., & Barron, H. V. (2000). Payer status and the utilization of hospital resources in acute myocardial infarction: A report from the National Registry of Myocardial Infarction 2. *Archives of Internal Medicine, 160*(6), 817-823.

Clemans-Cope, L. & Garrett, B. (2006). Changes in employer-sponsored health insurance sponsorship, eligibility, and participation: 2001-2005. Kaiser Commission on Medicaid and the Uninsured Report #7599.

Cunningham, P., & May, J. H. (2006). A growing hole in the safety net: physician charity care declines again. Center for Studying Health Systems Change Tracking Report.

Davidoff, A. J., & Kenney, G. (2005). Uninsured Americans with chronic health conditions: Key findings from the National Health Interview Survey. Retrieved from www.urban.org/publications/411161.html.

Doyle, J. J. (2005). Health insurance, treatment, and outcomes: Using auto accidents as health shocks. *Review of Economics and Statistics, 87*(2), 256-270.

Hadley, J. (2003). Sicker and poorer—the consequences of being uninsured: A review of the research on the relationship between health insurance, medical care use, health, work, and income. *Medical Care Research and Review, 60*(2 Suppl), 3S-75S.

Hadley, J. (2007). Insurance coverage, medical care use, and short-term health changes following an unintentional injury or the onset of a chronic condition. *Journal of the American Medical Association, 97*(10), 1073-1084.

Hadley, J., Holahan, J., Coughlin, T., & Miller, D. (2008). Covering the uninsured in 2008: Current costs, sources of payment, and incremental costs. *Health Affairs, 27*(5), w399-w415.

Himmelstein, D. U., Thorne, D., Warren, E., & Woolhandler, S. (2009). Medical bankruptcy in the United States, 2007: Results of a national study. *American Journal of Medicine, 122*(8), 741-746. Retrieved from www.pnhp.org/new_bankruptcy_study/Bankruptcy-2009.pdf.

Hoffman, C., & Schwartz, K. (2008a). Eroding access among nonelderly U.S. adults with chronic conditions: Ten years of change. *Health Affairs, 27*(5), w340-w348 (published online July 22, 2008).

Hoffman, C., & Schwartz, K. (2008b). Trends in access to care among working-age adults, 1997-2006. Kaiser Commission on Medicaid and the Uninsured Report #7824.

Institute of Medicine. (2009). *America's uninsured crisis. Chapter 3: Coverage matters.* Washington, D.C.: National Academy of Sciences.

Jacobs, P., & Claxton, G. (2008). Comparing the assets of uninsured households to cost sharing under high deductible health plans, *Health Affairs, 27*(3), w214-w221 (published online April 15, 2008).

Kaiser Family Foundation's Health Tracking Poll. (2009, August). Unpublished data.

Kaiser Commission on Medicaid and the Uninsured. (2009a). The uninsured: A primer. Report #7451-05. Table 5.

Kaiser Commission on Medicaid and the Uninsured. (2009b). Unpublished analysis of 2008 National Health Interview Survey data.

Kaiser Commission on Medicaid and the Uninsured and the Urban Institute. (2009). Unpublished analysis of 2009 ASEC Supplement to the Current Population Survey.

Kaiser Family Foundation and Health Research & Educational Trust. (2009). 2009 Kaiser/HRET Employer Health Benefits Survey. Retrieved from http//ehbs.kff.org.

Marks, C., Schwartz T., & Donaldson, L. (2009). State variation and health reform: A chartbook. Kaiser Commission on Medicaid and the Uninsured Report #7942.

National Association of Community Health Centers. (2008). Health centers and Medicaid. Fact sheet, August 2008.

National Association of Public Hospitals and Health Systems. (2009, May/June). 2007 Annual survey results highlight the importance of the nation's safety net hospitals and health systems. Research Brief.

National Center for Health Statistics. (2008). Summary health statistics for the U.S. population: National Health Interview Survey, 2007. Retrieved from www.cdc.gov/nchs/data/series/sr_10/sr10_238.pdf.

NewsHour with Jim Lehrer. (2003, March). Kaiser Family Foundation National Survey on the Uninsured.

Roetzheim, R. G., Pal, N., Gonzalez, E. C., Ferrante, J. M., Van Durme, D. J., & Krischer, J. P. (2000). Effects of health insurance and race on colorectal cancer treatments and outcomes. *American Journal of Public Health*, *90*(11), 1746-1754.

Schoen, C., et al. (2008). How many are underinsured? Trends among U.S. adults, 2003 and 2007. *Health Affairs Web Exclusive*, posted June 10, 2008.

CHAPTER 22

Policy Approaches to Address Health Disparities

Lauren A. Underwood and Antonia M. Villarruel

"Inequality is as dear to the American heart as liberty itself."

—William Dean Howells

Health disparities refer to differences in the incidence, prevalence, mortality, and burden of diseases and other adverse health conditions that may exist among specific population groups (P.L. 106-525, 2000; United States Department of Health and Human Services [U.S. DHHS], 2000). Health disparities have been documented between genders, among groups with different educational levels, and among different age groups. From a policy perspective, priority population groups in the United States include racial and ethnic minorities, persons from low socioeconomic backgrounds, women, children, older adults, and those living in rural areas (AHRQ, 2009). In this chapter we will discuss policies related to racial and health disparities.

HEALTH DISPARITIES REPORTS AND POLICIES

The *Report of the Secretary's Task Force on Black and Minority Health* by the U.S. DHHS Secretary's Task Force on Black and Minority Health (1985) led to a significant policy focus on health disparities. This landmark report identified disparities seen in U.S. blacks, Hispanic, Asian/Pacific Islander, and Native American populations. For example, 80% of excess mortality experienced by minority groups is linked to causes of death including cancer, cardiovascular disease, diabetes, infant mortality, unintentional injury, and chemical dependency. Importantly, the Task Force made eight specific recommendations that have served as a blueprint for subsequent policy to address these disparities (Box 22-1). Significant policy

initiatives stemming from this report include data requirements for federal data-collection systems to collect race and ethnicity data, the requirement to include racial and ethnic minorities in federally funded research (NIH, 1994), and the establishment of the Office of Minority Health within the Office of Secretary at the U.S. DHHS (Office of Minority Health, 2009).

Since the 1985 Secretary's Report, several additional key policy initiatives and reports have had a major impact in the effort to address health disparities. Perhaps the boldest policy initiative related to health disparities occurred with the unveiling of *Healthy People 2010: Understanding and Improving Health* (U.S. DHHS, 2000), a comprehensive set of disease prevention and health promotion objectives for the nation. As one of only two overarching goals for the decade, this initiative called for the elimination of health disparities. The *Healthy People 2010* goal is significant as it directed government-sponsored initiatives to monitor and address health disparities in their programs.

Another important report addressing disparities in health care was *Unequal Treatment: Confronting Racial and Ethnic Disparities in Health Care* (Smedley et al., 2003), issued by the Institute of Medicine. A key finding from the report was that "Racial and ethnic disparities in healthcare exist and, because they are associated with worse outcomes in many cases, are unacceptable" (p. 6). Notable findings from this report document that racial and ethnic minorities received lower-quality health care within the United States, even after controlling for insurance status, income, and other access factors (Smedley et al., 2003). The report presented multilevel recommendations to address health care disparities ranging from patient-provider interventions as well as

---

BOX 22-1 Recommendations from The Report of the Secretary's Task Force on Black and Minority Health (1985)

1. Outreach Campaign—Distribute health information targeting minority populations.
2. Patient Education—Ensure that all HHS programs and materials are sensitive to minority population needs, focusing on significant causes of death and disabilities in these populations.
3. Delivery and Financing of Health Services—Develop innovative models of health care delivery and financing to facilitate access to services by minority populations.
4. Developing Strategies Outside the Federal Sector—Collaborate with stakeholder groups to increase availability of health professionals in minority communities.
5. Developing Strategies Within the Federal Sector—Pursue avenues to allow HHS to work with other agencies to increase health access in minority communities.
6. Build the Capacity of the Non-Federal Sector to Address Minority Health Problems—Assist minority communities to define local health goals and develop action plans.
7. Improving and Fully Using Available Sources of Data—Utilize data resources to increase understanding of health status and needs of minority populations.
8. Research Agenda—HHS should adopt a research agenda prioritizing minority health focusing on risk factor identification, educational interventions, and socio-cultural influences.

---

interventions addressing the health system and federal policy.

To support the federal directive to monitor progress related to the elimination of disparities in health and health care, the Agency for Healthcare Research and Quality (AHRQ) annually publishes the *National Healthcare Disparities Report* (AHRQ, 2009). This report monitors the nation's progress toward eliminating disparities in health care, which are the differences in the quality of and ability to access health care services for different populations (AHRQ, 2004). Data are presented on quality measures including effectiveness, patient safety, timeliness, efficiency, and patient centeredness, as well as components of access to health care. The corresponding database NHQR-DRNet is publicly available on the AHRQ website (*nhqrnet.ahrq.gov*) to allow direct access to the dataset from which this report is based.

In addition to federal and state governments, private foundations have also prioritized the investigation and elimination of health disparities. For example, the Kaiser Family Foundation has sponsored a number of policy reports such as *Putting Women's Health Care Disparities on the Map: Examining Racial and Ethnic Disparities at the State Level* (James et al., 2009). This document describes the persistence of disparities domestically, providing a comprehensive state-level examination of disparities across race and ethnicity for a broad range of indicators of health and well-being.

HEALTH DISPARITIES IN INFANT MORTALITY: A CONTEMPORARY EXAMPLE

The complexity and challenges associated with eliminating racial disparities in health are evident by examining disparities in infant mortality. Hispanic, American Indian/Alaska Native, and African-American groups have all historically had elevated infant mortality rates compared with both non-Hispanic whites and the national average (National Center for Health Statistics [NCHS], 2008). While there have been dramatic decreases in infant mortality rates for whites, ethnic minority groups have not experienced similar decreases. A nation's infant mortality rate is considered a significant indicator of population health, given its relationship with and sensitivity to maternal health, public health services, access to quality health care, and socioeconomic status (MacDorman & Matthews, 2008).

The causes of infant mortality and related disparities are multifaceted and result from the intersection of genetic, environmental, and behavioral factors (Behrman & Butler, 2007). There are three main conditions that contribute to infant mortality: congenital abnormalities, Sudden Infant Death Syndrome (SIDS), and conditions related to short gestation and low birth weight (MacDorman & Matthews, 2008). Preterm birth, and low birth weight factors are potentially preventable during the prenatal period (Lang & Iams, 2009; Ashton et al., 2009; Lee et al., 2009). Consequently, policy solutions and evidence-based interventions predominantly focus on addressing low birth weight, preterm birth, and SIDS. Long recognized as a problem, particularly in African-American and other racial and ethnic minority populations regardless of socioeconomic status, there have been a variety of policy solutions offered by governmental and nongovernmental organizations at all levels to address the infant mortality disparities. We describe two policy interventions: the Nurse Family Partnership and the Children's Health Insurance Plan.

NURSE FAMILY PARTNERSHIP

The Nurse Family Partnership (NFP) is an evidence based program designed to improve pregnancy outcomes, improve child health and development, and improve parental life course (Olds, 2006). The program is structured around a series of home visits by registered nurses beginning in the first two pregnancy trimesters and ending with the child's second birthday. Outcomes of the program have included fewer verified cases of child abuse and neglect, lower numbers of subsequent pregnancies, fewer abortions, longer time between the births of the first and second child, and fewer months utilizing public assistance programs including welfare and food stamps (Olds, 2006). In 2003, an economic analysis of the NFP estimated costs to be approximately $8000 for 2.5 years of service, but the return on investment, as it relates to health outcomes and cost savings, is estimated at $17,000 (Olds, 2006; Olds et al., 2007).

The combination of improved infant and child outcomes, long-term cost savings, and popularity of the NFP across municipalities has led to federal support of the NFP and similar nurse home visitation programs. The president's FY 2010 budget request contains funding to support services to approximately 50,000 families, with plans to expand the program to some 450,000 families (U.S. DHHS, 2009; Administration for Children and Families, 2009). Continued federal support of programs to improve prenatal outcomes for high-risk and low- income individuals could lead to a substantial reduction in African-American infant mortality.

CHILDREN'S HEALTH INSURANCE PROGRAM

Since its congressional authorization in 1997, states across the country have utilized the Children's Health Insurance Program (SCHIP) as a tool to expand health insurance coverage for children, including infants in their first year of life (Centers for Medicare & Medicaid Services [CMS], 2009) (see Chapter 18). SCHIP covers pregnant women and children, facilitating access to health care services, including important health teaching and screening activities that can identify and reduce risk factors for SIDS and other sequela associated with preterm birth and low birth weight. SCHIP is a Medicaid expansion designed to provide health coverage to uninsured children whose families are in income brackets above Medicaid eligibility limits (Center for Children and Families, 2009). Basic eligibility is set by the federal government through the Medicaid program, and specific program eligibility standards are established by individual states to fit their unique needs, priorities, and funding abilities (CMS, 2009).

Reauthorized by Congress in 2009, the renamed Children's Health Insurance Program (CHIP) includes a new state option to cover pregnant women through 60 days postpartum (Center for Children and Families, 2009). Under this provision, states cannot impose preexisting condition limitations or enact waiting periods before pregnant women become eligible for care. Children born to women receiving pregnancy-related health care services through this option will be automatically enrolled in CHIP until that child turns one year old (Center for Children and Families, 2009). These policy stipulations will enable states to target high-risk pregnant women and connect them with the needed basic prenatal and supplementary services including case management and home visitation programs. States have flexibility in eligibility determination, outreach strategies, and reimbursement criteria, and they have the opportunity through the CHIP program to create a multiagency (e.g., CHIP, Medicaid, WIC) infrastructure to support community efforts to reduce infant mortality (Center for Children and Families, 2009).

SUMMARY

The issue of racial and ethnic health disparities is interwoven within a domestic history of discrimination and enacted laws meant to maintain privileges. As can be seen, efforts to address health disparities include broad public health policy in addition to targeted intervention-based programs for those most affected by health disparities. Moving forward, policy will need to focus on achieving health equity, a positive way to address disparity and inequality.

Health reform and the challenges of expanding access to health insurance to millions of uninsured individuals will need to simultaneously emphasize quality of health care as a way to reduce disparities. The renewed focus on primary care, investments in health information technology, and emphasis on evidence-based practices via comparative effectiveness policies are all federal attempts to improve the quality of health care across the country. Prevention and a reinvestment in public health will also likely address health disparities issues, particularly for disparities occurring as a result of environmental exposures, geographic location, and chronic disease.

Nursing expertise will be critical to implement the needed health system reforms, and our continued professional involvement with research, advocacy, community outreach, and policy will help ensure that even underserved populations' health challenges are addressed. However, to successfully eliminate health disparities, a broad range of policy solutions must be developed. Systemic efforts to increase the level of education, ensure meaningful work opportunities, and provide safe and secure housing are important ancillary policy areas that must be addressed for the sustained elimination of health disparities.

For a list of related websites, please refer to your Evolve Resources at http://evolve.elsevier.com/Mason/policypolitics/

REFERENCES

Administration for Children and Families. (2009). FY 2010 Justification of estimates for appropriations committees: Payments to states for home visitation. Retrieved from www.nursefamilypartnership.org/resources/files/PDF/Policy/ACF_budget_home_visitation.pdf.

Agency for Healthcare Research and Quality. (2004, February). National healthcare disparities report: Summary. U.S. Department of Health and Human Services. Retrieved from www.ahrq.gov/qual/nhdr03/nhdrsum03.htm#WhatAre.

Agency for Healthcare Research and Quality. (2009, March). National healthcare disparities report 2008. AHRQ National Healthcare Disparities Reports. U.S. Department of Health and Human Services. Retrieved from www.ahrq.gov/qual/nhdr08/nhdr08.pdf.

Ashton, D. M., Lawrence, H. C., Adams, N. L., & Fleischman, A. R. (2009). Surgeon General's conference on the prevention of preterm birth. *Obstetrics & Gynecology, 113*(4), 925-930.

Behrman, R. E., & Butler A. S. (2007). *Preterm birth: Causes, consequences and prevention.* Institute of Medicine. Washington, D.C.: National Academies Press.

Center for Children and Families. (2009, March). Children's Health Insurance Program Reauthorization Act of 2009: Overview and summary. Georgetown University Health Policy Institute. Retrieved from http://ccf.georgetown.edu/index/cms-filesystem-action?file=ccf%20publications/federal%20schip%20policy/chip%20summary%2003-09.pdf.

Centers for Medicare and Medicaid Services. (2009, September 25). Overview: National CHIP policy. U.S. Department of Health and Human Services. Retrieved from www.cms.hhs.gov/NationalCHIPPolicy.

James, C. V., Salganicoff, A., Thomas, M., Ranji, U., Lillie-Blanton, M., & Wyn, R. (June 2009). Putting women's health care disparities on the map: Examining racial and ethnic disparities at the state level. Henry J. Kaiser Family Foundation. Retrieved from www.kff.org/minorityhealth/upload/7886.pdf.

Lang, C. T., & Iams, J. D. (2009). Goals and strategies for prevention of preterm birth: An obstetric perspective. *The Pediatric Clinics of North America, 56*(3), 537-563.

Lee, E., Mitchell-Herzfeld, M. A., Lowenfels, A. A., Greene, R., Dorabawila, V., & DuMont, K. A. (2009). Reducing low birth weight through home visitation: A randomized controlled trial. *American Journal of Preventive Medicine, 36*(2), 154-160.

MacDorman, M. F., & Matthews, T. J. (2008). Recent trends in infant mortality in the United States. NCHS data brief, No. 9. Hyattsville, MD: National Center for Health Statistics. Retrieved from www.cdc.gov/nchs/data/databriefs/db09.pdf.

Minority Health and Health Disparities Research and Education Act of 2000, Pub. L. No. 106-525. 114. Stat. 2495 (2000). Retrieved from U.S. Government Printing Office, Federal Digital System.

National Center for Health Statistics (NCHS). (2008). *Health, United States, 2008.* Hyattsville, MD: Centers for Disease Control and Prevention. Retrieved from http://cdc.gov/nchs/data/hus/hus08.pdf.

National Institutes of Health. (1994, March 18). NIH guidelines on the inclusion of women and minorities as subjects in clinical research. *NIH Guide, 23*(11). Retrieved from http://grants.nih.gov/grants/guide/notice-files/not94-100.html.

Office of Minority Health. (2009, January 21). About OMH—Office of Minority Health. U.S. Department of Health and Human Services. Retrieved from http://minorityhealth.hhs.gov/templates/browse.aspx?lvl=1&lvlID=7.

Olds, D. L. (2006). The nurse-family partnership: An evidence-based preventive intervention. *Infant Mental Health Journal, 27*(1), 5-25.

Olds, D. L., Sadler, L., & Kitzman, H. (2007). Programs for parents of infants and toddlers: Recent evidence from randomized trials. *Journal of Child Psychology and Psychiatry, 48*(3-4), 355-391.

Secretary's Task Force on Black and Minority Health. (1985). *Report of the Secretary's Task Force on Black and Minority Health. U.S. Department of Health and Human Services.* Washington, D.C.: U.S. Government Printing Office. Retrieved from http://minorityhealth.hhs.gov/assets/pdf/checked/1/ANDERSON.pdf.

Smedley, B., Stith, A., & Nelson, A. (2003). *Unequal treatment: Confronting racial and ethnic disparities in health care.* Washington, D.C.: The National Academies Press.

U.S. Department of Health and Human Services. (2000). *Healthy People 2010: Understanding and improving health.* (2nd ed.). Washington, D.C.: U.S. Government Printing Office.

U.S. Department of Health and Human Services. (2009, May 9). Fiscal year 2010 budget in brief. Retrieved from www.hhs.gov/asrt/ob/docbudget/2010budgetinbrief.pdf.

CHAPTER 23

The Rural Health Care Tundra

Alan Morgan

"Both the ideal and the reality of rural community are hard to define"

—M. Troughton, 1999

Rural America is a vast, sparsely populated geographic location in which approximately 62 million people currently live. As much as 75% of the nation's geography is considered as being "rural and frontier" (Gamm & Hutchinson, 2005). The obstacles that health care providers and patients face in these rural areas are vastly different than those in urban areas. Rural Americans face a unique combination of factors that create significant disparities in health care— at levels often higher than in urban areas. To understand the rural health care system, one must first understand that rural is not simply a small version of urban. Rural America has specific defining characteristics that represent a distinctive health care delivery environment.

Economic factors, cultural and social differences, educational shortcomings, lack of recognition by policymakers, and the sheer isolation of living in remote rural areas all conspire to impede rural Americans in their struggle to lead a normal, healthy life. This unique health care environment requires a specialized health care approach to delivering care. Since rural health care providers often struggle to provide care while maintaining fiscal viability, it is a fragile health care system, and much like the Arctic tundra, it can be easily damaged by unintended state and/or federal health care policy actions.

This chapter looks at what makes rural different and discusses policy options to address these issues, which include the following three key characteristics of rural health:

- High health disparities within the patient population
- Geographic challenges that work to impede health
- Lack of health care resources

WHAT MAKES RURAL DIFFERENT?

Health care disparities in rural areas are higher than urban or suburban locations. This is a unique aspect that is a result of many factors, including education and poverty. Rural populations on average have relatively more elderly and children; unemployment and underemployment; and poor, uninsured and underinsured residents.

The fact that our private sector health insurance system is an employer-based system creates a financial barrier for many rural residents who do not access insurance through their employer. This is because many rural residents are either self-employed, work for small businesses that do not provide health insurance, or are unemployed. Rural people are less likely to have private health coverage, and the rural poor are less likely to be covered by Medicaid benefits than their urban counterparts. In addition, rural adults are more likely to be uninsured than urban adults, with un-insurance rates among rural Hispanic adults at more than 50%. Rural adults are more likely than urban adults to report having deferred care because of cost. On average, per capita income is $7000 lower in rural than in urban areas, and rural Americans are more likely to live below the poverty level (Gamm & Hutchinson, 2005).

The challenge of health care disparities among rural residents is significant, and it makes access to health care a paramount importance to rural communities. Included within the disparities facing rural residents are the following:

- Rural adults are more likely to be obese than urban adults, with particularly high rates of obesity among rural African Americans (Gamm & Hutchinson, 2005).
- Rural residents are less likely to receive an annual dental exam.

- Rural women are less likely than urban women to be in compliance with mammogram screening guidelines.
- Rural adults are more likely to have diabetes than urban adults.
- The death rate for people between the ages of 1 and 24 years old is 25% higher in rural areas than in urban areas (Bennett et al., 2008).

Rural residents have a significantly greater distance to travel to access health care on average than their urban counterparts. Of similar concern is the lack of public transportation within small towns and communities. This has a direct impact on patient care, follow-up care, and long-term outcomes. While the traditional goal of pre-hospital emergency medical services (EMS) has been to provide patients with immediate transportation to the nearest hospital, this role has greatly expanded in rural communities to serve in multiple patient transport roles. Very few small communities have paid EMS services. As of 2005, volunteer providers respond to medical emergencies in over 50% of the country (Gamm & Hutchinson, 2005).

Rural health care systems, with small numbers of providers and sparse resources, are tenuously balanced to meet the needs of residents while providing adequate income and quality of life to health care providers. Specialty care is delivered differently in rural areas, with a greater reliance on non-traditional staffing arrangements. The national shortage of nurses within our health care system has been well documented. In rural areas, nursing shortages are exacerbated by the rural employers' inability to compete with urban employers in terms of wages, start-up bonuses, and benefits that are offered (Gamm & Hutchinson, 2005).

DEFINING RURAL

The need to define "what is rural," remains a deceptively complex policy issue, and there is no single universally accepted definition. For the purposes of federal programs that target public resources toward rural communities, there are more than 15 program-specific rural designations that are currently used within various programs and over 70 federal definitions. The definition of *rural* remains a key issue of rural health care policy. The most widely used definitions of rural are based on either the federal Office of

Management and Budget (OMB) characterization of counties or the Census Bureau Urbanized Area categorization of census blocks and block groups.

The Census Bureau classifies rural as being all territory, population, and housing units located in non-urbanized areas and non-urban clusters. For the purposes of the Census Bureau, urbanized areas include populations of at least 50,000. Urban clusters include populations between 2500 and 50,000. The core areas of both urbanized areas and urban clusters are defined based on population density of 1000 per square mile (and then areas adjacent to them are added that have at least 500 persons per square mile).

The Office of Management and Budget classifies nonmetropolitan or rural counties as those counties outside the boundaries of metropolitan areas (50,000 or more). A metropolitan area must contain one or more central counties with urbanized areas. These nonmetropolitan counties are subdivided into two types; micropolitan areas and non-core counties. Micropolitan areas are urban clusters of at least 10,000 but fewer than 50,000.

By successfully defining rural, Medicare and Medicaid payment methodologies can be adjusted for the purposes of ensuring access to care in these geographic locations. Many rural communities have adverse economic conditions that limit a local health care provider's ability to furnish a broad array of necessary services. Therefore, payment policy interventions are often necessary to preserve rural patients' access to high-quality care.

Delivering care in rural areas is often represented by low volumes of patients, and they are often older and have significant underlying health care problems. This situation is further complicated by the lack of volume purchasing power, greater transportation costs, and higher health care needs in many situations. Efforts to define rural are based on efforts to specifically address this rural economic environment.

The National Rural Health Association (NRHA), a non-profit membership association, strongly recommends that definitions of rural be specific to the programmatic purpose in which they are used. According to the NRHA, these programs targeting rural communities, rural providers, and rural residents do so for particular reasons, and those reasons should be the guide for selecting the criteria for a programmatic designation. This position ensures that any rural designation is appropriate for a specific situation, and that it will best fit specific programs (National Rural Health Association [NRHA], 2005b).

Despite ongoing federal and state efforts to adequately address rural health, Medicare payments to rural hospitals and physicians remain less than those to their urban counterparts for equivalent services (Gamm & Hutchinson, 2005). The federal government has often responded to these rural financial realities by modifying the Medicare payment system by the means of rural payment "add-ons," or other payment enhancement methodologies that provide additional payment consideration for providers practicing in rural areas.

In addition, multiple federal grant programs have been established to target rural health. These grant programs are designed to assist the resource challenges faced by rural health care providers. Most often these grant programs target issues of workforce, infrastructure investment, and health care outreach.

RURAL POLICY, RURAL POLITICS

The political context for rural health policy is an ever-evolving process as politicians consider the political weight of a rural-voting block. Federal policymakers recognized the political and policy need for targeted rural legislation to address rural health care in the late 1990s. Since the Balanced Budget Act of 1997, federal legislation has not only recognized the importance of sustaining the rural health care safety net, but also utilizing its unique characteristics as a "learning lab" for successful systems of care.

Targeted rural Medicare provisions included within the Balanced Budget Act of 1997, and again within the Medicare Modernization Act of 2003, provided members of Congress the ability to tout a successful rural policy agenda to their constituents. Among these provisions was the establishment of new payment demonstration programs for rural hospitals and rural clinics, as well as new payment enhancements for rural home health care and increased payments for clinicians practicing in rural underserved areas.

Equally important in these payment reforms was the recognition from policymakers that rural health care systems are fragile, as they operate on slim margins, and that they possess limited resources. A loss of health care access in rural communities can have a significant adverse impact on the sustainability of the rural community itself.

Rural health care providers are usually part of small health systems, where response to health problems is easier to accomplish. This allows rural health to innovate and evolve easily, and this ability provides policymakers with opportunities to launch demonstration projects at a lower cost, with the potential for a meaningful and sustainable return on investment (Institute of Medicine [IOM], 2006).

This is the contradiction about rural health. It is a geographically defined area where the system is fragile, yet capable of innovation and adaptation. This makes it unique among our nation's health delivery settings. Inherent within this contradiction is why it is so appealing to many health care professionals to choose to practice in a rural setting.

THE OPPORTUNITIES AND CHALLENGES OF RURAL HEALTH

Ultimately, a key issue for rural health care policy and practice is the issue of access to care. With limited resources, the ongoing policy debate continues to center on the question of the appropriate level of care, provided in a timely manner, with the appropriate providers. This is particularly true for recruiting and retaining nurses. Nurses in rural areas are expected to be familiar with performing the expert generalist role. They must understand how to interface hospital services with community-based services and programs and be comfortable with rural social structures that can influence practice patterns. Rural social structures can include threats to confidentiality, problems associated with traditional gender roles, and, of course, geographic and professional isolation (Bushy, 2004).

However, the rural practice experience can be successful and rewarding for rural nurses, through increased professional experience and autonomy, quality of life outside the clinical setting, and the potential for federal support through grants that promote innovative rural nursing models of care. The small organizational structures in rural areas create an environment for creative solutions to address these challenges. To realize the opportunity, proper access to tools and information must be readily available.

Access to current and complete information to perform one's clinical responsibilities is a serious issue for rural professions. Because of rising printing costs, libraries of all types are providing fewer resources, and travel costs to attend continuing education courses are significant challenges. On-line courses are an emerging solution to this issue, but this remains a concern for recruitment and retention of health care providers.

Because of the limited number of physicians and the need for primary care practitioners, rural communities make widespread use of physician assistants (PAs) and advanced practice nurses (APRNs). These practitioners are well-qualified to improve access in rural locations.

From a national perspective, providing federally funded financial incentives for new graduates to practice in rural settings is a successful policy response to improve rural distribution of health care personnel. Loan forgiveness programs and the National Health Service Corps (NHSC) are prime examples of this policy effort. The NHSC offers programs to communities or specific employers to solicit community support for recruiting and retaining rural clinicians. Federal funding provides partial loan forgiveness, while the community provides partial financial support for the clinician's services for a specified period of time.

Health care providers most likely to serve in rural areas come from rural areas. Many of the 62 million Americans that choose to live and work in rural America do so for a cleaner environment, low crime rates, and a healthy environment to raise families. Health care students and professionals who work and live in rural communities feel appreciated by the communities in which they serve, and cite the benefit of knowing that they do make a difference in their rural community (NRHA, 2005a).

Rural communities provide wonderful opportunities as well as significant challenges to providing health care that best meets the needs of its people. A thorough understanding of their uniqueness can enhance the quality of life for both providers and recipients of care. The federal government's role in supporting innovative systems of care is critical.

For a list of related websites, please refer to your Evolve Resources at http://evolve.elsevier.com/Mason/policypolitics/

REFERENCES

Bennett, K., Olatosi, B., & Probst, J. C. (2008). *Health disparities: A rural-urban chartbook*. South Carolina Rural Health Research Center, 3. Retrieved from http://rhr.sph.sc.edu/report/SCRHRC_RuralUrbanChartbook_Exec_Sum.pdf.

Bushy, A. (2004). *Rural nursing: Practice and issues*. American Nurses Association Continuing Education module. American Nurses Association, 51.

Gamm, L. D., & Hutchinson, L. L. (Eds.) (2005). Healthy People 2010: A companion document for rural areas, Rural Healthy People 2010, Vol. 3. College Station, Texas: Health, Southwest Rural Health Research Center. Retrieved from www.srph.tamhsc.edu/centers/rhp2010/Volume_3/Vol3rhp2010.pdf.

Institute of Medicine. (2006). *Quality through collaboration: The future of rural health*. Washington, D.C.: Institute of Medicine.

National Rural Health Association. (2005a). Recruitment and retention of a quality health workforce in rural areas. Retrieved from www.ruralhealthweb.org/go/left/policy-and-advocacy/policy-documents-and-statements/issue-papers-and-policy-briefs.

National Rural Health Association. (2005b). Definition of rural. Retrieved from www.ruralhealthweb.org/go/left/about-rural-health/how-is-rural-defined.

CHAPTER 24

Long-Term Care Policy Issues

Charlene Harrington

"He who wants to warm himself in old age must build a fireplace in his youth."

—German proverb

The population of the United States is aging with the number of adults aged 65 and older almost doubling (from 37 million to over 70 million between 2005 and 2030) from 12% to almost 20% of the population by 2030 (Institute of Medicine [IOM], 2008). With the aging of the population, the demand for long-term care (LTC) and the need for nurses and other personnel to provide services is growing rapidly. The IOM predicts a major shortage of health workers with geriatric training to address the growing needs of the aging population. With total LTC expenditures of $190 billion in 2007 (Hartman et al., 2009), LTC is a critical sector (9% of total health spending), but one that receives little attention from the nursing profession.

This chapter focuses on some of the policy and political issues facing nursing in LTC. First, it reviews the problems with the quality of nursing home care, the poor enforcement of federal quality regulations, and a lack of ownership transparency (intelligibility). Second, it examines nursing home staffing and reimbursement policies. Third, it discusses the need for expanding home and community-based service (HCBS) programs. Finally, nurses are urged to become advocates for older and disabled people who need LTC services.

POOR QUALITY OF CARE AND WEAK REGULATORY ENFORCEMENT

Poor nursing home quality has been documented since the early 1970s and culminated in passage of the Omnibus Budget Reconciliation Act (OBRA) of 1987

to reform nursing home regulation (IOM, 2001). Although it was expected that OBRA 1987 would improve the survey and enforcement system and ultimately improve quality, these expectations have yet to be realized. A number of studies and reports have described the poor quality of some nursing homes (IOM, 1996, 2001, 2003). In 2008, over 90% of nursing homes received about 150,000 deficiencies for failure to meet federal regulations, for a wide range of violations of quality standards that result in unnecessary resident weight loss, pressure ulcers, accidents, infections, decline in physical functioning, and many other problems (Harrington et al., 2009). Almost 65,000 formal complaints were made to state regulatory agencies about poor nursing home quality, and 26% of nursing homes received deficiencies for causing harm or jeopardy to nursing home residents in the U.S. in 2008. Many studies during the past decade have documented the serious quality problems related to ongoing problems with the federal and state survey and enforcement system, including the complaint investigation process (U.S. General Accounting Office [U.S. GAO], 1999a, 1999b, 2002; 2003; U.S. Government Accountability Office [GAO], 2007, 2008).

State surveyors are often unable to detect serious problems with quality of care and allow most facilities to correct deficiencies without penalties (U.S. GAO, 2002; GAO, 2008). Some state survey agencies downgrade the scope and severity of deficiencies, and many states do not refer cases for intermediate sanctions (U.S. GAO, 2003; GAO, 2008). State surveys are problematic for reasons including the continued predictability of standard surveys and the inadequacy and lack of timeliness of consumer complaint investigations (U.S. GAO, 2003; GAO, 2008). Problems with poor state investigation and documentation of deficiencies and large numbers of inexperienced state surveyors in some states also occur, and federal oversight of state activities continues to be inadequate.

When violations are detected, few facilities have follow-up enforcement actions or sanctions taken against them (Harrington et al., 2004; Harrington, Tsoukalas, et al., 2008). The continued widespread variation in the number and type of deficiencies issued by states shows that states are not using the regulatory process consistently and are not following federal guidelines (U.S. GAO, 2003). Some state officials admit they are unable or are unwilling to comply with federal survey and enforcement requirements (Harrington et al., 2004). State enforcement problems are related in part to inadequate federal and state resources for regulatory activities, which have declined by 9% between 2002 and 2007 when adjusted for inflation (Harrington et al., 2004; GAO, 2009). U.S. Senate committees have held many hearings about nursing home survey problems and have repeatedly urged the Centers for Medicare and Medicaid (CMS) to improve the survey and enforcement process (U.S. GAO, 1999a, 1999b, 2002, 2003; GAO, 2007, 2008).

The federal-state nursing survey and certification process give the appearance that the government is doing something about the quality of care problems, but in reality the process does little to change or improve care. To ensure the safety of residents, strong improvement and increased funding for the survey and certification program are needed, and poor performing facilities should be terminated from Medicare and Medicaid.

INADEQUATE NURSING HOME STAFFING LEVELS

Low nurse staffing levels are the single most important contributor to poor quality of nursing home care in the U.S. Over the past 25 years, numerous studies have documented the important relationship between nurse staffing levels and the outcomes of care (IOM, 1996, 2001, 2003; Harrington, Zimmerman, et al., 2000). The benefits of higher staffing levels, especially RN staffing, can include lower mortality rates; improved physical functioning; fewer pressure ulcers, catheterized residents, and urinary tract infections; lower hospitalization rates; and less antibiotic use, weight loss, and dehydration (IOM, 1996, 2001, 2003). Three separate IOM reports have recommended increased nurse staffing in nursing homes, particularly RN staffing.

The average U.S. nursing home provides a total of 3.7 hours per resident day (hprd) of total RN and Director of Nursing, licensed vocational or practical nurse (LVN/LPN), and nursing assistant (NA) time (Harrington et al., 2009). Of the total time, most (62% or 2.3 hours) is provided by NAs, who have an average of 11 residents for whom to provide care with only 2 weeks of training. RNs provide only 36 minutes (0.6 hour) of time per patient day and must care for about 34 to 40 residents, although nurses usually have many more residents on nights, weekends, and holidays (Harrington et al., 2009). The most disturbing finding is that average RN staffing hours in nursing homes has declined by 25% since 2000, with RNs having been replaced by NAs (Harrington et al., 2009). This has reduced the quality of care at a time when nurse staffing levels are already inadequate to protect the health and safety of residents (CMS, 2001).

One study found widespread quality problems in most nursing homes: inadequate assistance with eating (only 4 to 7 minutes of assistance); verbal interactions during mealtime only 28% of the time; false charting (inaccurate documentation of feeding assistance, toileting, and repositioning); toileting assistance only 1.8 times on average in 12 hours; residents not turned every 2 to 3 hours; over one half of residents left in bed most of the day; walking assistance only one time a day on average; and widespread untreated pain and untreated depression (Schnelle et al., 2004). Comparing the results of the staffing study findings with studies of eight separate quality indicators (weight loss, bedfast condition, physical restraints, pressure ulcers, incontinence, loss of physical activity, pain, and depression), Schnelle and colleagues (2004) concluded that staffing levels were a better predictor of high-quality care processes than the eight quality indicators that were examined.

To ensure safe care, minimum staffing thresholds have been identified and need to be established in regulations. Schnelle and colleagues (2004) studied differences in the quality of care processes among selected California nursing homes with different staffing levels. They found that nursing homes in the top 10th percentile on staffing (4.1 hprd or higher) performed significantly better on 13 of 16 care processes implemented by NAs, compared with homes with lower staffing. Residents in the highest-staffed homes were significantly more likely to be out of bed and engaged in activities during the day and receive more feeding assistance and incontinence care.

A Centers for Medicare and Medicaid Services (CMS) (2001) report found that staffing levels for long-stay residents that are below 4.1 hprd result in harm or jeopardy for residents (if below 1.3 hprd for licensed nurses and 2.8 hprd of NA time). NA time should range from 2.8 to 3.2 hprd, depending on the care residents need, just to carry out basic care activities (CMS, 2001). This amounts to 1 NA per 7 or 8 residents on the day and evening shifts and 1 NA per 12 residents at night. When actual staffing levels were compared with the target goals recommended by the CMS report (2001), 97% of all facilities were found to be operating below the desired level in 2001. The recommended nurse staffing level in the CMS (2001) report was similar to the 4.5 hprd level recommended by experts (Harrington, Kovner, et al. 2000).

Unfortunately, CMS has not agreed to establish minimum federal staffing standards that would ensure that nursing facilities meet the 4.1 hprd, mostly because the potential costs were estimated to be at least $7 billion in 2000 (CMS, 2001). Most nursing homes are for-profit entities and are unlikely to voluntarily meet a reasonable level of staffing with regulatory requirements. If staffing levels are to improve, minimum federal staffing standards are needed, along with additional government funding to pay for the staffing. Some states have begun to raise their minimum staffing levels since 1999. California (3.2 hprd) and Delaware (3.29 hprd) have established high standards for direct care, and Florida established a 3.9 hprd total minimum standard (Harrington, 2008). These standards are improvements but are still well below the 4.1 hprd level recommended by the CMS 2001 report. Efforts to increase the minimum staffing standards that take into account resident acuity (case mix) should continue to have the highest priority at the state and federal levels.

NURSING FACILITY REIMBURSEMENT REFORM

Nursing home reimbursement methods and per diem reimbursement rates influence the cost of providing care. In 2007, Medicaid paid for 44% of the nation's total $131 billion nursing home expenditures; Medicare paid for 18%; consumers paid for 27%; and private insurance and other payers paid for 11%. Overall, the federal and state government paid for 62% of nursing home expenses (Hartman et al., 2009).

State Medicaid reimbursement policies have focused primarily on cost containment at the expense of quality and have established very low payment rates. The majority of states have adopted Medicaid prospective payment systems (PPSs) for nursing homes that set rates in advance of payments, which are successful in controlling reimbursement growth rates, but facilities tend to respond by cutting the staffing and quality levels (Grabowski et al., 2004).

To make matters worse, Congress passed Medicare PPS reimbursement for implementation starting in 1998 to reduce overall payment rates to skilled nursing homes (Medicare Payment Advisory Commission [MedPAC], 2009). Under PPS, Medicare rates are based in part on the resident case mix (acuity) in each facility to take into account the amount of staffing and therapy services that residents require. Skilled nursing homes, however, do not need to demonstrate that the amount of staff and therapy time actually provided is related to the payments allocated under the PPS rates.

As a result of Medicare PPSs, nursing home professional staffing decreased and regulatory deficiencies increased, showing the negative effect of Medicare PPSs (Konetzka et al., 2004). As noted previously, the level of RN staffing in U.S. nursing homes has declined by 25% since 2000 (Harrington et al., 2009). The average hours for licensed practical or vocational nurses held steady during the period, whereas the hours for NAs increased to replace the lost RN hours.

One policy option is to revise the Medicaid and Medicare PPS formulas to specify the minimum proportion of the payments that must be used for nurse staffing and therapy services. If the minimum amount of payments for nursing and therapy services were regulated, nursing homes would be prevented from cutting nurse staffing and using the funds for profit-making.

Despite the Medicare PPS rate cuts, excess profits have grown because Medicare does not limit the profit margins of nursing homes. A recent study showed that Medicare skilled nursing profit margins have exceeded 10% for the past 7 years and were 17.5% for for-profit facilities in 2007 (MedPAC,

2009). The median total margins for all payers were less (primarily because of low Medicaid payment rates). Facilities with very high profits appear to be taking profits at the expense of quality. Nursing homes with net income profit margins greater than 9% were found to have higher deficiencies and poorer quality of care, apparently because they were taking excess profits (O'Neill, et al., 2003). Strict limits on administrative costs and profit margins under Medicare and Medicaid PPS could be instituted to reduce the excess profit-taking by nursing homes.

Poor quality of care in nursing homes has been associated with low wages and benefits and high employee turnover rates (Harrington & Swan, 2003). Nursing home wages and benefits are substantially lower than those of comparable hospital workers (and lower than those in many jobs in the fast food industry and other unskilled jobs) and are generally well below the level of a living wage (CMS, 2001; Kaye et al., 2006). A CMS study (2001) found that NA wages and benefits need to be raised by 17% to 22% in order to retain employees and stabilize the workforce in long-stay facilities. Congress and CMS should ensure that state Medicaid rates include adequate amounts for nursing wages and benefits.

CORPORATE OWNERSHIP TRANSPARENCY

For-profit companies have owned the majority of the nation's nursing homes for many years and operate 66% of facilities compared to non-profit (28%) and government-owned facilities (6%) in 2007 (Harrington et al., 2009). Many studies have shown that for-profit nursing homes operate with lower costs and staffing, compared to non-profit facilities, which provide higher staffing and higher-quality care, and have more trustworthy governance (Harrington et al., 2001; Harrington, Zimmerman, et al., 2000; O'Neill et al., 2003; Schlesinger & Gray, 2005).

For-profit corporate chains emerged as a dominant organizational form in the nursing home field during the 1990s, promoted with the idea that they would be more efficient and have access to capital through the stock market. The proportion of chain-owned facilities increased from 39% in the 1990s to 52.5% of all nursing homes in 2008 (Harrington et al., 2009). The largest nursing home chains have been publicly-traded companies with billions in revenues. Research shows that shareholder value is pursued by such companies by using three interlinked strategies at the expense of quality: (1) debt-financed mergers, which place a burden on facilities to pay off their debts; (2) labor cost constraints including low nurse staffing levels and low wages/benefits to increase net income; and (3) noncompliance with regulatory requirements where regulatory sanctions are considered to be a normal cost of business (Kitchener et al., 2008). Many large nursing home chains own a number of related companies including residential care/assisted living facilities, home health agencies, hospices, pharmacies, staffing organizations, and other related companies. These related companies refer patients to each other and use their corporate interrelationships to maximum net revenues.

By 2007, private equity companies had purchased six of the largest chains with about 9% of nursing home beds; these companies have few reporting requirements (Duhigg, 2007). Shielded by private equity companies, the ownership of nursing homes has become so complex that it is increasingly difficult to identify the owners of nursing homes. Many large chains have multiple investors, holding companies, and multiple levels of companies involved, where property companies are separated from the management of facilities, largely designed to avoid litigation. The lack of transparency in the ownership responsibilities makes regulation and oversight by state survey and certification agencies problematic.

The new health care reform law begins to address these concerns. Nursing facilities receiving Medicare and Medicaid funding will have to disclose information regarding ownership, accountability requirements, and expenditures. This information must be made available to the public on the Medicare nursing home compare website (Kaiser Family Foundation, 2010). This provision was sponsored by the National Citizens Coalition for Nursing Home Reform (NCCNHR) and other advocacy organizations.

HOME AND COMMUNITY-BASED SERVICES

LTC services that are needed for long periods (more than 90 days) are focused on providing assistance with limitations in activities of daily living and supporting those with cognitive limitations and mental illness. About 13 million individuals (over half under age 65) living in the community in the U.S. received an average of 31.4 hours of personal assistance per week in 1995 (LaPlante et al., 2002). More recent data show that about 11 million living in the community receive assistance with activities of daily living and 92% of those individuals received informal help from family and friends, and only 13% received paid help (Kaye, Harrington et al., 2009).

The cost of nursing home care was almost six times as much as home- and community-based services (Kaye, Harrington, et al., 2009). One reason for the high institutional spending is the oversupply of institutional LTC beds and the undersupply of HCBS. Although the number of nursing home beds grew and the aged population increased over the past decade, it is surprising to note that the average certified nursing facility occupancy rates in states declined from 90% in 1995 to only 85% in 2008, creating an excess supply of nursing home beds in many states (Harrington et al., 2009). The reductions in nursing home facility occupancy rates are probably related to the growth in residential care and assisted living facilities as substitutes and to the rapid growth of HCBS.

There are increased pressures to expand HCBS, especially in the Medicaid program. The public increasingly reports a preference for LTC provided at home over services in institutions, and this is encouraged by reports of serious nursing home quality problems (Kitchener et al., 2005). In addition, the 1990 Americans with Disabilities Act (ADA) and the subsequent legal judgment in the 1999 Olmstead Supreme Court decision require that states must not discriminate against persons with disabilities by refusing to provide community services when these are available and appropriate.

In response to the increased demand, Medicaid HCBS programs increased by 46% and expenditures increased by 104% from 1999 to 2005 (Ng et al., 2008). Combined Medicaid home health and personal care services, and home- and community-based waiver programs served 2.8 million participants, and expenditures were $35 billion in 2005 (Ng et al., 2008).

The Affordable Care Act (ACA) of 2010 includes some important provisions regarding long-term care, specifically for HCBS. First, it establishes a national, voluntary self-funded insurance program for purchasing community living assistance services and supports (CLASS program), an initiative that was sponsored by Senator Edward Kennedy. The program is established through the workplace, and premiums would be paid through payroll reductions on a voluntary basis. After paying into the system for five years, individuals with functional limitations could receive a cash benefit of not less than an average of $50 per day to purchase the non-medical services and supports necessary to maintain community residence. The program becomes effective January 1, 2011 (Kaiser Family Foundation, 2010).

Second, the law extends the Medicaid Money Follows the Person Rebalancing Demonstration program through September 2016 and allocates $10 million per year for 5 years to continue the Aging and Disability Resource Center initiatives. In addition, it gives states new options for offering home- and community-based services through a Medicaid state plan rather than through a waiver. The program allows states to provide Medicaid coverage for individuals with incomes up to 300% of the Supplemental Security Income payment level to receive home- and community-based services after October 1, 2010 (Kaiser Family Foundation, 2010).

Third, it establishes the Community First Choice Option in Medicaid to provide community-based attendant supports and services to individuals with disabilities who require an institutional level of care. This provision would offer states an enhanced federal matching rate of 6 percentage points more than their current federal funds. In addition, it creates the State Balancing Incentive Program to provide enhanced federal matching payments to eligible states to increase the proportion of non-institutionally–based long-term care services for five years starting in October 2011 (Kaiser Family Foundation, 2010). These provisions to expand home- and community-based services under Medicaid were sponsored by ADAPT, an advocacy organization for individuals with disabilities, and a coalition of consumer advocacy groups.

But there is strong evidence that the current supply of HCBS is inadequate to meet current and future need. State Medicaid program directors report that many disabled groups are not served by existing HCBS programs and that state programs lack adequate funding and have waiting lists (Ng et al., 2008). In 2007, only 30 states had Medicaid personal care attendant programs, and many states have limited services under their HCBS waiver programs. The waiting lists for HCBS have increased from 192,447 reported in 2002 to 331,689 in 2007, with waiting periods of 9 to 26 months to access services (Ng et al., 2008).

Some states have rapidly expanded their HCBS programs, but others lag behind, relying heavily on institutional services. In spite of the steady growth in HCBS spending, the Medicaid program reported spending $58.99 billion (58.5% of total LTC) on institutional LTC services and $41.8 billion (41.5% of total LTC) on HCBS services in 2007 (Burwell et al., 2008). Medicaid HCBS programs urgently need more funding to expand access to care at home and to prevent institutionalization.

The main opposition to expanding HCBS is the potential costs if additional Medicaid participants request new LTC services. One study showed that states offering extensive HCBS had spending growth comparable to states with low HCBS spending (Kaye, LaPlante et al., 2009). States with well-established HCBS programs had much less overall LTC spending growth compared with those with low HCBS spending because these states were able to reduce institutional spending. There appeared to be a lag of several years before institutional spending declined. In contrast, states with low levels of HCBS expenditures had an increase in overall costs, as their institutional costs increased. Thus, states that expanded their HCBS programs have not had increased costs or have had a reduction in their total LTC costs over time.

PUBLIC FINANCING OF LONG-TERM CARE

As of 2010, the only segment of the U.S. population whose cost of LTC is covered consists of individuals who live below the poverty threshold and are enrolled in Medicaid. Except for short-term postacute care, the rest of the population must either pay for care out of pocket or resort to privately-purchased LTC insurance. The financially crippling cost of LTC (as much as $90,000 per year) is one of the great fears confronting persons who are otherwise self-supporting, and few persons have either the means or motivation to insure themselves privately. Only about 7 million private LTC policies were in force covering 3% of the population aged 20 and older in 2005 (Feder, et al., 2007). Thus, this does not appear to be a viable financing mechanism for the future (Wiener, 2009).

If individuals "spend down" to the poverty threshold, they can become Medicaid-eligible, making LTC a means-tested program. The spend-down requirements constitute a hardship to the patient, a social stigma, and dependence on public assistance that would be unnecessary if the entire population were insured.

A mandatory social insurance program for LTC offers distinct advantages over the current U.S. means-tested system. If everyone paid into the system, individuals would have access to coverage when they are chronically ill or disabled without the humiliation of having to become poor to receive services. By expanding the Medicare program to include LTC, the payment of LTC contributions early in a worker's life could "prefund" at relatively affordable LTC services that generally are required late in life. Thus, the financial risk could be spread across the entire population so that individual premium costs or taxes would be relatively manageable, in comparison with the costs of insurance purchased when individuals are older and at high risk of needing LTC. Countries in Scandinavia, Germany, and Japan have adopted mandatory public long-term insurance systems that can serve as models for the U.S. These countries generally provide protection and coverage for persons who need LTC (Wiener, 2009). The area of greatest concern for any type of new public LTC program is cost. The nation should focus on the public financing of LTC insurance that would ensure that all citizens have adequate, high-quality LTC when they need such services. The CLASS provision of the ACA may have limited success because it is voluntary.

SUMMARY

These policy changes for LTC that are embedded in PPACA would not have happened without major grassroots advocacy activities and a coalition of organizations supporting reforms for individuals with disabilities and those who are aged over a long period of time. This advocacy work did make a difference. Nurses and nursing organizations need to join forces with consumer groups to accomplish large-scale policy changes. These new long-term care reforms are major steps forward to the eventual goal of obtaining a comprehensive mandatory public long-term care insurance system for everyone in the U.S. who needs long-term care and supports.

But more needs to be done. We need a vision for advocacy in LTC that is multidimensional and long-range. Political efforts are needed at the local, state, and national levels. Community mobilization, public education, legislative reform, and legal actions are all needed to bring about policy changes to ensure access to high-quality LTC services. Consumer advocates and organizations, such as the National Citizens Coalition for Nursing Home Reform, ADAPT for disability rights, and the AARP, have taken a lead in reform efforts, but they need help to make progress. Nurses should join these organizations to work closely with consumer advocates.

For a list of related websites, please refer to your Evolve Resources at http://evolve.elsevier.com/Mason/policypolitics/

REFERENCES

Burwell, B., Sredl, K., & Eiken, S. (2008). *Medicaid LTc expenditures in FY 2007.* Thomson Medstat, September.

Centers for Medicare & Medicaid Services (CMS) (2001). *Appropriateness of minimum nurse staffing ratios in nursing homes.* Report to Congress: Phase II Final. Volumes I to III. Baltimore: CMS. (prepared by Abt Associates).

Duhigg, C. (2007). At many homes, more profit and less nursing. *New York Times, September 23,* A1-A20, A21.

Feder, J., Komisar, H. L., & Friedland, R. B. (2007). *Long-term care financing: Policy options for the future.* Washington, D.C.: Georgetown University. Retrieved from http://ltc.georgetown.edu/forum/ltcfinalpaper061107.pdf.

Grabowski, D. C., Angelelli, J. J., & Mor, V., 2004. Medicaid payment and risk-adjusted nursing home quality measures. *Health Affairs, 23*(5), 243-252.

Harrington, C. (2008). *Nursing home staffing standards in state statutes and regulations.* San Francisco, CA: University of California. Retrieved from www.pascenter.org/documents/Staffing_regulations_1_08.pdf.

Harrington, C., Carrillo, H., & Woleslagle Blank, B. (2009). *Nursing facilities, staffing, residents, and facility deficiencies, 2003-08.* San Francisco: University of California. Retrieved from www.pascenter.org/nursing_homes/nursing_trends_2008.php.

Harrington, C., Kovner, C., Mezey, M., Kayser-Jones, J., Burger, S., Mohler, M., et al. (2000). Experts recommend minimum nurse staffing standards for nursing facilities in the United States. *Gerontologist, 40*(1), 5-16.

Harrington, C., Mullan, J., & Carrillo, H. (2004). State nursing home enforcement systems. *Journal of Health Politics, Policy and Law, 29*(1), 43-73.

Harrington, C. & Swan, J. H. (2003). Nurse home staffing, turnover, and casemix. *Medical Care Research and Review, 60*(2), 366-392.

Harrington, C., Tsoukalas, T., Rudder, C., Mollot, R. J., & Carrillo, H. (2008). Study of federal and state civil money penalties and fines. *The Gerontologist, 48*(5), 679-691.

Harrington, C., Woolhandler, S., Mullan, J., Carrillo, H., & Himmelstein, D. (2001). Does investor-ownership of nursing homes compromise the quality of care? *American Journal of Public Health, 91*(9), 1452-1455.

Harrington, C., Zimmerman, D., Karon, S. L., Robinson, J., & Beutel, P. (2000). Nursing home staffing and its relationship to deficiencies. *The Journals of Gerontology. Series B, Psychological Sciences and Social Sciences, 55*(5), S278-S287.

Hartman, M., Martin, A., McDonnell, P., Catlin, A., and the National Health Expenditure Accounts Team. (2009). National health spending in 2007: Slower drug spending contributes to lowest rate of overall growth since 1998. *Health Affairs, 28*(1), 246-261.

Institute of Medicine (IOM), Committee on Improving Quality in Long-Term Care, Division of Health Care Services. In G. S., Wunderlich, & P., Kohler, (Eds.). (2001). *Improving the quality of long-term care.* Washington, D.C.: National Academies Press.

Institute of Medicine (IOM), Committee on the Adequacy of Nurse Staffing in Hospitals and Nursing Homes. In G. S., Wunderlich, F. A., Sloan, & C. K., Davis, (Eds.) (1996). *Nursing staff in hospitals and nursing homes: Is it adequate?* Washington, D.C.: National Academies Press.

Institute of Medicine (IOM), Committee on the Future Health Care Workforce for Older Americans. (2008). *Retooling for an aging America: Building the health care workforce.* Washington, D.C.: National Academy of Science Press.

Institute of Medicine (IOM), Committee on the Work Environment for Nurses and Patient Safety. (2003). In Page, A. (Ed.), *Keeping patients safe.* Washington, D.C.: National Academies Press.

Kaiser Family Foundation. (2010, March 26). Focus on health: Summary of new health reform law. Washington, D.C. Retrieved from www.kff.org/healthreform/upload/finalhcr.pdf.

Kaye, H. S., Chapman, S., Newcomer, R. J., & Harrington, C. (2006). The personal assistance workforce: Trends in supply and demand. *Health Affairs, 25*(4), 1113-1120.

Kaye, S. H., Harrington, C., & LaPlante, M. P. (2009). Long-term care in the United States: Who gets it, who provides it, who pays, and how much does it cost? *Health Affairs, 29*(1), 11-21.

Kaye, S. H., LaPlante, M. P., & Harrington, C. (2009). Do noninstitutional long-term care services reduce Medicaid spending? *Health Affairs, 29*(1), 262-272.

Kitchener, M., Ng, T., Miller, N., & Harrington, C. (2005). Medicaid home and community-based services: National program trends. *Health Affairs, 24*(1), 206-212.

Kitchener, M., O'Meara, J., Brody, A., Lee, H. Y., & Harrington, C. (2008). Shareholder value and the performance of a large nursing home chain. *Health Services Research, 43*(3), 1062-1084.

Konetzka, R. T., Yi, D., Norton, E. C., & Kilpatrick, K. E. (2004). Effects of Medicare payment changes on nursing home staffing and deficiencies. *Health Services Research, 39*(3), 463-487.

LaPlante, M., Harrington, C., & Kang, T. (2002). Estimating paid and unpaid hours of personal assistance services in activities of daily living provided to adults living at home. *Health Services Research, 37*(2), 387-415.

Medicare Payment Advisory Commission. (2009). A data book: Health care spending and the Medicare program. Washington, D.C. Retrieved from www.medpac.gov/june-0DataBook.pdf.

Ng, T., Harrington, C., & O'Malley, M. (2008). *Medicaid home and community based service programs: Data update.* (Report prepared for the Kaiser Commission on Medicaid and the Uninsured, August.) Washington, D.C.: Kaiser Commission on Medicaid and the Uninsured. Retrieved from www.kff.org/medicaid/upload/7720_02.pdf.

O'Neill, C., Harrington, C., Kitchener, M., & Saliba, D. (2003). Quality of care in nursing homes: An analysis of the relationships among profit, quality, and ownership. *Medical Care, 41*(12), 1318-1330.

Schlesinger, M., & Gray, B. H. (2005). *Why nonprofits matter in American medicine: A policy brief.* Washington D.C.: Aspen Institute.

Schnelle, J. F., Simmons, S. F., Harrington, C., Cadogan, M., Garcia, E., & Bates-Jensen, B. (2004). Relationship of nursing home staffing to quality of care? *Health Services Research, 39*(2), 225-250.

U.S. General Accounting Office (GAO). (1999a). *Nursing homes: Additional steps needed to strengthen enforcement of federal quality standards.* Report to the Special Committee on Aging, U.S. Senate. GAO/HEHS-99-46. Washington, D.C.: GAO.

U.S. General Accounting Office (GAO). (1999b). *Nursing homes: Complaint investigation processes often inadequate to protect residents.* Report to Congressional Committees. GAO/HEHS-99-80. Washington, D.C.: GAO.

U.S. General Accounting Office (GAO). (2002). *Nursing homes: Quality of care more related to staffing than spending*. Report to Congressional Requestors. GAO/HEHS-02-431R. Washington, D.C.: GAO.

U.S. General Accounting Office (GAO). (2003). *Nursing home quality: Prevalence of serious problems, while declining, reinforces importance of enhanced oversight*. Report to Congressional Requesters. GAO-03-561. Washington, D.C.: GAO.

U.S. Government Accountability Office (GAO). (2007). *Nursing home reform: Continued attention is needed to improve quality of care in small but significant share of homes*. GAO-07-794T, Washington, D.C.: GAO, May 2, 2007.

U.S. Government Accountability Office (GAO). (2008). *Nursing homes: Federal monitoring surveys demonstrate continued understatement of serious care problems and CMS oversight weakness*. GAO-08-517, Washington, D.C.: GAO, May 9, 2008.

U.S. Government Accountability Office (GAO). (2009). *Medicare and Medicaid participating facilities: CMS needs to reexamine state oversight of health care facilities*. GAO-09-64, Washington, D.C.: GAO, February 13, 2009.

Wiener, J. M. (2009). *Long-term care: Options in an era of health reform*. Washington, D.C.: RTI International.

CHAPTER 25

Home Care and Hospice: Evolving Policy

Jeannee Parker Martin

"Retain unwavering faith that you can and will prevail in the end, regardless of the difficulties, and at the same time have the discipline to confront the most brutal facts of your current reality."

—Jim Collins

There has never been a more exciting time in the United States to discuss policy and politics in home care; the Centers for Medicare and Medicaid Services (CMS), the Medicare Payment Advisory Commission (MedPAC), policymakers, and home care advocates all are involved. Each brings insight and influence to foster a common understanding of how home care can serve as a bridge in the health care delivery system and as a focal point for chronic and transitional care management. To challenge existing practices and to help formulate future health policy, these stakeholders examined the benefits—cost, quality, and access—and heard stories from hundreds of home care beneficiaries and providers. Home care nurses from 50 states were invited to tell their stories at a forum sponsored by Congressmen Jim McGovern (D-MA) and Walter Jones (R-NC), co-chairs of the House Home Health Working Group, underscoring the importance of home care (NAHC Report, 2009, May 13). President Barack Obama's grandmother received hospice care just days before his 2008 election causing some policymakers to focus on end-of-life care. Consumers invited congressional leaders into their homes to see first-hand how home care is provided. The National Association for Home Care & Hospice (NAHC), a key national home care association, launched a campaign, *HelpUsChooseHome.com,* to support findings that 9 out of 10 Americans prefer home care over institutional care (National Association for Home Care, 2009). The National Hospice and Palliative Care Organization (NHPCO), the largest hospice association, established a 501(c)(4) subsidiary corporation to lobby policymakers more directly.

These efforts paid off. On March 21, 2010, the Patient Protection and Affordable Care Act (H.R. 3590) was passed followed immediately by the Health Care and Education Affordability Reconciliation Act (H.R. 4872), signed into law days later by President Obama (Patient Protection and Affordable Care Act, 2010). Home care reductions were nearly 50% less than anticipated as a result of lobbying efforts.

Collaboration across health care sectors is crucial to the successful implementation of health care reform. Home care will serve as the bridge as patients transition from one care setting to another and will be core to the health care delivery system. Sutter Health, a $9 billion health system in California, already sees the benefit of home care in controlling costs by coordinating and managing chronically ill patients, according to Marcia Reissig, RN, MS, CHCE, and CEO of Sutter VNA & Hospice. According to Ms. Reissig, Sutter Health system executives increasingly acknowledge and indeed, embrace, the role of home care in reducing costs and improving access and quality for patients across its delivery system (Reissig, 2010).

THE HOME CARE INDUSTRY

The home care industry is composed of five segments: home health, hospice, home medical equipment (HME), home infusion pharmacy (HIP), and private duty. Collectively these home care services make up the care delivery system *surrounding* and bridging other health care segments—hospitals, long-term care services, and physicians. It is not just an adjunct; home care significantly reduces care delivery costs and in some instances substitutes for institutional care. Avalere Health LLC found that patients who received home care early were associated with a $1.71 billion reduction in Medicare posthospitalization spending in 2005-2006 for diabetes, COPD, and CHF (Aquilar et al., 2009). These savings demonstrate an opportunity to incorporate home care at the core of policy decisions and Value Based Purchasing (VBP), a pay-for-performance initiative that ties Medicare payment to quality measures (CMS Office of Public Affairs, 2009) and is included in health reform provisions for all health care sectors.

KEY INFLUENCERS

Home care has not always been a major focus of health policy discussions. Historically, this low-cost solution and its incumbent spending reductions have been overlooked by policymakers who are largely influenced by hospital and physician groups, supporting associations, and lobbyists. Former Senator Claude Pepper (D-FL), who served in both houses of Congress between 1936 and 1989, was a home care champion; former Senators Robert Dole (R-KS) and John Heinz (R-PA) pushed for the Medicare Hospice Benefit; few other legislators have had as strong an influence. By the early 2000s, the focus on home care by policymakers began to shift. Institutions dedicated to health care research—Avalere Health LLC, Brown University, California Healthcare Foundation, Dartmouth Institute for Health Policy and Clinical Practice, The Robert Wood Johnson Foundation, and others—released studies underscoring the economic and quality benefits of home care (Sutherland et al., 2009; Gozalo et al., 2002; Martin & English, 2008; Cole, 2006). MedPAC, in its capacity to analyze costs, dedicated a major section on home health and a chapter on hospice in its 2009 recommendations to Congress, an indication that home care's lower cost structure was drawing attention (MedPAC, 2009a). These studies suggest that more Americans will need home care, that chronically and terminally ill patients can be managed at home with significant savings to Medicare, and that rehospitalizations can be prevented with earlier home care interventions. The findings made home care a focal point of health care reform discussions.

Major home care institutions engaged in extensive lobbying efforts with policymakers. Nurses, as chief executives of many home care organizations, lobbied members of Congress, took congressional representatives on home visits, and spearheaded campaigns to influence decision-makers. In 2009, the most influential home care trade associations, NAHC, NHPCO, and VNAA, had a predominance of nurses as trustees and committee chairs. As members of trade associations and as executives of home care organizations, nurses have enormous influence on decision-making—a power that has been underutilized in the past and is increasingly recognized.

COMPONENTS OF HOME CARE

Home care is governed by state and federal mandates. Certain states require that all home care segments be licensed; others have licensure for some but not all segments. Payment is generally dictated by Medicare, Medicaid, and private insurance companies (HMOs, PPOs, and indemnity programs). Accrediting organizations, such as The Joint Commission, the Accreditation Commission for Health Care, and the Community Health Accreditation Program, provide enhanced standards that complement state licensure and federal payment regulations.

HOME HEALTH

Perhaps the most commonly known and most widely used segment, home health care services are provided to older adults, and to a lesser degree to children and other adults with chronic and debilitating diseases and immediate posthospitalization. In 2007, more than 3.1 million people received home health services (MedPAC, 2009b). Referred to as "skilled, intermittent services," its primary focus is postacute rehabilitation. Medicare, Medicaid, and private insurers pay care for patients with varying limitations, the most common being homebound status, requiring medically necessary nursing or therapy services. VBP, enhanced program integrity, hospital readmission measures, and independence at home demonstrations are provisions in health care reform that offer home health opportunities to strengthen its bridge to chronic care and transitional care management.

HOSPICE

Hospice and palliative care is in demand for care to adults and children with advanced and terminal illnesses. In 2008, more than 1.4 million people received hospice care. Hospice is provided in any setting including the home, inpatient, or institutional setting, and is most often considered during the last six months of life. Hospice's hallmark is its interdisciplinary approach to care delivery for myriad issues facing patients and caregivers. Physicians, nurses, social workers, therapists, counselors, aides, and volunteers together coordinate care delivery. Medicare, Medicaid, and private insurers pay for hospice, and generally follow the framework outlined in the Medicare conditions for coverage and participation (CMS, 2008a). Its most common limitation is too-late referrals to hospice, with 35.4% of patients receiving care for less than seven days (NHPCO, 2009). VBP, quality reporting, payment structure revision, and concurrent care demonstrations are provisions in health care reform impacting hospices.

HOME MEDICAL EQUIPMENT

Home medical equipment (HME; also known as durable medical equipment, DME) includes mobility devices; oxygen equipment; and incontinence, orthotic, and nutrition products. HME providers deliver equipment to the home or institutional residence and related retail stores. HME is paid out-of-pocket by patients, Medicare, or private insurers. To mitigate rising costs and concerns with quality and access, a controversial competitive bidding process was implemented in 2009 for DME, prosthetic, orthotics and supplies (DMEPOS). Under health care reform, the competitive bidding pricing timetable is accelerated and a controversial provision requires a face-to-face exam for all medical equipment items and services. The impact of these and other provisions (i.e., productivity adjustments, urban payment reduction, lower annual update) will be evaluated in the future based on policy goals focused on access, quality, and lower costs.

HOME INFUSION PHARMACY

Home infusion pharmacy involves administration of medications using intravenous, subcutaneous, and other routes by nurses in the home. Commonly administered therapies, including antibiotics, chemotherapy, pain management, and parenteral nutrition, are covered under Medicare Part D, and products, supplies, and nursing services are paid for under Medicare Part A, private insurers, and, to a lesser extent, by Medicaid. Efforts to close the gap between covered pharmaceuticals and products, supplies, and services is ongoing (NHIA, 2010).

PRIVATE DUTY

Private duty companies provide a range of services from medical and nursing care to bill paying and transportation. Their goal is to provide whatever is needed to keep an aged, ill, or disabled individual independent at home (PDHCA, 2009). Some states require licensure if nursing or therapy services are provided. Services are most frequently paid out-of-pocket, although some managed care organizations pay for services. Medicaid waiver programs in some states pay for long-term chronic care management at home, such as ventilator patient care.

RAPID GROWTH

Formalized home care services began in 1965 with the enactment of Medicare, although services have been available under the rubric of Visiting Nurse Associations for more than 115 years. Today, demand for home care is high. More than 45% of Americans have at least 1 chronic disease, and many home care patients have 5 to 6 chronic conditions. Nearly 2.5% of the U.S. population, 7.2 million people, receives home care services. This number is expected to increase rapidly by 2019 as the population over 65 increases. This is demonstrated dramatically by the growth in chronically disabled and severely mentally impaired war veterans. There have been more than 31,000 casualties in Iraq, many returning home with head injuries sustained during battle (Operation Iraqi Freedom, 2009). Improved helmets and combat techniques spare lives but not serious injuries. Likewise, in the frail elderly, many receive life-prolonging treatments but are left chronically impaired and in need of home care services.

IMPACT OF POPULATION CHANGES

From Medicare's inception, the U.S. population increased by 53%. By 2025, the U.S. population is estimated to be 357,452,000, of which 18% will be over 65 and 2.1% will be over 85. These numbers are staggering—more than 64 million over 65 years and 7.5 million over 85 years (U.S. Census Bureau, 2000). Chronic conditions will be prevalent and treatments to prolong life more accessible. Home care providers are experienced in managing chronically ill patients, making it a key solution to help control costs, quality, and access as demand increases.

COMPETITION FOR TALENT

Population growth has caused all health care segments to expand resulting in a demand for talent. Hospitals, long-term care, and home care providers all fight for the same nurses, aides, therapists, and social workers—as the supply decreases. Home care has nearly 1 million workers, approximately 79% clinical staff and 21% management and office support; this staff demand will escalate with home care growth. Advanced practice nurses will be critical to mitigating staff shortages by increasing capacity to manage chronically ill patients at home with more sophisticated clinical and technological interventions. This imbalance of patients to staff will require policymakers to look closely at who will care for patients and consider balancing compensation across all sectors to help assure an even distribution of talent.

REIMBURSEMENT

Since Medicare payment began, private insurers and Medicaid have generally followed Medicare's lead. Reimbursement focused only on home health until 1982, when hospice legislation passed. In 1986, states were given the option to include hospice under Medicaid. Other reimbursement distinctions have divided the industry. Until 1993, hospital-based agencies were reimbursed at a higher rate than freestanding agencies. (U.S. GAO, 1992). In a response to rapidly rising home health costs, the Balanced Budget Act of 1997 further impacted home health providers, authorizing the Interim Payment System, a temporary payment system that began the shift toward the Home Health Prospective Payment System (PPS), effective in 2000. Competitive bidding was implemented in 2009 for HME. Hospice providers had smaller more incremental changes between 1984 and 2009. Under provisions of health reform, all segments will be impacted by Medicare savings strategies.

QUALITY AND OUTCOMES MANAGEMENT

With the implementation of PPS Outcome and Assessment Information Set (OASIS) in 2000 and improvements implemented in 2010 (OASIS-C), quality and outcomes measures are in place for home health and results are available to consumers in Home Health Compare reports (U.S. DHHS, 2009). This outcomes data has improved the capacity to understand the impact of home health on certain disease conditions and related Medicare reimbursement changes and accountability for outcomes management.

No other home care segment has a similar quality measurement system that so closely aligns with outcomes. Hospices must comply with Quality Assessment and Performance Improvement (QAPI), but this more rudimentary approach is limited as a true outcomes measurement system (CMS, 2008b). More sophisticated data analysis will be expected with health care reform provisions, including payment, VBP, and concurrent care demonstrations.

Consumer satisfaction and preferences for home care also caught the attention of policy analysts, influencing decisions to include home care in CAHPS, the Consumer Assessment of Healthcare Providers and Systems (Harris Interactive, 2008). If a home health provider does not participate, Medicare imposes 2% penalties on the provider's Medicare payments.

NON-PROFITS VERSUS FOR-PROFITS

There are few indicators suggesting that a home care provider's tax status impacts quality of care or the amount or type of care provided. For hospices, longer lengths of stay have been attributed to some for-profits, but no generalizable research exists demonstrating a negative impact on patient care quality. Yet, the focus on reimbursement and outcomes measures resulted from the increase in for-profits. In 2009, approximately 53% of home health and 46.2% of hospice providers were for-profit (CMS, 2009). Profit margins exceeding 40% by some providers enhanced the concern and focus by MedPAC, policymakers, and researchers. Further research is needed to inform policymakers and to assure alignment of payment adjustments without regard for tax status.

REIMBURSEMENT REFORM

The focus on home care in health care reform discussions was driven largely by overall growth in: (1) the numbers of Medicare providers (home health 9800, hospice 3200), (2) related net income margins or profitability (more than 40% profit margins in some instances), (3) utilization (Medicare expenditures, patient numbers, lengths of stay), and (4) concerns about fraud and abuse. In deliberations, Congress was in large part influenced by trade associations, special interest groups and studies conducted on their behalf, insurance companies, and hospital utilization and readmission patterns.

THE ROLE OF ASSOCIATIONS

In any policy discussion, unified and disparate voices influence the discussion. In one attempt to nurture a common voice, five associations and two interest groups came together to design a common hospice agenda. Informally called *The Medicare Hospice Benefit Working Group,* the seven members included: NHPCO, NAHC, VNAA, Hospice and Palliative Care Nurses Association (HPNA), American Association of Hospice and Palliative Care Physicians (AAHPM), National Alliance for Hospice Access (NAHA), and National Hospice Work Group (NHWG). This "gang of seven"—each with its own strong executive and agenda—was unable to frame a common hospice reform proposal to MedPAC, causing their efforts to collapse. Their fragmentation distracted health care reform discussions by mixing messages and prioritizing different payment issues. Several of these same associations were, however, able to coordinate influential providers—both non-profits and for-profits— into alliances advocating on their behalf: the Alliance for Home Health Quality and Innovation by NAHC and the Alliance for Care at the End of Life by NHPCO. Each entity wanted to assure high-quality care and access and lower costs. Armed with provider data and research, they demonstrated Medicare savings, quality outcomes, and consumer satisfaction. Their efforts paid off resulting in nearly 50% less-than-anticipated payment reductions for home care providers.

THE ROLE OF INSURANCE COMPANIES

When asked which health care segments have the most political power, a panel of home care analysts indicated that first insurers, then hospitals, then physicians, followed last by home care (HCap, 2009). To every $1 spent by home care advocates others spent $10 or more. Yet, due to its ability to manage complex, chronically, and terminally ill patients and reduce hospital admissions, home care continues to be a key focus of health reform.

THE ROLE OF HOSPITAL UTILIZATION AND READMISSIONS

Since the announcement of readmission penalties on hospitals' Medicare reimbursement, home care providers have implemented aggressive measures in collaboration with hospitals to move patients from the acute to home setting more quickly. Chronic care management models are well-positioned to help align incentives across the continuum of care delivery. Two distinct programs demonstrate substantial cost savings and improvements in patient outcomes and satisfaction: Sutter Health's Advanced Illness Management Program (AIM) and University of Pennsylvania's Transitional Care Model (TCM). Sutter's AIM program, managed from its system-wide hospice provider, focused initially on transitioning hospice patients but gradually has taken on a system-wide focus of chronic care management (Reissig & Gornet, 2009). Likewise, the TCM is a care management intervention that is associated with significant improvements in health outcomes and reductions in care delivery costs among at-risk, chronically ill older adults (Naylor, 2009).

THE FUTURE OUTLOOK: HOME CARE LEADS THE HEALTH POLICY DISCUSSION

To borrow from Jim Collins who so aptly describes in *Good to Great* companies who succeed, we must confront the brutal facts of our current reality to succeed in changing our health care delivery system (Collins, 2001). Not only is home care the logical beginning, it is the logical end, enveloping all other elements of health care delivery. Ongoing and emerging trends—consumer desire for at home care, demographics, reimbursement reform, the fight for talent, chronic and transitional care management, technology acceleration, and end-of-life care—point to home care as the solution for sound U.S. health care policy in controlling costs, quality, and access. If home care is the solution, then how will it influence policymakers and what role will nurses play?

TECHNOLOGY ACCELERATION

With increasing population demand for health care and a shortage of staff, technology can accelerate home care delivery. Widely used examples include:

remote patient monitoring (RPM), point of care technology, online learning, telephony, and electronic data rooms. These and other innovations (e.g., Web-based cameras, electronic medical records, electronic pharmacy distribution, drop-ship supplies, robotics, and smart home monitoring) are key to home care's future utilization, quality, cost, and talent management. Such technology innovations will lead to cost savings: (1) more rapid communications and interventions resulting in improved patient outcomes and reduced hospitalizations and emergency department visits; (2) improvement in quality through more rapid communications and interventions; (3) improvement in talent management through more consistent education and training; and (4) improvement in utilization patterns by replacing some in-person visits with electronic interventions.

THE NURSES' ROLE

Home care is a resilient and growing segment of the health care industry and is a critical solution to decrease rising costs, improve consumer satisfaction, and reduce hospitalizations. Nurses, at the helm of key associations, home care organizations, and special interest groups, play a central role in policy discussions by using their deep-seated understanding of the home care environment and of the patient's socioeconomic, disease, and psychosocial needs. Nurses will continue to play a central role across home care's spectrum of services: providing direct care, assuring administrative oversight, conducting research, and advocating on behalf of patients to assure access to care at home, when the home setting is the most appropriate place to receive care.

For a list of related websites, please refer to your Evolve Resources at http://evolve.elsevier.com/Mason/policypolitics/

REFERENCES

Aquilar, C., Ahlstrom, A., Karaca Z., Dietz, K., & Lukens E. (2009). *Medicare spending and rehospitalization for chronically ill Medicare beneficiaries: Home health use compared to other post-acute settings.* Avalere Health, LLC, released May 11, 2009.

Centers for Medicare & Medicaid Services (CMS). (2008a). 42 CFR Part 418, Medicare and Medicaid Programs hospice conditions of participation; final rule, June 5, 2008. Retrieved from www.cms.hhs.gov/center/hospice.asp.

Centers for Medicare & Medicaid Services (CMS). (2008b). 42 CFR Part 418.58, Hospice conditions of participation: Quality assessment and performance improvement.

Centers for Medicare & Medicaid Services (CMS). (2009). Center for Information Systems, Health Standards and Quality Bureau.

Centers for Medicare & Medicaid Services (CMS). Office of Public Affairs. (2009, August 17). Press release: Medicare demonstrations show paying for quality health care pays off.

Cole, C. S. (2006, December). Home health and community based services. The Robert Wood Johnson Foundation.

Collins, J. (2001). *Good to great: Why some companies make the leap and others don't* (pp. 64-89). New York: HarperCollins.

Gozalo, P., Miller, S., & Mor, V. (2002). *Hospice in nursing homes: Factors influencing hospitalization and choice of hospice.* Academy for Health Services Research and Health Policy, *19,* 5.

Harris Interactive. (2008, August 19). Republican and Democratic voters view home care as a solution to rising Medicare spending, Harris Survey Finds, American Association for HomeCare press release.

Healthcare and Capital (HCap) Conference. (2009, November 17). 2010 Healthcare outlook: Reimbursement cuts, reform and regulatory changes. Jon Glaudemans, Avalere Health, Andrew Bressler, Bank of America Securities, Mark Francis, Houlihan Lokey, Bruce Fried, Sonnenschein Nath & Rosenthal. Mandarin Oriental Hotel, Washington, D.C..

Martin, J. P., & English, D. (2008, September). Issues brief: Collaborative care: Improving the hospice–nursing home relationship. California HealthCare Foundation.

Medicare Payment Advisory Commission (MedPAC) (2009a, March). Report to the Congress: Medicare payment policy, 190. Also see MedPAC transcripts 2007-2009 at http://medpac.gov/meetings.cfm.

Medicare Payment Advisory Commission (MedPAC) (2009b, March). Report to the Congress: Medicare payment policy, 185-200; 347-373. Also see MedPAC transcripts 2007-2009 at http://medpac.gov/meetings.cfm.

NAHC Report. (2009, May 13). In Celebration of National Nurses Week: Nurses from all 50 states to speak out on the need for home care.

National Association for Home Care (NAHC) (2009). Retrieved from www.helpuschoosehome.com.

National Home Infusion Association (NHIA) (2010). Retrieved from www.nhia.org/resource/medicare_ptd.

National Hospice and Palliative Care Organization (NHPCO) (2009). NHPCO Facts and figures: Hospice care in America. 2009 edition. Retrieved from www.nhpco.org.

Naylor, M. D. (2009). Roundtable on delivery system reform. United States Senate Committee on Finance, April 21, 2009. Washington D.C., 2. Retrieved from www.nursing.upenn.edu/news/Documents/Mary_Naylor_statement_4-17-09f.pdf.

Operation Iraqi Freedom. (2009). U.S. casualty status, November 2009. Retrieved from www.defenselink.mil/news/casualty.pdf.

Private Duty Home Care Association (PDHCA) (2009). An affiliate of the National Association for Home Care & Hospice. Retrieved from www.pdhca.org.

Reissig, M. (2010, March 23). Marcia Reissig, RN, MS, CHCE, and CEO of Sutter VNA & Hospice. E-mail communication to J. P. Martin.

Reissig, M., & Gornet, B. (2009). Sutter VNA & Hospice AIM Program. Presentation to the National Hospice Work Group. July 9, 2009. Napa, CA.

Sutherland, J. M., Fisher, E. S., & Skinner, J. S. (2009). Getting past denial—The high cost of health care in the United States. *New England Journal of Medicine, 361*(13), 1227-1230.

U.S. Census Bureau .(2000). Population Estimates Program, Population Division, U.S. Census Bureau. Retrieved from www.census.gov/popest/archives/1990s/popclockest.txt.

U.S. Department of Health and Human Services. (U.S. DHHS) (2009). Home Health Compare. Retrieved from www.medicare.gov/HHCompare.

U.S. General Accounting Office (U.S. GAO). (1992). Human Resources Division, Report B-245370, January 31, 1992, 5.

CHAPTER 26

Achieving Mental Health Parity

Freida Hopkins Outlaw, Patricia K. Bradley, and Marie Davis-Williams

"Of all the forms of inequality, injustice in health [mental health] is the most shocking and the most inhuman."

—Martin Luther King, Jr., at the Second National Convention of the Medical Community for Human Rights, Chicago, March 25, 1966

The fight for mental health parity has been long, protracted, and marked by many challenges, disappointments, and victories. Mental health parity refers to the equivalence of coverage for mental health treatment and clinical visits to medical and surgical benefits within an insurance plan (Peters, 2006). Historically, many insurance plans have legally placed limits on services for patients with mental health and/or substance abuse diagnoses, while requiring the patients to pay more out-of-pocket costs for selected services that are not required to be paid by patients who have medical conditions such as diabetes, asthma, or heart disease (Harvard Mental Health Letter [HMHL], 2009). Insurers and employers have been guarded about offering mental health and substance abuse coverage as they believe that these mental disorders are untreatable or are too expensive to treat (Barry, 2006). This disparity has had grave implications for those persons with mental health and substance abuse health care needs, such as late or missed diagnosis, inadequate care, or not seeking treatment for financial or social stigmatizing reasons. These behaviors may result in severe mental illness or suicide. The number of individuals, families, and society as a whole impacted by this disparity is substantial. It has been estimated that annually 54 million Americans experience a mental health disorder at a cost of $100 billion. This includes the cost of care as well as lost productivity (Marth, 2009).

This chapter will describe the historical struggle to achieve mental health and substance abuse parity,

gaps in the parity law, and challenges of implementing the law at both state and national levels.

HISTORICAL STRUGGLE TO ACHIEVE MENTAL HEALTH PARITY

Since the early 1970s, mental health advocates have been working in conjunction with federal legislators to secure the passage of mental health parity legislation (United States Department of Health and Human Services [USDHHS], 1999). Senators Paul Wellstone (D-WI) and Pete Domenici (R-NM) led the initial effort to achieve mental health parity. They spearheaded legislation in the U. S. Senate, as an amendment to a larger bill that required insurers to provide parity for mental health and physical health benefits. However, the U.S. House of Representatives, based on negative feedback from insurers, forced the parity language out of the final bill (Levinson & Druss, 2000).

Wellstone and Domenici's efforts in 1996 were not entirely thwarted as the senators were able to insert "partial parity" language that prevented insurance plans from being able to pay less to treat mental health disorders compared with what they paid to treat physical health conditions. Predictably, as a cost-containing measure, insurance companies found a loophole that weakened the parity law by limiting the number of days an individual could be covered for mental health treatment outpatient visits or days in the hospital (Levinson & Druss, 2000).

This first incremental step toward mental health parity was taken by the passage of the Mental Health Parity Act (MHPA) of 1996, which went into effect on January 1, 1998. The MHPA applied to two types of coverage—large group self-funded health plans and large group fully-insured group health plans. Although the passage of this 1996 Act was met with celebration, it was clear that further steps were needed to obtain more equitable coverage of mental health and addiction services.

One of the flaws of the 1996 Mental Health Parity Act was that it did not contain a substance abuse benefit, a fact that ignored that approximately 50% of individuals with a severe mental disorder have substance abuse issues as well as 37% of alcohol abusers and 53% of drug abusers have at least one serious mental illness (JAMA, 2009). Researchers have determined that when only one of the co-occurring disorders (mental illness or substance abuse disorder) is treated, both disorders usually get worse. In addition to the tremendous suffering that the individual with an untreated or poorly treated co-occurring disorder and their family experience, these individuals also use the most costly services, such as emergency rooms and inpatient facilities, and have the worse clinical outcomes (New Freedom Commission on Mental Health [NFCMH], 2003).

Committed to the belief that individuals need mental health equality in order to have comprehensive health care coverage, Senators Wellstone and Domenici were joined in 2001 in the House of Representatives by Patrick Kennedy (D-RI) and Jim Ramstad (R-MN) to try to pass a full and expanded mental health parity bill. Tragically, in 2002 as the broader bill was gathering support, Senator Wellstone was killed in an airplane crash. His son David continued to lobby after his death. Those efforts resulted in 2008 of passage of a more expansive parity bill, the Wellstone and Domenici Mental Health Parity and Addiction Equity Act of 2008 (MHPA 2008) that included a substance abuse benefit. Also, in 2008, Congress passed the Medicare Improvements for Patients Act, which supplements the mental health parity laws for Medicare recipients in every state except Idaho and Wyoming (HMHL, 2009).

MEANING OF PARITY FOR MENTAL HEALTH AND ADDICTION TREATMENT

The MHPA of 2008 affects large employers, Medicaid managed care plans, and State Children's Health Insurance Program (SCHIP) plans (HMHL, 2009). Specifically, it amends the Mental Health Parity Act (MHPA) of 1996 by stipulating businesses with 51 or more employees, who offer a health insurance plan with mental health and substance abuse coverage,

offer these benefits at the same level as what is offered in their medical and surgical coverage. It means that deductibles, co-payments, out-of-pocket expenses, outpatient visits, inpatient stays, and treatment limits must be the same for mental health and substance abuse treatment as they are for medical and surgical services (Melek, 2009).

In the 2008 MHPA, no requirement as to what conditions must be covered are imposed, but whatever is covered must be at parity with medical coverage. Benefits offered to out-of-network coverage will be extended so that a plan must offer out-of-network coverage for mental health and addiction services if it does so for medical/surgical services. The new law also preserves state parity and consumer laws. This legislation puts in place an oversight mechanism to determine if insurers are discriminating against certain conditions. It allows a cost-based exemption if the insurer can prove that parity raised their total plan costs by more than 2% or more in the first year after enactment (Melek, 2009).

The Wellstone-Domenici Act of 2008 became law on January 1, 2010. Interim final rules are scheduled to become effective on April 5, 2010, with comments from the public due on or before May 3, 2010. These new federal rules providing mental health parity are effective for insurance plans whose renewal date begins on or after July 1, 2010, and cover 82 million individuals in self-insured employer health plans that are not governed by state parity laws and an additional 31 million employees in plans that are subject to state regulations (HMHL, 2009).

GAPS IN THE MENTAL HEALTH PARITY LAW

Clearly the Mental Health Parity bill represents a step forward; however there are gaps that need to be addressed. For instance, the bill does not mandate mental health and substance abuse coverage, and services that are provided through most commercial plans do not include the recovery-based services for persons with severe and persistent mental illnesses. Recovery is defined by the New Freedom Commission on Mental Health (NFCMH, 2003) as the "process in which people [with serious mental illnesses] are able to live, work, learn, and participate fully in their communities" (p. 5). Recovery-based services in mental health treatment include those that encompass self-direction and empowerment; are holistic and strength-based; provide peer support;

and develop responsibility and hope. For example, researchers have noted that individuals with serious emotional illnesses, who have hope, usually linked with peer and family support, have higher rates of remission and recovery from their illness symptoms (SAMHSA, 2006).

Recovery-based services such as supportive housing and supported employment are not usually covered by the Medicaid program or commercial insurances as many of these services do not meet "medical necessity criteria." As a result, there is limited payment for services identified as essential for the treatment of the person's illness, injury, or condition. Medical necessity criteria often exclude anything deemed experimental or not yet proven. Ford (2000) suggests that the short-term challenge for advocates of mental health parity is to obtain the most acceptable and expansive definitions of medical necessity from third-party payers. The long-term challenge will be to develop a system that pays for the greatest number of high-quality evidence-based services for the greatest number of people in need, regardless of diagnosis.

STATE LEVEL IMPLEMENTATION

Understanding and navigating the provisions of the Wellstone-Domenici MHPA at state and federal levels can be challenging for patients and providers (HMHL, 2009). As of 2010, 34 states have enacted some mental health parity provisions. Wide variances exist, with some states such as Connecticut, Indiana, Kentucky, and Maryland following the federal laws and others such as South Carolina, West Virginia, and North Carolina limiting the benefit expansion to specific mental illnesses. Less comprehensive state laws will be replaced by the new federal law, and more comprehensive state laws will remain intact (HMHL, 2009). Garfield (2009) found in her research about the process of transformational policy change in four states that, in the end, states are primarily influenced by their own problems and the resources available to them, and are only guided by national efforts if they are congruent with their particular state's idiosyncrasies.

It is interesting to note that most insurers were concerned with the passage of parity legislation as they feared that health care costs would rise at an unsustainable rate. In fact, this has not been the case; health care costs have not increased significantly. For example, Pacula and Sturm (2000) found that those states that passed parity legislation did not experience a significant increase in the use of mental health services. According to Barry and colleagues (2006), the Congressional Budget Office is projecting a mere 0.4% on average increase in cost in total premiums after accounting for the offsetting impact of behavioral responses by health plans, employers, and workers. The authors also pointed out from a review of relevant research that parity implemented in the context of managed care would have little impact on mental health spending and would increase risk protection.

Mental health parity legislation may ameliorate many of the negative economic conditions for the states by increasing the work productivity of employees who need but have not been able to receive mental health and substance abuse services. As a result of the passage of the mental health and substance abuse parity law, effective and adequate treatment can be accessed, which will enable employees to remain in the workforce.

CHALLENGES IN IMPLEMENTING THE LAW

As insurers prepare to provide mental health and addiction services, they would be wise to implement those services that have been found to be evidence-based. The Institute of Medicine (IOM, 2001) defines evidence-based medicine as the integration of best researched evidence and clinical expertise with patient values. States can advance evidence-based practices by using dissemination and demonstration projects and create public-private partnerships to guide this implementation (NFCMH, 2003).

The "Bringing Science to Service" initiative is intended to make approaches that are supported by research widely available to patients and families (Isett et al., 2007). The first group of disseminated evidenced-based practices that support and enhance recovery-based psychiatric rehabilitation included assertive community treatment, supported employment, illness management and recovery, integrated treatment for co-occurring mental illness and substance abuse, family psychoeducation, and medication management. While by no means an exhaustive list of evidence-based practices, these represent those practices that the Center for Medicare and Medicaid Services (CMS) believes have undergone rigorous research and study and have proven outcomes.

CHALLENGES FOR THE FUTURE

In addition to the challenges of defining medical necessity and obtaining coverage for recovery-based services, a major challenge for the future involves having an adequate mental health workforce to provide care for the increased numbers of individuals with access to services. Mental health and addiction services struggle in most states to have a network of providers that are accessible and culturally and linguistically competent. The question remains about how network adequacy will be developed to meet the increased demand for services (Huckshorn, 2007; IOM, 2003).

The Institute of Medicine (IOM, 2001) addressed the issues of redesigning the health care system to be more inclusive of people with mental health issues and then followed up with a 2005 report on quality care for people with mental health and substance use problems (IOM, 2005). Both IOM reports are consistent with the New Freedom Commission on Mental Health report's identification of ways to transform the mental health system (NFCMH, 2003). This call to action requires clinicians to provide consumer- and family-driven services and to increase the consumers' coping and recovery. States will need to develop diversified, fully integrated continuums of care by expanding their own services, contracting with other health care organizations, affiliating with area providers, and including community and families.

IMPLICATIONS FOR NURSING: MENTAL HEALTH RELATED ISSUES AND STRATEGIES

Nurses, along with other health care professionals, can influence the knowledge, beliefs, and attitudes toward mental health and illness and the implementation of evidenced-based, culturally competent interventions for people with mental illness.

Issue: Consumers of mental health and substance abuse services and their families may not know or understand the extent of what mental health parity means for their health care.

Strategy: Psychiatric Mental Health nurses need to be knowledgeable about the law and regulations to ensure that consumers are receiving full benefits that promote recovery from mental illness and substance use disorders.

Issue: Gaps in the law remain relative to the vital services that are needed to support people with severe and persistent mental illness and substance use disorders.

Strategy: Psychiatric nurses need to continue to advocate for a wider array of services that are not currently covered by the parity law but that are effective for individuals with severe mental illness and substance use disorders.

Issue: As result of the new Mental Health Parity and Addictions Equity Act of 2008, an increased number of diverse individuals will have access to services, putting a strain on the existing inadequate network of providers.

Strategy: Psychiatric nurse educators must include emerging evidence-based practices in curriculum that support and enhance recovery-based psychiatric rehabilitation services.

Issue: The Mental Health Parity and Addictions Equity Act of 2008 provides a new mental health and substance benefit about which the general public will need more information.

Strategy: Psychiatric nurses need to be responsible for educating the public about eliminating discrimination in coverage for mental health and substance abuse services.

For a list of related websites, please refer to your Evolve Resources at http://evolve.elsevier.com/Mason/policypolitics/

REFERENCES

Barry, C. L. (2006). The political evolution of mental health parity. *Harvard Review of Psychiatry, 14*(4), 185.

Barry, C., Frank, R., & McGuire, T. (2006). The costs of mental health parity: Still an impediment? *Health Affairs, 25*(3), 623-634.

Ford, W. E. (2000). Medical necessity and psychiatric managed care. *Psychiatric Clinics of North America, 23*(2), 309-317.

Garfield, R. L. (2009). Mental health policy development in the states: The piecemeal nature of transformational change. *Psychiatric Services, 60*(10), 1329-1335.

Harvard Mental Health Letter (HMHL). (2009). Benefiting from mental health parity: Determining coverage, understanding the limits, and appealing decisions. *Harvard Mental Health Letter, 25*(7), 4-5.

Huckshorn, K. (2007). Building a better mental health workforce: 8 core elements. *Journal of Psychosocial Nursing & Mental Health Services, 45*(3), 24.

Institute of Medicine (IOM). (2001). *Crossing the quality chasm: A new health system.* Washington, D.C.: National Academies Press.

Institute of Medicine (IOM). (2003). *Health professions education: A bridge to quality.* Washington, D.C.: National Academies Press.

Institute of Medicine (IOM). (2005). *Improving the quality of health care for mental and substance abuse conditions.* Washington, D.C.: National Academies Press.

Isett, K. R., Burnam, M. A., Coleman-Beattie, B., Hyde, P. S., Morrissey J. P., Magnabosco, J., Rapp, C. A., Ganju, V., & Goldman, H. H. (2007). The state policy context of implementation issues for evidence-based practices in mental health. *Psychiatric Services, 58*(7), 914-921.

Journal of the American Medical Association (JAMA). (2009). Dual diagnosis and integrated treatment of mental illness and substance abuse disorder fact sheet. Retrieved from www.docstoc.com/docs/2602728/Journal-of-the-American-Medical-Association-JAMA.

Levinson, C. M., & Druss, B. G. (2000). The evolution of mental health parity in American politics. *Administration and Policy in Mental Health, 29*(2), 139-145.

Marth, D. (2009). Mental Health Parity Act of 2007: An analysis of the proposed changes. *Social Work in Mental Health, 7*(6), 556-571.

Melek, S. (2009). Preparing for parity: Investing in mental health. Retrieved from www.milliman.com/expertise/healthcare/publications/rr/pdfs/preparing-parity-investing-mental-WP05-01-09.pdf.

New Freedom Commission on Mental Health (NFCMH). (2003). *Achieving the promise: Transforming mental health care in America.* Final Report. DHHS Pub. No. SMA-03-3832. Rockville, MD: U.S. Department of Health and Human Services.

Pacula, R. L., & Sturm, R. (2000). Mental health parity legislation: Much ado about nothing? *Health Services Research, 35*(1 Pt 2), 263-275.

Peters, J. (2006). Mental health parity: Legislation and implications for insurers and providers. *The Heinz Journal, 3*(2), 1-9.

Substance Abuse and Mental Health Services Administration (SAMHSA). (2006). *National Consensus Statement on Mental Recovery.* Rockville, MD: USDHHS, CMHS.

U.S. Department of Health and Human Services. (USDHHS) (1999). Mental health: A report of the Surgeon General. Rockville, MD: National Institute of Mental Health.

CHAPTER 27

Integrative Health: Pathway to Health Reform and a Healthier Nation

Mary Jo Kreitzer

"Healing is a matter of time, but it is also sometimes a matter of opportunity."

—Hippocrates

In February 2009, the United States Senate Committee on Health, Education, Labor and Pensions held two hearings on integrative health as the early conversation on health care reform began in Washington. The titles of the hearings reflect the interest at a federal level in what is now commonly called *integrative health:* Integrative Health: Pathway to Health Reform; and Integrative Health: Pathway to a Healthier Nation (U.S. Senate Committee on Health, Education, Labor and Pensions, 2009). The hearings included evidence on consumer demand for expanded health care options and on clinical outcomes of integrated care.

The same week as these two senate hearings, the Institute of Medicine (IOM) and the Bravewell Collaborative convened a meeting to explore the science and practice of integrative medicine and examine ways that integrative approaches might shift the orientation of our health care system from the current sporadic, reactive, and physician-centric approach to one that fosters an emphasis on health, wellness, early intervention for disease, and patient empowerment (IOM, 2009).

Integrative health or *medicine* is the phrase increasingly used to describe the combination of conventional and complementary and alternative (CAM) treatments. The field commonly referred to as CAM is large, complex, and diverse. It is estimated to include over 1800 different therapies such as guided imagery, healing touch, and herbal medicine as well as culturally based systems of healing including traditional Chinese medicine, Ayurveda, homeopathy, and naturopathy. Even the title used to describe this continuum of healing approaches is laden with controversy and political considerations.

For many years, the term *alternative medicine* was used to describe these healing approaches. They were viewed as part of the "counterculture" and often used in lieu of conventional care. The term itself implies an "either-or" mentality. As it became more apparent that these healing approaches were used in conjunction with conventional care, the phrase *complementary medicine* began to emerge. Although accurate for some consumers, others would argue that complementary approaches for conditions such as pain and stress management are primary, and that the term *complementary* inaccurately and inappropriately deemphasizes their contribution and importance.

Within the discipline of medicine, the preferred term is *integrative medicine.* The Consortium of Academic Health Centers for Integrative Medicine (CAHCIM), an organization of 45 medical schools, defines *integrative medicine* as "the practice of medicine that reaffirms the importance of the relationship between practitioner and patient, focuses on the whole person, is informed by evidence, and makes use of all appropriate therapeutic approaches, health care professionals and disciplines to achieve optimal health and healing" (CAHCIM, 2009). This definition is broad in that it could refer to any type of practitioner and patient and it highlights the importance of relationship-centered and whole-person care. Within the nursing literature, *complementary* or *integrative therapies* and *healing practices* are the terms more commonly used. For many in nursing, the term *medicine* is associated with the discipline and practice of medicine and therefore is not an acceptable term for a broad range of healing approaches practiced by different types of health care professionals. In this chapter, the terms *integrative therapies, complementary therapies,* and *CAM* are used interchangeably, given that *CAM* is the acronym or phrase most commonly used in national policy documents as well as the National Institutes of Health (NIH).

Consumer demand for complementary therapies has increased dramatically over the past 15 years though remaining fairly stable since 2002. According to data released in 2009 by the National Center for Complementary and Alternative Medicine (NCCAM), approximately 38% of adults in the U.S. aged 18 years and over and nearly 12% of U.S. children aged 17 years and under use some form of CAM (Barnes, Bloom, & Nahin, 2008). The majority of people use CAM as a complement to conventional biomedicine, not as an alternative (Astin, 1998; Eisenberg et al., 1998; Barnes, Powell-Griner, McFann, & Nahin, 2004). Reasons commonly cited for using complementary therapies include compatibility with personal values, desire to be actively involved with decision-making regarding care, dissatisfaction with conventional care or a perception that conventional care cannot adequately address symptoms or health conditions, and a preference for care that is more attentive to the whole person—body, mind, and spirit.

With the growth in the use of complementary therapies, many policy issues have surfaced that include access to care and reimbursement for services, education and credentialing of providers, regulation of practice, funding of research, consumer education, and the creation of integrated care delivery systems.

USE OF COMPLEMENTARY THERAPIES WITHIN NURSING

Much of what is called "complementary therapy" has been within the domain of nursing for centuries. In her *Notes on Nursing* published in 1860, Florence Nightingale described nursing as a holistic and integrated pursuit. She advocated that the role of the nurse was to help the patient attain the best possible condition so that nature could act and self-healing could occur. She wrote about the importance of good hygiene and sanitation, fresh air, light, touch, diet, and spirituality (Dossey, 2000).

Although nursing has a long tradition of caring, healing, and wholeness, concerns have been raised about the visibility of nursing in the contemporary complementary therapies or integrative health movement. The noted absence of nursing leadership within many national initiatives, underrepresentation of nurses among investigators successfully obtaining funding from NIH, inadequate focus on complementary therapies in undergraduate and graduate curricula, reimbursement issues for nurses providing complementary therapies, and significant differences in how boards of nursing are addressing the inclusion of complementary therapies in nurse practice acts led a group of nurse leaders to convene the Gillette Nursing Summit in 2002 (Kreitzer & Disch, 2003). The proceedings described a set of strategies that focused on ways to better align and position nursing relative to the integrative health care movement, thus assuring a more visible presence in decision-making forums that are shaping the future of health care in the U.S.

NATIONAL INSTITUTES OF HEALTH

In response to growing public interest in and use of complementary therapies, U.S. Congress passed in 1991 Public Law 102-170, which provided $2 million to NIH to establish an office and an advisory panel to recommend a research program that would focus on promising unconventional medical practices. In 1993, as part of the NIH Revitalization Act, the Office of Alternative Medicine (OAM) was established within the Office of the Director of NIH. The purpose of the Office was to facilitate the evaluation of alternative medical treatment modalities and to disseminate information to the public via an information clearinghouse. In 1998, Public Law 105-277, the Omnibus Consolidated and Emergency Supplemental Appropriations Act, elevated the status and expanded the mandate of the OAM by authorizing the establishment of NCCAM. NCCAM is one of 27 institutes and centers that compose NIH. The mission of NCCAM is to explore CAM in the context of rigorous science, train CAM researchers, and disseminate authoritative information to the public and health professionals. Funding for NCCAM has increased significantly since its inception, as reflected in the fiscal year (FY) 2009 budget of $125.5 million.

THE WHITE HOUSE COMMISSION ON CAM POLICY

Since 2002, there have been two national policy initiatives on CAM: the White House Commission on Complementary and Alternative Medicine Policy (2002) and the Institute of Medicine (IOM) CAM Study Committee (2005). Nurses were appointed to serve as members of both groups, and nurses provided testimony in open hearings that were part of the deliberations of both groups. President William J. Clinton issued an executive order (Executive Order No. 13147) in March 2000 that established the White House Commission on Complementary and Alternative Medicine Policy (WHCCAMP). The primary task of the commission was to provide the Secretary of Health and Human Services (HHS) with legislative and administrative recommendations for "ensuring that public policy maximizes the potential benefits of CAM therapies to consumers" *(www.whccamp.hhs. gov/finalreport.html)*. The 20-member commission focused on the following four areas:

- Education and training of health care practitioners
- Coordination of research to increase knowledge about CAM products
- Provision of reliable and useful information on CAM to health professionals
- Provision of guidance on the appropriate access to and delivery of CAM

The 29 recommendations addressed CAM information development and dissemination, access and delivery of safe and effective CAM services, coverage and reimbursement, use of CAM to promote wellness and health, the importance of incorporating CAM information in the education of health professionals, and the need for coordinated federal efforts. The final recommendation was that the president, Secretary of HHS, or Congress create an office to coordinate federal CAM activities and to facilitate the integration into the nation's health care system of those complementary and alternative health care practices and products determined to be safe and effective. With a change in administration at the executive level and within Congress, there has not been a clear mandate for implementing the White House Commission recommendations, although a number of them are being reviewed and acted on incrementally within various public and private organizations and bodies at federal and state levels.

INSTITUTE OF MEDICINE REPORT ON CAM

In 2002, 16 NIH institutes, centers, and offices and the Agency for Healthcare Research and Quality (AHRQ) asked the IOM to convene a study committee to explore scientific, policy, and practice questions that arise from the significant and increasing use of CAM therapies by the American public. The report (National Academy of Sciences, 2005) emphasized that decisions about the use of specific CAM therapies should primarily depend on whether or not they have been shown to be safe and effective; it concluded that the goal should be the provision of comprehensive health care that does the following:

- Is based on the best scientific evidence available regarding benefits and harm
- Encourages patients to share in decision-making about therapeutic options
- Promotes choices in care that include CAM therapies when appropriate

The committee also cited the need for tools such as guidelines that would aid conventional practitioners' decision-making about offering or recommending CAM, where patients might be referred, and what organizational structures are most appropriate for the delivery of integrated care. In recommending the development of such tools, the Committee noted that the goal is to provide comprehensive care that is safe, effective, interdisciplinary, and collaborative. Recommendations were identified that would strengthen the Dietary Supplement Health and Education Act of 1994, expand research funding, promote teaching CAM content in health profession schools, and expand the number of providers able to work in integrated care.

EDUCATION OF HEALTH PROFESSIONALS

In both the IOM and WHCCAMP reports, recommendations on educating health professionals were linked to improving care. The IOM report specifically mentions nursing in advising that schools of the health professions incorporate sufficient information about CAM into the curriculum at the undergraduate, graduate, and postgraduate levels to enable licensed health professionals to competently advise patients about CAM. Similarly, the WHCCAMP report recommends that conventional as well as CAM practitioners receive education to ensure public safety, improve health, and increase the availability and collaboration among qualified practitioners.

The extent to which nursing programs have incorporated content on complementary therapies is unclear. As documented in the Gillette Nursing Summit (Kreitzer & Disch, 2003), the perception among nurse leaders was that this area has received limited explicit curricular emphasis. It was also noted that within some nursing programs, there is resistance to teaching what is perceived to be a fad or movement lacking in evidence that is being largely shaped and dominated by medicine. There are several nursing programs, however, that have been early leaders in integrating complementary therapies into nursing curricula. Three schools of nursing were recipients of NIH NCCAM R-25 CAM education grants: the University of Minnesota, the University of Washington, and Rush University College of Nursing. Each of these programs has extensive information on complementary therapies on its website. Content on integrative therapies has been more readily integrated into nursing continuing education programs.

Within medicine, a stronger and more-organized movement to integrate content on CAM is apparent. Eleven of 15 NIH NCCAM R-25 CAM education grants were awarded to schools of medicine. An additional grant was awarded to the American Medical Student Association to support the development of curricula that will be integrated into medical schools across the country. In 1999, CAHCIM was formed to advance medical schools' integrative efforts in education, research, and clinical care. Forty-four medical schools participate in the consortium.

It is likely that an increased focus on complementary therapies in nursing education will occur. A document prepared by the American Association of Colleges of Nursing (AACN) titled *The Essentials of Baccalaureate Education for Professional Nursing Practice* (2008) recognizes the importance of complementary and alternative therapies.

INTEGRATED CARE DELIVERY SYSTEMS

The IOM report (National Academy of Sciences, 2005) notes that in the U.S. there is a "distinct trend" toward the integration of complementary and alternative therapies within the conventional health care system. Evidence cited includes the increasing number of hospitals and health maintenance organizations offering CAM therapies, the increase in insurance coverage, and the growth in integrative medicine centers and clinics, many with close ties to medical schools and teaching hospitals.

According to American Hospital Association (AHA) surveys (Ananth, 2002), in 1998 only 7.9% of hospitals reported that they offered CAM services. By 2002 the number of hospitals offering CAM therapies had more than doubled to 16.6%. Seventy-five percent of hospitals offer community CAM education programs, and 49% offer CAM information on their hospital websites. Of those hospitals not currently offering CAM services, 24% indicated that they had plans to do so.

THIRD-PARTY REIMBURSEMENT

Although consumers are demanding access to CAM services and hospitals are increasingly offering CAM, reimbursement is a major policy issue. At present, access to CAM is largely limited to those who can afford to pay out-of-pocket. Reimbursement varies considerably region to region and is different based on the type of CAM services received. For example, Cleary-Guida, Okvat, Oz, & Ting (2001), in regional survey of insurance coverage, found that virtually all insurance carriers cover chiropractic care, and close to 40% cover acupuncture and 37% cover massage therapy. This pattern of reimbursement differs somewhat from that reported by Ananth (2002), who found in the AHA survey that CAM services most likely to be reimbursed included nutritional counseling (56%), chiropractic services (49%), and biofeedback (54%). Rather than provide across-the-board coverage for any type of CAM service, third-party payers seem more inclined to provide coverage for certain therapies for select conditions. For example, acupuncture may be reimbursed for people with chronic pain but not for a person wanting to use acupuncture to treat asthma.

In general, reimbursement is related to research evidence. As there is increased documentation of the safety, efficacy, and cost of a CAM therapy, there is an increased likelihood that it will be reimbursed. But there are two other trends in reimbursement that are important to note. Increasingly, third-party payers manage a portfolio of health plans that vary depending on the employer group. What a health plan covers and what it does not cover may depend more on the employer, who determines benefit coverage, than on the third-party payer who is managing the health plan. This has important implications for consumers who are advocating for increased reimbursement of CAM. Rather than lobby the health plan for changes, it may be more important to have input into decisions that the employer makes regarding selection of the health plan and what constitutes covered benefits.

Finally, over the past 5 years there has been an increase in the growth of health savings accounts (HSAs) and health care spending accounts. Individuals may establish HSAs that work much like independent retirement accounts (IRAs) but are directed toward medical expenses. Employers are also offering employees the option of establishing a health or medical savings account as part of their benefit package. The employee or employer makes contributions to the account, and it may be used to pay for unreimbursed health care expenses. Funds are controlled and owned by the account holder, and savings are rolled over every year and are portable. In some cases, these accounts can be used to reimburse expenses associated with accessing complementary therapies. Health care spending accounts work in a similar manner. Employees can set aside pretax money to use for paying health-related bills, but generally all of the money must be spent within the fiscal year.

From a nursing perspective, when complementary therapies are provided in hospitals as part of nursing care, third-party reimbursement is not an issue, as the cost is folded into the overall cost of the hospitalization or these services are financially supported through philanthropy. Although this may enrich the role responsibilities of nurses and be beneficial to patients, adding this care component likely increases time demands for nurses and may not be associated with a commensurate increase or adjustment in staffing. Advanced practice nurses such as nurse practitioners who are providing complementary therapies as part of their primary care practice in outpatient settings face the same challenges and constraints as physician colleagues—that is, the services may or may not be reimbursed depending on the health plan, the patient's condition, and the type of service provided.

Both the White House Commission and the IOM reports addressed the policy issue of CAM coverage and reimbursement. The White House Commission recommended that insurers and managed care organizations offer purchasers (usually employers) the option of health benefit plans that incorporate coverage of safe and effective CAM interventions provided by qualified practitioners. The IOM recommendations were less prescriptive and focused on the importance of generating research that addresses the outcomes and costs of combinations of CAM and conventional medical treatments and models that deliver such care.

REGULATION OF PRACTICE

As nurses work within interdisciplinary teams that include CAM practitioners, it is important to understand how CAM practitioners are regulated as well as how state boards of nursing regulate the practice of nurses who incorporate the use of complementary therapies into their practice. States vary considerably in the regulatory frameworks established to govern the practice of complementary therapies. From a policy perspective, what is often weighed is protection of public safety versus assuring the public access to complementary approaches to healing. As detailed in the White House Commission report, some states such as Minnesota provide almost unlimited freedom to practice, thus assuring consumers broad access to services. Unlicensed CAM practitioners in Minnesota must inform clients of their education, experience, and intended treatments, as well as possible side effects or known risks of treatments. Clients must sign an informed consent statement and are informed that complaints may be filed with the state department of health. In contrast, the state of Washington has adopted a much more tightly regulated environment. Washington provides licensure, registration, or exemption for various categories of CAM professionals. Regulations delineate the standards of practice; scope of practice; education and training requirements for licensure, registration, or exemption; and required professional oversight.

State boards of nursing have also varied in how they have approached the practice of complementary therapies by nurses. In a survey of boards of nursing, Sparber (2001) found that 47% of the boards permitted nurses to practice a range of CAM therapies, and an additional 13% were in the process of discussing whether or not to allow nurses to practice such therapies. Minnesota (Minnesota Board of Nursing, 2003) is an example of a state that has adopted a formal statement on the use of integrative therapies in nursing practice. Rather than specify what therapies nurses can and cannot provide, the document states that nurses who employ integrative therapies in their nursing practice are held to the same accountability for reasonable skill and safety as they are with the implementation of conventional treatment modalities.

RESEARCH

To advance the integration of complementary therapies, it is clear from a policy perspective that it is most critical to further develop the evidence base. Access to services is clearly tied to reimbursement, and reimbursement, in turn, is related to evidence. As noted in the IOM report (National Academy of Sciences, 2005), decisions about the use of complementary therapies should primarily depend on whether or not such therapies have been shown to be safe and effective. In addition to clinical research, basic science and health services research is necessary to help elucidate the mechanism of action underlying various complementary therapies and the cost-effectiveness and outcomes associated with various models of care delivery that integrate CAM with conventional care.

Other NIH centers and institutes fund research in complementary therapies including the National Institute for Nursing Research (NINR). Although funding for NCCAM, NINR, and CAM overall has increased over the past 5 years, in 2008 total NIH funding for CAM research was estimated to be $298 million, which constitutes less than 1% of the overall NIH budget (NCCAM, 2009).

As consumer demand for access to complementary therapies continues to grow, it is clear that access will be related to reimbursement and in turn, reimbursement directly linked to evidence. Thus, research is a critical political tool to change policy.

For a list of related websites, please refer to your Evolve Resources at http://evolve.elsevier.com/Mason/policypolitics/

REFERENCES

American Association of Colleges of Nursing (AACN). (2008). *The essentials of baccalaureate education for professional nursing practice.* Washington D.C.: American Association of Colleges of Nursing.

Ananth, S. (2002). *Health Forum/AHA 2000-2001 Complementary and Alternative Medicine Survey.* Chicago: Health Forum.

Astin, J. A. (1998). Why patients use alternative medicine: Results of a national study. *Journal of the American Medical Association, 279*(19), 1548-1553.

Barnes P. M., Bloom B., Nahin R. (2008, December 10). *CDC National Health Statistics report #12. Complementary and alternative medicine use among adults and children: United States, 2007.*

Barnes, R., Powell-Griner, E., McFann, K., & Nahin, R. (2004, May 27). Complementary and alternative medicine use among adults: United States, 2002. Advance data from vital and health statistics (no. 343). Data from the 2002 National Health Interview Survey (NHIS), conducted by the Centers for Disease Control and Prevention's (CDC) National Center for Health Statistics (NCHS). *Advance Data, May 27*(343), 1-19.

Cleary-Guida, M. B., Okvat, H. A., Oz, M. C., & Ting, W. (2001). A regional survey of health insurance coverage for complementary and alternative medicine: Current status and future ramifications. *Journal of Alternative and Complementary Medicine, 7*(3), 269-273.

Consortium of Academic Health Centers for Integrative Medicine (CAHCIM) (2009). Definition of integration medicine. Retrieved from www.imconsortium.org/about/home.html.

Dossey, B. M. (2000). *Florence Nightingale: Mystic, visionary, healer.* Springhouse, PA: Springhouse.

Eisenberg, D. M., Davis R. B., Ettner, S. L., Appel, S., Wilkey, S., Van Rompay, M., & Kessler, R. C. (1998). Trends in alternative medicine use in the United States, 1990-1997: Results of a national follow-up survey. *Journal of the American Medical Association, 280*(18), 1569-1575.

Institute of Medicine. (2005). *Complementary and alternative medicine in the United States.* Washington, D.C.: National Academies Press.

Institute of Medicine. (2009). Retrieved from www.iom.edu/integrativemedicine.

Kreitzer, M. J., & Disch, J. (2003). Leading the way: The Gillette Nursing Summit on Integrated Health and Healing. *Alternative Therapies in Health and Medicine Special Supplement, 9*(1), S2-S9.

Minnesota Board of Nursing. (2003). *Statement of accountability for utilization of integrative therapies in nursing practice.* Minnesota Board of Nursing. Retrieved from www.nursingboard.state.mn.us.

National Academy of Sciences. (2005). *Complementary and alternative medicine in the United States.* Retrieved from www.nap.edu.

National Center for Complementary and Alternative Medicine (NCCAM). (2009). *Expanding horizons in medical care: Strategic plan 2005-2009.* NIH Publication No. 04-5568. Washington, D.C.: U.S. Department of Health and Human Services, National Institutes of Health.

Sparber, A. (2001). State boards of nursing and scope of practice of registered nurses performing complementary therapies. *Online Journal of Issues in Nursing, 6*(3), 10.

U.S. Senate Committee on Health, Education, Labor and Pensions. (2009). Hearings and Executive Sessions. Retrieved from http://help.senate.gov/Hearings.html.

White House Commission on Complementary and Alternative Medicine Policy. (2002). Final report. Retrieved from www.whccamp.hhs.gov/finalreport.html.

CHAPTER 28

Nursing's Influence on Drug Development and Safety

Ruth Merkatz and Elyse I. Summers

"Get to the table and be a player, or someone who does not understand nursing will do that for you."
—Loretta Ford, EdD, RN, PNP, FAAN, FAANP

Americans take a lot of medicine. Pharmaceutical drugs are available because of a robust research infrastructure that works in tandem with the United States Food and Drug Administration's (FDA's) review and approval process and allows for new, innovative treatments to become available to a populace clamoring for cures for life-threatening or chronic illnesses. As this chapter explains, with so many drugs being used by so many people, it is of paramount importance that the safety and efficacy of these products be demonstrated and monitored over time. Nurses help assure the safety and welfare of research participants and patients during development, early-phase use, and the postapproval monitoring periods of these life-enhancing and life-saving products.

For decades, Americans have been enthusiastic consumers of the thousands[1] of drugs approved for use in this country. And, as we moved from the late twentieth century into the first decade of the twenty-first century, U.S. prescription drug use continued to grow. The Centers for Disease Control and Prevention's (CDC's) National Center for Health Statistics (NCHS) National Health and Nutrition Examination Survey (NHNES) surveyed individuals regarding their "prescription drug use in the past month," during the years 1988 to 1994. In this survey, almost 40% of the American populace had used a prescription drug in the course of a month's time (NHNES, 2008). By the

agency's most recent survey, 2001 to 2004, the figure had grown to close to 50% (NHNES, 2008).

Regardless of the survey time frame, the most significant factor in prescription drug usage is age. From 1988 to 1994, almost 74% of individuals 65 years and older reported drug use (NHNES, 2008); from 2001 to 2004, it was 87% for this same cohort (NHNES, 2008). Moreover, between 1988 and 1994 and between 2001 and 2004, the elder group increased the number of medications they were using. Just over 35% of this cohort reported using three or more prescription drugs in the earlier time frame, a figure that rose to almost 60% in the early 2000s (NHNES, 2008).

The trend in U.S. medication is clear. In any given week, a solid majority of the population (81% of adults) will take at least one prescription or non-prescription medication; many will use at least one prescription drug (50% of adults), and some will take five or more (7% of adults) (Kaufman et al., 2002).

HISTORICAL BACKGROUND

For drugs to be available to American consumers, they are to be safe and effective. However, this was not always the case. The central role the FDA now occupies on the bench-to-bedside continuum took years to establish and is, in some ways, ever-evolving. The oldest comprehensive consumer protection agency in the U.S. federal government, the FDA's activities trace back to the mid-1800s when a section within the Patent Office began carrying out chemical analyses of agricultural products (U.S. Food and Drug Administration [FDA], n.d.-a).

The 1906 Wiley Act was the first U.S. law to prohibit interstate commerce of adulterated and misbranded food and drugs. However, it wasn't until

---

[1]More than 2400 prescription drugs are listed in the *2010 Physician's Desk Reference*, 64th ed. Available at *www.pdrbookstore.com*.

after the 1937 sulfanilamide tragedy that the FDA gained meaningful authority to ensure drug safety. Elixir of Sulfanilamide, marketed as a new sulfa wonder drug that children could ingest easily, was actually prepared with a highly toxic chemical analogue of anti-freeze that led to the deaths of more than 100 children (Ballentine, 1981). The result of this tragedy and subsequent public exposure was the Food, Drug, and Cosmetic Act of 1938. This law mandated premarket approval of all new drugs based on a demonstration of safety to the FDA; it authorized FDA inspection of manufacturing facilities; and, it granted FDA authority over cosmetics and medical devices. In 1962, the thalidomide disaster, centered in Europe, prompted the expansion of the FDA's regulatory purview to also include "effectiveness." Outside the U.S., thalidomide had been marketed as another "wonder drug," but its use by pregnant women resulted in the birth of thousands of severely deformed babies (phocomelia defect). Alarmed by the European experience, U.S. Senator Estes Kefauver held hearings on the American drug approval process, pushed for, and ultimately secured passage of the Kefauver-Harris Amendments (FDA, n.d.-b).

The Kefauver-Harris Amendments required the FDA to assess the efficacy of all drugs introduced since 1938; instituted stricter agency control over drug trials (including formal introduction of the concept of and requirement for patient informed consent in drug trials); transferred to the FDA from the Federal Trade Commission regulation of prescription drug advertising; established good manufacturing practices as a drug industry requirement; and granted the FDA greater powers of inspection and enforcement.

CURRENT DRUG APPROVAL FRAMEWORK

Since the 1962 amendments, new drug development has become an increasingly costly, time-consuming endeavor (DeMasi, Hansen, & Grabowski, 2003). Estimates on the amount of time it now takes for a new compound to reach approval are as high as 12 to 13 years (Figure 28-1).

Generally speaking, new drug discovery and development proceeds in a sequence of phases, sometimes overlapping (DeMasi et al., 2003). Prior to any human testing, a new drug's sponsor, typically a pharmaceutical company, but sometimes, a non-governmental organization or government agency, tests a new compound in assays and animal models. If encouraged by the results, the sponsor submits to the FDA

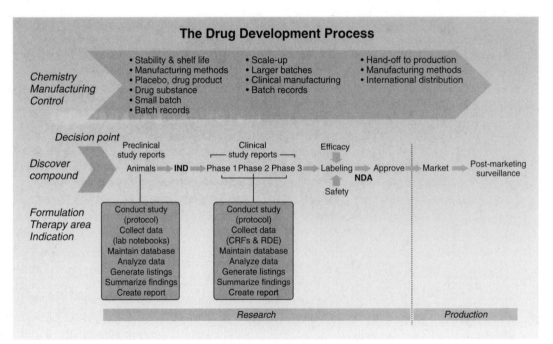

FIGURE 28-1 The drug development process.

an investigational new drug application (IND) that contains all known information about the compound, including manufacturing information to demonstrate that the test article can be produced consistently with high quality. The IND also specifies the clinical research plan and protocol for phase 1 studies. Unless the FDA affirmatively objects, the IND is automatically allowed after 30 days, and human clinical trials can begin. In accordance with federal regulations, local institutional review boards (IRBs) charged with protecting research participants must approve these trials (FDA Protection of Human Subjects Regulations, 1980; FDA Institutional Review Board Regulations, 1981). IRBs review protocols relative to their scientific merit, risks and benefits, and procedures for gaining informed consent. They are also expected to review plans for recruiting volunteers to avert inappropriate incentives or coercive tactics (FDA Protection of Human Subjects Regulations, 1980; FDA Institutional Review Board Regulations, 1981).

A drug's premarket clinical testing must proceed through three successive phases consistent with the required safety and efficacy standards. In Phase 1, a small number of usually healthy volunteers are given the drug to establish safe dosages, and characterize the absorption, distribution, metabolic effects, and excretion (ADME) of the drug. These data help determine the drug's pharmacokinetic (PK) profile (the way the body processes a drug), its tolerability and safety profile, and pharmacodynamics (PD), the way the drug works in the body. Phase 2 trials include a few hundred volunteers who have the targeted disease or condition to determine an effective dose and to begin to evaluate efficacy and short-term risks. In Phase 3, studies are conducted to evaluate safety and efficacy in several hundred to several thousand patients or volunteers at risk for the drug's targeted condition (e.g. a new female contraceptive is tested in women at risk for pregnancy; a colon cancer treatment is tested in people with this condition). Depending on a drug's indication, testing occurs in hospitals and/or outpatient settings. Phase 3 studies are usually randomized, controlled multicenter trials with results of the new drug tested against an approved standard therapeutic agent (sometimes referred to as the "gold standard"). The goal of these studies is to gather precise information on a drug's effectiveness for specific indications, determine whether or not the drug produces a broader range of adverse events (AEs)

than those exhibited in the smaller Phase 1 and 2 study populations, and identify the best way to administer and use the drug for its intended purpose. These studies also can uncover infrequent side effects.

Once a sponsor has finished preclinical and clinical testing, analyzed the data, and written reports in accordance with regulatory guidelines, it can compile and submit a new drug application (NDA) to the FDA, which will assess it for completeness before filing and initiating its review. In addition to the aforementioned components, the NDA must also include detailed chemistry, manufacturing and quality controls (CMC) documentation to ensure that the marketed product will adhere to consistent safety and purity standards.

In accordance with a time frame mandated by the Prescription Drug User Fee Act (PDUFA) that took effect initially in 1993, the FDA must complete its review in a timely fashion. The approval process for most new drugs takes 12 months on average, while priority applications are generally reviewed within 6 months.

During the review period, the FDA may seek clarification of data contained in the NDA or ask for new information. To augment its internal review, the FDA sometimes will convene an advisory "expert" panel to discuss the NDA publicly and advise the agency regarding the new drug's approvability. These panels are comprised of health professionals with expertise in the therapeutic area applicable to the drug under review, including statisticians and/or epidemiologists, and generally a consumer and industry representative. Historically and currently, physicians compose the majority of health professional representatives to these panels. On occasion, nurses are invited to serve, but often as consumer representatives who may or may not be voting members.

As part of the approval process, information gleaned during the phases of drug testing forms the basis for product labeling information. The FDA's guidance on drug labeling ensures that package inserts include the same types of information in a standardized format, although the titles may vary according to manufacturer preference. Developing this label is a lengthy process that often includes heated negotiation between sponsor representatives and FDA staff regarding the exact wording of an approved drug label. Every single word is important. Adding an indication or removing a contraindication can have a several-million-, even billion-dollar impact for a sponsor as well as significant health consequences for the medication-taking public. The addition of a "black box" warning (the strongest warning the FDA issues in its drug labeling) on antidepressants prescribed to children and adolescents, for example, not only reduced prescriptions for selective serotonin reuptake inhibitors (SSRIs) by an estimated 22% in the U.S., but also was associated with reducing aggregate rates of diagnosis and treatment of pediatric depression (Gibbons et al., 2007; Libby et al., 2007). A label's contents, therefore, are of paramount importance to nurses who care for patients and/or are responsible for updating other nurses on labeling changes.

POSTMARKETING SURVEILLANCE

Participants in clinical trials prior to marketing must meet strict inclusion/exclusion criteria to minimize safety risks and to increase the likelihood of achieving reliable results. Consequently, clinical trial populations may not necessarily represent typical users of drugs once approved and released into the marketplace. Eligibility criteria for clinical trial volunteers, for example, often require confirmation of normal kidney and liver function as measured through serum chemistries such as creatine clearance, blood urea nitrogen, SGOT (AST), and SGPT (ALT). Abnormalities of these functions can limit participation, especially among older adults and those with chronic conditions who may fail to meet eligibility criteria. Given that most drugs are metabolized through the liver or kidneys, which affects drug metabolism and excretion and influences concentration of drugs in the tissues, eliminating such groups during clinical trials can result in biased or incomplete results relative to both safety and efficacy, and may mask toxicities (Benet, Massoud & Gambertoglio, 1984; Rowland & Tozer, 1995). Also, the relative size of trials included in the development process is small (e.g., 300 to 3000 volunteers) compared to the much larger number of individuals who will take a drug once available— another factor that can limit wide generalizations of clinical trial results. And due to the limited duration of trials, data from volunteer usage of a new drug generally cannot reveal long-term effects. Once marketed, a new drug may also be prescribed for unapproved uses not specified on the drug label and/or

TABLE 28-1 Chronology of Significant U.S. Drug Withdrawals (2000-2009)

Year	Drug	Reason for Withdrawal
2009	Efalizumab (Raptiva)	Increased risk of progressive multifocal leukoencephalopathy
2008	Aprotinin (Trasylol)	Increased risk of death
2007	Tegaserod (Zelnorm)	Increased risk of serious cardiovascular adverse events
2007	Pergolide (Permax)	Risk of heart valve damage
2006	Gatifloxacin (Tequin)	Liver damage
2005	Natalizumab (Tysabri)	Progressive multifocal leukoencephalopathy
2005	Pemoline (Cylert)	Liver toxicity
2005	Hydromorphone extended-release (Palladone)	High risk of accidental overdose when taken with alcohol
2004	Rofecoxib (Vioxx)	Increased risk of CV events, including MI and stroke
2001	Rapacuronium (Raplon)	Risk of fatal bronchospasm; unexplained fatalities
2001	Cerivastatin (Baycol)	Risk of fatal rhabdomyolysis
2000	Phenylpropanolamine (i.e., Dexatrim)	Risk of hemorrhagic stroke
2000	Cisapride (Propulsid)	Risk of serious cardiac arrhythmias and death
2000	Alosetron (Lotronex)	Risk of fatal complications of constipation
2000	Troglitazone (Rezulin)	Risk of irreversible liver damage and liver failure

Source: *www.fda.gov.*

prescribed along with other medications that can alter the known PK and PD. While sponsors typically study the way a new drug interacts with certain other types of drugs, it is impossible to identify all potential interactions. Ultimately, all of these scenarios compound risks that could not have been identified easily during the time-sensitive drug-approval process, but then emerge post-marketing. That is why evidence is accumulating for vigilant post-marketing surveillance and why a number of drugs either have received strict safety warnings after approval, including the black box warning, or been withdrawn from the market (Table 28-1).

The situation with Avandia illustrates how wider distribution following approval can alter a specific drug's safety profile. Approved in 1999, Avandia seemed the perfect replacement to a predecessor and chemically related Type II diabetes treatment, Rezulin (troglitazone), which had been prescribed widely. In March 2000, the manufacturer removed Rezulin from the market following 63 confirmed deaths from liver failure, case reports of acute hepatotoxicity, and strong urging from the FDA (Avorn, 2007).

Since Avandia's approval, however, numerous investigators and practitioners have identified cardiovascular risks, and results from a meta-analysis suggest a 43% increase in the rate of heart attacks among study participants (Nissen and Wolski, 2007). This information prompted the FDA to issue a safety alert, and convene a meeting of its Endocrinology and Metabolic Drugs, and Drug Safety and Risk Management Advisory Committees to review the data and determine an appropriate course of action. Subsequently, in November 2007, FDA "officially" required black box labeling for Avandia. Despite these actions, questions about Avandia have persisted, including mounting controversy about adverse event (AE) reporting and another FDA advisory panel was convened in July 2010 (DeAngelis & Fontanarosa, 2010; Nissen, 2010). Following testimony and presentation of currently available data, the 33 panelists voted 20-12 (with 1 abstention) to keep the drug on the market. The majority's opinion was that the risks were not severe enough to justify removing a drug used by hundreds of thousands of patients. Ten members, however, called for stricter prescribing limitations. The FDA generally follows the advice of its advisory panels, and a final decision by the agency was pending in Fall 2010 (American Heart Association, 2010).

The story of Avandia, as well as safety concerns of other widely publicized drugs, highlights the relevancy of recommendations made by the Institute of Medicine Committee on the Assessment of the U.S. Drug Safety System (Institute of Medicine [IOM], 2006a). That committee, chaired by Sheila Burke, MPA, RN, urged that the FDA needed the leadership and authority to require manufacturers to conduct high-quality postmarketing trials of selected drugs. The committee also shed light on several other FDA shortcomings that required action or change. Subsequent to the publication of the 2006 IOM report, Congress passed the Food and Drug Administration Amendments Act of 2007 (FDAAA), which derives much of its content from the IOM report (Box 28-1). Rather than requesting drug manufacturers to *voluntarily* comply with

---

BOX 28-1 Institute of Medicine Committee on the Assessment of U.S. Drug Safety System: Major Recommendations

- Urged labeling requirements and advertising limits for new medications
- Clarified authority and additional enforcement tools for the FDA
- Reiterated the FDA's role in gathering and communicating additional information on marketed products' risks and benefits
- Advised mandatory registration of clinical trial results for public access to drug safety information
- Pushed for an increased role for the FDA's drug safety staff
- Advocated a significant boost in agency funding and staffing

Source: Institute of Medicine. (2006). *The future of drug safety: Promoting and protecting the health of the public.* Washington, D.C.: Institute of Medicine of the National Academies, National Academies Press.

---

postmarketing commitments, the FDAAA gave the agency the authority to *require* postmarketing studies following approval of certain new drugs. Between implementation of the FDAAA in 2007 and the end of 2008, the FDA approved 29 drugs for which sponsors are now required to conduct formal postmarketing safety studies (Hamburg, 2009; FDA makes postmarket safety evaluation comprehensive for all NMEs, BLAs, 2009).

Other sections of the FDAAA specified that following approval of a new drug, sponsors must (1) prepare labeling changes based on new safety information that emerges post-marketing, (2) develop risk evaluation and mitigation strategies (REMS) to be implemented upon marketing a new drug, (3) continue to notify the FDA within 15 days of hearing about any serious adverse events (SAEs), as under already existing regulations, and (4) provide quarterly safety reports to the FDA for the first 3 years after a drug is approved, followed by annual reports after that. These reports include analysis and summary of adverse events and any new information from studies initiated as a result of these events. Additionally, the FDAAA gave the FDA authority to impose civil penalties, among other enforcement tools, for violations to FDAAA requirements. The FDA also established a new Office of Drug Safety and changed one of the FDA's most criticized practices, whereby drug reviewers responsible for product approvals maintained sole responsibility for their continued oversight, even when safety issues arose. Viewed as a conflict of interest, the FDA's Office of Drug Safety now pursues postmarketing safety concerns with the aid of those initial reviewers and others.

NURSES AS ADVOCATES TO IMPROVE DRUG SAFETY

With inherent limitations to data collected during premarketing clinical trials (as described above), an overstretched FDA confronting necessities for change, drug companies racing to develop and sell products as quickly as possible, and patients eager to try new therapies to improve their health status, it ultimately comes down to grassroots practitioners and policymakers to identify and prevent potential drug safety problems. Nurses can play a prominent role by overseeing their own practices and establishing policies that include exercising a major voice in local, state, and federal efforts to promote safety for patients. A 2006 report by another IOM committee, also co-chaired by a nurse, Linda Cronenwett, estimated that 1.5 million preventable adverse drug events occur each year (IOM, 2006b). As a result, policymakers have been exploring interventions to improve drug safety and nurses play a pivotal role, A nursing perspective is important during clinical trials prior to drug approval, in health care settings as new drugs are introduced and use is broadened, and as part of committee proceedings when policy and even legislation is being formulated.

During drug development, nurses often are the "face" of clinical trials to participants. They may serve as study coordinators with responsibility for obtaining potential participants' informed consent, a critical task consistent with professional obligations to protect research participants (American Nurses Association [ANA], 2001). A thorough understanding of all aspects of a study protocol for an investigational drug is required to explain and determine if participants are informed adequately about risks, benefits, and participation requirements. As described earlier, before a study begins, a local IRB will review and must approve the protocol. Nursing representation on IRBs is important. During reviews, a nursing perspective can help ensure clarity of information in all sections of study protocols, including procedures to be followed and readability of the informed consent document. A solid informed consent procedure can enhance protocol adherence and, in turn, the usefulness of trial results. The process should empower participants with knowledge, and open channels of communication with health care providers, especially in relation to timely reporting of AEs and SAEs. To maximize the benefits to all stakeholders, both providers and participants must work in partnership to identify and report both AEs and SAEs (Basch, 2010). This information will be critical to the FDA for decisions about drug approvals and labeling. For nurses to be effective in AE identification and reporting, they must utilize observational, interviewing, and clinical skills and must also track and understand implications of changes in biochemical (laboratory) assessments. Nurses may be the first to identify potential investigational drug toxicities and report these to investigators, IRBs, and regulatory authorities in accordance with regulatory requirements and professional obligations.

AE occurrences are hardly confined to clinical trials. Reporting must continue postmarketing, especially for newly released drugs. In the 1990s, it was estimated that 3% to 11% of hospital admissions resulted from adverse drug events (Couig & Merkatz, 1993). More recent data suggest that AEs cause 3.6 million physician's office visits per year, 700,000 emergency department visits, and 117,000 hospitalizations (Budnitz et al., 2006; Zhan et al., 2005). Patient age is a major factor. Among emergency department visits, ages older than 65 or younger than 5 placed patients at a much greater risk for AEs (IOM, 2008), most likely related to the number of medications taken and the risk for drug-drug interactions.

The issue of identifying postmarketing safety issues prompted the FDA Commissioner in 1993, David Kessler, to launch MedWatch and its accompanying database, the Adverse Event Reporting System (AERS). This system encourages health care professionals and patients to report AEs to the FDA using a standardized format. Today, the FDA receives more than 400,000 AE reports annually from providers and consumers. Providers seem more aware of the importance and process for AE reporting (IOM, 2007). Still, the FDA estimates that only 1 in 10 AEs is reported (IOM, 2007) with nurses contributing 11% of health care provider–submitted AE reports (Trontell, 2004). While the FDA's AE reporting systems are always evolving and improving, the success of active or voluntary surveillance rests with vigilant health care providers, especially nurses, who are knowledgeable about their patients' conditions and their treatments. They must be aware and utilize information on drug labels to identify expected or unexpected side effects and report these appropriately and quickly (IOM, 2007).

Nurses must also be cognizant of patients' understanding about their medications. It is well known that even simplified labeling can pose comprehension problems for patients (IOM, 2008). Approximately 46% of patients across all literacy levels misunderstand one or more dosage instructions, and 54% misunderstand one or more auxiliary warnings, (e.g., "Take with Food") that stand out separately on medication packaging (IOM, 2008). Nurses can identify and help to clarify such instructions with patients. Concurrently, nurses can educate patients regarding known side effects and stress the importance of reporting AEs promptly.

NURSING LEADERSHIP: POLICY AND PRACTICE

No drug will ever be proven risk-free. Additionally, no breadth of reform will create a regulatory agency or collection of agencies that can identify all risks prior to drug approvals or prevent SAEs from occurring. Nevertheless, nursing policies can be strengthened and implemented that contribute to national efforts to reduce drug toxicities. We must endorse strong policies, even reform, in both nursing education and practice related to aspects of drug development and postmarketing surveillance aimed at safeguarding patients and the public at large. The following efforts are recommended:

1. Nursing policies should encourage contributions by nurses during drug development, such as representation on IRBs and active collaboration and leadership by nurses in conducting clinical trials. The recent ANA policy statement, Promoting Safe Medication Use in the Older Adult, advocates nursing research in a number of areas, including pharmacodynamics and pharmaceutics in older adults across the continuum of care (ANA, 2009a). Research of this nature is also needed for specific population groups such as children and pregnant women, who historically have been excluded from clinical trials (Merkatz, Temple, Sobel, Feiden, & Kessler, 1993). FDA guidances encourage studies in both of these groups as well as pharmacokinetic studies in pregnant women (FDA, 2004). Support from the National Institute of Nursing Research and other NIH institutes for this type of pharmacologic research by nurse investigators, inclusive of interdisciplinary approaches, is essential.

2. Nursing curriculums at all levels must include and strengthen content related to pharmacology. Nurses need to know how drugs are developed and marketed, and they must be familiar with the effects that patient-specific characteristics (e.g., age, sex, and polypharmacy) may have on a drug's PK and PD (Merkatz et al., 1993). They must be knowledgeable about reading drug labels.

3. Nurses must understand and fulfill their professional responsibility to report AEs and must take a leadership role in all patient care settings, including the home, to track and report systematically drug-related SAEs and AEs. Working in partnership with their patients, they should encourage self-reporting to enhance timely alerts of safety problems. During clinical trials, the informed consent process should include clear instructions on how and to whom AEs should be reported, and postmarketing policies must be in place to ensure appropriate and timely AE reporting. Expanded use of electronic medical records is advocated to facilitate this process (Thiede, 2010; ANA, 2009b). Additionally, it is recommended that states offer continuing medical education programs that include information about reporting AEs and SAEs, including the mechanics of reporting. State licensing boards might even consider mandating such programs.

4. Policies should be in place in all patient care settings to ensure that nurses can access reliable new information about marketed drugs. Using modern methods of communication technology, drug alerts should be distributed for newly approved drugs along with the most current information about their AEs. While news about drug problems and withdrawals is often covered in popular press, such information is not always accurate and often is limited in scope. Reliable sources should be used for broad dissemination. For example, the FDA's Office of Special Health Issues (OSHI) serves as a liaison between the FDA and health professional organizations, dispatching alerts regularly. The OSHI encourages and supports active participation of these groups in forming FDA regulatory

policy, which serves as the cornerstone to the FDA's new Safe Use Initiative, launched in November 2009. More information about this initiative is available at *www.fda.gov/Drugs/DrugSafety/ucm187806.htm.*

5. Finally, it is recommended that nurses play an active role in collaborating with the FDA in its mission to ensure that drugs are safe and effective. While nurses have and continue to hold leadership positions at the agency, heightened outside influence from nursing organizations is required. Whether acting alone or through nursing organizations, nurses should utilize the full panoply of opportunities to take part in FDA public processes including, but not limited to: developing and submitting comments in response to proposed rules and guidances published in the Federal Register; providing meaningful testimony during public comment portions of advisory committee meetings, such as the Avandia advisory committee meeting held July 13-14, 2010 (speakers included 9 physicians, 1 patient, and presidents from 2 different organizations focused either on consumers or women and families; there was no testimony given on behalf of a nursing organization or by a nurse); and preparing written correspondence that could then be followed by face-to-face meetings with FDA leaders. Such meetings can provide opportunities to advocate for specific measures to promote safe use of medications and, importantly, to advocate for enhanced nursing participation as voting members on advisory committees. Currently there are 16 advisory committees in the Center for Drug Evaluation and Research (CDER) that have, on average, 12 to 13 voting members each. A mere two of these several dozen voting advisory committee members currently are nurses. As the largest group of caregivers in our nation, this situation must change. Nursing leaders should begin in earnest to nominate qualified colleagues to serve on FDA advisory committees and set into motion a series of measures to encourage a stronger, more influential relationship with the nation's agency charged with ensuring safe and effective use of medications.

For a list of related websites, please refer to your Evolve Resources at http://evolve.elsevier.com/Mason/policypolitics/

REFERENCES

American Nurses Association. (2001). 3.3: Protection of participants in research. *The code of ethics for nurses with interpretive statements.* Retrieved from http://nursingworld.org/ethics/code/protected_nwcoe813.htm#3.3.

American Nurses Association. (2009a). Promoting safe medication use in the older adult. Retrieved from www.nursingworld.org/NursingPractice.

American Nurses Association. (2009b). Electronic health record: position statement. Retrieved from www.nursingworld.org/NursingPractice.

American Heart Association. (2010). Advisory Committee recommends that U.S. Food and Drug Administration keep rosiglitazone (Avandia) on the market, continue clinical trial of safety and efficacy. Retrieved from www.newsroom.heart.org/index.php?s=43&item=1081.

Avorn, J. (2007). Keeping science on top in drug evaluation. *New England Journal of Medicine, 357*(7), 633-635. Retrieved from http://content.nejm.org/cgi/content/full/357/7/633.

Ballentine, C. (1981). Taste of raspberries, taste of death: The 1937 elixir sulfanilamide incident. *FDA Consumer Magazine, 15*(5). Retrieved from www.fda.gov/AboutFDA/WhatWeDo/History/ProductRegulation/SulfanilamideDisaster/default.htm.

Basch, E. (2010). The missing voice of patients in drug-safety reporting. *New England Journal of Medicine, 362*(10), 865-869. Retrieved from http://content.nejm.org/cgi/content/full/362/10/865.

Benet, L. Z., Massoud, N., & Gambertoglio, J. G. (1984). *Pharmacokinetic basis for drug treatment.* New York: Raven Press.

Budnitz, D. S., Pollock, D. A., Weidenbach, K. N., Mendelsohn, A. B., Schroeder, T. J., & Annest, J. L. (2006). National surveillance of emergency department visits for outpatient adverse drug events. *Journal of the American Medical Association, 296*(15), 1858-1866.

Couig, M. P., & Merkatz, R. B. (1993). From FDA Nurses: MedWatch: The new medical products reporting program. *American Journal of Nursing, 93*(8), 65-68. Retrieved from www.jstor.org/pss/3464254.

DeAngelis, C. D., & Fontanarosa, P. B. (2010). Ensuring integrity in industry-sponsored research. *Journal of the American Medical Association, 303*(12), 1196-1198. Retrieved from http://jama.ama-assn.org/cgi/content/full/303/12/1196?home#REF-JED05016-1.

DeMasi, J. A., Hansen, R. W., & Grabowski, H. G. (2003). The price of innovation: New estimates of drug development costs. *Journal of Health Economics, 22*(2), 151-185.

FDA makes post-market safety evaluation comprehensive for all NMEs, BLAs. (2009). *The Pink Sheet, 71*(42), 18-19.

Gibbons, R. D., Brown C. H., Hur, K., Marcus, S. M., Bhaumik, D. K., Erkens, J. A., Herings, R. M., & Mann J. J. (2007). Early evidence on the effects of regulators' suicidality warnings on SSRI prescriptions and suicide in children and adolescents. *American Journal of Psychiatry, 164*(9), 1356-1363.

Hamburg, M. A. (2009, July 31). Report to Congress: Changing the future of drug safety: FDA initiatives to strengthen and transform the drug safety system.

Institute of Medicine. (2006a). *The future of drug safety: Promoting and protecting the health of the public.* Washington, D.C.: Institute of Medicine of the National Academies, National Academies Press.

Institute of Medicine. (2006b). *Preventing medication errors: quality chasm series.* Washington, D.C.: Institute of Medicine of the National Academies, National Academies Press.

Institute of Medicine. (2007). *Workshop summary of adverse drug event reporting: The roles of consumers and health-care professionals, forum on drug discovery, development, and translation.* Washington, D.C.: Institute of Medicine of the National Academies, National Academies Press.

Institute of Medicine. (2008). *Standardizing medication labels: Confusing patients less, workshop summary.* Washington, D.C.: Institute of Medicine of the National Academies, National Academies Press.

Kaufman, D. W., Kelly, J. P., Rosenberg, L., Anderson, T. E., & Mitchell, A. A. (2002). Recent patterns of medication use in the ambulatory adult population of the United States: The Slone survey. *Journal of the American Medical Association, 287*(3), 337-344.

Libby, A. M., Brent, D. A., Morrato, E. H., Orton, H. D., Allen, R., & Valuck, R. J. (2007). Decline in treatment of pediatric depression after FDA advisory on risk of suicidality with SSRIs. *American Journal of Psychiatry, 164*(6), 884-891.

Merkatz, R. B., Temple, R., Sobel, S., Feiden, K., & Kessler, D. K. (1993). Women in clinical trials of new drugs—A change in Food and Drug Administration Policy. *New England Journal of Medicine, 329*(4), 292-296.

National Center for Health Statistics. Centers for Disease Control and Prevention. (2008). *National Health and Nutrition Examination Survey.*

Nissen, S. E. (2010). Setting the RECORD straight. *Journal of the American Medical Association, 303*(12), 1194-1195. Retrieved from http://jama.ama-assn.org/cgi/content/full/303/12/1194?ijkey=af1095e0628ad51b44613efa30055423c2f2bc7a&keytype2=tf_ipsecsha.

Nissen, S. E., & Wolski, K. (2007). Effect of rosiglitazone on the risk of myocardial infarction and death from cardiovascular causes. *New England Journal of Medicine, 356*(24), 2457-2471. Retrieved from http://content.nejm.org/cgi/content/full/NEJMoa072761.

Rowland, M., & Tozer, T. N. (1995). *Clinical pharmacokinetics: Concepts and applications* (3rd ed.). Philadelphia: Lippincott, Williams & Wilkins.

Thiede, L. (2010). Informatics: Electronic health records: A boon or privacy nightmare? *Online Journal of Issues in Nursing, 15*(2). Retrieved from www.nursingworld.org/MainMenuCategories/ANAMarketplace/ANAPeriodicals/OJIN/TableofContents/Vol152010/No2May2010/Electronic-Health-Records-and-Privacy.aspx.

Trontell, A. (2004). Expecting the unexpected—Drug safety, pharmacovigilance, and the prepared mind. *New England Journal of Medicine, 351*(14), 1385-1387.

U.S. Food and Drug Administration. (2004). Guidance for industry pharmacokinetics in pregnancy—Study design, data analysis, and impact on dosing and labeling. Retrieved from www.fda.gov/downloads/Drugs/GuidanceComplianceRegulatoryInformation/Guidances/ucm072133.pdf.

U.S. Food and Drug Administration. (nd-a). About FDA—History. Retrieved from www.fda.gov/AboutFDA/WhatWeDo/History/default.htm.

U.S. Food and Drug Administration. (nd-b). About FDA—FDA history—Part III. Retrieved from www.fda.gov/AboutFDA/WhatWeDo/History/Origin/ucm055118.htm.

U.S. Food and Drug Administration Department of Health & Human Services Food and Drugs Protection of Human Subjects Regulations, 21 C.F.R § 50 (1980).

U.S. Food and Drug Administration Department of Health & Human Services Food and Drugs Institutional Review Board Regulations, 21 C.F.R § 56 (1981).

Zhan, C., Arispe, I., Kelley, E., Ding, T., Burt, C. W., Shinogle, J., & Stryer, D. (2005). Ambulatory care visits for treating adverse drug effects in the United States, 1995-2001. *The Joint Commission Journal on Quality and Patient Safety, 31*(7), 372-378.

CHAPTER 29

Chronic Care Policy: Medical Homes and Primary Care

Susan Apold

"Change will not come if we wait for some other person or some other time. We are the ones we've been waiting for. We are the change that we seek."

—Barack Obama

Chronic conditions are the leading cause of death in the world and have replaced specific acute episodic disease as the number one cause of mortality and morbidity in the United States. (Yach, Hawkes, Gould, & Hofman, 2004; Centers for Disease Control and Prevention [CDC] & the Merck Company Foundation, 2007). Almost half of all adults in this country are living with at least one chronic condition (Robert Wood Johnson Foundation, 1996). This tectonic shift in the health profile of Americans has evolved over the last century as the result of an aging population; advances in public health; increasing knowledge of genetics; and improvements in pharmacology, research, and technology.

Because of the changing epidemiology of the nation, policymakers are beginning to reform the health care system by supporting innovative mechanisms to provide quality, cost-effective care, with an emphasis on management of chronic illness.

THE EXPERIENCE OF CHRONIC CARE IN THE UNITED STATES

Chronic illness is illness that continues indefinitely, limits activity, and requires ongoing activities and response from patients and caregivers (Larsen, 2009; Robert Wood Johnson Foundation, Partnership for Solutions, 2002). It is a relatively new phenomenon. In the early 1900s, the leading causes of mortality in the U.S. were tuberculosis, pneumonia, and gastritis/enteritis. The average life expectancy then was 47 years (National Center for Health Statistics, 1909). *Health care* was an oxymoron as diagnosis and treatment of disease were the only tools in the health care armamentarium. With only a rudimentary comprehension of the major causes of mortality and without antibiotics, insulin, and imaging ability, the sick were identified late in their illness (or not at all) and either got better or died. The care of the day was *illness care.* The system that was developed to handle disease was based on face-to-face encounters with physicians who provided a service in exchange for a fee. That fee-for-service system with an emphasis on illness management remains central to health care policy today.

A century later, life expectancy is 78.9 years (Social Security Online Actuarial Tables, 2010) and the first baby boomers are Medicare-eligible, challenging the nation's ability to effectively and efficiently manage the growing prevalence of chronic illness. Seven out of 10 deaths among Americans each year are a result of chronic disease (CDC, 2009). The most common chronic diseases in the U.S. are hypertension, chronic mental conditions, respiratory diseases, arthritis, eye disorders, asthma, cholesterol disorders, and diabetes. Among children, eye disorders, emotional/behavioral disorders, asthma, and other respiratory diseases account for the top four chronic problems (CDC & the Merck Company Foundation, 2007). One quarter of people with chronic conditions have activity limitation (Agency for Health Care Quality and Research, 1998).

Eighty percent of the causes of chronic illness are lifestyle-related and thus preventable. DeVol and colleagues (2007) estimate that if the health care system targeted prevention, the economic impact of chronic disease could be reduced by 27%. The CDC identifies preventable causes of chronic disease as: lack of physical activity, poor nutrition, tobacco use, and alcohol consumption. All of these are modifiable and with appropriate health counseling can prevent the majority of chronic disease (Robert Wood Johnson Foundation, 2002). Treatment of chronic disease accounts for more than 75% of the nation's health care budget. The financial impact on the U.S. economy of treatment and lost productivity caused by chronic illness is more than $1.3 trillion per year, with projections of an increase to $5.7 trillion by 2050 (Centers for Medicare and Medicaid Services, 2008). Lowering obesity rates alone would avoid $60 billion in treatment expenses (CDC, 2009; Dall, et al., 2010). While the majority of people with a chronic disease are under 65 years of age, the likelihood of having more than one chronic disease increases with age; 83% of all Medicare beneficiaries report at least one chronic condition (Anderson, 2005), and 23% of Medicare beneficiaries with five or more conditions account for 68% of the program's funding (DeVol et al., 2007).

Increases in health care spending have not translated into improvements in health care quality. In a fee-for-service episodic care model, research shows that care is fragmented and illness-based; patients frequently do not get the care that they want or need (Coleman, Austin, Brach, & Wagner, 2009; Mattke, Seid, & Ma, 2007). Neither federal entitlement programs nor private insurances have provided coverage for prevention or care management.

A CALL FOR CHRONIC CARE DELIVERY REFORM

Periodically, efforts have been made to manage cost and sporadically test models of care management. The earliest effort at cost control emerged in 1980 with the implementation of a prospective payment system utilizing diagnosis-related groups (DRGs). This shift from payment for any service consumed to regulated payment for specific diagnoses appears to have somewhat curbed Medicare spending, however prospective payment is rooted in an illness model and does not address disease management (Coulam & Gaumer, 1991).

In the early 1990s, Wagner determined that an orientation to acute episodic illness and lack of a system to educate patients regarding self management were barriers to quality chronic disease management. He developed the Chronic Care Model (CCM) and outlined the elements essential to high-quality chronic illness management (Wagner, 1998). The Robert Wood Johnson Foundation authorized a comprehensive evaluation of the CCM in the Improving Chronic Illness Care initiative and demonstrated that implementing the model in primary care practices improves chronic care outcomes (Nutting et al., 2009; Bodenheimer, Wagner, & Grumbach, 2002). However, reimbursement has been based on an episodic illness model.

In March, 2010, President Barack Obama signed HR 3590, The Affordable Care Act (ACA). This first major change in health care finance and delivery provides the seeds for overhauling the existing system, developing evidence-based models of prevention and chronic care provision, and testing a reimbursement infrastructure that will support health care for the majority of Americans.

MEDICAL HOMES

The initiative that has gained the most traction in blending quality and reimbursement has been the development of the Patient-Centered Medical Home. The concept of the "medical home" was first advanced by the American Academy of Pediatrics (AAP) in 1967 as a place where all medical information about a patient would be located (Sia, Tonniges, Osterhus, & Taba, 2004). The concept has since expanded and is defined as "a health care setting that provides patients with timely, well-organized care and enhanced access to providers" (Beal, Doty, Hernandez, Shea, & Davis, 2007, p. ix) and must be "patient centered." Gerteis and colleagues (2003) identified eight dimensions of patient-centered care (Box 29-1). Central to the success of a medical home is whole-person orientation and the relationship between a regular, accessible provider and an informed patient or family caregiver.

Building on the AAP concept of the Medical Home, the American College of Physicians (ACP) proposed the development of the "advanced medical home," a care delivery model that would not only provide for a location of patient records, but also provide patient-centered care based on the principles of the Chronic Care Model and include reimbursement incentives for the management and coordination of care (Barr & Ginsburg, 2006). The

---

BOX 29-1 Dimensions of Patient-Centered Care

1. Respect for patients' values, preferences, and expressed needs
2. Information and education
3. Access to care
4. Emotional support to relieve fear and anxiety
5. Involvement of family and friends
6. Continuity and secure transition between health care settings
7. Physical comfort
8. Coordination of care

From Gerteis, M., Edgman-Levitan, S., Daley, J., & Delbanco, T. L. (2003). *Through the patient's eyes: Understanding and promoting patient-centered care.* San Francisco: Jossey-Bass.

BOX 29-2 Key Elements of the Advanced Medical Home

1. Use evidence-based medicine and clinical decision support tools to guide decision-making at the point of care.
2. Organize the delivery of that care according to the Chronic Care Model, but leverage the core functions of the CCM to provide enhanced care for all patients with or without a chronic condition.
3. Create an integrated, coherent plan for ongoing medical care in partnership with patients and their families.
4. Provide enhanced and convenient access to care not only through face-to-face visits but also via telephone, e-mail, and other modes of communication.
5. Identify and measure key quality indicators to demonstrate continuous improvement in health status indicators
6. Adopt and implement the use of health information technology to promote quality of care, to establish a safe environment in which to receive care, to protect the security of health information, and to promote the provision of health information exchange.
7. Participate in programs that provide feedback and guidance on the overall performance of the practice and its physicians.

From Barr, M., & Ginsburg, J. (2006). *The advanced medical home: A patient-centered, physician-guided model of health care.* Policy monograph of the American College of Physicians, p. 4.

---

advanced medical home model requires that a physician, most often a primary care physician, lead a team of health care professionals. The key attributes of the advanced medical home are listed in Box 29-2. Reimbursement in this model would support system-based versus volume-based care; that is, payment based on a process of care delivery that assures positive outcomes rather than the volume of patients seen by a given provider. As well, reimbursement would acknowledge the value of providing coordinated care in a system that incorporates the elements of the CCM. In order to qualify as an advanced medical home, a practice would be required to be meet the National Committee for Quality Assurance (NCQA) guidelines for a medical home. The NCQA's 9 standards (with 10 "must pass" elements) are listed in Box 29-3.

In 2006, IBM, seeking to explore cost-effective models of health care delivery, partnered with the ACP, the American Association of Family Physicians (AAFP), and other primary care groups to establish an advocacy group for the implementation of the medical home model in primary care practice. The Patient Centered Primary Care Collaborative (PCPCC) was created to facilitate improvements in patient-clinician relationships and create a more effective and efficient model of health care delivery. With a membership of over 100 employers and professional organizations, the PCPCC is the major developer and advocate for the patient-centered medical home.

THE ROLE OF NURSING IN MEDICAL HOMES

Larsen (2009) differentiates chronic disease from chronic illness: "chronic disease" refers to specific changes in structure and function, while chronic "illness refers to how the disease is perceived, lived with, and responded to by individuals and their families" (p. 4). It is the response to chronic illness that has challenged the health care system, not its identification. Every viable solution proposed to manage what is essentially a positive outcome of advances in science and medicine—longevity—involves prevention and management of disease through provider-patient relationships that approach the patient as a whole person at the center of the relationship.

Nursing has always held the core values inherent in patient-centered care. An orientation to the whole

---

BOX 29-3 NCQA Standards with "Must Pass" Elements of a Patient-Centered Medical Home

Standard I. Access and communication
Access and communication processes
Access and communication results
Standard II. Patient tracking and registry functions
Organizing clinical data
Identifying important conditions
Standard III. Care management guidelines
Guidelines for important conditions
Standard IV. Patient self-management support processes
Self-management support
Standard V. Electronic prescribing
Standard VI. Test tracking
Test tracking and follow-up
Standard VII. Referral tracking
Referral tracking
Standard VIII. Performance reporting and improvement
Measures of performance
Reporting to physicians
Standard IX. Advanced electronic communication

From National Committee for Quality Assurance. (n.d.). Physician practice connections®—Patient-centered medical home™. Retrieved from *www.ncqa.org/tabid/631/default.aspx*.

---

person; consideration of the patient's emotional, social, and educational needs; and coordination of care across multiple community and health care agencies are fundamental nursing skills. The American Nurses' Association's definition of nursing provides the best evidence that the profession of nursing has both opportunities and responsibilities as a driving force in the development of health care reform, chronic care policy, and implementation of new models of care delivery:

Nursing is the protection, promotion, and optimization of health and abilities, prevention of illness and injury, alleviation of suffering through the diagnosis and treatment of human response, and advocacy in the care of individuals, families, communities, and populations. (2003, p. 3)

The paradigm shift that is essential to the adoption of visionary and sustainable health care policy is a move from a medical to a nursing model.

Recognizing the need to educate and mobilize the entire health care workforce in pursuit of health care quality in a reformed health care delivery system, recommendations from major thought leaders and advisors identified not an individual professional, but a skill set necessary for implementation of new care models. The Institute of Medicine (IOM, 1996) identifies clinicians appropriate to deliver primary care as "individual[s] who use a recognized scientific knowledge base and has the authority to direct the delivery of personal health care services to patients." The IOM further asserts that a primary care clinician can be "a physician, nurse practitioner, or physician assistant" (p. 24). In its 2008 Report to Congress, the Medicare Payment Advisory Commission listed physicians, physician assistants, and nurse practitioners (NPs) as professionals likely to provide primary care. The literature is replete with evidence that use of advanced practice registered nurses (APRNs) in the workforce will control cost (McCauley, Bixby, & Naylor, 2006; Brooten et al., 2003; Blue, et al., 2001) and provide effective primary care and chronic disease management (Boville, et al., 2007; Seale, Anderson, & Kinnersley, 2006; Mackey, Cole, & Lindenberg, 2005: Naylor et al., 2004; Pioro et al., 2001).

The natural fit between the nursing profession and the concepts underpinning the chronic care model led the advanced practice nursing community to lobby for a name change from *medical home* to *health home*. A health home reframes the context of care from pathology (medicine) to health and supports the IOM focus on the process of care and not any one type of provider. However, legislation requiring the implementation of demonstration projects designed to test this method of health care delivery (Tax Relief and Health Care Act [S.1796], 2006) codified the term *medical home* in federal statute, although the new ACA includes both phrases.

While evidence supports utilization of APRNs in advanced medical homes, the concept has been controversial with the greatest concerns emerging from the medical community. The Joint Principles of the Patient-Centered Medical Home (PC-MH) (Table 29-1), written and adopted in 2007 by major physician organizations (American College of Physicians, the American Academy of Family Practitioners, AAP, and American Osteopathic Society), allow only those practices led by a physician to be recognized and certified as advanced medical homes. The NCQA,

TABLE 29-1 Joint Principles of the Patient-Centered Medical Home

Principle	Elaboration
The option to develop an ongoing relationship with a personal physician	Each patient has an ongoing relationship with a personal physician trained to provide first contact, continuous, and comprehensive care
Physician-directed medical practice	The personal physician leads the team who take collective responsibility for the ongoing care of patients
Whole-person orientation	The personal physician provides for all the patient's health care needs or takes responsibility for arranging care with other qualified professionals
Coordinated care across the health system	Care is facilitated by registries, IT, and other means in a culturally and linguistically appropriate manner
Ongoing, voluntary pursuit of quality and safety	Care planning process is driven by robust relationships between physicians and patients where physicians are accountable for continuous quality improvement and patients actively participate in decision-making
Enhanced access to care	Access is improved through open scheduling, expanded hours, and new options for communication
Payment recognizing the value added	Payment system recognizes the value added to patients who have a patient-centered medical home

Adapted from Patient Centered Primary Care Collaborative. (n.d.). Joint principles of the patient-centered medical home. Retrieved from *www.pcpcc.net/content/joint-principles-patient-centered-medical-home*.

adopting the Joint Principles of the PC-MH, would not certify advanced medical homes led by NPs as of June 2010. In July 2007, representatives from the American College of Nurse Practitioners were invited to provide testimony to the NCQA regarding the qualifications and abilities of APRNs in leadership positions in medical home practices. Subsequent communications between the NCQA and the National Nurse Practitioner Roundtable indicate that the NCQA is developing criteria for the certification of nurse practitioner–led medical homes.

Nursing has had some measure of success in influencing policy specific to the inclusion of advanced practice nurse-led medical home practices. While the terminology "medical home" remains part of HR 3590, grassroots efforts among NPs influenced members of the Senate Finance Committee to recognize NPs as leaders of medical home demonstration projects. Support for a technical amendment to the S.1796 emerged from Senators Bingaman (D-NM), Harkin (D-Iowa), Murkowski (R-Alaska), and Collins (R-Maine), who read a colloquy on the Senate floor that spoke to inclusion of NPs as leaders of medical homes (Congressional Record, 2008).

In July 2008, representatives from the ACP and the Nurse Practitioner Roundtable[1] met to discuss the ACP's policy on NPs. As a result of this meeting, the ACP published a policy monograph that recognizes the role of NPs in primary care and advocates for testing nurse practitioner–led medical homes (ACP, 2009). Conversations between the leadership of nursing organizations and the leadership of the PCPCC have resulted in that organization's substitution of the word *clinician* for *physician* in much of their literature (although the Joint Principles still require that the medical home be physician led).

These victories, while seemingly small, provide the foundation for greater change in health care delivery and increase opportunities for patients in the U.S. to receive quality prevention and chronic care delivery from NPs and other providers best able to meet health care needs. While progress has been made, there is still work to be done. NPs are identified in some sections of HR3590 as acceptable lead providers in some chronic care models of delivery. NPs are identified as lead providers in Independence at Home Medical Demonstration Programs. Like medical homes, these demonstration projects are designed to improve care and reduce costs of care for Medicare beneficiaries with chronic disease by bringing health care to their homes. HR3590, Section 3024 states: "nothing in this section shall be construed to prevent a nurse practitioner . . . from participating in or leading a home

---

[1]In 2009, the Nurse Practitioner Roundtable was composed of the American College of Nurse Practitioners (ACNP); the American Academy of Nurse Practitioners (AANP); the National Organization of Nurse Practitioner Faculties (NONPF); and, the National Association of Pediatric Nurse Practitioners (NAPNAP). NP attendees at the 2008 ACP meeting included representatives from ACNP, AANP, and NONPF.

based primary care team as part of an independence at home medical practice" (p. 287).

The ACA does provide a state option to provide "health homes" for Medicaid enrollees with chronic conditions. Language describing health home providers is provider neutral, specifically "the term health home means a designated provider ... selected by a(an) eligible individual with chronic conditions to provide health home services" (HR 3590, Section 2703, p. 203).

SUMMARY

Prevention and management of chronic disease is the number-one driver of health care policy in the U.S. Cost-effective quality strategies to provide care are dependent upon the development of health care policy that supports a paradigm shift from "diagnose and cure" to "prevent and manage." The advanced medical home is a viable model within which to provide patient-centered preventive and management services. Thought leaders and policymakers have identified that NPs possess the skill set required to lead medical homes. Research on access, quality, and management of primary and chronic care supports utilization of NPs in a medical home model. While some health care leaders have interpreted the call for primary and chronic care management as a physician-only initiative, advanced practice nursing has made some progress. The ACA identifies NPs as lead providers in independence at home medical home demonstration projects and allows for provider neutral language in the definition of health homes. NCQA is reexamining the criteria for medical home certification and is expected to include medical homes led by nurses.

For a list of related websites, please refer to your Evolve Resources at http://evolve.elsevier.com/Mason/policypolitics/

REFERENCES

Agency for Healthcare Quality and Research. (1998). Medical Expenditure Panel Survey. Retrieved from www.ahrq.gov/about/cj2000/cjmeps00.htm.

American College of Physicians. (2009). *Nurse practitioners in primary care.* Washington, D.C. Policy monograph of the American College of Physicians.

American Nurses' Association. (2003). *Nursing's social policy statement* (2nd ed.). Silver Springs, MD: American Nurses' Association.

Anderson, G. F. (2005). Medicare and chronic conditions [electronic version]. *New England Journal of Medicine, 343*(3), 305-309.

Barr, M., & Ginsburg, J. (2006). *The advanced medical home: A patient-centered, physician-guided model of health care* (pp. 1-22). A policy monograph of the American College of Physicians.

Beal, A., Doty, M., Hernandez, S., Shea, K., & Davis, K. (2007). Closing the divide: How medical homes promote equity in health care. Results from the Commonwealth Fund 2006 Health Care Quality Survey. Retrieved from www.commonwealthfund.org/Content/Surveys/2006/The-Commonwealth-Fund-2006-Health-Care-Quality-Survey.aspx.

Blue, L., Lang, E., McMurray, J. J., Davie, A. P., McDonagh, T. A., et al. (2001). Randomised controlled trial of specialist nurse intervention in heart failure. *British Medical Journal, 323*(7315), 715-718.

Bodenheimer, T., Wagner, E. H., & Grumbach, K. (2002). Improving primary care for patients with chronic illness. *The Journal of the American Medical Association, 288*(14), 1775-1779.

Boville, D., Saran, M., Salem, J. K., Clough, L., Jones, R. R., et al. (2007). An innovative role for nurse practitioners in managing chronic disease. *Nursing Economic$, 25*(6), 359-364.

Brooten, D., Younblut, J., Deatrick, J., Naylor, M., & York, R. (2003). Patient problems, advanced practice nurse (APN) interventions, time and contacts among five patient groups. *Journal of Nursing Scholarship, 35*(4), 73-79.

Centers for Disease Control and Prevention. National Center for Chronic Disease Prevention and Health Promotion. (2009). Retrieved from www.cdc.gov/chronicdisease/overview/index.htm.

Centers for Medicare and Medicaid Services (CMS). (2008). National health expenditures 2008 highlights. Retrieved from www.cms.hhs.gov/NationalHealthExpendData/downloads/highlights.pdf.

Centers for Disease Control and Prevention & the Merck Company Foundation. (2007). *The state of aging and health in America 2007.* Whitehouse Station, NJ: The Merck Company Foundation.

Coleman, K., Austin, B., Brach, C., & Wagner, E. (2009). Evidence on the chronic care model in the new millennium. *Health Affairs, 28*(1), 75-85.

Congressional Record, July 9, 2008, S6485-S6486.

Coulam, R. F., & Gaumer, G. L. (1991). Medicare's prospective payment system: A critical appraisal. *Health Care Finance Review, Annual Supplement, 1991,* 45-77.

Dall, T., Zhang, Y., Chen, Y., Quick, W., Yang, W., & Fogli, J. (2010). The economic burden of diabetes. *Health Affairs, 29*(2), 297-303.

DeVol, R., Bedrossian, A., Charuworn, A., Chatterjee, A., Kim, I. K., Kim, S., et al. (2007). *An unhealthy America: The economic burden of chronic disease: Charting a new course to save lives and increase productivity and economic growth.* Santa Monica, CA: Milken Institute Publications. Retrieved from www.milkeninstitute.org.

Gerteis, M., Edgman-Levitan S., Daley J., & Delbanco, T. L. (2003). *Through the patient's eyes: Understanding and promoting patient-centered care.* San Francisco: Jossey-Bass.

Institute of Medicine. (1996). *Primary care: America's health in a new era.* Washington, D.C.: National Academy Press.

Larsen, P. D. (2009). Chronicity. In P. D. Larsen & I. M. Lubkin (Eds.), *Chronic illness: Impact and intervention* (7th ed.), (pp. 3-23). Sudbury, MA: Jones & Bartlett.

Mackey, T. A., Cole, F. L., & Lindenberg, J. (2005). Quality improvement and changes in diabetic patient outcomes in an academic nurse practitioner primary care practice. *Journal of the American Academy of Nurse Practitioners, 17*(12), 547-553.

Mattke, S., Seid, M., & Ma, S. (2007). Evidence for the effect of disease management: Is $1 billion a year a good investment? (electronic version). *American Journal of Managed Care, 13*(12), 670-676.

McCauley, K. M., Bixby, M. B., & Naylor, M. D. (2006). Advanced practice nurse strategies to improve outcomes and reduce cost in elders with heart failure. *Disease Management, 9*(5), 302-310.

Medicare Payment Advisory Commission. (2008). *Report to the Congress: Reforming the delivery system.* Washington, D.C.: MedPAC.

National Center for Health Statistics. Mortality Statistics 1909 Tenth Annual Report. Retrieved from www.cdc.gov/nchs/products/vsus.htm.

Naylor, M. D., Brooten, D. A., Campbell, R. L., Maislin, G., McCauley, K. M., & Schwartz, J. S. (2004). Transitional care of older adults hospitalized with heart failure: A randomized, controlled trial. *Journal of the American Geriatrics Society, 52*(5), 675-684.

Nutting, P., Miller, W., Crabtree, B., Jaen, C. T, Steward, E., & Stange, K. (2009). Initial lessons from the first national demonstration project on practice transformation to a patient-centered medical home. *Annals of Family Medicine, 7*(3), 254-260.

Patient-Centered Primary Care Collaborative. Retrieved from www.pcpcc.net/content/about-collaborative.

Patient-Centered Primary Care Collaborative. Retrieved from www.pcpcc.net/content/joint-principles-patient-centered-medical-home.

The Patient Protection and Affordable Care Act of 2010, Rangel, C. (D-NY), Retrieved from www.thomas.gov.

Pioro, M. H., Landefeld, C. S., Brennan, P. F., Daly, B., Fortinsky, R. H., et al. (2001). Outcomes-based trial of an inpatient nurse practitioner service for general medical patients. *Journal of Evaluation in Clinical Practice, 7*(1), 21-33.

Robert Wood Johnson Foundation, Partnership for Solutions. (2002). Chronic conditions: Making the case for ongoing care. Retrieved from www.rwjf.org/reports/npreports/betterlives.htm.

Robert Wood Johnson Foundation. (1996). *Chronic care in America: A 21st century challenge.* San Francisco: The Institute for Health & Aging, University of California. Retrieved from www.rwjf.org/files/publications/other/ChronicCareinAmerica.pdf.

Seale, C., Anderson, E., & Kinnersley, P. (2006). Treatment advice in primary care: A comparative study of nurse practitioners and general practitioners. *Journal of Advanced Nursing, 54*(5), 534-541.

Sia, C., Tonniges, T. F., Osterhus, E., & Taba, S. (2004). History of the medical home concept. *Pediatrics, 113*(5 Suppl), 1473-1478.

Social Security Online Actuarial Tables (2010). Retrieved from www.ssa.gov/OACT/STATS/table4c6.html.

Tax Relief and Health Care Act of 2006, Section 204 of HR 6111, Baucus, M. (D-MT), Retrieved from www.thomas.gov.

Wagner, E. H., (1998). Chronic disease management: What will it take to improve care for chronic illness? *Effective Clinical Practice, 1*(1), 2-4.

Yach, D., Hawkes, C., Gould, C. L., & Hofman, K. J. (2004). The global burden of chronic disease. *The Journal of the American Medical Association, 291*(21), 2616-2622.

CHAPTER 30

Family Caregiving and Social Policy

Karen M. Robinson and Susan C. Reinhard

"No government can love a child, and no policy can substitute for a family's care. But at the same time, government can either support or undermine families as they cope with moral, social and economic stresses of caring. ..."

—Hillary Rodham Clinton

It is well established that the American population is aging. The oldest of 79 million baby boomers, born between 1946 and 1964, will reach age 65 in just a few years. With the graying of the population, family caregivers will be needed more than ever to provide services to persons with chronic illness for increasingly long periods of time (Stevenson, 2008). Family caregivers play a valuable, irreplaceable role in our society, particularly in supporting people who have long-term needs for services and supports.

UNPAID VALUE OF FAMILY CAREGIVING

Family caregivers' contributions have great enormous value not only to their loved ones, but also to the United States health care system. Caregivers provide high-quality care at low cost, including care that is consistent with patient preferences. National estimates indicate that 44 million Americans over the age of 18 provide support to older adults with chronic illnesses who live in the community. In 2007, the economic value of family caregiving reached $375 billion—more than the total national spending for Medicaid, including federal and state contributions and medical and long-term care that totaled $311 billion in 2006 (Gibson & Houser, 2008).

Among noninstitutionalized persons needing assistance with activities of daily living, two-thirds depend solely on family and friends, and another one-fourth supplement family care with services from paid providers (Liu, Manton, & Aragon, 2000). The work of family caregivers is essentially irreplaceable, mainly because providing an alternate source of care is difficult and costly. There are not enough long-term care workers to replace contributions of family caregivers (Maslow, Levine, & Reinhard, 2006). Family caregiving provides an unpaid workforce critical to maintaining the long-term care system. The value of this unpaid care is stunning, but it exacts a high, often hidden cost on the health of caregivers. The risk related to caregiving is enormous, even to caregivers who are initially in good health.

CAREGIVING AS A STRESSFUL BUSINESS

The association between physical and mental health and being a family caregiver are well established (Pinquart & Sorensen, 2007). Caregiving has all the features of a chronic stress experience as it creates physical and psychological strain over an extended period of time. Caregiving situations are accompanied by high levels of unpredictability and uncontrollability. Thus, caregiving has the capability to create secondary stress in multiple domains of life, such as in work and family relationships. Caregiving fits the definition for chronic stress so well that it is used as a model for studying the health effects of chronic stress (Schulz & Sherwood, 2008).

Evidence indicates that most caregivers are not prepared for caregiving and often provide care with little or no support (National Alliance for Caregiving [NAC] & AARP, 2009; Family Caregiver Alliance [FCA], 2006). More than one-third of caregivers provide intense care to others while suffering from poor health themselves (Navale-Waliser, et al., 2002). An influential factor in a caregiver's decision to relocate a loved one to a nursing home is the caregiver's own failing physical health (Buhr, Kuchibhatia, & Clipp, 2006).

Related to mental health, caregivers consistently report higher levels of depressive symptoms and mental health problems when compared to their non-caregiving peers (Pinquart & Sorensen, 2003). Estimates identify that between 40% and 70% of caregivers have clinically significant symptoms of depression, with approximately one-quarter to one-half of these caregivers meeting the diagnostic criteria for major depression (FCA, 2009).

Research not only documents negative physical and mental health, but also negative outcomes from caregiving. Caregivers report that they suffer from high levels of stress and frustration (Pinquart & Sorensen, 2003), with resultant feelings of anger, guilt, exhaustion, and helplessness as a result of providing care (Center for Aging Society, 2005). Caregiving can also result in a loss of self-identity, with less time for leisure and enjoyable activities. Constant worry or feelings of uncertainty are identified as caregivers experience less control over their lives when compared to non-caregivers (Pinquart & Sorensen, 2003).

Women compose about two-thirds of all unpaid caregivers (Johnson & Wiener, 2006; NAC & AARP, 2009). In a national survey on caregiver health, about 1 in 5 (24%) women surveyed had mammograms less often because of caregiving (NAC & Evercare, 2006). They also reported higher levels of depression and anxiety, and lower levels of subjective well-being, life satisfaction, and physical health when compared to male caregivers. Evidence identifies that women caregivers fare worse than their male counterparts (Pinquart & Sorensen, 2006).

A 2009 survey (NAC and AARP, 2009) found almost one-third (34%) of caregivers were men; in 1997, 27% were men. Reasons for the increased number of men who take on caregiving were smaller families, longer life spans, more women working outside the home, and greater geographic distance among family members. More male caregivers were working full-time (60%) compared to women (41%).

As family caregivers struggle to care for their loved ones, their own physical and mental well-being is put at risk. Overall caregiver health is quickly becoming a public health issue that requires focused attention from health professionals, policymakers, and caregivers themselves to improve the health and quality of life of family caregivers who are dedicated to the care of others (Talley & Crews, 2007; FCA, 2009). Because of public interest in health care reform, the role of informal caregivers must receive more attention in public policy initiatives regarding how to better support family caregivers.

SUPPORTING FAMILY CAREGIVERS

Long-term family caregiving is risky business. Caregivers make great sacrifices to provide this care, enduring negative effects on their physical and mental health, as well as burnout, strain, and depletion of financial resources. More than one-half of caregivers caring for someone 50 years of age and older spend more than 10% of their income on expenses—an average of $5531. Caregivers (34%) were forced to use some of their savings to cover expenses (NAC, 2009). Caregivers (78%) say more help and information is needed. The demand for caregiving information has increased since 2004 (77% versus 67% in 2004). Of six national policies and programs (tax credits, vouchers to pay minimum wage for some caregiving hours, respite services, transportation, assessment, and paid leave of absence from work) presented to caregivers as potential help, the most popular was a tax credit of $3000. The majority of caregivers (56%) rated the tax credit as their preferred policy strategy (NAC & AARP, 2009). State and federal investments in family caregiver support are needed now more than ever. A number of policy solutions could help; some of these solutions are embedded in larger reform areas, and some are more specific to family caregivers. Table 30-1 summarizes several high-priority recommendations (Reinhard, Montgomery, & Gibson, 2008).

HEALTH CARE HOMES

Caregivers need support, for their own sake and for the sake of sustaining their essential work for as long as it is desirable and possible to do so. An example of how practice and policy solutions for family caregivers can be embedded in larger system reform is the movement toward "medical home" or "health care home" as it is named in Minnesota Statutes §256B.0751 (Minnesota Department of Health, 2010, p. 4). The core feature of these models is that each patient has a health care professional who leads a coordinated and integrated team, where patient and caregiver are viewed holistically (FCA, 2009). In the

TABLE 30-1 High-Priority Policy Recommendations to Support Family Caregivers

Categories of Support	Federal	State
Direct Services, such as Respite, Information, and Referral		
Ensure that all publicly funded log-term care programs cover services, such as respite care and adult day services, that supplement caregiving by family, friends, and others	X	X
Provide adequate funding for the Lifespan Respite Care Program	X	
Expand funding for the National Family Caregiver Support Program	X	
Increase state and federal funding for respite care	X	X
Offer additional services geared to special needs of caregivers, such as support groups and mental health counseling	X	X
Ensure that services and supports reflect needs of diverse caregiver populations	X	X
Assessment of Caregivers' Needs		
Stimulate development and delivery of caregiver assessment protocols across all care settings to develop effective support plans for both care recipient and caregiver	X	X
Require assessment of caregiver's willingness and ability to provide care prior to hospital discharge	X	X
Reimburse health care professionals for family caregiver assessment, care management, and training	X	X
Education and Training		
Direct caregivers to appropriate training opportunities, particularly to ensure a safe transition from hospital to home or nursing home to home; funding training for caregivers	X	X
Financial Relief		
Establish and coordinate policies to pay relatives and friends who care for people with disabilities as part of a plan of services and supports		X
Permit payment of family caregivers through consumer-directed models in publicly funded programs		X
Expand programs that permit caregivers to direct the services that are offered to them (consumer direction for caregivers' services)		X
Amend Supplemental Security Income rules so they do not reduce benefits for caregivers living with family members	X	
Assure continued health insurance benefits for caregivers forced to leave employment or during leaves of absence due to caregiving duties	X	X
Create incentives for increased public awareness about existing programs and policies		X
Tax Implications		
Provide a refundable Long-Term Services and Supports tax credit for caregivers to give some relief from the high costs of caregiving	X	X
Encourage employers to take advantage of existing tax incentives, such as flexible spending accounts for dependent care, to provide dependent- or family-care benefits	X	
Workplace Flexibility, Including Family and Medical Leave Act		
Extend the Family and Medical Leave Act to provide paid leave and cover more workers for longer periods	X	
Provide paid family leave for caregiving	X	X
Caregiver Rights; Legal Protection		
Ensure that caregivers as well as patients are aware of the patient's right to appeal hospital discharge, skilled nursing facility, and Medicare home health care decisions	X	X

From Reinhard, S. C., Montgomery, R., Gibson, M. J. (2008). Informal caregivers: Sustaining the core of long-term services and supports. Commissioned for "Building Bridges: Making a difference in long term care. Fifth Annual Long Term Care Colloquium sponsored by the Commonwealth Fund and conducted by Academy Health, Washington, D.C., June 7, 2008.

health care home concept, a team of health professionals is organized to address the specific health care needs of the individual and caregiver. All health professionals involved with patient care talk to one another (and with the individual and caregiver) about existing care needs. The online medical history of the individual and the caregiver is available at any time of the day or night to all health professionals involved in the care situation. Patient-specific health information is readily available because of the unified information technology system, whereby all team members can access needed information and keep in frequent touch about ongoing needs. Thus members of the health care home can be in different locations. Regulations that specify the need to include family caregivers in designing and implementing care, in cases where family care is embraced by the patient and essential to the patient's well-being, should be carefully crafted and implemented.

CARE COORDINATION

State, federal, and private sector efforts to better coordinate care should explicitly include attention to the family caregiver's core role in navigating the health and long-term care system. Care coordination for persons with multiple chronic illnesses can cut costs, eliminate waste, and improve quality of health care. Most caregivers report that the patient's care coordination among various service providers was "very" to "somewhat" easy, although 1 in 4 (25%) reported some difficulty with coordination (NAC & AARP, 2009).

Care coordination should include comprehensive assessment of the care recipient, as well as assessment of the needs of the family caregiver. The plan of care should be developed and implemented in collaboration with the patient, family caregivers, physicians, advanced practice registered nurses, other medical personnel, home care providers, and social service providers. Care coordination can ease the burden on family caregivers by helping develop and implement plans of care that make sense to them, and communicate effectively and efficiently with all the interdisciplinary health care providers and social service providers involved in the care. Another outcome of care coordination is support and education to navigate the health care system, access needed services, and anticipate and plan for future needs by recognizing that caregivers have separate needs from that of the care recipient.

HOME AND COMMUNITY-BASED SERVICES

Caregivers need education and support services to sustain their critical role as care providers. Frequently caregivers do not know where to turn for help. When assistance is sought, many community agencies cannot provide assistance due to budget constraints and outdated policies. The federal government can take steps to ensure that all family caregivers have access to caregiver assistance and to practical, high-quality, and affordable home and community-based services. The Medicare and Medicaid programs must be updated to better support family caregivers through home and community-based services. Supporting family caregivers is one of the most cost-effective long-term care investments to be made. When caregivers can continue as providers of care, they are often able to delay costly nursing home admission and reduce reliance on programs such as Medicaid (Reinhard, Montgomery, & Gibson, 2008).

FUND CAREGIVER ASSESSMENT

To help support more people with chronic illnesses in the community, the needs of both the ill individual and the family caregiver must be assessed. Federal and state programs, such as Medicare and Medicaid, should pay providers to conduct family caregiver assessments if we expect these caregivers to provide substantial care. This is particularly true during hospital discharge, transitional care, and postacute care (FCA, 2009). Both the family caregiver's needs as well as the care recipient's needs must be made part of a "safe and adequate discharge" (FCA, 2009, p. 1). Assessment of the family caregiver's health, willingness to provide care, and training and support needs will promote family-centered care and will help assure the health and safety of Medicaid beneficiaries who are served in the community rather than in nursing homes.

For a list of related websites, please refer to your Evolve Resources at http://evolve.elsevier.com/Mason/policypolitics/

REFERENCES

Buhr, G. T., Kuchibhatia, M., & Clipp, E. C. (2006). Caregivers' reasons for nursing home placement: Clues for improving discussions with families prior to the transition. *The Gerontologist, 46*(1), 52-61.

Center for Aging Society. (2005). *How do family caregivers fare? A closer look at their experiences.* (Data Profile, Number 3). Washington, D.C.: Georgetown University.

Family Caregiver Alliance. (2006). *Caregiver assessment: Principles, guidelines and strategies for change.* Report from a National Consensus Development Conference (vol. 1). San Francisco: Author.

Family Caregiver Alliance. (2009). *2009 National policy statement.* FCA National Center on Caregiving (FCC).

Gibson, M. J., & Houser, A. (2008). *Valuing the invaluable: The economic value of family caregiving 2008 Update.* Washington, D.C.: AARP.

Johnson, R. W., & Wiener, J. M. (2006). *A profile of older Americans and their caregivers* (Occasional paper number 8). Washington, D.C.: The Urban Institute.

Liu, K., Manton, K. G., & Aragon, C. (2000). Changes in home care use by disabled elderly persons: 1982-1994. *Journal of Gerontology: Series B, Psychological Sciences and Social Sciences, 55B,* S245-S253.

Maslow, K., Levine, C., & Reinhard, S. (2006). Assessment of family caregivers: A public policy perspective. In *Voices and views from the field* (Vol. II). Report from a National Consensus Development Conference. San Francisco: Family Caregiver Alliance.

Minnesota Department of Health. (2010). Health Care Homes (aka Medical Homes)—Adopted Rule. Retrieved from www.health.state.mn.us/healthreform/homes/standards/AdoptedRule_January2010.pdf.

National Alliance for Caregiving (NAC). (2009). The Evercare Survey of the economic downturn and its impact on family caregiving. Retrieved from www.caregiving.org/data/EVC_Caregivers_Economy_Report%20FINAL_4-28-09.pdf.

National Alliance for Caregiving (NAC) and AARP. (2009). *Caregiving in the US: A focused look at those caring for someone age 50 or older.* Washington, D.C.: Author.

National Alliance for Caregiving (NAC) and Evercare. (2006). *Evercare study of caregivers in decline: A close up look at the health risks of caring for a loved one.* Bethesda, Md. National Alliance for Caregiving and Minnetonka, MN: Evercare.

Navale-Waliser, M., Feldman, P. H., Gould, D. A., Levine, C. L., Kuerbis, A. N., & Donelan, K. (2002). When the caregiver needs care: The plight of vulnerable caregivers. *American Journal of Public Health, 92*(3), 409-413.

Pinquart, M., & Sorensen, S. (2003). Differences between caregivers and non-caregivers in psychological health and physical health: A meta-analysis. *Psychological Aging, 18*(2), 250-267.

Pinquart, M., & Sorensen, S. (2006). Gender differences in caregiving stressors, social resources, and health: An updated meta-analysis. *Journal of Gerontology & Psychological Social Sciences, 61*(1), P33-P45.

Pinquart, M., & Sorensen, S. (2007). Correlates of physical health of informal caregivers: A meta-analysis. *Journal of Gerontology & Psychological Social Sciences, 62*(2), P126-P137.

Reinhard, S. C., Montgomery, R., Gibson, M. J. (2008). Informal caregivers: Sustaining the core of long-term services and supports. Commissioned for "Building Bridges: Making a difference in long term care. Fifth Annual Long Term Care Colloquium sponsored by the Commonwealth Fund and conducted by Academy Health, Washington, D.C., June 7, 2008.

Schulz, R., & Sherwood, P. C. (2008). Physical and Mental health effects of family caregiving. *The American Journal of Nursing, 108*(9), 23-27.

Stevenson, D. G. (2008). Planning for the future—long term care and the 2008 election. *New England Journal of Medicine, 358*(19), 1985-1987.

Talley, R., & Crews, J. E. (2007). Framing the public health of caregiving. *American Journal of Public Health, 97*(2), 224-228.

CHAPTER 31

Retail Health Care Clinics: Filling a Gap in the Health Care System

Donna L. Haugland and Patricia J. Hughes[1]

"There's a way to do it better—find it."
—Thomas Edison

It was a long wait that evening in 1999 when Rick Krieger needed diagnosis and treatment for his son's sore throat (Agency for Healthcare Research and Quality, 2008). With limited choices for after-hours care, he sat in an urgent care center for over 2 hours. He became frustrated with the wait, the slow service, the cost, and the overengineered processes for a common, simple throat infection. One year later, he and his business associates opened a walk-in clinic at a strip mall under the name QuickMedx (now MinuteClinic, L.L.C. [MinuteClinic]) and created a whole new sector in the health care industry—retail clinics. Christensen (2007) hailed creation of the retail clinic as one of the top 10 disruptive innovations of the decade. The retail clinic has reshaped the health care marketplace through the core concepts of disruptive innovation: simplicity, accessibility, convenience, and affordability. This shift in the health care marketplace also has produced a new model of nurse-led service delivery.

A NEW APPROACH TO ACCESSING CARE

The term "retail clinic" certainly sounds a bit strange. However, it appropriately communicates the fact that the care is delivered at medical clinics located in retail outlets, such as pharmacies, groceries, and mass merchandisers. The typical retail clinic or convenient care clinic is usually 200 to 500 square feet large, located near the business's pharmacy, sparsely furnished to accommodate 15-minute appointments, and staffed by a nurse practitioner (NP) or physician assistant (Scott, 2006). Retail clinics do not offer the full array of acute, chronic, and preventive services found in primary care or urgent care. The focus is on common acute illnesses, such as sore throat and urinary tract infection, as well as vaccinations and limited screenings, such as cholesterol testing. But, the 10 most common conditions managed in retail clinics account for 12% of emergency department (ED) visits (Mehrotra, Wang, Lave, Adams & McGlynn, 2008).

The term *retail clinic* connotes retail principles that are at the core of the concept—consumer focus, competitive pricing, convenience, efficient service, extended operating hours, and products with consistent quality. These clinics are open during evenings and weekends, usually offer short wait times, require no appointment, and post the menu and prices of their limited offerings. This is a radically different approach from the way health care historically has been delivered in the United States, requiring trips to medical campuses away from the person's daily routine, limiting office visits to weekday business hours, and enduring wait times of up to several days for an episodic illness.

Price transparency also is not seen in traditional health care settings since they typically do not post the cost of services. Yet, in the consumer-driven health care marketplace, the overall cost—not just out-of-pocket cost—is an important consideration in choosing a provider (Fronstin & Helman, 2009). Retail clinics usually can provide a bargain for the

[1]Although previous nursing leaders at MinuteClinic, L.L.C., the views opinions and recommendations in this chapter are solely those of the authors and do not necessarily reflect the opinion of MinuteClinic, L.L.C., its parent organization, CVS Caremark Corporation, or their employees, officers, or directors.

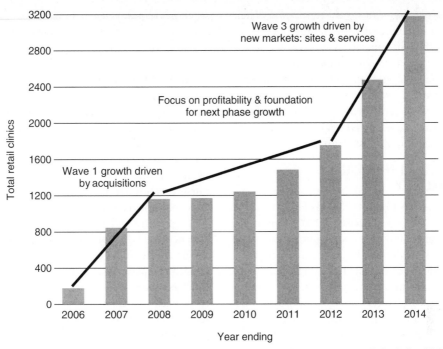

FIGURE 31-1 Estimated growth and growth phases of retail clinics. (From Keckley, P. H., Underwood, H. R., & Gandhi, M. [2009]. *Retail clinics: Update and implications.* [p. 5]. Washington, D.C.: Deloitte Center for Health Solutions. Copyright © 2009 Deloitte Development LLC. Reprinted with permission.)

health care shopper. Low overhead costs from their small spaces, lack of expensive equipment, minimal or no support staff, and lower salaries for non-physician providers allow retail clinics to offer lower costs for the services that they offer—approximately 30% to 40% less than in a physician's office and 80% less than in an emergency department (Mehrotra et al., 2009).

CONSUMER RESPONSE

Since its debut in 2000, the retail health care sector has grown to over 1100 clinics located in 38 states and the District of Columbia (Retail Clinics, 2009) (Figure 31-1). This expansion has been attributed to the consistently favorable response to and growing adoption of the retail clinic model on the part of consumers (Keckley, Underwood, & Gandhi, 2009). One recent survey indicates that 16% of respondents have sought care at a retail clinic within the past 2 years (Deloitte Center for Health Solutions, 2009), representing millions of patient visits. About 90% of these visits were for 10 simple acute illnesses, including upper respiratory tract infection, pharyngitis, sinusitis, conjunctivitis, otitis media, and urinary tract infection

(Mehrotra et al., 2008). Nearly two-thirds of customers cited the convenient hours and locations as major factors in choosing retail clinics instead of other sources of care (Tu Ha & Cohen, 2008). Overall satisfaction rate has been 90%, with some retail clinic operators reporting rates higher than 95% (New WSJ. com, 2008; Hunter, Weber, Morreale, & Wall, 2009). This contrasts starkly with patient satisfaction rates of 71% for primary care physicians (Deloitte Center for Health Solutions, 2009).

Despite this high satisfaction, more than three-fourths of those surveyed believed the retail clinic is appropriate only for basic medical care when a person's regular provider is unavailable. Nearly two-thirds of consumers have reported concerns about staff qualifications and the possibility that serious problems might be missed or diagnosed incorrectly (New WSJ.com, 2008). What remains unclear is whether these concerns stem from unfamiliarity with a new and evolving model, lack of consumer awareness about NPs and their scope of practice, or a combination of both. The level of concern has decreased slightly between 2005 and 2008 (New WSJ.com, 2008). However, the public still has limited awareness of NPs and what they can do (Green, 2007). Their understanding is confounded by the many kinds of nurses, each with different nomenclature and scope of practice. For NPs, role confusion also is fostered by the state-by-state variation in professional designations and degree of physician oversight. Whether or not retail clinics can serve as a vehicle for promoting the image and acceptance of NPs as autonomous care providers remains an open question.

REACTIONS FROM THE HEALTH CARE COMMUNITY

While a few business futurists, such as Harvard Business School's Clayton Christensen (2007), embraced the change as an "innovative disruption," initial reactions from stakeholders in health care varied from tepid to negative. However, as retail clinics continue to strengthen a foothold in the marketplace, some segments have accepted the model as a positive indicator of future solutions for health care reform.

Third-Party Payers. The original retail clinics operated on a fee-for-service, cash payment basis. However, in response to the demands of their members for more voice in consumer-directed health care, major health plans began to add retail clinics to their provider networks. Early on, they applied urgent care or emergency department co-payments, but some have reduced or waived them as retail clinics demonstrated a cost-savings proposition (Scott, 2007). For example, Blue Cross and Blue Shield of Minnesota decided to waive co-payments after its study of claims showed that a retail clinic visit cost half as much as a visit at a primary care office (Krizner, 2006), saving the company more than $1.25 million in health care costs during 2007 (Wilson, 2009). Employers, too, discounted co-payments in an effort to capitalize both on cost savings and the reduced time employees were away from work due to illness (Silva, 2007). Currently, almost all retail clinics accept insurance and Medicare fee-for-service reimbursement, and only 16% of patients pay out-of-pocket for their visits (Mehrotra et al., 2008; Rudavsky, Pollack, & Mehrotra, 2009).

However, coverage issues still present challenges to the growth of the retail clinic industry. Some plans continue to require a larger co-payment than that for primary care providers. Many payers limit coverage only to services they deem appropriate for the retail setting instead of reimbursing the full menu of clinics'

services (Kantor, 2007). Finally, for some insurers, clinic operators must renegotiate contracts whenever a new service is offered, even though it falls within an NP's scope of practice and skill set.

Nurse Practitioners. Nurse practitioner leaders initially complained that the limited number of minor conditions managed in the retail clinic represented an oversimplified practice that not only failed to utilize the full potential of the NP's education and skills, but also ran the risk of distorting the public's perception of the NP role (Green, 2007). However, professional nurse practitioner associations have collaborated on principles for retail clinics that support nurse practitioner practice and now see it as a way to expand and enhance the NP profession and help to educate the public about nurse practitioner practice (American Academy of Nurse Practitioners, 2007).

Physicians. Many of the most vocal critics of the retail health care model have been from physicians. As Sage (2009, p. 8) asserted, "physicians would prefer to label and hopefully control retail clinics … using familiar narratives of quackery, corporatization, profit-seeking, and conflict of interest." The official stance of major physician organizations, such as the American Medical Association, the American Academy of Family Physicians (AAFP), and the American Academy of Pediatrics, was disapproval of retail clinics. As the number of retail clinics grew, the AAFP formed a Retail Medicine Workgroup in 2005 that collaborated with the largest retail health companies "to shape the emerging retail clinics in a way that could benefit patients" (Sullivan, 2006, p. 68) through development of desirable attributes and principles, such as limited scope of services, support of the medical home, collaborative relationships with local medical providers, and use of electronic medical records. Other medical organizations then promulgated similar guidelines. Operators of retail clinics endorsed these standards because they reflected practices consistent with quality and patient safety, and, in many cases, already were in place in most retail clinic environments. Subsequently, the Convenient Care Association (CCA), which represents more than 20 of the largest operators, published even more stringent quality and safety standards that its members have committed to meet (Table 31-1). MinuteClinic, a CCA member, set the benchmark with its Joint Commission accreditation in 2006 and reaccreditation in 2009. Accreditation was an important

TABLE 31-1 **Convenient Care Association (CCA)**

What CCA is:	Trade association of the companies and health systems that provide retail health care
Membership:	95% of the retail health care industry
Founded:	October 2006
CCA Quality and Safety Standards:	• Credentialed providers • Ongoing quality monitoring, including peer review, collaborative physician review, use of evidence-based guidelines, outcome measurement, and patient satisfaction assessment • Continuity of care through relationships with other health care providers • Use of electronic health records • Appropriate referrals for follow-up care or for conditions outside the scope of the clinic's services • Encouraging patients to establish a relationship with a primary care provider • Compliance with applicable standards for quality care and patient safety, including those of the Occupational Safety and Health Association (OSHA), Clinical Laboratory Improvement Act (CLIA), Centers for Disease Control and Prevention (CDC), and Americans with Disabilities Act (ADA) • Provision of self-care and prevention instructions and educational materials • Established protocols for emergency response and care • Patient empowerment through price transparency

Adapted from *Convenient Care Association Quality and Safety Standards*. Copyright © 2008. Convenient Care Association.

milestone for retail clinics because it demonstrated adherence to the same rigorous standards and quality requirements applicable to prominent health care facilities operating within the more traditional medical system.

A growing body of evidence does not support the early concern of physician groups about the quality of care provided in retail clinics. For example, the 2006 Minnesota Community Measurement Health Care Quality Report showed that MinuteClinic outperformed all other medical practices in the state for prescribing antibiotics only when a strep test was positive. On this measure, MinuteClinic scored 100%, while the average rating was 83% (Herrick & Goodman, 2007). In the first study to compare retail clinics with other settings, the quality of care was at least as good as the same services rendered in physician offices and urgent care centers (Mehrotra et al., 2009). This study found no differences among the three settings in the rate of follow up visits, prescription costs, or receipt of preventive care within the ensuing 3 months.

There have also been concerns about disruption of the relationship between patients and their primary care providers (PCPs). Retail clinic data indicate that as many as 60% of their patients have reported that they do not have a primary care provider (Mehrotra et al., 2008). Nationally, almost 19% of non-elderly adults and 6% of children have reported no usual source of care or medical home (National Center for Health Statistics, 2009a, 2009b). With the increasing shortage of physicians entering primary care, almost 60 million Americans (almost 20%) will lack access to primary care (National Association of Community Health Centers, 2009). Retail clinics can ease the strain on primary care and offer a less costly alternative to emergency department visits for an estimated 13.5 million patients (Mehrotra et al., 2008) and are an affordable option for those who need acute care while traveling or who are between providers due to health plan changes.

Many retail clinic organizations work to promote a medical home for those who do not have one by providing a list of practices in the area that are accepting new patients. They also encourage the ongoing relationship with the PCP by sending electronic or faxed copies of visit records to the provider.

Research indicates that consumers value low cost and quick access more than the care setting when they have a minor illness (Ahmed & Fincham, 2010). In response to retail clinic success in meeting the demand for increased access, physician practices are increasingly offering same-day appointments as well as expanding office hours to include evenings and weekends (Bachman, 2006).

LEGISLATIVE AND REGULATORY ISSUES

Evidence does not support concerns about quality or overprescribing, but some states have pursued regulatory and legislative avenues to define retail clinic operations. Bills have been considered relating to physician oversight, ownership, facility licensure, marketing and advertising, referral requirements, Medicaid participation, and practice issues (Scott, 2007; Takach & Witgert, 2009a). Commenting on a complex bill introduced in the state legislature, Illinois Representative Elaine Nekritz (Takach & Witgert, 2009a, p. 9) characterized the purpose of this legislative activity as impeding growth of retail clinics so they would be "no longer viable."

Although many of the bills failed, there have been examples of increased legislation to regulate the practice in retail clinics. Florida passed a statute limiting primary care physician supervision to no more than four NPs. Massachusetts became the first state to specifically regulate retail health care by enacting in 2008 new Department of Public Health regulations that delineate what medical conditions and age groups may be treated at retail clinics. Originally, the proposed regulation included a requirement for prescreening by the Department of Public Health of all forms of advertising, but this was stricken after feedback from the Federal Trade Commission (FTC) indicated that it could be interpreted as anticompetitive and anticonsumer since prescreening applied only to retail clinics and not other types of clinics or practices (FTC, 2007).

The FTC also issued a formal opinion that certain provisions of an Illinois bill competitively disadvantaged retail clinics and limited health care access. Provisions of this failed bill included prohibitions against retail clinics within stores that sell tobacco products, negotiated copayments lower than for primary care practices, and advertising that compares clinic fees to those of other facilities (FTC, 2008).

BARRIERS TO SUCCESS

While the retail clinic model is cutting edge and exciting in many ways, it has faced barriers on the road to growth and success. Most of the challenges stem from market forces such as supply, demand, and barriers to entry.

FINANCIAL

Despite 65% average annual industry growth from 2000 through 2007 (Keckley, Underwood, & Gandhi, 2009), the financial hurdles to profitability have proven difficult. Retail clinics operate on a fixed-cost

model with approximately 85% of the costs committed to employee pay, leases, and general administration such as technology support and marketing (Scott, 2007), estimated at $600,000 per 450 square-foot clinic during 2006 (Keckley, Underwood, & Gandhi, 2008). With high fixed costs and low profit margins, profitability depends upon a high volume of patients. To break even, each clinic would need an estimated 200 to 230 patient visits every week (Keckley, Underwood, & Gandhi, 2008). Operators needed to invest heavily in marketing clinic openings in new markets to stimulate the broad consumer awareness that drives visit volumes (Armstrong, 2008). Additionally, one of the most significant barriers to financial success is the emphasis on simple acute conditions. This model favors clinic visits in the months during which upper respiratory illnesses are prevalent, making revenue seasonal. Thus, it has taken 1 to 2 years for a clinic to break even (Costello, 2008; Keckley, Underwood, & Gandhi, 2009). Some of the smaller companies, such as SmartCare Health Clinics and Corner Care Clinic, have withdrawn from the market because their capital investments were insufficient to carry them through the long interval to the break-even point (Keckley, Underwood, & Gandhi, 2008; Scott, 2007). Others have slowed expansions and even closed some of their clinics (see Figure 31-1).

LIMITED AVAILABILITY OF PRACTITIONERS

A limiting factor in the growth of retail clinics is the supply of health care providers. In the retail health industry, most of the staff are nurse practitioners. Generally, practitioners with a specialty in family medicine (FNPs) are hired since they can provide care across all age groups. Keckley and colleagues (2009) have estimated that staffing each retail clinic requires the equivalent of 2.5 full-time NPs. As of 2005, there were approximately 82,622 primary care NPs practicing in the U.S., but this number included adult and pediatric NPs in addition to those in family medicine (Steinwald, 2008). Of the recently graduated FNPs, 42% entered specialty practice instead of primary care (Allen & Viens, 2006). Further, the FNPs who might opt for practice in a retail clinic are not uniformly distributed. The available pool varies across geographic regions and even across communities within a state or region. The potential difficulty recruiting sufficient staff constrains expansion within current and new markets.

REGULATORY

State corporate practice of medicine (CPM) laws affect costs and business efficiencies. The CPM doctrine was created by the American Medical Association (Huberfeld, 2004) and has since been incorporated into some state laws to ensure that only those licensed to do so may legally practice medicine. In the states that have them, CPM laws mainly prohibit lay entities, such as business corporations, from (a) employing physicians, (b) owning the organization providing physician services, and, in some cases, (c) receiving a share of the physicians' fees (Huberfeld, 2004). In many states, CPM laws do not include NPs, but retail clinic operators must ensure that their business structures legally accommodate any oversight services provided by physicians (LeGros & Robison, 2008; Mullin, 2009).

Facility licensing also may impede or delay new clinic openings. It can become costly for multiclinic operations in states, such as Florida, that license and relicense on a per-clinic basis. In a very small number of states, such as Rhode Island, the physical space and privacy requirements make it difficult for many operators to enter the state with their current models (LeGros & Robison, 2008; Takach & Witgert, 2009b).

Another influencing factor is the state-by-state variation in NP practice regulations. Requirements for physician oversight range from none to on-site supervision. In the more restrictive states, there are increased costs associated with recruiting enough supervising physicians and with paying physicians to be on-site. There also is lack of uniformity in scope of NP practice across the country. For national or regional chains, there is a significant expenditure of resources in ensuring that existing and added services fall within the scope of practice in each state where clinics are located (LeGros & Robison, 2008). The result of these regulations is that operators may concentrate their business in states friendly to NP practice and to shy away from others.

FUTURE DIRECTIONS AND POLICY IMPLICATIONS

There is no doubt that retail clinics have significantly impacted the health care delivery system by providing patients with convenience, choice, control, and cost-effectiveness. The leadership of the retail health industry has spurred many traditional providers to expand their operating hours or provide open-access scheduling. The health care literature increasingly includes discussions about consumerism and a competitive marketplace in health care. Despite recent clinic closings, industry analysts expect continued growth, perhaps by as many as 4000 clinics by 2015 (see Figure 31-1). The opportunity to refine the business model is unmistakable as the retail clinic industry enters its next iteration (Keckley, Underwood, & Gandhi, 2009).

Retail clinic organizations are reaching out to medical systems, health plans, and employers to help solve the problem of fragmentation of care. Multiple convenient locations provide easy access, and multiple providers could utilize retail clinics to help them meet their patients' goals. They may become a venue for helping to monitor and manage patients with chronic diseases, which would also help the medical home build a medical neighborhood (Friedsam & Pfefferkorn, 2009) with multiple access points that allow patients to receive the right care in the lowest cost setting. Working collaboratively with PCP partners, retail health care centers could contribute to these robust medical homes through provision of services supporting standards of care to be accomplished and communicated real time to PCPs. A key example of this development was the agreement reached between MinuteClinic and Cleveland Clinic in February 2009. According to the Bureau of National Affairs (2009), MinuteClinic would provide more coordinated care for Cleveland Clinic patients, including two-way electronic record sharing. This kind of interconnectedness has been viewed as a positive step for health care delivery in reducing fragmentation and improving quality. However, Herrick and Goodman (2007) suggest that true integration, in which primary care and retail clinics derive mutual financial benefit from the efficiencies of a shared practice, may require changes to the federal Stark Laws that prohibit referral to a clinic in which a physician has a financial interest. Regulatory barriers to a systems approach for health care, such as the corporate practice of medicine laws, would need to be resolved (Scott, 2006).

There also is the opportunity to support current health care reform efforts by expanding access to lower-cost care for those who are underinsured or uninsured. Many do not have a usual source of care and are three times more likely than those with insurance to go without the care they need (Lugo, Giorgianni, & Zimmerman, 2006). Retail clinics typically provide a lower-cost alternative to physician practices and the emergency department for acute episodic care, and they currently have the capacity for 17 million visits a year (Bureau of National Affairs, 2009). To help broaden access, state Medicaid plans must lift restrictions such as the requirement for a referral from the primary care provider to use a retail clinic or reimbursement to retail clinics only for urgent and emergent care.

Retail clinics also have opportunities to promote population health in collaboration with the traditional public health system (Salinsky, 2009). The customer outreach generated by the clinics' retail partners, such as advertising and in-store campaigns, can drive awareness of health promotion and disease prevention campaigns. The holistic paradigm of NPs and physician assistants who staff retail clinics fosters an environment for discussion of risk factors such as elevated blood pressure, tobacco use, and missed immunizations. The widespread availability of clinics also increases access points for mass immunizations or prophylaxis in the event of epidemics. Since most retail clinics use electronic medical records, easy data access can be helpful for disease surveillance. However, this would be facilitated only when the health care community produces a nationwide platform for data exchange.

For sustainability and to fulfill a public health role, Harlow (Bureau of National Affairs, 2009) has suggested that retail clinics need to expand services. Already some retail clinic companies are offering screenings and wellness services, such as blood pressure checks, cholesterol screenings, and tobacco cessation. Since approximately 44% of people with chronic conditions do not get the care recommended by evidence-based guidelines (McGlynn et al., 2003), broadening services to address chronic diseases can help meet the needs of millions of consumers. Regulatory and reimbursement structures, however, need the changes that would permit NPs in retail settings to engage in a more expanded scope of practice.

The retail clinic model continues to evolve, and its ultimate impact on health care delivery in America is yet to be determined. Unquestionably, this innovative model has spurred changes in the health care delivery system in response to consumers' demands for convenience, accessibility, and price transparency. But, will retail health clinics prove to be a "transformational force" (Mullin, 2009, p. 533) in the health delivery systems of the future? Or, will professional, payer, and regulatory pressures force retail clinics to mold themselves into more traditional models of care? Since the topic of health care reform is sure to be with Americans for the foreseeable future, it is exciting that new and innovative models are being tested to help solve the nation's health care crisis.

For a list of related websites, please refer to your Evolve Resources at http://evolve.elsevier.com/Mason/policypolitics/

REFERENCES

Agency for Healthcare Research and Quality. (2008, April 14). *Innovation profile: Retail walk-in clinics provide easy access to low-cost primary care services.* Rockville, MD: Author. Retrieved from www.innovations.ahrq.gov/content.aspx?id=1772.

Ahmed A., & Fincham, J. E. (2010). Physician office vs retail clinic: Patient preferences in seeking care for minor illnesses. *Annals of Family Medicine, 8*(2), 117-123.

Allen, P. J., & Viens, D. C. (2006). Employment characteristics of recent FNP graduates. *American Journal for Nurse Practitioners, 10*(10), 13-26.

American Academy of Nurse Practitioners. (2007). *Standards for nurse practitioner practice in retail based clinics.* Austin, TX: Author.

Armstrong, D. (2008, May 7). Health clinics inside stores, likely to slow their growth. *Wall Street Journal.* Retrieved from www.wakeupwalmart.com/news/article.html?article=1553.

Bachman, J. (2006, May). What do retail clinics mean for family medicine? *Family Practice Management, 13*(5), 19-20.

Bureau of National Affairs. (2009, April 20). *Efforts to regulate retail clinics slow, as industry finds its place* (Health policy report 17 HCPR 599). Arlington, VA: Author.

Christensen, C. (2007, Oct 26). A decade of disruption. *Forbes.* Retrieved from www.forbes.com/2007/08/31/christensen-disruption-kodak-pf-guru_in_cc_0904christensen_inl.html.

Convenient Care Association quality and safety standards. (2008). Philadelphia: Convenient Care Association. Retrieved from www.ccaclinics.org/index.php?option=com_content&view=article&id=6&Itemid=13.

Costello, D. (2008). A checkup for retail medicine. *Health Affairs, 27*(5), 1299-1303.

Deloitte Center for Health Solutions. (2009). *2009 Survey of health care consumers: Key findings, strategic implications.* Washington, D.C.: Author.

Federal Trade Commission. (2007, September 27). *Health care Federal Trade Commission staff comment to LouAnn Stanton, Massachusetts Department of Health* [Letter]. Retrieved from www.ftc.gov/os/2007/10/v070015massclinic.pdf.

Federal Trade Commission. (2008, May 29). *FTC staff comment to Representative Elaine Nekritz of the Illinois General Assembly* [Letter]. Retrieved from www.ftc.gov/os/2008/06/V080013letter.pdf.

Friedsam, D., & Pfefferkorn, B. (2009, March). *Medical homes and retail clinics: Policy considerations for accountable health care* (Issue brief, vol. 9 no. 1). Madison, WI: University of Wisconsin Population Health Institute.

Fronstin, P., & Helman, R. (2009, July). *The 2009 Health Confidence Survey: Public opinion on health reform varies; strong support for insurance market reform and public plan option, mixed response to tax cap* (Issue brief no. 331). Washington, D.C.: Employee Benefit Research Institute.

Green, R. (2007). Rationale against NPs in retail-based clinics. *Journal for Nurse Practitioners, 3*(8), 528-529.

Herrick, D. M., & Goodman, J. C. (2007, February). *Why you don't know the price; why you don't know the quality; and what can be done about it* (Report no. 296). Dallas: National Center for Policy Analysis.

Huberfeld, N. (2004). Be not afraid of change: Time to eliminate the corporate practice of medicine doctrine. *Health Matrix, 14*(2), 243-291.

Hunter, L. P., Weber, C. E., Morreale, A. P., & Wall, J. H. (2009). Patient satisfaction with retail health clinic care. *Journal of the American Academy of Nurse Practitioners, 21*(10), 565-570.

Kantor, A. (2007, September/October). The retail health clinic: A revolution in convenience. *America's Health Insurance Plans.* Retrieved from www.ahip.org/content/default.aspx?bc=31%7C130%7C136%7C21129%7C21131.

Keckley, P. H., Underwood, H. R., & Gandhi, M. (2008). *Retail clinics: Facts, trends and implications.* Washington, D.C.: Deloitte Center for Health Solutions.

Keckley, P. H., Underwood, H. R., & Gandhi, M. (2009). *Retail clinics: Update and implications.* Washington, D.C.: Deloitte Center for Health Solutions.

Krizner, K. (2006, December 1). Health plan networks slowly embrace nurse practitioners. *Managed Healthcare Executive.* Retrieved from http://managedhealthcareexecutive.modernmedicine.com/mhe/Hospitals+&+Providers/Health-plan-networks-slowly-embrace-nurse-practiti/Article Standard/Article/detail/389263.

LeGros, N., & Robison, A. (2008, September). Retail clinics—coming soon to a store near you. *Health Lawyer News,* 32-39.

Lugo, N. R., Giorgianni, S. J., & Zimmerman, P. A. (2006, April 17). *Nurse practitioner services in retail locations: A white paper by the Nurse Practitioner Healthcare Foundation.* Bellevue, WA: Nurse Practitioner Healthcare Foundation.

McGlynn, E. A., Asch, S. M., Adams, J, Keesey, J., Hicks, J., DeCristofaro, A., & Kerr, E. A. (2003). The quality of health care delivered to adults in the United States. *New England Journal of Medicine, 348*(26), 2635-2645.

Mehrotra, A., Liu, H., Adams, J. L., Wang, M. C., Lave, J. R., Thygeson, N. M., Solberg, L. I., & McGlynn, E. A. (2009). Comparing costs and quality of care at retail clinics with that of other medical settings for 3 common illnesses. *Annals of Internal Medicine, 151*(5), 321-328.

Mehrotra, A., Wang, M. C., Lave, J. R., Adams, J. L., & McGlynn, E. A. (2008) Retail clinics, primary care physicians, and emergency departments: A comparison of patients' visits. *Health Affairs, 27*(5), 1272-1282.

Mullin, K. (2009). Considering retail health clinics. *Journal of Nursing Administration, 39*(12), 531-536.

National Association of Community Health Centers. (2009, March). *Primary care access: An essential building block of health reform.* Bethesda, MD: Author.

National Center for Health Statistics. (2009a). *No usual source of health care among adults 18-64 years of age, by selected characteristics: United States, average annual 1997-1998, 2001-2002, and 2006-2007.* Atlanta: Centers for Disease Control and Prevention. Retrieved from www.cdc.gov/nchs/health_policy/adults_no_source_health_care.htm.

National Center for Health Statistics. (2009b). *No usual source of health care among children under 18 years of age, by selected characteristics: United States, average annual 1997-1998, 2001-2002, and 2006-2007.* Atlanta: Centers for Disease Control and Prevention. Retrieved from www.cdc.gov/nchs/health_policy/children_no_source_health_care.htm.

New WSJ.com/Harris Interactive study finds satisfaction with retail-based health clinics remains high. (2008, May 21). *Harris Interactive.* Retrieved from www.harrisinteractive.com/news/allnewsbydate.asp?NewsID=1308.

Retail Clinics. (2009). Arlington, VA: Association of State and Territorial Health Officials. Retrieved from www.astho.org/Programs/Access/Primary-Care/Retail-Clinics-Fact-Sheet.

Rudavsky, R., Pollack, C. E., & Mehrotra, A. (2009). The geographic distribution, ownership, prices, and scope of practice at retail clinics. *Annals of Internal Medicine, 151*(5), 315-320.

Sage, W. M. (2009, February 2). Out of the box: The future of retail medical clinics. *Harvard Law and Policy Review Online, 3,* 1-11. Retrieved from http://hlpronline.com/new/wp-content/uploads/2009/11/Sage_HLPR_020209.pdf.

Salinsky, E. (2009). Medicine, big business, and public health: Wake up and smell the Starbucks. *Preventing Chronic Disease, 6*(2), A75-A79.

Scott, M. K. (2006). *Healthcare in the express lane: The emergence of retail clinics.* Oakland, CA: California HealthCare Foundation.

Scott, M. K. (2007). *Healthcare in the express lane: Retail clinics go mainstream.* Oakland, CA: California HealthCare Foundation.

Silva, C. (2007, April 15). One-minute drill: Black & Decker finds MinuteClinic drills down costs. *Employee Benefit News.* Retrieved from http://ebn.benefitnews.com/news/one-minute-drill-black-decker-finds-39958-1.html.

Steinwald, A. B. (2008, February 12). *Primary care professionals: Recent supply trends, projections, and valuation of services* (Publication no. GAO-08-472T). Washington, D.C.: U.S. Government Accountability Office.

Sullivan, D. (2006, May). Retail health clinics are rolling your way. *Family Practice Management, 13*(5), 65-72.

Takach, M., & Witgert, K. (2009a). *Retail clinics: Six state approaches to regulation and licensing.* Oakland, CA: California HealthCare Foundation.

Takach, M., & Witgert, K. (2009b). *Analysis of state regulations and policies governing the operation and licensure of retail clinics.* Portland, ME: National Academy for State Health Policy.

Tu Ha, T., & Cohen, G. R. (2008). *Checking up on retail-based health clinics: Is the boom ending?* (publication no. 1199). *48,* 1-11. New York: The Commonwealth Fund.

Wilson, C. (2009, March 5). Growing retail clinic industry could impact self-pay collections volume. *InsideARM.* Retrieved from www.insidearm.com/index.cfm?objectID=D6F6FF6E-D754-50F9-FF63B9107B547566&print=1.

CHAPTER 32

Nurse-Managed Health Centers

Tine Hansen-Turton and Ann Ritter

"The innovation point is the pivotal moment when talented and motivated people seek the opportunity to act on their ideas and dreams."

—W. Arthur Porter

Nurse-managed health centers (NMHCs) have been established by innovative health care providers who are eager to extend the reach of community health services. These health centers represent a promising delivery model for high-quality primary and preventive care, especially for low-income and vulnerable populations. In addition, they serve an important role in nursing education, acting as clinical education sites for nurses and other health professionals throughout the United States. By supporting increased funding and enhanced reimbursement for this model of care, policymakers can encourage the sustainability of existing nurse-managed primary care access points *and* improve clinical education opportunities for the next generation of nurses.

Since its creation in 1996, the National Nursing Centers Consortium (NNCC) has worked with its health center members to pursue national- and state-level policy reform efforts that will increase the capacity of NMHCs to educate students and serve patients. (See Box 32-1 for more on the NNCC.) This chapter provides an overview of the NMHC model, the policy barriers that threaten NMHCs, and examples of recent state and federal policy initiatives designed to encourage their growth and development.

THE NURSE-MANAGED HEALTH CENTER MODEL

NMHCs are community-based health centers led by advanced practices registered nurses. Although predominantly staffed by nurse practitioners (NPs), these health centers employ a team-based approach to care that often includes social workers,

health educators, registered nurses, outreach workers, collaborating physicians, and other health professionals. While the roots of the model are in public health nursing, most modern NMHCs were created beginning in the 1980s, as NPs saw their professional authority to provide care evolve, and new governmental funding sources allowed for the creation of NMHCs (King, 2008). Today, the founders of several NMHCs have been designated as "Edge Runners" by the American Academy of Nursing because their centers represent innovative models of care for which there are excellent clinical and financial outcome data (Box 32-2).

Despite some ongoing confusion among the public, NMHCs are not nursing homes. In fact, relatively few NMHCs provide care exclusively to senior populations, and less than 10% of NMHCs' payer mix can be attributed to Medicare (Hansen-Turton, Line, O'Connell, Rothman, & Lauby, 2004). NMHCs serve a diverse patient population, both in terms of racial and ethnic make-up, as well as age. A number of NMHCs serve exclusively pediatric patients, while most provide care to adult patients of all ages. Overall, there are approximately 250 NMHCs located throughout the country in 40 states (National Nursing Centers Consortium [NNCC], 2008). According to NNCC member data from 2010, the Northeast, the Southeast, and the Midwest are the regions of the country with the greatest numbers of NMHCs.

NNCC members vary in services but fall into two broad categories. *Nurse-managed primary care centers* offer a broad scope of primary care services and can serve as designated primary care providers for patients. The services provided by these clinics are comparable to those provided by federally-qualified health centers (FQHCs), and some nurse-managed primary care centers are part of the FQHC program. (See Box 32-3 for more on FQHCs.) *Nurse-managed wellness centers* serve as crucial entry points into the

BOX 32-1 National Nursing Centers Consortium (NNCC)

The NNCC works to advance nurse-led health care through policy, consultation, programs and applied research to reduce health disparities and meet people's primary care and wellness needs. The NNCC has published two toolkits designed to help nurses start and sustain primary care and wellness health centers. The first, entitled *Community and Nurse-Managed Health Centers: Getting Them Started and Keeping Them Going*, was published in 2005 and was selected as the American Journal of Nursing's Best Book of the Year. The second, entitled *Nurse-Managed Wellness Centers: Developing and Maintaining Your Center*, was published in 2009. Both are available from Springer Publications. For more information about the NNCC, its members, and its current policy initiatives, visit *www.nncc.us*.

Source: *www.nncc.us*.

BOX 32-2 American Academy of Nursing (AAN) Edge Runners

A number of NNCC members have been recognized for their innovative work through the AAN Edge Runners project. To learn more about these outstanding health centers (and the nurses who direct them), visit the following sites:

- Eleventh Street Family Health Services of Drexel University (Patricia Gerrity, PhD, RN, FAAN): *www.drexel.edu/cnhp/11thstreet/home.asp*
- Harambee Nursing Center (Kay T. Roberts, EdD, MSN, ARNP, FAAN): *http://louisville.edu/nursing/harambee*
- Living Independently for Elders (LIFE) Center (Eileen Sullivan-Marx, PhD, CRNP, FAAN): *www.lifeupenn.org*

but also innovative approaches to lifestyle, community, and environmental issues that can significantly impact patients' health. One such example of this kind of service integration can be found at Eleventh Street Family Health Services of Drexel University, an NMHC serving public housing residents in Philadelphia. This nationally-recognized health center provides an array of services to the community, including comprehensive primary care and integrated behavioral health services. A team of social workers, educators, nurses, outreach workers, and others conduct health screenings, group exercise and cooking classes, and outreach programs to prevent lead poisoning and reduce asthma complications in children (Ferrari & Rideout, 2005). In addition, the health center has recently developed an outdoor garden on-site to increase access to nutritious food and further address the social determinants of health in its community (Drexel University, 2009).

QUALITY OF CARE IN NURSE-MANAGED HEALTH CENTERS

Comprehensive, team-based care and enabling services in NMHCs result in excellent outcomes for patients. Studies have shown that NPs provide high-quality primary care with outcomes similar to those of physicians (Mundinger et al., 2000; Lenz, Mundinger, Kane, Hopkins, & Lin, 2004). An evaluation of 11 NMHCs in Pennsylvania (funded by the Centers for Medicare and Medicaid Services) found that NMHCs also had higher patient retention rates and lower patient hospitalization rates when compared with similar safety-net providers (i.e., physician-managed community health centers) (Hansen-Turton et al., 2004, p. 5). NMHCs consistently receive high patient satisfaction ratings, with patients giving especially high marks in areas such as "being treated with respect" and "explaining things to you" (Benkert, George, Tanner, Barkauskas, Pohl, & Marszalek, 2007, p. 107).

THE ROLE OF NURSE-MANAGED HEALTH CENTERS IN HEALTH WORKFORCE DEVELOPMENT

In addition to providing services directly to clients, NMHCs also play an important role in health professions education. More than 85 nursing schools operate NMHCs that provide care to patients and enhance learning and practice opportunities for

primary care system for many patients. Nurses provide health screenings, vaccinations, direct care for minor acute problems, health education, and counseling services. They also provide community-based health promotion programs to address problems such as smoking, obesity, and poor nutrition, all with the goal of improving patients' quality of life.

NMHCs also provide support, outreach, and counseling services that are integrated into the larger community. This approach takes into account not only diagnosis of disease and medication therapies,

BOX 32-3 Federally Qualified Health Centers (FQHCs)

Throughout the United States, federally qualified health centers (FQHCs) provide health care to medically underserved communities and vulnerable patients. Often referred to as community health centers, these community-based providers offer primary care and other health services to patients regardless of their ability to pay. The FQHC designation was created by the federal government more than 40 years ago, and health centers that are part of the FQHC program are able to access enhanced reimbursement and federal grant funding streams that are not available to other safety net providers. The FQHC program has specific requirements for participation and is administered by the U.S. Health Resources and Services Administration (HRSA) Bureau of Primary Health Care, which is part of the U.S. Department of Health and Human Services. There are currently 1200 FQHCs in the U.S., serving more than 20 million people each year.

For more information about the funding requirements of the Federally Qualified Health Center Program, visit the website of the HRSA Bureau of Primary Health Care at *bphc. hrsa.gov.* For more information on Federally Qualified Health Centers generally, visit the website of the National Association of Community Health Centers at *www.nachc.org.*

Source: *www.nncc.us.*

students and faculty (NNCC, 2009a). A member survey conducted by NNCC in 2009 found that the largest percentage of health professions students completing clinical rotations in NMHCs were bachelors-level nursing students (49% of all students), followed by masters-level NP students (22%) (NNCC, 2009b). These centers also provided clinical opportunities to students in associates degree and doctoral nursing programs. Also, hundreds of students in medicine, social work, pharmacy, and dentistry programs complete clinical rotations annually in NMHCs (Institute for Nursing Centers, 2008).

CHALLENGES TO SUSTAINABILITY

AVAILABILITY OF FEDERAL FUNDING

NMHCs are safety net providers for patients regardless of their ability to pay. About 35% to 40% of NMHC patients are uninsured (Institute for Nursing Centers, 2008). NMHCs use a sliding fee scale to collect payment from uninsured patients, but these contributions alone do not cover the actual cost of care. As a result, they rely heavily on charitable grants in order to make up the difference, which translates into greater year-to-year budget instability for many health centers. Lack of access to predictable governmental funding and inconsistent reimbursement from insurers compounds the problem, leaving hundreds of thousands of low-income and vulnerable patients throughout the country at risk of losing their primary source of health care.

Many NMHCs in the U.S. were initially launched with start-up grants from the Health Resources and Services Administration (HRSA) Bureau of Health Professions' Division of Nursing. Recognizing the important role that NMHCs could play in providing clinical education placements for nursing students and faculty, the Division of Nursing funded NMHCs through its "special projects" program (King, 2008, p. 14). However, these grants were nonrenewable and many schools found themselves unable to identify and secure sustainable long-term funding once the grant period had ended. As a result, many NMHCs closed their doors after Division of Nursing funding dried up. Meanwhile, the remaining health centers focused on acquiring funding from private foundations and improving reimbursement from third-party payers, all with varying degrees of success.

A small minority of the surviving academic NMHCs have been able to achieve fiscal sustainability by becoming part of the FQHC program, administered by the HRSA Bureau of Primary Health Care (a separate administrative entity from the HRSA Bureau of Health Professions). However, this was not an option for many academic NMHCs. The fact that many NMHCs are affiliated with schools of nursing often prevents them from qualifying for FQHC program funding because they cannot meet the program's governance requirements.[1] Inability to qualify for the FQHC program threatens the sustainability of NMHCs, because it prevents them from accessing the

---

[1]Specifically, the HRSA Bureau of Primary Health Care requires that more than half of the Directors of an FQHC are community members served by the health center. Since schools of nursing are controlled by the trustees of their larger college or university, they cannot meet this requirement. Although most academic nurse-managed health centers have community advisory boards, this is not enough to meet the governance requirements of the FQHC program.

many benefits that the government makes available to FQHCs. For example, FQHCs are able to receive enhanced reimbursement for services provided to Medicaid beneficiaries. FQHCs were also able to qualify for special funding opportunities through the American Recovery and Reinvestment Act of 2009 (e.g., for capital improvement projects or increased staffing) that were unavailable to non-FQHCs. Without access to ongoing federal support (like that provided to FQHCs by the Bureau of Primary Health Care), NMHCs struggle to provide care to uninsured patients while remaining financially solvent.

INSURER POLICIES REGARDING NURSE PRACTITIONERS

Lack of access to federal funding is not the only barrier to NMHC sustainability. Although many patients seen by NMHCs are uninsured, a significant proportion has publicly-funded or commercial insurance that could provide reimbursement for services. Unfortunately, many insurers do not recognize NPs as primary care providers and will not reimburse them directly. A 2008 study of managed care policies conducted by NNCC found that only 53% of insurers credential NPs as primary care providers (Hansen-Turton, Ritter, & Torgan, 2008). While some of these restrictive insurer policies appear to be attributable to a lack of understanding about NPs' ability to provide high-quality primary care to patients, the problem is compounded by confusing state regulations regarding the legal authority of NPs to work in NMHCs with off-site physician involvement (Hansen-Turton, et al., 2008). Even though NPs are able to serve as primary care providers in all 50 states, insurers are considerably less likely to recognize NPs as primary care providers when state laws contain language requiring physician "supervision" or "delegation" for NP practice (Hansen-Turton et al., 2008). As a result, many NMHCs are not reimbursed by insurers for the care that they provide to patients, and they are less able to attract insured patients who could offset the cost of providing care to the uninsured. Recognizing that insurer policies like these result in fewer primary care access points for patients, lawmakers in Massachusetts recently passed new legislation requiring insurers to contract with NPs as primary care providers, which could serve as a model for other states (Craven & Ober, 2009).

EXPANDING THE REACH OF NURSE-MANAGED HEALTH CENTERS

STATE-LEVEL APPROACHES TO SUPPORT NURSE-MANAGED HEALTH CENTERS

There are a variety of state laws and policies that can impact NMHCs and their ability to serve patients (Ritter & Hansen-Turton, 2008). Because they are managed and staffed by advanced practice nurses, scope of practice, licensing, and physician collaboration laws can all have a big impact on care provided in NMHCs. Meanwhile, state laws regarding managed care insurers can either encourage or discourage patients from selecting a NMHC as his or her primary care home. In addition, some state governments with an interest in improving health care have made additional funding and other resources available to primary care practices through "medical home" demonstration projects and other quality improvement initiatives. These initiatives may or may not include nurse-led models.

One example of a recent effort that provided additional support and recognition for NMHCs is Pennsylvania Governor Edward G. Rendell's *Prescription for Pennsylvania* health reform plan (Hansen-Turton, Ritter, & Valdez, 2009). Launched in 2006, this multifaceted policy initiative was designed to increase access, reduce costs, and improve health care quality by implementing an array of strategies touching a broad cross-section of the health care industry (including insurers, hospitals, providers, and others) (Commonwealth of Pennsylvania, 2009). Some of the first components of *Prescription for Pennsylvania* to be implemented successfully were three bills designed to improve the practice environment for NPs, certified nurse midwives, and clinical nurse specialists. These laws removed long-standing barriers to efficient advanced nursing practice by granting NPs the authority to order home health and hospice care, granting certified nurse midwives prescriptive authority, and, for the first time, defining the specific education and training requirements needed to practice as a clinical nurse specialist (Hansen-Turton et al., 2009, p. 9). In subsequent years, the Governor's Office of Health Care Reform also spearheaded efforts to implement a medical home pilot project in southeastern Pennsylvania that is inclusive of nurse-led practices, and also inserted language into its Medicaid managed care Request for Proposals (RFP) encouraging insurers to better utilize NPs and other non-physicians in their provider networks (Pennsylvania Department of Public Welfare, 2008). Although they have not removed all barriers to independent advanced nursing practice, this combination of cost-effective policy efforts, driven by both the executive and legislative branches and championed by Governor Rendell throughout his tenure, has made it easier for NMHCs in Pennsylvania to continue providing care to low-income and vulnerable patients.

FEDERAL-LEVEL APPROACHES TO SUPPORT NURSE-MANAGED HEALTH CENTERS

Providing access to predictable, adequate public funding is the best way to support non-profit health centers that provide care to high percentages of uninsured patients. As explained above, lack of access to stable funding is one of the most challenging aspects of maintaining an NMHC. As a result, NNCC has conducted a variety of policy advocacy and education efforts with the goal of creating a dedicated funding stream for NMHCs within HRSA.

NMHC advocates have worked with Congressional health staffers to introduce the Nurse-Managed Health Clinic Investment Act in 2007 and 2009. While these bills would not provide NMHCs immediate access to the enhanced reimbursement available to FQHCs, they would define NMHCs as a recognized entity in federal statute, provide access to a new dedicated federal funding stream, and set the stage for improved reimbursement in the future.

The Nurse-Managed Health Clinic Investment Act (S. 2112) was first introduced in the Senate by Senators Daniel Inouye (D-HI) and Lamar Alexander (R-TN) in 2007. This piece of legislation would have created a $50 million grant program to support NMHCs, to be administered by HRSA's Bureau of Primary Health Care. Ultimately, this bill died in committee, but it helped lay the groundwork for reintroduction of the bill.

The Nurse-Managed Health Clinic Investment Act was reintroduced in early 2009 in the Senate by Senators Alexander and Inouye (S. 1104) and in the House of Representatives by Congresswoman Lois Capps (D-CA) and Congressman Lee Terry (R-NE) (H.R. 2754). Recognizing the opportunity that the Obama administration's health reform efforts presented,

Congressional staff in both chambers worked with NNCC advocates to insert language from this bill into the Patient Protection and Affordable Care Act of 2010. The new law authorizes $50 million for 2010 and additional funding as needed through fiscal year 2014, but this funding is not mandated and must be appropriated every year by Congress. Given concerns about the federal deficit, securing this appropriation will be challenging. However, NMHCs also have the opportunity to apply for funding opportunities for expanding community-based health centers for which funding is mandated and is not subject to the annual appropriations process. As the nation recognizes that it must expand its capacity for community-based primary care and wellness services, NMHCs offer an infrastructure that could be expanded to meet this need if the financial and development support is available.

SUMMARY

Because of their unique dual role as training sites for health professionals and health care homes for vulnerable patients, NMHCs are an especially critical component of our health care system. NMHCs must be better supported to ensure that we have enough qualified providers to guarantee access to health care for all Americans and enough safety net providers to take care of vulnerable people with complex needs. Policymakers at all levels of government are beginning to understand the untapped potential of advanced practice nurses and NMHCs to improve care for patients throughout the country.

For a list of related websites, please refer to your Evolve Resources at http://evolve.elsevier.com/Mason/policypolitics/

REFERENCES

Benkert, R., George N., Tanner, C., Barkauskas, V., Pohl, J., & Marszalek, A. (2007). Satisfaction with a school-based teen health center: A report card on care. *Pediatric Nursing, 33*(2), 103-109.

Commonwealth of Pennsylvania. (2009). Prescription for Pennsylvania. Retrieved from www.rxforpa.com.

Craven, G., & Ober, S. (2009). Massachusetts nurse practitioners step up as one solution to the primary care access problem: A political success story. *Policy, Politics and Nursing Practice, 10*(2), 94-100.

Drexel University. (2009, November 4). Drexel University's Eleventh Street Health Services recognized as national model of innovative health care [Press Release]. Retrieved from www.drexel.edu/cnhp/11thstreetnews. asp.

Ferrari, A., & Rideout, B. (2005). The collaboration of public health nursing and primary care nursing in the development of a nurse managed health center. *Nursing Clinics of North America, 40*(4), 771-778.

Hansen-Turton, T., Line, L., O'Connell, M., Rothman, N., & Lauby, J. (2004). *The Nursing Center Model of Health Care for the Underserved.* Submitted to the U.S. Centers for Medicare and Medicaid Services (CMS), June 2004. (Available from the National Nursing Centers Fairman Consortium, 260 S. Broad Street, 18th Floor, Philadelphia, PA 19102.)

Hansen-Turton, T., Ritter, A., & Torgan, R. (2008). Insurers' contracting policies on nurse practitioners as primary care providers: Two years later. *Policy, Politics, and Nursing Practice, 9*(4), 241-248.

Hansen-Turton T., Ritter, A., & Valdez, B. (2009). Developing alliances: How nurse practitioners became part of the Prescription for Pennsylvania. *Policy, Politics, and Nursing Practice, 10*(1), 7-15.

Institute for Nursing Centers. (2008). Highlight report from the Data Warehouse, October 2008. Retrieved from www.nursingcenters.org/PDFs/INC%20Highlight%20Report%2010_6_08.pdf.

King, E. S. (2008). A 10-year review of four academic nurse-managed centers: Challenges and survival strategies. *Journal of Professional Nursing, 24*(1), 14-20.

Lenz, E. R., Mundinger, M. O., Kane, R. L., Hopkins, S. C., & Lin, S. X. (2004). Primary care outcomes in patients treated by nurse practitioners or physicians: Two-year follow-up. *Medical Care Research and Review, 61*(3), 332-351.

Mundinger, M. O., Kane, R. L., Lenz, E. R., Totten, A. M., Tsai, W., et al. (2000). Primary care outcomes in patients treated by nurse practitioners or physicians: A randomized trial. *Journal of the American Medical Association, 283*(1), 59-68.

National Nursing Centers Consortium. (2008). *Comments regarding notice of proposed rulemaking—Designation of medically underserved populations and health professional shortage areas.* Submitted to United States Health Services and Resources Administration (HRSA), May 23, 2008. (Statement of Tine Hansen-Turton, Executive Director, National Nursing Centers Consortium). (Available from the National Nursing Centers Consortium, 260 S. Broad Street, 18th Floor, Philadelphia, PA 19102.)

National Nursing Centers Consortium. (2009a). *Colleges and Universities with Affiliated Nurse-Managed Health Centers.* (Available from the National Nursing Centers Consortium, 260 S. Broad Street, 18th Floor, Philadelphia, PA 19102.)

National Nursing Centers Consortium. (2009b). *Student Education in Nurse-Managed Health Centers.* (Available from the National Nursing Centers Consortium, 260 S. Broad Street, 18th Floor, Philadelphia, PA 19102.)

Pennsylvania Department of Public Welfare. (2008). Physical Health Southwest (PHSW)—RFP #34-08, Part II. Retrieved from www.dpw.state.pa.us/omap/rfp/PHSW/PHSWrfpPart2.asp.

Ritter, A., & Hansen-Turton, T. (2008). The primary care paradigm shift: An overview of the state-level legal framework governing nurse practitioner practice. *The Health Lawyer, 8*(4), 21-28.

CHAPTER 33

Community Health Centers: Successful Advocacy for Expanding Health Care Access

Alice Sardell

This chapter is dedicated to the life and memory of Senator Edward M. Kennedy (1932-2009), who was the legislative "father" of the community health center program in 1966 and its most steadfast and eloquent champion for the rest of his life.

In 2010, there were more than 1200 community health centers (CHCs) serving more than 20 million people at 8000 clinical sites all over the United States (National Association of Community Health Centers, 2010a). These programs provide medical, dental, mental health, and substance abuse services, nutrition counseling, outreach, transportation, and other social services to uninsured patients as well as those with Medicaid, Medicare, Children's Health Insurance Program (CHIP), and even private health insurance. Community health centers also include programs serving migrant workers and the homeless.

CHCs are located in areas designated by the federal government as medically underserved and provide care without regard to insurance status or ability to pay. They are primarily funded by a mix of public insurance and federal grants. Patients served by CHCs are poorer, sicker, and much more likely to live in a rural area and to be persons of color than the general U.S. population (National Association of Community Health Centers, 2010a).

CHCs are unique health service institutions in several important ways. First, they are a community-oriented, culturally sensitive model of health care services integrated with social and educational services. Second, they are governed by consumer boards that by federal law must have a majority of members who are patients at the health center. Third, they are "safety net providers," caring for people who do not have health insurance.

These health care institutions were first funded as "neighborhood health centers" as part of the War on Poverty in 1965, one aspect of President Lyndon B. Johnson's Great Society program. They were created by activist physicians and federal government officials—"policy entrepreneurs"—who believed that disparities in health status were intimately linked to social, economic, and political inequalities. Health centers were to treat whole communities, not just individuals, and to provide jobs as well as health services. Although these programs were products of the policy environment of the 1960s, they survived the end of the War on Poverty and subsequent political challenges during the more conservative Nixon and Reagan Administrations. Not only did they overcome these challenges, but they became institutionalized as part of the federally funded health care system. In fact, health centers were the only domestic social program (other than abstinence-only health education) that was expanded during President George W. Bush's tenure in office.

The policy history of the CHC program explains how a program providing care to communities with very few political resources and therefore little political influence was able to survive and grow in an era in which less and less attention was paid to problems such as poverty and inequality. This occurred because supporters within federal executive agencies and Congress nurtured the program during its first decade until an effective national advocacy organization was built. This national organization, its state partners, and local health centers then successfully created broad support for health centers that is bipartisan and exists across ideological boundaries. The story of the survival of the CHC program is a story about the creation of a "policy network" supportive of CHCs. The story of its expansion is a tale of skilled policy advocates who have been able to frame the argument for health center funding in a way that fits within a political environment vastly different from the one in which it was born.

THE CREATION OF THE NEIGHBORHOOD HEALTH CENTER PROGRAM

The first neighborhood health centers were funded in 1965 as demonstration programs by the Community Action Program established by the Economic Opportunity Act (EOA) of 1964. The goal of this legislation was to eliminate the causes of poverty in the United States. Health was not initially one of the areas in which programs were to be established, but early on it became clear that participants in the educational and training programs that were established (e.g., Head Start and the Jobs Corps) suffered from lack of access to health care. The very first health programs were created by two medical educators, Dr. H. Jack Geiger and Dr. Count Gibson, of Tufts University Medical School.

The model of the two centers that they established, one in a Boston housing project and one in a poor rural area of Mississippi, was based on a public health–social medicine approach. It combined comprehensive health services, community development, and the training and employment of community residents. Health center staff in Mississippi found that children in the community had recurring episodes of malnutrition and dysentery. In response they organized residents who decided to construct wells and establish a farm cooperative to feed themselves and their children. Other health centers funded under this program, which was authorized by an amendment to the EOA by Senator Edward Kennedy (D-MA), also provided community development and employment opportunities as well as health care services. For example, a neighborhood health center in Brooklyn, New York, gave preference in hiring to local residents, and health center staff facilitated the creation of a

community organization to rehabilitate housing in the area.

By the end of 1971, 100 neighborhood health centers had been funded under Kennedy's 1966 amendment. The original neighborhood health center model contained four elements: social medicine, community-based care, community economic development, and community participation. From the social medicine perspective, health status is shaped by the physical and social environment, and treatment includes intervention in that environment. Health care was to be community based by offering services to all of the residents of a specific geographic catchment area (rather than to those who fit within certain disease or health insurance categories) and by employing community residents to serve as a bridge between patients and professional staff. These workers, often called *family health workers,* made home visits and provided health education and advocacy services along with health care. The recruitment, training, and employment of these workers were also an example of the way in which neighborhood health centers were venues for community economic development.

Finally, "maximum feasible participation" of the poor was required of all programs funded under the EOA. The operationalization of this concept in the health center case included conflict between project administrators, many of whom were employed by hospitals, medical schools, and health departments, and health center consumers during the program's early years. When health centers received a separate federal program authorization in 1975, community governance became a central component that defined the program (Sardell, 1988).

Policy innovation in the United States most often requires that one or more individuals "invest their resources—time, energy, reputation, and sometimes money" in advocating for a new policy idea. John Kingdon calls these advocates "policy entrepreneurs" (Kingdon, 1995). Policy advocacy is most successful when entrepreneurs in and outside of government work together to support a new policy or program. This is what happened in the case of the creation of the neighborhood health center program. Activist physicians and federal Office of Economic Opportunity (OEO) officials worked together to create a policy that would increase health care access to low-income populations and to provide services that were different from those offered by "mainstream" medical institutions. In addition, Senator Edward M. Kennedy (D-MA) acted as an advocate for the program within Congress, deflecting opposition to both antipoverty programs and to "socialized medicine."

When President Nixon took office, the political environment changed; Nixon was not supportive of the social programs initiated by the Johnson Administration. Yet during the Nixon Administration, sympathetic federal agency officials protected the program until its advocates outside of government grew stronger (Sardell, 1988).

PROGRAM SURVIVAL AND INSTITUTIONALIZATION

Beginning in 1968, the public health service (PHS) within the Department of Health, Education and Welfare (DHEW) also provided funding for the establishment of about 50 comprehensive health centers in low-income areas. The involvement of the PHS in primary health services had been historically limited to the funding of categorical disease programs. However, the 1960s was a period in which socially concerned health professionals, administrators, and social scientists joined the agency as an alternative to serving in the military during the Vietnam War. Some of these individuals became policy entrepreneurs within the PHS for comprehensive health service programs for underserved populations. They were supported in their efforts by top DHEW officials appointed by President Johnson.

Although the Nixon Administration did not support the neighborhood health center program, there were civil servants in the PHS, as well as the OEO, who acted to protect it. As the OEO was phased out, decisions as to the timing of the transfers of individual programs to the PHS were made in ways that would protect more politically vulnerable programs, such as those in the south. In addition, agency officials awarded technical assistance grants to newly formed state health center associations and (in 1973) to the National Association of Neighborhood Health Centers, an organization created in 1970. Key congressional leaders such as Senator Kennedy and Congressman Paul Rogers (D-FL) also supported the health center program during the presidencies of Richard Nixon and Gerald Ford.

In 1972, the DHEW announced that it planned to phase out federal grants to health centers on the assumption that they would be funded through Medicaid. However in 1974 and 1975, in opposition to the Nixon and Ford Administrations, Congress enacted legislation that specifically described "community health centers" and authorized grant funding for them. The legislation was vetoed by both presidents, but in 1975 Congress overrode President Ford's veto. The creation of the program took place within the wider context of intense conflict between presidents who aimed to reduce the role of the federal government in social policy and a liberal democratic Congress that wanted to preserve the social programs of the Great Society. This congressional action was a critical point in the history of the program because it now had its own legislative authority that defined its characteristics.

A CHC has to have a governing board with a consumer majority. This board establishes general policies for the center, has fiduciary responsibility, and appoints its executive director. A majority of board members have to be consumers who use its services. When enacted, this was the most rigorous community participation provision in any health service program up to that time. This legislative provision, reaffirmed many times (including the program's last reauthorization in 2008), has meant that community-based primary care programs that don't have such a governing board structure, such as those run by hospitals, cannot receive federal grants as CHCs. This provision has also enabled advocates to frame CHCs as embodying "local control," an aspect of the program that has appealed to Republicans as well as Democrats.

The Ford Administration (1974 to 1977) attempted to reduce CHC program funding and to end categorical grant programs in health. Within that political environment, federal program officials initiated changes that helped to expand congressional support. New program monitoring systems were established that provided measurable performance criteria for the health centers so that congressional concern with efficiency was addressed. In addition, "rural health initiatives," smaller-scale basic medical programs were funded. More centers could be funded because they required fewer resources than the large urban centers. Rural, white congressional districts could potentially become a part of the health center constituency. These changes were part of the "institutionalization" of the health center program (Sardell, 1988). Over time, the cost-effectiveness of CHCs has been one of the major arguments made for increasing support for this model of care. Further, since the 1980s, members of Congress from rural districts and states have been important health center champions.

At the same time that federal agency officials were making programmatic decisions that would ultimately strengthen congressional support for CHCs, the National Association of Community Health Centers (NACHC) began to focus on educating members of Congress about the value of CHCs. A policy analyst was hired, a weekly newsletter on policy events was published, and the association initiated an annual "policy and issues forum" in Washington, D.C. which brought together health center consumers and staff to learn about policy issues and the policy process. In 1976, a Department of Policy Analysis was created. During the following decades, membership in NACHC grew, as did the organizational infrastructure. Today this organization is one of the most effective advocacy organizations in Washington.

CONTINUING POLICY ADVOCACY

During the next two decades, under both Republican and Democratic Presidents, the health center community strengthened its advocacy efforts and Congress continued to increase funding for the program. While Jimmy Carter was President (1977-1981), the rural health initiative concept of smaller centers was extended to urban areas and the focus on management efficiency continued. President Ronald Reagan's attempt to end the community health center program as a separate federal grant program was rejected by Congress in 1981. An important shift in health center funding occurred as a result of legislation initiated by the staff of Senator John Chafee (R-RI) and NACHC to deal with the problem of low Medicaid and Medicare reimbursement rates for services delivered at CHCs. Under the Federally Qualified Health Center (FQHC) program, which became part of Medicaid in 1989 and Medicare in 1990, CHCs and "look-alikes" (clinics that did not get federal grant monies under the CHC program but had the characteristics of CHCs) would have special Medicaid and Medicare reimbursement rates that were closer to actual costs than regular per-visit rates paid by Medicaid in many states. As a result, health centers were able to collect higher reimbursements for

Medicaid and Medicare patients, and Medicaid replaced federal grants as the major source of revenue for health centers. From 1990 to 1998, the proportion of health center revenues from federal grants substantially decreased from 41% to 26%.

THE EXPANSION OF CHCS UNDER A CONSERVATIVE PRESIDENT

Republican George W. Bush was elected president in 2000 as a conservative who would look to outside government for the solutions to social problems. Yet he embraced CHCs, a program created by liberal Democratic President Lyndon Johnson in the 1960s. In 2001, in his first year in office, President Bush proposed a 5-year initiative to expand health center sites to serve 6.1 million new patients. Congress supported funding for this initiative, and throughout his two terms in office President Bush acted to fulfill his promise to expand the community health center program. Each time that Congress did not approve his full request for health center funding, the president would add the missing funds to his request for the following year (Hawkins, 2009). While the Bush Administration was promoting the expansion of health centers, it was slashing spending for a wide variety of domestic programs including food stamps, home energy assistance, training grants for health professions, veterans' benefits, and Medicaid (Pear, 2005). The CHC program was only one of two domestic public health programs that grew during the Bush Administration, but the money budgeted for the other program (abstinence-only sex education) was far less than the amount appropriated for the health center program.

In addition, during the effort to reauthorize the CHC program during 2007 and 2008, the Bush Administration was "quietly supportive." It helped to get the votes of some Republican members of Congress, in spite of conservative opposition to expansions of federal funding for social programs. Along with the president, a bipartisan coalition of members of Congress was supportive of the program's expansion and, for the first time, the CHC authorization contained "hard numbers," that is, explicit amounts were targeted for the program, rather than leaving funding amounts to the appropriations process as previously (Hawkins 2009). The Health Care Safety Net Act of 2008 (PL 110-355) authorized a total of

$13 billion for 5 years, increasing each year: $2.2 billion in fiscal year (FY) 2008 and $ 3.3 billion in FY 2012. Although this includes funding for the National Health Service Corps, most of the money goes to expand the health center program (BNA, 2008). What explains the support that CHCs (programs serving ethnic minorities and the poor) had from President George W. Bush, a Republican conservative?

First are the data-based policy arguments that show that health centers provide access to high-quality health care for underserved populations in a cost-effective way. For example, studies comparing uninsured patients who receive care at CHCs with uninsured patients who do not receive care have found that CHC patients are more likely to report having a usual source of care and receiving preventive health counseling, and are less likely to wait to see providers. Low-income minority women who are uninsured or have Medicaid are more likely to have had cancer screening tests if they are patients at health centers than similar women who are not health center patients (Proser, 2005). Health centers are also central in efforts to reduce ethnic and racial disparities in health status. One way in which this occurs is through the provision of enabling services such as health and nutrition education, central to the management of chronic diseases, and outreach services, such as translation and transportation.

Second is the expansion of the policy network to include conservative members of Congress, so the network now includes an ideologically diverse set of policymakers. Beginning as early as the 1980s, policy staff at NACHC worked with moderate and conservative Republicans as well as Democrats on issues of concern to health centers. This process of building relationships on a bipartisan basis became critical when the Republicans gained control of Congress in 1994 and then in 2000 when Bush was elected president. In addition to the liberal Democrats and moderate Republicans who were program supporters in its formative years, health center champions in Congress during Bush's first term in office included powerful Republican conservatives such as Senators Orin Hatch of Utah (R), Christopher "Kit" Bond of Missouri (R), and Representative Henry Bonilla (R) of Texas. In fact, Senator Bond and Congressman Bonilla educated George W. Bush on the value of the health center model during his first campaign for the presidency (Hawkins, 2005).

Third, it is the long experience and high levels of skill of the officials and staff of the CHC advocacy community that has successfully wedded policy arguments with grassroots political activity. In 2010, NACHC's Department of Policy Analysis and Research has 17 full-time and two part-time staff members. Primary care associations at the state and regional levels, together with the NACHC, have successfully met a series of policy challenges to the program's continued existence and growth and have helped to create the very broad support enjoyed by the CHC program 45 years after its creation.

COMMUNITY HEALTH CENTERS IN THE OBAMA ERA

The election of a liberal Democratic president who began his professional life as a community organizer (and who was famously endorsed during the Democratic presidential primary by Senator Edward M. Kennedy, long-time champion of community health centers) suggested that the CHC program would continue to enjoy presidential support.

The American Recovery and Reinvestment Act (ARRA), signed into law in February 2009, included an almost $2 billion investment in community health centers for both new sites and the expansion of existing sites. Three quarters of the funding ($1.5 billion) was allocated for CHC construction, renovation, and equipment, while the rest was to help fund the operation of the centers (Bureau of Primary Health Care, 2010). The CHC program was the only direct health services program to receive money under the ARRA.

When Congress was beginning to consider this legislation, two CHC "champions"—Congressman David Obey (D-WI), Chair of the House Appropriations Committee, and Senator Tom Harkin (D-IA), Chair of the Senate Appropriations Subcommittee for Labor-HHS programs—included funding for CHCs in the House and Senate bills. Health centers presented data to members of Congress about the many newly unemployed workers seeking care at CHCs, the cost savings achieved when disparities in access to care were reduced and chronic disease was effectively managed, and the fact that health centers were engines of job creation and community economic development.

The $2 billion authorized for community health centers in the ARRA was *more* than that recommended by either the House ($1.5 billion) or the Senate ($1.87 billion). Usually, when the Senate and House negotiate on final legislation, the amount of funding for a program is a compromise. But in the case of funding for community health center expansion in the Recovery Act, those negotiating the final bill—Democratic party leaders from both Houses, representatives from the Obama Administration, one conservative Democrat (Ben Nelson of Nebraska), and a small group of Republicans supporting the stimulus package (Susan Collins and Olympia Snowe of Maine and Arlen Spector of Pennsylvania, then a Republican)—agreed to actually raise the amount (Hawkins, 2009). Clearly, support for CHCs comes from both parties and from members of Congress across the liberal/conservative ideological spectrum—from socialist Bernie Sanders to conservative Orin Hatch.

Community health center advocates were very active in the process of formulating health care reform legislation during 2009, arguing that expanding health insurance alone is not sufficient to create access to high-quality preventive and primary health care. Senator Bernard Sanders (I-VT) and the House Majority Whip James Clyburn (D-SC) were key congressional champions for including funding for health centers in the health reform bills (Hawkins, 2009).

The health reform legislation enacted in March 2010 (The Reconciliation Act of 2010 and HR 3590, the Patient Protection and Affordable Care Act) emphasizes public health initiatives and preventive and primary health services as means to improve health outcomes, reduce health care disparities, and save money. The legislation continues federal support for expansion of the numbers of community health centers and the services that they provide. Eleven billion dollars in new funding is authorized for the CHC program over a period of 5 years, beginning in FY 2011, both to serve an additional 20 million patients and to increase medical, dental, and mental health services. While most of the funds will be spent on providing services, $1.5 billion of the authorization is for new construction and renovation of existing facilities.

Other provisions of the new health reform legislation also affect the operations of health centers. Federal eligibility for Medicaid is expanded (to all those with an annual income less than 133% of the federal poverty level), and this will provide health insurance coverage to 16 million more people, some of whom were previously treated as "self-pay" patients at CHCs, and some of whom probably did not seek primary care. The legislation also seeks to protect the financial viability of health centers within the new health insurance system. Additionally, $1.5 billion is authorized for the National Health Service Corps (NHSC) which provides educational scholarships and loans to primary care providers who agree to serve in provider shortage areas. In addition, new grant programs are established for the development of teaching and residency programs at community health center sites (National Association of Community Health Centers, 2010b).

LESSONS LEARNED

The policy history of CHCs illustrates several aspects of the advocacy process for health care innovation.

1. First is the crucial importance of understanding the general political environment and framing policy solutions in ways that fit that environment. Socially concerned health professionals and others created neighborhood health centers as part of the War on Poverty, and health center advocates today frame their policy arguments in terms of current health policy concerns such as reducing health care disparities and cost-effectiveness.

2. Second is that program survival and institutionalization during the 1970s was the result of the actions of federal officials who were ideologically and personally committed to health center programs and helped to create a nongovernmental advocacy organization to represent them. The resulting health center policy community or policy network consisted of federal agency officials, members of Congress, and the NACHC.

3. Third, the expansion of health centers as a central plank of Bush Administration health policy was the result of the development of long-term relationships between health center advocates and members of Congress from across the political and ideological spectrum and policy arguments made in terms of access, reduction of health disparities, and cost-effectiveness of the program.

For a list of related websites, please refer to your Evolve Resources at http://evolve.elsevier.com/Mason/policypolitics/

REFERENCES

BNA's Health Care Policy Report, "Public health/bush signs Community Health Center Bill; reauthorized program receives $13 billion." (2008, October 20).

Bureau of Primary Health Care. (2010). The Health Center Program: Recovery Act grants. Retrieved from www. bphc.hrsa.gov/recovery.

Hawkins, D. R. Jr. (2005, October 31). Phone interview with Daniel R. Hawkins, Jr., Senior Vice President, Public Policy and Research, NACHC.

Hawkins, D. R. Jr. (2009, October 23). Phone interview with Daniel R. Hawkins, Jr., Vice President for Federal, State, and Public Affairs, NACHC.

Kingdon, J. (1995). *Agendas, alternatives, and public policies.* (2nd ed.). New York, HarperCollins.

National Association of Community Health Centers. (2010a). U.S. fact sheet. Washington, D.C. Retrieved from www.nachc.com/client/documents/United%20States%20FSv2.pdf.

National Association of Community Health Centers. (2010b). Community Health centers and health reform. Washington, D.C. Retrieved from www.nachc.com/client/Summary%20of%20Final%20Health%20Reform%20Package.pdf.

Pear, R. (2005, February 8). Domestic programs subject to Bush's knife: Aid for food and heating. *New York Times,* A22.

Proser, M. (2005). Deserving the spotlight: Health centers provide high-quality and cost-effective care. *Journal of Ambulatory Care Management, 28*(4), 321-330.

Sardell, A. (1988). *The U.S. experiment in social medicine: The Community Health Center Program, 1965-1986.* Pittsburgh: The University of Pittsburgh Press.

CHAPTER 34

TAKING ACTION
Setting Health Care in Its Social Context

Interview with Ruth Watson Lubic by Diana J. Mason

"There is no doubt that it is around the family and the home that all the greatest virtues, the most dominating virtues of human society, are created, strengthened and maintained."

—Winston Churchill

Ruth Watson Lubic, EdD, CNM, has been a pioneer in advancing new models of maternal and child health services in the United States. She founded and directed three childbearing centers: the nation's first out-of-hospital birth center at the Maternity Center Association (now Childbirth Connections) on East 92nd Street in Manhattan, the Morris Heights Childbearing Center in the southwest Bronx, and the Family Health and Birth Center (FHBC) in northeast Washington, D.C. The first nurse recipient of the prestigious MacArthur Foundation Fellowship (so-called "Genius" Award), Dr. Lubic has dedicated her life to promoting the health of families, particularly ethnic minorities living in poor communities, through a model of empowerment.

She co-founded the American College of Nurse Midwives Foundation, the American Association of Birth Centers, and the Community Based Nurse-Midwifery Education Program Consortium for the distance education of new nurse-midwives. In 2001, she received the Gustav O. Lienhard Award from the Institute of Medicine for "pioneering work in the development of humane and innovative services for childbearing and childrearing families."

In 2009, Diana Mason interviewed Dr. Lubic in her apartment in Washington, D.C., where she stays when she's working—at the age of 83—as the interim general director of the FHBC. Her primary home is in New York City, where she lives with husband, Bill, a lawyer who plans to retire when she does.

DM: Ruth, you've dedicated your life to developing new models of childbirthing services. Why have we needed new models of care?

RL: Originally it was to try to provide young families who were disenchanted with in-hospital childbirthing experiences with what they were seeking to meet their needs. So we set up the first birth center demonstration project in New York in 1975. We tried to find out from them what it was that they didn't like: They didn't like being separated; they didn't like the threat of the Caesarean section; they didn't like having the baby taken away. Some hospitals had "rooming in," but it was always somebody else's house—it wasn't their house. And so we thought we would see if home birth might meet their needs. But home birth is really expensive if you institutionalize it. If we had tried to set up a home birth service that was providing birth at home with New York City being as large as it is, we would have needed a number of midwives on call at one time. But Maternity Center had done that when it opened the first school of nurse midwifery in 1931. They had run it that way because they couldn't run it any other way. They wanted to meet the needs of immigrant families, or poor families from the South who knew midwives and still believed that hospitals were places you go to die. A hospital had that "taint" on it. They had run that home birth service from 1931 until about 1958 or 1959. And it had gotten to the point where there weren't enough people coming for home births anymore. I mean the idea of *hospital* birth had pretty much taken hold, especially after World War II; it became more institutionalized. The people that the midwives did see were largely affluent and could afford anything; they didn't want to leave their homes, go to the hospital, and they wanted to be more in control.

I think that the control idea with childbearing is very important, because if a woman feels she's in control of her birth—not meaning that she's alone with her birth or that she's dictating to professionals, but that her wishes are taken into consideration—that's a preparation for motherhood that can't really be imitated anywhere else. Let me just tell you an anecdote about when I had become a midwife and I went to work at Flower Fifth Avenue Hospital [in Manhattan]. There was no midwifery service there. So I was just teaching expectant parents part-time and working there. And I remember one time a woman coming up to me and saying—on the postpartum floor this is— "Can you tell me the name of the nurse who was with me during my labor?" And I said, "Well, I can find out. But why do you want to know?" She said, "Well, I think I bit her. I think that I was cursing her, but I'm not sure." But she wanted to apologize to the nurse. The reason that that happened was because in those days, women were given usually Demerol and Scopolamine (Scopolamine being an amnesiac), so they would forget what happened in labor. Then they would be put in a bed with padded side rails raised because they were often not under control of themselves or their emotions, having been given those medications. So that to me was a real sadness that a woman would be thinking that she had behaved badly in labor, when labor is really a time for empowerment to take place. It's not pain-free, but when you teach a woman how to manage the discomfort that she's feeling and you assist her in doing that, and you encourage her, it's a totally different experience.

Earlier in the day, Dr. Lubic had introduced Dr. Mason to Joan Brickhouse at the Family Health and Birth Center. Ms. Brickhouse gave birth at the Center and became a breastfeeding "peer counselor," encouraging women to breastfeed and helping with problems and questions that may arise. The breastfeeding rate for women who deliver at the Center is 100%.

RL: Joan Brickhouse is a breastfeeding peer counselor. I took her with me when I went to testify in the capitol building. Representative Steve Cohen [D-TN] had brought people in from Memphis, from the large city hospital there, and they were talking about all their problems—you know, the numbers of deliveries and how many deliveries they had and how many babies went to the NICU and so forth. We listened to all of that. Then I got up and gave the statistics from the birth center, which were very different. Of course people looked at them, sort of with disbelief, because they were so different [from those of the Memphis hospital] and we had been able to reduce the disparities associated with birth so remarkably. So then I said, "But I would like you to meet one of our mothers, Joan Brickhouse." Joan got up to the microphone and she said, "I wasn't delivered. I gave birth." The audience was blown away. That's the way we want women to feel about the birth experience because that sets the tone for mothering. And if you enter mothering with that feeling of 'I did something wrong', 'I wasn't a nice girl', you know, and all that guilt that the use of drugs, and so forth, sets up in the hospital setting, then you're going to be very uncertain of yourself where mothering is concerned. And of course, in the days where all those drugs were being used, fathers were excluded; so you didn't have the support of your mate to advocate and assist you.

There is a difference between the midwifery approach and the obstetrical approach. Midwives feel that bearing a child is not just a medical situation, or a biological situation. It's a situation that has important implications—social, emotional, and medical, true, but even religious and political implications. When I talk about that, I usually cite an example from the birth center that we started in the South Bronx. One woman who came from a Muslim country gave birth at the center, and people from her mosque came in afterward and formed a big circle in the reception area. It happened at night, although if it had happened in the daytime, we would have encouraged the same thing. The cultural dictate was for the baby to be passed around among mosque members. And each person spoke the words of Allah into the baby's ear. So that's an example of a religious dimension of childbirth.

But, childbirth is also political. Moses was saved from Pharaoh's wrath by the midwives who took him into the bulrushes and hid him because Pharaoh had dictated that all Hebrew males be killed.

And the empowerment—when we were on 92nd Street in New York, even though the families were empowered at the center, they were mostly middle-class, well-educated people. We had some racially mixed couples who felt themselves upwardly mobile. In other words, they weren't low-income families who suffer from lack of self-esteem and depression because of where they live and their hopelessness that they can never get out of that. We went to the South Bronx to serve a low-income population because we felt that we could do a lot for their outcomes. At that time, the Bronx had the second highest infant mortality in the country, with only Washington, D.C., having worse outcomes. It was when we were in the Bronx that I really became aware of the empowerment factor, and how effective it was to do simple little things like have every women test her own urine, weigh herself, and write it on her chart—which she saw and she got the test results, and so forth. We really believed that it was her health, not our health. And we felt that every woman should have access to her chart. So, every woman did. When she came into the unit, she would pick her chart out of the chart drawer, and then she would begin doing her own self-care. Now, she did that with some oversight if she had any trouble. But when you treat women that way, you're saying, "We think that you're intelligent enough to do this; we think you have the ability, the interest to do this. And, we think you can do it."

In coming down to Washington, I wanted to replicate this empowerment idea. And then coming here expanded into what it is now a collaborative effort. I looked for partners because we were not into being the "Golden Arches" of birth centers, in other words. There had been at least one obstetrician who came to us in New York wanting to franchise birth centers. We just wanted to set something up and have someone in the community keep it going as we had done in the Bronx where we formed a partnership between the Morris Heights Health Center and the Maternity Center Association. And we made it a good deal for them, in the sense that we said that if it's successful, programmatically and fiscally, we will give it to you. And then we raised the money to renovate the space, and so forth. It was another demonstration project, and that center is operating today.

I came to Washington to replicate the birth center in the South Bronx. But when I got down here, I met with the woman who was running Healthy Babies Project at the time—Dolores Farr—which is a case management, home visiting, educational sort of organization. They were really surviving on donations and foundation grants. We partnered with Healthy Babies because they weren't doing any clinical care and we needed to find a place to put these services. I had my

stipend from the MacArthur Award, but we didn't have any money other than that and we needed a building. But Dolores said, "Well, I know where there's a building." And she then took me to show me the building that we're in today, which at the time was a derelict former Safeway supermarket. And when she showed it to me, it was sitting in the neighborhood, sort of at the top of a rise, and everyone coming out of the housing project behind it must have walked past it every day. I took a look at the size of it and exclaimed, "Oh, Dolores, we could have child care in there as well." And we do.

Under the umbrella of the Developing Family Center, we have the Family Health and Birth Center, which does clinical care, maternity care, pediatrics, family planning, and well-women gynecology, and then we have the Healthy Babies project, which does the home visiting. They do a lot of education. For example, they have a program that is called Effective Black Parenting, which is a curriculum that came out of California. Right now they lost their funding for a fathers' group called Developing Dads. And there's Early Childhood Development in the building. Babies 6 weeks to 3 years can be cared for there. So it's "one-stop shop," as the saying goes. But more than that, it's what we like to say: "It's setting health care in its social context."

We're eager to get older women to come. Typically, older, low-income women don't come in for care. And we did some focus groups on that. I spoke to women in the housing project behind us and said, "Look, we're all women, I know what it's like to be flat on my back with my legs in the air and it's not fun. We're gentle. We know what it feels like, and so forth. So, come and see us because there's a high rate of cervical cancer and that sort of thing." It turns out that because so often they are matriarchs in their families, the reason they don't go for care, as they expressed it, is "if there's something wrong with me, I don't want to know about it." It's not typical of only low-income women. We meet women over all economic levels who have the sense that, "If I have cancer, I don't want to find it. I don't want to look for it." So, we're not doing as much "GYN-ing" as we like, although it's improved a lot over the period of time that we've been there.

The pediatric nurse practitioners in the District can take care of young people up to age 21. But we don't see many adolescents coming in for preconceptions. We see them mainly when they're already known to be pregnant. And one of the reasons for that is that the pediatric rooms of which we have two are decorated for small children. So you can just see a strapping 16-year-old boy sitting in there amongst all the little animals, and so forth. One year as a community service, we did physicals on young men in nearby Spingarn High School, who were coming out for football. The coach said they were having trouble getting physical exams for the young men who didn't have any coverage. So we said we would do physicals on them and we did. That year it was just a few, maybe four or five young men, and already one of them had hypertension. The life expectancy of black males in this ward of D.C., where we are—Ward 5—the last I heard it was 56 years, which is worse than Kenya. So, one of my favorite sayings is, "Come home, Bill Gates—there's a little in your backyard that needs to be taken care of too!"

DM: So now you have this Family Health and Birth Center in Ward 5 of Washington, D.C. What are the clinical outcomes and financial outcomes?

RL: Well, we have been able to reduce the disparities among African Americans. In 2005, we were able to save over a million dollars because of lower preterm birth; lower low birth rate and lower Caesarean section. This was at a time when our operating expenses were $1,007,400. So we saved more money for the system than it cost us to operate, but we were unable to realize those savings because the savings all went to Medicaid and to managed care companies and their stockholders because they're for-profit entities. This is a major weakness in the system.

We don't know what our infant mortality rate is because we haven't had the funds to follow the families to find out how many babies might die between 6 weeks and 1 year of age. So what we're doing is estimating our infant mortality rate, although we never say what we think it is because we're not sure. But the infant mortality rate would be dependent on these precursors to infant mortality, and preterm birth is the largest precursor. Preterm babies are born before 37 weeks of pregnancy. Low birth rate babies are born below $5\frac{1}{2}$ pounds, even though they may be 40 weeks of gestation. So there are two different approaches there. But when you do something that runs against the common thread,

you're always suspect. So the folks who have been doing it and getting poor results don't have to explain what they're doing, but those of us who are doing it and getting good results have to prove that we're getting good results.

DM: There are about 200 birth centers across the country that provide a beginning infrastructure for making childbearing centers the frontline of maternity care. With the clinical and financial outcomes that you have, it's stunning that you continue to have to do battle just to sustain childbearing centers financially, let alone promote them. What are the major barriers to being able to ramp this up and have it be the model for the country?

RL: From my point of view, the major barriers are that we are flying in the face of generally accepted patterns of care, for example, with organized medicine and hospitals.

DM: So over the years, you fought against organized medicine, which tried to claim that the outcomes for free-standing childbirthing centers and outcomes nurse-midwives in general were not comparable to outcomes from hospital-based deliveries and obstetricians. Now, recently, you've had the American College of Obstetrics and Gynecologists [ACOG] come out as supporting accredited childbirthing centers. Do you still have resistance from organized medicine?

RL: I think so, though we try to be friends. We try to reach out. But in terms of organized medicine, I have invited representatives of ACOG to come out and see us, and they're always too busy. It's very difficult not to have the impression that organized medicine would wish that we would go away, never bother them again. But my position is that the health care professions exist to improve the care of families. And if you're not doing that, then you need to put your tail between your legs and go away.

DM: Now at the Family Health and Birth Center there is Linda Randolph, who plays a key role and she's a physician.

RL: She's actually the president of the umbrella organization, which is called the Developing Families Center. We wanted to be very sure that people understood that we were not physician-haters and that we welcome any kind of physician input into what we were doing, but that the opinions of the families mattered to us more than the opinions of organized medicine.

DM: You also, over the years, have fought the issue of reimbursement of services, payment of services. Maybe you can talk a minute about how that battle has gone. I remember back when you were at Maternity Center Association how you fought and fought to get Medicaid and Blue Cross Blue Shield reimbursement for deliveries. You were successful then. Do you still have issues with getting paid for services?

RL: At the Maternity Center Association in the early days, about 5% of our clients were eligible for Medicaid. So, it wasn't a big deal, except it was an important policy issue. So we fought to get Medicaid reimbursement and we got it. In going to the Bronx, it's a different deal because almost everybody was coved by Medicaid. And that's true in Washington as well. But the Medicaid reimbursement is not always dependable, in the sense that Medicaid programs, after covering birth centers for their facilities fees [for overhead] for something like 22 years, withdrew that fee at the end of the Bush administration. It has since been restored under the Affordable Care Act, but it's an example of hardball tactics that are not in the best interest of the nation; the facility fee that a birth center needs is perhaps a quarter of the facility fee that a hospital needs. And now, there is a bill in Congress to ensure that birth centers are paid a facility fee. It's so poignant that the facility fee that a birth center gets is like a quarter of the facility fee that a hospital gets. So, suppose you don't pay the birth center their facility fee. Suppose you make them close down, which I think some groups would like to see happen. You drive the women into hospital births, and the Medicare program has to pay 3 to 4 times what it would have paid if the women had been cared for in a birth center—to say nothing of her personal empowerment and her ability to mother. Then in 2008, it was withdrawn in South Carolina, Florida, Alaska, and the state of Washington.

DM: And the argument was that Medicaid bureaucrats realized that it wasn't required by law to pay the fee to childbearing centers but it was for hospitals. So, that in itself is a lesson about the importance of having a policy that's clear in statute and not relying on the kindness of strangers, if you will, who write or interpret regulations. Let me provide another frame for this and that is that it's also about empowerment of women and families and providing really high-quality childbearing services and

getting families off to a healthy start for the whole country.

RL: To me, you make the decision based on which system is most supportive to families. Because, I have to ask the question: How are we going to compete in a global economy if about 16% of our population is not able to realize its potential? And that's what's happening with the African-American community. Whatever health care is given should ensure the fact that African-American families feel capable of making health care decisions and implementing those health care decisions. And that's what we're all about. One of the things that my husband exhorts me about is you should not focus solely on low-income African-American families. What is happening is good for any American family, whether they're low-income black, low-income Hispanic, or low-income anything; or whether they're middle income; or whether they're upper income even, because we know that people who have a high level of income don't necessarily have important opportunities to strengthen their families.

DM: So if you were going to ensure that their childbirthing centers are a framework and part of the infrastructure of our health care system, we need to require a sustainable facility fee, but what else needs to happen from a policy perspective?

RL: I would like to see the United States of America take a position similar to that of France, which is "the protection of mothers and babies." Not *aid to,* not *assistance for,* but *protection of.* It's a whole different mindset. And so I work to try to affect that mindset, because to me it's very important to the health and strength of the country. I think that it's very important that physicians and midwives work together as a team and they provide what the families need at any given point in time. And that means that not every family needs physician care. Many families need more than midwifery care. But we need to work together as a team. And that's not always easy to effect, but I would work for as long as I can for that to happen.

DM: And what are the policy approaches to support that?

RL: I think that Congress has to be able to say "We want our families strengthened," and this is one route that has been proven to some extent and we need to support it, for the future. We need funding that will support this model of care. And supporting it will save money in the long run. Because of what I mentioned in the past that if all Medicaid supported births were managed on the model that we have presented, it would save billions a year. I think that nowhere in the whole health care reform effort will there be the payoff that you would get from personalized, supportive, empowering, maternity services. Because it's not just that birth, it's what goes on through the whole life of the family. If you're going to make change in this country, you have to start with childbearing families.

For a list of related websites, please refer to your Evolve Resources at http://evolve.elsevier.com/Mason/policypolitics/

CHAPTER 35

TAKING ACTION
Reimbursement Issues for Nurse Anesthetists: A Continuing Challenge

Frank Purcell

"I was taught that the way of progress is neither swift nor easy."

—Marie Curie

A number of federal initiatives since 1980 have had a significant impact on the nurse anesthesia profession. Three federal reimbursement policies significantly affected the American Association of Nurse Anesthetists (AANA) and its 40,000 members. This chapter explores how federal policy can affect the economics of a profession, raise or lower barriers to practice, and cause or remediate inefficiencies in the delivery of anesthesia services. It also highlights that conflict can occur when two professional groups—in this case, Certified Registered Nurse Anesthetists and anesthesiologists—have overlapping scopes of practice and major stakes in policy outcomes.

NURSE ANESTHESIA PRACTICE

Certified registered nurse anesthetists (CRNAs) are educated in the specialty of anesthesia at the masters or doctoral level in an integrated program of academic and clinical study, and must pass a national certifying exam to practice anesthesia. In addition, they must meet the requirements of recertification every 2 years. CRNAs are eligible to receive reimbursement for their services directly from Medicare, from most Medicaid programs, from TRICARE (the United States Department of Defense health program),

and from most private insurers and managed care organizations.

CRNAs, working with surgeons, anesthesiologists, and, where authorized, podiatrists, dentists, and other health care providers, administer 32 million anesthetics annually in the U.S. CRNAs provide anesthesia for every age and type of patient using the full scope of anesthesia techniques, drugs, and technology that characterize contemporary anesthesia practice, as well as interventional pain management services. They work in every setting in which anesthesia is delivered: tertiary care centers, community hospitals, labor and delivery rooms, ambulatory surgical centers (ASCs), diagnostic suites, and outpatient settings. Predominant in rural America, CRNAs are the sole anesthesia providers in most rural hospitals, affording anesthesia and resuscitative services to these medical facilities for surgical, obstetric, and trauma care.

NURSE ANESTHESIA REIMBURSEMENT

Nurse anesthetists gained direct Medicare reimbursement in 1986. Medicare Part A establishes the regulations by which hospitals and ambulatory care facilities are reimbursed for services, supplies, drugs, and equipment used in the care of Medicare patients. Medicare Part B sets forth the payment regulations for health care professionals who are eligible to receive direct reimbursement through the Medicare program. With the advent of the Medicare program in 1965, payment for the anesthesia services provided by nurse anesthetists was provided through both Part A and

This updates a chapter originally developed by John Garde, CRNA, MS, FAAN and Rita Rupp, RN, MA and draws substantially upon their excellent work.

Part B of the Medicare program. For the services provided by CRNAs who were hospital employed, the hospitals were reimbursed under Part A for "reasonable costs" of anesthesia services. For the services provided by CRNAs who were employed by anesthesiologists, the anesthesiologists who employed and supervised CRNAs could bill under Part B as if they personally had administered the anesthesia. These forms of payment were in effect until 1983, when Congress enacted the Prospective Payment System (PPS) legislation to control Medicare hospital costs. The law provided that all services by providers, other than those reimbursed through Medicare Part B, would be bundled into a hospital diagnostic-related group (DRG) payment. The legislation created serious problems relative to the payment for nurse anesthesia services. Hospitals would have been required to pay for their CRNA employees from the fixed DRG payment, jeopardizing their ability to recoup actual costs and creating a disincentive for hospitals to employ CRNAs. Further, because the PPS precluded the unbundling of services, anesthesiologists who employed CRNAs would have been forced to contract with hospitals to get the CRNA portion of the DRG. Simply put, CRNA services were effectively non-reimbursable.

In addition, hospitals that accrued Medicare cost savings by using the services of CRNAs stood to be hurt the most by the move to a DRG payment system. Hospitals using more physicians for such services did not need to take the costs from the DRG payment; physician services were reimbursed from Medicare Part B. Further, for every $1 paid to CRNAs, anesthesiologists were being paid $3 to $4. If the substitution of anesthesiologists for CRNAs were to increase, the cost of anesthesia care to Medicare beneficiaries could be expected to escalate (Garde, 1988).

ADVOCACY ISSUES IN ANESTHESIA REIMBURSEMENT

Because of the potential negative effect of the PPS legislation on nurse anesthetists, AANA advocated several legislative changes, most notably that the Omnibus Budget Reconciliation Act (OBRA) of 1986 should include direct reimbursement for CRNAs (to become effective January 1, 1989, with extension of the two temporary provisions to the effective date of the legislation).

The mission of AANA was to convince Congress and the Health Care Financing Administration (HCFA, renamed the Centers for Medicare and Medicaid Services [CMS] in 2001) that CRNAs were concerned about health care costs as well as equitable reimbursement for their services. Even though the American Society of Anesthesiologists (ASA) opposed the direct reimbursement legislation, AANA's message was understood because use of CRNAs in the provision of anesthesia services represents substantial cost savings from several standpoints. On average, the income of CRNAs is one-third that of anesthesiologists. Also, for providing the same high-quality of anesthesia care, the educational cost of preparing CRNAs is significantly less than that needed to prepare anesthesiologists. Congress passed the legislation granting CRNAs direct Medicare reimbursement, with two payment schedules incorporated in the law: one for CRNAs not medically directed by anesthesiologists and the other for CRNAs working under anesthesiologists' medical direction (Gunn, 1997). As a result of this legislation, all CRNAs, regardless of whether they are employed or are in independent practice, now have the ability to receive reimbursement from Medicare directly or to sign over their billing rights to their employers. In addition to Medicare direct reimbursement, CRNAs were reimbursed through many health plans. Although CRNAs still face a variety of practice barriers in some facilities and health plans, they can and do serve as exclusive providers for the full range of anesthesia services at hospitals and ambulatory surgical facilities.

TEFRA: DEFINING MEDICAL DIRECTION

Congress enacted the Tax Equity and Fiscal Responsibility Act of 1982 (TEFRA) to, among other provisions, control escalating Medicare costs for hospital-based services including anesthesiology, pathology, and radiology. Among the many cost concerns that TEFRA addressed was a need to ensure that an anesthesiologist provided specified services when billing Medicare for medical direction when a CRNA was administering the anesthesia. Before enactment of TEFRA, an anesthesiologist could bill for services in conjunction with supervision of hospital-employed CRNAs, without demonstrating that the anesthesiologist had provided specific services to qualify for such payment.

In 1983, the HCFA published the final rules implementing TEFRA relative to payment for anesthesiology physician services, limiting medical direction payment to an anesthesiologist to no more than four concurrent procedures administered by CRNAs. The rules implemented seven conditions that an anesthesiologist must satisfy in each case to obtain reimbursement for medical direction (U.S. Department of Health and Human Services [USDHHS], 1983). Interestingly, the TEFRA regulations also increased health care costs by providing incentives for the additional involvement of anesthesiologists in cases that could otherwise be provided by a CRNA as non-medically directed. Medicare Part B did not require the involvement of anesthesiologists in CRNA services, except to the extent than an anesthesiologist submits a claim for medical direction.

In the early 1990s, in the course of the Physician Payment Review Commission (PPRC) study of anesthesia payments (which was intended to examine ways to reduce anesthesia team payments in cases involving both anesthesiologists and CRNAs), government-related study groups and individual research studies reported the need for changes in TEFRA. The 1992 Center for Health Economics Research (CHER) report to the PPRC recommended the following: "Refinements to the TEFRA provisions should be considered in view of the reductions in payments to the anesthesia care team. In particular, opportunities for increasing the flexibility of role functions should be reviewed. ... [W]ith the implication of a capped payment, the HCFA should consider whether to review the TEFRA requirements to see if modifications of the TEFRA rules would permit greater efficiencies without decreasing the quality of care" (PPRC, 1993). The PPRC concluded that "the use of the anesthesia care team seems to be determined by individual preferences for that practice arrangement. There appears to be no demonstrated quality of care differences between the care provided by the solo anesthesiologist, solo CRNA, and the team." No longer could anesthesiologists argue that medical direction of CRNAs by anesthesiologists and the TEFRA conditions under which medical direction is provided represent any safer or higher standard of care than the care provided by a CRNA practicing alone or an anesthesiologist practicing alone. The

final conclusion reached by PPRC on anesthesia payment represented a milestone in the recognition of anesthesia services provided by nurse anesthetists. A single payment methodology for anesthesia services was recommended by PPRC and adopted by Congress, which resulted in a policy that the payment for anesthesia services—whether provided by a CRNA-anesthesiologist team, by a solo anesthesiologist, or by a solo CRNA providing non-medically directed services—would be the same. In the case of medically directed services, the payment would be split so that each practitioner received 50% (PPRC, 1993).

In 1998, the AANA initiated a regulatory advocacy program to revise the TEFRA medical direction conditions. In a joint meeting in 1998 with the ASA, AANA, and HCFA, proposals were advanced by both AANA and ASA for revisions in the seven conditions of payment for physician medical direction. The ASA and AANA reached consensus on a revised recommended set of medical direction requirements. However, a publication entitled "Anesthesia Answer Book—Action Alert" (1998) indicated that the ASA had second thoughts about the agreed-on revisions. The HCFA's response to the concerns posed by ASA membership and several state anesthesiologist societies was to retain the current requirements established in 1983 (USDHHS, 1998b). The HCFA did decide that the medically directing physician must be present at induction and emergence for general anesthesia and present as indicated in anesthesia cases not involving general anesthesia, and that the medically directing anesthesiologist alone must attest in any claim for Medicare reimbursement of medical direction to having performed the seven medical direction tasks in each case (USDHHS, 1998b). The HCFA announced plans to study the medical direction issue further, welcomed comments, and suggested that it might propose changes in the future (USDHHS, 1998b). The AANA's influence on the development of medical direction policy helped secure the following:

- A published statement by the HCFA that medical direction should not be considered a quality-related standard, but a payment criterion
- Adoption of a 50% split in payment by the anesthesiologist and CRNA for a case as long as the ratio of medical direction does not exceed 1:4
- A 50% split in payment between the anesthesiologist and CRNA when the medical direction is 1:1.

(Before this change, the physician received 100% of the payment.)

Non-medically directed CRNA services represent an important value to patients, ensure a high quality of anesthesia service indistinguishable from more costly practice modalities, and create savings by comparison with medically directed services even though both are reimbursed identically under Medicare Part B. Box 35-1 shows an example of this comparison.

PHYSICIAN SUPERVISION OF CRNAS: MEDICARE CONDITIONS OF PARTICIPATION

Medicare regulations in 2010 require physician supervision of CRNAs as a condition for hospitals, ASCs, and critical access hospitals (CAHs) to receive Medicare payment, except where the state has opted out of this requirement. These regulations do not require that a CRNA be supervised by an anesthesiologist.

During the 1990s, AANA pursued a revision of these Medicare conditions of participation that would remove the physician supervision requirement for CRNAs. In December 1997, the HCFA released for comment the proposed revisions in the Medicare Conditions of Participation for Hospitals, ASCs, and CAHs, which would eliminate the requirement for physician supervision of CRNAs, deferring instead to state law. The HCFA's proposal to remove the physician supervision requirement was opposed by the ASA, whose main message was that if the rule was implemented, patients would die. To counter the claims, AANA pointed to the extensive published literature documenting the safety of CRNA care, and commissioned a survey of Medicare beneficiaries in October 1999 by an independent research firm, Wirthlin Worldwide. The survey revealed that 88% of Medicare beneficiaries surveyed would be comfortable if their surgeon chose a nurse anesthetist to provide their anesthesia care; 81% surveyed preferred a nurse anesthetist or had no preference between a CRNA or anesthesiologist when it came to their anesthesia care (American Association of Nurse Anesthetists, 2000). From the time that the proposed rule was announced, AANA implemented a number of key activities to advocate its position on this supervision issue. Box 35-2 shows AANA strategies used in advocacy on this issue.

BOX 35-1 Comparison of Cost of Four Types of Delivery of Anesthesia Services

Suppose that there are four identical cases: (a) has anesthesia delivered by a non-medically directed CRNA, (b) has anesthesia delivered by a CRNA medically directed at a 4:1 ratio by a physician overseeing four simultaneous cases and attesting fulfillment of the seven conditions of medical direction in each; (c) has anesthesia delivered by a CRNA medically directed at a 2:1 ratio; and (d) has anesthesia delivered by a physician personally performing the anesthesia service. Further suppose that the annual pay of the anesthesia professionals approximate national market conditions in 2007, $145,000 for the CRNA and $380,000 for the anesthesiologist (American Society of Anesthesiologists, April 2007 newsletter).

Under the Medicare program and most private payment systems, practice modalities (a), (b), (c), and (d) are reimbursed the same. Moreover, the literature indicates that the quality of medically directed vs. non-medically directed CRNA services is indistinguishable. However, the annualized labor costs (excluding benefits) for each modality vary widely. The annualized cost of (a) equals $145,000. For case (b), it is $145,000 + (0.25 × $380,000), or $240,000 per year. For case (c), it is $145,000 + (0.50 × $380,000), or $335,000 per year. Finally, for case (d), the annualized cost equals $380,000 per year.

Anesthesia Payment Model	FTEs/Case	Clinician Costs per Year/FTE
(a) CRNA non-medically directed	1.00	$145,000
(b) Medical direction 1:4	1.25	$240,000
(c) Medical direction 1:2	1.50	$335,000
(d) Anesthesiologist only	1.00	$380,000

If Medicare and private plans pay the same rate whether the care is delivered according to modalities (a), (b), (c), or (d), some part of the health care system is bearing the additional cost of the medical direction service—most likely hospitals and other health care facilities, and, ultimately, patients, premium payers, and taxpayers. In the interest of patient safety and access to care, these additional costs imposed by medical direction modalities more than justify the public interest in continuing to recognize and reimburse fully for non-medically directed CRNA services within Medicare, Medicaid, and private plans, in the same manner that physician services are reimbursed.

BOX 35-2 AANA Strategies Used in Advocacy on the Supervision Issue

- AANA representatives met with key government personnel to advocate on behalf of CRNAs on the issue of supervision. Meetings were held with HCFA analysts, the Administrator of HCFA (Nancy-Ann DeParle), members of Congress and their staffs, the Secretary of Health and Human Services, staff members of the Clinton White House, the staff of the Office of Management and Budget, and others.
- As the ASA's opposition to the proposed rule increased, together with the delay in HCFA's announcement of the final rule, the AANA called on Senator Kent Conrad (D-ND) and Representative Jim Nussle (R-IA) to introduce legislation requiring HCFA to implement the proposed regulation related to deleting physician supervision of CRNAs in the hospital, ASC, and CAH as conditions for receiving Medicare payment.
- The AANA retained legislative consultants to assist in the promotion of its legislative initiatives.
- The AANA's public relations endeavors focused on increasing the public's awareness of the issues and advocating the position of the vital role that CRNAs play in anesthesia delivery in the country. Efforts included advertising in many news publications, including Capitol Hill newspapers and *USA Today;* assisting with media training for AANA officers and staff to increase their effectiveness on radio programs and in interviews; and developing radio advertisements in Washington, D.C. to garner support for the AANA's position.
- The AANA retained grassroots political action consultants to assist in gaining letters of support for the new proposed regulations from key members of Congress.
- The AANA solicited a broad base of support from the nursing organization community, national hospital associations, related health professional associations, civic organizations, individual nurses, physicians, and the general public.

These advocacy efforts yielded an extensive base of support from all sectors. AANA gained support for the proposed rule changes from the American Hospital Association; VHA, Inc.; Premier, Inc.; National Rural Health Association; Federation of American Health Systems; St. Paul Fire and Marine Insurance Company; Kaiser Permanente Central Office; California and Oregon Kaiser System; and numerous rural hospitals across the country. On January 18, 2001, the HCFA published a final rule in the Federal Register, removing the federal physician supervision requirement for nurse anesthetists and deferring to state law on the issue. The HCFA refuted all major arguments advanced by the ASA opposition. Examples of several conclusions the HCFA reached in its study of the supervision issue are as follows:

- States have constitutionally and traditionally acted in matters of licensure and scope-of-practice and have not been found to be negligent in their exercise of this authority.
- There is no research that conclusively demonstrates a need for this federal requirement, nor demonstrates that physician or anesthesiologist supervision makes a difference in anesthesia outcomes. The HCFA stated in the final rule that studies purported by the ASA to demonstrate such findings had serious limitations and did not support the ASA's conclusions. Furthermore, the HCFA stated that it cannot agree with the ASA's belief that anesthesia administration is the practice of medicine and therefore can be done only after medical school training.
- The HCFA's rule noted the safety of anesthesia as reported by the Institute of Medicine (IOM) (IOM Committee on Quality of Health Care in America, 2000).
- The flexibility resulting from the rule change would provide increased access to services in some areas and broaden the opportunity for providers to implement professional standards of practice that improve quality of care and promote more efficacious models of care delivery for anesthesia services.

However, on January 20, 2001, the incoming Bush administration placed a 60-day moratorium on all regulations published in the final days of the Clinton administration. This action was not unexpected; every new administration takes the opportunity to review pending regulations that are not yet in effect.

The AANA took its case to HHS Secretary Tommy Thompson in 2001 and continued to urge the 107th Congress to leave the final regulation published by HCFA on January 18, 2001, in place, while the ASA proposed legislation calling for continuation of the supervision requirements pending a study on supervision. Following extensions of the implementation moratorium, on July 5, 2001, the CMS published its new proposed rule (66 FR 35395-35399), which, if implemented, would replace the January 18 rule. The proposed rule would enable states to "opt out" of (or seek an exemption from) the federal supervision requirement for CRNAs. Hospitals, ASCs, and critical access hospitals in a particular state would be exempted from the requirement if the governor submitted a letter to the CMS requesting the exemption. The letter would need to attest that the governor consulted with the boards of medicine and nursing about issues related to access to and quality of anesthesia services in the state; concluded that it is in the best interests of the state's citizens to opt out of the physician supervision requirement; and determined that opting out was consistent with state law. It would also have the Agency for Healthcare Research and Quality (AHRQ) design and conduct a prospective study to assess only CRNA practices with input from the CMS, anesthesiologists, and CRNAs or, alternatively, establish a registry to monitor only CRNA practice.

The AANA expressed concern that the proposed rule would potentially allow state medical boards to dictate how nurse anesthetists would be regulated on a state-by-state basis. In addition, the governors would be the targets of intense lobbying by organized medicine, and any exemption from supervision could be removed at any time because of this political pressure, creating a constant state of legal and professional limbo for CRNAs and the facilities they serve. The AANA's response to the CMS in response to the July 5 proposed rule urged the agency to revert to the January 18, 2001, final rule and defer to state law concerning anesthesia services regarding the issue of physician supervision of CRNAs.

The CMS ultimately adopted a final rule on November 13, 2001 (66 FR 56762), closely mirroring the July 5 proposed rule. As of February 2010, 15 states had exercised the process authorized to opt out of the Medicare physician supervision requirement for nurse anesthetists: Alaska, California, Idaho, Iowa, Kansas, Minnesota, Montana, Nebraska, New Hampshire, New Mexico, North Dakota, Oregon, South Dakota, Washington, and Wisconsin. To date, AHRQ had not undertaken the study authorized by the final rule, which the agency already had authority to undertake. Anesthesia services continued to be delivered safely as the nurse anesthesia profession had promised, as measured by trends in nurse anesthetists' medical liability premiums to the extent that such premiums are a market proxy to measure relative risk. The largest insurer of CRNAs in 2005 announced its first premium increases since 2002 for policies effective in 2006. Increases averaged 8% for the 4-year period. Premium increases in states that had opted out of the Medicare physician supervision mandate were lower, averaging 6% (Fetcho, 2005). The increases approximate the consumer price index (CPI) for the period and were considerably below medical liability premium increases reported by the medical community.

SUMMARY

The primary impetus for seeking direct reimbursement legislation was the problem created by a new Medicare payment system that had threatened the viability of the nurse anesthesia profession. However, the AANA saw a clear opportunity to seek this legislation to expand and secure patient access to care, and to establish a more equitable market in which to promote CRNA services as fully qualified anesthesia providers. As of February 2010, 40 states do not have a physician "supervision" requirement for CRNAs in nursing or medical laws or regulations. Clearly this is an indication that many states, as a matter of public policy, believe it is unnecessary to require physician supervision of CRNAs.

The AANA has learned from its experience in the political and legislative arena that politics is the use of power for change. Although politics may not always be nice or fair, health care professionals must engage in the political process. As has been illustrated in the federal policy initiatives discussed in this chapter, there are generally other forces at work to attempt to influence policy decisions that can have a detrimental impact on one's patients and profession. Therefore the choice of whether or not to engage should be a simple one. The achievements won in the federal policy arena by the AANA could not have been possible without the commitment and dedication of its members.

However, it is very rare for a single group to be able to promote legislation or to effect major policy change. In the case of the federal supervision requirement for nurse anesthetists, networking with other groups, especially with nursing organizations, has been critical to achieving support on Capitol Hill and in communications with the executive branch. The message to legislators has been loud and clear: Remove restrictive barriers to practice when it is in the public's interest and is sound health care policy.

For a list of related websites, please refer to your Evolve Resources at http://evolve.elsevier.com/Mason/policypolitics/

REFERENCES

American Association of Nurse Anesthetists (AANA). (2000). Nine out of 10 Medicare patients are comfortable with nurse anesthesia care. *Roll Call*.

Fetcho, J. (2005). CNA requests rate increases. *AANA NewsBulletin, 59*(6), 34.

Garde, J. F. (1988). A case study involving prospective payment legislation, DRGs, and certified registered nurse anesthetists. *Nursing Clinics of North America, 23*(3), 521-530.

Gunn, I. P. (1997). Nurse anesthesia. In J. J. Nagelhout & K. L. Zaglaniczny (Eds.), *Nurse anesthesia*. Philadelphia: Saunders.

Institute of Medicine (IOM) Committee on Quality of Health Care in America. (2000). In L. T. Kohn, J. Corrigan, & M. S. Donaldson (Eds.), *To err is human: Building a safer health system*. Washington, D.C.: National Academies Press.

Physician Payment Review Commission (PPRC). (1993). *PPRC report to Congress. Payments for the anesthesia care team*. Washington, D.C.: PPRC.

U.S. Department of Health and Human Services (USDHHS). (1983, March 2). Federal Register, 48, FR 8928.

U.S. Department of Health and Human Services (USDHHS). (1998a, June 5). Federal Register, 63, FR 30818.

U.S. Department of Health and Human Services (USDHHS). (1998b, November 2). Federal Register, 63, FR 58813.

U.S. Department of Health and Human Services (USDHHS). (2001a, January 18). Federal Register, 66(12), FR 4674.

U.S. Department of Health and Human Services (USDHHS). (2001b, July 5). Federal Register, 66(129), FR 35395.

U.S. Department of Health and Human Services (USDHHS). (2001c, November 13). Federal Register, 66(219), FR 56762.

CHAPTER 36

The Role of Foundations in Improving Health Care

Susan Hassmiller and John Lumpkin

"Philanthropy is commendable, but it must not cause the philanthropist to overlook the circumstances of economic injustice which make philanthropy necessary."

—Martin Luther King, Jr.

A patient was asked about her experience as part of the discharge process during a recent hospital visit. She responded, "Do you mean did I notice that the same nurse took care of me every day? Yes, I noticed, and it was wonderful. The last time I was here, I had a different nurse every day." The impetus to develop a consistent working relationship between individual nurses and patients came from the regular quality-improvement meetings of the staff on the hospital unit participating in a Robert Wood Johnson Foundation (RWJF)–funded program called "Transforming Care at the Bedside" (TCAB). In this innovative program, frontline nurses are empowered to work with other frontline staff to develop and present ideas to improve the quality of patient care and their own satisfaction with the work that they do. In several of the TCAB units, the time that floor nurses spent doing nursing tasks (e.g., assessing patient status) as opposed to non-nursing tasks (e.g., hunting for supplies and equipment or emptying garbage cans) on the experimental unit went from 35% to almost 70%, and turnover dropped to near zero—and this was in 2006, before nurses were holding onto their jobs due to the economic downturn that began in 2008. Many of the TCAB units in the original 13 participating hospitals had waiting lists to work there. For many of the nurses in the program, it was the first time that they felt as though their needs, concerns, and ideas were valued by management at the hospital.

By 2010, TCAB had spread to hundreds of hospitals in the United States and globally. This is just one example of the role that foundations can play in providing the financial, technical, and knowledge-related resources to help nurses change their environment and improve the quality of care.

The mission of the RWJF is to improve the health and health care for all Americans. Following in the footsteps of Robert Wood Johnson II, the RWJF has been engaged in programs to strengthen nursing, from support for nurse education to the development of interdisciplinary training vehicles in quality improvement at academic health centers. Recognizing the critical nature of the nurse staffing shortage and the central role that nurses play in the delivery of health and health care services, the RWJF made nursing one of eight focus areas in 2002, and it is still a major funding area today. The goal was to reduce the shortage in nurse staffing and to improve the quality of nursing-related care by transforming the way care is delivered at the bedside. The TCAB program has remained an integral piece of a nursing effort that has included work to improve hospital work environments in an effort to improve nurse satisfaction and ultimately the quality of patient care. The foundation has since expanded its funding to address the nurse faculty shortage. With funding support over $200 million, the foundation has been addressing nursing programs in four areas, including: (1) building leadership capacity, (2) addressing the nurse and nurse faculty shortage, (3) stimulating research that links nursing care to high-quality and safe outcomes, and (4) identifying solutions to more effectively and efficiently deploy nurses to meet the demands of a reformed health care system. The Institute of Medicine (IOM) recently released a report on the Future of Nursing as part of the RWJF Initiative on the Future of Nursing. See *www.thefutureofnursing.org* for further details on the IOM recommendations and the RWJF Future of Nursing national campaign. Additionally, to further leverage the foundation's investment in nursing, the RWJF founded the National Nurse Funders Collaborative, a group of approximately 90 organizations nationwide committed to engaging new funding partners so that nursing issues across the spectrum may be strategically addressed.

FOUNDATIONS: WHAT THEY ARE AND WHAT THEY FUND

A foundation is an organization that is established as a non-profit corporation or a charitable trust under state law, with a principal purpose of making grants to unrelated institutions or entities or to individuals for scientific, educational, cultural, religious, health-related, or other charitable purposes (Schlandweiler, 2004). Foundations are regulated by the Internal Revenue Code—refer to 501(c)3 status—and most can give grants only to non-profit charitable organizations, and sometimes to individuals in the form of scholarships. By federal law, most foundations must spend at least 5% of their average assets each year. Although foundations can use their funds to inform or educate on any issue, lobbying or engaging in political activities is significantly restricted and, in the case of private foundations, it is prohibited.

In general, foundations have great freedom to fund what they want, consistent with their mission. The mission is generally established by the wishes of the individual or individuals who donated resources to the foundation, the original charter, the direction of its board of directors, or a combination of these three. Some foundations are sharply limited in the categories they can fund or the geography they can serve by the enabling donation or at the direction of their board. They are instrumental in funding ideas that are new, innovative, and otherwise untested. If it were not for foundations, many of our country's most pressing social problems, such as improving the quality of care for those at the end of life, would never get the attention they deserve. Most of the philanthropic dollars in this country go to causes that support education (25%), but health care gets the second largest number of dollars at 20% (Foundation Center, 2009).

There are over 75,000 grant-making foundations in the U. S. that generally fall into one of the following four categories (Indiana Grantmakers Alliance, n.d.).

See Box 36-1 for more suggestions about working with foundations.

PRIVATE FOUNDATIONS

This category includes family foundations created by individuals and families as vehicles for carrying out their charitable vision. The Packard Foundation and the Bill and Melinda Gates foundations are examples. Other private foundations are independent foundations that often were originally organized as family foundations, but over a period of time family involvement in the leadership declined. The Ford Foundation is an example. Some foundations maintain very close relationships with the industry that was built by their founder. For example, the Annie E. Casey Foundation has a board of directors largely composed of former UPS corporate leaders. Corporate foundations are another type of private foundation whose assets are derived primarily from contributions of a for-profit or not-for-profit company. The contributions may be from an initial endowment, periodic contributions, or both. Many maintain their ties to the parent corporation despite their existence as an independent entity. Hospital-related foundations that provide funding for community projects are an example.

PUBLIC FOUNDATIONS

These foundations receive at least one-third of their income from the general public or sources outside of the main funder. The Pew Charitable Trusts (n.d.) is a public charity and the sole beneficiary of seven individual charitable funds established between 1948 and 1979 by two sons and two daughters of Sun Oil Company founder Joseph N. Pew and his wife, Mary Anderson Pew. Another type of public foundation is the community foundation, which is organized to serve specific geographic regions and receives its support from a variety of donors. The New York Community Trust is an example. Some public foundations are set up to collect funds from donors for a specific issue such as health or the arts. The National Endowment for the Arts is an example.

OPERATING FOUNDATIONS

These foundations are generally not grant-making organizations but primarily provide information about and analysis of health care issues to policymakers, the media, and the general public. The Kaiser

---

BOX 36-1 Important Things to Remember When Working with a Foundation

- Know your own program and funding needs. Does the entire program need funding? Are there any partners that can be brought on to help fund segments?
- Do not chase money for money's sake. Know what you want to accomplish, and do not let a foundation or other funder dictate your mission. Foundations can have constructive ideas about shaping a program, but it should be your program.
- Be familiar with the foundation's website and the possibility of a programmatic match before making any contacts. Understand the funders' needs and expectations.
- Know who you want to talk to, their funding priorities, and their areas of expertise.
- Prepare a sound byte version, a paragraph version, and a one-page version of what you hope to accomplish with foundation support. The foundation will ask for a full proposal if they want it.
- Know the following about your proposal off the top of your head: intent, anticipated outcomes, measures of success, approximate funding required, duration, deliverables, potential for matching or in-kind funds, and sustainability plans.
- If you submit a proposal, have someone who knows nothing about the topic read it and then describe in three sentences what you are asking the foundation to do. If they cannot, you have probably written it in "nurse" jargon instead of English.

- Never turn in any piece of work without first having a trusted editor review it.
- Nurture foundation relationships. Be of service to the foundation; let them see your talents and skills by serving on advisory panels or reviewing papers if you are asked. Foundations are always "trying out" experts to see who might be useful for meeting their objectives. Foundations want to be successful, and just like any other organization they prefer to work with someone with a track record of success.
- Think about what else local funders offer besides money—for example, access to political or business leaders, technical assistance workshops for prospective grantees, convening capacity, and so on. Talk with the people you identify.
- Always look locally for funding first. If you can pilot something with local funding, you are in a better position to get national funding to bring your model to scale. Think about and work with others in the community on the same issue, as evidence of collaboration is always considered a plus by funders.
- "Toot your own horn" about your agency and its good work. It's better for the funder to hear about what you have been doing before they get the proposal.
- Don't give up. You may not be funded the first time around, but following the above recommendations will definitely get you closer to your goal.

Family Foundation is one example of an operating foundation, and their Chartbook on Medicare is an example of one of their many contributions. It is available at *www.kff.org/medicare/7284.cfm*.

CORPORATE GIVING PROGRAMS

Corporate giving programs are grant-making programs established and administered within a for-profit corporation and are often administered by marketing or public relations staff. Grants made by these entities are often closely related to the parent company's profitability and business cycles. Gifts from corporate giving programs go directly to the receiving organization and are generally free from the reporting and other requirements of foundations.

Many foundations have started in the last two decades as a result of the conversion of not-for-profit health care providers or insurers into for-profit organizations or less commonly, through sales, mergers,

joint ventures, or corporate restructuring. Because non-profit organizations' assets are considered to be held in the public trust, state attorneys general have overseen many of these conversions. Conversion foundations are charged with funding health-related activities in their communities. The converted assets are to be used in a manner consistent with the original non-profit organization's mission. For example, the Colorado Trust has assets of over $191 million from the sale of PSL Healthcare Corporation for accessible and affordable health care and programs that strengthen families (The Colorado Trust, n.d.).

HOW FUNDERS MAKE DECISIONS

Each foundation is different and has its own unique process for making funding decisions. Some generalizations can be made, however.

WHAT IS FUNDED?

Foundations will generally state up front on their website what they will and will not fund. National foundations will screen proposal "fitness" before determining if the proposal is worthy of funding. For example, at the RWJF we state clearly on our website that we do not fund bricks-and-mortar types of projects. A proposal to construct a building to house a new nursing school will be rejected without further review. Some foundations will accept unsolicited grants only at certain times during the year, and those dates will be on the website. Some foundations solicit proposals as part of a developed program or in a specific content area. Proposals outside that content area will be rejected. Finally, many foundations restrict the size of the initial inquiry to a set number of pages. Proposals beyond that size may be rejected without further review.

EVALUATING THE PROPOSAL

Once a proposal passes the "does it fit with what we do" screen, it will be reviewed by foundation staff related to the substance of the proposal. If it is a small foundation without significant staff, the proposal may go right to the board of trustees for a decision. A proposal will be reviewed based on the following preliminary and basic questions:

- Do the applicants seem to have expertise in the area, and do they have the ability to do what they want to do?
- Is the project going to make a difference that lasts beyond the funding period (a concept that is called *sustainability*)?
- Does the applicant's organization have the organizational capacity and leadership structure to do what is proposed?
- Is the budget appropriate to what is being proposed (not too big and not too small)?

Foundations look on potential grantees as partners in effecting social change or, at the very least, partners to create action to solve a community problem. The applicant must know the subject matter and be able to explain how the proposal fits with what is known in the field. Larger foundations have content matter experts for their areas of interest available for consultation. Often foundations look for applicant teams that include individuals who are known in their field. Other times, foundations look for people with new approaches or want to broaden the numbers of partners they work with. Regardless, the proposal needs to demonstrate that the applicants know the territory.

WHAT'S THE IMPACT?

National foundations may want to have an impact on a field. Frequently we look for programs that are innovative by addressing a new aspect of a problem, addressing a problem in a different way, or applying a new or tested approach to newly affected or difficult-to-serve populations. Proposals that address an old problem in a way that has been proven to work tend to be less attractive. Many national foundations are willing to make a multiple-year commitment to a project but tend to see projects as having a beginning and an end. The project should have clearly stated goals, reasonable approaches to achieving those goals, and a clear plan to disseminate the findings or sustain the changes implemented without foundation funding. Most foundations are no longer interested in funding a good program that will fade away when the funding ends. Our goal is to make a lasting difference for society.

WHAT'S THE APPLICANT'S CAPACITY?

As part of the fiscal due diligence process, each foundation will want to make sure that the organization has the capacity to complete the tasks proposed. We do realize that in some communities and programmatic areas organizational capacity is a problem and may include building organizational capacity as part of the grant. It is important for applicants to be direct about what they can and cannot do and where they need help.

A BUDGET THAT WORKS

Finally, foundations review the budget for a project. This can be a show stopper. At one extreme, the amount requested may be more than the foundation is willing to invest in the type of project. At the other extreme, the foundation may feel that the applicant underestimates what it will take to accomplish what is proposed. Either case will lead to a rejection of the project. The foundation's staff will be looking to see if the funds requested seem reasonable and consistent with what is being proposed. They become proficient at identifying core costs versus extravagant costs.

After a review of the four areas, each proposal is assigned to a program staff person and goes through an internal review process and sometimes external reviews. But if we like the project and it stands up to the tests and we have the funds, we will fund it.

DEVELOPING A FUNDING STRATEGY: HOW TO WORK WITH FOUNDATIONS

Let's assume that you are very interested in trying to find funding to start a mentorship program for new nurses. Foundations get many more proposals than they can possibly fund, so creating a funding strategy is very important. The two components that you have to know well from the onset are your own programmatic needs and a list of all the foundations that may be interested in funding your project. A list of health care foundations both nationally and in your region can be found at the Grantmakers in Health website *(www.gih.org)*. For grants of any kind, including health care grants, go to the Foundation Center website at *http://foundationcenter.org*.

Once you determine which foundations match your topic area, go to their Websites to assess the specificity of their funding. For example, you might find a number of foundations interested in the topic of "nursing" but only a very small percentage that might actually be interested in a mentorship program for new nurses. However, a foundation might be interested in nurse retention, and you could frame your proposal for a mentorship project in terms of that priority. Foundations do tend to adopt specific areas within a topic, and these can change from year to year. If a website is unclear as to whether your topic might be of interest to the organization, then either e-mailing them or calling might be helpful. Many foundations also have helpful ways for you to get answers to your questions, such as a letter-of-intent process. The most important thing to remember is that you should never send a large, multipage proposal to a number of foundations on a random basis without first determining a foundation's specific needs and your actual chances of getting funded. You should always keep a record of where you sent a letter of intent and with whom you have had a conversation.

Foundations always seek to create the greatest leverage for turning project or demonstration work into actionable results. In this regard, you must have an idea ahead of time of how you will help foundations with this goal, including the identification of key stakeholders or people who will help turn results into action and policy. Knowing who your key stakeholders are and engaging them early, including the identification of an advisory committee, will be important. Throughout the lifespan of a project, especially those that are more long-term and key to foundation strategy, foundations will use a host of mechanisms to engage key stakeholders and inform policymakers, such as newsletters; listservs; invitations to presentations; inclusion of stakeholders in opinion polls (both formal and informal); use of video, Internet presentations, and postings on the Foundation's website; and blast e-mails. Engaging the media will also be important and will include press releases and press briefings. Foundations are also adopting new social media, such as Facebook, Twitter, LinkedIn, and other similar sites.

Foundations know that the more people and groups are engaged in an area and the more money invested, the greater the likelihood that action will be taken and policies will be changed. Thus, they will often give preference to those projects that have partnerships built in and extra sources of funding—either matching funds or in-kind resources. Funders know that with each additional key partner comes a potential layer of added influence that can only broaden and deepen the sustainability of the work. For example, as the RWJF seeks to bring recognition to nurses and their role in improving the quality of patient care, we apply a variety of approaches from building the capacity of nurse leaders through leadership and media development activities, conducting and disseminating research that links nursing outcomes to quality of care and convening activities that bring nurses in contact with other key influencers of health care.

The RWJF and other foundations also engage in demonstration projects in an effort to test and learn from potential good ideas. Examples of demonstration projects that went on to inform health care policy include the computerization of childhood vaccine records, simplifying the paperwork to enroll eligible people for Medicaid and Children's Health Insurance Program, the 911 emergency call system, and support for the development of the nurse practitioner role, including prescriptive authority.

Once you get into the process, it will be the relationship you develop with a foundation officer that will help you most. Never make the mistake of believing that a foundation is an entity from which you might receive just money. Foundations are also important organizations with regard to intellectual capital. They are extremely thoughtful about the areas that they fund and many times are experts in your topic, so consider them partners in achieving your goals. Even if they are not experts themselves, they generally know the experts in your area. Your program is always your program, but an experienced program officer can help you improve and/or fine-tune your approach.

For a list of related websites, please refer to your Evolve Resources at http://evolve.elsevier.com/Mason/policypolitics/

REFERENCES

The Colorado Trust. (n.d.). About the Trust. Retrieved from www.coloradotrust.org/about.

Foundation Center. (2009). Highlights of foundations giving trends. Retrieved from www.foundationcenter.org/gainknowledge/research/pdf/fgt09highlights.pdf.

Indiana Grantmakers Alliance. (n.d.). Retrieved from www.indianagrantmakers.org/s_inga/sec.asp?CID=14069&DID=31690.

Pew Charitable Trusts. (n.d.). History. Retrieved from www.pewtrusts.org/about_us_history.aspx?page=a4.

Schlandweiler, K. (Ed.). (2004). *Foundations fundamentals: A guide for grant-seekers* (7th ed.). New York: Foundation Center.

CHAPTER 37

Social Security: Key to Economic Security

Carroll L. Estes, Catherine Dodd, and Eva Williams

"…it is well that we pause to celebrate one of the great peacetime achievements of the American people; namely, the enactment of the Social Security Act."

—Harry Truman

This chapter[1] describes the economic and social conditions under which Social Security was constructed during the 1930s, equating them with the economic conditions of the first decade of this century. The chapter reaffirms the nursing profession's ongoing commitment to the eradication of health disparities and establishment of economic security for all people as an essential "determinant" of health and reveals the precarious position of many nurses as women who are most economically vulnerable in old age. Protecting and improving Social Security as it exists today protects the economic security of hundreds of thousands of "baby-boomer generation" nurses who are currently retiring or nearing retirement without adequate sources of other income. Notably, less than half of retirees and of working Americans have private employer-sponsored pensions (which are also increasingly tied to risky defined contribution plans), and women are least likely to have these sources of retirement income (United States Department of Labor [DOL] & U.S. Bureau of Labor Statistics [BLS], 2009; U.S. Social Security Administration [SSA], 2010).

This chapter distinguishes between Social Security policy formulation and Social Security policy enactment, both historically and amidst today's major battles over the future of this most successful social insurance program in our nation's history. As exemplified by overviews of the program's development and basic benefits, Social Security is positioned within the American ideology of *self-reliance*, since individuals earn Social Security by paying into the program during their working years. Furthermore, Social Security insurance protects individuals and families from economic calamity in old age or in younger age in the event of disability as well as surviving dependents in the case of the death of a parent or a family's breadwinner. The potential peril in curtailing or privatizing Social Security is set forth as a call to action for the nursing profession to protect all people from economic and health insecurity.

A BRIEF OVERVIEW OF THE DEVELOPMENT OF SOCIAL SECURITY

The concept of social insurance is not new; it arose with the emergence of industrially based economies and the growing dependence of workers and their families on earnings for economic security should the ability to earn income be curtailed. Simply put, social insurance is a system whereby members of a society collectively contribute payments into the system, thus insuring any member against a number of unforeseen risks that may result in earnings losses. In the U.S., the demand for social insurance peaked during the Great Depression of the last century when large-scale economic forces drove the development of policy formulation and the creation of the most important social program in our country's history.

Early in his first presidential term, Franklin Delano Roosevelt launched a period of federal government expansion, promising a "New Deal" for the American people in response to increasing rates of poverty and despair. Initially, the design and passage of New Deal legislation provided *economic relief* by creating temporary and long-term government programs that

---

[1]The authors gratefully acknowledge Shirley S. Chater, PhD, RN, for her contributions to this version of the chapter.

ensured a minimum standard for quality of life. However, Roosevelt soon realized that bringing about an *economic recovery* required more than economic relief; thus, the design of subsequent New Deal programs focused on job creation. Jobs and projects created work for the vast number of unemployed, including work in hospitals, schools, and public health departments for thousands of unemployed nurses (Pollitt & Reese, 1997). Nurses not only benefitted by employment but also exerted influence on program implementation through the strength of professional organizations like the National Organization for Public Health Nurses and the American Nurses Association (Kalisch & Kalisch, 1995).

Social Security, the longest-lasting program of Roosevelt's New Deal with the American people, ensured economic security for those who could not work, such as older adults, blind persons, and single mothers with young children. In a 1934 message to Congress, President Roosevelt announced his intention to create a "social security" program. By executive order, he organized the cabinet-level Committee on Economic Security (CES) to study the problem of economic insecurity and make legislative recommendations. Through appointments of nursing leaders and public health experts to advisory committees, the input of nursing professionals was added to final CES recommendations to Congress that formed the basis for the legislative proposal that ultimately became the Social Security Act of 1935.

UNDERLYING CONCEPTS THAT CONTRIBUTE TO SOCIAL SECURITY'S SUCCESS

In this second decade of the twenty-first century, the people of the United States are yet again confronted with unprecedented economic problems. At the time of Social Security's enactment, only 6 million people (less than 15% of the population) were covered by any kind of retirement income. Since 1977, 93% of all people 65 and older have been eligible for Social Security retirement income. Although many Americans have worked to develop a retirement supported by a combination of Social Security, savings, and private pensions, achievement of that goal is challenged by the economic climate of today. The vital importance of keeping Social Security benefits intact and keeping the program vigorous cannot be overemphasized.

Robert Ball (2009) describes nine principles as pivotal in a framework that keeps Social Security strong. At the framework's core lie the American ideology of self-reliance and the principle of Social Security as an *earned right* that entitles workers and their families to Social Security benefits by virtue of their having paid into it and having earned it. As an earned right, Ball maintains that Social Security is a positive experience, underscored by *wage-related benefits:* A worker can easily visualize the connection between his or her present income and standard of living and the benefit level necessary for future financial security during retirement.

Social Security is also predicated on a framework that acknowledges intergenerational chains of exchange and shared societal risks across generations (Williamson & Watts-Roy, 1999). Contributions from all workers and employers are the most efficient and affordable way to insure coverage for all families and generations across the entire population. Such shared coverage is necessary because of many vicissitudes for which no individual can appropriately plan or insure against. Major societal risks (and the death and disability among younger or older adult workers) for which no individual can adequately prepare are wars (Iraq and Afghanistan), terrorist attacks (9/11), natural disasters (Hurricane Katrina), and chronic or catastrophic health events. By spreading the risk over a large pool of people, social insurance offers protection against devastating loss of income through the death of a parent or spouse, the acquisition of a disability, or the simple act of retirement. The uncertainty and presence of such adverse life events illustrates the importance of the program to all Americans. The nation requires the universal social insurance system of Social Security, a system that ensures our responsibility to ourselves, to our families, and to one another, and that ensures social and economic stability.

THE BENEFITS OF SOCIAL SECURITY[2]

The success of Social Security is attributed to its significant positive effect in reducing poverty in old age. The facts speak for themselves, as shown in Figure

---

[2]The Social Security Act was amended in 1965 to include Medicare. See Chapter 17.

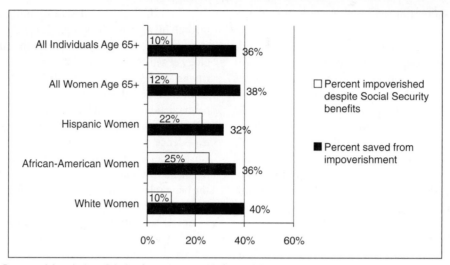

FIGURE 37-1 Percent of female beneficiaries (ages 65 and older) saved from impoverishment by Social Security in 2005, by race. (Adapted from Wu, K. B. [2007, November]. Sources of income for women age 65 and older. *Data Digest, 161*, 2. Washington, D.C.: AARP Public Policy Institute.)

37-1: Without Social Security, 46% of Americans age 65 and older would be poor, including an astonishing 61% of African-American women and 54% of Hispanic women.

The monthly benefit for Social Security is modest (an average of $1153 in 2008), with 40% of African Americans, 43% of Hispanics, 33% of Asian beneficiaries, and 19% of whites aged 65 and older receiving *all* of their income from Social Security. Nearly two-thirds (63%) of whites receive one-half of their income from Social Security (Table 37-1).

Social Security is a family program based on the simple concept that if you work, you pay taxes into the system. When you retire, or if you become disabled or die, then you, your spouse, your dependent children, or your survivors receive monthly benefits that are based on your earnings. Most people think of Social Security as a retirement program only, but of the 50.9 million people who received benefits from Social Security in 2008, 35 million are retired workers and family members, 6.5 million are survivors, and 7.4 million are disabled persons. Most notably, owing to retirement, survivor, and disability benefits earmarked for children of American workers, more children (nearly 3.3 million in 2008) are covered by benefits from Social Security than by any other government program except the earned income tax credit.

The Social Security program is financed by a "pay as you go" system, with present-day workers paying

TABLE 37-1 Importance of Social Security: Percentage of Income from Social Security for Population Age 65(+) by Race

Race	At least 50% of Income from Social Security	100% of Income from Social Security
White	63%	19%
Asian	65%	33%
Black	73%	40%
Hispanic	77%	43%

Adapted from U.S. Social Security Administration. (2009). *Income of the population 55 or older, 2006* (SSA Publication No. 13-11871), p. 300.

for present-day beneficiaries. Each worker pays Social Security taxes of 7.65% (6.2% for Social Security and 1.45% for Medicare) on gross salary (up to $106,800 gross salary in 2009).[2] Employers pay a matching 7.65% amount. Both parts of the payroll tax are paid by self-employed workers, and half is a tax-deductible business expense. By law, these taxes are paid into the Social Security Trust Fund.[3] Excess funds not needed for immediate payment to beneficiaries or

---

[3]Social Security actually has two separate trust funds that are jointly regarded as the combined Old-Age and Survivors and Disability Insurance (OASDI) Trust Fund: the Old-Age and Survivors Insurance (OASI) Trust Fund for retirement and survivors payments and the Disability Insurance (DI) Trust Fund for disability payments.

administrative expenses are invested with interest in U.S. government bonds.

The Social Security Act limits trust fund expenditures to benefits and administrative costs.

Eligibility for Social Security coverage is acquired by earning *credits* for working and paying into the system. The dollar amount of earnings required per credit is established annually (since 2008, 1 credit per quarter for $1090 earned, up to 4 credits per year of $4360). Most workers need 40 quarters to qualify for benefits. Fewer credits are needed for younger people to qualify for disability or for family members to be eligible for survivor benefits.

How much workers pay into the system and how long they work determines benefit amounts. While high-wage earners may receive higher benefits than low-wage earners, the benefit formula is weighted in favor of the low-wage earner by providing about 57% of preretirement earnings compared with replacement of 43% for average earners and 35% for high-income earners.

Since 1975, Social Security benefit amounts have been adjusted annually for inflation, based on cost-of-living adjustments (COLAs) linked to the Consumer Price Index (CPI). COLAs do not occur if the CPI falls, as was the case in 2008 to 2009; so while the COLA for 2009 was 5.8%, the COLA in 2010 will be *zero* by virtue of the CPI's drop.

RETIREMENT BENEFITS

Social Security Amendments of 1983 contained a provision that gradually (over a 22-year period) changed the full retirement age from 65 to 67 for those born in 1938 and later. For people retiring in 2009, the full retirement age was 66 and the average monthly benefit a modest $1153. Early retirement at age 62 remains an option, but with a slight permanent reduction in monthly benefits to provide for a longer period of lifetime benefits. Conversely, working beyond full retirement age adds earnings to the worker's record, increasing the eventual monthly benefit.

During the time a worker receives retirement benefits, a spouse can receive benefits on the worker's record if the spouse is 62 years of age or older and can subsequently receive benefits at retirement age on his or her own work record. A spouse who never worked can receive up to one-half of the retired worker's full benefit. Other benefits may be paid to family members who meet certain requirements, as in Box 37-1.

BOX 37-1 Retirement Benefits for Other Family Members Who Meet Certain Requirements

- A spouse of *any age* who is caring for a worker's child (if the child is less than 16 years old or disabled and is entitled to Social Security benefits on that worker's record)
- Children up to age 18
- Children age 18 to 19 who still attend elementary or secondary school, full-time
- Children age 18+ with severe disabilities that existed prior to the age of 22
- If the worker becomes a parent after benefits have begun (includes by adoption), the SSA must be notified so that the child's eligibility can be determined

---

Certain limits exist for how much money a family may receive. First, the full amount of the worker's benefit is provided. Then, if the benefits of all other family members exceed the limit, they are adjusted proportionately, keeping the total equal to the limit set by law.

Penalties affect monthly benefit amounts. If a worker chooses early retirement and continues to work, a $1 deduction penalty reduces benefits for each $2 in earnings above an annually established limit. Similarly, during the months of the year in which the worker reaches full retirement age, he or she is penalized $1 for every $3 earned over an annually established limit. After reaching full retirement age, the worker can work as much as he or she likes without penalty.

SURVIVOR BENEFITS

Survivors of deceased workers account for 13% of total benefits paid by Social Security. When a family member who has worked and paid into Social Security dies, his or her survivors, including widows, widowers (as well as divorced widows and widowers), children, and dependent parents, may qualify for benefits. This life insurance benefit helps to keep families together after the breadwinner dies. Widows or widowers receive full benefits at full retirement age or reduced benefits as early as age 60. Widows or widowers who are raising children under age 16 or children with disabilities can get full benefits *at any age*. Surviving children below the age of 18 (up to age 19, if still in school) are also eligible for benefits. Dependent parents age 62 or older also qualify. Under a special ruling, benefits are paid to a worker's surviving spouse and children, even if the deceased worker worked only 1.5 years in a 3-year period prior to death.

DISABILITY INSURANCE

Amendments to the Social Security Act, beginning in 1954, initiated the disability insurance program of Social Security and furnished the American people with further protections against economic insecurity. While initial measures only froze benefits so that future benefits were not lost during the period of disability, subsequent amendments added monetary benefits for disabled workers (age 50 to 64) and adult children. In 1960, disability payments were extended to workers of all ages and their dependents. Today, disabled workers and their dependents account for 18% of total benefits paid under the Social Security program.

There has been a drop in the average age of disabled worker beneficiaries currently receiving benefits since 1960. Age 57.2 was the average age for disabled workers in 1960, dropping to an average of 52.6 by 2008. A large majority of workers in the private sector (69%) do not receive (or pay out-of-pocket for) long-term disability insurance through their employer (DOL & BLS, 2009). Estimates for today's 20-year-old workers predict that 3 out of every 10 will be disabled by age 67. Notably, it is through Social Security that the majority of workers age 21 to 64 (about 91%) and their families are protected in the event of long-term disability.

Since 2010, Social Security provides disability benefits for younger individuals with health conditions so serious those disability standards apply. A list of *compassionate allowances* rapidly identifies diseases and health conditions like early-onset Alzheimer's disease, thus qualifying individuals (using minimal objective medical information) for disability benefits.

THE SUPPLEMENTAL SECURITY INCOME PROGRAM (SSI)

The Social Security Administration's responsibilities expanded in the 1970s by the addition of the Supplemental Security Income (SSI) program. As a federal and state public assistance program, SSI provides cash benefits to the neediest, to people who are age 65 and older, blind, or disabled, and to children who are blind or disabled. To qualify, recipients must have little income and own very few assets. Many SSI

TABLE 37-2 Gender Differences in Social Security Recipients

Age Group	Female Recipients	Male Recipients	Total Recipients
Age 62 to 69	8,418,000	7,230,000	15,648,000
Age 70 to 84	11,585,000	9,115,000	20,700,000
Age 85+	3,462,000	1,640,000	5,102,000
Total age 62+	23,465,000	17,985,000	41,450,000

Adapted from "Number of beneficiaries by age," Social Security Online, 2009. See *www.ssa.gov/OACT/ProgData/byage.html*.

beneficiaries also receive food stamps and Medicaid. SSI is funded from *general revenue*—money from the Social Security program is never used to pay for the SSI program.

SOCIAL SECURITY: A PROGRAM ESPECIALLY IMPORTANT FOR WOMEN

Any attempt to privatize Social Security would have an extraordinarily large effect on the financial security of older women (Table 37-2). The disparity between the income for men and the income for women is astonishing by the age of 65(+), with women more likely to be impoverished at about twice the rate of men (Harrington Meyer, 2009). Compared to older men, older women are more likely to be single, live alone, and be less likely to receive a private pension (and when they do, the average pension amount is half that of the men). While older women are just as likely as older men to be a Social Security beneficiary, those benefits tend to average 75% that of men's (Harrington Meyer, 2009). Women receive substantially less Social Security than men for several reasons. Women's wages are lower than men's, and women spend fewer years in the workforce while they care for children or aging parents. Women average 32 years in the paid workforce compared to 44 years for men (Reno & Lavery, 2007). Minority women tend to fare even more poorly according to Harrington Meyer (2009).

SOCIAL SECURITY: ESPECIALLY IMPORTANT FOR ETHNIC AND RACIAL MINORITIES

Today, about one-third of Americans are members of a minority group (Stanford & Nelson, 2009), with the largest group of minority elders being African Americans; however, due to lower male life expectancy, this group is not expected to grow as rapidly as other ethnic groups. Hispanics, the fastest-growing group among older adults, will compose 16% of older adults by 2050 (Federal Interagency Forum on Aging-Related Statistics, 2008). A big issue is the rapid growth of Hispanic baby boomers who remain a "hidden population" but one of major import (Gassoumis, Wilber, & Torres-Gil, 2008). Kochhar (2004) demonstrates that fully one-fourth of Hispanic households have negative or no net worth. In relation to lack of net worth, the SSA (2008) reports that 63% of unmarried Hispanic older adults and 39% who are couples are dependent on Social Security for at least 90% of their income.

Racial and ethnic minorities (throughout the life course and into old age) are poorer than their white counterparts, with the exception of some Asian-American groups. People of color experience not only lower socioeconomic and educational status, but also experience higher risks of earlier morbidity and mortality compared to same-age whites (Angel & Hogan, 2004). Their higher rates of disability, acute and chronic illness, exposure to environmental risks, and added stresses of discrimination and prejudice (Miles, 1999) are compounded by decreased access to health care and social resources to cope with them (Jackson & Govia, 2009).

These poverty figures and data about health and social disparities dramatically emphasize the importance of Social Security benefits for low-wage workers. Evidence presented by Hacker (2007) shows that less than one-half of working Americans have a private pension and that minority older adults have, by far, the worst private pension coverage of all older adults. As long as our society continues to be stratified by race and ethnicity in education, employment, and housing, it will be necessary to assure that policies do not disproportionately worsen the economic security of racial and ethnic minorities. Additionally, racial and ethnic minority groups have worse health outcomes, higher health costs, and, in most cases, shorter life expectancy than their white counterparts (Suthers, 2008), raising further concerns about policy proposals to increase the retirement age, which clearly will disadvantage minority communities the most.

BOX 37-2 The Debate in Resolving the Social Security Shortfall

No Cuts to Benefits Necessary	Serious Cuts to Benefits Necessary
• Adjust or remove the cap on wage income that workers contribute to Social Security • Include all future state and federal workers in Social Security (some government employees are in separate retirement systems) • Dedicate estate taxes to the Trust Fund	• Privatize • Raise the retirement age • Change wage indexing to price indexing • Make participation voluntary

---

SOCIAL SECURITY: FUND SOLVENCY

Recent annual Trustees Reports indicate that Old-Age, Survivors, and Disability Insurance (OASDI) funds will cover full scheduled benefits until 2037. Without legislative interventions, present tax revenues will be sufficient to pay about 75% of full benefits after trust fund exhaustion. Opposing positions exist for resolving the shortfall between fund revenues and expenditures. Many experts, including former Social Security commissioner Robert Ball and national organizations like AARP and the NCPSSM (National Committee to Preserve Social Security and Medicare), maintain that the gap is easy to solve, while other experts contend that serious cuts to beneficiaries are essential. These opposing viewpoints are summarized in Box 37-2.

SOCIAL SECURITY: POLITICS AND POLICY

Since the 1980s, political conflict concerning Social Security, its viability, and its future has intensified. The supporters of Social Security as an entitlement earned by workers remain dedicated to the values on which it is based: the interdependence of the generations and collective responsibility. Yet opponents of Social Security continue to portray Social Security as economically "unsustainable," requiring cuts and privatization. They extol the superiority of the "free market," saying that demographics and economics require us to modify or abandon the nation's commitment to Social Security and the underlying social contract between the American people and their government that has been in place for more than 75 years. The social contract is based on the commitment that we each take responsibility and contribute to this universal, earned benefit through our wages in order to insure ourselves and our families against the unpredictable events of death of a parent or spouse, or being orphaned, disabled, or retired.

The attention of policymakers, economists, and the media to the conflicts and challenges facing Social Security has shaken the confidence of many Americans who want Social Security to be there for future generations of young people. Nevertheless, there is consensus that Social Security is crucial, especially during tough economic times.

SUMMARY

The vital importance of Social Security in preventing and reducing poverty is underscored by the recent Wall Street, banking, and insurance crisis; dramatic losses in the savings and private pensions of millions; a subprime mortgage bust in which millions of Americans have lost their homes and millions more have lost the equity value in their homes; and very high double-digit jobless rates. The effects of The Great Recession of 2008-onward will shape the life chances of all current and future generations of Americans well into the second decade of the twenty-first century.

In a time of great economic uncertainty, Social Security was created to provide economic security for the most vulnerable: those unable to earn an income. It lifted millions of older adults, younger disabled persons, and surviving family members out of poverty. A bipartisan fiscal commission, created by President Obama's executive order, will now address debt reduction and the future of this essential base of social insurance as well as the Medicare and Medicaid entitlement programs. Nurses understand the importance of "economic security" as a crucial determinant of health status, morbidity, and mortality. It is, therefore, imperative to protect the most vulnerable in our society—the aged, persons with disabilities, and children—through the Social Security program. As a profession and as individuals, nurses today must take

up the historical leadership responsibilities demonstrated by nurses nearly a century ago and use their political clout to shape the development of policies that strengthen Social Security. In 2008, the American Nurses Association took a first step in that direction and passed a resolution for supporting and strengthening Social Security.[4]

For a list of related websites, please refer to your Evolve Resources at http://evolve.elsevier.com/Mason/policypolitics/

REFERENCES

Angel, J. L., & Hogan, D. P. (2004). Population aging and diversity in a new era. In K. E. Whitfield (Ed.), *Closing the gap: Improving the health of minority elders in the new millennium* (pp. 1-12). Washington, D.C.: Gerontological Society of America.

Ball, R. M. (2009). Social insurance and the right to assistance. In L. Rogne, C. L. Estes, B. R. Grossman, B. A. Hollister, & E. Solway (Eds.), *Social insurance and social justice: Social Security, Medicare, and the campaign against entitlements* (pp. 15-24). New York: Springer.

Federal Interagency Forum on Aging-Related Statistics. (2008). *Older Americans 2008: Key indicators of well-being*. Washington, D.C.: Government Printing Office.

Gassoumis, Z. D., Wilber, K. H., & Torres-Gil, R. (2008). Latino baby boomers: A hidden population (Latinos & Social Security Policy Brief No. 3). Retrieved from the University of California, Los Angeles, Chicano Studies Research Center website at www.chicano.ucla.edu/press/briefs/documents/LSS PB3July08rev.pdf.

Hacker, J. S. (2007). *The great risk shift: The new economic insecurity and the decline of the American dream*. New York, NY: Oxford University Press.

Harrington Meyer, M. (2009). Why all women (and most men) should support universal rather than privatized Social Security. In L. Rogne, C. L. Estes, B. R. Grossman, B. A. Hollister, & E. Solway (Eds.), *Social insurance and social justice: Social Security, Medicare, and the campaign against entitlements* (pp. 149-164). New York: Springer.

Jackson, J. S., & Govia, I. O. (2009). Quality of life for ethnic and racial minority elders in the 21st Century: Setting a research agenda. In P. Stanford & T. C. Nelson (Eds.), *Diversity & aging in the 21st century: Let the dialogue begin*. Washington, D.C.: AARP.

Kalisch, P. A., & Kalisch, B. J. (1995). *The advance of American nursing* (3rd ed.). Philadelphia: Lippincott.

Kochhar, R. (2004). *The wealth of Hispanic households: 1996-2002*. Washington, D.C.: Pew Hispanic Center. Retrieved from http://pewhispanic.org/files/reports/34.pdf.

Miles T. P. (Ed.). (1999). *Full-color aging: Facts, goals and recommendations*. Washington, D.C.: Gerontological Society of America.

Pollitt, P., & Reese, C. N. (1997). Nursing and the New Deal: We met the challenge. *Public Health Nursing, 14*(6), 373-382.

Reno, V., & Lavery, J. (2007). *Social Security and retirement income adequacy* (Social Security Brief 25). Retrieved from www.ncpssm.org/pdf/nasi-report.pdf.

[4]The resolution called on the Congress and president to oppose privatization, assure solvency for future generations, and add a caregiver credit for workers who must leave the workforce to care for children or aged/disabled family members; it urged that affiliate associations advocate for Social Security's protection.

Stanford P. & Nelson T. C. (Eds.). (2009). Introduction. In *Diversity & aging in the 21st century: Let the dialogue begin* (pp. 2-6). Washington, D.C.: AARP.

Suthers, K. (2008). *Evaluating the economic causes and consequences of racial and ethnic health disparities* (Issue Brief). Retrieved from American Public Health Association website at www.apha.org/NR/rdonlyres/26E70FA0-5D98-423F-8CDF-93F67DE319FE/0/CORRECTED_Econ_Disparities_Final2.pdf.

U.S. Department of Labor, & U.S. Bureau of Labor Statistics. (2009). *National Compensation Survey: Employee benefits in the United States, March 2009* (Bulletin 2731). Retrieved from www.bls.gov/ncs/ebs/benefits/2009/ebbl0044.pdf.

U.S. Social Security Administration. (2008). *Social Security is important to Hispanics* [Fact Sheet]. Baltimore: Author. Retrieved from www.ssa.gov/pressoffice/factsheets/hispanics-alt.pdf.

U.S. Social Security Administration. (2009). *Income of the population 55 or older, 2006* (SSA Publication No. 13-11871). Retrieved from www.ssa.gov/policy/docs/statcomps/income_pop55/2006/incpop06.pdf.

U.S. Social Security Administration. (2010). *Annual statistical supplement to the Social Security Bulletin, 2009* (SSA Publication No. 13-11700). Retrieved from www.ssa.gov/policy/docs/statcomps/supplement/2009/supplement09.pdf.

Williamson, J. B., & Watts-Roy, D. M. (1999). Framing the generational equity debate. In J. B. Williamson, D. M. Watts-Roy, & E. R. Kingston (Eds.), *The Generational Equity Debate* (pp. 3-37). New York: Columbia University Press.

Wu, K. B. (2007, November). Sources of income for women age 65 and older. *Data Digest, 161*, 2. Washington, D.C.: AARP Public Policy Institute. Retrieved from http://assets.aarp.org/rgcenter/econ/dd161_income.pdf.

CHAPTER 38

The United Kingdom's Health System: Myths and Realities

Dame June Clark

"The evidence that insurance and the access to care it facilitates improves health, particularly for vulnerable populations (due to age or chronic illness, or both) is as close to an incontrovertible truth as one can find in social science."

—Austin Frakt

"Socialized medicine" is not a phrase that British people would use to describe their health care system, and many are puzzled by the rather contemptuous tone in which it is often spoken by those who do use it. British people are more likely to describe the UK National Health Service (NHS) as a core public service, alongside other public services such as schools or the fire service, and to see health care as a citizen's right rather than as a commodity to be sold for profit to those who can afford to buy it. However, this does not mean that the British health care system does not include private practice or that the market plays no part in publicly funded services. In 2010, the UK NHS is no longer (if it ever was) a monolith in which all components are centralized, all facilities are government-owned or run, and all health care providers are government employees. Since its inception more than 60 years ago, the NHS has been subjected to a constant process of organizational reforms and restructurings, boom and bust expenditures, and constant criticisms and "scandalous exposures" in the media. The NHS is a top issue in every general election, and a top priority for every government of whatever party.

FUNDAMENTALS: PHILOSOPHY AND VALUES

What it does mean is that the fundamental principles upon which the NHS was based in 1948 remain, and are now deeply embedded in the British psyche. Even the British Medical Association, which strongly opposed its establishment, is now a strong supporter of its principles, however much it may carp at some of the details. Any attempt to undermine these principles provokes public outcry reflected in newspaper headlines such as "Hands off our NHS!"

The founding principles were that the NHS should provide the following type of services:
- Universal: available to all citizens based on clinical need and not ability to pay
- Comprehensive: all types of services—hospital and community-based, preventive as well as curative, from "cradle to grave"
- Free at the point of delivery
- Funded from general taxation

In July 2008, the Health Ministers of the four countries of the UK reaffirmed their commitment to these core principles, issuing a Statement of Common Principles that affirms the following: (All UK health ministers affirm commitment to core principles of NHS, 2008):
- The NHS belongs to all the people of England, Scotland, Wales, and Northern Ireland.
- The NHS provides a comprehensive service, available to all.
- Access to NHS services is based on clinical need, not an individual's ability to pay.
- The NHS aspires to high standards of excellence and professionalism.
- NHS services must reflect the needs and preferences of patients, their families, and their caregivers.
- The NHS works across organizational boundaries with other organizations in the interests of patients, communities, and the wider population.

- The NHS is committed to providing the best value for taxpayers' money, making the most effective and fair use of finite resources.
- The NHS is accountable to the public, communities, and patients that it serves.

MYTHS

The concept of the NHS as "socialized medicine" contains many myths that were made visible in the debate about health care reform in the United States. Perhaps the silliest example was the story published in the *Investor's Business Daily* and on television that "People such as scientist Stephen Hawking wouldn't have a chance in the UK, where the National Health Service would say the life of this brilliant man, because of his physical handicaps, is essentially worthless." In fact, Stephen Hawking is British, does live in the UK, and is sustained by the services provided by the NHS. Hawking himself responded via the UK newspaper *The Guardian*: "I wouldn't be here today if it were not for the NHS; I have received a large amount of high-quality treatment without which I would not have survived."

Other myths include:
- The government tells doctors and nurses who we can care for, when we can care for them, how we can care for them, and what care we can provide for them.

The UK countries' governments do set national policy priorities; and, at the local level, health authorities (Primary Care Trusts in England, Local Health Boards in Scotland and Wales) do plan services for their populations based on assessment of need. But at the level of the individual patient, clinical freedom is demanded and given, both by nurses and by doctors—and is probably greater than in a system in which insurance companies specify what they will and will not pay for.

The organization that appears to perpetuate the myth to U.S. audiences is the National Institute for Health and Clinical Excellence *(www.NICE.org.uk)*, which, in fact, was originally modeled on the U.S. Agency for Healthcare Quality and Research. This organization, established in 1999, is the independent organization responsible for providing national guidance on the best (and most cost-effective) treatment (including drugs) for specific diseases and conditions. NICE guidance is developed using the expertise of health care professionals, patients and caregivers, industry, and the academic world. Health organizations are not compelled to follow its guidance, but they usually do; problems arise primarily when a new and expensive drug (often for the treatment of the terminal stages of cancer) is not recommended by NICE, and is therefore not provided by a particular health care agency.

- Patients have to wait a long time to receive treatment.

In the past, waiting times for non-urgent hospital treatment were unacceptably long, and waiting was used as a form of rationing. Over the past decade, waiting times have been dramatically reduced; in 2008 in England the median waiting time between referral by a primary care or general practitioner (GP) and admission to hospital was 8.3 weeks, and the accepted maximum was 18 weeks. For an urgent condition, the waiting time is much less. A consultation with a GP is usually achieved within 48 hours. Access to an emergency department is immediate; after initially being seen by a triage nurse, patients must receive treatment within 4 hours.

- Patients have no choice about which doctor, which hospital, or which treatment.

Every UK citizen has the right to "register" with a GP of his or her choice. About 96% of the population do so, although there are sometimes difficulties for some mobile or homeless people. Patients often remain with the same GP from birth until death or until they move to another locality, although they may change their GP at any time, subject to the GP's willingness (usually limited only by geographical practicalities) to accept them on his or her "list." Except for access to the hospital emergency department, the GP is the point of first contact for people needing health care and acts as "gatekeeper" to other services to which he or she refers patients as necessary. Patients will usually accept the advice of their GP about treatment and about which hospital specialist is most appropriate, but every patient has the right to a second opinion and at least a limited choice of which hospital. (In England, patients may choose any hospital, but for most patients, especially outside the big cities, choice is limited by practicalities such as nearness to home, travel facilities, and so on.) Currently there is debate about the right of UK patients to receive treatment in any country of the European Union (EU).

REALITIES

There is no such thing as free health care. The debate is about the source of funding and the way in which the money is collected and distributed. There are various funding models used in different countries, but there is no consensus among analysts about which one is best. The choice among the various options depends on a country's history, culture, and political ideology.

The UK system of financing health care is based on achieving equity and social justice through the concepts of social solidarity and risk pooling. *Risk pooling* in health care means spreading the risks and costs of ill health across society—from poor to rich and from ill to well. The basic principle is that the cost burden is shared by everyone, even though not everyone will need to receive its benefits. This idea is deeply embedded in European culture and in stark contrast to the American ideology of individualism and commitment to a free market. It explains the choice of funding health care from general taxation or compulsory universal social insurance in order to ensure that health care is available to all who need it and free at the point of need.

The UK NHS is funded primarily (approximately 95%) from taxes, including a small proportion from the national insurance scheme, which is compulsory for all employers and employees; approximately 5% is derived from co-payments, mainly for drugs (only in England) and dental and ophthalmic services. In the NHS, the only third-party payer is the government. In 2001, at the height of the "New Labour" impetus to "modernize" the NHS, the UK government commissioned Sir Derek Wanless to undertake a review of the NHS, including possible funding models (NHS Confederation, 2009). He described one of the report's conclusions to journalists (Hall & Martin, 2001):

> *The current message by which health care is financed through general taxation is both a fair and efficient one ... There is no evidence that any alternative financing method to the UK's would deliver a given quality of health care at a lower cost to the economy ... Indeed other systems seem likely to prove more costly. Nor do alternative balances of funding appear to offer scope to increase equity.*

From the patient's point of view, health care is free. There are some exceptions, such as dental treatment and eye testing, although in both of these cases the NHS pays the full cost for older adults, children, and those receiving social welfare benefits and pays a contribution for all others. But hospital care (including diagnostic procedures and drugs) and home health care are totally free and there is no charge to see a primary care physician, through whom hospital care will be arranged if needed. Drugs prescribed outside hospital are free in Wales and Scotland, and this arrangement is soon to be extended to England.

The assumption made in 1946 that once the "backlog" of disease had been dealt with, the costs of the NHS would become less, turned out to be a major mistake; as in all western countries, the costs of health care have risen inexorably, and in Britain, as in most countries, cost constraint is a major preoccupation. Until the late 1990s, expenditure on health care was low in the UK compared with other European countries, but the Labour government elected in 1997 was elected on a commitment to increase it to at least the European average.

In 2002, the Wanless Report included a number of recommendations (Box 38-1) and called for a review of the progress being made in improving the NHS and a reassessment of its future needs in 2007. The government accepted the recommendations, and by 2007 most of them had been achieved. Although the review applied only to England, similar reviews, with similar recommendations, were undertaken in Scotland, Wales, and Northern Ireland. The 5 years following 2002 witnessed unprecedented levels of government investment in the NHS. Over that period, NHS spending rose by nearly 50%—a total increase of £43.2 billion—while the proportion of the UK's GDP devoted to health care spending grew to 9.2%, which is close to the estimated average EU health care proportion spent on health (although little more than half of the U.S. expenditure).

It was always recognized that this level of expansion could not be sustained, but the 2009 global recession meant that the investment could not go on increasing and there were likely to be future cuts in all public spending including health care. In fact, after the general election in 2010, the new coalition government announced major cuts in all public services, including the NHS.

BOX 38-1   Select Recommendations from the Wanless Report of 2002

- An increase in health spending from £68bn in 2002 to £184 billion by 2022
- Proportion of GDP spent on health to rise from 7.7% at present to 12.5% by 2022
- NHS spending to increase by 7.7% over the next 5 years reaching £96 billion by 2007
- A one-third increase in the number of nurses, and a two-thirds increase in the number of doctors
- A maximum 2-week waiting time for hospital appointments by 2022
- Improvements to NHS pay and new financial incentives to encourage staff to improve services
- Increase in staff productivity from 2% a year at present to 2.5% a year in the first 10 years if improvements are to be made
- A doubling of spending on information technology
- A major increase in the building program for new hospitals
- Redistribution of tasks between NHS staff, with health assistants taking over some of the work of nurses and nurses taking over some of the responsibilities of doctors
- A look at whether or not patients should be charged for missing NHS appointments
- Greater patient involvement in the running of the NHS
- A review of the policy on prescription charges
- The introduction of charges for non-clinical services
- Greater cooperation between the NHS and the private sector
- Financial incentives to reduce bed-blocking in NHS hospitals
- More self-care by patients
- Greater integration between the NHS and social services

From *NHS funding and reform: The Wanless Report* (2002). London: The House of Commons.

PRIVATE VERSUS PUBLIC

As part of the negotiations to establish the NHS in 1948, the doctors insisted that they must be allowed to undertake private practice in addition to working for the NHS. The services for which this facility is used are mainly in elective surgery and services such as IVF or cosmetic surgery which may not be provided within the NHS, or for which the patient is not prepared to wait. The services may be provided either in private hospitals or in private beds in NHS hospitals. NHS commissioning authorities may commission services from private providers as well as from NHS Trusts. There are approximately 300 private hospitals and Private Patient Units in the UK, providing just over 11,000 acute beds (compared with approximately 200,000 beds in the NHS). Both public and private sectors are now reducing bed numbers as inpatient treatment is replaced wherever possible by ambulatory services. Most of the UK's hospice care is provided through independent charitable organizations, which are, however mainly funded through the NHS. There is very little private practice in primary care, although in England, where the government is keen to promote "new models" of delivering care, private organizations and "social enterprises" are beginning to develop. Around 11% of the population has some private health care insurance, but the cover provided can be limited, and is often "tailor-made" to cover only circumstances or conditions in which NHS care is thought to be deficient. Patients can also pay directly for services.

The cardinal difference between private health care in the UK and private health care in the U.S. is that in the UK private health care is seen as a supplement to the NHS and not a substitute for it. People who use private health care remain entitled to use the NHS, and would almost always use it for expensive, long-term, or highly specialist services such as trauma care and posttrauma rehabilitation.

The one area in which care is dominated by the private sector is long-term care of frail older people. During the 1980s and 1990s, under the Thatcher government and as a result of policies initially introduced to change the basis of Social Security payments, this sector was almost entirely privatized. There are now approximately 200,000 beds in private facilities for long-term care of frail older adults—more than the total number of beds in the NHS—and about one-third of nurses in the UK work in this sector. Paying for long-term care for older adults is a major political issue in the UK. The recommendations of a Royal Commission on Long Term Care were rejected by the government in 2000, and the problem remains.

Part of this same problem is the distinction made between health care and social care and between nursing care and personal care. Care that is defined as "health care" is provided through the NHS and is therefore free at the point of delivery; care that is defined as "social care" is provided through local government social services and is means tested. "Nursing care" is defined as part of "health care"; "personal care" is defined as social care. These distinctions and the consequent budgetary arrangements create enormous problems for patients and their families as well as for nurses. In 2010, the governments in both England and Wales began consultations with a view to improving the funding arrangements; in Scotland this care is already provided free to the patient at the point of use.

POLITICS SHAPING THE NHS STRUCTURE AND ORGANIZATION

Three significant "NHS reorganizations" have shaped how it works today.

THE 1974 REORGANIZATION OF THE NHS

In the early 1970s, there was an attempt to integrate three separate branches of the NHS—the hospital services that were run by regional hospital boards, the community health services and public health that were run by local authorities, and the GPs, who practiced as independent contractors. The GPs again fought for and won the right to retain their independent contractor status, but hospital, community, and public health services were brought together under newly created health authorities, while in local authorities, which now ceased to provide health care, new social services departments were established to provide what became known as "social care," including child protection and services for frail older adults. This distinction between the NHS, which is centrally controlled and provides services free at the point of use, and local authority social services, which are locally controlled and subject to means testing (i.e., eligibility based on income), continues to be a major tension in health policy, especially in the issues of long-term care.

THE 1990 THATCHERITE REFORMS

In 1979, the election of a new right-wing conservative government under the leadership of Margaret Thatcher began a series of changes in the health care system (and many other aspects of British society) that were ideological as well as organizational, and more radical than anything that had happened since the end of World War II. The 1980s saw a sequence of changes that were introduced as "efficiency improvements" but that in their effects constituted radical cultural as well as organizational changes. The most significant for nursing was the introduction in 1983, on the recommendation of Sir Roy Griffiths, of the concept of general management to replace the system of functional management by the traditional triumvirate of doctor, nurse, and administrator. This meant that nurses no longer managed the nursing service or controlled its budget. Many senior nurses retired or lost their jobs, provoking a loss of leadership from which the nursing profession took a long time to recover. At the same time, the view that care in the community was cheaper as well as better than hospital care led to major reductions in the number of hospital beds, especially in psychiatric hospitals and hospitals providing long-term care. Health care began to become redefined as acute medical care. Many of the support services that had previously been provided "in-house" were contracted out to commercial agencies. The long-term care of frail older adults was gradually transferred to private nursing homes, which proliferated, causing a reconfiguration of the nursing workforce that had previously been employed almost exclusively in the NHS.

The changes were confirmed in new legislation in 1990. The core component of the 1990 NHS reforms was the introduction of an *internal market* through changes in the roles of the health authorities, hospitals, and community health agencies to create a "purchaser/provider split." Instead of using their money to run facilities themselves, the Health Authorities were to use it to purchase services for their resident population from the provider agencies that were now reconstituted as self-governing not-for-profit organizations called NHS Trusts. Some of the money was made available to GPs who chose to become "fundholders" to directly purchase certain services for their patients from Trusts and other agencies. The idea was that Trusts would compete with one another (and with the private sector agencies) for contracts with health authorities and fundholders, and the government believed that this competition would drive down costs and improve quality.

These changes produced a great change in the organizational culture of the NHS. On the one hand, it undoubtedly became more cost-conscious at all levels, and therefore probably more efficient. Quality assurance and outcome measurement became much more important. But clinicians of all disciplines complained that commercial pressures interfered with clinical freedom. Services that were regarded as uneconomic were cut or responsibility transferred to other sectors. Commercial competitiveness prevented the sharing of good practice. Most seriously, the negotiation by some general practitioners of contracts that gave preferential terms for their patients produced for the first time in the history of the NHS a "two-tier" service that violated the basic principle of access on the basis of need alone.

THE EFFECTS OF POLITICAL DEVOLUTION

In the 1997 general election, in which the NHS was a major election issue, the Conservative government was heavily defeated, and power moved to the "New Labour" government led by Tony Blair, among whose election commitments was "restoration" of the NHS. Within a few months of the election, the new government's proposals were published in a White Paper entitled *The New NHS—Modern, Dependable* (Department of Health, 1997). However, the new government's second major commitment—to political devolution for Scotland, Wales, and Northern Ireland—was soon to have a much greater influence on health care in the next decade.

From 1999 onwards, responsibility for the provision of health care was devolved to the new governments in Scotland and in Wales (because of continuing political turbulence, Northern Ireland has moved in and out of devolution). Since this time, the health care systems of the four countries of the UK have gradually diverged, although the core principles of a comprehensive health care system, funded by general taxation, provided to all citizens on the basis of clinical need, and free of charge at the point of use, remain sacrosanct. The organizational structures through which services are delivered are different in the four countries. The relative emphasis given to various aspects of health policy and the policy priorities also differ, with each country reflecting its own particular health problems and political ideologies.

In particular Scotland, Wales, and Northern Ireland "all stand apart from England in their commitment to communities and participation rather than markets and technical solutions" (Greer & Rowland, 2008). Scotland and Wales have rejected the market model and have reverted to systems similar to that which operated throughout the UK before 1990. The National Assembly for Wales has explicitly stated: "We firmly reject the privatisation of NHS services or the organisation of such services on market models. We will guarantee public ownership, public funding

---

> **BOX 38-2 Health Services Offered by All UK Countries**
>
> While each of the four countries of the UK is responsible for the way health care is delivered, they all provide the following:
>
> - Acute hospital services, including emergency services
> - Community-based nursing services
> - Maternity services (hospital and community-based)
> - Mental health services (hospital and community-based)
> - Child health services (including parental support, immunizations, developmental surveillance programs, and school health services)
> - Various preventive health programs, including screening programs
> - Public health services
> - Primary care, provided by GPs and their associated nurses
> - Community-based pharmaceutical services
> - Community-based opticians
> - Dental services (limited, and subject to co-payment)
> - A 24/7 telephone helpline (called *NHS Direct* in England and Wales and *NHS24* in Scotland), which is staffed by nurses and provides health information and advice to all callers, including referral to other services

and public control of this vital public service" (Welsh Assembly Government, 2007). In both countries, geographically defined health boards both plan and provide services for their defined populations. England, on the other hand, has retained and developed the market model of the 1990s, and as a result its health care system is now much more complex and diverse than those of the other UK countries. All four countries, however, provide for the services listed in Box 38-2.

While the details of the organization and structure of the NHS may shift with the political winds, the UK remains committed to the core values that undergird it.

REFERENCES

All UK health ministers affirm commitment to core principles of NHS. (2008). National electronic Library for Medicine. Retrieved from www.nelm.nhs.uk/en/NeLM-Area/News/2008-July/505495/505503.

Department of Health. (1997). *The new NHS—Modern, dependable.* Retrieved from www.archive.official-documents.co.uk/document/doh/newnhs/newnhs.htm.

Greer, S. L., & Rowland, D. (2008). *Devolving policy, divergent values?* London: Neuffield Trust. Retrieved from www.nuffieldtrust.org.uk/publications/detail.aspx?id=0&PRid=307.

Hall, C., & Martin, N. (2001). Tax-funded NHS "offers fair and first value way ahead." *Telegraph*, November 29. Retrieved from www.telegraph.co.uk/finance/2743774/Tax-funded-NHS-offers-fairest-and-best-value-way-ahead.html.

NHS Confederation. (2009). *The NHS handbook, 2009-10*. London: The NHS Confederation.

NHS funding and reform: The Wanless Report. (2002). London: The House of Commons. Retrieved from www.parliament.uk/documents/commons/lib/research/rp2002/rp02-030.pdf.

Welsh Assembly Government. (2007). *A healthy future*. Retrieved from http://wales.gov.uk/about/programmeforgovernment/1wales/ahealthyfuture/?lang=en.

CHAPTER 39

Science, Policy, and Politics

Mary W. Chaffee

"Pretending that politics and science do not coexist is foolish, and cleanly separating science from politics is probably neither feasible nor recommended."

—Madelon Lubin Finkel

Politics and science often reside together quietly, and their close relationship is not readily apparent. However, conflicts involving the two occur occasionally and draw the attention of the media, the public, and policymakers. This chapter explores how science and politics interact with and influence each other as well as how science can influence policy. This exploration dispels the myth that science is free from political influence. It also illustrates the concept that science can be used productively, or it can be ignored or misused (intentionally or inadvertently) in policymaking. Recognizing the intricate relationships among science, politics, and policy is the first step in making sense of the influence they can exert on each other. To assist, a model is presented that displays the relationships (Figure 39-1). The model depicts the "supply" side of science (research) and the "demand" side of science (science users). It is important for nurses and other health professionals involved in advocacy and policymaking to understand how to use science to shape good policy—as well as to understand how political forces may influence scientific data.

American science is second to none in its productivity, scope, scale, and budget. Since World War II, the scientific community has received extensive resources from the United States government (i.e., the citizens) and has become the world's greatest scientific enterprise (Greenberg, 2007). Table 39-1 presents some U.S. government agencies involved in the production and regulation of science; this provides a glimpse at the broad scope of scientific activities carried out or supported by the U.S. government.

Scientific knowledge informs the practice of the clinical disciplines, drives organizational and administrative practices in the health system, and influences access initiatives, cost-control measures, and quality improvement strategies. Pioneering research has led to great benefits for health, wealth, and the nation's defense, but the corporate presence in science has caused concern, and unscrupulous activities are not unknown (Greenberg, 2001, 2007).

POLITICS AND SCIENCE: THE DEFINITIONS

Politics has been defined as the process of influencing the allocation of scarce resources, and *policy* is a deliberate course of action. *Science* is the study, documentation, and collection of evidence pertaining to observable, naturally occurring objects, processes, and phenomena in ways that can be objectively reproduced to verify the results (Shrake, Elfner, Hummon, Janson, & Free, 2006). *Research* is a process of systematic inquiry using disciplined methods to solve problems or answer questions. Simply put, research is the process of building and refining scientific knowledge (Polit & Beck, 2008). Research develops *evidence* through numerous methods including case studies, randomized controlled trials, surveys and polls, systematic reviews, meta-analyses, and data mining of existing data sources (Diers & Price, 2007).

THE RELATIONSHIPS AMONG SCIENCE, POLITICS, AND POLICY

Research is expensive and the process of funding it is an inherently political one. Research scientists, including nurses, often compete with others for funding by having their research proposals evaluated. Based on proposal reviews, federal agencies,

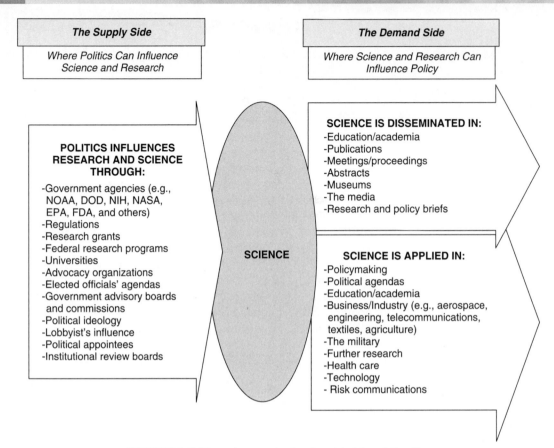

FIGURE 39-1 Politics, science, and policy: A model of the relationships.

universities, and private organizations award research funding. This is a political process because research funds are a scarce resource allocated according to predetermined criteria. The political influences on science may not always support the selection of the best proposals to receive funding. Greenberg sums up the clash of science and politics by describing science as "a deliberately nonpolitical enterprise embedded in a political system of rewards for vote gathering and campaign fund-raising" (Greenberg, 2001, p. 1). Hegde and Mowery (2008) assert there is political influence on some award decisions by the National Institutes of Health through complex congressional appropriations. There have been broad allegations of presidential meddling in the nation's science agenda, and interest groups have been accused of using sophisticated political tactics to discredit, suppress, or advance research on potential human health hazards (McGarity, 2006).

EXAMPLES OF COLLISIONS BETWEEN POLITICS AND SCIENCE

Many examples exist that illustrate how politics and science sometimes collide; the cases that follow are a sampling.

PHENYLPROPANOLAMINE (PPA)

PPA was an over-the-counter drug used as an appetite suppressant and decongestant. Reports of strokes in women who had used PPA occurred over a 20-year period, and the Food and Drug Administration (FDA) raised questions about the drug's safety. The trade association representing PPA's manufacturers used scientists and lobbyists to prevent PPA's removal from the market. Finally, the drug manufacturers and the FDA agreed to select an investigator to design a study of PPA; the findings indicated PPA causes

TABLE 39-1 Select U.S. Government Agencies and Organizations That Conduct Research, Fund Science, or Provide Oversight

Government Science Agency or Organization	Mission or Role
Agency for Healthcare Research and Quality, Rockville, MD	To improve the quality, safety, efficiency, and effectiveness of health care for all Americans
Argonne National Laboratory, Argonne, IL	One of the U.S. Department of Energy's oldest and largest national laboratories for science and engineering research
Consumer Product Safety Commission, Bethesda, MD	To protect the public from risk of serious injury or death from consumer products
Defense Advanced Research Projects Agency, Arlington, VA	Research and development arm of the U.S. Department of Defense; mission is to maintain technological superiority of the U.S. military and prevent technological surprise from harming national security
Environmental Protection Agency, Washington, D.C.	To protect human health and the environment
Federal Advisory Committees	To provide advice on matters ranging from research funding priorities and awards to strategic planning for federal investment in research
Federal Aviation Administration, Washington, D.C.	To provide the safest, most efficient aerospace system in the world
Food and Drug Administration, Silver Spring, MD	To protect the public health by assuring the safety, efficacy, and security of drugs, biologic products, medical devices, the food supply, cosmetics, and other products
House of Representatives Committee on Science and Technology, Washington, D.C.	Committee's jurisdiction includes all non-defense federal scientific research and development at a number of federal agencies and has special authority to review and study on a continuing basis laws, programs, and government activities relating to non-military research and development
Los Alamos National Laboratory, Los Alamos, NM	One of the largest science and technology institutions in the world; conducts multidisciplinary research on national security, space, renewable energy, medicine, and nanotechnology
National Academy of Sciences, Washington, D.C.	Brings together committees of experts in all areas of scientific and technological endeavor; includes the Institute of Medicine
National Aeronautics and Space Administration, Washington, D.C.	To pioneer the future in space exploration, scientific discovery, and aeronautics research
National Highway Transportation Safety Administration, Washington, D.C.	To save lives, prevent injuries, and reduce economic costs due to road traffic crashes, through education, research, standards, and enforcement
National Institutes of Health, Bethesda, MD	Primary agency of the U.S. government responsible for biomedical and health-related research
National Institutes of Standards and Technology, Gaithersburg, MD	To promote U.S. innovation and industrial competitiveness by advancing measurement science, standards, and technology in ways that enhance economic security and quality of life
National Renewable Energy Laboratory, Golden, CO	Part of the U.S. Department of Energy; the United States' primary laboratory for renewable energy and energy efficiency research and development
National Science Board, Washington, D.C.	To establish the policies of the National Science Foundation within the framework of policies set forth by the president and Congress
National Science Foundation, Arlington, VA	To support fundamental research and education in all the non-medical fields of science and engineering
U.S. Army Medical Research Institute of Infectious Disease, Ft. Detrick, MD	To conduct basic and applied research on biologic threats and medical solutions to protect warfighters
U.S. Geologic Survey, Reston, VA	Multidisciplinary science organization that focuses on biology, geography, geology, geospatial information, and water; dedicated to the study of the landscape, natural resources, and natural hazards
White House Office of Science and Technology and Policy, Washington, D.C.	To advise the president and others in the Executive Office of the President on the effects of science and technology on domestic and international affairs

stroke. But, instead of removing the drug from the market, the manufacturers used a product-defense firm to criticize the study. The FDA finally ordered PPA off the market in 2000 (Michaels, 2005).

EVOLUTION AND INTELLIGENT DESIGN

In 2005, the clash of politics and science played out in dramatic fashion in Dover, Pennsylvania. Eight members of a school board were sued for requiring that intelligent design be included in the Dover school system's biology curriculum as an alternative to evolution. Concerned residents challenged the incumbent school board members. Ultimately, all eight members of the school board were voted out of office and replaced by a group of challengers, including nurse Bernadette Reinking, who campaigned against the intelligent design agenda (Goodstein, 2005). The newly elected board members rescinded the intelligent design policy two weeks after Judge John E. Jones III ruled the policy was unconstitutional. Jones stated the concept of intelligent design is religious, not scientific (Raffaele, 2006).

MAMMOGRAM GUIDELINES

Controversy erupted in 2009 when a government panel abruptly changed mammogram screening guidelines. The U.S. Preventive Services Task Force recommended routine mammogram screening for women begin at age 50, not age 40 as recommended for the previous 25 years, and that mammograms be done every 2 years rather than annually (Agency for Health Care Quality and Research, 2009). Government guidelines are powerful because they influence the behavior of patients, health care providers, and insurers. In this case, the data may actually support the altered recommendation. Trials in Sweden that monitored 265,000 women found virtually no benefit from mammograms for women under age 55 (Crewdson, 2009). Despite this, the push back has been robust and was fueled by media coverage that failed to explore the potential dangers of unnecessary mammograms. The American Cancer Society has refused to change its recommendation to reflect the new federal guidelines (American Cancer Society, 2009). The Society of Breast Imaging president released a statement that the recommendations are a "step backward and represent a significant harm to women's health" (Steenhuysen, 2009). Allegations have flown back and forth like tennis volleys and have

left some women and health professionals confused about how best to proceed, but the task force was clear that the decision should be made between the patient and provider.

HEALTH DISPARITIES

Policymakers had recognized in 2004 that disadvantaged minority groups received poorer health care and often have poorer health outcomes. Despite this, a draft report by the Agency for Healthcare Quality and Research (AHRQ) providing evidence of health disparities was ordered rewritten, and researchers were directed to drop their conclusion that racial disparities are pervasive in the U.S. health care system. The rewrite downplayed the researchers' conclusions and "broke with the weight of scientific opinion" (Bloche, 2004). Disgruntled government staff members leaked the altered draft reports. Secretary of Health and Human Services Tommy Thompson ultimately called the episode a mistake and said that the goal had been to produce a report that was more positive (Bloche, 2004). In an analysis of the controversy, Bloche noted, "The affair was embarrassing because Americans expect scientific rigor, not aggressive advocacy, from federal research agencies" (2004).

LYME DISEASE CLINICAL PRACTICE GUIDELINES

Kraemer and Gostin (2009) chronicled a troubling conflict between the Infectious Diseases Society of America (IDSA) and the Connecticut attorney general. IDSA issued clinical practice guidelines for management of Lyme disease in 2006. The guidelines did not recommend antibiotic treatment for nonspecific symptoms (fatigue, headache, and others) that persist after standard antibiotic treatment. The IDSA guidelines also did not recommend the use of alternative diagnostic tests (the Centers for Disease Control and Prevention and the Food and Drug Administration had deemed the tests invalid). The Connecticut attorney general initiated an investigation and alleged the IDSA had violated state antitrust law by recommending against the use of long-term antibiotics to treat "chronic Lyme disease." Despite developing guidelines that were based on scientific evidence, the IDSA was forced to settle the case after spending more than $250,000 on legal fees (Kraemer & Gostin, 2009).

PREMENSTRUAL DYSPHORIC DISORDER

Controversy has emerged over the existence of premenstrual dysphoric disorder (PMDD). The American Psychiatric Association is debating whether to add PMDD to the *DSM-5* (the fifth edition of its diagnostic manual) due to be published in 2013 (American Psychiatric Association, 2010). Part of the controversy involves whether or not scientific evidence exists to support inclusion of PMDD as a diagnosis. Including PMDD in the *DSM-5* would increase the chances that health insurers would cover the cost of PMDD treatment and may encourage further research and development of new therapies (Chen, 2008).

THE DEATH OF AHCPR AND THE BIRTH OF AHRQ

The Agency for Healthcare Quality and Research (AHCPR) was established in 1989. Its mission was to use outcomes research to develop practice guidelines to improve health care cost and quality. Only 6 years later, it was on the brink of closure due to several political realities: A special-interest group launched an attack, the agency had fewer powerful political allies in Congress, it was criticized for inefficiency, and it was target for partisan political attack (Gray, Gusmano, & Collins, 2003). AHCPR published practice guidelines in 1995 supporting nonsurgical treatment for low back pain. The North American Spine Society, an association of spine surgeons, protested the guidelines and underlying research. The Society formed an advocacy organization devoted to shutting down AHCPR (Deyo & Psaty, 1997). Their efforts gained significant traction. After having its budget "zeroed out" by the House of Representatives in 1996, it was resuscitated, given a new name and an altered mission. The new Agency for Healthcare Quality and Research, launched in 1999, would no longer produce practice guidelines and the word *policy* was removed from its name. The agency's story illustrates the complexities of mixing politics and research.

CONTROVERSIES DURING THE GEORGE W. BUSH ADMINISTRATION

Many controversies plagued President George W. Bush's administration, including perceived manipulation of science and science policy. The Democratic staff of the House Government Committee on Oversight and Government Reform assessed the handling of science and scientists by the Bush Administration and released a report that stated the administration's "political interference with science has led to misleading statements by the President, inaccurate responses to Congress, altered Web sites, suppressed agency reports, erroneous international communications and the gagging of scientists" (U.S. House of Representatives Committee on Oversight and Government Reform, 2003). A Bush political appointee, George Deutsch, resigned after he prevented reporters from interviewing the leading climate scientist at the National Aeronautics and Space Administration (NASA) and instructed a NASA scientist to insert the word *theory* in discussions of the Big Bang because NASA should not discount the possibility of intelligent design by a creator. Deutsch lied about having a nonexistent undergraduate degree, which led *The Washington Post* to state in an editorial, "The spectacle of a young political appointee with no college degree exerting crude political control over senior government scientists and civil servants with many decades experience is deeply disturbing" (The Politics of Science, 2006).

While other allegations regarding the Bush administration's possible manipulation of science policy arose, few were as dramatic as those raised by former U.S. Surgeon General Richard Carmona who served from 2002 to 2006. In testimony before the House Committee on Oversight and Government Reform, Carmona stated that public health reports were withheld unless they praised the administration and that he was prevented by political appointees within the Department of Health and Human Services from speaking out on scientific evidence concerning stem cell research, contraception, and sex education. Carmona testified "Anything that doesn't fit into the political appointee's ideological, theological, or political agenda is often ignored, marginalized or simply buried" (Vergano, 2007). He added that "The problem with this approach is that in public health, as in a democracy, there is nothing worse than ignoring science or marginalizing the voice of science for reasons driven by changing political winds" (Lee, 2007). The White House denied political interference; spokesman Tony Fratto stated that it was disappointing Carmona "failed to use his position to the fullest extent in advocating for policies he thought were in the best interest of the nation" (KaiserNetwork.org, 2007).

GLOBAL WARMING

Climate science has generated significant interest since global warming emerged as a potential threat. This science has become embroiled in particularly ugly politicization efforts. "Warmists" believe the evidence of heating in the stratosphere and other types of man-made climate change is compelling (Begley, 2009). "Deniers" contend global warming is an alarmist, political crusade. One particular controversy in the ongoing battle between global warming believers and skeptics concerned "Climate-gate"—the theft of some British climate scientists' e-mail and the attempt to use them to discredit the science. Hackers stole about 1000 e-mails from scientists in the University of East Anglia's Climate Research Unit and posted them online. Some of the scientists' language in the messages was used by skeptics who argued the scientists were engaging in manipulation of their findings to support global warming. The second of three investigations into allegations of research misconduct cleared the scientists; investigators did note the scientists could have used more rigorous statistical procedures (Adam & Eilperin, 2010).

QUESTIONS RAISED BY THE UNION OF CONCERNED SCIENTISTS

The Union of Concerned Scientists (UCS) is a nonprofit group that combines research and action to urge responsible change in government policy, corporate practices, and consumer choices to promote a healthy environment and safer world (Union of Concerned Scientists, 2010a). The UCS has identified problems in the relationships between science and politics and has proposed solutions. The UCS published the *A to Z Guide to Political Interference in Science*. This website, using a periodic table–like graphic, presents dozens of cases of perceived political interference in science (Union of Concerned Scientists, 2010b). The Union also published findings from surveys they conducted of government scientists from 2005 to 2007. Participants reported political interference in federal science including direction to alter the reporting of scientific findings, fear of retaliation for speaking out, and being pressured to remove certain language from their communications (Union of Concerned Scientists, 2009).

HOW CAN SCIENCE BE USED TO SHAPE HEALTH POLICY?

Evidence should be used to inform policy debates and shape policy choices. To do this effectively requires an understanding of the policy process. Research findings can play a powerful role in the first step of the policy process—getting attention for particular problems and moving them to the policy agenda. Research can be valuable in defining the size and scope of a problem (Diers & Price, 2007); this can help to obtain support for a particular policy option and in advocating for support.

WHAT CAN BE DONE TO ENSURE A HEALTHY PARTNERSHIP BETWEEN SCIENCE AND POLITICS?

A variety of strategies can be employed to see that reliable and valid research is used in policymaking and to prevent inappropriate political influence in science and research. Several strategies are discussed here; additional strategies appear in Table 39-2.

CRITIQUE RESEARCH FINDINGS

The ability to critically analyze research findings is essential to ensure good science is used to shape health policy, to advocate for specific policy choices, and to evaluate claims made by advocates. Best (2001) declared, "We need statistics; we depend upon them to summarize and clarify the nature of our complex society" (p. 5). However, he cautions that some statistics are "born bad" (due to dubious data) and others mutate; some findings are distorted and lead to poor policy choices. Users of scientific findings must be able to critically evaluate the research methods, interpret the findings, and assess whether or not they can be considered reliable and valid. If data are flawed, the study will not produce useful evidence (Polit & Beck, 2008). Note who funded the research and the authors' affiliations and any stated disclosures of relationships.

MAINTAIN SCIENTIFIC INTEGRITY

Scientific integrity is the foundation of the scientific enterprise. Ensuring integrity requires firm and clear rules, penalties for not complying, and expert observers as well as established procedures for investigating

TABLE 39-2 Strategies to Foster Healthy Partnerships Between Science and Politics and to Support the Use of Research in Policymaking

Strategy	Description
Appoint unbiased government panel members	The judgment of the scientific community is injected into policymaking through scientific advisory panels. Allegations have been made that panel members sometimes represent industries regulated by the government. Policymaking would benefit from uncompromised scientific opinion from government advisory panels (Sneyd, 2009).
Assess the source of attempts to discredit research findings	Because absolute certainty can rarely be achieved in science, industry groups sometimes attempt to inject "manufactured uncertainty" into the analysis of scientific findings to undermine the findings (Michaels, 2005).
Assess the source of funding for research studies	Evaluate the source of funding to determine if the funding entity might have a reason to desire a certain finding. Some industry groups have attempted to manipulate scientific findings to suit their goals.
Assess the source of scientific assertions	When science or scientific findings become mired in political controversy, assess the source of the data and who is using it as a political tool.
Communicate scientific findings clearly	Communicating effectively bridges the gap between data and application. Scientific information should be carefully considered as to the type of data and the presentation approach to use so it is persuasive to the audience and scientifically defensible (Nelson et al., 2009).
Demand scientific integrity	Maintaining high standards of integrity ensures the soundness of the scientific product and the public's confidence in research findings.
Recognize actual and spurious claims of "junk science"	Term describes an advocate's claims about scientific data, research, or analyses that appear to be spurious; conveys a connotation that the advocate is driven by political, ideologic, financial, or other unscientific motives (Wikipedia, 2010).
Protect peer review from interference	Peer review, if done in a balanced and effective manner, can play a powerful role in separating politics from science. If done well, it can keep norms and values in their appropriate places and cause researchers to be explicit about their research premises (Bloche, 2004).
Recognize the influence of values on science	The values of scientists are infused into the research process. Values and ethics are an integral, though generally hidden, aspect of decision-making in science (Nelson et al., 2009).
Scrutinize the commercialization of academic research relationships with industry partners	The academic-industrial research system produces beneficial results, but concern exists about the penetration of commercialism at some universities (Greenberg, 2007).
Use data to raise awareness of problems	One of the most powerful uses of data to increase awareness of a problem came from the publication of the Institute of Medicine's report "To Err is Human: Building a Safer Health System" in 1999. A key statistic reported (that 44,000 to 98,000 persons died each year because of preventable medical errors) became an extremely influential research finding. The report, which chronicled the scope of health care errors, generated extensive response and focused the media's and public's attention on the problem.
Use metaphors to communicate statistical data to audiences and improve comprehension	Metaphors can transform health data into something people can understand and connect to their own lives (Nelson et al., 2009):"College students consumed enough alcohol to fill 3,500 Olympic-sized swimming pools" (Wallack, Dorfman, Jernigan, & Themba, 1993)."Each year, more than 1 million children begin smoking; this is the equivalent of 33,000 classrooms per year or 90 classrooms every day" (Nelson et al., 2009).

offenses and good citizenship by all in the scientific community (Greenberg, 2007).

TRANSLATE RESEARCH FINDINGS SO THEY CAN BE APPLIED IN POLICYMAKING

Scientists, and scientific data, are generally highly regarded and viewed to be credible. But conducting rigorously designed and conducted research is not always enough in the policy arena. For researchers, communicating findings so they can be understood and utilized is vitally important. Cornelia Dean (2009) has written a book that provides guidance to scientists on how they can most effectively connect with audiences, tell stories that illuminate their findings, and communicate them clearly to the media.

USE APPROPRIATE DATA TO SHAPE POLICY

Policymakers are influenced by many factors, and while scientific data does matter, it may not matter as much as scientists and health professionals desire. Descriptive data can be valuable when communicating the scope of a problem or providing evidence that a problem exists. Findings from analyses of trends, risk estimates, and cost studies are often successfully used to raise awareness of issues. Cause-and-effect analyses are generally found in intervention, evaluation, or related studies. Relative risk (e.g., "a four times greater risk of complication if treated with the drug") can be a helpful way to communicate findings as well as using meta-analyses and reviews of evidence (Nelson, Hesse, & Croyle, 2009). The power of data shouldn't be underestimated. Scientific findings provided the foundation for major legal or regulatory action against manufacturers of tobacco, asbestos, the Dalkon Shield intrauterine device, and others (Wagner & Steinzor, 2006).

SUMMARY

Science is not free from the influence of politics. Pielke (2008) argues that science and politics will always be intermixed in the practice of governance. He also contends that an attempt to separate them would be doomed to failure and would create conditions that would encourage the pathologic politicization of science. Science, politics, and policy will continue to co-exist, but science should not be compromised by political ideology (Finkel, 2007).

For a list of related websites, please refer to your Evolve Resources at http://evolve.elsevier.com/Mason/policypolitics/

REFERENCES

Adam, K., & Eilperin, J. (2010). Academic experts clear scientists in "climate-gate." *The Washington Post*, April 15. Retrieved from www.washingtonpost.com/wp-dyn/content/article/2010/04/14/AR2010041404001.html.

Agency for Health Care Quality and Research. (2009). Screening for breast cancer—Recommendation statement. Retrieved from www.ahrq.gov/clinic/uspstf09/breastcancer/brcanrs.htm.

American Cancer Society. (2009). American Cancer Society responds to changes to USPSTF mammography guidelines. Retrieved from www.cancer.org/docroot/med/content/med_2_1x_american_cancer_society_responds_to_changes_to_uspstf_mammography_guidelines.asp.

American Psychiatric Association. (2010). DSM-5 Development. Retrieved from www.dsm5.org.

Begley, S. (2009, December 5). The truth about "Climategate." *Newsweek*. Retrieved from www.newsweek.com/id/225778.

Best, J. (2001). *Damned lies and statistics: Untangling numbers from the media, politicians, and activists*. Berkeley, CA: University of California Press.

Bloche, M. G. (2004). Health care disparities—Science, politics and race. *New England Journal of Medicine, 350*(15), 1568-1570.

Chen, I. (2008). A clash of science and politics over PMS. *The New York Times*, Retrieved from health.nytimes.com/ref/health/healthguide/esn-pms-ess.html.

Crewdson, J. (2009). Rethinking the mammogram guidelines. *The Atlantic*, November.

Dean, C. (2009). *Am I making myself clear? A scientist's guide to talking to the public*. Boston: Harvard University Press.

Deyo, R., & Psaty, M. (1997). The messenger under attack—Intimidation of researchers by special interest groups. *New England Journal of Medicine, 336*(16), 1176-1180.

Diers, D., & Price, L. (2007). Research as a political and policy tool. In D. Mason, J. Leavitt, & M. Chaffee (Eds.), *Policy and politics in nursing and health care* (pp. 195-207). St. Louis: Elsevier.

Finkel, M. (2007). *Truth, lies, and public health—How we are affected when science and politics collide*. Westport, CT: Praeger.

Goodstein, L. (2005). Evolution slate outpolls rivals. *The New York Times*. Retrieved from www.nytimes.com/2005/11/09/national/09dover.html.

Gray, B., Gusmano, M., & Collins, S. (2003). AHCPR and the changing politics of health services research. *Health Affairs*, 283-307. Retrieved from content.healthaffairs.org/cgi/content/full/hlthaff.w3.283v1/DC1.

Greenberg, D. (2001). *Science, money, and politics: political triumph and ethical erosion*. Chicago: University of Chicago Press.

Greenberg, D. (2007). *Science for sale—The perils, rewards, and delusions of campus capitalism*. Chicago: University of Chicago Press.

Hegde, D., & Mowery, D. C. (2008). Politics and funding in the U.S. public biomedical R&D system. *Science, 322*(5909), 1797-1798.

KaiserNetwork.org. (2007). Former Surgeon General Carmona says Bush administration blocked him from speaking about certain issues. *Kaiser Daily HIV/AIDS Report*, (July 11). Retrieved from www.kaisernetwork.org/daily_reports/rep_index.cfm?DR_ID=46127.

Kraemer, J., & Gostin, L. (2009). Science, politics, and values—The politicization of professional practice guidelines. *Journal of the American Medical Association, 301*(6), 665-667.

Lee, C. (2007). Ex-Surgeon General says White House hushed him. *The Washington Post*, (July 11). Retrieved from www.washingtonpost.com/wp-dyn/content/article/2007/07/10/AR2007071001422_pf.html.

McGarity, T. (2006). Defending clean science from dirty attacks by special interests. In W. Wagner & R. Steinzor (Eds.), *Rescuing science from* politics—*Regulation and the distortion of scientific research* (pp. 24-45). New York: Cambridge University Press.

Michaels, D. (2005). Doubt is their product. *Scientific American, 292*(6), 96-101.

Nelson, D., Hesse, B., & Croyle, R. (2009). *Making data talk—Communicating public health data to the public, policy makers, and the press.* New York: Oxford University Press.

Pielke, R., Jr. (2008). Science and politics—Accepting a dysfunctional union. *Harvard International Review, Summer,* 36-41.

Polit, D., & Beck, C. (2008). *Nursing research: generating and assessing evidence for nursing practice* (8th ed.). Philadelphia: Lippincott Williams & Wilkins.

The politics of science. (2006, February 9). *The Washington Post.* Retrieved from www.washingtonpost.com/wp-dyn/content/article/2006/02/08/AR 2006020801991.

Raffaele, M. (2006). Intelligent-design policy rescinded. *MSNBC.com.* Retrieved from www.msnbc.msn.com/id/10698535.

Shrake, D., Elfner, L., Hummon, W., Janson, R., & Free, M. (2006). What is science? *Ohio Journal of Science, 106*(4), 130-135.

Sneyd, M. (2009, March 23). Rescuing science from politics. *The Cleveland Plain Dealer.*

Steenhuysen, J. (2009). Experts question motives of mammogram guidelines. *Business & Financial News.* Retrieved from www.reuters.com/assets/print?aid=USTRE5AF5)S20091116.

U.S. House of Representatives Committee on Oversight and Government Reform. (2003). About politics and science—The state of science under the Bush Adminstration. Retrieved from http://oversight.house.gov/features/politics_and_science/index.htm.

Union of Concerned Scientists. (2009). Voices of federal scientists—Americans' health and safety depends on independent science. Retrieved from www.ucsusa.org/assets/documents/scientific_integrity/Voices_of_Federal_Scientists.pdf.

Union of Concerned Scientists. (2010a). About us. Retrieved from www.ucsusa.org.

Union of Concerned Scientists. (2010b). The A to Z guide to political interference in science. Retrieved from www.ucsusa.org/scientific_integrity/abuses_of_science/a-to-z-guide-to-political.html.

Vergano, D. (2007, August 7). Science v. politics gets down and dirty. *USA Today.* Retrieved from www.usatoday.com/news/washington/2007-08-05-science-politics_N.htm.

Wagner, W. & Steinzor, R. (Eds.). (2006). *Rescuing science from politics—Regulation and the distortion of scientific research.* New York: Cambridge University Press.

Wallack, L., Dorfman, L., Jernigan, D., & Themba, M. (1993). *Media advocacy and public health—Power for preventon.* Newbury Park, CA: Sage.

Wikipedia. (2010). Junk science. Retrieved from en.wikipedia.org/wiki/Junk_science.

CHAPTER 40

Research as a Political and Policy Tool

Lynn Price

"We are drowning in information but starved for knowledge."

—John Naisbitt

That research has any nexus to politics or policy may strike one as curious, if not an outright oxymoron. Research, using any methodology, is carefully considered, designed, implemented, and interpreted. Politics is, well, messy. Policy is birthed from political process—and is therefore often complex and messy in its own right. Yet, research is a powerful lever in the world of politics and policymaking. In the last few decades, research has come to play an increasingly influential role in the crafting of both political messages and policy declarations, in nursing and health generally.

SO WHAT IS POLICY?

Policy is usually thought of as formal "rules," set by Congress, state legislatures, or various agencies at city, county, state, or federal levels. But it is also made by private entities. Clinics and long-term and acute-care settings have infection-control policies, visitation policies, and other rules pertaining to the work. Nursing schools craft policies about student dress codes for clinical settings and academic progression. Insurance companies create policies about how much of the physician's rate for services will be paid to advanced practice registered nurses (APRNs). The private policy sources often look to evidence in the same manner as do public policymakers.

In both venues, research alone is not responsible for producing policy. The rules for the use of data are the same, but as policy and political actors change, so do considerations about research, and how best to utilize findings, or even what research question to ask.

One can think of this as the "political ecology" of policymaking—that is, the many subtle and sometimes overt influences that surround the making of any policy.

WHAT IS RESEARCH WHEN IT COMES TO POLICY?

Research in policymaking venues involves a roundup of all the usual suspects in quantitative methodology, including the randomized controlled trial, though the opportunities for using this "gold standard" are fewer than in bench science. Meta-analysis has tremendous potential in the world of policy. A meta-analysis is a "study of the studies," sifting, distilling, and analyzing quantitative data gathered from multiple studies on the same topic. It produces a solid summary of evidence in one package—efficient for both advocates and policymakers. Meta-analyses can also "refocus attention" on key policy points (Aiken, 2008, p. 75). Qualitative methods are increasingly invoked for use within the policy realm (Brazier, Cooke, & Moravan, 2008).

Data-mining, the use of data collected through large health care entities and government agencies, offers a strong nexus between problems and policy solutions as well (Cheung, Moody, & Cockram, 2002). Diers has been a proponent of data-mining of clinical databases for nursing's benefit, such as how patient acuity influences nursing's work (Diers & Potter, 1997; Heslop, Gardner, Diers, & Poh, 2004; Diers, 2007; Duffield, Diers, Aisbett, & Roche, 2009). Using "secondary data" is challenging, but rewarding given its immense scope in time and data points, compared to what most researchers can accomplish in traditional data collection (Garmon Bibb, 2007).

And then there are a few surprises when it comes to what qualifies as research in policymaking. Policymakers are interested in data, "hungry … for new solutions and new ideas for addressing old and new health care challenges" (Fitzpatrick, 2004, p. 71). Reports from expert panels, foundations, and government research agencies can all carry great weight, if introduced in the context of moving an issue forward (Goldstein, 2009; Aiken, 2008; Winkelstein, 2009). Op-ed pieces by experts, and position papers generated by legislative staff or others can also be powerful. The point is that one must be wide open to sources when looking for evidence to support or oppose a policy position.

In *presenting* data to policymakers, it behooves the advocate to be short and to the point. Legislators and other policy-generators deal with a tremendous number of issues across economic, health, and social terrains. Keeping the focus on one's issue requires policy briefs that are short and specific to the problem and the policy solution (McDonough, 2001; Jennings, C. P., 2002; Jennings, B. M., 2003; Goldstein, 2009).

Narrative—that is, the telling of a pertinent story to bring the issue to life—also has its place in the process (McDonough, 2001). Deborah Stone, a prominent observer of policymaking, refers to what she calls "causal stories" as necessary to the very genesis of a policy initiative. She notes that "[S]ocial problems do not exist 'out there,' waiting to be discovered by careful empirical observation and analysis." Rather, people have to view any particular trend, experience, or event as problematic and capable of solution; stories are the mechanism for crafting this view (Stone, 2006, p. 127). Narrative data must meet the standards of rigor expected of other data: truthful, verifiable, and representative of the problem or solution it is put forward to illustrate (Steiner, 2007).

THE CHEMISTRY BETWEEN RESEARCH AND POLICYMAKING

Research can be extremely useful in casting light on a problem and nudging policymakers to action, which is easier when the problem is non-controversial, such as violence against women (Moodie, 2009). Nursing has a distinguished lineage of nurses affecting policy through the use of data, from Nightingale's Crimean data to American midwives who accomplished great things for their practice by persistent and consistent

collection of ordinary practice data (Diers & Burst, 1983). Today, health care research examines how intricately intertwined in practice are the pieces of the health care puzzle: delivery, providers, procedures, patients, families, cultures, reimbursement, and so on. One consequence of this examination is a growing acknowledgement by non-nurse researchers of nursing's contributions (Ginsburg, 2008; Needleman, 2008).

Breaking through professional and disciplinary silos is critical for research *and* policymaking, particularly as care has become both interdisciplinary in nature and under intense financial scrutiny (Talsma, Grady, Feetham, Heinrich, & Steinwachs, 2008). Pay-for performance policies recently implemented by Medicare and several large private payers highlight the need for nursing to work across party lines to ensure a voice in the ongoing discussion about this financing approach (Kurtzman & Buerhaus, 2008). It is equally important that decision-makers be aware that nursing is absolutely essential to meaningful health care, from cradle to grave; for rich or poor; during prevention, secondary, or tertiary care alike. But neither our constancy nor our work is universally acknowledged when it comes to implementing policies in these systems.

USING RESEARCH TO CREATE, INFORM, AND SHAPE POLICY

An example of how research can vitalize policy decisions (and of the benefit of outside advocacy for nursing services) comes from Australia. Early in this decade, a body of Australian research found that the risk for death in some rural communities was over 300 times that in a city. Armed with this initial research, the Clinical Oncological Society of Australia (a physician specialty association) issued a report in early 2006, mapping available services across the continent (and documenting the paucity of services by doing so); nursing services were fortunately part of the mapping and were clearly in short supply (Clinical Oncology Society of Australia, 2006). By August 2006, the Australian Government Department of Health and Ageing had funded and directed implementation of a national effort to "direct the long-term workforce development of nurses specialized in cancer care" based on this report (Piggott, 2006, p. 33).

We have a powerful mapping project in our own country, undertaken by an advanced practice nurse, which illustrates the utility of casting a wide net in nursing research. Each year over the past several decades, Linda Pearson has provided an updated snapshot of nurse practitioner (NP) practice across the United States by state. She has never endeavored to describe the clinical practice itself—a practice that remains consistent across state boundaries as it is driven by the patient populations for whom the NP provides care, and by current standards of care. Pearson is instead describing the political state of practice—what NPs can and cannot do according to state law and regulation. Despite curricula adhering to national standards, and national certifying exams for each recognized NP specialty, advanced nursing practice is contradictory from state to state in legally-allowed scope. Pearson's annual update catalogs which states sanction fully autonomous practice without mandatory physician presence, require physician supervision or have a compromise position between the two.

Pearson cleverly added two other descriptors recently. She now presents data from the National Practitioner Data Bank illustrating the rates of malpractice actions against NPs compared to the rate against physicians. She also includes data from the Healthcare Integrity and Protection Data Bank, capturing the rates of "accumulated adverse action reports, civil judgments, and criminal conviction reports" for physicians and NPs (Pearson, 2009). Nurses score quite well in these rankings. Advocates are using the data to lobby for removal of unnecessary restrictions on APRN practice.

Equally important to breaking through professional silos in creating research is the need for nurses to present its research in non-nursing forums. It may be that those looking for research on a particular topic (including policy researchers and policymakers) overlook or discount nursing's role, or vice versa. The public's health will be best served when the two communities of health policy research and nursing better understand their common interests. The expertise residing in each will produce a stronger base of evidence from which to launch policies on which the two communities, and the public, agree.

Although nurses continue to score high in public opinion, many in the policy world and elsewhere do not understand what it is we really do—a fact of which we have been aware for some time (Fagin & Diers, 1983) and which continues. A 2009 article in a leading health policy journal lumped NPs together with physician assistants and concluded that only 42% of visits to this combined group involve primary care, even though 66% of NPs practice in primary care settings (Bodenheimer, Chen, & Bennett, 2009; American Academy of Nurse Practitioners, 2009). Lack of accurate understanding about the contributions of advanced practice nursing to patient access and health outcomes makes it extremely difficult to advocate for moving that practice forward.

RESEARCH AND POLITICAL WILL

The key to moving any issue into the public or institutional eye is transforming it into a political issue—that is, casting the issue as problematic enough to make public or private policymakers want to fix it. Effective research casts the problems it exposes as bad, even immoral, situations that must be addressed (Stone, 2006). But how will any particular issue be perceived, among the numerous issues competing for attention? Sometimes political leaders themselves offer the issue as important, as has been the case with health care reform under the Obama administration. Other times, the issue comes to the fore because of the general social environment, as with the financial regulation efforts in the wake of a major recession. An issue can also be presented via a compelling summary of the research on the problem; the Institute of Medicine's reports on patient safety and health disparities come to mind. Framing the policy question at hand is also important, because it is fundamental to setting up the argument. So, the strategic use of research will anticipate the viewpoints of other stakeholders.

Highlighting a problem and getting it on the agenda is not enough to advance policy in most instances. There must be enough "political will" to devote attention, time, and effort to solve the problem, particularly when the problem is pervasive or longstanding. Complex problems are challenging because it is difficult to capture a single framing perspective, leading to many differing opinions about what the real problem is and a subsequent dilution of political will about the issue. Health disparities have been extremely well-documented, for example, and embraced by several presidential administrations as an issue that needs fixing. The ultimate measure of eliminating these disparities is improved health status, but it is enormously complex figuring out exactly what leads to good health. Thus it is difficult to propose a straightforward solution to ending disparities and hard to capture sustained political will to undertake the work of eliminating this form of discrimination (Stone, 2006).

This interplay of research, political will, and policymaking frequently frustrates action-oriented people such as nurses, who want to see change happen more directly and in a timely manner. Forty years of outcomes research documenting that advanced practice nurses are safe, competent providers is now coupled with a current policy environment that is trying to solve the primary care provider shortage. It seems pretty straightforward, right? Several factors intervene that make the progress to full autonomous practice nationwide slow, sometimes agonizingly so. Nursing and, in particular, advanced practice nursing is not well understood outside of the outdated (and questionable) paradigm of "working under physician orders." It is surprising how many legislators, even those whose personal provider *is* a nurse practitioner, have no idea that we are diagnosing and prescribing on our own, and quite safely.

THE STRATEGIC RESEARCHER

Changing the worldview of policymakers and others is not a quick or linear process. But it is crucial—it means that a researcher must first examine his or her own assumptions. Frederick Grinnell, a cell biologist, notes that "[r]eal-life scientists begin their work situated within particular interests and commitments" (2009, p. ix). He later describes how his own discoveries in cell function were impeded by his dogged fidelity to his original assumptions, which took him many years to question. Long before Grinnell, Butterfield (1957) noted that scientific knowledge is due not so much to new or additional evidence, as much as it has to do with "the art of handling the same bundle of data as before, but placing them in a new system of relations … by giving them a new framework" (p. 13). Policymakers are no different, nor are any of us really. We all come to the table with predefined assumptions about health care, nursing, outcomes, and so on. So ascertaining what assumptions already exist is fundamental to making a case for a new policy in any setting. Research that offers new perspectives or that

assuages doubts about abandoning preconceived notions is equally vital to the policy process. In fact, sometimes the very act of researching can lift the veil from one's eyes, and from there others can be educated (Smith, 2002).

But back to advanced practice nursing. There is a second reason policymakers often do not jump readily toward removing barriers to practice. Often a very powerful stakeholder (e.g., organized medicine in one form or another) sits at the table, opposing any further entry into its "world" by nursing or other professionals. And like it or not, this is a potent disincentive for policymakers to move off the dime on an issue.

So there must be a compelling story to engage legislators in advancing full autonomous nursing practice. In the past, the theme has been access to health care in rural areas. A quick look at the states who first achieved APRN practice independent of physician involvement (e.g., Alaska, Maine, and New Mexico) reveals that they have large rural populations in need of competent providers. Lately, the theme is turning to the decreased number of physicians entering or staying in primary care practice—something we know from research into health care workforce distribution. Organized medicine often has a hand in causing this research to exist as part of a strategy to increase medical education dollars and resources. Nursing could turn this research into a successful foray for independent practice by offering competent APRN providers right here and now, without the need for additional resources or expenditure. And these providers cannot fill primary care needs unless barriers such as collaborative agreements or inadequate insurance reimbursement schemes are removed (Hansen-Turton, Ritter, Rothman, & Valdez, 2006).

Further research is needed, however. In 1994, in the context of an earlier perceived crisis in primary care, Sekscenski and colleagues (1994) published a study examining whether or not state practice environments had any impact on the number of NPs and physician assistants available. Strong correlations were found between environments that sanctioned APRN autonomy and higher numbers of practicing NPs. An update to this research in the current climate would be quite useful. Policy researchers investigating the state of practice for the Arkansas legislature found some intriguing possible associations between states with independent practice and lower rates of teen births, infant mortality, and other state health indicators (Bureau of Legislative Research, 2008); additional research on these questions would also be handy to have in one's pocket while advocating to remove barriers to nursing practice.

So in addition to setting the scene for policy intervention by illuminating a problem, research has a vital role in creating an atmosphere conducive for policymakers to step up to the plate, especially when the issue is likely to be controversial. Ginsburg (2008) offers some valuable insights about nursing in the hospital setting and the research necessary to capture policymakers' interest in nursing intensity and hospital payment, for instance. Moodie (2009) suggests that researchers interested in moving policy forward pay attention to what policymakers need answered, as well as the constituencies to which they have to answer, a theme also echoed by the September 2009 Briefing Paper from the Overseas Development Institute (ODI).

Moodie and the ODI are looking at research from a "marketing" viewpoint: the researcher is using data to persuade a policymaker that a certain policy answer is the one called for, based on the evidence. Moodie (2009) describes the various "ecologic" factors that a researcher should assess before designing any particular research with an eye toward influencing policy. The ODI paper (2009) also emphasizes Moodie's point that research needs to be mindfully performed *and* presented. "Simply presenting information to policymakers and expecting them to act upon it is very unlikely to work" (ODI, p. 1). ODI sets forth five other lessons for "policy entrepreneurs" who want to involve policymakers in evidence-based decisions. This advice from non-nurse policy researchers recognizes that in addition to highlighting a problem, research can enhance, perhaps even shape the political climate in which change can occur; this is valuable advice to nursing as it continues its political and policy evolution. And along these lines, there is one other way research is influencing the policy context—through artful dissemination in documentaries seen on television and in movie theaters.

RESEARCH—NOT JUST FOR JOURNALS

In 2005, David Satcher (former Surgeon General in the Clinton Administration), with a host of esteemed public health and academic colleagues, published a study entitled "What If We Were Equal? A Comparison of the Black-White Mortality Gap in 1960 and 2000." One of those esteemed colleagues was Dr. Adewale Troutman, whose most recent appointment in a distinguished career is Director of the Louisville, Kentucky, Metro Health Department. The study concluded that annually we could prevent more than 83,000 "excess deaths" in the African-American community if we addressed health disparities, and their consequent gulag effect on access to care for minority populations.

This research, and other health disparity documentation, was picked up and studied again, journalistically, by Larry Adelman in 2008. He produced a 7-hour series called "Unnatural Causes," which aired on PBS later that year. During the segment entitled "In Sickness and in Wealth," Dr. Troutman offers a compelling visual tour of both the physical and sociological realities of his city, vividly illustrating the interplay of poverty, social class, and health outcomes in what could be a new frontier of compelling qualitative research, which seeks to engage the public (and policymakers) directly through visual and narrative data. It is worth noting how effective such documentaries can be at getting an issue out into public discourse while bypassing special interests.

Nursing's future rests on the clear and convincing record of research on nursing work. Moving our future forward requires that we and others understand our role in the complex and dynamic world of health and health care (Kurtzman, 2009). As nursing is increasingly recognized as a vital pillar in the temple of health care, we must continue to document and broadcast who we are, what we do, and why it matters to patients, to policymakers, to budgets, and to the delivery of meaningful health care to all.

For a list of related websites, please refer to your Evolve Resources at http://evolve.elsevier.com/Mason/policypolitics/

REFERENCES

Adelman, L. (Producer), Stange, E. (Director), & Rutenbeck, J. (Director). (2008). *Unnatural causes* (Documentary). Retrieved from www.unnaturalcauses.org.

Aiken, L. H. (2008). Economics of nursing. *Policy, Politics, & Nursing Practice, 9*(2), 73-79.

American Academy of Nurse Practitioners. (2009). Nurse practitioner facts. Retrieved from www.aanp.org/NR/rdonlyres/32B74504-2C8E-4603-8949-710A287E0B32/0/AANP_NPFactsLogo709.pdf.

Bodenheimer, T., Chen, E., & Bennett, H. D. (2009). Confronting the growing burden of chronic disease: Can the U.S. health care workforce do the job? *Health Affairs, 28*(1), 64-74.

Brazier, A., Cooke, K., & Moravan, V. (2008). Using mixed methods for evaluating an integrative approach to cancer care. *Integrative Cancer Therapies, 7*(1), 4-17.

Bureau of Legislative Research. (December 18, 2008). Advanced practice nursing: Interim study proposal 2007-2008. Retrieved from www.arna.org/SNAS/AR/APN/APNs-A-Strategy-that-is-Working-2010(2)10.pdf.

Butterfield, H. (1957). *The origins of modern science* (rev. ed.). New York: MacMillan.

Cheung, R. B., Moody, L. E., & Cockram, C. (2002). Data mining strategies for shaping nursing and health policy agendas. *Policy, Politics, & Nursing Practice, 3*(3), 248-260.

Clinical Oncology Society of Australia. (2006). Mapping rural and regional oncology services in Australia. Retrieved from www.cosa.org.au//PublicationsPositionStatements/Publications.htm.

Diers, D. (2007). Finding midwifery in administrative data systems. *Journal of Midwifery and Women's Health, 52*(2), 98-105.

Diers, D. & Burst, H. V. (1983). Effectiveness of policy-related research: Nurse-midwifery as a case study. *Image: The Journal of Nursing Scholarship, 15*(3), 68-74.

Diers, D. & Potter, J. (1997). Understanding the unmanageable nursing unit with case-mix data. *Journal of Nursing Administration, 27*(11), 27-32.

Duffield, C., Diers, D., Aisbett, C., & Roche, M. (2009). Churn: Patient turnover and case mix. *Nursing Economics, 27*(3), 185-191.

Fagin, C., & Diers, D. (1983). Nursing as metaphor. *New England Journal of Medicine, 309*(2), 116-117.

Fitzpatrick, J. (2004). Translating clinical research into health policy. *Applied Nursing Research, 17*(2), 71.

Garmon Bibb, S. C. (2007). Issues associated with secondary analysis of population health data. *Applied Nursing Research, 20*(2), 94-99.

Ginsburg, P. B. (2008). Paying hospitals on the basis of nursing intensity. *Policy, Politics, & Nursing Practice, 9*(2), 118-120.

Goldstein, H. (2009). Translating research into public policy. *Journal of Public Health Policy, 30*(Suppl 1), S16-S20.

Grinnell, F. (2009). *Everyday practice of science: Where intuition and passion meet objectivity and logic.* New York: Oxford University Press.

Hansen-Turton, T., Ritter, A., Rothman, A., & Valdez, B. (2006). Insurer policies create barriers to health care access and consumer choice. *Nursing Economics, 24*(4), 204-211.

Heslop, L., Gardner, B., Diers D., & Poh, B. C. (2004). Using clinical data for nursing research and management in health services. *Contemporary Nurse, 17*(1-2), 8-18.

Jennings, B. M. (2003). A half-dozen health policy hints. *Nursing Outlook, 51*(2), 92.

Jennings, C. P. (2002). The power of the policy brief. *Policy, Politics, & Nursing Practice, 3*(3), 261-263.

Kurtzman, E. T. (2009). Planning a national nursing quality and safety alliance: Strengthening nursing's policy voice. *Journal of Nursing Administration, 39*(3), 47-50.

Kurtzman, E. T., & Buerhaus, P. I. (2008). New Medicare payment rules: Danger or opportunity for nursing? *American Journal of Nursing, 108*(6), 30-35.

McDonough, J. E. (2001). Using and misusing anecdote in policy making. *Health Affairs, 20*(1), 207-212.

Moodie, R. (2009). Where different worlds collide: Expanding the influence of research and researchers on policy. *Journal of Public Health Policy, 30*(S1), 33-37.

Needleman, J. (2008). Is what's good for the patient good for the hospital? Aligning incentives and the business case for nursing. *Policy, Politics, & Nursing Practice, 9*(2), 80-87.

Overseas Development Institute (ODI). (2009, September). *Briefing paper 53: Helping researchers become policy entrepreneurs.* London: Overseas Development Institute.

Pearson, L. J. (2009). The Pearson report. *American Journal for Nurse Practitioners, 13*(20), 8-82.

Piggott, C. (2006). Access to cancer nursing is crucial for remote Australia. *Australian Nursing Journal, 14*(2), 33.

Satcher, S., Fryer, G. E., McCann, J., Troutman, A., Woolf, S. H., & Rust, G. (2005). What if we were equal? A comparison of the black-white mortality gap in 1960 and 2000. *Health Affairs, 24*(2), 459-464.

Sekscenski, E. S., Sansom, S, Bazell, C., Salmon, M. E., & Mullan, F. (1994). State Practice Environments and the Supply of Physician Assistants, Nurse Practitioners, and Certified Nurse-Midwives. *New England Journal of Medicine, 331*(19), 1266-1271.

Smith, S. M. (2002). Nursing as a social responsibility: Implications for democracy from the life perspective of Lavinia Lloyd Dock (1858-1956). Unpublished dissertation, Louisiana State University. Retrieved from http://etd.lsu.edu/docs/available/etd-0903102-190634/unrestricted/Smith_dis.pdf.

Steiner, J. F. (2007). Using stories to disseminate research: The attributes of representative stories. *Journal of General Internal Medicine, 22*(11), 1603-1607.

Stone, D. (2006). Reframing the racial disparities issue for state governments. *Journal of Health Politics, Policy and Law, 31*(1), 127-152.

Talsma, A., Grady, P., Feetham, S., Heinrich, J., & Steinwachs, D. (2008). The perfect storm: Patient safety and nursing shortages within the context of health policy and evidence-based practice. *Nursing Research, 57*(1S), S15-S21.

Winkelstein, W. (2009). The development of American public health, a commentary: Three documents that made an impact. *Journal of Public Health Policy, 30*(1), 40-48.

CHAPTER 41

Health Services Research: Translating Research into Policy

Patricia W. Stone, Arlene M. Smaldone, William M. Enlow, and Robert J. Lucero

"Research is formalized curiosity. It is poking and prying with a purpose."

—Zora Neale Hurston

The high cost of health care, large numbers of uninsured Americans, uncontrolled health care spending, and an unstable economy have led to the most recent efforts to reform health care in the United States. Most health policy experts agree that the nation must control health care costs, improve efficiency, increase access to health care, and improve the quality of care. However, it is often unclear how best to make these improvements. A strong evidence base is needed to inform decision-makers on what does and does not work to improve the health care system. Research that attempts to provide this evidence is often called "health services research" (HSR).

DEFINING HEALTH SERVICES RESEARCH

AcademyHealth, the preeminent professional society for health services researchers, defines HSR as "the multidisciplinary field of scientific investigation that studies how social factors, financing systems, organizational structures and processes, health technologies, and personal behaviors affect access to health care, the quality and cost of health care, and ultimately our health and well-being. Its research domains are individuals, families, organizations, institutions, communities, and populations" (AcademyHealth, 2008). The Agency for Healthcare Research and Quality (AHRQ), a primary funding organization for this type of research, states that, "Health services research examines how people get access to health care, how much care costs, and what happens to patients as a result of

this care. Health services research aims to identify the most effective ways to organize, manage, finance, and deliver high-quality care; reduce medical errors; and improve patient safety" (Helping the nation with health services research, 2002).

A recent focus of HSR, based on the Comparative Effectiveness Research Act of 2008, is the conduct and synthesis of research comparing the benefits and harms of various interventions and strategies for preventing, diagnosing, treating, and monitoring health conditions in real-world settings (Conway & Clancy, 2009). The purpose of comparative effectiveness research (CER) is to improve health outcomes by developing and disseminating evidence-based information to patients, clinicians, and other decision-makers about interventions that are most effective for patients under specific circumstances (Iglehart, 2009; Volpp & Das, 2009). The Department of Health and Human Services (DHHS) as part of the American Recovery and Reinvestment Act of 2009, provided $400 million of financial support for CER. In June 2009, the Institute of Medicine recommended 100 national priorities for CER (Committee on Comparative Effectiveness Research Prioritization, 2009). Of the top 25 priorities, the following may be of particular interest to nurses: (1) "Compare the effectiveness of various primary care treatment strategies...and (2) Compare the effectiveness of literacy-sensitive disease management programs and usual care in reducing disparities in children and adults with low literacy and chronic disease." The Patient Protection and Affordable Care Act authorizes CER and a number of demonstration projects that will depend on the use of HSR methods.

Dougherty and Conway (2008) developed a model intended to accelerate implementation of innovations

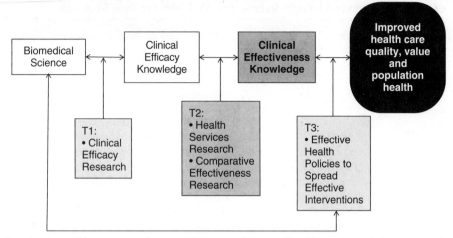

FIGURE 41-1 Transforming health care across the research spectrum. (Adapted from Dougherty, D., & Conway, P. H. [2008]. The "3T's" road map to transform US health care: The "how" of high-quality care. *Journal of the American Medical Association, 299*[19], 2319-2321.)

in clinical settings to address the "how" of health care delivery (Figure 41-1). This transformational model suggests that basic science and its translation into clinical practice is only the first step to achieve effective, safe delivery of high-quality care (translation 1 or T1). Translation 2 (T2) processes focus on the translation of clinical efficacy knowledge into clinical effectiveness, and the policy changes needed to improve outcomes is addressed in T3 activities. Health services research and CER are the necessary population-based research activities at the T2 level and serve as the foundation for effective health policy.

HSR METHODS

HSR researchers use both quantitative and qualitative research methods, and these methods are not unique to the field. However, it is the use of these methods to generate knowledge to inform health policy development and changes that is the hallmark of HSR. Edwardson (2007) reported on the theories and conceptual frameworks used by HSR nurse researchers in studies funded by AHRQ between 2000 and early 2005. A total of 28 different frameworks were identified in the 49 studies reviewed. The frameworks most often used were Donabedian's quality paradigm (Donabedian, 1966) (i.e., structure-process-outcome), Rogers Diffusion of Innovation Theory (Rogers, 2003), Reason's Theory of Human Error (Reason, 1990), and Andersen and Aday's Model of

Healthcare Access (Aday & Andersen, 1974). The common theoretical underpinning among these frameworks is their conceptualization of variables at the system level rather than the individual level.

QUANTITATIVE METHODS AND DATA SETS

Using quantitative multivariate methods, HSR researchers sometimes analyze data from administrative data sets, such as hospital discharge data, and national survey data to examine health care access and quality, regional differences in care delivery patterns, health behavior patterns, and health outcomes from a population perspective. Various types of data are available to HSR researchers through the federal agencies in the DHHS including the Centers for Disease Control and Prevention, and AHRQ. Additionally, population census and employment data are available through the U.S. Census Bureau and the Bureau of Labor Statistics. Table 41-1 provides examples of some of the available national and state data available to HSR researchers through free public websites or by paying a fee to have access to data in a useable format for research.

Often researchers must combine data from multiple sources or over multiple years. The researcher must become familiar with the data set methodology report and list of variables with their respective definitions to ascertain how variables are categorized, the sampling methodology employed, and how missing data were handled. National surveys often use

TABLE 41-1 Examples of Publicly Available Data for Use in Health Services Research

Agency	Data	Access	Fees
U.S. Department of Health and Human Services	Hospital Consumer Assessment of Healthcare Providers and Systems	Hospital Compare: *www.hospitalcompare.hhs.gov*	Free
	Area Resource File	Health Resources and Services Administration: *www.arfsys.com*	$500.00
Centers for Disease Control and Prevention	Behavioral Risk Factor Surveillance System	Behavioral Risk Factor Surveillance System: *www.cdc.gov/brfss*	Free
	National Health and Nutrition Examination Survey	National Center for Health Statistics: *www.cdc.gov/nchs/nhanes.htm*	Free
	National Immunization Survey	National Center for Health Statistics: *www.cdc.gov/nis*	Free
	National Survey of Ambulatory Surgery	National Center for Health Statistics: *www.cdc.gov/nchs/nsas.htm*	Free
	National Survey of Children with Special Health Care Needs	National Center for Health Statistics: *www.cdc.gov/nchs/slaits/cshcn.htm*	Free
	National Survey of Children's Health	National Center for Health Statistics: *www.cdc.gov/nchs/slaits/nsch.htm*	Free
Agency for Healthcare Research and Quality	Nationwide Inpatient Sample	Healthcare Cost and Utilization Project: *www.hcup-us.ahrq.gov/nisoverview.jsp*	Fees vary
	Kids' Inpatient Database	Healthcare Cost and Utilization Project: *www.hcup-us.ahrq.gov/kidoverview.jsp*	Fees vary
	State Inpatient Databases	Healthcare Cost and Utilization Project: *www.hcup-us.ahrq.gov/sidoverview.jsp*	Fees vary
	Nationwide Emergency Department Sample	Healthcare Cost and Utilization Project: *www.hcup-us.ahrq.gov/nedsoverview.jsp*	Fees vary
	State Ambulatory Surgery Database	Healthcare Cost and Utilization Project: *www.hcup-us.ahrq.gov/sasdoverview.jsp*	Fees vary
American Hospital Association	Annual Survey Database	AHA Data: *www.ahadata.com/ahadata_app/index.jsp*	Fees vary
American Nurses Association	National Database of Nursing Quality Indicators	NDNQI: *http://ndnqi@kumc.edu*	Fees vary
Dartmouth	Healthcare Utilization Data of Medicare Patients	The Dartmouth Atlas of Health Care Project: *http://dartmouthatlas.org/index.shtm*	Free

complex sampling frames and employ sampling weights enabling generalizability of survey findings to the population at large. To effectively use data sets that employ weighted sampling requires expertise in use of statistical analysis software such as SAS (SAS Institute Inc., Cary, NC) that allows for incorporation of sampling weights into the data analysis process. A few sources of publicly available data are discussed in greater detail.

Area Resources File (ARF). As part of the DHHS, the Health Resources and Services Administration (HRSA) maintain the ARF. The ARF is a county-specific database made of more than 50 sources of data. The ARF contains more than 6000 variables that

can be used to describe each county including information on health facilities, medical and dental professionals, population characteristics, health care utilization, as well as socioeconomic and environmental characteristics. The basic ARF file also contains geographic codes and descriptors, thereby facilitating linkage with other data set files. The ARF is designed to be used by planners, policymakers, HSR researchers, and others to evaluate the health care delivery system and other factors that impact health status in the U.S. To date, there are no standard methods being used to monitor the number of nurses and nursing schools across regions to include these data in the ARF.

Hospital Consumer Assessment of Healthcare Providers and Systems (HCAHPS). The HCAHPS ("HCAHPS fact sheet," 2009) is the first national standardized, publicly reported patient survey of hospital care quality and has only recently become publically available to researchers. The HCAHPS survey contains 27 questions, 18 of which elicit the perspectives of recently hospitalized patients regarding 8 key areas: communication with physicians, communication with nurses, responsiveness of hospital staff, management of pain, communication about medicines, receipt of discharge information, cleanliness of the hospital environment, and quietness of the hospital environment. Using data from HCAHPS, a hospital quality survey (conducted by the research team), and the American Hospital Association, Kutney-Lee and colleagues (2009) designed a cross-sectional study using multivariate regression modeling techniques to examine the relationship between nurse staffing levels and patient perceptions of their nursing care across 430 hospitals in 4 states (California, New Jersey, Pennsylvania, and Florida). Higher nurse-patient ratios and better work environments were associated with greater patient satisfaction. These findings demonstrate that appropriate staffing levels are important to patient satisfaction and support ongoing efforts to improve hospital performance.

National Health and Nutrition Examination Survey (NHANES). First administered in 1971, the NHANES ("About the National Health and Nutrition Examination Survey," n.d.) has enabled researchers to assess the health and nutritional status of adults and children in the U.S. and observe survey trends over time. The NHANES is unique because it combines interviews, physical examinations, and laboratory data for each survey participant. Using current census information, the NHANES selects participants through a complex multilevel statistical sampling of randomly selected households. The NHANES survey data have been instrumental in tracking the prevalence of health problems such as obesity and diabetes over time and examining factors that may be associated with changes in prevalence. Using 24-hour dietary recall data from two cross-sectional NHANES surveys (NHANES III 1988-1994 and NHANES 1999-2004), researchers examined national trends in sugar-sweetened beverage consumption among adults 20 years of age or older (Bleich, Wang, Wang, & Gortmaker, 2009). During this study period, both the percentage of adults who consumed sugar-sweetened beverages (58% versus 63%) and daily caloric intake from these beverages (239 versus 294 calories) increased and accounted for a significant proportion of daily caloric intake. The taxation of sugar-sweetened beverages has received increasing interest as a policy option to fund obesity prevention efforts (Brownell & Frieden, 2009).

Healthcare Cost and Utilization Project (HCUP). The HCUP is a federal-state-industry partnership sponsored by AHRQ. Through the HCUP, a set of databases and software tools have been developed to inform health care decision-making efforts at the national, state, and local levels. The National Inpatient Sample (NIS), released yearly, provides uniform data on hospitalizations from 1044 hospitals in 40 states. These data can be used to analyze changes over time in health care access, utilization, and quality. Using longitudinal NIS data (1990-1995) combined with data from the American Hospital Association Annual Survey, the ARF, and Centers for Medicare and Medicaid Services, researchers (Mark, Harless, McCue, & Xu, 2004) examined the effects of changes in registered nurse (RN) staffing on quality of care in a sample of 422 hospitals from 11 states. The quality of care was based on measures of inpatient mortality and three nurse-sensitive outcomes: hospital acquired pneumonia, urinary tract infection, and pressure sores. Hospitals were stratified by level of RN staffing. The magnitude of effect of a one-unit increase in RN staffing on inpatient mortality was greater for hospitals at the 25th percentile of staffing compared to the 75th percentile of staffing, suggesting a nonlinear relationship between RN staffing and inpatient mortality. There may be a staffing threshold that dictates an optimal level of staffing to improve patient outcomes. The evidence supports administrators to develop nurse staffing plans, and policymakers to advance nurse staffing legislation.

National Database of Nursing Quality Indicators (NDNQI). The University of Kansas Medical Center School of Nursing is contracted by the American Nurses Association (ANA) to manage the NDNQI. This proprietary database collects unit-specific nurse-sensitive data from over 1000 hospitals across the nation. The ANA has expressed interest in making these longitudinal data more available to researchers.

Dartmouth Atlas. This Dartmouth University project uses Medicare data to provide comprehensive information and analysis about national, regional, and local markets, as well as individual hospitals and their affiliated providers. This database has been used by researchers to highlight regional variations in health care. They can access the data tools used in the Dartmouth Atlas online and produce individualized reports. Indeed, data from the Dartmouth Atlas on hospital spending and quality informed policies was cited by President Obama as evidence for implementing a range of policy incentives to reward hospital administrators for improving efficiency.

QUALITATIVE METHODS

The use of rigorous qualitative research methods by HSR researchers has increased over the past decade. Qualitative methods may be used in mixed-methods research, in the development of survey questionnaires, and in research where the aim is to gain the perspective of stakeholders regarding a particular topic. For example, researchers (Elder et al., 2007) conducted focus groups using a sample of African-American adults housed temporarily in South Carolina hotels following Hurricane Katrina to identify why New Orleans residents decided to either remain in their homes or heed local warnings to evacuate. The use of focus groups led to the discovery of a number of themes, including misperceptions about the severity of the hurricane because of miscommunication, and evacuation barriers related to poverty and concern about neighborhood crime. Future disaster preparedness plans targeted at underserved minority communities should consider the importance of culturally sensitive approaches.

PROFESSIONAL TRAINING IN HEALTH SERVICES RESEARCH

HSR has a tradition of training that emphasizes multidisciplinary education. Providing answers to complex health and health care problems requires a diverse research skill set. Traditional clinical research approaches (i.e., epidemiology, biology, chemistry) coupled with social and economic sciences use a combination of quantitative and qualitative methodologies to address health and health care problems. From randomized controlled trials to qualitative case studies, there is a strong emphasis on research that addresses health service policy needs. Health services research promotes the use of interdisciplinary collaborations to address system-level problems.

COMPETENCIES

Fourteen core competencies for doctoral-prepared HSR researchers have been proposed (Forrest, Martin, Holve, & Millman, 2009). The competencies for nurse HSR researchers build upon these and are listed in Table 41-2.

A research doctorate (e.g., PhD) is the usual educational pathway to become an HSR researcher and develop knowledge that influences policymaking. Few schools of nursing have the capacity to train nurses to become health services researchers; therefore, it is important to identify a university that has an HSR training program. Health services research training takes place in a number of disciplines, including nursing, public health, business, and public policy. Schools of nursing that offer HSR training often provide interdisciplinary opportunities through partnerships with the disciplines described earlier in the chapter. This is key to developing the competencies of an HSR researcher.

EDUCATIONAL FUNDING

Funding for training in HSR comes from a variety of sources including government-funded institutional and individual training grants. In the past, AHRQ has been the primary funder of health services research; their website lists available training and educational opportunities. Of the 28 universities that have training grants, none are based in schools of nursing; but, nurses have successfully competed for individual HSR dissertation awards (R36) and postdoctoral research training awards.

Although not the primary mission of the National Institutes of Health (NIH), increasingly it is interested in funding HSR. For example, the National Institute of Nursing Research (NINR) recently announced two separate calls for research proposals that address cost-effectiveness analysis, which is an important method in HSR (04-NR-101 and RFA-NR-09-005). The NINR allows universities to compete for institutional training grants. These funds are given directly to schools of nursing to provide qualified students with stipends for living expenses, funds for tuition and

TABLE 41-2 Nursing Health Services Research Doctoral-Level Core Competencies and Associated Learning Objective Content Area

Core Competency	Associated Learning Objective Content Areas
1. Interdisciplinary collaboration including application and knowledge of theories and concepts from relevant disciplines	Economics Epidemiology Informatics Management research Operations research Political science Psychology Sociology Statistics
2. Knowledge of the structures, performance, quality, policy, and environmental context of health and health care to formulate solutions for health policy problems	Access and use Financing of health care Health Health economics Health policy Organization of health care Quality of care
3. Use of appropriate research design	Study design for interventions Observational study design Qualitative research
4. Assemble needed primary and/or secondary data	Survey research Qualitative research Primary data acquisition and quality control Secondary data acquisition and quality control
5. Appropriate analytic methods	Advanced statistics Economic evaluation Decision sciences Qualitative methods
6. Effectively communicate the findings and implications through multiple modalities including technical, lay, and stakeholder audiences	Dissemination Community participatory research Translating research into practice and policy

From Forrest, C. B., Martin, D. P., Holve, E., & Millman, A. (2009, June 25). Health services research doctoral core competencies. *BMC Health Services Research, 9*, 107.

fees, as well as limited travel to scientific meetings. Additionally, doctoral students who have matriculated can apply for individual National Research Service Awards (NRSA), which provides similar funding to institutional training grants.

JOURNALS

There are a number of scientific journals that focus on health services research (e.g., *Health Affairs, Health Services Research, Medical Care,* and *Policy, Politics, & Nursing Practice*). As a source for scientific dissemination, AcademyHealth has become the primary interdisciplinary professional association for HSR researchers. As a component of AcademyHealth, the "Interdisciplinary Research Group on Nursing Issues (IRGNI)" provides a forum for researchers interested in promoting and supporting the development of HSR that focuses on nursing practice, workforce, and delivery of care. These important resources have become important mechanisms to disseminate evidence for policy development and to guide the field of HSR.

For a list of related websites, please refer to your Evolve Resources at http://evolve.elsevier.com/Mason/policypolitics/

REFERENCES

About the National Health and Nutrition Examination Survey. Retrieved from www.cdc.gov/nchs/nhanes/about_nhanes.htm.

AcademyHealth. (2008). What is HSR? Retrieved from www.academyhealth.org/About/content.cfm?ItemNumber=831&navItemNumber=514.

Aday, L. A., & Andersen, R. (1974). A framework for the study of access to medical care. *Health Services Research, 9*(3), 208-220.

Bleich, S. N., Wang, Y. C., Wang, Y., & Gortmaker, S. L. (2009). Increasing consumption of sugar-sweetened beverages among US adults: 1988-1994 to 1999-2004. *American Journal of Clinical Nutrition, 89*(1), 372-381.

Brownell, K. D., & Frieden, T. R. (2009). Ounces of prevention—The public policy case for taxes on sugared beverages. *New England Journal of Medicine, 360*(18), 1805-1808.

Committee on Comparative Effectiveness Research Prioritization, Institute of Medicine. (2009). Initial national priorities for comparative effectiveness research. Retrieved from www.iom.edu/Object.File/Master/71/107/CER%20report%20brief%206%2030%2009.pdf.

Conway, P. H., & Clancy, C. (2009). Comparative-effectiveness research—Implications of the Federal Coordinating Council's report. *New England Journal of Medicine, 361*(4), 328-330.

Donabedian, A. (1966). Evaluating the quality of medical care. *Milbank Memorial Fund Quarterly, 44*(Suppl. 3), 166-206.

Dougherty, D., & Conway, P. H. (2008). The "3T's" road map to transform US health care: The "how" of high-quality care. *Journal of the American Medical Association, 299*(19), 2319-2321.

Edwardson, S. R. (2007). Conceptual frameworks used in funded nursing health services research projects. *Nursing Economic$, 25*(4), 222-227.

Elder, K., Xirasagar, S., Miller, N., Bowen, S. A., Glover, S., & Piper, C. (2007). African Americans' decisions not to evacuate New Orleans before Hurricane Katrina: A qualitative study. *American Journal of Public Health, 97*(Suppl. 1), S124-S129.

Forrest, C. B., Martin, D. P., Holve, E., & Millman, A. (2009, June 25). Health services research doctoral core competencies. *BMC Health Services Research, 9*, 107.

HCAHPS fact sheet. (2009). Retrieved from www.hcahpsonline.org/files/HCAHPS%20Fact%20Sheet,%20revised1,%203-31-09.pdf.

Helping the nation with health services research. (2002). Retrieved from www.ahrq.gov/news/focus/scenarios.pdf.

Iglehart, J. K. (2009). Prioritizing comparative-effectiveness research—IOM recommendations. *New England Journal of Medicine, 361*(4), 325-328.

Kutney-Lee, A., McHugh, M. D., Sloane, D. M., Cimiotti, J. P., Flynn, L., Neff, D. F., et al. (2009). Nursing: A key to patient satisfaction. *Health Affairs (Millwood), 28*(4), w669-w677.

Mark, B. A., Harless, D. W., McCue, M., & Xu, Y. (2004). A longitudinal examination of hospital registered nurse staffing and quality of care. *Health Services Research, 39*(2), 279-300.

Reason, J. (1990). *Human error.* Cambridge, UK: Cambridge University Press.

Rogers, E. (2003). *Diffusion of innovations* (5th ed.). New York: Free Press.

Volpp, K. G., & Das, A. (2009). Comparative effectiveness—Thinking beyond medication A versus medication B. *New England Journal of Medicine, 361*(4), 331-333.

CHAPTER 42

Politics and Evidence-Based Practice and Policy

Sean P. Clarke

"The union of the political and scientific estates is not like a partnership, but a marriage. It will not be improved if the two become like each other, but only if they respect each other's quite different needs and purposes. No great harm is done if in the meantime they quarrel a bit."

—Don K. Price

Health care has been a conservative field characterized by deep investments in tradition. Evolution of treatment approaches and facility and service management often has been very gradual, punctuated by occasional breakthroughs. For many years, it was said that nearly 2 decades could pass between the appearance of research findings and their uptake into practice. While this is a statement that bears revisiting in the era of evidence-based practice and in the Internet age, disconnects between evidence and care practices are still common, as are inconsistencies in practice and variations in patient outcomes across providers and institutions. It is clear that bringing research findings to "real world" settings remains a slow and uneven process.

Clinicians, researchers, and policymakers are well aware of poor uptake of research evidence and lost opportunities to improve service, spurring an interest in clinical practice and more recently, health care policy, driven by high-quality scientific evidence. An often-cited definition of evidence-based practice is "the conscientious, explicit, and judicious use of current best evidence in making decisions about the care of individual patients" (Sackett et al., 1996). Evidence-based policy is an extension or extrapolation of the tenets of evidence-based practice to decisions about resource allocation and regulation by various governmental and regulatory bodies. Awareness of the scale of investments in both health and social service programs and on research around the world, the enormous stakes of providers and clients in the outcomes of policy decisions, and increasing demands for transparency and accountability have influenced its rise:

Evidence-based policy has been defined as an approach that "helps people make well informed decisions about policies, programmes and projects by putting the best available evidence from research at the heart of policy development and implementation" (Davies, 1999). This approach stands in contrast to opinion-based policy, which relies heavily on either the selective use of evidence (e.g., on single studies irrespective of quality) or on the untested views of individuals or groups, often inspired by ideological standpoints, prejudices, or speculative conjecture (Davies, 2004, p. 3)

Controversies in clinical care and policy development are sometimes very strong. Furthermore, political forces can greatly influence the types of research evidence generated, whose hands evidence works its way into, how it is interpreted in the context of other data and values, and, most significantly, how it is used (if at all) in influencing practice. This chapter will review the politics of translating research into evidence-based practice and policy, from the generation of knowledge to its synthesis and translation.

THE PLAYERS AND THEIR STAKES

Translating research into practice involves many stakeholder groups. *Health care professionals* are often directly influenced by practice changes based on evidence. Many are quite invested in particular clinical methods or work practices and structures of practice, or, put otherwise, in the status quo in terms of treatment approaches they use and the way their care is organized. They often have preferences, pet projects, and passions and may even have visions for health care and their profession's role that might be advanced or dashed by change. There can be issues of protecting working conditions, as well as turf issues with other professions, notably the protection of services or programs that are lucrative for particular professions.

There are often direct financial consequences for *industries* connected with health care when research drives adoption, continued use, or rejection of specific products, such as pharmaceuticals and both consumable (e.g., dressings) and durable (e.g., hospital beds, information technology) medical supplies, but also less visible (but equally expensive and important) products, such as consulting services.

Managers, administrators, and ultimately *policymakers* have stakes in delivering services in their facilities or organizations or jurisdictions in certain ways or within specific cost parameters. In general, administrators would prefer to have as few constraints as possible in managing health care services and thus may be less than enthusiastic about regulations as a method of controlling practice; however, changes that increase available resources may be better accepted.

For *researchers,* wide uptake of findings into practice is one of the most prestigious forms of external recognition, particularly if mandated by some sort of high-impact policy or legislation. This is especially the case for researchers working in policy-relevant fields where funding and public profile are mutually reinforcing. Researchers and academics involved in the larger evidence-based practice movement also have stakes in the enterprise. There are researchers, university faculty, and other experts who have become specialists in synthesizing and reporting outcomes and have interests in ensuring that distilled research in particular forms retains high status. Furthermore, funding agency advisers and bureaucrats may also be very much invested in the legitimacy conferred by the use of evidence-based practice processes.

The *general public,* especially subgroups that have stakes in specific types of health care, wants safe, effective, and responsive health care. They want to feel as if their personal risks, costs, and uncertainties are minimized, and they may or may not have insights or concerns about broader societal and economic consequences of treatments or models of care delivery. Expert opinions and research findings tend to carry authority, but for the public, these are filtered through the media, including Internet outlets.

Elected politicians and *bureaucrats* want to maintain appearances of being well-informed and responsive to the needs of the public and interest groups, while conveying that their decisions balance risks, benefits, and the interests of various stakeholder groups. Elected politicians are usually concerned about voter satisfaction and their prospects for reelection. They, like the public, receive research evidence filtered through others, sometimes by the media but often by various types of civil servants. Non-elected bureaucrats inform politicians, manage specialized programs, and implement policies on a day-to-day basis. They may be highly trained and come to be quite well-informed about research evidence in particular fields. And top bureaucrats serve at the pleasure of elected officials, so are sensitive to public perceptions, opinions, and preferences.

THE ROLE OF POLITICS IN GENERATING EVIDENCE

Health care research is often a time- and cost-intensive activity involving competition for scarce resources and rewards. Much is on the line for many stakeholders. What projects are attempted, what is generated, and what is reported from completed studies are all very much affected by political factors at multiple levels.

Much research likely to influence practice or policy requires financial support from outside institutions. Researchers write applications to funders for grants to pay for the resources required to carry out their work. Before agreeing to underwrite projects, external funders must believe that a topic being researched is important and relevant to the funding mission, the research approach is viable, and the proposed research team is able to carry out the project as proposed. Funders are often governmental or quasi-governmental agencies, but research can also be subsidized by producers or marketers of specific products or services. When research is supported by suppliers of particular medications, products, or services, funders may have overtly-stated or implicit interests in the results of the studies, and researchers may face pressures around the framing of questions, research approaches, and how, where, and when findings are disseminated. Only recently has the full extent of potential conflicts of interest related to industry-researcher partnerships come to light. However, not-for-profit and government agencies funding also have stakes and preferences in what types of projects are funded as well, and their decisions are also influenced by public relations and political considerations.

Researchers must also please their employers with evidence of their productivity (e.g., successful research grants and high-profile publications). Not surprisingly, researchers choose to pursue certain types of projects over others and gravitate toward topics they believe will help them secure funding. They may also defend or try to increase the profile of their particular approaches or topics through their influences as reviewers or members of editorial boards for journals, grant review committees, and appointments to positions of real or symbolic power. There can be a great disincentive to move away from research and research approaches that have garnered support and recognition in the past. Nonetheless, research topics and approaches go in and out of style over time—subjects become especially relevant or capture the public's or professionals' imaginations and then often fade. As a result, academic departments, funding bodies, institutions, and dissemination venues become the locales where specific tastes and priorities emerge or disappear. This also applies to methodologies and theoretical stances within research fields.

Some subject matter areas or theoretical stances for framing subjects are so inherently controversial that securing funding and carrying out data collections is extremely challenging. Anything touching on reproductive health or sexual behavior tends to be potentially volatile, especially in a conservative political climate, but the questioning of the effectiveness or cost-benefit ratio of a health service much beloved by providers, the public, or both as potentially wasteful can also encounter a good deal of resistance.

COMPARATIVE EFFECTIVENESS STUDIES

Research that compares the effectiveness of different clinical approaches or different approaches to managing services is of course the most relevant for shaping practice and making policy. However, there are a variety of reasons comparative effectiveness research is difficult to carry out. To get access to health care settings and to ethically conduct studies exposing patients or communities to different approaches, a freely acknowledged state of uncertainty regarding the superiority of one approach over another is needed. In order to conduct meaningful research, the interventions or approaches in question need to be sufficiently standardized and researchers must be able to rigorously measure outcomes across sufficient numbers of patients across enough clinical settings. On the whole, comparative intervention research is complicated, demanding, and expensive work to carry out. It is also likely to plunge researchers into debates that can be quite politically sensitive. Thus, it may not be surprising that, because of the practical challenges and political pitfalls involved in evaluating or testing interventions, many researchers in health care are engaged in research intended mainly to inform understandings of health-related phenomena that will enable the design of interventions that are likely to work. Unfortunately, history has shown that many widely accepted treatments have been shown to be ineffective and needlessly increase both health care costs and risks to the public when careful evaluations are carried out. Funding for comparative effectiveness research, which many hope will stimulate this essential type of inquiry, is included in the Patient Protection and Affordable Care Act of 2010.

THE POLITICS OF RESEARCH APPLICATION IN CLINICAL PRACTICE

INDIVIDUAL STUDIES

To stand any chance of influencing practice or policy, findings must be disseminated and read by those in a position to make or influence either clinical or policy decisions. Individual research papers may or may not receive much attention depending on timeliness of the topic, whether or not findings are novel, the profile of the researchers, and the prestige of a journal or conference where results are presented.

Of course, a key principle of evidence-based practice and policy is that one study alone never establishes anything as incontrovertible fact. In theory, if not always in practice, single studies are given limited credence until their findings are replicated. Despite evidence that dramatic findings in "landmark" studies, especially using non-randomized or observational research designs, are rarely replicated under more rigorous scrutiny (Ioannidis, 2005), there is still often an appetite for novel findings and a drive to act on them. As a result, single studies, particularly ones with findings that resonate strongly with one or more interest groups, can receive a great deal of attention and even influence health policy, even though their findings are preliminary.

Journalists must find the most newsworthy of the findings in research reports and make them understandable and entertaining to their audiences. In contrast, for scientists, legitimacy hinges on integrity in reporting findings. Use of simplistic language or terminology or the reworking of complex scientific ideas into laymen's terms in the popular press may result in broad statements unjustified by the findings at hand. Being seen as a "media darling," especially one whose work is popularized without careful qualifiers, can be damaging to a researcher's scientific credibility. Furthermore, given that reactions and responses (and backlashes) can be very strong, researchers seeking media coverage of their research must be cautious. It is generally best to avoid popular press coverage of one's results before review by peers and publication in a venue aimed at research audiences. In addition, avoiding overstating results and ensuring that key limitations of study findings are clearly described is essential, particularly if a treatment or approach has been studied in a narrow population or context or without controlling for important background variables.

SUMMARIZING LITERATURE AND THE POLITICS OF GUIDELINES AND SYNTHESES

Despite the appeal of single studies with intriguing results, the principles of evidence-based practice and policy dictate that before action is taken, some type of synthesis of available research results be carried out. Studies with larger, more representative samples and tighter designs are granted more weight in such syntheses.

Conducting and writing systematic reviews and practice guidelines are labor-intensive exercises requiring skill in literature searching, abstracting key elements of relevant research, and comparisons of findings. The process is expensive and time-consuming, often requiring by investments stakeholder groups to ensure completion. The work is often conducted in teams to make it manageable and to increase the quality of the products, including

perceptions of balance and fairness in the conclusions. The procedures used to identify relevant literature are now almost always described in detail to permit others to verify (and later update) the search strategy. It is worth noting that except in contexts such as the Cochrane Collaboration (where all procedures are extremely clearly laid out and designed to be as bias-free as possible), the grading of evidence and the drafting of syntheses are often somewhat subjective and reflect rating compromises.

Political forces will influence what topics, clienteles, or areas of science or practice are targeted for synthesis or guidelines—often high-volume or high-cost services or services where clients are at high risk. Who compiles synthesis documents and under what circumstances will also reflect research and professional politics as well as influences from funders and policymakers. In the end, the credibility of syntheses or guidelines hinges on the scientific reputation of those responsible for writing and reviewing them. There is some debate regarding whether or not subject matter expertise is required of those conducting a synthesis and whether or not having conducted any research in an area creates a vested interest that can jeopardize integrity of a review. Interestingly, different individuals tend to be involved in conducting research versus carrying out reviews. Key investigators in the area may not want to take the time away from their research to be involved, but may feel a need to defend their studies or protect what they believe to be their interests. Often, recognized experts are brought in at the beginning or end of a search and synthesis exercise to ensure that relevant studies have not been omitted and that results of studies have been correctly interpreted.

Systematic reviews, disseminated by authoritative sources, can be especially influential on both clinical practice and health policy. When a treatment's usefulness for recipients is brought into question or it is suggested that some diagnostics or treatments are superior to others, it is very likely that the creators, manufacturers, or researchers involved with the "losers" will bring their resources together to fight. In 1995, the Agency for Health Care Policy and Research (AHCPR), the federal entity that was the precursor of the AHRQ (Agency for Healthcare Research and Quality), released a practice guideline dealing with the treatment of lower back pain that stated spinal fusion surgery produced poor results (Gray, Gusmano,

& Collins, 2003). Lobbyists for spinal surgeons were able to garner sympathy from politicians averse to continued funding for the agency. In the face of other political enemies and threats, the result was the threatened disbanding of the agency. AHCPR was reborn in 1999 as AHRQ, with a similar mandate to focus on "quality improvement and patient safety, outcomes and effectiveness of care, clinical practice and technology assessment, and health care organization and delivery systems" *(www.ahrq.gov)* but without practice guideline development in its portfolio.

Clearly, skepticism is warranted when reading literature syntheses involving the standing of a particular product or service that have either been directly funded by industry or interest groups or had close involvement by industry-sponsored researchers (Detsky, 2006). Guidelines and best practices to reduce bias in literature synthesis and guideline creation are now being circulated (IOM, 2009; Palda, Davis, & Goldman, 2007) in much the same way as parameters, checklists, and reporting requirements for randomized trials and observational research (e.g., the CONSORT guidelines at *www.consort-statement.org*) were first created and disseminated a number of years ago.

THE POLITICS OF RESEARCH APPLIED TO POLICY FORMULATION

Distilling research findings and crafting messages to allow research evidence to influence policy can be even more complex and daunting than translating research related to particular health care technologies or treatments. Direct evidence about the consequences of different policy actions is often sparse, and much extrapolation is necessary to link available evidence with the questions at hand. Nevertheless, attempts have been made in the U.S. and elsewhere, often through non-profit foundations such as the Robert Wood Johnson Foundation *(www.rwjf.org)* and the Canadian Health Services Research Foundation *(www.chsrf.ca)*, to educate the public and policymakers about relevant health services research findings. The political challenges in implementing health policy change are also considerable. The amounts of money are often higher, and symbolic significance of the decisions is even greater, which

---

BOX 42-1 Pearls and Pitfalls in Using Research in Policy Contexts

Pearls

- Before trying to link research with a policy issue, understand the underlying policy issue as well as possible to determine how results in question add to a debate.
- Consider the way "opponents" of a particular policy stance will interpret the study findings, and consider adjusting messages accordingly.
- Be aware of major limitations in the study findings (e.g., weaknesses or "Achilles heels" such as lack of randomization in an evaluation study or a failure to consider an important confounder), and be prepared to respond to them and explain why results are relevant anyway.
- Refer to bodies of similar or related research rather than individual studies, where possible, and acknowledge controversies.

Pitfalls

- Assuming policymakers and journalists are familiar with or interested in research method details.
- Writing research results with needlessly biased or strong language and/or citing such research in policy without reservations.
- Exaggerating the magnitude of effects and ignoring all weaknesses or inconsistencies, especially those that can be skewered by educated nonspecialists.
- Citing research and/or researchers without checking credibility or verifying scientific quality of the results
- Failing to recognize that research findings are only one component of wider policy debates.

---

makes conflict across the same types of stakeholder interests discussed throughout this chapter potentially even more dramatic. Box 42-1 shows "pearls and pitfalls" of using research in a policy context.

Glenn (2002) explores the role of scientific evidence in policymaking with respect to "ultimate" and "derivative" values and their relationships to each other. He frames "ultimate" values as those held without real justification (or need for justification) with facts. For instance, notions that patient suffering is bad and is to be avoided at all costs, that health care is a right (and that society has a duty to help those in need), or that patients deserve care free of errors could all be considered as ultimate values. Ultimate values are by nature ill-suited to scientific investigation—and in addition to "value judgments," they may be fundamental political views about the role of government or even religious beliefs. "Derivative" values result from (or are derived from) the combination of an ultimate value with a stance about the realities of the world. A specific example: Some may argue that because low nurse staffing leads to higher error rates (an interpretation of research offering a testable insight about the clinical world) and their belief that patients should, when possible, be exposed to as few errors as possible (an ultimate value), that low staffing should be avoided (or legislated against) through the use of minimum nurse staffing ratios (a derivative value).

In Glenn's words "...science can assess the validity of the beliefs about reality that link derivative to ultimate values" (p. 69). Verifying statements about reality—not defending either ultimate or derivative values—is its role. Researchers are expected to remain objective and fair: to use "the rules of evidence" for scientific inquiry properly, clearly reporting facts that contradict their impressions or hypotheses as well as ones consistent with their and others' ultimate and derivative values. However, several forces, namely, a tendency to resist admitting having drawn incorrect or overly simplified conclusions in the past, as well as social and political pressures from one's "fan base" (what Glenn calls the researcher's "significant others") can create problems with keeping these boundaries clear. Researchers may be accused of bias, or worse, promulgating "junk science." Journalists have commented on inflated estimates of prevalence or impacts of various diseases or conditions using research data (using loose definitions, questionable assumptions, or data with limited potential to be verified) (Greve, 2005) used to lobby for increased funding for research, treatment initiatives, or policy actions.

Of course, when research findings collide with the interests of stakeholder groups in a policy debate, the responses can be extreme. The ethical integrity, scientific competence, or motivations of the researchers involved (or all three) can be called into question by stakeholders whose interests are in conflict with particular results. Late in 2009, controversy emerged when e-mails exchanged between prominent U.K. climate researchers were made public. These scientists' work is often cited to document claims of global warming and ultimately, to justify tighter vehicular, industrial emissions, and environmental controls.

The content of the e-mails was considered by some to show clear evidence of departures from objectivity, as well as data massaging, and even politicking to reduce the impact of conflicting findings from competing scientists (Booker, 2009; Sarewitz & Thernstrom, 2009).

The "culture of critique" and a media appetite for sensationalism, fuelled by rapid dissemination of news stories through the Internet, have certainly decreased the mystique of objectivity in research and highlighted the political aspects of research. Whether or not the scientific claims or conclusions of any researchers are "correct" or even whether "objectivity" can ever exist in research is probably immaterial to the discussion here. Today, researchers, like politicians, will be assumed to have vested interests unless proven otherwise. Good scientific practice is the best defense against claims of bias or worse, but it doesn't confer immunity from accusations. Nurse researchers aspiring to policy relevance and politically active nurses seeking to use research findings in their endeavors should be aware of the pitfalls and consequences. It's often useful for researchers and activists to identify potential winners and losers under proposed policy changes and anticipate their likely interpretations of research findings. In the case of making policy from the research literature tying outcomes to nurse staffing levels, opposing stakeholders at their extremes either cast managers and executives as untrustworthy when it comes to decisions where the "bottom line" and patient safety might collide, or nurses, their associations, and collective bargaining units as self-interested and prepared to see hospitals bankrupt by having unnecessarily high staffing levels and/or expensive staffing models.

In the end, it is probably wise to avoid exaggerating the ultimate influence of research findings on shaping policy. Policy victories attributed to research evidence may be more about skill and luck in turning opinion than the research evidence itself and how it is "spun" in various forums. Furthermore, policy changes stimulated by or defended by research can be short-lived. The balance between various political forces and interest groups can and often do influence the outcomes of many policy debates as much—or more than—thoughtful application of research evidence. Resistance from organized medicine to expanded scope of practice for advanced practice nurses is one example of where a critical mass of evidence supports a change but political forces have conspired against it (Hughes, Clarke, Sampson, Fairman, & Sullivan-Marx, 2010).

By applying the best methods for studying care and outcomes, researchers can increase the likelihood of influencing policy by designing studies that will yield the clearest possible answers to questions with policy relevance and carefully framing their results as honestly, humbly, and objectively as possible, even when findings disappoint or there is a temptation to oversimplify and trumpet. Researchers and lobbyists alike would do well to remember the multiple influences on public opinion and political decisions and avoid overstating research findings.

For a list of related websites, please refer to your Evolve Resources at http://evolve.elsevier.com/Mason/policypolitics/

REFERENCES

Booker, C. (2009, November 28). Climate change: This is the worst scientific scandal of our generation. *The Telegraph*. Retrieved from www.telegraph.co.uk/comment/columnists/christopherbooker/6679082/Climate-change-this-is-the-worst-scientific-scandal-of-our-generation.html.

Davies, P. (2004, February 19). Is evidence-based government possible? Jerry Lee lecture, 2004. Presented at the 4th Annual Campbell Collaboration Colloquium, Washington, D.C. National School of Government (UK). Retrieved from www.nationalschool.gov.uk/policyhub/downloads/Jerry LeeLecture1202041.pdf.

Davies, P. T. (1999). What is evidence-based education? *British Journal of Educational Studies, 47*(2), 108-121.

Detsky, A. S. (2006). Sources of bias for authors of clinical practice guidelines. *Canadian Medical Association Journal, 175*(9), 1033, 1035.

Glenn, N. (2002). Social science findings and the "family wars." In J. B. Imber (Ed.), *Searching for science policy* (pp. 67-82). New Brunswick, NJ: Transaction.

Gray, B. H., Gusmano M. K., & Collins S. R. (2003 Jan-Jun). AHCPR and the changing politics of health services research. *Health Affairs*, Suppl Web Exclusives, W3-283-307.

Greve, F. (2005, April 24). Sicker by the numbers. *The Philadelphia Inquirer*, C1, C3.

Hughes, F., Clarke, S. P., Sampson, D. A, Fairman, J., & Sullivan-Marx, E. M. (2010). Research in support of nurse practitioners. In M. D. Mezey, D. O. McGivern, & E. M. Sullivan-Marx (Eds.), *Nurse practitioners: The evolution and future of advanced practice* (5th ed.). New York: Springer.

Ioannidis, J. P. (2005). Contradicted and initially stronger effects in highly cited clinical research. *Journal of the American Medical Association, 294*(2), 218-228.

Institute of Medicine (IOM). (2009). Conflicts of interest and development of clinical practice guidelines. In B. Lo & M. J. Field (Eds.), *Conflict of interest in medical research, education, and practice*. Washington, D.C.: National Academies Press. Retrieved from www.ncbi.nlm.nih.gov/bookshelf/picrender.fcgi?book=nap12598&blobtype=pdf.

Palda, V. A., Davis, D., Goldman, J. (2007). A guide to the Canadian Medical Association handbook on clinical practice guidelines. *Canadian Medical Association Journal, 177*(10), 1221-1226.

Sackett, D. L., Rosenberg, W. M. C., Gray, J. A. M., Haynes, R. B., & Richardson, W. S. (1996). Evidence based medicine: what it is and what it isn't. *British Medical Journal, 312*(7023), 71-72.

Sarewitz, D., & Thernstrom, S. (2009, December 16). Climate change e-mail scandal underscores myth of pure science. *Los Angeles Times*. Retrieved from http://articles.latimes.com/2009/dec/16/opinion/la-oe-sarewitzthernstrom16-2009dec16.

CHAPTER 43

The Society for Women's Health Research: Using Evidence-Based Policy to Improve Health

Irma Goertzen and Suzanne Stone

"True science investigates and brings to human perception such truths and such knowledge as the people of a given time and society consider most important."

—Leo Tolstoy

The Society for Women's Health Research (SWHR), established in 1990, has changed the way research is conducted in the United States. Because of the SWHR's efforts, women are included in medical research and scientists are investigating the different ways health and disease affect men and women as well as the reasons why. The SWHR attributes its advocacy success to four factors: demonstrating evidence-based policy needs (each of the SWHR's campaigns to effect change has begun with documentation of the problem sought to be corrected), including multipronged education efforts, involving a mix of health care providers and policymakers, and extending lobbying beyond legislators and regulators. The SWHR's advocacy includes education of federal legislators and their staff members; scientists employed by the federal government, in academia, and in industry; and the public.

FOUNDING OF THE SOCIETY FOR WOMEN'S HEALTH RESEARCH

The SWHR remains, 20 years after its founding, the only organization dedicated to exploring differences in research as it relates to men and women. It was the idea of Florence Haseltine, PhD, MD. When she first started working at the National Institutes of Health (NIH) in 1985, Haseltine was advised her role was "to champion the field of obstetrics and gynecology,"

which at that time was underrepresented in research. Near that time, Congresswoman Patricia Schroeder said, "There are three gynecologists and 39 veterinarians at NIH," highlighting the lack of focus on women's health in the research community (Haseltine, 2006).

THE BIRTH OF AN ADVOCACY ORGANIZATION

In 1989, Dr. Haseltine gathered individuals from medical and scientific organizations to meet in Washington, D.C. Those gathered agreed on the need for more women's health research at NIH, but they also agreed that women's health generally lacked sufficient research focus. From this discussion, the Society for Women's Health Research was born (Box 43-1).

To validate its belief that the health of American women was at risk due to biases in biomedical research, the all-volunteer members of SWHR's first Board of Directors worked with the Congressional Caucus for Women's Issues and its Executive Director Leslie Primer and Congressman Henry Waxman (D-CA). They requested the Government Accountability Office (GAO) (then called the General Accounting Office) to study NIH's policies and practices concerning the inclusion of women and minorities in clinical trials. The GAO report was released at an NIH reauthorization hearing in June 1990. It concluded that the NIH policy (NIH, 1986) announced in October 1986 to encourage the inclusion of women in clinical trials had not been well communicated or understood within NIH or the research community, was applied inconsistently across institutes, and only

> **BOX 43-1 The Mission and Goals of the Society for Women's Health Research**
>
> **Mission:** To improve the health of women through research.
>
> **Goals:**
> 1. To identify those areas of research that will have an impact on the health of women,
> 2. To effect changes in policies and behavior to improve the health of women based on research outcomes.

was applied to extramural research. The GAO report concluded that there was "… no readily accessible source of data on the demographics of NIH study populations" (U.S. GAO, 1990). So at that time it was impossible to determine if NIH was enforcing its own recommendations.

Haseltine found this to be a "tipping point" that spurred significant advocacy efforts that would result in major policy changes over many years. Throughout the advocacy work, the SWHR leaders sought evidence to support their initiatives. They used an Institute of Medicine (IOM) report that demonstrated federal funding for research in obstetrics and gynecology to be inadequate as the tool to garner additional evidence in the form of the GAO audit.

CONGRESSIONAL ADVOCACY

The SWHR's first policy efforts were addressed almost exclusively at lobbying members of Congress to change policies and regulations at federal agencies that affected women's equity in health research. Shortly after release of the 1990 GAO audit, the NIH published guidelines that required women be included in clinical research and established the Office of Research in Women's Health. Because these guidelines were not fully implemented, the SWHR advocated for passage of the 1993 NIH Revitalization Act, which codified these requirements and also required that Phase III clinical trial results be analyzed by sex. This act permanently established the NIH's Office of Research on Women's Health.

Next came important changes at the U.S. Food and Drug Administration (FDA). Following the successful tactic of securing information via a GAO review, the

SWHR asked members of Congress to request that the GAO examine the inclusion of women in the clinical trials used by the FDA in evaluating drugs for marketing approval. The resulting 1993 report found that while women were sometimes included in drug trials, they were significantly underrepresented (U.S. GAO, 1993). Even when women were included, data were not analyzed to determine if women's responses to drugs differed from those of men. The report found an insufficient number of women were included in preapproval clinical trials of drugs and charged the FDA with improving women's representation. It concluded by recommending that the FDA ensure that drug companies consistently include "sufficient numbers of women in drug testing to identify gender-related differences in drug response and that such sex differences are explored and studied" (U.S. GAO, 1993). Later in 1993, the FDA reversed its 1977 guidelines and published a new *Guideline for the Study and Evaluation of Gender Differences in the Clinical Evaluation of Drugs* that encouraged the inclusion of women in Phase I and II (safety and dosing) studies and required their inclusion in efficacy studies. The guideline also requires analysis of data on sex differences, as well as race and ethnicity.

CONTINUING SEX AND GENDER INEQUITIES FOUND

At the SWHR's urging, the GAO was asked to review the NIH's practices again. In 2000, the GAO issued a follow-up report concluding that "NIH has made less progress in implementing the requirement that certain clinical trials be designed and carried out to permit valid analysis by sex, which could reveal whether interventions affect women and men differently." Another GAO report sought by SWHR concluded "The FDA has not effectively overseen the presentation and analysis of data related to sex differences in drug development" (U.S. GAO, 2001).

THE IMPORTANCE OF INTEGRATED PROFESSIONAL ACTION

To have success with government entities, it was important that the SWHR's voice represent a broad spectrum of health care researchers, providers, and policymakers. In 1999, the SWHR established the

Women's Health Research Coalition. It now comprises more than 600 advocates from a broad range of academic, health care, and scientific institutions. The SWHR reaches out to health care providers including nurses and researchers in many fields when invited to provide testimony at government hearings and to present briefings. These briefings inform policymakers about contemporary women's health issues, the need for increased research funding for women's health, and the need to study biological sex differences affecting the prevention, diagnosis, and treatment of disease.

EXPANDING THE UNDERSTANDING OF SEX AND GENDER DIFFERENCES IN HEALTH AND DISEASE

As a non-profit entity, the SWHR functions under the governance of a board of directors. Within 5 years of being hired, the SWHR chief executive officer Phyllis Greenberger formed a team of administrative, fundraising, government relations, and scientific staff, whose efforts gradually replaced much of the work that had been accomplished by the all-volunteer board. Board members still were called on to represent the SWHR, particularly in scientific venues, and to network to advance advocacy efforts. Second, the findings from studies that included women in clinical trials corroborated the SWHR's belief that, in matters of health and disease, men and women are different. Now, scientists needed to be convinced of this so they would design studies to explain these differences. The SWHR response to this challenge was multipronged. It sought and received independent, unbiased validation of research on sex differences, hosted interdisciplinary conferences on sex differences in biology, and successfully sought funding for novel interdisciplinary sex differences research.

DOES SEX MATTER? ABSOLUTELY

Greenberger led a 6-year campaign to secure funding for the formation of an IOM "Committee on Understanding the Biology of Sex and Gender Differences." The strength of long-term relationships that she had forged through the years was instrumental in securing the necessary funding from private and public sources for this initiative. The SWHR submitted a proposal to the IOM to validate the concept of sex differences. In 2001, the IOM published a landmark report generated by this committee, *Exploring the Biological Contributions to Human Health: Does Sex Matter?* This IOM report pointed out that every cell has a sex, sex begins in the womb, and sex affects behavior and perception. The IOM report concluded the following:

> There is now sufficient knowledge of the biological basis of sex differences to validate the scientific study of sex differences and to allow the generation of hypotheses with regard to health... Naturally occurring variations in sex differentiation can provide unique opportunities to obtain a better understanding of basic differences and similarities between and within the sexes. (Institute of Medicine, 2001, p. 3)

The SWHR sponsored five regional Scientific Advisory Meetings to educate scientists and policymakers about the 2001 IOM report. From 2000 to 2006, the SWHR convened conferences on Sex and Gene Expression (SAGE) that explored how the biological variable of sex influences the expression of genetic information from embryonic development through adulthood. The SAGE conferences brought together leading established researchers and new researchers in biochemistry; genetics; and molecular, developmental, and cellular biology. Working with the SWHR staff, these leaders in sex differences research founded the Organization for the Study of Sex Differences (OSSD) in 2006.

Other advocacy efforts within the scientific community include analyzing sex differences research efforts at the NIH. In 2005, the SWHR released a report showing the NIH's support of research on biological health differences between women and men is less than the growing evidence of the importance of sex differences warrants. It also showed that the institutes with the largest budgets appeared to be supporting the least research on sex differences. Several of the NIH institutes have recognized the need for sex differences research and have established programs to fund research on sex differences. Success in this arena shows how the SWHR has worked within the legislative arena, by advocating for research funding for research in sex and gender differences, and outside that arena, by advocating directly with researchers.

PUBLIC EDUCATION

The SWHR's first public educational effort was the "Woman Can Do" campaign, to educate and recruit more women to become involved in medical research. After regulatory changes mandating women's participation as research subjects, the SWHR learned researchers had difficulty finding women to participate in research studies. The SWHR continues to advise researchers, research organizations, and the FDA about ways to eliminate barriers to recruiting and retaining women in research. The SWHR conducts other consumer education campaigns on a variety of topics, has a press service distributing news on women's health to over 10,000 media outlets, conducts periodic media briefings and roundtables, and holds workshops for clinicians. The SWHR has published the first consumer book discussing sex differences: *The Savvy Woman Patient: How and Why Sex Differences Affect Your Health.*

In addition to disseminating research on conditions that affect women differently from men, the SWHR's education program emphasizes women need to become advocates for themselves and their families. The SWHR is founded on the belief that health can be improved through research efforts and that this new knowledge must be communicated and translated into individual care, which requires an up-to-date, current exchange of information between health care providers and patients.

CURRENT CHALLENGES AND OPPORTUNITIES

The efforts by the SWHR have borne fruit; increasingly, those who fund biomedical research have become interested in sex as a biologic variable. Researchers have found sex differences in every tissue and organ system (Becker et al., 2007). The SWHR is working to ensure women's health remains a high priority on the national agenda and that sex differences become more widely recognized as vital to health care treatment options. Both the size of the SWHR's staff and the roster of volunteer leaders have grown over time to assist in these efforts. Experts from a wide range of disciplines have been involved with the SWHR's efforts, including founding the Isis Fund interdisciplinary research networks. Staff can now call on OSSD officers and members, current and past members of Isis Fund Networks, authors of chapters in *The Savvy Woman Patient,* and presenters from past SWHR conferences, as well as board members for the clinical and technical knowledge that informs advocacy efforts. The SWHR will continue to work with a wide range of health care providers and policymakers to gather scientific evidence and to encourage that it be used to shape policy.

For a list of related websites, please refer to your Evolve Resources at http://evolve.elsevier.com/Mason/policypolitics/

REFERENCES

Becker, J. B., Berkley, K. J., Geary, N., Hampson, E., Herman, J. P., & Young, E. (Eds.). (2007). *Sex differences in the brain: from genes to behavior.* New York: Oxford University Press.

Haseltine, F. (2006). Foreword in J. Wider, P. Greenberger, and the Society for Women's Health Research (Eds.). *The savvy woman patient: How and why sex differences affect Your health.* Herndon, VA: Capital Books.

Institute of Medicine. (2001). Exploring the biological contributions to human health: Does sex matter? Retrieved from www.nap.edu/openbook.php?record_id=10028&page=3.

National Institutes of Health. (1986). *NIH guide for grants and contracts.* Bethesda, MD: National Institutes of Health.

U.S. Government Accounting Office. (1990). *National Institutes of Health: Problems in implementing policy on women in study populations.* Rep. GAO/T-HRD-90-50. Washington, D.C.: United States Government Accounting Office.

U.S. Government Accounting Office. (1993). *Women's health: FDA needs to ensure more study of gender differences in prescription drugs testing.* Rep. GAO-HRD-93-17. Washington, D.C.: United States Government Accounting Office.

U.S. Government Accounting Office. (2001). *Women sufficiently represented in new drug testing, but FDA oversight needs improvement.* Rep. GAO-01-754. Washington, D.C.: United States Government Accounting Office.

CHAPTER 44

Using Research to Advance Healthy Social Policies for Children

Sally S. Cohen, Sandra Bishop-Josef, and Louise Kahn

"Children are the world's most valuable resource and its best hope for the future."

—John F. Kennedy

Over the past decade, policymakers have increasingly recognized the importance of children's issues. This heightened awareness has been due to new research findings on the relationships among factors such as early brain development, stressful environments, and poor outcomes in later life. Moreover, researchers and professionals who work with families with young children are noting the significance of conceptualizing child health policy broadly, so as to encompass the many aspects of social policy that affect children's well-being. The purposes of this chapter are to identify major themes pertaining to social policies for children, explain how research has enhanced such policies, describe remaining gaps in children's social policy and research, and explain how nurses can make meaningful contributions to advancing healthy social policies for children.

Many social policies affect children's mental, physical, emotional, and spiritual health, especially children of racial minorities in low-income families who rely on public policies more than their more advantaged counterparts. Millions of children, disproportionately from ethnic or racial minorities, depend on welfare, foster care, and juvenile justice systems, which unfortunately too often fail to provide developmentally appropriate services and adequate oversight that children require to grow and thrive. Millions of middle- and upper-income families also rely on social policies to ensure children's health. This is especially true during tough economic times when unemployment and other family social benefits become critical parts of the social policy fabric for families with young children.

RESEARCH INFORMING SOCIAL POLICIES FOR CHILDREN

Many research studies have contributed to policy outcomes. We focus on research pertaining to early brain development, social determinants of health, obesity, childhood indicators, framing of children's policy issues, and the Nurse-Family Partnership program.

RESEARCH ON EARLY BRAIN DEVELOPMENT

Child advocates and researchers have connected child development and social policy for the past 40 years. New evidence about infant brain development in the 1990s further propelled children's advocates and researchers to push for earlier intervention with young children and families. The groundbreaking report, *From Neurons to Neighborhoods: The Science of Early Childhood Development* (Shonkoff & Phillips, 2000), provided important findings about the effects of genetics, environment, and early stress on brain architecture. Policymakers and children's advocates continue to use this report to inform children's policies.

In the early 2000s, with new neuroimaging technology and research, scientists demonstrated the impact of neurophysiologic and neurodevelopmental stress, trauma, and neglect on children. Their findings pointed to the need for safe, predictable, and enriched environments for young children (Perry, 2002) and strengthened advocates' arguments for better funding of early childhood education, prevention of child and abuse neglect (including home visitation programs), child protection and foster care, and mental health treatment. Advocacy groups such as Zero to Three (Gebhard, 2009) used the brain research to develop science-based policy agendas for improving children's physical and social-emotional health, through physical health, family leave, child welfare, home visiting, and early care and education.

RESEARCH ON SOCIAL DETERMINANTS OF HEALTH AND HEALTH DISPARITIES

Research on the link between social determinants of health and health disparities has proliferated in recent years. One of the most widely cited policy reports on social determinants of health was issued by the World Health Organization (WHO) (2005). It included a definition of social determinants of health:

> The social determinants of health are the conditions in which people are born, grow, live, work and age, including the health system. These circumstances are shaped by the distribution of money, power and resources at global, national and local levels, which are themselves influenced by policy choices... (WHO, 2005)

Several major national and international reports have reached similar conclusions about the relationship between social determinants of health and health outcomes. Specifically, the WHO final report (WHO, 2009), *Healthy People 2020* (USDHHS, 2010), and a landmark Institute of Medicine study on health disparities (Smedley, Stith, & Nelson, 2003) all explain how social determinants often play a larger role in determining health outcomes than clinical interventions.

Regarding children, several major themes emerge from the plethora of recent reports in this area. Specifically, children of low socioeconomic and minority status experience significant shortfalls in their health compared to other children (Egerter et al., 2008). Disadvantaged and minority families have the highest rates of infant mortality. Similarly, compared to children in families with higher income, those in poor, near-poor, or middle income families were more likely to be in less than optimal health. Children from poor, racially segregated neighborhoods also have more challenges than other children in accessing services needed to maintain good health (Acevedo-Garcia, Osypuk, McArdle, & Williams, 2008).

Studies on social determinants of health and the factors that contribute to health disparities have enabled policymakers and professionals on the frontlines of care to recognize the importance of including issues such as poverty, housing, neighborhood safety, transportation, and environmental stress when developing strategies for improving child health outcomes. Such research has also highlighted the importance of integrating education and child development with child health care because of the intrinsic connection between educational attainment and health outcomes later in life. Research on social determinants of health and health disparities also points to the importance of social structures in determining many aspects of personal health and to the pervasiveness of racial discrimination across many sectors of society.

RESEARCH RELATED TO CHILDHOOD OBESITY

Minority children and poor children also suffer disproportionately from obesity, putting them at greatly increased lifetime risk of diabetes, and cardiovascular, respiratory, mental health, social and occupational problems. Although the rise in childhood obesity over the past several decades impacts the entire population, research has shown that Hispanic, non-Hispanic Black, and Native-American children and adolescents are disproportionately affected (Koplan, Liverman, & Kraak, 2005). Differential access to healthy foods in low-income communities is a major contributor to health disparities in diet-related chronic diseases and obesity (Story, Hamm, & Wallinga, 2009).

Using this research, advocates for children across various disciplines are developing strategies to focus on social and environmental determinants of obesity, rather than on individual behavior or predisposition (Robert Wood Johnson Foundation, 2010). A new focus has emerged on the "built environment," which encompasses people's living and working conditions and how they impact opportunities for physical activity and recreation, healthy food, and neighborhood safety. Increasingly, affected communities are involved in becoming places where safe physical activity and healthy eating are possible. For example, nursing students in New Mexico were involved in assessing the "walkability" of low-income neighborhoods, through a CDC Project Achieve (Action Communities for Health, Innovation and Environmental Change) project (CDC, 2010). In February, 2010, Michelle Obama announced the "Let's Move" initiative, a collaboration between the White House and the federal Departments of Health and Human Services, Agriculture, and Education. "Let's Move" aims to "to end the American plague of childhood obesity in a single generation" (White House, 2010).

RESEARCH ON CHILDHOOD INDICATORS

The Annie E. Casey Foundation has long been a leader in providing data and analyzing how policies are meeting (or failing to meet) the needs of children and families. The annual release of the *KIDS COUNT* data book, which includes state data for 10 leading indicators, receives extensive media attention and is often a catalyst for policy development (Annie E. Casey Foundation, 2009a). Other foundations and organizations publish similar compilations of child and family indicators. These indicator data have played a vital role in defining the problems that social policies are then designed to ameliorate.

RESEARCH ON "FRAMING THE PROBLEM"

Since the late 1990s, researchers and child advocates have become increasingly savvy about how to communicate research findings and thereby move public policy, primarily using frame theory. Frame theory suggests that people organize the world by using preexisting frames that guide their thoughts and feelings on an issue (FrameWorks Institute, 2001). Frames are strongly influenced by the media and can be very resistant to change. The FrameWorks Institute has been the leader in this area, conducting research to determine current frames around child and family issues and subsequently designing strategic communications to change these frames (i.e. "reframing") to facilitate policy development. These efforts have advanced children's policy, particularly in the area of child care, now reframed as "early care and education" (ECE).

Early framing research on child care (Nall Bales, 1998) found that the predominant frames were safety (i.e., importance of children being safe; dangers associated with bad child care) and work (i.e., child care as a service that allows mothers, especially those on welfare, to work). Neither of these frames focused on child development or child care as a setting to promote optimal development (Brauner, Gordic, & Zigler, 2004). Further, framing child care as a safety or work issue results in the public and policymakers seeing it as an individual, parental responsibility, rather than a public policy issue.

In an effort to advance child care on legislative and other public agendas, advocates hired consultants to help reframe the issue. The culmination of this work, which included extensive public opinion surveys,

focus groups, and other research, was that advocates eventually reframed their issue as early childhood education (Gruendel & Aber, 2007). In particular, in line with the education frame, they began to focus on prekindergarten for 3- and 4-year-olds about to enter school. Partially as a result of these reframing efforts, the pre-k movement has taken off, with most states increasing funding for preschool, thereby increasing children's access to these services (Clothier & Poppe, 2007).

One of the most effective frames for children's policies is in terms of the economic benefits current investments in children will yield in the future. A RAND study (Karoly et al., 1998) provided the impetus for other analyses of how funding ECE programs would be cost-effective. These studies eventually led economists and researchers from the Minnesota Federal Reserve Bank to endorse such policies and form partnerships with early childhood programs (Early Childhood Research Collaborative, 2010).

RESEARCH ON THE NURSE-FAMILY PARTNERSHIP PROGRAM

One major success in linking research and policy that spans many of the issues discussed earlier in the chapter is the Nurse Family Partnership (NFP), internationally recognized as a highly effective home visiting intervention with young parents and their infants. The NFP was first developed and implemented in 1977 by David Olds, MD, a pediatrician and psychiatrist, and Harriet Kitzman, PhD, RN, FAAN, at the University of Rochester. The program partners low-income, first-time mothers with maternal and child health nurses during pregnancy and continuing until the child's second birthday. Trusting relationships between the nurses and mothers have resulted in benefits to both mothers and children (Olds et al., 1997).

Randomized, controlled trials in Elmira, New York (1977), Memphis, Tennessee (1988), and Denver, Colorado (1994) have demonstrated impressive and sustained results, with the strongest effects on improved prenatal health and later school readiness, decreases in childhood injuries and mother's subsequent pregnancies, and increases in maternal intervals between births and employment rates. Researchers documented other positive outcomes in at least one of the clinical trials, including reductions in child arrests at age 15, child abuse and neglect, and language delays, and improvement in achievement test scores at grades 1 to 3 among the low-resource group (Eckenrode et al., 2010).

Evaluations of the NFP and other home visitation models convinced President Barak Obama in 2009 to initiate a multibillion dollar federal program to expand nurse home visitation. A home visitation provision was included in the Affordable Care Act (ACA), the federal health care reform legislation that was enacted in March 2010. The legislation will provide $1.5 billion over 5 years to states, tribes, and territories to develop and implement one or more evidence-based Maternal, Infant, and Early Childhood Visitation models. These are excellent opportunities for nurses to become involved in advocacy and consultation at state and community levels. As an example, because of her expertise as a nurse practitioner and children's advocate, one of the chapter authors (Kahn) was recently appointed to the New Mexico home visiting task force.

SHORTCOMINGS IN LINKING RESEARCH AND SOCIAL POLICIES FOR CHILDREN

Although research has contributed to policy and programs on behalf of children and their families, children's outcomes remain unsatisfactory, in many areas, including those discussed in this chapter. For example, the reframing of child care as early education and the subsequent expansion of prekindergarten has not benefited infants and toddlers. Prekindergarten expansion has also not included advocacy on workplace issues, such as parental leave policies, which could provide additional relief from parenting stress. Although the infant mortality rate in the United States has dropped significantly since 1960 (from 26.0 to 6.9 per 1000 live births), progress on this indicator has slowed since 2000 and the U.S. lags behind other industrialized countries (Annie E. Casey Foundation, 2009b). Furthermore, discrepancies exist between what research indicates is needed for healthy development and what society delivers. For example, we are not able to ensure that most children receive the quality of child care that is commensurate with brain development research findings. Nor do we ensure that all children have adequate coverage and are able to access good quality physical and mental health care.

Further, overall financial investments in programs for children are still relatively low. In 2008, only 10% of the U.S. federal budget was spent on children, compared to 38% on older adults and disabled persons (Isaacs, Vericker, Macomber, & Kent, 2009). Moreover, the percentage of federal expenditures directed toward children has actually declined over time (from 20% in 1960 to 15% in 2008). During the first 2 years of the Obama presidency (2009-2010), laws were enacted that included substantial funding increases for the Child Care and Development Block Grant, Nurse-Family Partnerships, and the Child Health Insurance Program Reauthorization Act. This infusion of funding will be an important start to improving children's health and developmental outcomes.

WHO SPEAKS FOR CHILDREN?

Gaps in linking research and policy for children prompt questions about what advocacy for children's policies is most effective. Certainly, data, framing, and political will are essential. Additionally, it is important to consider how to widen the advocacy community involved in children's issues. The addition of well-known economists to ECE advocacy has been tremendously valuable in garnering political support for these issues. The work of Fight Crime, Invest in Kids, a national organization focused on linking the crime enforcement community with ECE, has also been important (Cohen, 2001). Nonetheless, advocacy remains difficult because the constituents themselves—children and parents—are not easily mobilized due to the realities of their daily lives. Children from families with low socioeconomic status and from racial and ethnic minority groups are particularly disadvantaged. But being raised in a middle- or upper-income family is no guarantee of attaining good health or educational outcomes.

Political realities also figure prominently here. Historically, children and families have not been high policy priorities. Moreover, with a tight economy and limited government resources, policymakers have limited capacities to assist families with children. Also, children's advocates compete with those representing other groups, such as older adults.

National and state nursing organizations have much untapped potential in terms of educating the public and policymakers, testifying on behalf of children and joining other coalitions. In so doing, it is important for nurses to be mindful of research and policy linkages and to keep abreast with the types of resources provided in this chapter. Nurses can synthesize research and present their own findings so as to enhance the connections between research and policy. As discussed here, though, it is important to remember that data alone cannot change policies. In advancing children's policies, other factors are valuable such as careful framing, working with professionals from other disciplines, keeping in mind the needs of the whole child, widening the policy community, and remaining hopeful that policy change can occur.

For a list of related websites, please refer to your Evolve Resources at http://evolve.elsevier.com/Mason/policypolitics/

REFERENCES

Acevedo-Garcia, D., Osypuk, T. L., McArdle, N., & Williams, D. R. (2008). Toward a policy-relevant analysis of geographic and racial/ethnic disparities in child health. *Health Affairs (Millwood), 27*(2), 321-333.

Affordable Care Act of 2010. H.R. 3590, Public Law No. 111-148.

Annie, E., Casey Foundation. (2009a). The 2009 KIDS COUNT data book. Retrieved from http://datacenter.kidscount.org/databook/2009/Default.aspx.

Annie, E., Casey Foundation. (2009b). *KIDS COUNT indicator brief—Reducing infant mortality.* Baltimore, MD: Author. Retrieved from www.aecf.org/~/media/Pubs/Initiatives/KIDS%20COUNT/K/KIDSCOUNTIndicatorBrief ReducingInfantMortalit/ReducingInfantMortality.pdf.

Brauner, J., Gordic, B., & Zigler, E. (2004). Putting the child back into child care: Combining care and education for children ages 3-5. *Social Policy Report, XVIII*(III).

Centers for Disease Control and Prevention. (2010). ACHIEVE Communities. Retrieved from www.cdc.gov/healthycommunitiesprogram/communities/achieve.htm.

Clothier, S., & Poppe, J. (2007). Preschool rocks: Policy makers around the country are investing in preschool. National Council of State Legislatures. Retrieved from www.ncsl.org/Portals/1/documents/magazine/articles/2007/07SLJan07_Preschool.pdf.

Cohen, S. S. (2001). *Championing child care.* New York: Columbia University Press.

Early Childhood Research Collaborative. (2010). Retrieved from www.earlychildhoodrc.org/partners.cfm.

Eckenrode, J., Campa, M., Luckey, D., Henderson, C., Cole, R., et al. (2010). Long-term effects of prenatal and infancy nurse home visitation on the life course of youths: 19-year follow-up of a randomized trial. *Archives of Pediatric and Adolescent Medicine, 164*(1), 9-15. Retrieved from http://archpedi.ama-assn.org/cgi/reprint/164/1/9.pdf.

Egerter, S., Braverman, P., Pamuk, E., Cubbin, C., Dekker, M., et al. (2008). *America's health starts with healthy children: How do states compare?* Princeton, N.J.: Robert Wood Johnson Foundation Commission to Build a Healthier America. Retrieved from www.commissiononhealth.org/Report.aspx?Publication=57823.

FrameWorks Institute. (2001). *A five minute refresher course in framing.* Washington, D.C.: author. Retrieved from http://frameworksinstitute.org/assets/files/eZines/five_minute_refresher_ezine.pdf.

Gebhard, B. (2009). *Early experiences matter policy guide.* Washington, D.C.: Zero to Three National Center for Infants, Toddlers, and Families. Retrieved from www.zerotothree.org/site/DocServer/Policy_Guide.pdf?docID=8401.

Gruendel, J., & Aber, J. L. (2007). Bridging the gap between research and child policy change: The role of strategic communications in policy advocacy. In. J. L. Aber, S. J. Bishop-Josef, S. M. Jones, K. T. McLearn, & D. A. Phillips (Eds.), *Child development and social policy: Knowledge for action.* Washington, D.C.: American Psychological Association.

Isaccs, J. B., Vericker, T., Macomber, J., & Kent, A. (2009). *Kids' share: An analysis of federal expenditures on children through 2008.* Washington, D.C.: Urban Institute and Brookings. Retrieved from www.brookings.edu/~/media/Files/rc/reports/2009/1209_kids_share_isaacs/1209_kids_share_isaacs.pdf.

Karoly, L., Greenwood, P., Everingham, S., Hoube, J., Kilburn, R., et al. (1998). *Investing in our children: What we know and don't know about the costs and benefits of early childhood interventions.* Santa Monica, CA: Rand Corporation.

Koplan, J., Liverman, C. T., & Kraak, V. A. (Eds.). (2005). *Preventing childhood obesity—Health in the balance.* Washington, D.C.: National Academies Press.

Nall Bales, S. (1998). Early childhood education and the framing wars. In *Effective language for discussing early childhood education and policy.* Washington D.C.: Benton Foundation.

Olds, D., Eckenrode, J., Henderson, C., Kitzman, H., Powers, J., et al. (1997). Long-term effects of home visitation on maternal life course and child abuse and neglect: Fifteen-year follow-up of a randomized trial. *Journal of the American Medical Association, 278*(8), 637-643. Retrieved from http://jama.ama-assn.org/cgi/reprint/278/8/644.

Perry, B. D. (2002). Childhood experience and the expression of genetic potential: What childhood neglect tells us about nature and nurture. *Brain & Mind, 3*(1), 79-100.

Robert Wood Johnson Foundation. (2010). Childhood obesity. Retrieved from www.rwjf.org/childhoodobesity.

Shonkoff, J. P. & Phillips, D. A. (Eds.). (2000). *From neurons to neighborhoods: The science of early childhood development.* Washington, D.C.: National Academies Press.

Smedley, B. D., Stith, A. Y., & Nelson, A. R. (Eds.). (2003). *Unequal treatment: Confronting racial and ethnic disparities in health care.* Washington, D.C.: National Academies Press. Retrieved from www.nap.edu/openbook.php?isbn=030908265X.

Story, M., Hamm, M., & Wallinga, D. (2009). Food systems and public health: Linkages to achieve healthier diets and healthier communities. *Journal of Hunger & Environmental Nutrition, 4*(3), 219-224.

U.S. Department of Health and Human Services. (2010). Healthy People 2020: The road ahead. Retrieved from www.healthypeople.gov/hp2020.

White House, Office of the First Lady. (2010). First Lady Michelle Obama launches Let's Move: America's move to raise a healthier generation of kids. Retrieved from www.whitehouse.gov/the-press-office/first-lady-michelle-obama-launches-lets-move-americas-move-raise-a-healthier-genera.

World Health Organization (WHO) Commission on Social Determinants of Health. (2005). Social determinants of health. Retrieved from www.who.int/social_determinants/en.

World Health Organization (WHO) Commission on Social Determinants of Health. (2009). Final report: Closing the gap in a generation: Health equity through action on the social determinants of health. Retrieved from www.who.int/social_determinants/thecommission/finalreport/en/index.html.

CHAPTER 45

TAKING ACTION
Reefer Madness: The Clash of Science, Politics, and Medical Marijuana

Mary Lynn Mathre

"If you want to make enemies, try to change something."

—Woodrow Wilson

A DRUG WITH AN IMAGE PROBLEM

It's a drug with an image problem—a drug that has been shown to help certain patients but whose use is forbidden by federal law. We know it as *dope, pot, reefer, grass, weed,* or *ganja.* In its clinical form, cannabis, it is a valuable therapeutic aid. However, the Drug Enforcement Administration (the federal agency responsible for placing drugs in categories on the controlled substances schedule) has refused to move cannabis to a less restrictive schedule, while allowing a synthetic form of the primary psychoactive substance (THC) in cannabis to be placed at a less restrictive level. Cannabis (marijuana) and natural THC (the primary psychoactive substance in cannabis) remain in Schedule I, while dronabinol (Marinol®), the synthetic form of THC, has since been reassigned to Schedule III (less controlled and more available) due to its safety and lack of activity as a "diverted" drug.

In 1999, at the request of the White House, the Institute of Medicine (IOM) completed an 18-month study on therapeutic cannabis (Joy, Watson, & Benson, 1999). The study team found that cannabis is not highly addictive, is not a "gateway" drug, and has therapeutic value. It recommended that until pharmaceutical grade products become available, cancer and AIDS patients should be allowed to smoke the crude plant material for up to 6 months. The IOM also recommended that physicians should be able to conduct "N-of-1" studies on the patients whom they believe could benefit from cannabis and that research should be conducted on alternative delivery systems. This report has largely been ignored by the federal government, but research is going forward on the therapeutic use of cannabis in the United States and other countries. Despite the barriers and social bias against cannabis, 14 states have passed laws permitting the medical use of the drug. However, in June 2005, the U.S. Supreme Court ruled that federal authorities have the power to prosecute individuals for possession and use of medical marijuana even in the states that permit it (Tierney, 2005). How did this once-legal drug become the socially shunned problem child of the pharmaceutical industry and a political hot potato? The saga of cannabis in the U.S. health system is a story of the clash of politics, opinion, fear, emotion, and science.

ONCE UPON A TIME, CANNABIS WAS LEGAL

Prior to the U.S. Congress passing the Marihuana Tax Act of 1937, cannabis was a medicine commonly used by physicians for a variety of ailments. Originally *Cannabis sativa* and *Cannabis indica* plant material were imported to this country for use in medical products. As time went on, *Cannabis americana* was grown in the U.S. to provide access to fresh plant

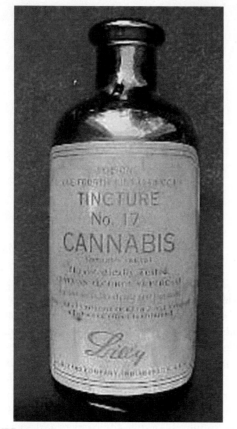

FIGURE 45-1 Historical Photo. Tincture of Cannabis No. 17 produced by Eli Lilly. (The Cannabis Museum, Elliston, VA.)

> **BOX 45-1 Cannabis Terms**
>
> *Cannabis*—A plant genus that is unique in the plant kingdom in that it contains a group of chemicals known as *cannabinoids*
>
> *Cannabis indica*—A species of the cannabis plant that has short, broad leaflets
>
> *Cannabis sativa*—a species of the cannabis plant that has long, narrow leaflets
>
> *Cesamet®*—Nabilone, a synthetic derivative of THC that is available in Europe, Canada, and the United States
>
> *Marijuana/marihuana*—The obsolete pejorative Mexican name for cannabis, used by the federal government in their efforts to prohibit the use of the cannabis plant
>
> *Marinol®*—A registered trademark of Unimed Pharmaceuticals. It is the commercial name for dronabinol (the synthetic form of delta-9-tetrahydrocannabinol), which is formulated with sesame oil and encapsulated in soft gelatin capsules. When first on the market, it was a Schedule II medication for use in the treatment of nausea and vomiting caused by chemotherapy, as well as appetite loss caused by AIDS.
>
> *Sativex*—A cannabis extract oro-mucosal spray developed by GW Pharmaceuticals in the UK and first on the market in Canada in 2005 for use by patients with multiple sclerosis
>
> *THC*—Delta-9-tetrahydrocannabinol, the primary psychoactive ingredient in cannabis/marijuana; one of more than 60 cannabinoids

material to avoid the degradation that occurred when it was brought overseas on slow-moving ships. Cannabis tinctures (Figure 45-1), elixirs, salves, and even smokeable products were available. It was listed in the U.S. Pharmacopoeia until 1940.

HOW AND WHY DID THE PROHIBITION BEGIN?

After Prohibition (the U.S. alcohol prohibition in the 1930s) ended in failure, the Bureau of Narcotics and Dangerous Drugs and its leader, Harry Anslinger, needed to find something for the department to do or it would be dissolved. Anslinger targeted a drug used by "Negro" jazz musicians in the American South and Mexicans in the Southwest. The drug was cannabis, but was called *reefer* by the African-American population and *marijuana* (or marihuana) by the Hispanic population (Box 45-1).

THE DESCENT INTO "REEFER MADNESS"

In 1936, the film *Reefer Madness* was released (a reefer being a marijuana cigarette) to warn the American population of the dangers of using marijuana. The film's plot involves tragic events that ensue when high school students are lured by drug pushers into using marijuana. A "Reefer Madness" mentality was adopted by some government agencies, individuals, and media moguls like William Randolph Hearst. Few people realized at the time that this dangerous "new" drug was the same as the cannabis medicine that physicians prescribed.

MY INTRODUCTION TO THE PROBLEM OF MEDICAL CANNABIS USE

In the early 1980s, I was working in a small hospital in Washington state, when the Director of Nursing approached me with a problem. A cancer patient was going to be admitted who had experimental "marijuana" pills from the University of Washington. What should we do? I suggested we lock it up in the narcotics cabinet and dispense it as prescribed. No problems were encountered, and I began learning about Marinol® (Figure 45-2), the synthetic "marijuana" pill. At about the same time, I came across a flyer about an organization called the Alliance for Cannabis Therapeutics (ACT). It was started by a glaucoma patient, Robert Randall, and his wife. In 1976, Randall had gained legal access to federally grown marijuana under the Compassionate Use Investigational New Drug (IND) program following a series of court battles because no other medicine could control his intraocular pressure. He formed ACT, a nonprofit organization, to let others know about the therapeutic benefits of cannabis and how patients could get a legal, federally-approved supply of it. I was drawn to the issue.

After moving to Ohio to complete graduate school at Case Western Reserve University in 1983, I conducted a survey on marijuana disclosure to health care professionals using the membership of the National Organization for the Reform of Marijuana Laws (NORML) as my survey population (Mathre, 1985). The thrust of my thesis was to determine if health care professionals asked patients about the use of cannabis and whether or not the survey subjects would disclose their use patterns. I received some surprising responses that led me to consider the therapeutic potential of cannabis. In a final question that asked the subjects to identify their concerns regarding the use of cannabis from a list of health problems, numerous respondents noted in the "other" option that they used it as medicine for stress, migraines, spasticity, pain, and other ailments (Mathre, 1988).

AN OPPORTUNITY FOR EDUCATION

I accepted the position of Director of the NORML's Council on Marijuana and Health. By 1990, there

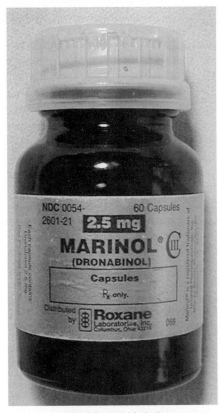

FIGURE 45-2 Marinol.

were five patients who had legal access to marijuana through the Compassionate IND program. I was serving on the planning committee for the annual NORML conference and suggested that we have the patients present their cases in a panel presentation. The patients were eager to tell their stories and were excited to meet others with similar issues. Their presentations were aired on C-SPAN and garnered national attention. We had each patient interviewed and videotaped by a volunteer professional videographer. Over the next 2 years, excerpts from the interviews were used to create an 18-minute video called Marijuana as Medicine (Byrne & Mathre, 1992), which was designed to be a teaching aid. Following the airing of the patients' panel, the U.S. Food and Drug Administration (FDA) received many requests for IND access to marijuana, especially from HIV/AIDS patients. The Secretary of the U.S. Department of Health and Human Services (HHS), Dr. Louis Sullivan, responded by shutting down the IND access to marijuana in 1992. At that time, 15 patients were receiving marijuana, over 30 patients had been approved and were waiting for their medication to be delivered, and hundreds of applications were waiting for review (Randall & O'Leary, 1998). Only the 15 current patients would be allowed to continue in the program, closing the door to all others. Also at this time, one of the legal patient's supply of marijuana was cut off. Corinne Millet, a widow and glaucoma patient, sought help from her congressman to regain her supply of medicine, but during the 6 weeks she spent without her medication, she lost 80% of her peripheral vision (Byrne & Mathre, 1992).

These events made me feel that it was important to end the prohibition on the use of cannabis in the U.S. My perspective was that there was no justifiable reason for the marijuana prohibition. It has therapeutic value, it is safe, and patients benefit from it. I saw this as a problem that required patient advocacy and that had ethical implications. I believed it to be a professional responsibility to end the cannabis prohibition and make this medicine legally available to patients.

The more I learned, the more determined I became. I embarked on a more than 20-year fight, met countless barriers, and often felt like David taking on the Goliath of the federal government. Colleagues have questioned me over the years as to why I'm still trying to change the laws, but the answer is always the same: Patients still do not have access to a safe and legal supply of this medicine.

BARRIERS AND STRATEGIES

Over the years, I've encountered many barriers and tried various strategies; often the same strategies have been used under different circumstances. Barriers that I've encountered include misinformation presented as facts, censorship of information, intimidation, laws and regulations that prevent research, an image based on racism and ideology rather than science and reality, and pharmaceutical industry pressure to prevent potential competition. I've used strategies such as finding a strong mentor; building a support system; mobilizing grassroots support; reframing the problem; partnering with patients; building a coalition; starting a nonprofit organization; providing continuing accredited education for health care professionals about cannabis; using the

Internet effectively; playing by the government's rules; teaching others; conducting research, disseminating research findings; and educating the public through publications, the press, and the media.

HIDING THE TRUTH

In the years following the Marihuana Tax Act of 1937, cannabis was removed from the U.S. Pharmacopoeia, it was no longer included in medical school curricula, and health care professionals learned about marijuana only in the context of substance abuse. The Controlled Substances Act of 1970 further condemned the drug when officials wrongly, in my opinion, placed marijuana in Schedule I of the Controlled Substances Schedule—the category of drugs that are highly addictive, are not safe for medical use, and have no therapeutic value (Box 45-2).

By the 1960s and 1970s, the average American had little knowledge of cannabis but had been taught about the dangers of marijuana. The legal consequences for possession of marijuana became so severe (up to a life sentence for a single "joint") that people who used it medicinally kept their use a secret. Thus the "stoned" teenager became the public image of a marijuana user (Sean Penn in *Fast Times at Ridgemont High* exemplified this image).

FINDING THE TRUTH

I knew cannabis had therapeutic value after searching for and reviewing historical records that included national studies and patient studies conducted in the late 1970s and early 1980s. For studies conducted prior to the Marihuana Tax Act of 1937, I had to search using the terms *cannabis* and *hemp*. I initially depended upon others in the field to gain access to rare copies of studies that validated the efficacy of cannabis. I found some published reports with negative results, but on close review the studies were either flawed or not accurately reported.

A POWERFUL MENTOR

I was lucky to meet an influential nursing leader, Melanie Dreher, PhD, RN, FAAN, who at the time was Dean of the University of Florida School of Nursing in Miami. Her doctorate was in anthropology, and her research was on "ganja" (marijuana) use

---

BOX 45-2 Schedule of Controlled Substances in the United States

21 U.S. Code §812(b) specifies the following classification system for drugs in the U.S. based on the purpose, safety, and effectiveness of the drug:

Schedule I Drugs

a. The drug or other substance has a high potential for abuse.
b. The drug or other substance has no currently accepted medical use in treatment in the U.S.
c. There is a lack of accepted safety for use of the drug or other substance under medical supervision.

Schedule I drugs include marijuana (cannabis), heroin (diacetylmorphine), ecstasy (MDMA), psilocybin, GHB (gamma-hydroxybutyrate), LSD, mescaline, and peyote.

Schedule II Drugs

a. The drug or other substance has a high potential for abuse.
b. The drug or other substance has a currently accepted medical use in treatment in the United States or a currently accepted medical use with severe restrictions.
c. Abuse of the drug or other substance may lead to severe psychological or physical dependence.

Schedule II drugs are only available by prescription, and distribution is carefully controlled and monitored by the DEA. Schedule II drugs include cocaine, methylphenidate (Ritalin®), most pure opioid agonists, meperidine, fentanyl, opium, oxycodone, morphine, short-acting barbiturates such as secobarbital, methamphetamine, and PCP.

Schedule III Drugs

a. The drug or other substance has a potential for abuse less than the drugs or other substances in Schedules I and II.
b. The drug or other substance has a currently accepted medical use in treatment in the U.S.
c. Abuse of the drug or other substance may lead to moderate or low physical dependence or high psychological dependence.

Schedule III drugs are available only by prescription, though control of wholesale distribution is somewhat less stringent than for Schedule II drugs. Schedule III drugs include Marinol®; anabolic steroids; intermediate-acting barbiturates such as talbutal; preparations that combine codeine or hydrocodone with aspirin or acetaminophen; ketamine; and paregoric.

Schedule IV Drugs

a. The drug or other substance has a low potential for abuse relative to the drugs or other substances in Schedule III.
b. The drug or other substance has a currently accepted medical use in treatment in the U.S.
c. Abuse of the drug or other substance may lead to limited physical dependence or psychological dependence relative to the drugs or other substances in Schedule III.

Schedule IV control measures are similar to those for Schedule III; drugs on this schedule include benzodiazepines such as alprazolam (Xanax®), chlordiazepoxide (Librium®), and diazepam (Valium®); long-acting barbiturates such as phenobarbital; and some partial agonist opioid analgesics, such as propoxyphene (Darvon®) and pentazocine (Talwin®).

Schedule V Drugs

a. The drug or other substance has a low potential for abuse relative to the drugs or other substances in Schedule IV.
b. The drug or other substance has a currently accepted medical use in treatment in the U.S.
c. Abuse of the drug or other substance may lead to limited physical dependence or psychological dependence relative to the drugs or other substances in Schedule IV.

Schedule V drugs are sometimes available without a prescription; drugs on this schedule include cough suppressants containing small amounts of codeine and preparations containing small amounts of opium, used to treat diarrhea.

Source: Title 21 United States Code (USC) Controlled Substances Act. Retrieved from *www.deadiversion.usdoj.gov/21cfr/21usc/802.htm#32a.*

---

by pregnant women in Jamaica and fetal outcome (Dreher, Nugent, & Hudgins, 1994; Dreher, 1997). She taught me a great deal and validated my understanding of the benefits of cannabis.

GAINING SUPPORT

I began collecting signatures on a petition to demand that cannabis be removed from Schedule I of the Controlled Substances to make it available for patient use. Many people agreed with the idea but were afraid to put their name on a public document. Although I and others collected tens of thousands of signatures, it became apparent that this approach was not cost-effective or time-effective.

By getting the first five legal patients together, I had helped them develop a lasting bond, and they in turn trusted me. This bond empowered them to speak out about the injustice of the prohibition of cannabis use. The video, *Marijuana as Medicine* (Byrne & Mathre, 1992), has served as a powerful teaching tool with other health care professionals, the public, and legislators. I began to approach nursing organizations and to show them the video. Following the video presentation, I urged them to pass a resolution that I had drafted in support of cannabis. My initial success began with resolutions passed by the Virginia Nurses Society on Addictions (1993), the Virginia Nurses Association (1994), and the National Nurses Society on Addictions (1995). During these presentations, the proper name for the plant—cannabis—was used in an attempt to change the negative image of the drug. By getting professional organizations to formally support patient access to therapeutic cannabis, individual members had a stronger voice on the issue.

"PATIENTS OUT OF TIME"

In 1995, following the deaths of a young couple with AIDS who were in the IND program, my husband and I felt the need to take this issue more seriously. With the help of several patients with legal access to cannabis and other health care professionals, we founded a national nonprofit organization, *Patients Out of Time*. We kept our mission simple: to educate the public and health care professionals about the therapeutic use of cannabis. Initially we focused on getting professional organizations, including the American Public Health Association (APHA), to issue resolutions in support of patient access to cannabis. I submitted a proposed resolution to the APHA, and it was passed at their annual meeting in California in 1995. I sent out copies of the Virginia Nurses Association's resolution and a letter to the leadership of all the state nurses associations. Colorado, Mississippi, and New York were among states that took action. The California Nurses Association had passed a resolution in 1994. We posted a list of these organizations on our website *(www.medicalcannabis.com)*, which we continually updated as more organizations joined. We verify accuracy before placing any organization on our list. In 2002, I received a call from a New York nurse who was drafting a resolution on therapeutic cannabis to present at the American Nurses Association (ANA) 2003 House of Delegates meeting. I assisted in developing its content and went to the convention to speak on behalf of the resolution. It easily passed. I believe the ANA resolution most clearly encompasses the issues of concern regarding the marijuana prohibition.

CHALLENGES IN DISSEMINATING INFORMATION ABOUT CANNABIS

In 1993, I sent a manuscript on the ethical and legal dilemmas for nurses related to therapeutic cannabis to the *American Journal of Nursing (AJN)* to try to increase professional awareness on this issue. *AJN* rejected it saying it wasn't appropriate. I called Mary Mallison, the AJN editor-in-chief, and she suggested I submit a second article on cannabis dosing. Upon receipt of that manuscript, I received a letter from the editorial director, Martin DiCarlantonio, which stated: "We'd like to accept your manuscript and run it as soon as marijuana is moved to Schedule II category (if that day ever comes)."

In 1995, I was asked by Mary Gorman, RN, to write a manuscript for *AJN*'s substance abuse column on the medical use of marijuana. I submitted it with a projected publication date of 1996. Again it was considered too controversial and remained in the journal's files for more than a year until a change in editorial staff occurred. It was published in November 1997. Several positive letters to the AJN editor were printed in 1998. I was told that no negative letters to the editor had been received.

In 1999, I decided to submit another article to *AJN* after reading an editorial by Dr. Diana Mason, *AJN*'s new editor-in-chief, in which she urged nurses to work to influence health policy. This manuscript was published in 2001, and again, only positive letters to the editor were received. In 2004, I was asked to submit a manuscript to *Nursing 2004* on therapeutic cannabis. It was accepted for publication, but in 2005 I received a letter stating that it would not be published because they could not get anyone to submit an opposing view.

BIRTH OF A BOOK AND DEATH OF A JOURNAL

In 1995, I began work on a cannabis book and began finding experts on various topics who were willing to contribute a chapter. *Cannabis in Medical Practice* was published in 1997 by McFarland, containing the work of 17 contributing authors (Mathre, 1997). The book received great reviews. Dr. Geoffrey Guy, a physician and drug researcher in the UK, read the book and reported that it motivated him to start a pharmaceutical company to develop cannabis-based pharmaceuticals *(www.gwpharm.com)*. Because of my book, I was invited to serve on the editorial board of a new quarterly journal, *The Journal of Cannabis Therapeutics*, which premiered in 2001, published by Haworth Press. Unfortunately, due to the continued illegal status of cannabis, this journal was not purchased by many university libraries or individual subscriptions, and the publication ceased by 2004. I served as co-editor along with Ethan Russo, MD, and Melanie Dreher, RN, PhD, FAAN, on *Women and Cannabis: Medicine, Science and Sociology*, a double-issue that was also published as a monograph in 2002.

RAISING AWARENESS AT PROFESSIONAL CONFERENCES

In 1995, I went to the continuing education department at the University of Virginia Health System and asked if they would host a national conference on cannabis therapeutics. My proposal was considered by the administration, where it was immediately rejected. I countered with a request to limit it to a statewide nursing conference on the topic, since the 1994 VNA resolution called for the "education of Virginia Nurses on evidence-based use of cannabis." I was then informed by the director of the Continuing Education department that they wouldn't support such a conference because "it still had the same political issues." In 1996, my proposal for the 100th Anniversary Convention of the ANA to present *Therapeutic Cannabis & the Law: Ethical Dilemma for Nurses* was accepted, and in 2002 I presented "Evidence Based Support for Cannabis Therapeutics" as part of a lecture series at the ANA convention.

THE FIRST NATIONAL CLINICAL CONFERENCE ON CANNABIS THERAPEUTICS

In 1999, Dr. Dreher, who was now the Dean of the College of Nursing at the University of Iowa (and also on the board of directors for Patients Out of Time), was able to gain support to hold a national conference at the University of Iowa. *Patients Out of Time* managed the agenda and faculty. In 2000, Patients Out of Time held *The First National Clinical Conference on Cannabis Therapeutics* with the University of Iowa's Colleges of Nursing and Medicine as

co-sponsors. We had an international conference faculty that included researchers, clinical experts, patients, and patients' care providers, and the conference was teleconferenced to seven other sites. One of them was in Oregon sponsored by the Oregon Public Health Department, since their new law allowed patient use of cannabis under a physician's recommendation that was regulated by the Health Department. The Oregon Public Health Department broadcast the conference throughout its system, which led them to co-sponsor the second conference in Oregon with the Oregon Nurses Association in 2002. Since the first conference, we continue to hold biennial conferences. The audience feedback has been very positive, and the faculty has been very impressed with the "nursing" approach for the conference content.

At the third conference in 2004, co-sponsored by the University of Virginia Schools of Medicine, Nursing, and Law, we applied for and received grant funding to provide scholarships to legislators and health care professionals in leadership positions to attend the conference. Some of these scholarships went to nurses representing state nurses associations. These nurses took this information back to their leadership and had articles published in their state newsletters. Subsequently, the nurses from Illinois and Connecticut were able to get resolutions passed by their state associations, and the nurse representing the Virginia nurses convinced the association to reaffirm their support of the issue with the passage of a second resolution supporting therapeutic cannabis. Laurie Badzek, director of the ANA's Center for Ethics and Human Rights, was one of the scholarship recipients and informed me that she hoped to attend our fourth conference so she could keep ANA up-to-date on the issue. Our fourth conference was in April 2006 in Santa Barbara, California, and our fifth conference was in April 2008 in Monterey, California. Badzek presented "Nursing, Ethics and Cannabis" at the 2008 conference.

THE NEED FOR EVIDENCE

In 2001, Patients Out of Time received grant funding from John Gilmore, Preston Parish, the Zimmer Family Foundation, and the Multidisciplinary Association for Psychedelic Studies to conduct an in-depth review of the chronic effects of cannabis on four of the surviving legal medical marijuana patients. These patients offered a unique opportunity for study because they had been receiving and using a known quality and quantity of cannabis provided by the federal government. The study was led by Ethan Russo, a pediatric neurologist and expert in cannabis therapeutics, and conducted in Missoula, Montana. Study findings indicated that the patients were gaining great benefit from cannabis treatment, had been able to substantially reduce the amounts of other medications they required, and had little evidence of harmful side effects as a result of their use (Russo et al., 2002).

TAKING ON THE U.S. DRUG ENFORCEMENT ADMINISTRATION

Attempts have been made to change the federal prohibition of cannabis, and all have failed. Even the state initiatives that have been passed to allow patients to use cannabis medicinally under the recommendation of a physician have been thwarted by the federal government's prohibition. In 2002, Jon Gettman, PhD, submitted a *Petition to Reschedule Cannabis* to the U.S. Drug Enforcement Administration (DEA) on behalf of a coalition of cannabis patients. Patients Out of Time is a prominent member of that coalition and serves as the lead voice (*DrugScience.org,* 2005). The Controlled Substances Act dictates that a drug in its natural form cannot be assigned to a more restricted schedule than its active constituent (*DrugScience.org,* 2005). Synthetic THC (Marinol®) was placed in Schedule II in 1985 and was approved for use as an antiemetic and appetite stimulant. By 1999, due to a lack of diversion and its safety record, it was moved to the less restrictive Schedule III. Following the prescribed rules, whole cannabis extracts should be placed in a Schedule III or an even less restrictive category. The DEA accepted the rescheduling petition as a legitimate request and, according to protocol, passed it on to HHS for review in 2005. This review could take up to 3 years. By the fall of 2008, a response from HHS was overdue, but we felt they were stalling. Based on legal advice and the strong ideologic approach to policies by the Bush Administration, our coalition decided to wait until after the 2008 presidential election when there would be a change of leadership at HHS.

PROGRESS

The public's awareness and acceptance of therapeutic cannabis has increased over the years to 70% to 80% approval per public opinion polls (*Medical Marijuana ProCon.org,* 2005; NORML, 2005). Despite the federal prohibition, nine states and the District of Columbia have passed voter initiatives supporting patient use of therapeutic cannabis and five states that have passed similar laws through legislative action. Eric Holder, the U.S. Attorney General, issued a statement in 2009 clarifying that the federal government will no longer interfere with medical marijuana patients in states that have medical marijuana laws. President Obama made a statement in his inaugural address announcing that his administration would make policy changes based on science rather than ideology. These were viewed as initial steps toward ending the cannabis prohibition. The recent discovery of an endogenous cannabinoid system (ECS) has spawned much research. Pharmaceutical companies are now conducting research into cannabis-based products. In 2005, an oro-mucosal cannabis extract spray, Sativex®, developed by GW Pharmaceuticals in the UK, was approved as medicine in Canada. Clinical trials began in the U.S. in 2007 investigating the use of Sativex® in cancer patients suffering intractable pain unresponsive to opiate treatment. In 2004, Dr. Ethan Russo wrote an article proposing that various conditions such as migraines, fibromyalgia, and irritable bowel syndrome may actually be the result of a clinical endocannabinoid deficiency (CECD).

In April of 2010, a documentary on cannabis called "What if Cannabis Cured Cancer" premiered at the Sixth National Conference on Cannabis Therapeutics. The filmmaker, Len Richmond, worked with Patients Out of Time to gain access to some of our video footage as well as researchers. The hour-long film documents the emerging research on theECS and explains how cannabis may help prevent cancer and other diseases.

On July 22, 2010 the U.S. Department of Veterans Affairs issued a new directive (Directive 2010-035 Medical Marijuana) in which it provides guidance on access to and the use of cannabis by veterans. Veterans are allowed to use medicinal cannabis if they receive a recommendation from a civilian physician in one of the states permitting its use. The VA directive states that VA policy "does not prohibit

Veterans who use medical marijuana from participating in Veterans Health Administration substance abuse programs, pain control programs, or other clinical programs where the use of marijuana may be considered inconsistent with treatment goals" (Petzel, 2010). In a letter to the Director of the VMMA, Dr. Robert Petzel, Under Secretary of Health of Veterans Affairs stated that VA doctors should treat cannabis like "any other medication" *(www. veteransformedicalmarijuana.org).*

LOOKING AHEAD

The ECS appears to be vital to maintaining homeostasis, and with the increase in environmental toxins and processed foods, humans may need cannabis and cannabinoid medicines not only to manage symptoms and combat disease processes, but as a maintenance medication to prevent disease. This new science needs to be incorporated into the curricula for schools of nursing and disseminated to practicing nurses. Also, due to the emerging science on the endocannabinoid system, I and a small group of nurses have begun the process of creating a new specialty organization in nursing, the American Cannabis Nurses Association.

For a list of related websites, please refer to your Evolve Resources at http://evolve.elsevier.com/Mason/policypolitics/

REFERENCES

Byrne, A., & Mathre, M. L. (1992). *Marijuana as medicine* (video). Retrieved from www.medicalcannabis.com.

Dreher, M. (1997). Cannabis and pregnancy. In M. L. Mathre (Ed.), *Cannabis in medical practice: A legal, historical and pharmacological overview of the therapeutic use of marijuana*. Jefferson, NC: McFarland.

Dreher, M. C., Nugent, K., & Hudgins, R. (1994) Prenatal marijuana exposure and neonatal outcomes in Jamaica: An ethnographic study. *Pediatrics*, *93*(2), 254-260.

DrugScience.org. (2005). The Cannabis Rescheduling Petition. Retrieved from www.drugscience.org.

Joy, J. E., Watson, S. A., & Benson, Jr., J. A. (1999). *Marijuana and medicine: Assessing the science base*. Washington, D.C.: Institute of Medicine, National Academy Press.

Mathre, M. L. (1985). *Disclosure of marijuana use to health care professionals*. Unpublished master's thesis. Cleveland, OH: Case Western Reserve University.

Mathre, M. L. (1988). A survey on disclosure of marijuana use to health care professionals. *Journal of Psychoactive Drugs, 20*(1), 117-120.

Mathre, M. L. (Ed.) (1997). *Cannabis in medical practice: A legal, historical and pharmacological overview of the therapeutic use of marijuana*. Jefferson, NC: McFarland.

Mathre, M. L. (2001). Therapeutic cannabis: A patient advocacy issue. *American Journal of Nursing, 101*(4), 61-68.

Mathre, M. L. (2002, July 2). Evidence-based support for cannabis therapeutics. Part of the NOLF Lecture Series at the American Nurses Association's 2002 Biennial Convention and Exposition in Philadelphia.

Medical Marijuana ProCon.org. (2005). Voting/polling on medical marijuana: 2000 to present. Retrieved from www.medicalmarijuanaprocon.org/pop/votes2000.htm.

National Organization for the Reform of Marijuana Laws (NORML). (2005). Favorable medical marijuana polls. Retrieved from www.norml.org/index.cfm?Group_ID=3392.

Petzel, R. A. (2010). *Medical Marijuana (VHA Directive 2010-2035)*. Washington, DC: Department of Veterans Affairs, Veterans Health Administration. Retrieved from www1.va.gov/vhapublications/ViewPublication.asp?pub_ID=2276.

Randall, R. C., & O'Leary, A. M. (1998). *Marijuana Rx: The patient's fight for medicinal pot*. New York: Thunder's Mouth Press.

Russo, E. (2004). Clinical endocannabinoid deficiency (CECD): Can this concept explain therapeutic benefits of cannabis in migraine, fibromyalgia, irritable bowel syndrome, and other treatment-resistant conditions? *Neuroendocrinology Letters, 25*(1-2), 31-39.

Russo, E., Dreher, M., & Mathre, M. L. (Eds.). (2003). *Women and cannabis: Medicine, science, and sociology*. Binghamton, NY: Haworth Integrative Healing Press.

Russo, E., Mathre, M. L., Byrne, A., Velin, R., Bach, P., et al. (2002). Chronic cannabis use in the compassionate investigational new drug program: An examination of the benefits and adverse effects of legal clinical cannabis. *The Journal of Cannabis Therapeutics, 2*(1), 3-57.

Tierney, J. (2005, August 27). Marijuana pipe dreams. *New York Times*. Retrieved from www.mapinc.org/drugnews/v05/n134/a03.html?295921.

CHAPTER 46

TAKING ACTION

The Journey into the Hallowed Halls of Politics: How Nurse Practitioners Changed Pennsylvania Policy

Norma Alicea-Alvarez and Susan D. Hellier

"There is nothing more difficult to take in hand, more perilous to conduct, or more uncertain in its success, than to take the lead in the introduction of a new order of things."

—Niccolo Machiavelli

We were merely completing an assignment during the second year of our Doctor of Nursing Practice program at Waynesburg University in Pennsylvania—or so we thought. We had conducted a pilot study on a high school screening program for Chlamydia. We both had an interest in adolescent health and worked in the same county. Our professors had given us the go-ahead to work on a practicum assignment together.

THE PILOT STUDY

A literature review revealed that Chlamydia is prevalent in sexually active adolescents with rates ranging from 3% to 12.4% among 15- to 19-year-old adolescents (Wang, Burstein, & Cohen, 2002). Chlamydia is known as the silent epidemic; more than 75% of cases are asymptomatic. Up to 40% of cases that are untreated or undertreated will result in pelvic inflammatory disease with the risk of infertility, pelvic pain, ectopic pregnancy, and abscess. We also learned that the screening rate for Chlamydia in the United States was 41.6% and that Pennsylvania's was 39% (CDC, 2009). Protecting the reproductive health of young women and the prevention of sequela were the goals of our screening program.

We first had to find a school for a study site, gain approval for screening for a sexually transmitted disease (STD)—viewed as a "sensitive" topic by many parents and teachers, and arrange for an educational session for the school prior to the actual screenings. Finding a laboratory to take the samples was a challenge. Some labs charged up to $80 per sample, but after many phone calls we found one that charged $12.50.

The study site was grades 10 through 12 at the vocational high school in the rural county where we worked. Before we could walk through the doors of the school, our study had to be approved by the Institutional Review Board, the director of the high school, the principal, the school board, the teachers, the school nurse, and parents of the students who would consent to participate in the study. The process was completed with the help of our collaborating physician Dr. Carlos I. Flores and the director of the vocational school, who was also a doctoral student at a different university. We were on our way!

Grant writing was a challenge that we met both head-on and with trepidation. We found the appropriate organization and began the elaborate process of writing a grant to cover the cost of the urine screening for Chlamydia. We wrote and rewrote the grant several times. We had two conference calls with the director of the organization and our program director, and we had to defend our study, present the literature, and explain why we needed the grant. After several months, we were finally informed that due to the economy, the organization had decided not to provide funds to any applicants for the fiscal year but had they decided to give money away, we would have received it.

We entered through the doors of the high school and were handed badges from the principal's office. We presented a PowerPoint lecture about Chlamydia and its etiology, treatment, and prevention, and then we spoke about our study. This took place in the lunchroom, which doubled as the auditorium. Students were aware that parents had to consent to the study in order for them to be screened. Screening would take place by a urine sample that was sent to an independent laboratory and tested for Chlamydia. We mailed 165 consents and waited, expecting to get about 3 back. We received 51 consents! The mailbox was full each day for a week.

On 2 separate days, we went to the school and collected urine samples from the students. They provided some basic demographic information. Of the 51 girls, 2 received positive results, and we later found out that 1 was also pregnant. Parents were informed first, and then the students were informed. The adolescent girls were aware of this protocol, as it was a requirement by the school board for participating in the study.

THE CAPSTONE PROJECT

Once our pilot study was completed, we hoped that two Capstone Project ideas would emerge for our final year as doctoral students. We met again with our professor to ask for guidance, and she recommended that we work together and take the pilot study to the next level. We weren't really sure what the "next level" was, and being doctoral students she obviously wanted us to decipher her "coded" language. The Early and Periodic Screening, Diagnosis, and Treatment Program (EPSDT), a medical assistance program for children from infancy to 21 years, did not require yearly urine screening for any STD. The screening for STDs in the EPSDT program was based on symptoms. Since the majority of Chlamydia cases are asymptomatic, this was the "light-bulb moment" that acted as the springboard for the Capstone Project. We decided to change the current policy of the EPSDT program and require the state's Medicaid program to adopt a new policy that requires adolescents, regardless of sexual history, to be screened for Chlamydia.

We also wanted to disseminate information about the risks of Chlamydia to health care providers and the community.

We became educated in the legislative process and politics; policy change theories; and orchestrating the collaboration of politicians, colleagues, and the community to influence patient care outcomes. We used Kingdon's Agenda Setting Theory to ground our policy aims in theory. Kingdon's Theory seeks to develop structure for successful policy change and explain the political factors that influence legislative action and how an advocate of a cause can bring attention to a societal problem.

Our pilot study metamorphosed into a Capstone Project with three aims: (1) a policy change to increase Chlamydia screening for 15- to 21-year-old adolescents enrolled in a Medicaid program, (2) the support of House Bill 1163: The Healthy Youth Act (making all public high schools teach a comprehensive sex education class), and (3) the institution of Chlamydia Awareness Day in Pennsylvania to bring attention to the disease (Figure 46-1).

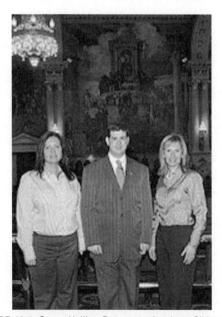

FIGURE 46-1 Susan Hellier, Representative Jaret Gibbons, and Norma Alicea-Alvarez in the Pennsylvania House of Representatives on the day they were recognized by the House and Chlamydia Awareness Day was voted upon.

THE POLITICAL ARENA

To accomplish these aims, we collected over 300 signatures from health care providers supporting the policy change and shared them with legislators as a reflection of what their constituents wanted. Over the course of several months, we gained invaluable legislative experience and knowledge of the legislative process through the one-on-one meetings with each state legislator.

Our first meeting was especially successful as we spearheaded the process of instituting Chlamydia Awareness Day in Pennsylvania by acquiring the support of Representative Jaret Gibbons. We were required to write a resolution, which was to be presented to the House of Representatives. This was also a new undertaking for us, as the resolution requires a very specific format. We were asked to choose a date for Chlamydia Awareness Day, and we chose February 11, 2010, since it was close to Valentine's Day and Cupid was aiming his arrows.

We were thrilled when Representative Gibbons informed us that we had been invited to the House floor to be recognized for our research and advocacy work. The resolution was introduced to the House of Representatives in Harrisburg as HR 582. On February 8, 2010, Representative Charelle Parker read the resolution. She made quite an impact as the statistics were revealed. It was a surreal experience as we heard our research and resolution echo from the microphone. As Representative Gibbons introduced us separately, we each stood in front of the entire House and the Speaker of the House. All 194 representatives voted "yes," and February 11, 2010, was declared the first Chlamydia Awareness Day in Pennsylvania.

The overall metrics of implementing a policy change in EPSDT for inclusion of Chlamydia screening was more challenging. With the help and support of the executive director of the Pennsylvania Coalition of Nurse Practitioners (PCNP), we met with Dr. David K. Kelley, the Chief Medical Officer of the Office of Medical Assistance Program in Pennsylvania. He fully supported our evidence regarding the need to change the current policy to include yearly screening for Chlamydia and offered to present our research and proposal to the EPSDT Task Force Committee later that month. We also offered our assistance and presence at this meeting.

Susan Schrand, executive director of PCNP, wrote a letter on behalf of the PCNP stating the organization's full support of the inclusion of yearly urine screenings to augment the EPSDT program. She specifically addressed our research, which supported the policy change, the proposal, Chlamydia Awareness Day, and our advocacy work.

One of our doctoral committee members, Dr. Carlos Flores, is a delegate of the Pennsylvania Medical Society (PMS) and recommended that we present our research to the group in the form of the resolution previously written to gain support for improved Chlamydia screening. The regional representatives of the PMS were in full support of the inclusion of yearly urine Chlamydia screening for adolescents enrolled in a Medicaid program. However, due to timing, the resolution could not be included in the agenda at the meeting of the society. The PMS representative encouraged resubmission of the resolution as part of next year's agenda.

Despite having the full support of legislators, the CMO of the Office of Medical Assistance Program of Pennsylvania, and PCNP, the Department of Public Welfare stated that the intervals of screening currently in place were based on guidelines from the American Academy of Pediatrics (AAP). They conducted discussions with representatives of the Pennsylvania AAP and the national AAP. They concluded that at the time the AAP did not recommend that all women be screened for Chlamydia. Our literature review and pilot study provided the evidence, which supports the screening of all female adolescents regardless of sexual activity. Also, the literature supports age-based screening because most cases of Chlamydia are asymptomatic. Untreated cases can result in serious reproductive organ sequela to young women who are unaware they are infected. Therefore, we do not agree with the current guidelines provided by the AAP, as many cases of Chlamydia among female adolescents and young women are currently missed and will continue to be missed.

Our Capstone Project has laid the groundwork for ongoing research on screening for Chlamydia among asymptomatic women. As researchers and advocates of this cause, we will continue to present evidence and conduct clinical research that supports effective intervention and improved health care outcomes. We will continue to develop our political knowledge and skill, as well. We were recipients of The Nurses In Washington Internship grant awarded by the National Association of Pediatric Nurse Practitioners (NAPNAP), which supported our attendance at a conference in Washington D.C. to learn more about the legislative, political, and economic forces driving health care policy. The Grassroots Advocacy Award is given by NAPNAP in recognition of sustained effort in advocacy in the area of child health policy at the local, state, or national level. We received the award at the National NAPNAP Conference in 2010.

For a list of related websites, please refer to your Evolve Resources at http://evolve.elsevier.com/Mason/policypolitics/

REFERENCES

Centers for Disease Control and Prevention. (2009, April 17). Chlamydia screening among sexually active young female enrollees of health plans—United States, 2000-2007. Retrieved from www.cdc.gov/mmwr/preview/mmwr html/mm5814a2.htm?s_cid=mm5814a2_e.

Wang, L., Burstein, G., & Cohen, D. (2002). An economic evaluation of a school-based sexually transmitted disease program. *Sexually Transmitted Diseases, 29*(12), 737-745.

CHAPTER 47

Policy and Politics in the Contemporary Work Environment

Pamela Thompson, Laura Caramanica, Elaine Cohen, Patricia Reid Ponte, and Rose Sherman

"Far and away the best prize that life offers is the chance to work hard at work worth doing."

—Theodore Roosevelt

The most important contemporary issues in the health care workplace are ultimately related to the ability of the health care system and practitioners to provide high-quality and safe care. There are several key elements that capture the essence of these issues. First, the drivers that demonstrate how we know we are providing safe and high-quality care are the measurable outcomes. Second, the delivery of consistent and sustainable quality outcomes is dependent on the performance of the health care team. Third, technology is quickly becoming a critical element that can support the health care team to achieve the desired outcomes. Finally, all of these issues come together when we consider the financial implications of providing quality care.

This chapter will explore some of the major policy issues in the workplace related to these key elements. Who decides what "quality" is and how it is done? How do we create and maintain environments that support high-reliability teams? How is nursing engaged in the deployment of technology? And how do we blend the control of cost by expenditure reduction with the ethics of delivering appropriate care?

ASSURING QUALITY, SAFETY, AND RELIABILITY

AGENCIES LEADING QUALITY AND SAFETY EFFORTS

Quality and safety in health care have emerged as a key focus of consumer attention since the Institute of Medicine (IOM) reports about medical errors (2000, 2001, 2004) drew attention to medication error rates and prevention, patient safety, and quality. In the wake of these events, local and national regulatory agencies, insurers, health plans, and state and federal payers such as The Joint Commission (TJC), the Center for Medicare and Medicaid Services, and Blue Cross & Blue Shield have set new quality and safety standards. The goal of these standards is to assure positive patient outcomes by guiding providers, clinicians, and organizational performance. National quality and safety associations, funding agencies, and discipline-specific boards and agencies, such as the National Quality Forum (NQF), the National Patient Safety Foundation, the American Organization of Nurse Executives (AONE), the Agency for Healthcare Research and Quality (AHRQ), the American Medical Association (AMA), the American Nurses Association (ANA), and, most recently, the National Alliance for Nursing Quality and Safety (NQSF), have committed their constituencies to develop new knowledge and disseminate evidenced-based best practices in quality, safety, and patient outcomes (Kurtzman, 2009).

Quality and safety have also become a focus for organizations dedicated to educating clinicians. Academic institutions are beginning to integrate quality and safety topics into undergraduate curriculums using the content identified by the Quality and Safety Education for Nurses (QSEN) project (QSEN, 2010). Continuing education for current providers has also been addressed. Organizations such as the Institute for Health Improvement and Intermountain Health Care, whose missions include the development and teaching of best practices for effective, efficient, patient-centered, equitable, safe, and timely care delivery, have developed state-of-the-art provider- and clinician-directed training programs (IOM, 2001). These programs use the fundamental and foundational work of early industrial engineers such as Shewhart (1938), Deming (1982, 1986), and Juran (1951), and the groundbreaking health quality work of Donabedian (1980, 1982, 1985). These individuals developed theory and content on waste and variation reduction related to structure, process, and outcomes that were first applied to industry and later to health care services. General Electric's Six Sigma program (General Electric, 2009) and Toyota's Lean program (Liker, 2004) are examples of their application in industry.

AWARD PROGRAMS

Additionally, award programs for excellence in organizational performance have embraced measures and criteria related to quality and safety as core requirements for recognition. Examples of such award programs include the American Nurses Credentialing Center's Magnet Recognition Program (American Nurses Credentialing Center, 2010), the American Association of Critical Care Nurses' Beacon Award (American Association of Critical Care Nurses, 2009), and the Baldrige National Quality Program's Malcolm Baldrige National Quality Award (National Institute of Standards and Technology, 2010). Finally, consumer organizations such as the AARP and the Institute for Family-Centered Care have begun to provide strong coalitions of patients, families, and citizens that demand a voice in assuring quality and safety in health care organizations.

All of these factors have set the stage for a highly interactive and inclusive culture that places quality and safety at the highest level of value during a decade fraught with commensurate increases in the cost of care. Consumers understand and want the safest and highest-quality care and related outcomes. Providers, clinicians, health organizations, insurers, and government want to deliver this high-quality care. However, the costs of care continue to soar due to inefficiencies, heavy administrative cost structures, and high numbers of uninsured Americans. This will require complex changes in policy and health care delivery processes.

On March 23, 2010, President Barack Obama signed into law the Affordable Care Act (ACA). This reform bill is the largest change to the health care system since the creation of Medicare and Medicaid. The bill addresses coverage, insurance reform, key delivery system reforms, workforce education, wellness and prevention, and payment reform. Cost and quality are key components in most aspects of the legislation. Implementation of all of the elements in the legislation will not take place until 2014, but it is clear that there will be significant and profound changes over the coming years.

HEALTH CARE TEAMS: COMMUNICATION AND PATIENT SAFETY

The second organizing concept to assure the attainment of meaningful and healthy patient outcomes involves coordination: among patient, family, and health care providers; between patient and caregiver; between nurse and physician, and among every member of the interdisciplinary team. The importance of forging these relationships is the basis of the IOM 2001 report, *Crossing the Quality Chasm: A New Health System for the 21st Century,* which focuses on the value that teamwork, collaboration, and effective communication have on positive patient outcomes. National efforts to put into operation the IOM aims of safe, timely, effective, efficient, and equitable care have resulted in a powerful partnership with the Robert Wood Johnson Foundation and the Institute for Healthcare Improvement (IHI) to improve hospital work environments. Their joint involvement led to the development of the Transforming Care at the Bedside (TCAB) model, which includes four elements: Safe and Reliable Care; Vitality and Teamwork; Patient-Centered Care; and Value-Added Care Processes (Rutherford et al., 2004, 2008) (see Chapter 54). The American Organization of Nurse Executives (AONE) has made TCAB a major initiative and added nurse manager leadership development, shared decision making, and nurse ownership of practice as additional key design themes.

Recognizing the importance of communicating accurate information to meet patient safety goals, TJC 2009 National Patient Safety Goals recommend developing a standardized approach to multiple types of "hand-off" communication (TJC, 2008a). Through their Nurse Manager Fellowship, AONE laid the foundation for the importance of collaboration and communication on a broader level (AONE 2008).

BOX 47-1 **Communication Methodologies**

SBAR: The use of a standard communication formula of describing the *S*ituation, *B*ackground of situation, *A*ssessment of what is happening, and *R*ecommendation for what is needed to address the situation. Following the SBAR streamlines clinician dialogue around patient care.

Intentional Rounding: Patient rounding to explore safety issues by asking staff if they see any issues that relate to safety.

Safety Huddles: Unit staff meeting for short sessions on a routine basis to discuss safety issues that have been observed.

Various academic partnerships use the principles of TCAB in their curriculum (AHRQ/TeamSTEPPS, 2007) to engage students to promote safe and reliable care. Various communication methodologies aimed at improving the safety of patients are being used in the clinical environments (Box 47-1). These are examples of promoting and ensuring connectedness and coordination of care, good communication, and positive patient outcomes.

TEAMWORK AND TEAM TRAINING

Hamman (2004) demonstrated that team training is an effective tool to improve operational performance of team members. Team training is a complex set of processes that requires an organizational commitment. Organizations must provide skill building and agreement by team leaders and members to be successful. Those that do are more likely to improve care delivery processes and outcomes.

The team training models in health care have arisen from the aviation experience with teamwork measurement aimed at preventing and mitigating error. The training approach draws on early educational theory and involves the systemic acquisition of *knowledge* (what we think), *skills* (what we do), and *attitudes* (what we feel)—known as "KSAs"—and leads to ideally improved performance. Cronenwett, Sherwood, and Gelmon (2009) used this approach in their framework for developing undergraduate nursing curriculum for quality and safety, in which interdisciplinary teamwork and collaboration are major components.

Team training approaches often include a method for task analysis of the team's work within the given practice, the development of behavioral standards and expectations related to closed-loop communication and decision-making approaches and parameters, practice tools that help facilitate standardized processes of communication, mechanisms for ongoing team maintenance, and team building and team development (QSEN, 2010). Team training approaches consist of simulation exercises and the development or use of standardized measures of team effectiveness. These measures or markers may consist of team process attributes such as (1) information sharing; (2) inquiry; (3) assertion; (4) intentions shared; (5) teaching; (6) evaluation of plans; (7) workload management; (8) vigilance/environmental/situational awareness; (9) teamwork overall; and (10) leadership (Thomas, Sexton, and Helmrich, 2004; Burke, Salas, Wilson-Donnelly, & Priest, 2004; Hamman, 2004).

IMPACT ON POLICY

The development and implementation of these initiatives all beg the overarching policy question of how we incentivize the creation of a practice environment that ensures safe, effective, reliable, and equitable patient care. A culture that supports collaborative working environments through interprofessional communication and teamwork prohibits behaviors, including lateral violence, that endanger the safety of the patient and health care team alike. Through sponsorship by the American Association of Critical Care Nurses, Vital Smarts and Crucial Conversations, a nationwide study was conducted that demonstrated how essential interpersonal communication is among health care teams to ensure patient safety and quality of care. The authors of this work, entitled *Silence Kills,* defined seven elements that are challenging to talk about but if handled well can potentially decrease errors, improve patient safety and quality of care, increase staff satisfaction and productivity, and sustain healthy work environments (Maxfield, Grenny, McMillan, Patterson, & Switzler, 2005) (Box 47-2).

These types of situations have shown to build staff resentment and complacency, which eventually leads to poor patient outcomes. The importance of developing effective and good care teams cannot be overstated. The opposite can lead to erosion of trust in the integrity of the professionals involved, distrust in the delivery of appropriate patient care, and job turnover (see Chapter 56).

Creating organizational cultures that support healthy and safe work environments where individuals are comfortable speaking up and expressing their

---

BOX 47-2 Silence Kills: The Seven Elements

1. *Broken Rules:* Team members taking shortcuts in their clinical care processes that may put the patient in jeopardy (e.g., not following evidence-based policies and procedures)
2. *Mistakes:* Colleagues showing poor clinical judgment (e.g., missing vital information during patient assessments)
3. *Lack of Support:* Staff refusing to assist team members in care delivery or when team members ask for needed assistance
4. *Incompetence:* Colleagues expressing concerns regarding their fellow team members' ability to carry out their care responsibilities resulting in harm to the patient
5. *Poor Teamwork:* Team members engaging in splitting behaviors, thereby eroding the foundation of the team itself (e.g., a team member refusing to take his or her share of the workload)
6. *Disrespect:* Staff who display rude and condescending behavior toward one another
7. *Micromanagement:* Team members who abuse their authority and bully others into providing care that may not be correct for the patient or family

From Maxfield, D., Grenny, J., McMillan, R., Patterson, K., & Switzler, A. (2005). Silence kills: The seven crucial conversations for healthcare. VitalSmarts, L.C. Retrieved from *www.silencekills.com*.

BOX 47-3 Silence Kills: Recommendations

1. Gain full organization-wide support and engagement so that health care team members will have the ability to become comfortable with challenging interpersonal communication (American Association of Critical Care Nurses, 2005).
2. Conduct focus groups and surveys to establish baseline data for outcome measurement and to identify barriers to communication at all levels of the organization.
3. Take an active role in teaching, training, and mentoring staff in interprofessional communication and assisting with improvement opportunities.

From Maxfield, D., Grenny, J., McMillan, R., Patterson, K., & Switzler, A. (2005). Silence kills: The seven crucial conversations for healthcare. VitalSmarts, L.C. Retrieved from *www.silencekills.com*.

---

concerns is indeed possible and vital for patient safety. When the conversation is about poor teamwork, the concomitant results of team members who are able to confront their colleagues is higher morale, more efficient work processes (decreased workarounds), positive work environments, and more unit/service/team loyalty (Maxfield et al, 2005). Recommendations from this study identify several ways to address our policy question in the beginning of this segment (Box 47-3).

LEVERAGING TECHNOLOGY

Recent technological advances have the potential to improve patient safety, enhance quality outcomes, and reduce workload demands. Examples include electronic documentation systems with the capability to capture information from other systems such as the laboratory and pharmacy, and equipment, such as cardiac monitors and intravenous smart pumps. Despite the availability of advanced technology, which could be leveraged to improve care, health care organizations have lagged behind other industries in the implementation of information technologies. Recent health reform policy discussions at the national level have focused on the slow implementation of information systems and a lack of interconnectedness, which has resulted in considerable information duplication and unnecessary health care expenditures. As part of the American Recovery and Reinvestment Act passed in 2009, $20 billion was allocated to aid in the development of a robust and integrated IT infrastructure for health care and to assist providers and other entities in adopting and using IT (Health Information Management Systems Society [HIMSS], 2009). Beginning in 2010, this bill also contains provisions to establish incentive payments through Medicare for the meaningful use of certified electronic health record technology by eligible professionals and hospitals (HIMSS, 2009). It is hoped that reimbursement by Medicare will assist hospitals that are financially challenged to make technology investments and convert systems that demonstrate leverage potential.

OPPORTUNITIES FOR IMPROVEMENT

There are many opportunities in the current system to improve care with updated technology. Inpatient medication management is an example of a complex process with multiple handoffs involving different departments. There is a potential for error at any stage in the process. Medication bar coding, pioneered by the Department of Veterans Affairs on a national level, has resulted in a decrease in the number of incorrect medication administrations at the point of care. Software called *electronic medication administration (eMAR)* with bar coding has now been implemented in 23% of hospitals nationwide, while more than 50% of the remaining hospitals plan to implement it in 3 years (Turisco & Rhodes, 2008). Organizations such as the Leapfrog Group and the IOM have strongly advocated the adoption of computerized physician order entry (CPOE) as an avenue to decrease medical errors. Movement toward CPOE on a national level has been slow as organizations evaluate the best practice strategies to implement this transformational technology.

Breakdown in communication plays a significant role in sentinel events (TJC, 2008a) and has the potential to be avoided with updated technology. Typically, nurses use multiple modes of communication, many of which are fixed devices, whereas nurses are mobile. Voice over Internet Protocol (VoIP) technologies that tap into the hospital's wireless network have been implemented in some medical centers and allow for point-to-point communication and connectivity with communication systems and medical equipment (Turisco & Rhodes, 2008). In busy patient care environments, locating providers and necessary equipment can be time-consuming. An increasing number of hospitals now use real-time location systems (RTLS) that use radio frequency identification (RFID) technology to locate equipment, patients, and staff. Robots, which have a long track record of working well in pharmacies and laboratories, are now being piloted as delivery assistants for nursing in some settings (California Health Care Foundation, 2008). Remote intensive care management, better known as the tele-ICU, is a growing trend in the nation's hospitals, which struggle to improve care in ICUs while coping with a severe shortage of intensive care medical specialists. Studies done with patients who are hospitalized in tele-ICUs have found a decline in mortality and length of stay in ICUs where bedside care is supplemented by remote monitoring, but the cost-benefit of these expensive systems has not been studied (Sapirstein, Lone, Latif, Fackler, & Pronovost, 2009).

THE ROLE OF NURSING

The future work of nurses will be in a high-technology environment. Parker (2005) predicted that we are at the dawn of the digital hospital. Integrated electronic health records, telehealth, robotics, "cyber" home visits, and smart equipment with decision support will be commonplace. There is great potential with technology to better leverage the scarce resources available in the health care delivery system today, but there are caveats. The Joint Commission outlined the guiding principles for the hospital of the future. Nurse leaders were urged to recognize that the sheer volume of new technologies has made health care more complex and often presents unforeseen opportunities for error (TJC, 2008b).

A key policy question is the role of nursing in the design and deployment of technology in the clinical setting. Leaders in the Alliance for Nursing Informatics (Fortner, 2009) have advised that the electronic health record must support the delivery of nursing care and patient information exchange wherever nurses work and patients receive nursing care. Nurse leaders play a critical role in the selection, evaluation, and implementation of information systems to ensure that the systems support and leverage the work of nursing. The AONE has assumed a key role in the discussion with the development of guiding principles to define the role of the nurse executive in technology acquisition (AONE, 2007). Guidance is provided for all phases of the process including pre-acquisition, acquisition, contract negotiations, implementation, and evaluating the return on investment. With the rapid changes in technology, nurse executives and other nurse leaders need to consider the policy implications of technology implementation and stay informed about state and national policy initiatives related to technological advances.

BALANCING FINANCIAL CONSIDERATIONS WITH QUALITY

The 2010 ACA expanded support for clinical effectiveness and strengthened primary care by advocating for the use of interdisciplinary care teams and medical homes. This act identified measurements for quality outcomes and aligned fiscal incentives among providers, health care organizations, insurers, and employers. The basis for this radical shift will be assuring high-quality, effective, equitable, timely, efficient, and safe patient- and family-centered care (IOM, 2001). This new focus on primary care will be significant for

Advanced Practice Registered Nurses (APRNs). There is a growing shortage of primary care physicians, and it is predicted that there will not be enough to care for the millions of individuals who will have coverage in the future. Certainly, coverage does not ensure access, and APRNs will be in high demand to meet this increased demand for primary care providers.

The Center for Medicare and Medicaid Services (CMS) has collaborated with a wide range of public and private agencies and organizations with a common goal of improving health care quality and decreasing unnecessary costs. Many pay-for-performance initiatives that are currently being piloted or that exist in the new legislation for future piloting seek to determine if they are reliable methodologies for measurement and reporting of quality care. For instance, a pilot program is currently underway to test a population-based model of disease management in which participating organizations are paid a monthly fee per beneficiary to manage a population of chronically ill beneficiaries with advance congestive heart failure and/or complex diabetes. The disease management groups and insurance companies must guarantee the CMS a savings of the monthly fees compared to similar populations of beneficiaries (Cromwell, McCall, & Burton, 2008).

There is a widespread support by providers, insurers, employers, and advocacy groups to provide consumers with information about the quality of health care that they seek. Quality reports include consumer ratings, clinical performance measures, or both. These reports are available through employers, health plans, hospitals, nursing homes, and community health clinics.

The intense interest in aligning payment with performance has significant implications for providers. We know that health care outcomes are linked to the practice of nursing. To the extent that research continues to link nursing practices, staffing, and other characteristics (e.g., number of hours staff work or their educational preparation) to the quality of patient care outcomes, the transparency and contribution of nursing to health care will be made evident.

There is concern by many that consumers will not be able to discern the complexity of reporting performance measures. Health care delivery is still fragmented; performance still varies widely, and data is not always organized in a way that the layperson understands. CMS is leading the way to define pay for performance as "the use of payment methods and other incentives to encourage quality improvement and patient focused high value care" (Lanos, Rothstein, Dyer, & Bailit, 2007).

Through the 2010 ACA, the United States will expand health care to more than 31 million people. The regulations will outline the details about how this will happen. Determining how we will blend cost control by expenditure reduction with the ethics of delivering appropriate care will be critical as the regulations are developed (Fogoros, 2008).

SUMMARY

It is reassuring that contemporary health care policy is aligning with the quality and safety of the care provided to patients and families. These elements have long been foundational to nursing practice. However, the congressional partisanship and lack of collaboration continues to be a barrier to progress. It is essential that health care advocates keep a keen focus on the key elements outlined in this chapter. Quality and safety are deemed present when care is measured by standardized metrics that are linked to desired outcomes. These outcomes are directly linked to the health care team that plans, delivers, and evaluates the care. Creating the environments that support these highly reliable teams is critical. These teams require training to gain the skills that produce the best outcomes. The role of leadership at all levels cannot be underestimated in achieving these goals. Although the health care environment is extraordinarily complex, there are important leverage points that can dramatically increase system capacity for safety-technology being one of the key levers. All of this must fit within a new financial reality of limited resources and changing payment systems. Learning to operate with less while striving to achieve optimal quality will be an ongoing challenge. The need to balance the ethical delivery of care with ever-increasing financial constraints will be a significant challenge in the future. It will best serve all consumers of health care if we create the cultures in our work environment that will assure that safety and quality are the foundation.

For a list of related websites, please refer to your Evolve Resources at http://evolve.elsevier.com/Mason/policypolitics/

REFERENCES

Agency for Healthcare Research and Quality. (n.d.). *Quality and patient safety.* Retrieved from www.ahrq.gov/qual.

Agency for Healthcare Research and Quality. (2007). *TeamSTEPPS curriculum tools and materials.* Instructor Guide. Rockville, MD.

American Association of Critical Care Nurses. (2005). *AACN Standards for establishing and sustaining healthy work environments: A journey to excellence.* Retrieved from www.aacn.org/WD/HWE/Docs/HWEStandards.pdf.

American Association of Critical Care Nurses. (2009). *Welcome to the Beacon Award for critical care excellence.* Retrieved from www.aacn.org/wd/beaconapps/content/mainpage.pcms?menu=beaconapps.

American Medical Association. (2010). *Advocacy.* Retrieved from www.ama-assn.org/ama/pub/advocacy.shtml.

American Nurses Association. (2009). *National database of nursing quality indicators.* Retrieved from www.nursingquality.org.

American Nurses Association. (2010). *Patient safety & nursing quality.* Retrieved from http://nursingworld.org/MainMenuCategories/ThePracticeofProfessionalNursing/PatientSafetyQuality.aspx.

American Nurses Credentialing Center. (2010). ANCC Magnet Recognition Program. Retrieved from www.nursecredentialing.org/Magnet.aspx.

American Organization of Nurse Executives. AONE and the Robert Wood Johnson Foundation. (2008). Partnering to disseminate Transforming Care at the Bedside (TCAB). Retrieved from www.aone.org/aone_app/aonetcab/index.jsp.

American Organization of Nurse Executives. (2007). AONE guiding principles for defining the role of the nurse executive in technology acquisition and implementation. Retrieved from www.aone.org.

Blue Cross Blue Shield Association. (2009). *Blue distinction.* Retrieved from www.bcbs.com/innovations/bluedistinction.

Burke, C. S., Salas, E., Wilson-Donnelly, K., & Priest, H. (2004). How to turn a team of experts into an expert medical team: Guidance from the aviation and military communities. *Quality and Safety in Health Care, 13*(Suppl 1), i86-i104.

California Health Care Foundation. (2008, December). Equipped for efficiency: Improving nursing care through technology. Retrieved from www.chct.org/topics/view.cfm?itemID=133816.

Center for Medicare and Medicaid Services. (2009). *Quality of care center.* Retrieved from www.cms.hhs.gov/center/quality.asp.

Cronenwett, L., Sherwood, G., & Gelmon, S. B. (2009). Improving quality and safety education: the QSEN learning collaborative. *Nursing Outlook, 57*(6), 304-312.

Cromwell, J., McCall, N., & Burton, J. (Fall 2008). Evaluation of Medicare Health Support Chronic Disease Pilot Program. *Healthcare Financing Review, 3*(1), 47-60.

Deming, W. E. (1982). *Quality productivity and competitive position.* Cambridge, MA: MIT Press.

Deming, W. E. (1986). *Out of the crisis.* Cambridge, MA: MIT Press.

Donabedian, A. (1980). *Explorations in quality assessment and monitoring, Volume I: The definition of quality and approaches to its assessment.* Ann Arbor, MI: Health Administration Press.

Donabedian, A. (1982). *Explorations in quality assessment and monitoring, Volume II: The criteria and standards of quality.* Ann Arbor, MI: Health Administration Press.

Donabedian, A. (1985). *Explorations in quality assessment and monitoring, Volume III: The methods and findings of quality assessment and monitoring: An illustrated analysis.* Ann Arbor, MI: Health Administration Press.

Fogoros, R. (2008, June 11). *The right way to think about medical ethics* (weblog post). Retrieved from http://covertrationingblog.com/medical-ethics/the-right-way-to-think-about-medical-ethics.

Fortner, P. (2009, December 15). Nurses claim their seat at the Health IT decision-making table. *iHealthBeat.* Retrieved from www.allianceni.org.

General Electric. (2009). *What is six sigma?* Retrieved from www.ge.com/en/company/companyinfo/quality/whatis.html.

Hamman, W. R. (2004). The complexity of team training: What we have learned from aviation and it applications to medicine. *Quality and Safety in Health Care, 13*(Suppl 1), i72-i79.

Health Information Management Systems Society. (2009, July 1). The American recovery and reinvestment act of 2009: Summary of key health technology provisions. Retrieved from www.himss.org/content/files/HIMSS_SummaryOfARRA.pdf.

Institute for Family-Centered Care. (2010). *Institute for Family-Centered Care: About us.* Retrieved from www.familycenteredcare.org/about/index.html.

Institute for Healthcare Improvement. (n.d.). *About us.* Retrieved from www.ihi.org/ihi/about.

Institute of Medicine. (2004). *Keeping patients safe: Transforming the work environment of nurses.* Washington, D.C.: National Academies Press.

Institute of Medicine. (2001). *Crossing the quality chasm: A new health system for the 21st century.* Washington, D.C.: National Academies Press.

Institute of Medicine. (2000). *To err is human: Building a safer health system.* Washington, D.C.: National Academies Press.

Institute of Medicine, Committee on Quality of Health Care in America. (2001). *Crossing the quality chasm: A new health system for the 21st century.* Washington, D.C.: National Academies Press. Retrieved from www.nap.edu/books/0309072808/html.

The Joint Commission. (2008a). 2009 *National patient safety goals—Hospital program.* Oakbrook Terrace, IL. Retrieved from www.jointcommission.org?PatientSafety/NationalPatientSafetyGoals/09_hap_npsgs.htm.

The Joint Commission. (2008b). *Health care at the crossroads: Guiding principles for development of the hospital of the future.* Retrieved from www.jointcommission.org/NR/rdonlyres/1C9A7079-7A29-4658-B80D-A7DF8771309B/0/Hosptal_Future.pdf.

The Joint Commission. (2010). *Patient safety.* Retrieved January from www.jointcommission.org/PatientSafety.

Juran, J. M. (1951). *Quality control handbook.* New York: McGraw-Hill.

Kurtzman, E. T. (2009). Planning a National Nursing Quality and Safety Alliance: Strengthening nursing's policy voice. *Journal of Nursing Administration, 39*(2), 47-50.

Lanos, K., Rothstein, J., Dyer, M. B., & Bailit, M. (2007, March). Physician pay-for-performance in Medicaid: A guide for states. Retrieved from www.chcs.org/usr_doc/Physician_P4P_Guide.pdf.

The Leapfrog Group. (2008). The *Leapfrog Group: Informing choices, rewarding excellence.* Retrieved from www.leapfroggroup.org.

Liker, J. (2004). *The Toyota way.* New York: McGraw-Hill.

Maxfield, D., Grenny, J., McMillan, R., Patterson, K., & Switzler, A. (2005). *Silence kills: The seven crucial conversations for healthcare.* VitalSmarts, L.C. Retrieved from www.silencekills.com.

National Institute of Standards and Technology. (2010). *Baldrige National Quality Program.* Retrieved from www.baldrige.nist.gov.

Parker, P. J. (2005) Technology in the crystal ball. *Nursing Administration Quarterly, 29*(2), 123-124.

Quality and Safety Education for Nurses. (2010). *About QSEN.* Retrieved from www.qsen.org/about_qsen.php.

Robert Wood Johnson Foundation. (2009). *Aligning forces for quality (AF4Q).* Retrieved from www.forces4quality.org.

Rutherford, P., Lee, B., & Greiner, A. (2004). *Transforming care at the bedside.* Cambridge, MA: Institute for Healthcare Improvement. IHI Innovation Series white paper. Retrieved from www.ihi.org/IHI/Results/WhitePapers/TransformingCareattheBedsideWhitePaper.htm.

Rutherford, P., Phillips J., Coughlan P., Lee, B., Moen, R., et al. (2008). *Transforming care at the bedside. How-to guide: Engaging front-line staff in innovation and quality improvement.* Cambridge, MA: Institute for Healthcare Improvement.

Sapirstein, A., Lone, N., Latif, A., Fackler, J., & Pronovost, P. J. (2009). Tele ICU: Paradox or panacea? *Best Practices & Research Clinical Anaesthesiology, 23*(1), 115-126.

Shewhart, W. A. (1938). *Application of statistical methods to manufacturing problems.* Murray Hill, NJ: Bell Telephone Laboratories.

Thomas, E. J., Sexton, J. B., & Helmrich, R. I. (2004). Translating teamwork behaviors from aviation to healthcare: Development of behavioral marker for neonatal resuscitation. *Quality and Safety in Health Care, 13*(Suppl 1), i57-i64.

Turisco, F., & Rhodes, J. (2008) *Equipped for efficiency: Improving nursing care through technology.* (Report). California Healthcare Foundation. Retrieved from www.chcf.org/topics/view.cfm?itemID=133816.

CHAPTER 48

Quality and Safety in Health Care: Policy Issues

Ellen T. Kurtzman and Jean E. Johnson

"If a physician make a large incision with an operating knife and cure it…he shall receive ten shekels in money. …If a physician make a large incision with the operating knife, and kill him…his hands shall be cut off."

—Code of Hammurabi, Code of Laws, No. 215, 218; ca 1760 BC

Beginning in the 1990s, the public was besieged with accounts of the United States health system's failures. Landmark reports including the President's Advisory Commission on Consumer Protection and Quality in the Health Care Industry, *Quality First: Better Health Care for All Americans* (1998), and the Institute of Medicine (IOM), *Health in Transition: Protecting and Improving Quality* (1994), along with media accounts of preventable mistakes (Millenson, 1997; Gibson & Singh, 2003) resulted in a greater awareness among consumers of the prevalence of medical errors and the significant gaps in quality. These accounts were closely followed by the media's sensationalism of health care's woes (Knox, 1995; Berens, 2002). Subsequent and ongoing reports of escalating cost (*The High Cost of Health Care,* 2007)—an increasing investment by the United States and by consumers for mediocre results—caused a public outcry.

In the decade after these events, problems continue to plague the best resourced and technologically advanced health care system in the world. While some of the sensation has dulled, reports continue to portray a system in chaos. IOM reports (Kohn, Corrigan, & Donaldson, 2000; IOM, 2001) have described the U.S. health care system as one that "…harms too frequently and routinely fails to deliver its potential benefits" (IOM, 2001, p. 1). Although some progress has been made, health care continues to be suboptimal, inconsistent, and error-prone in every setting and for all patients.

Annual reports issued by the Agency for Healthcare Research and Quality ([AHRQ] 2009a, 2009b), The Joint Commission (TJC) (2008), and the Commonwealth Fund (2008) reveal only modest improvements among certain populations and clinical conditions. In some cases, outcomes are actually worsening. McGlynn and colleagues (2003) discovered, for example, that among adults receiving care for the most common chronic conditions including asthma, breast cancer, diabetes, and lower back pain, nearly half fail to receive basic recommended care. Dismal performance exists among a handful of the ranking conditions, with adult patients receiving only 11%, 23%, and 25% of recommended care for alcohol dependence, hip fractures, and atrial fibrillation, respectively. For those who are most vulnerable—children and older adults—care is marginal. Fewer than 50% of children (Mangione-Smith, et al., 2007) and 52% of older adults (Asch, et al., 2006) receive recommended care. Alarmingly, quality lapses persist among patients in long-term care settings including nursing homes, home health care agencies, and hospices (AHRQ, 2009b).

This chapter will review a decade of federal policymaking intended to address health care value with a particular focus on the implications for nurses and the nursing profession. We will describe the critical factors above and beyond the inadequacies in quality that have contributed to the current political context, and we will discuss key organizations involved in the quality enterprise and their contributions. We will also provide examples that include Medicare's hospital-acquired conditions rule and the emergence of public-private partnerships such as the Nursing Alliance for Quality Care (NAQC).

THE ENVIRONMENTAL CONTEXT

While ongoing underperformance has garnered the attention of consumers, providers, policymakers, and payers, there are other environmental influences that have motivated and enabled a 10-year stretch of policy setting. Most notably, shortfalls in quality have been accompanied by a growing, excessive investment in the health care system—more than $2.3 trillion and an estimated 16.2% of the gross domestic product (GDP) in 2008, up from 15.9% in 2007 (Hartman, Martin, Nunccio, Catlin, and the National Health Expenditures Account Team, 2010). By 2018, analysts estimate that health care spending in the U.S. is expected to nearly double from current levels, reaching $4.3 trillion and consuming 20.3% of the nation's GDP (Sisko et al., 2009). Notable for 2008 was that the rate of growth of health care (4.4%) was the lowest in nearly 50 years due primarily to the recession. But, as the economy improves, the rate of cost increases is expected to accelerate again.

Undoubtedly, these investments have led to advancements in knowledge, technology, and innovation; however, while the U.S. surpasses other developed countries in spending and may outshine these nations in scientific advancements, outcomes lag for key indicators such as preterm births, infant mortality, and life expectancy (Hussey, et al., 2004; Reinhardt, Hussey, & Anderson, 2004). The nation simply cannot afford to keep paying exponentially more for health care without an equivalent improvement in quality.

Threats to health care access, quality, and costs have not been lost on patients, their families, or the public. Since the 1980s, the U.S. has experienced a rise in consumerism, generally, and a growth in consumer-driven health care, specifically (U.S. Congress, Office of Technology Assessment, 1988; Robinson & Ginsburg, 2009). Product information is more readily available than ever before. The growth of electronic media and performance ratings has led to a public that is a highly informed purchaser of supplies and products. The richness in performance data and the speed in which these data migrate through distribution channels have enabled activists to demand the same for health care.

The dissemination of performance results is a natural extension of this consumerism and an intentional response by policymakers to the growing problems. The 1998 President's Advisory Commission on Consumer Protection and Quality in the Health Care Industry viewed consumers as central players in improving quality and driving value. In its report, the Commission recommended that, "mobilizing the full power of the marketplace to improve health care quality requires that the power of the individual consumer be maximized" (p. 115). The result has been a proliferation of provider-level performance reports that enable competitive comparisons (Marshall, Shekelle, Davies, & Smith, 2003). Health care, like other goods and services, is now seen as a commodity, and consumer choice is a vehicle to drive selection.

THE POLICY CONTEXT: VALUE-DRIVEN HEALTH CARE

Value-driven health care or *high-value health care* are terms that typically refer to improving the quality of care while lowering or stabilizing its costs. In technical terms, value is "a specified stakeholder's... preference-weighted assessment of a particular combination of quality and cost of care performance" (National Quality Forum [NQF], 2009, p. 61). In simple terms, value is obtaining more quality for the same investment. In recent years, intentions have shifted from merely improving the state of health care quality and safety to improving the value and efficiency of care. For the federal government, which operates Medicare—the nation's largest health insurance program covering more than 45 million Americans (The Boards of Trustees, Federal Hospital Insurance and Federal Supplementary Medical Insurance Trust Funds, 2009)—achieving value is dependent on the government moving "from a passive payer of services into an active purchaser of higher-quality, affordable care" (U.S. Department of Health and Human Services [USDHHS], 2009).

In the years that have elapsed since the Commission's report was published, the federal government has taken deliberate steps in this transformation. On August 22, 2006, then-President George W. Bush's signed Executive Order 13410 (2006) to "...promote quality and efficient delivery of health care through the use of health information technology, transparency regarding health care quality and price, and better incentives for program beneficiaries, enrollees, and providers." The Order effectively directed federal agencies to gather cost and quality outcomes and to publicly report performance results to their beneficiaries and enrollees. The government's "value" agenda has relied on a three-pronged strategy embodied in this Executive Order and referred to as the *quality enterprise:* transparency in cost and quality, accountability for performance, and performance-based incentives to stimulate quality improvement.

Within the health care context, *transparency* and *accountability* are terms that typically refer to activities aimed at measuring and publicly disclosing provider performance along with a complementary set of tools that reward—typically through financial payments—high performance (USDHHS, 2009; JCAHO, 1994). Taken together, transparency and accountability are approaches to drive quality improvement and stimulate consumer choice. And while the Executive Order of 2006 placed a spotlight on efforts to drive higher value, the building blocks of transparency and accountability—performance measurement, public reporting, and value-based purchasing—were already in place. Table 48-1 provides a list of these building blocks and the key milestones in their development. A brief description follows.

PERFORMANCE MEASUREMENT

Transparency is dependent on performance measures that accurately portray the features of the health care system. Because public reporting and performance-based incentives cannot exist in the absence of cost and quality outcomes on which they are based, performance measurement is a precursor to public reporting and accountability.

Health care performance measurement is not a new phenomenon. Florence Nightingale, the mother of contemporary nursing, had, in fact, recognized the virtues of measurement in her effort to explain inpatient mortality rates following the Crimean War (Nightingale, 1863). It was Nightingale who pioneered the systematic collection and analysis of hospital mortality rates that enabled comparative reporting and quality improvements in the UK's public health system (McDonald, 2001). She was the first to use a pie chart to organize and display data collected on mortality to convince others of the need

for change in care procedures. Her legacy was perpetuated by more contemporary proponents of performance measurement including Ernest Codman, Walter Shewhart, W. Edwards Deming, Joseph Juran, and Avedis Donabedian.

Performance measurement is foundational to high-value health care. The IOM's report, *Performance Measurement: Accelerating Improvement,* noted: "Many proposals have been offered to improve and reform the functioning of the health care marketplace. … While each of these proposals is based on a different set of assumptions and values … all would require performance measures to achieve their goals." (2006, p. 30). Since recognizing its virtues and acknowledging its necessity, hundreds of quality measures have been developed by government agencies (e.g., Centers for Medicare & Medicaid Services [CMS], Agency for Healthcare Research and Quality [AHRQ]), accreditation organizations (e.g., TJC, National Committee on Quality Assurance), professional societies and certification boards (e.g., American Medical Association-Physician Consortium for Performance Improvement, American Board of Medical Specialties), quality improvement organizations, and private organizations.

Nursing has made a significant investment in and contribution to performance measurement. Measures that portray nurses' contributions to high-quality inpatient care, referred to as "nursing-sensitive measures," have been developed, tested, and implemented by organizations such as the American Nurses Association, Veterans Health Administration, and Association of periOperative Registered Nurses (Kurtzman, Dawson, & Johnson, 2008). Consensus has been achieved among diverse stakeholders on the usefulness of measuring nursing's contribution to quality as evidenced by the adoption of nursing-sensitive measures by the CMS and TJC.

PUBLIC REPORTING

Measurement alone is not a remedy to the nation's aforementioned problems. In fact, it is widely acknowledged that improvements in quality are motivated, if not driven, by public disclosure of performance results (Lansky, 2002). As a result, a sizable increase in the number of provider-level performance reports has been realized (Schneider & Lieberman, 2001; Marshall et al., 2003; Epstein, 1998). As of 2009, the AHRQ listed over 200 examples of performance

TABLE 48-1 Decade of Emphasis on High-Value Health Care: Key Milestones

1997	Clinton Advisory Commission on Consumer Protection and Quality in the Health Care Industry delivers *Quality First*
1998	The Joint Commission introduces ORYX initiative
1999	National Quality Forum (NQF) is established
2000	IOM releases the report, *To Err Is Human*
2001	IOM releases the report, *Crossing the Quality Chasm*
	HHS announces the Hospital Quality Initiative
	CMS launches Dialysis Facility Compare
2002	Joint Commission–accredited hospitals begin collecting data on standardized (i.e., "core") performance measures
	Public-private partnerships emerge (HQA—2002, AQA—2004, PQA—2006)
	Nursing Home Compare is launched by CMS
2003	Medicare Prescription Drug, Improvement and Modernization Act (MMA) of 2003 and Reporting Hospital Quality Data or Annual Payment Update (RHQDAPU) are introduced
	CMS launches Home Health Care Compare
2004	NQF endorses 15 voluntary consensus standards for nursing-sensitive care
2005	Deficit Reduction Act of 2005 expands RHQDAPU
	CMS launches Hospital Compare
	IOM releases the report, *Performance Measurement: Accelerating Improvement*
	Massachusetts launches Patients First, a public website that portrays the quality of hospital care among Massachusetts hospitals including the portrayal of nursing-sensitive performance measures
2006	Executive Order 13410, Promoting Quality and Efficient Health Care, is issued
	Quality Alliance Steering Committee (QASC) is established
	IOM releases the report, *Rewarding Provider Performance: Aligning Incentives in Medicare*
	Maine statute through 22 M.R.S.A. §8708-A, Chapter 270 requires public reporting of nursing-sensitive performance measures
2007	Physician Quality Reporting Initiative (PQRI) is launched
	Report to Congress on hospital value-based purchasing is submitted
2008	HCAHPS data are included in Hospital Compare
	CMS's hospital-acquired conditions policy is implemented
	National Priorities Partnership (NPP) announces national goals to transform health care
2009	Barack Obama is inaugurated as 44th president of the United States
	Stand for Quality is released
	Health care reform efforts begin
2010	LTQA is launched
	NAQC is launched
	Health reform legislation stalls and then is enacted

AQA, Formerly the Ambulatory Care Quality Alliance; *CMS,* Centers for Medicare & Medicaid Services; *HCAHPS,* Hospital Consumer Assessment of Healthcare Providers and Systems; *HHS,* U.S. Department of Health and Human Services; *HQA,* Hospital Quality Alliance; *IOM,* Institute of Medicine; *LTQA,* Long Term Quality Alliance; *MMA,* Medicare Modernization Act; *NAQC,* Nursing Alliance for Quality Care; *NPP,* National Priorities Partnership; *NQF,* National Quality Forum; *PQA,* Pharmacy Quality Alliance; *PQRI,* Physician Quality Reporting Initiative; *QASC,* Quality Alliance Steering Committee; *RHQDAPU,* Reporting Hospital Quality Data for Annual Payment Update.

reports in its online Health Care Report Card Compendium. A growing number of reports are available through websites created and sustained by the CMS including Hospital Compare, Nursing Home Compare, Home Health Compare, and Dialysis Compare. Some states, regional collaboratives, managed care organizations, commercial health insurers, and professional organizations and societies also provide performance reports with the intended purpose of enabling provider-level comparisons. So too has the demand for high-value health care led to public reporting of performance by such sponsors as HealthGrades and Consumer Reports, which have appealed to the consumer audience.

It is notable that a number of publicly disclosed performance reports are specific to the value of nursing. At least two states publicly report hospital-level nursing-sensitive performance on measures. In the case of Maine, state statute 22 M.R.S.A. §8708-A, Chapter 270, requires uniform statewide reporting of data related to health care quality including nursing-sensitive measures. A voluntary initiative undertaken by the Massachusetts Hospital Association and Massachusetts Organization of Nurse Executives, and referred to as Patient's First, led to the public disclosure of hospital-level nursing-sensitive measures. While these are public reporting initiatives that are specific to nursing care, other reports—including the CMS's Hospital Compare—include at least one or more measures that have been specified as nursing-sensitive.

While the CMS does not devote a dedicated public report to nursing care quality per se, several measures that address nursing care have been incorporated into Hospital Compare. In 2008, for example, performance results from the Hospital Consumer Assessment of Healthcare Providers and Systems (HCAHPS), which includes several measures related to nursing care, were posted to the website. In 2009, "failure to rescue" was added as a required measure under the Reporting Hospital Quality Data or Annual Payment Update (RHQDAPU) program. Since the CMS typically draws measures for public reporting on Hospital Compare from those that are required through the RHQDAPU, failure to rescue is likely to be publicly reported in the future.

The proliferation of performance measures and the growth in public reporting led, at least in part, to the need for and the establishment of the National Quality Forum (NQF). The NQF was established in 1999 as a voluntary consensus standards-setting organization as defined by the National Technology Transfer and Advancement Act of 1995 and the Office of Management and Budget's (OMB) Circular A-119. In its early years, NQF work focused on the identification, examination, and consensual endorsement of uniform health care measurement and reporting standards (Kizer, 2001). It is in this spirit that the NQF endorsed a set of national voluntary consensus standards for nursing-sensitive care (2004) that reflect nursing's contribution to high-quality inpatient care. Since its inception, the NQF's role has expanded beyond the endorsement of measurement and reporting standards to one in which it also establishes national priorities for quality and safety and works with stakeholders to systematically implement the measures.

Despite these substantial efforts to standardize measurement and reporting, evidence is equivocal about the direct link between disclosure of health care performance and improvements in quality of care. A 2009 systematic review, for example, found a number of studies across settings in which reporting stimulated quality improvement activities but found no associations or mixed associations between public reporting and provider selection, greater effectiveness, safety, and patient-centeredness (Fung, Lim, Mattke, Damberg, & Shekelle, 2008). Studies of post-acute care (Werner et al., 2009; Werner, Konetzka, & Kruse, 2009) found that public reporting has resulted in some improvements in selected quality measures, but there is evidence of widening gaps between high and low performers and declining quality scores on other measures. The 2006 IOM report on performance measurement acknowledged the absence of strong evidence linking performance measurement and reporting to value and recommended a greater federal investment for evaluation.

PERFORMANCE-BASED INCENTIVES

A central component of high-value health care is the use of incentives—"arrangements that reward both those who offer and those who purchase high-quality, competitively-priced health care" (USDHHS, 2009)—that typically take the form of pay-for-performance or consumer-directed rewards programs.

In June 2003, the Medicare Advisory Payment Commission (MedPAC) examined the need to accelerate improvements in care and concluded that Medicare must lead efforts to improve quality through financial incentives (MedPAC, 2003). Since MedPAC issued its report, there has been a growth in performance-based incentive programs. While many of these programs have been initiated in the private sector (Baker & Carter, 2004-2005), the Medicare Program has taken the lead in pursuing performance-based payment with a goal of fostering clinical and financial accountability. Demonstrations have been conducted in hospitals, physician offices, and dialysis facilities, as well as in chronic care and long-term care (IOM, 2007). A 2007 report to Congress described a Medicare hospital pay-for-performance program that would incentivize hospitals for improvements in quality and sustained performance (CMS, 2007).

More contemporary applications of performance-based incentives include Medicare's existing hospital-acquired conditions policy and innovations enacted under health reform including bundled payments, the patient-centered medical home, and accountable care organizations (ACOs). Bundled payments are also referred to as *episode-based payment* or *case rates.* Conceptually, a bundled payment provides a single payment that covers all services related to a condition or treatment. This could include physician visits, laboratory tests, hospitalization, and any other service needed. Under health reform legislation, demonstration projects were authorized to evaluate the use of bundled payments for Medicare beneficiaries that include a hospitalization and concurrent physician services. The bundled payment approach is a significant departure from the current system in which every service and provider is billed separately and is intended to provide incentives to providers to eliminate care that has limited to no benefit. The patient-centered medical home, a concept introduced by the American Academy of Pediatrics (AAP) and promoted by the AAP, the American Academy of Family Physicians, the American College of Physicians, and the American Osteopathic Association (2007) extends the concept of primary care to include an emphasis on improving outpatient care and engaging patients in health care decision making. Health reform legislation also enacts a shared savings program through ACOs. ACOs are groups of providers, including practitioners and suppliers who have an established shared governance arrangement operating in group practice arrangements, networks, or joint ventures, that are responsible for the quality, cost, and overall care of the assigned Medicare fee-for-service beneficiaries. ACOs are an effort to improve the efficiency through better care coordination, investment in infrastructure, and redesigned care processes. Those that deliver better care will receive financial bonuses (Devers & Berenson, 2009). While the details of each are unique, they effectively shift payment away from rewarding volume with the intention of stimulating more efficient use of resources, cost efficiencies, and more coordination within and across providers. The government's swift adoption of performance-based payment policy is not yet matched with definitive results of its effectiveness. A number of studies and systematic reviews of the relationship between hospital pay-for-performance and quality (Rosenthal & Frank, 2006; Christianson, Leatherman, & Sutherland, 2008; Mehrotra, Damberg, Sorbero, & Teleki, 2009) have discovered significant, positive effects that have been somewhat mitigated by design limitations (e.g., small sample size, lack of comparison group, measure selection). Despite the equivocal nature of the evidence, the federal government is proceeding with its plan to reward high and penalize low performers.

The Affordable Care Act of 2010 includes provisions designed to stimulate high-value health care, including the development of performance measures and public reporting infrastructures. Demonstration and pilot projects will test approaches to bundled payments, ACOs, performance-based incentives, care coordination, transitional care, comparative effectiveness research, workforce capacity-building, nurse-managed health centers, and prevention and wellness. The aim is clearly to maintain and expand the existing value-driven health care agenda.

THE ROLE OF PUBLIC-PRIVATE PARTNERSHIPS

Public-private partnerships have emerged to facilitate the role of the federal government in driving a high-value agenda by avoiding the protracted rule-making process. A number of these partnerships, referred to as quality "alliances," exist and actively participate in the quality enterprise. Their role ranges from developing and testing performance measures (or contracting for those activities) to adopting implementation measures for public reporting and promoting quality improvement initiatives and the use of measures to support these improvement activities.

The Hospital Quality Alliance (HQA), established in 2002, was the first of these partnerships. Its membership includes hospitals, purchasers, government agencies, health plans, quality groups, and consumers for the purpose of making "meaningful, relevant, and easily understood information about hospital performance accessible to the public and to [inform] and [encourage] efforts to improve quality" (Hospital Quality Alliance, n.d.). Since its establishment, a number of other quality alliances have been established. These include the AQA (formerly known as the Ambulatory Care Quality Alliance), the Pharmacy Quality Alliance, the Alliance for Pediatric Quality, the Cancer Quality Alliance, the Surgical Quality Alliance, and the Kidney Care Quality Alliance.

In 2010, the NAQC was launched to provide a policy voice for nursing in the transparency and accountability agenda. The NAQC is a bold partnership among the nation's leading nursing organizations to "advance the highest quality, safety, and value of consumer-centered health care for all individuals—patients, families, and communities." To achieve this aim, the NAQC works to strengthen the visibility of nursing in performance measurement and public reporting activities, serves as a resource to federal partners in health care delivery and payment reform, and builds nursing's capacity to serve in leadership roles that advance consumer-centered, high-quality health care. While the NAQC is a new public-private partnership, significant gains will be realized from having an informed and persuasive nursing presence.

VALUE-DRIVEN HEALTH CARE AND NURSING

As is evident, an enormous commitment in the quality enterprise has been made and has resulted in an infrastructure for transparency and accountability. While this infrastructure is not specifically designed to recognize nursing's contributions nor align with it, nurses both impact and are impacted by this infrastructure and its by-products.

Most importantly, based on every indication, the policy directions of the last decade will be perpetuated and possibly accelerated. There will be more pressure on providers to provide higher *value* care. Nurses are exceedingly well positioned to deliver on that expectation. First, nurses are the single largest provider of health care in the U.S. (Bureau of Labor Statistics, n.d.) and frequent points of patient contact in many care settings. By sheer size, nurses represent a sizable workforce that could alter the value equation. Beyond size, however, associations between nursing and high-value health care have been demonstrated. A growing evidence base substantiates that nurse staffing effects outcomes in acute care settings (Kane, Shamliyan, Mueller, Duval, & Wilt, 2007). Researchers have begun to look at the effect of hospital nursing on economic indicators with signs of positive impact (Needleman, Buerhaus, Stewart, Zelevinsky, & Mattke, 2006; Dall, Chen, Seifert, Maddox, & Hogan,

2009); and a number of rigorous studies recognize the value of advanced practice nurses in primary care settings (Horrocks, Anderson, & Salisbury, 2002; Laurant et al., 2005; Eibner, Hussey, Ridgely, & McGlynn, 2009).

Restructuring the quality enterprise in such a way that it takes advantage of nursing's contributions is an obvious solution; however, it will require continued development of nursing-sensitive measures, public reporting of these data, and advocacy by nurses for the inclusion of these performance measures in transparency and accountability initiatives. It is especially important to note that because the components of the existing infrastructure that reflect nursing have emphasized inpatient care, nursing should advocate or assume responsibility for the development and implementation of measures that reflect high value across settings, including care delivered by postacute, primary, long-term, and public health providers.

Second, while no federal performance-based payment program targets nurses per se, Medicare's hospital-acquired conditions policy represents a value-based purchasing initiative that reflects the care delivered by hospital nurses and provides a "glimpse" into how future policies are likely to affect nursing. The policy eliminates certain Medicare payments for the occurrence of preventable and costly inpatient complications including several nursing-sensitive outcomes, and effectively creates a link between hospital revenue and nursing care. This link and the policy on which it is based present both an opportunity and threat for hospital nurses. A range of responses to the policy have been described in the literature (Wachter, Foster, & Dudley, 2008; Rosenthal, 2007). On the positive side, it can be argued that better nursing care results in higher Medicare reimbursement, and this is likely to be viewed favorably by hospital executives and give nurses more economic clout. On the other hand, hospitals experiencing reductions in Medicare revenue may take cost-saving measures that ultimately weaken the ability of nurses to maintain quality on the very outcomes for which reimbursement is being modified. Blaming behaviors directed at nurses who may be assumed to be responsible for these conditions could render the workforce incapable of teamwork, cooperation, or shared accountability (Kurtzman, 2007).

Recent evidence supports this possibility. Nurses who were surveyed about the effects of this hospital-acquired-conditions policy reported some positive effects—greater emphasis on prevention and surveillance activities and additional education and training. However, the nurses also identified negative effects including additional work and blame directed at them for the occurrence of these events (Buerhaus, Donelan, DesRoches, & Hess, 2009). These early warning signals suggest that this performance-based payment policy could weaken the nursing workforce and should be closely monitored and swiftly mitigated by (among other strategies) using data to substantiate nursing's economic contributions, emphasizing a nonpunitive environment through "just culture" and structured teams, and systematic adoption of evidence-based nursing care to early identify and treat complications (Kurtzman & Buerhaus, 2008).

Finally, emphasis on value-driven health care by policymakers demonstrates the importance of nurses as active collaborators and contributors to policy development. Studies have found that nurses' vivid anecdotes from first-hand involvement in health care are reported to be extremely powerful—making nurses very persuasive advocates (Gebbie, Wakefield, & Kerfoot, 2000). However, multiple barriers (e.g., socialization to the political process, time constraints) prevent nurses from contributing meaningfully (Winter & Lockhart, 1997). Findings from a national poll of opinion leaders conducted by the Gallup Organization in 2009 confirm these findings. Despite these leaders' views of nurses as trusted sources of health information, they considered nursing's influence on health policy to be eclipsed by that of government officials, insurance and pharmaceutical executives, health care executives, physicians, and patients (Gallup, Inc., 2010).

The administration's ongoing commitment to the quality enterprise heightens the need for a stronger nursing presence. The NAQC and other advocacy groups should actively pursue a course that will awaken nursing's interest in these policy directions and stimulate policymakers' reliance on nurses.

For a list of related websites, please refer to your Evolve Resources at http://evolve.elsevier.com/Mason/policypolitics/

REFERENCES

Advisory Commission on Consumer Protection and Quality in the Health Care Industry. (1998). *Quality first: Better health care for all Americans.* Washington, D.C.: U.S. Government Printing Office. Retrieved from www.hcqualitycommission.gov/final.

Agency for Healthcare Research and Quality. (2009a, March). *2008 National Healthcare Disparities Report.* Rockville, MD: U.S. Department of Health and Human Services.

Agency for Healthcare Research and Quality. (2009b, March). *2008 National Healthcare Quality Report.* Rockville, MD: U.S. Department of Health and Human Services.

American Academy of Family Physicians, American Academy of Pediatrics, American College of Physicians, American Osteopathic Association. (2007). *Joint principles of the patient-centered medical home.* Washington, D.C.: Authors.

Asch, S. M., Kerr, E. A., Joan, K., Adams, J., Setodji, C. M., et al. (2006). Who is at greatest risk for receiving poor-quality health care? *New England Journal of Medicine, 354*(11), 1147-1156.

Baker, G., & Carter, B. (2004-2005). *Provider pay-for-performance incentive programs: 2004 national study results.* San Francisco: Med-Vantage.

Berens, M. J. (2002, July 21). Infection epidemic carves deadly path across America. *Chicago Tribune.*

The Boards of Trustees, Federal Hospital Insurance and Federal Supplementary Medical Insurance Trust Funds. (2009, May 12). *The 2009 annual report of the boards of trustees, federal hospital insurance and federal supplementary medical insurance trust funds.* Washington, D.C.: Author.

Buerhaus, P. I., Donelan, K., DesRoches, C., & Hess, R. (2009). Registered Nurses' perceptions of nurse staffing ratios and new hospital payment regulations. *Nursing Economics, 27*(6), 372-376.

Bureau of Labor Statistics (BLS), U.S. Department of Labor (DOL). (n.d.). *Occupational outlook handbook, 2006-07 edition, registered nurses.* Retrieved from www.bls.gov/oco/ocos083.htm.

Centers for Medicare & Medicaid Services (CMS), HHS. (2007, November 21). *Report to Congress: Plan to implement a Medicare hospital value-based purchasing program.* Washington, D.C.: Centers for Medicare & Medicaid Services. Retrieved from www.cms.hhs.gov/AcuteInpatientPPS/downloads/HospitalVBPPlanRTCFINALSUBMITTED2007.pdf.

Christianson, J. B., Leatherman, S., & Sutherland, K. (2008). Lessons from evaluations of purchaser pay-for-performance programs: A review of the evidence. *Medical Care and Research Review, 65*(6 Suppl), 5S-35S.

Commonwealth Fund. (2008, July). *Why not be the best? Results from a national scorecard on U.S. Health system performance, 2008.* New York: The Commonwealth Fund.

Dall, T. M., Chen, Y. J., Seifert, R. F., Maddox, P. J., & Hogan, P. F. (2009). The economic value of professional nursing. *Medical Care, 47*(1), 97-104.

Devers, K., & Berenson, R. (2009). *Can accountable care organizations improve the value of health care by solving the cost and quality quandaries? Timely analysis of immediate health policy issues.* Washington, D.C. and Princeton, NJ: Urban Institute and The Robert Wood Johnson Foundation.

Eibner, C., Hussey, P., Ridgely, M. S., & McGlynn, E. A. (2009). *Controlling health care spending in Massachusetts: An analysis of options.* Santa Monica, CA: RAND Corporation.

Epstein, A. M. (1998). Rolling down the runway: The challenges ahead for quality report cards. *Journal of the American Medical Association, 279*(21), 1691-1696.

Exec. Order No. 13410, 71 FR 51089, August 28, 2006.

Fung, C. H., Lim, Y. W., Mattke, S., Damberg, C., & Shekelle, P. G. (2008). Systematic review: The evidence that publishing patient care performance data improves quality of care. *Annals of Internal Medicine, 148*(2), 111-123.

Gallup, Inc. (2010, January 20). *Nursing leadership from bedside to boardroom: Opinion leaders' perceptions top line report.* Princeton, NJ: Author. Retrieved from www.rwjf.org/files/research/nursinggalluppolltopline.pdf.

Gebbie, K. M., Wakefield, M., & Kerfoot, K. (2000). Nursing and health policy. *Journal of Nursing Scholarship, 32*(3), 307-315.

Gibson, R., & Singh, J. P. (2003). *Wall of silence.* Washington, D.C.: LifeLine Press.

Hartman, M., Martin A., Nunccio, O., Catlin, A., & the National Health Expenditures Account Team. (2010). Health spending growth at a low in 2008. *Health Affairs, 29*(1):147-155.

The High Cost of Health Care (editorial). (2007, November 25). New York Times. Retrieved from www.nytimes.com/2007/11/25/opinion/25sun1.html.

Horrocks, S., Anderson, E., & Salisbury, C. (2002). Systematic review of whether nurse practitioners working in primary care can provide equivalent care to doctors. *British Medical Journal, 324*(7341), 819-823.

Hospital Quality Alliance (HQA). (n.d.). Improving care through information. Retrieved from www.hospitalqualityalliance.org/hospitalqualityalliance/index.html.

Hussey, P. S., Anderson, G. F., Osborn, R., Feek, C., McLaughlin, V., et al. (2004). How does the quality of care compare in five countries? *Health Affairs, 23*(3), 89-99.

Institute of Medicine (IOM). (1994). *America's health in transition: Protecting and improving quality.* Washington, D.C.: National Academies Press.

Institute of Medicine (IOM). (2001). *Crossing the quality chasm: A new health system for the 21st century.* Washington, D.C.: National Academies Press.

Institute of Medicine (IOM). (2006). *Performance measurement: Accelerating improvement.* Washington, D.C.: National Academies Press.

Institute of Medicine (IOM). (2007). *Rewarding provider performance: Aligning incentives in Medicare.* Washington, D.C.: National Academies Press.

The Joint Commission. (2008). *Improving America's hospitals: The Joint Commission's annual report on quality and safety.* Chicago: The Joint Commission. Retrieved from www.jointcommission/assets/1/18/2008_Annual_Report.pdf.

Joint Commission on the Accreditation of Healthcare Organizations (JCAHO). (1994). *Framework for improving performance: From principles to practice.* Oakbrook Terrace, IL: Joint Commission on the Accreditation of Healthcare Organizations.

Kane, R. L., Shamliyan, T., Mueller, C., Duval, S., & Wilt, T. J. (2007 March). Nursing staffing and quality of patient care. *Evidence Report/Technology Assessment, 151,* 1-115. Rockville, MD: Agency for Healthcare Research and Quality.

Kizer, K. W. (2001). Establishing health care performance standards in an era of consumerism. *Journal of the American Medical Association, 286*(10), 1213-1217.

Knox, R. A. (1995, March 23). Doctor's orders killed cancer patient: Dana-Farber admits drug overdose caused death of *Globe* columnist, damage to second woman. *Boston Globe.*

Kohn, K. T., Corrigan, J. M., & Donaldson, M. S. (Eds.). (2000). *To err is human: Building a safer health system.* Washington, D.C.: National Academies Press.

Kurtzman, E. T. (2007). *A summary of the impact of reforms to the Hospital Inpatient Prospective Payment System (IPPS) on nursing services.* Washington, D.C.: George Washington University, Department of Nursing Education, School of Medicine and Health Sciences.

Kurtzman, E. T., & Buerhaus, P. I. (2008). New Medicare payment rules: Danger or opportunity for nursing? *American Journal of Nursing, 108*(7), 30-35.

Kurtzman, E. T., Dawson, E. M., & Johnson, J. E. (2008). A current state of nursing performance measurement, public reporting, and value-based purchasing. *Policy, Politics, & Nursing Practice, 9*(3), 181-191.

Lansky, D. (2002). Improving quality through public disclosure of performance information. *Health Affairs, 21*(4), 52-62.

Laurant, M., Reeves, D., Hermens, R., Braspenning, J., Grol, R., & Sibbald, B. (2005). Substitution of doctors by nurses in primary care. *Cochrane Database Systematic Review, 18*(2), CD001271.

Mangione-Smith, R., DeCristofaro, A. H., Setodji, C. M., Keesey, J., Klein, D. J., et al. (2007). The quality of ambulatory care delivered to children in the United States. *New England Journal of Medicine, 357*(15), 1515-1523.

Marshall, M. N., Shekelle, P. G., Davies, H. T., & Smith, P. C. (2003). Public reporting on quality in the United States and the United Kingdom. *Health Affairs, 22*(3), 134-148.

McDonald, L. (2001). Florence Nightingale and the early origins of evidence-based nursing. *Evidence-Based Nursing, 4*(3), 68-69.

McGlynn, E. A., Asch, S. M., Adams, J., Keesey, J., Hicks, J., et al. (2003). The quality of health care delivered to adults in the United States. *New England Journal of Medicine, 348*(26), 2635-2645.

Medicare Payment Advisory Commission (MedPAC). (2003, March). *Report to the Congress: Medicare payment policy.* Washington, D.C.: MedPAC.

Mehrotra, A., Damberg, C. L., Sorbero, M. E., & Teleki, S. S. (2009). Pay for performance in the hospital setting: What is the state of evidence? *American Journal of Medical Quality, 24*(1), 19-28.

Millenson, M. L. (1997). *Demanding medical excellence.* Chicago: The University of Chicago Press.

National Quality Forum (NQF). (2004). *National voluntary consensus standards for nursing-sensitive care.* Washington, D.C.: Author. Retrieved from www.qualityforum.org/pdf/nursing-quality/txNCFINALpublic.pdf.

National Quality Forum (NQF). (2009). *Measurement framework: Evaluating efficiency across patient-focused episodes of care.* Washington, D.C.: National Quality Forum.

Needleman, J., Buerhaus, P. I., Stewart, M., Zelevinsky, K., & Mattke, S. (2006). Nurse staffing in hospitals: Is there a business case for quality? *Health Affairs, 25*(1), 204-211.

Nightingale, F. (1863). *Notes on hospitals.* London: Longman, Green, Longman, Roberts & Green.

Reinhardt, U. E., Hussey, P. S., & Anderson, G. F. (2004). U.S. health care spending in an international context. *Health Affairs, 23*(3), 10-25.

Robinson, J. C., & Ginsburg, P. B. (2009). Consumer-driven health care: Promise and performance. *Health Affairs, 28*(2), w272-w281.

Rosenthal, M. B. (2007). Nonpayment for performance? Medicare's new reimbursement rule. *New England Journal of Medicine, 357*(16), 1573-1575.

Rosenthal, M. B., & Frank, R. G. (2006). What is the empirical basis for paying for quality in health care? *Medical Care and Research Review, 63*(2), 135-157.

Schneider, E. C., & Lieberman, T. (2001). Publicly disclosed information about the quality of health care: Response of the US public. *Quality Health Care, 10*(2), 96-103.

Sisko, A., Truffer, C., Smith, S., Keehan, S., Cylus, J., et al. (2009). Health spending projections through 2018: Recession effects add uncertainty to the outlook. *Health Affairs, 28*(2), w346-w357.

U.S. Congress, Office of Technology Assessment. (1988). *The quality of medical care; information for consumers, OTA-I-I-386.* Washington, D.C.: U.S. Government Printing Office.

U.S. Department of Health and Human Services (DHHS). (2009). Value-driven health care. Retrieved from www.hhs.gov/valuedriven.

Wachter, R. M., Foster, N., & Dudley, R. A. (2008). Medicare's decision to withhold payment for hospital errors: The devil is in the details. *Joint Commission Journal on Quality and Patient Safety, 34*(2), 116-123.

Werner, R. M., Konetzka, R. T., & Kruse, G. B. (2009). Impact of public reporting on unreported quality of care. *Health Services Research, 44*(2 Pt 1), 379-398.

Werner, R. M., Konetzka, R. T., Stuart, E. A., Norton, E. C., Polsky, D., & Park, J. (2009). Impact of public reporting on quality of postacute care. *Health Services Research, 44*(4), 1169-1187.

Winter, M. K., & Lockhart, J. S. (1997). From motivation to action: Understanding nurses' political involvement. *Nursing and Health Care Perspectives, 18*(5), 244-250.

CHAPTER 49

The Nursing Workforce

Mary Lou Brunell and Angela Ross

"If we want affordable, patient-centered health care in this country, then we have to make a renewed commitment to nurses, who carry out such important work."
—Representative Tom Latham, R-Iowa,
March 12, 2009

The supply of nurses in the United States is made up of all licensed practical/vocational nurses (LPNs), registered nurses (RNs), and advanced registered nurse practitioners (ARNPs). Those with active licenses that are clear (without disciplinary or other limitation) are eligible for employment and represent the *potential* nurse employment pool. The actual *nursing workforce* is composed of those working in the practice of nursing or those whose job requires a license. To demonstrate the significance of these distinctions, Figure 49-1 illustrates the breakdown of licensed RNs, including ARNPs, in Florida, compared to those that define Florida's potential nursing workforce, and then to those that are actually working (Florida Center for Nursing [FCN], 2009).

Successful planning requires knowing the real workforce supply numbers. As shown in Figure 49-1, there is a difference of nearly 85,000 RNs (34.4%). Using the wrong base number could make it appear that a shortage does not exist—on paper—when reality says otherwise. Forecasting models project demand based on the current supply of nurses and the reported need (employment) for nurses. Demand exists when the supply does not meet the need. If there is a need for 200,000 nurses, a supply of 246,707 indicates no demand, while a supply of 161,778 implies a demand for nearly 40,000 nurses.

CHARACTERISTICS OF THE WORKFORCE

The U.S. nursing workforce is the largest potential nursing workforce in the world and is still predominately female and White/Non-Hispanic, with only 6.6% of surveyed respondents reporting as male and 16.8% reporting as Non-White/Hispanic (U.S. Department of Health and Human Services [USDHHS], Health Resources and Services Administration [HRSA], 2010). These nurses are the frontline providers of care for many health care consumers.

In 2006, the USDHHS HRSA projected a shortage of 1 million full-time-equivalent (FTE) RNs by 2020—with RNs working full-time counted as 1 FTE and RNs working part-time counted as one-half of an FTE (USDHHS, Bureau of Health Professions, 2004). A nursing shortage exists because demand, or need, exceeds the supply. Demand is expected to increase more rapidly than the supply as the Baby Boomer cohort of the U.S. population reaches retirement age. In 2007, the U.S. entered a severe economic recession. Buerhaus, Auerbach, & Staiger (2009) evaluated the impact of this economic recession on the projected nursing shortage. The authors found that in 2007 and 2008 combined, hospital RN employment increased by 243,000 FTE RNs—the largest 2-year increase in their 30-year dataset. In addition to representing increased education capacity over the previous several years, this influx is probably attributable to delayed retirements by older nurses, increases in hours worked, and re-entry of younger nurses to the workforce following spouse layoffs or reduction in work. Thus, even with record-setting growth in the nursing workforce, this report states that the country is still expected to see a shortage of 260,000 FTE RNs by 2025.

It is no surprise that the current nursing shortage is not its first. During the 1980s, the country faced two marked nursing labor shortages, caused primarily by wage controls and cost-cutting approaches. They were essentially resolved through wage increases and increased funding for nursing education. What makes the current shortage different is that it isn't driven by the cyclic nature of the economy. A significant portion of the nursing workforce is approaching retirement age, and there are not enough younger nurses entering the profession to replace them. The average age of the RN population was 46.8 in 2004. Figure 49-2 details how the average age of nurses has climbed upward on every HRSA survey since 1980 (USDHHS, 2006).

This exodus of experienced nurses has grave implications for patients, nurses, and employers. Studies have corroborated the intuitive idea that when nurses are understaffed, patient safety suffers and medical errors increase (Kane, Shamliyan, Mueller, Duval, &

Wilt, 2007; Mark Harless, McCue, & Xu, 2004; Aiken, Clarke, Sloane, Sochalski, & Silber, 2002; Needleman, Buerhaus, Mattke, Stewart, & Zelevinsky, 2002). Understaffing also leads to nurse burnout (Aiken et al., 2002), which, of course, causes increased turnover and more nurse burnout. The demand for nurses is expected to dramatically increase as consumers are living longer with more chronic diseases; a significant portion of the population is approaching retirement age, creating increased need for health care services. As patients, these consumers will require a level of care that is best provided by an appropriate balance of nurses—those with years of hands-on experience and knowledge along with new nurses fresh from the education system.

Recent estimates put the cost of nurse turnover at up to 200% of a nurse's annual salary (Robert Wood Johnson Foundation [RWJF], 2006; Hayes et al., 2006; Jones, 2004, 2005; Waldman, Kelly, Arora, & Smith, 2004). The costs associated with turnover and understaffing have a powerful impact on the economy. In an article analyzing the economic value of RNs, Dall and colleagues (2009) found significant economic value when even a single RN was added to an understaffed unit. The authors calculated the costs of patient mortality due to understaffing and evaluated the benefits of adding 133,000 FTE RNs to the acute care hospital workforce—the number needed to improve staffing at hospitals with low to medium staffing

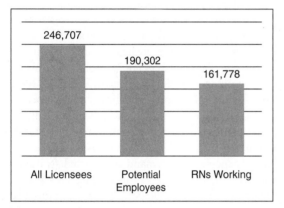

FIGURE 49-1 RNs and ARNPs in Florida in 2008. (From Florida Center for Nursing (2009). *Estimation of the RN workforce in Florida as of January 2009.*)

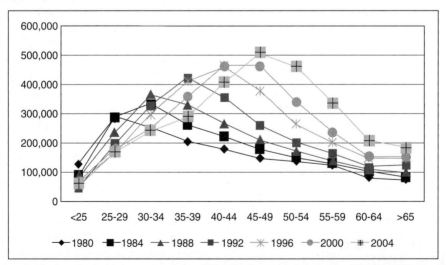

FIGURE 49-2 Age distribution of registered nurse population 1980-2004. (From U.S. Department of Health and Human Services, Bureau of Health Professions (2006). *The registered nurse population: Findings from the March 2004 National Sample Survey of Registered Nurses.*)

levels. Increasing these nurses could save 5900 patient lives each year, with a productivity value of $1.3 billion annually. They also found that this increase in workforce would reduce hospital stays by 3.6 million days and thus generate additional productivity value of $231 million annually and $6.1 billion in annual medical savings. In Florida alone, the Florida Center for Nursing found that the cost of turnover for LPNs and RNs exceeded $1.6 billion in fiscal year 2006-2007 (FCN, 2008a).

This research makes a compelling case to address nurse supply needs by not only expanding the workforce, but also by retaining current nurses. Although continuing to expand education capacity and produce new nurses is important, more needs to be done. As with the nursing workforce in general, the educator workforce is also aging and a mass wave of faculty retirements is anticipated within the next decade. There is already a faculty shortage, making it impossible for nursing education programs to accept the number of students needed to meet the demand. More than 49,000 qualified applicants were turned away from baccalaureate and graduate nursing programs in 2008 due to limited funding for faculty, lack of clinical sites, and lack of qualified faculty applicants (American Association of Colleges of Nursing [AACN], 2009a). Even if education capacity could be expanded to meet demand, there will still be a lapse before an adequately experienced workforce is operational. Policy initiatives must take a multipronged approach by focusing on expanding both the general nursing and faculty workforce, increasing diversity, and retaining workers.

EXPANDING THE WORKFORCE

Nursing education programs must be expanded to facilitate growth in the nursing workforce. Successful expansion should be measured—not just by increased admissions, but also by increased graduations and successful passage of the National Council Licensure Examination for Registered Nurses (NCLEX). Lack of funding to hire additional faculty members and lack of qualified faculty applicants are consistently identified as reasons why programs turn away qualified applicants (AACN, 2009a). Increased funding for graduate education is an essential first step toward increasing capacity. Funding for graduate education

could help expand the faculty pipeline while also expanding the pool of candidates for other hard-to-fill nursing positions. Through HRSA, the federal government has a variety of grant programs that offer loan repayment for nurses (USDHHS, 2009).

Another key reason for lack of faculty applicants is the wide discrepancy between clinical and educational salaries. Nurses can often earn significantly more in clinical practice than in teaching. Kaufman (2007) suggests that this salary difference may be a chief reason for the faculty shortage. Funding aimed at increasing salaries for nurse faculty in entry-level programs (associate and baccalaureate) would have considerable impact on reducing the faculty shortage where doctoral education may not be provided for faculty positions. Many employers partner with local colleges to develop faculty sharing programs; employers pay for salary and benefits and then donate 50% to 100% of the nurse's time to the school. These programs have been quite successful, enabling educational institutions to expand admissions while providing faculty who are familiar with the clinical sites and policies. Employers may also offer tuition reimbursement for nurses seeking an advanced degree; this not only serves as a retention strategy for the employer, but may expand the pool of potential nurse educators. Private donations are another source of additional funding for educational programs.

Strategic utilization of scarce resources is a critical component of effectively expanding education capacity. Lack of access to clinical sites ranks as a barrier to expansion. As a result, simulation technology is being used as a highly effective method for hands-on experience with a wide range of clinical scenarios. Though the cost of simulation technology is still high, collaboration among educational programs may be the most beneficial. Some examples of collaboration include the following:

- In Colorado, the state's nursing workforce center developed the Colorado Work, Education, and Lifelong Learning Simulation (WELLS) Center *(www.wellssimulationcenter.org)*. This single facility provides state-of-the-art patient simulation tools and curricula to educate nursing students, faculty, and practicing nurses and physicians throughout the state. Not only does the simulation center provide clinical space for students, it also serves as a resource for continuing education for faculty members and clinical practitioners.

- The Florida Center for Nursing, with funding from the Blue Foundation for a Healthy Florida in 2009, has explored the feasibility of regional simulation centers. Uncovering how simulation resources can be pooled will enable smaller nursing education programs to benefit from simulation technologies and in turn help expand capacity for more programs.
- In 2004, the Oregon Center for Nursing developed the StudentMAX® system; the California Institute for Nursing & Health Care developed a similar program for the nine-county San Francisco Bay area. These Web-based, centralized clinical placement software systems improve the process for placing nursing students at clinical sites and improve efficiency by identifying underutilized clinical sites, thus increasing placement capacity.

Critical to expanding the nursing workforce is the successful entry of new graduates into work settings. Residency programs may help ease the transition from education to clinical practice, strengthen commitment to the profession, and improve retention for first-year nurses. Increasing the availability of specialized training for experienced nurses may also help produce a workforce with qualified applicants to enter hard-to-fill positions such as critical care and front-line management.

INCREASING DIVERSITY

As the U.S. population continues to grow and increase its diversity, it is important that the nursing workforce reflect these changes to effectively meet patient care needs and ensure cultural competency. Nursing is a predominately female profession; only 6.6% of the national nursing workforce is composed of men, though men make up nearly 50% of the population. To address this issue, several state nursing workforce centers have launched campaigns to recruit men into nursing. The Oregon Center for Nursing (www. oregoncenterfornursing.org) launched the "Are You Man Enough to be a Nurse?" campaign in 2002; this campaign received local and national coverage and was replicated in other states with success. Increasing the visibility of men in nursing is a crucial first step toward attracting more male applicants. The same is true for improving the appeal of nursing to ethnic and racial minorities. In 2004, the Oregon Center for Nursing launched a separate campaign, "Caring Knows No Boundaries," aimed at recruiting racial and ethnic minorities into nursing. Stereotypical views of nurses as white women may be limiting the entry of men and minorities into the field; however, if these obstacles could be overcome, men and Hispanics alone could add enough RNs to the workforce to resolve the projected shortage by 2025 (Buerhaus, Auerbach, & Staiger, 2009).

Increasing diversity in the nursing workforce also requires increasing diversity in the education pipeline. Utilizing alternative recruitment strategies to target male and minority students as well as providing funding incentives may help create the pipeline that will lead to a more inclusive nursing workforce. Ensuring a diverse nursing education faculty is also key to attracting and maintaining a diverse student population; currently, only about 10% of nursing faculty members are from minority backgrounds compared to 34% for the national population (AACN, 2009b). To address diversity, the American Association of Colleges of Nursing (AACN) established a minority scholarship program. The AACN also launched an initiative to improve the ability of new graduate nurses to provide culturally competent care (AACN, 2009b).

RETAINING WORKERS

Policy efforts to address the shortage must include a focus on retention both in the public and private sectors. At the national level, grants have been given by the HRSA for demonstration programs that can be evaluated and replicated. Foundations have given grants to pilot regional initiatives, and employers have used different types of retention approaches. The Partners Investing in Nursing's Future (PIN) grants, for example, sponsored by the Robert Wood Johnson Foundation (RWJF) and the Northwest Health Foundation, provide funding for localized initiatives and encourage regional collaboration. By requiring a dollar-for-dollar commitment from a local funder, the PIN program also seeks to encourage a framework for collaborative efforts addressing the shortage. The RWJF has also commissioned numerous reports, including *Wisdom at Work: Retaining Experienced Nurses* and *Wisdom at Work: The Importance of Older and Experienced Nurses in the Workplace.*

Retention of nurses is also a key issue for state nurse workforce centers. The Florida Center for Nursing, for example, provides small grants to focus on retention and recruitment. The Center has successfully shared the results with schools and employers throughout the state. In the 2009 round of grants, there was a return-on-investment of $13.92 for every dollar the Florida Center for Nursing invested.

Several of the state workforce centers sponsor nursing leadership development programs to not only enhance the professional image of nursing but also to improve training for frontline managers. The Colorado Center for Nursing Excellence has implemented a 5-year project to replicate one hospital's model of collaborative process improvement and nurse empowerment. Through the Colorado Consortium for Nurse Retention (*coloradonursingcenter.org*), the Center has successfully worked in other rural and urban sites throughout the state.

With research showing that job satisfaction is an indicator of turnover (Hayes et al., 2006), improving the work environment at the facility level is perhaps the most effective strategy for improving the retention of both new and experienced nurses. An important and effective first step toward improving nurse retention is ensuring that the organization's leadership clearly values nurses. The Magnet Recognition Program administered by the American Nurses Credentialing Center is one example of a process that supports nursing work (see Chapter 60). It provides a focus on improved collaboration, increased autonomy/accountability for nurses, improved decision-making abilities, safe staffing levels, effective leadership, and improved access to professional development opportunities. Another highly successful initiative is Transforming Care at the Bedside (TCAB), a quality improvement program led by the RWJF and the Institute for Healthcare Improvement. One of its goals is to increase the amount of time nurses spend in direct care, thereby improving the work environment and reducing turnover (see Chapter 47). The American Organization for Nurse Executives helps implement TCAB in 68 hospitals across the country.

In addition to visible leadership at the organizational level, effective nurse managers can have a significant impact on turnover. To ensure that frontline managers are both a good fit and adequately trained, some organizations have divided the traditional role into two—one focused on clinical and the other on administrative and management. Separating the roles not only helps reduce what was previously an overwhelming workload for one manager, but enables nurses with strong clinical skills to lead without being responsible for management. A Florida Center for Nursing 2008 grant recipient implemented the Clinical Nurse Leader®, and initial results indicated improvements in nurse retention and satisfaction (FCN, 2008b). Identifying new roles is an important step in developing career pathways, which may improve retention. Lack of clear opportunities for professional advancement can also increase turnover (Hayes et al., 2006). Developing new roles, such as patient liaison or admissions counselor, is an important step toward retaining older nurses while also reducing the workload for staff nurses (RWJF, 2006).

To keep a safe mix of new and experienced nurses, nurse employers must implement strategies specifically aimed at retaining older nurses. In addition to the improved benefit to patients, the expertise that older and experienced nurses bring to the workplace is invaluable. This expertise is particularly beneficial when older nurses are paired with new nurses in mentorship programs. Not only do experienced nurses possess extensive clinical knowledge from years of hands-on experience, they also possess a strong knowledge of the organizational culture. Mentorship initiatives help organizations facilitate the transfer of the institutional knowledge to new nurses. New graduates in particular benefit from mentorships, to help ease the transition from school to real-life clinical work. Strategies aimed at retaining older nurses may also serve to improve retention among others groups, including working mothers or inactive nurses. These strategies include implementing tools to reduce the physical demands of the job, offering alternative shorter shifts and reduced workweeks, enhancing retirement benefits, and rewarding loyalty by creating incentives for longevity (RWJF, 2006).

PUBLIC AND PRIVATE EFFORTS TO ADDRESS THE NURSING SHORTAGE

To address the nursing shortage on a local level, many states have established nursing workforce centers.

Though these centers vary, in general they focus on collecting, analyzing, and reporting state-level nursing workforce data while also serving as a source of information related to the shortage and identifying strategies for resolution. Because these centers collect data at a state level, they are typically able to produce more accurate information than previously published by national groups. The 2007 Florida Center for Nursing survey of primary nurse employers (hospitals, skilled nursing facilities, home health agencies, hospices and public health departments) asked responders to identify the top five most difficult to fill positions. In each case, for each industry the most difficult to fill positions required advanced experience, advanced education, or both (FCN, 2008c).

Nursing workforce centers also focus on workforce planning within the state, and they serve a key role in presenting recommendations and educating state legislators and policymakers about the shortage. For example, in 2006 the Mississippi Office of Nursing Workforce participated in the successful passage by the state legislature of a $12,000 increase (over 2 years) in base faculty salaries. With salaries in clinical practice far outpacing nurse faculty salaries, this increase has had a significant impact in addressing the faculty shortage (see Chapter 69).

In 2005, several of the state nursing workforce centers came together to establish the Forum of State Nursing Workforce Centers (Forum). With 33 participating centers (as of 2009), the Forum seeks to ensure the strategic and effective resolution of the nation's nursing shortage by sharing research and best practices. Many of these centers have established data-collection methods and are producing extremely accurate state-level information. However, there are substantial differences in both the methods and metrics used for collecting nursing workforce data, making it nearly impossible to produce an accurate national picture of the nursing shortage. After evaluating data-collection practices, the Forum initiated the Minimum Dataset Project to standardize the collection of state-level nursing workforce data and to create a national repository of data. The goal is to enable state and national workforce planners to identify and implement accurate and timely approaches to resolve the shortage. Planners and policy analysts will be able to benchmark progress and improve accuracy in forecasting the future workforce supply and demand.

In addition to state nursing workforce centers, private foundations, consumer groups, and professional practice associations have collected information and made recommendations for policy changes in the public arena as well as in the workplace. One major funder of nursing, the RWJF, has provided millions of dollars in funding for a broad range of nursing research and nursing workforce retention initiatives. The RWJF partnered with the AARP to create the Center to Champion Nursing in America, which focuses on expanding nursing education capacity and retaining the existing nursing workforce (see Chapter 84). The RWJF has also partnered with the Northwest Health Foundation to institute the PIN program, which provides grants to advance nursing initiatives at a local level.

The Institute of Medicine (IOM), an arm of the National Academy of Sciences, has produced research critical to understanding the impact of the nursing shortage, including *To Err is Human: Building a Safer Health System, Keeping Patients Safe: Transforming the Work Environment of Nurses,* and *Crossing the Quality Chasm: A New Health System for the 21st Century*. In 2009, the IOM partnered with the RWJF to lead a major study on the future of nursing. The 2-year initiative seeks to create an actionable agenda for changes at the local, state, and national levels to address the nursing shortage.

Numerous professional practice associations have initiated efforts to address the shortage, particularly efforts to improve the work environment and enhance the image of nursing. The American Nurses Association, the American Association of Colleges of Nursing, the Center for American Nurses, the American Hospital Association, and the National League for Nursing have made the shortage a priority issue. The Joint Commission (TJC) has a Nursing Advisory Council on initiatives to resolve the nursing shortage.

At the federal level, the HRSA conducts the National Sample Survey of Registered Nurses every 4 years to evaluate the state of the nursing workforce and to provide grants for a wide range of nursing initiatives. The HRSA also distributes funding for Nursing Workforce Development Programs through Title VIII of the Public Health Service Act; in fiscal year 2009, funding for these programs totaled over $171 million. Through the American Recovery and Reinvestment Act of 2009 (ARRA), the HRSA dedicated $200 million to provide grants, loans, loan repayments, and scholarships to expand training within the health care profession; $39 million of these funds were specifically for nurses and nurse faculty. The U.S. Department of Labor (DOL) provided funding for workforce initiatives, including funding the 2008 and 2009 Education Capacity Summits presented by the Center to Champion Nursing in America. The DOL dedicated ARRA funds to the health care profession, including $220 million for high-growth industries with a priority on training workers within the health care sector. The DOL actively sought projects in nursing that facilitated progression along the nursing career pathway. In 2003, the Congressional Caucus on Nursing was founded by a nurse member of Congress, Lois Capps (D-California), to better educate members of Congress about nursing (see Chapter 76). The Caucus has focused specifically on the shortage and workforce issues. It also serves as a clearinghouse for information and a sounding board for ideas brought forth by the nursing community.

SUMMARY

The uniqueness of the current shortage is related to a variety of factors that require new solutions. Increasing salaries and expanding education capacity alone will not assure an adequate, qualified workforce to meet health care needs in the coming decades. Strategic resolution must include strategies that will (1) increase education capacity by addressing the nurse faculty shortage and clinical space limitations; (2) retain the current nursing workforce by improving the work environment, addressing age-related challenges, and valuing nurses' contributions; and (3) collect necessary data as the base for accurate forecasting and evaluation of interventions. The Forum of State Nursing Workforce Centers provides a vehicle to bring state-level data and resolution strategies to the national level.

Continued sharing of information, collaboration to successfully implement programs, and funding are critical to effectively resolve the nursing shortage. Good policy requires good data, and this is particularly evident in developing policy surrounding the nation's nursing shortage.

For a list of related websites, please refer to your Evolve Resources at http://evolve.elsevier.com/Mason/policypolitics/

REFERENCES

Aiken, L. H., Clarke, S. P., Sloane, D. M., Sochalski, J., & Silber, J. H. (2002). Hospital nurse staffing and patient mortality, nurse burnout, and job dissatisfaction. *Journal of the American Medical Association, 288*(16), 1987-1993.

American Association of Colleges of Nursing. (2009a). *Fact sheet: Nursing faculty shortage.* Retrieved from www.aacn.nche.edu/Media/FactSheets/FacultyShortage.htm.

American Association of Colleges of Nurses. (2009b). *Fact sheet: Enhancing diversity in the nursing workforce.* Retrieved from www.aacn.nche.edu/Media/FactSheets/diversity.htm.

Buerhaus, P. I., Auerbach, D. I., & Staiger, D. O. (2009). The recent surge in nurse employment: Causes and implications. *Health Affairs, 28*(4), w657-w668. Retrieved from http://content.healthaffairs.org/cgi/content/abstract/hlthaff.28.4.w657.

Dall, T. M., Chen, Y. J., Seifert, R. F., Maddox, P. J., & Hogan, P. F. (2009). The economic value of professional nursing. *Medical Care, 47*(1), 97-104.

Florida Center for Nursing. (2008a). The economic benefits of resolving Florida's nursing shortage. Retrieved from www.flcenterfornursing.org/files/Econ_Benefits.pdf.

Florida Center for Nursing. (2008b). 2008 Retention & recruitment funded projects. Retrieved from www.flcenterfornursing.org/retention/funded_2008.cfm.

Florida Center for Nursing. (2008c). Statewide vacancies and job growth expectations in nursing-intensive healthcare settings. Retrieved from www.flcenterfornursing.org/files/Vacancies_Job_Growth.pdf.

Florida Center for Nursing. (2009). Estimation of the RN workforce in Florida as of January 2009. Retrieved from www.flcenterfornursing.org/files/Workforce_Estimation.pdf.

Hayes, L. J., O'Brien-Pallas, L., Duffield, C., Shamian, J., Buchan, J., et al. (2006). Nurse turnover: A literature review. *International Journal of Nursing Studies, 43*(2), 237-263.

Jones, C. B. (2004). The costs of nurse turnover, part 1: An economic perspective. *Journal of Nursing Administration, 34*(12), 562-570.

Jones, C. B. (2005). The costs of nurse turnover, part 2: Application of the nursing Turnover Cost Calculation Methodology. *Journal of Nursing Administration, 35*(1), 41-49.

Kane, R. L., Shamliyan, T. A., Mueller, C., Duval, S., & Wilt, T. J. (2007). The association of registered nurse staffing levels and patient outcomes: Systematic review and meta-analysis. *Medical Care, 45*(12), 1195-1204.

Kaufman, K. (2007). Compensation for nurse educators: Findings from the NLN/Carnegie National Survey with implications for recruitment and retention. *Nursing Education Perspectives, 28*(4), 223-225.

Mark, B. A., Harless, D. W., McCue, M., & Xu, Y. (2004). A longitudinal examination of hospital registered nurse staffing and quality of care. *Health Services Research, 39*(2), 279-300.

Needleman, J., Buerhaus, P., Mattke, S., Stewart, M., & Zelevinsky, K. (2002). Nurse staffing levels and the quality of care in hospitals. *The New England Journal of Medicine, 346*(22), 1715-1722.

Robert Wood Johnson Foundation. (2006, June). *Wisdom at work: The importance of the older and experienced nurse in the workplace.* Princeton, NJ: Robert Wood Johnson Foundation.

U.S. Department of Health and Human Services. (2009). News release: Secretary Sebelius makes Recovery Act funding available to expand health professions training. Retrieved from www.hhs.gov/news/press/2009pres/07/20090728c.html.

U.S. Department of Health and Human Services, Bureau of Health Professions. (2004). *What is behind HRSA's projected supply, demand, and shortage of registered nurses?* Retrieved from ftp://ftp.hrsa.gov/bhpr/workforce/behindshortage.pdf.

U.S. Department of Health and Human Services, Health Resources and Services Administration. (2006). *The registered nurse population: Findings from the*

March 2004 National Sample Survey of Registered Nurses. Retrieved from ftp://ftp.hrsa.gov/bhpr/workforce/0306rnss.pdf.

U.S. Department of Health and Human Services, Health Resources and Services Administration. (2010). The registered nurse population: Initial findings from the 2008 National Sample Survey of Registered Nurses. Retrieved from http://bhpr.hrsa.gov/healthworkforce/rnsurvey/initialfindings2008.pdf.

Waldman, J. D., Kelly, F., Arora, S., & Smith, H. L. (2004). The shocking cost of turnover in health care. *Health Care Management Review, 29*(1), 2-7.

CHAPTER 50

Nursing Education Policy: The Unending Debate over Entry into Practice and the New Debate over Doctoral Degrees

Elaine Tagliareni and Beverly L. Malone

"In the ongoing improvisation of leadership—in which you act, assess, take corrective action, reassess, and intervene again—you can never know with certainty how an intervention is received unless you listen over time."

—R. A. Heifetz and M. Linsky, *Leadership on the Line: Staying Alive through the Dangers of Leading.*

The issue of educational entry level into nursing practice has been debated for decades. The old debate about entry into professional nursing at the prelicensure level and the latest debate about doctoral education and entry into advanced nursing practice are two specific issues that have emerged. Both debates stimulate the expression of strong beliefs by leaders in nursing education and nursing practice. The early debate focused on entry at the prelicensure level, more specifically, the movement of professional nursing practice into the academic setting. The current debate moves the dialogue to consideration of doctoral education, challenging the position of the traditional research-focused doctorate, calling for the Doctor of Nursing Practice (DNP) to be the profession's accepted credential for the advanced practice of nursing. Both debates concern the transformation of nursing practice in the midst of changing health care system and practice demands (Box 50-1).

The belief that a nurse's educational entry point impacts the quality and competence of the nurse's work has fueled both debates. This notion, that entry affects practice, has resulted in numerous position statements from professional organizations describing the nature of education needed for the future. The first of these statements, the American Nurses Association (ANA) 1965 "First Position on Education for Nursing" (ANA, 1965) sought to change the trajectory of nursing education and move education out of the service sector and into academic settings. The paper's authors saw a future with two levels of nursing—technical and professional; 2-year colleges would provide "minimum preparation for beginning technical nursing practice" (Committee on Nursing Education, 1965, p. 108), and 4-year programs would prepare graduates for beginning professional practice. This document also called for practical nursing programs to eventually be replaced by technical programs. Its publication created controversy and debate in the nursing education and practice community. Since 1965, other nursing organizations have published position statements calling for the baccalaureate degree to be entry level into professional nursing (e.g., American Association of Critical-Care Nurses [AACN], American Organization of Nurse Executives [AONE]).

Following the 1965 ANA position paper, colleges and university nursing programs created specialized masters programs. This educational approach became the norm, and credentialing and licensing of advanced practice roles recognized the masters degree as entry into advanced practice. The 2004 position paper of the American Association of Colleges of Nursing (AACN), which called for the establishment of the DNP, proposed that study for advanced practice roles—as midwives, nurse anesthetists, clinical nurse specialists, or nurse practitioners—should no longer

---

BOX 50-1 Concerns Voiced by the Nursing Community about the DNP

1. *The place for schools that do not have the option or the desire to offer a doctorate degree.* Many programs had successfully offered nurse practitioner programs at the masters degree level. How would these programs survive if the DNP was mandated for advanced practice?

2. *The premature release of the AACN document prior to adequate analysis and support from the nursing community.* Deans who voiced concern about the timing of the release also questioned the validity of diverting their energy away from discussions about the critical shortage of nurses and national policy decisions about new models of care delivery to a debate about a new degree. "The timing for developing, implementing, and evaluating this degree is, in a nutshell, disastrous to the potential involvement of nurses to make a substantial difference in the safety and quality of healthcare" (Meleis & Dracup, 2005).

3. *The separation of practice and research in the program's curriculum.* Opponents of the DNP argued that nursing had worked tirelessly to bridge the schism between research, practice, theory, and policy, and now the profession was proposing a separate research and practice doctorate. The thinking was that nursing requires more integration rather than fragmentation (Meleis & Dracup, 2005; Donley & Flaherty, 2002).

4. *The research-intensive environment of higher education.* Nursing faculty struggle in an environment that requires substantial acquisition of resources and, in particular, funding through research. A decrease in research-intensive doctorally prepared faculty might negatively affect the ability of deans and their faculty to maintain the research productivity that has become a standard for survival.

---

exist on the masters level. The DNP was, as proposed, now viewed as the clinical path into specialized advanced practice (Donley and Flaherty, 2002). This was a radical departure from specialized masters programs and represented a new form of entry into advanced roles in nursing.

Both debates occurred at unique times, in the framework of complex and evolving health care environments. Both debates placed new emphasis on shifting the educational trajectory of the nursing workforce. The intent of both debates was to elevate the status of nurses and improve patient care. Certainly, the most viable vision for nursing education must be nestled within the vision for the nation's health care system. This intent does not minimize nursing/education contributions of a strong, diverse workforce of well-prepared health care providers to the vision; it only reinforces and strengthens nursing's unique focus on patient-centered, community responsive care. But both debates sought to achieve this vision through new entry requirements, which has the appearance of self-enhancement, rather than focus decision making on the nation's health care needs. This may be the most powerful lesson learned from nursing's unending debates over entry into practice.

THE ENTRY INTO PRACTICE DEBATE

HISTORICAL PERSPECTIVE

Following World War II, an increased demand for nurses occurred because many nurses returning from military service did not reenter the workforce. Also, changes in health care, including hospital-based births, surgical procedures, and anesthesia, necessitated more nurses working in hospitals (Haase, 1990). In 1946, Congress passed the Hill-Burton Act, which provided federal grants and guaranteed loans to improve the physical plant of the nation's hospitals, nursing homes, and other health care facilities. In return, these agencies agreed to provide a reasonable volume of services to persons unable to pay and to make their services available to all persons residing in the facility's area, making the demand for nurses more urgent. At the time, hospital diploma programs were the primary source of new nursing graduates. Baccalaureate programs produced only 15% of the new nurses each year and could not meet the increasing demand for graduate nurses (Orsolini-Hahn & Waters, 2009).

In 1948, the Carnegie Foundation commissioned a sociologist, Dr. Esther Lucille Brown, to study nursing education and to address the critical nursing shortage in the United States due to a decreased supply of nurses and an increased demand following World War II. Brown's report, *Nursing for the Future*, called for nurses to be educated in colleges and universities instead of hospital-based programs (Brown, 1948). The ANA and the National League for Nursing

(NLN) supported the Brown report and urged the nursing education community to move nursing education into the college environment (Orsolini-Hahn & Waters, 2009). Simultaneously, President Harry Truman convened a National Commission on Higher Education, which called for the expansion of community colleges. In response to both documents, NLN representatives arranged a meeting with the Association of Community Junior Colleges (AAJC), now known as the American Association of Community Colleges (AACC), to explore the idea of teaching nursing in 2-year community college programs (Haase, 1990).

While these events transpired on a national level, faculty at Teachers College, Columbia University, were engaged in the exploration of new models of nursing education. A doctoral student, Mildred Montag, proposed in her dissertation that nurses be educated at community colleges as nursing technicians (Montag & Gotkin, 1959). Montag was influenced by a study group at Teachers College, chaired by Eli Ginzburg, which proposed two levels of nurse practitioners, a practical or technical level and a professional level. Dr. Montag's dissertation, entitled, *"Education for Nursing Technicians,"* received funding to conduct research on this new model, and in 1952, under her leadership, faculty from seven original associate degree programs created the 2-year technical program. Although the course of study was referred to as *technical and terminal,* a term used at the time to signify that the entire course of study could be accomplished in a set time-frame, faculty in the new programs viewed their mandate as more than development of a shortened traditional program; they envisioned a program of learning that would revolutionize nursing education. The curriculum was no longer based on a "map of the hospital" (Waters, 2007). Rather, the concept of nursing was patient-centered (not disease-centered), and the curriculum was based on broader structures like fundamental concepts and adult nursing considerations (Haase, 1990). By 1980, associate degree programs were educating approximately 20% of new graduate nurses (Orsolini-Hahn & Waters, 2009). Simultaneously, professional nursing programs developed in baccalaureate programs, but not at the same pace as community college programs (Haase, 1990). The extraordinary growth of associate degree nursing education from the midpoint of the last century is compelling. Today associate degree nursing graduates account for slightly over 60% of new RN graduates each year (NLN, 2008) from over 900 associate nursing degree programs nationally.

UPHEAVAL WITHIN THE PROFESSION

Controversy followed the associate degree programs from their inception. For one reason, the educational model was not consistent with the way associate degree graduates were utilized in practice. Dr. Montag had proposed this new model based on a two-level system of nursing care delivery. She intended that associate degree graduates would function on teams led by baccalaureate prepared nurses. As noted, she used the term *terminal* course of study and never intended that programs would articulate, due to the significant difference in technical and professional education. But the practice environment used the new associate degree graduate almost immediately in management and leadership positions, where they performed satisfactorily (Orsalini-Hahn & Waters, 2009). By the 1970s, associate degree graduates were actively encouraged to pursue advanced study in baccalaureate programs in order to advance their career options.

The response of the nursing community to this education/practice role confusion was to engage in differentiation of practice debates. For almost 50 years, nursing attempted to define and articulate differences between graduates of the two types of nursing programs. Because these debates focused on practice in acute care both at the bedside and in management, where roles of both graduates were blurred and overlapped, they failed to clearly define differences (Haase, 1990). Waters (2007) reports that at a meeting in California in the 1980s faculty from baccalaureate and associate degree programs met to distinguish curricula and were unsuccessful in creating a document that delineated distinctive core content. In both education and practice, no clear distinctions between the two levels emerged.

As early as 1965, organized nursing attempted to bring clarity to the differentiation debate. The ANA convened the Committee on Education to study nursing education, practice, and scope of responsibilities, due to the increasing complexity of health care and changes in practice. The study group recommended that the minimum preparation for beginning professional nursing practice should be the baccalaureate degree. The Committee on Education's statement became ANA's "position paper" and contained a description of three levels of nursing education: baccalaureate education for beginning professional nursing practice, associate degree education for beginning technical nursing practice, and vocational education for assistants in the health service occupations (ANA, 1965). The authors of the 1965 position statement also recommended that associate degree programs replace practical nursing programs, further alienating vocational and practical nurses and faculty. During the same year, the NLN published *Resolution 5,* a document that called for examination of the differentiated functions of the two levels of nursing education (Haase, 1990). Subsequently, the 1965 ANA position paper was reaffirmed by a 1978 ANA House of Delegates resolution that resulted in the recommendation that by 1985 the minimum preparation for entry into professional practice would be the baccalaureate degree.

In 1969, the AACN was established to advance nursing education at the baccalaureate and graduate levels. Since the 1970s, the organization called for quality standards for bachelor's and graduate degree nursing education and actively promoted public support of baccalaureate and graduate education, calling for the baccalaureate degree in nursing as the educational basis for the profession. In 1982, the NLN published *Position Statement on Nursing Roles—Scope and Preparation,* emphasizing that professional nursing practice required a baccalaureate degree and that preparation for technical nursing practice be accomplished through associate degree or diploma education (Kaiser, 1983). The designation of two levels of nursing practice, professional and technical, was reaffirmed by NLN, at a time when both ANA and AACN called for the baccalaureate degree as the minimum entry for professional nursing practice. The nursing education community envisioned an orderly transition to professional entry at the baccalaureate level and an educational system of two levels with subsequent differentiated practice. This never occurred.

What did happen was a divided health and nursing community (Donley & Flaherty, 2002). Many associate degree nurse educators became disillusioned with the ANA and NLN, leaving both organizations to start a new organization in 1986, the National Organization for the Advancement of Associate Degree Nursing, which later became the National Organization for Associate Degree Nursing (N-OADN). The NLN established separate councils for associate degree and baccalaureate educators. The councils rarely interacted, and strained relationships developed between faculty in both types of programs. This resulted in few opportunities for constructive dialogue about ways to create articulation between programs and build a more educated workforce, which had been the primary intent of the Brown report, the ANA 1965 position statement, and the NLN early documents. The central focus of the early debate to move nursing education to higher education, away from hospital-based certificate programs, had been to improve educational preparation, elevate the status of nurses, and ultimately improve the quality and safety of patient care, thereby addressing nursing's long-held vision. Yet nursing had become mired in differentiation debates that only served to sidetrack the discussion. As a result, over 50 years later, the need for a more educated workforce remains at the core of the entry into practice debate.

CURRENT CLIMATE: THE REALITIES OF THE WORKFORCE

In adopting the 1965 ANA Position Statement, the nursing community declared that they were ready to set their own standards, apart from those dictated by the physician-driven (or led) hospital system. ANA commission members clearly determined that professional nurses must be grounded in science and critical thinking, and not merely follow ritualistic practices (Donley & Flaherty, 2002). Nurse leaders were also making the case that more educated nurses would improve patient care and have a greater impact on the health care system. This same belief lies at the foundation of nursing's current debate about the educational level that best prepares nurses to deliver safe and efficient nursing care.

The current health care reform agenda, led by the Obama administration, calls for new models of chronic care delivery and a greater focus on health promotion and disease prevention. This will require knowledge of research, centralized care coordination, outcomes management, risk assessment, and quality improvement—educational core content traditionally assigned to the baccalaureate curriculum. Furthermore, new models of service delivery will require a systems approach to address the consequences of disparities in access to health care services that preclude quality care for all individuals. These approaches require advanced study and practice implementation.

Yet the most recent workforce data (U.S. Department of Health and Human Services [USDHHS], 2006) reveal that too few nurses are pursuing graduate degrees needed to assume advanced roles. These data show that about 6.4% of those initially educated in associate degree programs and 11.7% of those prepared in diploma programs had obtained post-RN graduate degrees in nursing or related fields. Additionally, only 22.1% of nurses prepared initially in a baccalaureate program had obtained post-RN masters or doctoral degrees. Comprehensive analyses of these same data 4 years later were not available at the time of publication. But preliminary data indicate that the number of RNs with masters and doctorate degrees rose by 46% from 2004, suggesting that, finally, more nurses are progressing to advanced practice roles. This slow movement to advanced practice may be an unintended consequence of the differentiation wars that occurred over the past 50 years.

Debates about entry into practice at the prelicensure level have been divisive and counterproductive. Nurses enter the profession today from a wide variety of access points: LPN progression programs; generic pre-licensure programs in diploma, associate degree, and baccalaureate programs; accelerated baccalaureate programs for graduates of non-nursing disciplines; and entry-level masters programs. All of these options contribute to the diversity and expanding numbers of RNs available to meet the current nursing shortage. Certainly, one of the strengths of the current nursing education system is the multiple entry points currently available to individuals who desire to pursue a nursing career. In fact, it is our belief that recognition of multiple access points to the profession is not in conflict with the current need for a more educated nursing workforce.

To make this happen, innovative and expanded educational opportunities must be available and utilized by increasing numbers of nurses currently employed in the RN workforce. This is the heart of the current entry into practice debate: How will the nursing community improve patient care and increase the educational level of its workforce while accepting multiple educational access points?

A critical goal for the nursing profession must be to sidestep the old argument of baccalaureate entry and move to the option of RN to BSN or RN to MSN (not based on entry but for lifelong learning) and take fullest advantage of the diversity offered by multiple progression points. The NLN contends that creative approaches need to be conceptualized and implemented so that the capacity of baccalaureate and masters programs to accommodate all RNs who would be required to earn the advanced academic degree is addressed. Current efforts to seek federal and state funding to offer tuition reimbursement and/or loan repayment options are actively supported by members of nursing's Tri-Council—ANA, NLN, AACN, and AONE. The nursing community has begun to come together around this issue and, rather than focus on entrance to the profession, are working collaboratively to improve patient care and address the needs for a more educated workforce.

In 1965, nurse leaders made a clear statement of autonomy (Donley & Flaherty, 2002) by declaring the need for a more educated nurse. For the next 50 years, the nursing community became sidetracked about how to achieve that goal, and the differentiation debates diverted nursing's productive energy away from its fundamental vision to meet the needs of a changing practice environment. It is imperative now that the nursing community return to this original intent and that a new conversation emerge—one centered on improving health care through active dialogue about progression within the profession.

THE ENTRY INTO ADVANCED PRACTICE DEBATE

HISTORICAL PERSPECTIVE

Advanced practice nursing emerged as a response to the physician shortage in the late 1950s (Joelle, 2002). By the mid-1960s, nurse practitioner programs existed throughout the U.S. as postbaccalaureate certificate programs of varying length (O'Sullivan, Carter, Marion, Pohl, & Werner, 2005). In 1990, the National Organization of Nurse Practitioner Faculties (NONPF) published *Advanced Nursing Practice: Nurse Practitioner Curriculum Guidelines* and called for nurse practitioner education to be grounded in graduate-level programs (NONPF, 1990). Within the next decade, the shift away from certificate nurse practitioner programs was complete, with less than 1% of all nurse practitioner programs representing non-masters education tracks (O'Sullivan, Carter, Marion, Pohl, & Werner, 2005).

Since that time, a growing movement within nursing emerged to reconsider nurse practitioner educational preparation; the practice doctorate was discussed as a means to meet the demand for increased knowledge and skills. The following societal changes and emerging health care trends sparked this movement:

- In the late 1990s, nurse-managed health centers emerged as safety net providers for underserved populations, extending the range of primary care services offered by nurse practitioners in autonomous practice settings (Hansen-Turton & Kinsey, 2001). These centers were operated and managed by advanced practice nurses and offered both primary care services as well as wellness-based health promotion and disease prevention services. These centers provided new opportunities for advanced practice nurses to create comprehensive models to serve vulnerable populations and helped to offset the decreasing numbers of physicians interested in primary care careers (O'Sullivan, Carter, Marion, Pohl, & Werner, 2005).
- The nursing community recognized that the demand for new models of care to manage complex chronic co-morbidities, specifically of an aging population, required movement away from illness management to non-traditional approaches to case management involving multiple intersecting systems of care. Nurse leaders raised the question of whether or not these new models could be addressed adequately in the current advanced practice masters curriculum.
- Nurse faculty teaching in nurse practitioner programs called for parity with other allied health professions. These disciplines (e.g., pharmacy, audiology, and physical therapy) had expanded their masters degree programs and created practice doctorates in response to the need for advanced practice professionals to work within complex systems, advocating for evidence-based quality care in an interdisciplinary environment. Nursing leaders argued that parity for nursing was not simply a matter of status but a necessary credential for credibility in leadership and policy positions (Lenz, 2005).

- The Institute of Medicine (IOM) proposed changes in practice (IOM, 2003) calling for a reduction of medical errors and an increase in competencies necessary to deliver quality health care, including utilization of informatics, understanding of quality improvement, a focus on patient-centered care, wide acceptance of evidence-based practice, and movement to interdisciplinary care models. Changes in practice would require new approaches to the education of advanced practice health care professionals, including courses in health care finance and policy, process, and outcomes measurement and analysis and use of evidence-based methods to plan and implement care (O'Sullivan, Carter, Marion, Pohl, & Werner, 2005). As these new educational demands resulted in increased clinical and classroom hours in nurse practitioner programs, the credit allotment had not increased commensurately. It became apparent to faculty in nurse practitioner programs that nursing may be under-credentialing its advanced practice graduates to the point where they far surpassed requirements for masters programs in other clinical disciplines (Lenz, 2005).

EMERGENCE OF THE DNP: THE EARLY DEBATE

In 2004, AACN members endorsed a position statement on the *Practice Doctorate in Nursing* (AACN, 2004). This document was a response to calls for a change in masters-level advanced practice nursing programs and advocated for moving entry into advanced nursing practice from the masters to the doctorate level by the year 2015. The Doctor of Nursing Practice (DNP), as the new entry level would be termed, was viewed as a viable alternative to the research-focused doctorate in nursing for nurses who desired to pursue excellence in nursing practice.

After a 2-year consensus-building process, AACN member institutions voted to endorse the *Essentials of Doctoral Education for Advanced Nursing Practice* (AACN, 2006a). The DNP Essentials were purposely developed to incorporate *The Essentials of Master's Education for Advanced Practice Nursing* (AACN, 2006b) and to further expand and increase the level of this content. In this way, proponents of the new program of study sought to establish parity with other health care professionals with whom NPs collaborate in providing health care. Competencies for nurse practitioner education had already been developed and published in 2002 by the NONPF (NONPF, 2002). These competencies were refined and clarified in 2006, and the *Practice Doctorate Nurse Practitioner Entry-Level Competencies* were distributed nationally (NONPF, 2006). There was significant synergy between the AACN Essentials and the NONPF Competencies; both documents built on the current masters-level advanced practice programs and expanded practice to include such areas as evidence-based practice, quality improvement, and systems thinking (AACN, 2006a, 2006b).

Yet despite the collaboration between the NONPF and the AACN, the publication of the AACN documents (AACN, 2004, 2006a) generated considerable debate within the nursing community. Additionally, *The Essentials of Doctoral Education for Advanced Nursing Practice* (AACN, 2006a) suggests that individuals who acquire the DNP will "seek to fill roles as educators and will use their considerable practice expertise to educate the next generation of nurses" (p. 7). In its Reflection and Dialogue series, the NLN (2007) voiced a concern that the foundational essentials for the DNP curriculum design did not include courses related to pedagogy, evaluation, academic role issues and elements, and educational theory. The NLN questioned the ability of graduates of DNP programs to manage the complex and specialized knowledge intrinsic to the advanced specialty role of the academic nurse educator. Faculty who are not educated in pedagogy, evaluation, and educational theory reasoned that the NLN may not be in a position to engage meaningfully in nursing education research or make evidence-based contributions to nursing education reform. The overall concern of the NLN continues to be the shortage of faculty and the need for significant educational reform in these complex times. Graduates of DNP programs may help to alleviate the faculty shortage as the number of graduates increases, but to achieve curriculum reform and knowledge of teaching, faculty need the specialized knowledge that is fundamental to the advanced specialty role of nurse educator.

Proponents of the DNP cite the value of the DNP for contemporary practice. The benefit to advanced practice nurses of balancing the playing field in terms of status and authority between nursing and other health care professionals with doctorates has already been noted. Additionally, it has been suggested that the development of DNP programs will inevitably reflect the range of nursing roles that typify nursing practice, and the increasing complexity of health care will necessarily shape the direction of DNP practice, both in clinical settings and in nursing education. This natural evolution, it is argued, will lead to a synergy between DNP graduates and their PhD colleagues and provide new ways to foster research expertise, leading to the advancement of nursing science and improved patient care.

It is too early to know the outcome of the entry into advanced practice debate. Essential questions to be addressed by nursing leadership include the following:

- Will the move lead to greater confusion about nursing education than is already experienced by the public, other health professionals, and even nurses themselves (Dracup & Bryan-Brown, 2005)?
- Will the existence of DNP programs siphon off badly needed enrollment in traditional research-focused doctoral programs (Dracup, Cronenwett, Meleis, & Benner, 2005)?
- Will the DNP curricula combine educational theory and curriculum instruction with practice requirements in order to meet the needs of the significant number of graduates seeking faculty positions?

LESSONS LEARNED FROM NURSING'S JOURNEY

There are at least five major areas of learning from the profession's protracted journey in nursing education: Vision, Inclusion, Diversity, the Practice and Education Bridge, and the Politics of Connection: Allies, Partners and Champions (Box 50-2). These are not unknown areas of learning for nursing; they are frequently the forgotten and discounted priorities as change is pursued. As time moves us forward, to achieve not only change but transformation of a system, these priorities must be acknowledged and consistently implemented as essential components of the nursing education agenda.

SUMMARY

Donley and Flaherty (2002) raise the question about the long-term achievements of the 1965 ANA position paper. The document called for all nursing education

BOX 50-2 Lessons Learned from Nursing's Journey

Vision

Dr. Gloria Smith describes the vision for nursing education and for the American people in her article "Commentary: In Pursuit of the American Dream" (Smith, 2009). The new health care system for the twenty-first century "... would be both patient centered and community responsive; it would be culturally sensitive, accessible, affordable, and cost effective. It would use health personnel more effectively and would value public health and primary prevention" (p. 67). By refusing to become distracted by old and new arguments related to entry, rather than focus on being responsive to a new vision for the nation's health care system, nursing/education today has the opportunity for leadership into a new era of lifelong learning and progression, claiming a stake in the vision without the perception of exclusive professional self-enhancement (sometimes referred to as *tribalism*). The vision requires a nursing workforce that meets current and future demands for quality and safety. The vision is the overarching umbrella that allows space for dialogue, reflection, and debate that can exceed our individual/professional differences, leading to creative pathways of collaboration and transformation.

Inclusion

Nursing's history is replete with vivid examples describing the exclusion of nursing as a legitimate profession. Challenged on every front frequently by other health care providers, nurses have had to demonstrate and verify their competence from taking blood pressures to delivering anesthesia services. However, from the early days of Florence Nightingale as she turned Mary Seacole (a black British nurse) away from the opportunity to work with her in the Crimean War zone, we, the nurses, have worked from a model of exclusion, particularly with one another.

It would seem that having been the recipient of a model of exclusion, we would be especially sensitive and proactive to dispel it within our ranks. Even at this time of twenty-first century enlightenment, the nursing profession still clearly disallows space for the licensed practical nurse (LPN) and the health care assistant (HCA). The question is not whether they are professional registered nurses—which they are not; it is more whether they are involved in nursing practice— which they are. The majority of nursing care delivered in nursing homes and many community centers is delivered by these two groups of care providers. Therefore, our older adults and some of our most fragile population are primarily being cared for by LPNs and HCAs. Their exclusion can be noted in our professional organizations, our policy initiatives, and our professional development activities, with the exception, to some degree, of groups like the Black Nurses Association and the NLN. For nursing not to claim our relationship to our colleagues and to exclude nurses from a

variety of entry points for both prelicensure and postlicensure programs is shortsighted of the patient-centered, community responsive care vision that a reformed health care system can offer.

Diversity

The NLN's (2008) definition of diversity is as follows: "A culture of diversity embraces acceptance and respect. We understand that each individual is unique and recognize individual differences which can be along the dimensions of race, ethnicity, gender, sexual orientation, socio-economic status, age, physical abilities, religious beliefs, political beliefs or other ideologies. A culture of diversity is about understanding ourselves and each other and moving beyond simple tolerance to embracing and celebrating the richness of each individual. While diversity can be about individual differences, it also encompasses institutional and system-wide behavior patterns."

To focus on the vision, diversity has to be broader than race and ethnicity. Yet to be true to the vision for this nation with its multicultural people, race and ethnicity must be a focus. From 1990 to 2000, the percentage of minorities graduating from our nursing programs remained flat, with African Americans having the highest at about 7%. Even into the twenty-first century, African Americans remain the highest at approximately 11% of those graduating from basic RN programs, followed by Hispanics at 6.5%, Asians at 5.3%, and American Indians at approximately 1%. One especially troubling aspect of this is the growth in Hispanics, totaling 13% of the country's population, and the lack of adequate representation in the nursing workforce. The old and new debates infrequently discuss these issues. Strategic efforts are still lacking in making a difference in diversity. Gutmann (2009) states, "to transform, there must be desire." For a culture of diversity within the nursing/education workforce and workplace, there must be the desire, the will to envision, create, plan, and implement and to move to a culture of inclusiveness.

The Practice and Education Bridge

It would seem that the more recent debate on the DNP learned from the earlier debate on entry for education and practice. The effort to work together as reflected by the involvement of the NONPF with the AACN provided a link between education and practice. However, nursing's practice world has more sectors than one organization, and, in addition, the practice/education connection, which started as a primary base of the DNP, changed as practice took priority over development of nurse educator competencies and education receded into the background.

The new learning involves an ongoing relationship between practice and education—one that does not begin with a new project or initiative but is simply how the profession deliberates, strategizes, implements, and evaluates its vision—still nestled

BOX 50-2 **Lessons Learned from Nursing's Journey—cont'd**

within the larger health care system vision. This means a redesigning of both our nursing education and clinical organizations to be more inclusive of one another. The resounding question is "How can one think about a nursing education or clinical issue without practice or education playing a primary role in understanding the question and helping to determine the answer?"

The Politics of Connection

Allies, Partners and Champions: From these nursing education debates of old and today, there is the message that nursing cannot stand alone or that even sectors of nursing cannot stand alone. Without allies, partners, and champions, we become so internally focused that we repeatedly lose sight of the vision. Allies are those in friendly association with nursing; partners are united or associated with nursing in an activity or a sphere of common interest; champions are those who will fight for nursing.

There are internal and external allies, partners, and champions. For example, the Tri-Council for Nursing mentioned earlier in the chapter fits all three definitions and yet is internal to nursing. It does provide a forum for dialogue and reflection as well as a political/governmental agenda that directs the organization's attention to the vision. However, it is the external allies, partners, and champions such as the Robert Wood Johnson Foundation, the Gordon and Betty Moore Foundation, the Johnson and Johnson Foundation, the W. K. Kellogg Foundation, and the Center for Championing Nursing that consistently challenge nursing to stay focused on the vision. The vision of a transformed health care system that is patient-centered and community responsive is the lifeline for the nursing profession. Nursing education, with all of its twists and turns through time, has consciously and unconsciously worked to create a strong diverse nursing workforce to heal the world.

to take place in colleges and universities; today over 90% of prelicensure nursing programs exist in community colleges and bachelors degree–granting institutions. In that sense, the position paper had a profound effect on changing the trajectory of nursing education. However, if you consider the document to be a call for a more educated workforce, then the mandate was less successful. Similarly, if you consider the major outcome of the DNP to be parity for advanced practice nursing with other allied health disciplines, then the nursing profession is well on its way to establishing leadership and policy credibility. However, if the intent is to advance excellence in nursing practice and nursing education to address the vision of a transformed health care system that is patient centered and community responsive, the outcome is presently unknown.

For a list of related websites, please refer to your Evolve Resources at http://evolve.elsevier.com/Mason/policypolitics/

REFERENCES

American Association of Colleges of Nursing (AACN). (2004). *Position statement on the practice doctorate in nursing.* Retrieved from www.aacn.nche.edu/DNP/DNPPositionStatement.htm.

American Association of Colleges of Nursing (AACN). (2006a). *The essentials of doctoral education for advanced nursing practice.* Retrieved from www.aacn.nche.edu/DNP/pdf/Essentials.pdf.

American Association of Colleges of Nursing (AACN). (2006b). *The essentials of master's education for advanced nursing practice.* Retrieved from www.aacn.nche.edu/Education/pdf/MasEssentials96.pdf.

American Nurses Association (1965). *A position paper.* New York: American Nurses Association.

Brown, E. L. (1948). *Nursing for the future: A report prepared for the National Nursing Council.* New York: Russell Sage Foundation.

Committee on Nursing Education, American Nurses Association. (1965). American Nurses Association's first position on education for nursing. *American Journal of Nursing, 65*(12), 106-107.

Donley, R., & Flaherty, M. J. (2002, May 31). Revisiting the American Nurses Association's First Position on Education for Nurses. *Online Journal of Issues in Nursing, 7*(2), manuscript 1. Retrieved from http://nursingworld.org/MainMenuCategories/ANAMarketplace/ANAPeriodicals/OJIN/TableofContents/Volume72002/No2May2002/RevisingPostiononEducation.aspx.

Dracup, K., & Bryan-Brown, C. W. (2005). Doctor of nursing practice—MRI or total body scan? *American Journal of Critical Care, 14*(4), 278-281.

Dracup, K., Cronenwett, L., Meleis, A. I., & Benner, P. E. (2005). Reflections on the doctorate of nursing practice. *Nursing Outlook, 53*(4), 177-182.

Gutmann, D. (2009). *From transformation to transformaction: Methods and practices.* London: Karnac.

Haase, P. T. (1990). *The origins and rise of associate degree nursing.* Durham, NC: Duke University Press.

Hansen-Turton, T., & Kinsey, K. (2001). The quest for self-sustainability: Nurse-managed health centers meeting the policy challenge. *Policy, Politics, & Nursing Practice, 2*(4), 304-309.

Institute of Medicine. (2003). *Health professions education: A bridge to quality.* Retrieved from http://books.nap.edu/openbook.fhp?record_id=10681.

Joelle, L. (2002). Education for entry into nursing practice: revisited for the 21st century. *Online Journal of Issues in Nursing, 7*(2). Retrieved from www.nursingworld.org/MainMenuCategories/ANAMarketplace/ANAPeriodicals/OJIN/TableofContents/Volume72002/No2May2002/EntryintoNursingPractice.aspx.

Kaiser, J. E. (Ed.) (1983). *The associate degree nurse: Technical or professional?* New York: National League for Nursing.

Lenz, E. R. (2005). The practice doctorate in nursing: An idea whose time has come. *Online Journal of Issues in Nursing, 10*(3).

Meleis, A., & Dracup, K. (2005). The case against the DNP: History, timing, substance, and marginalization. *Online Journal of Issues in Nursing, 10*(3).

Montag, M. L., & Gotkin, L. G. (1959). *Community college education for nursing: An experiment in technical education for nursing: Report of the cooperative* research project in junior-community college education for nursing. New York: McGraw-Hill.

National League for Nursing. (2007). *Reflection and dialogue: Academic/professional progression in nursing*. Retrieved from www.nln.org/aboutnln/reflection_dialogue/refl_dial_2.htm.

National League for Nursing (2008). *Nursing data review, academic years 1990-2006. Baccalaureate, associate and diploma degree programs*. New York: National League for Nursing.

National Organization of Nurse Practitioner Faculties. (1990). *Advanced nursing practice: Nurse practitioner curriculum guidelines*. Author.

National Organization of Nurse Practitioner Faculties. (2002). NONPF clinical doctorate initiative. NONPF Practice Doctorate Resource Center. Retrieved from www.nonpf.org/cdstratinitiative.htm.

National Organization of Nurse Practitioner Faculties. (2006). *Advanced nursing practice: Curriculum guidelines and program standards for nurse practitioner education*. Washington, DC: Author.

Orsolini-Hahn, L., & Waters, V. (2009). Education evolution: A historical perspective of associate degree nursing. *Journal of Nursing Education, 48*(5), 266-271.

O'Sullivan, A., Carter, M., Marion, L., Pohl, J., & Werner, K. (2005). Moving forward together: the practice doctorate in nursing. *Online Journal of Issues in Nursing, 10*(3). Retrieved from www.nursingworld.org/MainMenuCategories/ANAMarketplace/ANAPeriodicals/OJIN/TableofContents/Volume102005/No3Sept05/tpc28_416028.aspx.

Smith, G. (2009). Commentary: In pursuit of the American Dream. In H. Bessent (Ed.), *Minority nurses in the new century*. New York: National League for Nursing.

Waters, V. (2007). Reflecting on revolutions: A half-century in nursing education. In P. M. Ironside (Ed.), *On revolutions and revolutionaries: 25 years of reform and innovation in nursing education* (pp. 163-168). New York: National League for Nursing.

U.S. Department of Health and Human Services (HRSA, BHPr). (2006). *The Registered Nurse population: Findings from the March 2004 National Sample Survey of Registered Nurses*.

CHAPTER 51

The Politics of Advanced Practice Nursing

Eileen T. O'Grady and Loretta C. Ford

"We shall be what we determine to be."
—Margareta Madden Styles, Nurse leader
and legend (1930-2005)

Advanced Practice Registered Nurses (APRNs) have achieved unprecedented growth and recognition over the last four decades; political activism and social justice have always been at the heart of all four APRN roles. This chapter explores the major political issues facing APRNs with suggestions from the authors about ways to increase their political competence, visibility, and political power to impact the larger health policy context.

APRN DEFINITION

The term *Advanced Practice Registered Nurse* is an umbrella term comprising four advanced practice nursing roles: nurse anesthetists, clinical nurse specialists, nurse midwives, and nurse practitioners. APRNs are licensed independent practitioners who are expected to practice within standards established or recognized by a licensing body. Although all APRNs are educationally prepared to provide care to patients across the health wellness-illness continuum, the practice emphasis within each APRN role varies. The defining factor for all four APRN roles is that a significant component of the education and practice focuses on the direct care of individuals Box 51-1 (National Council of State Boards of Nursing [NCSBN], 2008).

THE POLITICAL ISSUES

Until 2008, there were no common standards for state licensing for APRNs. While education, accreditation, and certification are necessary components of an overall approach to preparing APRNs for practice, the state licensing boards are the final arbiters of who is recognized to practice within a given state. Each state independently determines the APRN legal scope of practice, the roles that are recognized, the criteria for entry, and the certification examinations required. A consensus among all of the various stakeholders was needed to establish stronger internal cohesion within the APRN movement. This high degree of variability around practice created significant barriers for APRNs to easily move from state to state, decreased access to care, and created confusion among policymakers. Barriers to practice in many states include: requiring physician supervision, limiting reimbursement, and restricting prescriptive privileges (Pearson, 2010). The lack of national standards has made APRNs vulnerable to criticism from those who oppose their independence, such as the AMA. There was much disagreement in the APRN community about the definition of APRNs. For example, clinical nurse specialists (CNSs), who blend advanced practice and specialty nursing practice, have a high degree of variability in their educational programs. They did not uniformly define their role as direct care providers; most are not nationally certified and often do not have a standardized curriculum (Gray, 2001). Certified Nurse Midwives (CNM) created another quandary. They include non-nurses, under the rubric of "midwives" since they credential non-nurse midwives. This decision allows midwives to practice in 14 states provided they hold a bachelors degree, complete an education program in midwifery, and pass a certification exam (Gray, 2001). The practice and/or educational variability of CNSs and CNMs to be included under the APRN umbrella created a particular

---

BOX 51-1 APRN Criteria

1. Completes an accredited graduate-level program in one of the four roles, to be at the Doctor of Nursing Practice (DNP) level by 2015.
2. Passes a national certification exam that measures APRN role and population-focused competencies and maintains continued competence through recertification.
3. Possess advanced clinical knowledge preparing one to provide direct care to patients.
4. Is educationally prepared to assume responsibility and accountability for all health promotion and/or maintenance as well as the assessment, diagnosis, and management of patient problems including the use of prescription pharmacological and nonpharmacological interventions.
5. Has significant breadth and depth of clinical experience to reflect the intended license.
6. Obtained a license to practice as an APRN in one of the four APRN roles: certified registered nurse anesthetist (CRNA), certified nurse-midwife (CNM), clinical nurse specialist (CNS), or certified nurse practitioner (CNP).

From National Council of State Boards of Nursing. (2008). *Consensus model for APRN regulation: Licensure, accreditation, certification & education.*

---

challenge. As any practice field evolves, a common language is required for guiding and evaluating practice, standardizing educational programs and certification requirements so that states can create sensible regulations to protect public safety.

The history of physician opposition to APRNs is a long one, but was not present when the first NP program was developed, according to Loretta Ford. The early partnership between nurse practitioners (NPs) and pediatricians was built on mutual respect, collaboration, and shared values and goals for patients. However this relationship deteriorated into turf battles as medical organizations sought to control the NP's expanding scope of practice. The belief that physicians were "Captains of the Ship" fueled a growing animosity between nursing and medical organizations.

Politics introduces divisive and self-interested agendas into the policymaking process. This resistance to APRNs by some organized physician groups is a quintessential definition of politics—the struggle for ascendency or dominance among groups with different power relationships and agendas. One strategy to level the playing field is for organizations to use the power of government to achieve what they cannot alone.

A COMMON LICENSURE: LACE

It is within this context that APNs have made a significant achievement with the publication of the *Consensus Model for APRN Regulation: Licensure, Accreditation, Certification and Education* (hereafter referred to as *LACE*) (NCSBN, 2008). This document and the 3-year process that brought together over 70 organizational stakeholders is one of the most important, cutting-edge, and visionary achievements in decades Box 51-2. The LACE document establishes clear, professionally-endorsed, national expectations for APRN licensure, accreditation, certification, and education (Stanley, 2009). It has strengthened the position of APRNs to confront resistance. It creates clear national standards for state regulators to adapt a framework for modernizing their state nurse practice acts across the nation.

The core educational criteria for all four APRN roles includes the "three *P*s": intensive study in advanced **p**hysical assessment, **p**athophysiology, and **p**harmacology. LACE lays out how the State Boards of Nursing must have complete control of licensure for APRN roles, which assures independent practice, full prescriptive authority, titling, and compact agreements for interstate licensure and practice mobility. Sub-specialization, such as pediatric oncology, requires competence in one of the roles and population foci, and certification by the corresponding specialty board (Figure 51-1).

The implementation of LACE recommendations must be incorporated as each state modernizes its Nurse Practice Act. All APRN stakeholders, including educational institutions, certifying bodies, and regulators are challenged to incorporate the recommendations.

The late Margareta Madden Styles (2008), in her challenge to nursing specialization and credentialing, offers some sage advice applicable to APRNs. She asked, "How is this pulled together so that it can be said that the profession is self-regulating, self-determining? If we truly understand the importance of [licensing and] credentialing to profession-building, we must realize that the integrity of our professional structure is threatened [when we do not have consistent, standardized, licensing, accreditation, certification and educational requirements across the country]" (p. 57).

BOX 51-2 Organizations Participating in the APRN Consensus Process

1. Academy of Medical-Surgical Nurses
2. American College of Nurse-Midwives Division of Accreditation
3. American Academy of Nurse Practitioners
4. American Academy of Nurse Practitioners Certification Program
5. American Association of Colleges of Nursing
6. American Association of Critical Care Nurses Certification
7. American Association of Neuroscience Nurses
8. American Association of Nurse Anesthetists
9. American Association of Occupational Health Nurses
10. American Board for Occupational Health Nurses
11. American Board of Nursing Specialties
12. American College of Nurse-Midwives
13. American College of Nurse-Midwives Division of Accreditation
14. American College of Nurse Practitioners
15. American Holistic Nurses Association
16. American Nephrology Nurses Association
17. American Nurses Association
18. American Nurses Credentialing Center
19. American Organization of Nurse Executives
20. American Psychiatric Nurses Association
21. American Society of PeriAnesthesia Nurses
22. American Society for Pain Management Nursing
23. Association of Community Health Nursing Educators
24. Association of Faculties of Pediatric Nurse Practitioners
25. Association of Nurses in AIDS Care
26. Association of PeriOperative Registered Nurses
27. Association of Rehabilitation Nurses
28. Association of State and Territorial Directors of Nursing
29. Association of Women's Health, Obstetric and Neonatal Nurses
30. Board of Certification for Emergency Nursing
31. Council on Accreditation of Nurse Anesthesia Educational Programs
32. Commission on Collegiate Nursing Education
33. Commission on Graduates of Foreign Nursing Schools
34. District of Columbia Board of Nursing
35. Department of Health
36. Dermatology Nurses Association
37. Division of Nursing, DHHS, HRSA
38. Emergency Nurses Association
39. George Washington University
40. Health Resources and Services Administration
41. Infusion Nurses Society
42. International Nurses Society on Addictions
43. International Society of Psychiatric-Mental Health Nurses
44. Kentucky Board of Nursing
45. National Association of Clinical Nurse Specialists
46. National Association of Neonatal Nurses
47. National Association of Nurse Practitioners in Women's Health, Council on Accreditation
48. National Association of Pediatric Nurse Practitioners
49. National Association of School of Nurses
50. National Association of Orthopedic Nurses
51. National Certification Corporation for the Obstetric, Gynecologic, and Neonatal Nursing Specialties
52. National Conference of Gerontological Nurse Practitioners
53. National Council of State Boards of Nursing
54. National League for Nursing
55. National League for Nursing Accrediting Commission
56. National Organization of Nurse Practitioner Faculties
57. Nephrology Nursing Certification Commission
58. North American Nursing Diagnosis Association International
59. Nurses Organization of Veterans Affairs
60. Oncology Nursing Certification Corporation
61. Oncology Nursing Society
62. Pediatric Nursing Certification Board
63. Pennsylvania State Board of Nursing
64. Public Health Nursing Section of the American Public Health Association
65. Rehabilitation Nursing Certification Board
66. Society for Vascular Nursing
67. Texas Nurses Association
68. Texas State Board of Nursing
69. Utah State Board of Nursing
70. Women's Health, Obstetric & Neonatal Nurses
71. Wound, Ostomy, & Continence Nurses Society
72. Wound, Ostomy, & Continence Nursing Certification

LACE is a foundation for APRN profession-building; therefore planning for political action to implement the recommendations is essential. Styles issued a warning that "unilateral decisions, tinkering with the contemporary configuration, even today's remedy will have no solid future without a process to sustain it" (p. 58). The foundational building block in this regulatory model is licensure (see Figure 51-1). All nursing organizations within a state, especially APRN groups, must create a comprehensive plan to update their state nurse practice acts by addressing the issues of titling, standards, independent practice, and prescriptive authority so that they are consistent with the LACE framework.

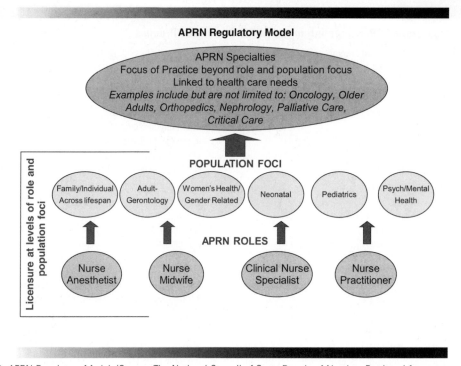

FIGURE 51-1 APRN Regulatory Model. (Source: The National Council of State Boards of Nursing. Retrieved from *www.ncsbn.org/08_APRN_Roundtable_Update.pdf* .)

Many of the political issues confronting current APRN practice are in some way addressed in the LACE framework. For example, as organized physician groups (external forces) increase resistance to expanded scopes of practice, the LACE recommendation calls for nursing to regulate itself, which will require unity among various nursing stakeholders (internal force in nursing). The degree of unity required to implement LACE is significant and necessary in order for APRNs to become a force within health care.

APRN PAYMENT ISSUES

Comparable worth, also called *pay equity,* is the principle of equal pay for equal value. One of the very first laws that President Barack Obama signed during his first week in office was the *Lilly Ledbetter Fair Pay Act of 2009,* which protects those with wage discrimination due to race, sex, or national origin. This amendment to the Civil Rights Act addresses comparable worth and the Obama Administration's bold attempt to achieve pay equity across gender and race.

For APRNs, the difference in Medicare reimbursement can be considered such an issue. Current Medicare payment for NPs is set at 85% of the physician rate, a payment disparity that the APRN community has quietly accepted. The Medicare Advisory Payment Commission (MedPAC), an independent advisory commission to Congress on Medicare, determined that there is no analytic foundation for these payment differentials (2002). Medicare payment for treating otitis media by a nurse practitioner, for example, is 15% less than when the same condition is treated by a physician. Payors will likely be paying for services without regard to provider type as evidenced by the 2010 health reform provision, which increased the Medicare reimbursement rate for Certified Nurse-Midwives from 65% of the rate paid when a physician performs the service, to the full rate.

APRNs have not aggressively pursued 100% reimbursement or publicly marketed the reduced payments as a cost-saving measure. There is a paradox in this payment differential. Providers should be paid the same rate for the same service, and APRNs can provide high-quality care at a lower rate than physicians—both of which are true. In addressing the issue, MedPAC Commissioners asked whether physicians and APRNs produce the same product. They determined that not enough research had been con-ducted on the case mix and outcomes between APRNs and MDs regarding their "product" (MedPAC, 2002, p. 13). In principle, Medicare should recommend equal pay if both physicians and APRNs provide the same service and reimburse at the lowest cost, that is, to pay the provider who uses the least resources to provide the service (MedPAC, 2002).

MedPAC recommends that Medicare pay for resources used, not provider type, for payment to physician specialists. The physician fee schedule does not differentiate among specialties, although higher payments are made for more complex services to account for the additional time, effort, skill, and stress that may be required to provide care. MedPAC (2002) concluded that payment rates should adequately account for differences in resource costs among ser-vices, and that "paying different amounts for services when they are provided by NPs may not be justified" (MedPAC, 2002, p. 8).

APRNs with their knowledge and skill set are uniquely positioned to serve as highly effective alter-natives to traditional physician care. The emergence of DNP-prepared APRNs will strengthen and expand the role significantly. APRNs have been ambivalent about using the argument of comparable worth. It does create problems when the emphasis in the policy arena is to seek lower costs. On the other hand, adher-ing to an 85% payment standard limits income, espe-cially for private practices, and communicates APRNs as "less-than."

However, the best approach may be avoiding both positions. Instead, the emphasis needs to be on creat-ing a delivery system that is patient-centered, longi-tudinal, relationship-based, available 24/7 in person and online, and delivered by content providers that use evidence-based care. It is likely that in the future, care will be delivered by high-functioning teams of providers and payments will be bundled. Payment incentives will spur innovative strategies for coordi-nated care to improve quality and satisfaction among patients and providers.

OPPORTUNITIES UNDER HEALTH REFORM

The health reform legislation passed in 2010. The Patient Protection and Affordable Care Act (PPAC) presents a number of astonishing opportunities for APRNs. The bill is full of provider-neutral language,

opening up highly favorable circumstances for APRNs to engage and fully participate in high-value health systems, such as Accountable Care Organizations and health care homes. There are opportunities for nurse-managed health centers, school-based health centers, and faculty and nursing workforce centers to demonstrate how to measure and improve quality and reduce costs. If carried out with exceptional skill and unity, the reform initiatives could position APRNs as central to any future improved health care delivery effort.

In 2008 under Medicare Part A, the federal govern-ment paid hospitals $9 billion to cover the costs of medical residency training (MedPAC, 2009). MedPAC determined that payment for physician training (Graduate Medical Education [GME]) is not aligned with Medicare's goals to ensure beneficiary access to care. They recommend de-linking hospital payments based on the number of physician trainees, which creates a perverse incentive to increase the supply of physicians, rather than improve the quality of care. The PPAC 2010 goes a step further and mandates increased flexibility in laws and regulations that govern GME funding to promote training in outpatient settings. The legislation mandates devel-opment of training programs that focus on primary care models such as medical homes, team management of chronic disease, and those that inte-grate physical and mental health services (Kaiser Family Foundation, 2010).

Bolder still, the 2010 health reform legislation appropriates $50 million per year from 2012 through 2015 to establish a graduate nurse education demon-stration program in Medicare. Up to five eligible hos-pitals will receive Medicare reimbursement for the educational costs, clinical instruction costs, and other direct and indirect costs of an eligible hospital's expenses attributable to the training of advanced practice nurses with the skills necessary to provide primary and preventive care, transitional care, chronic care management, and other nursing services appro-priate for the Medicare-eligible population. The legislation is intended to encompass hospitals that will partner with community-based care settings (e.g., federally qualified health centers and rural health clinics) and accredited schools of nursing to under-take the demonstration program (Kaiser Family Foundation, 2010). This demonstration, if carried out with methodological rigor, presents an enormous opportunity for APRNS to demonstrate high-value care and gain a foothold on Medicare dollars for APRN education for generations to come.

Nursing education funding is administered by the Health Resources and Services Administration (HRSA), which supports nursing education, practice, and retention with scholarships, grants, and loans to students, graduate nurses, and faculty. In addition, Medicare paid $300 million for hospital costs of operating approved training programs for nurses, including hospital-based nursing diploma programs (MedPAC, 1999, p. 6) (see Chapter 63). As Medicare reform unfolds, there are few who agree that the federal government should be supporting diploma nursing programs, and it is the work of the entire nursing community to get this funding redirected to baccalaureate or graduate nursing programs.

Naylor and colleagues (2004, 2005) have firmly established the cost savings and quality improvements when APRNs are directing care transitions, especially with frail older adults. The research on transitional care models is so compelling; it led to the "Independence at Home Demonstration" program for chronically ill Medicare beneficiaries as part of the 2010 health reform legislation. It will test a payment incentive and service delivery system that utilizes physician-directed and nurse practitioner–directed home-based primary care teams aimed at reducing costs and improving health outcomes. Those practices that spend *less* than established spending targets are eligible for incentive payments.

EXPANDING THE USE OF APRN SKILLS

As health reform unfolds and millions of people obtain health insurance coverage, states will look for creative strategies to lower health care costs and improve quality, yet a considerable segment of the APRN workforce remains underutilized because of state laws and regulations that govern APRN practice. For example, an analysis of how nurse practitioner regulations in each state and the District of Columbia impact consumers revealed state regulations that ranged from exceedingly restrictive for nurse practitioners and their patients to unimpeded professional autonomy and consumer access (Rudner, O'Grady, Hodnicki, & Hanson, 2007). These results suggest that the wide differences reflect the lack of an evidence-base in APRN regulation, which may limit innovative care approaches and access to care. Although the regulation of health professions is intended to protect

public safety, some of the restrictions on practice can have the opposite effect, not only impeding consumer access but also creating patient safety hazards. For example, some states permit nurse practitioners to prescribe only a 7-day course of medication, creating a potential for incomplete treatments, drug-resistant microbes, and poor quality.

In recent years, states such as Pennsylvania and California have developed plans to expand access to care. As part of those reform proposals, the governors recognized the need to remove unnecessary restrictions, such as physician supervision, and expand prescriptive authority before reform proposals could be implemented. The Institute of Medicine (2001) calls these inconsistencies in state regulations "outdated" and "counter to best practices which must be resolved over time" (p. 217). With the enormity of the need for more providers and to allow for innovations to emerge, one sensible policy solution would be to maximize APRNs by eliminating unfounded restrictive regulations.

OVERCOMING INVISIBILITY

As health care becomes increasingly measured by quality and outcomes, and care becomes more collaborative and interdisciplinary, it is critical that the care given by APRNs is identified and evaluated. Flattening the educational and cultural silos between medicine and nursing education does not equate to APRN invisibility in patient care. It is crucial that APRNs are separated out as distinct provider types in all interdisciplinary research, administrative, and clinical datasets (O'Grady, 2008). It may take the nursing profession decades to untangle nursing's unique role and value within the hospital and decouple professional registered nursing from the "hotel costs" of a hospital stay. RNs have historically been characterized as a cost center rather than a highly valued revenue source within hospitals. If all professional nursing activity was billed separately, such as is done with physicians, the value of nursing would be clear.

As the evidence-base for interdisciplinary teams is created, APRNs must not become invisible on the health team. Building a research base to demonstrate APRN effectiveness will require adherence to methodological quality and identification of APRN contributions within an interdisciplinary context (O'Grady & Johnson, 2008). Moreover, APRNs must be made distinct and visible in all national data sets used in health services research. For example, APRNs have not been included in federal demonstrations looking at health care home models (Centers for Medicare and Medicaid [CMS], 2010). Whether this is due to political marginalization or lack of education about the work of APRNs, APRNs must overcome this invisibility and demand to be identified.

Another serious issue about invisibility is the Medicare payment mechanism of "incident-to" billing. When services provided by some APRNs are billed as "incident-to" the professional services of a physician, the physician is paid the full fee as though he or she personally performed the service. The bill is then submitted to Medicare as a physician visit, and the practice is reimbursed at the 100% of the physician rate, thus increasing revenue to the practice. When APRNS bill Medicare, they are paid 85% of the physician rate, so there is a financial disincentive for NPs to be "visible" in the care they are delivering. Politically, the APRN community has taken a strong stance against APRNs billing as "incident-to," rendering the APRN invisible in the care transaction. However, in actual practices when NPs work with physicians, "incident-to" is widely practiced because of the financial gain to practices, even though the physician may have never seen the patient. "Incident-to" billing is fraught with problems and may often be considered fraud when not in compliance with all of the Medicare requirements defining "incident-to" billing.

FUTURE CHALLENGES AND OPPORTUNITIES: MAKING LACE OUR PREFERRED FUTURE

HARNESSING THE POWER OF THE APRN

There are at least seven national organizations representing NPs, as well as national organizations representing CNSs; CRNAs; CNMs; and hundreds of local, state, and regional APRN groups. These organizations have worked together occasionally, but, more often, advocate separately. What is needed is a unified APRN coalition that is sharing resources and educating policymakers about their roles and connecting the appropriate groups with particular issues. In addition, there should be support for helping practicing APRNs join the group that is most appropriate, instead of competing for members. Competition for members and

garnering of support by separate organizations has diluted political power and does not serve APRNs well. To be sure, there are many examples of the nursing and APRN community coming together with a single message on important policy topics, however, more sharing of resources and stronger, more cohesive political power is needed.

In addition, APRN organizations must create opportunities for APRNs to be appointed to public and private advisory commissions that develop quality-improvement measures. APRN organizations must also identify key corporate boards and insurance companies and develop long-term strategies and political capital to get APRNs appointed to these influential boards. These groups are increasingly influential as payors as well as consumers who seek to know more about what they are getting for their health care dollar. It is critical to broaden the base of stakeholders and policy communities knowledgeable about APRNs as competent providers committed to improving quality and access and lowering health care costs. Certainly the commitment of groups such as the AARP and the positive response of the convenient care industry will go a long way in getting the support of the business community (see Chapter 84).

EXPANDING MEDIA AND RESEARCH BEYOND THE NURSING AUDIENCE

Research and media stories about APRN practice must be published in wider venues (e.g., the public media) to reach a broader policymaking and public audience. Key policymakers as well as the public must be made more aware of the contributions that APRNs make in reducing health care costs and improving access and quality of care. Achieving broader recognition, reducing invisibility, and removing barriers to practice will be contingent on expanding research that is methodologically sound and produces results that can be applied across states and to the larger delivery system.

SUMMARY

The LACE document presents 28 recommendations to guide states in revising their practice acts for APRNs. It clearly outlines the standards for APRN titling, program accreditation, national certification, and educational requirements, including licensing APRNs as independent practitioners with no requirements for collaboration, direction, or supervision. Arguably, these LACE recommendations create the strongest leverage for APRNs to confront state policymakers with the need to modernize antiquated state practice acts. The LACE recommendations could become the APRN political force to overcome the economic threats voiced by some physician groups.

The rapid growth and success of the APRN movement has been described as a *disruptive innovation* in that APRNs can, in many ways, provide the same or better care than physicians, at a lower cost in more convenient settings (Christensen, Bohmer, & Kenagy, 2000). This disruption has contributed to professional turf battles and sharpened the political opposition to APRNs. The LACE document enables APRNs to use a process that demonstrates their success as providers. Making LACE a reality for the future will necessitate fierce energy, laser-beam focus, and unity among all APRN stakeholders.

APRNs can do much more to create policy leverage. Strategies proven to strengthen coalitions, including working more effectively with consumer groups, think tanks, policy groups, and the media, would significantly strengthen the political power of APRNs. Moreover, unifying APRN organizations will expand their political power. When Florence Nightingale defined the role of the nurse, she saw patient advocacy in its broadest sense and considered influencing and educating policymakers as foundational to the role. As we follow her example, it is imperative to advocate on behalf of our patients with one strong voice.

For a list of related websites, please refer to your Evolve Resources at http://evolve.elsevier.com/Mason/policypolitics/

REFERENCES

Centers for Medicare and Medicaid (CMS). (2010). *Factsheet on CMS health care home demonstration projects.* Retrieved from www.cms.hhs.gov/demoprojectsevalrpts/downloads/medhome_factsheet.pdf.

Christensen, C., Bohmer, R., & Kenagy, J. (2000). Will disruptive innovations cure health care? *Harvard Business Review, 78*(5), 102-112, 199.

Gray, M. (2001). Advanced practice roles in nursing: Preparation and scope of practice. In N. Chaska (Ed.), *The nursing profession: Tomorrow and beyond* (pp. 515-526). Thousand Oaks, CA: Sage Publications.

Institute of Medicine. (2001). *Crossing the quality chasm: A new health system for the 21st century.* Washington, D.C.: National Academies Press.

Kaiser Family Foundation. (2010). *Focus on heath reform: Summary of health reform legislation.* Retrieved from www.kff.org/healthreform/upload/8061.pdf.

MedPAC. (2002). Report to Congress: Medicare payment to advanced practice nurses and physicians' assistants. Retrieved from www.medpac.gov/publications/congressional_reports/jun02_NonPhysPay.pdf.

MedPAC. (June 1999). Report to Congress: Rethinking Medicare's payment policy for graduate medical education and teaching hospitals. Retrieved from www.medpac.gov/publications/congressional_reports/august99.pdf.

MedPAC. (June 2009). Report to Congress: *Medical education in the United States: Supporting long-term delivery system reforms.* Retrieved from www.medpac.gov/chapters/Jun09_Ch01.pdf.

National Council of State Boards of Nursing. (2008). *Consensus model for APRN regulation: Licensure, accreditation, certification & education.* Retrieved from www.ncsbn.org/7_23_08_Consensue_APRN_Final.pdf.

Naylor, M. D., Brooten, D. A., Campbell, R. L., Maislin, G. M., McCauley, K. M., & Schwartz, J. S. (2004). Transitional care of older adults hospitalized with heart failure: A randomized clinical trial. *Journal of the American Geriatrics Society, 52*(5), 675-684.

Naylor, M. D., Stephens, C., Bowles, H. K., Bixby M. B. (2005). Cognitively impaired older adults: From hospital to home. *American Journal of Nursing, 105*(2), 52-62.

O'Grady, E. T. (2008). Advanced practice registered nurses: The impact on patient safety and quality. In R. G. Hughes (Ed.). *Patient safety and quality: An evidence-based handbook for nurses.* Retrieved from www.ahrq.gov/qual/nurseshdbk/docs/O'GradyE_APRN.pdf.

O'Grady E. T., & Johnson, J. (2008). Health policy issues in changing environments (Chapter 22). In A. B. Hamric, J. A. Spross, & C. M. Hanson (Eds.). *Advanced practice nursing: An integrative approach* (4th ed.). St. Louis: Elsevier-Saunders.

Pearson, L. (2010). The Pearson Report 2010: Annual state by state legislative update. *The American Journal for Nurse Practitioners, 14*(2), 49-53.

Rudner, N., O'Grady, E. T., Hodnicki, D., & Hanson, C. (2007). Ranking state regulation: Practice environment and consumer health care choice. *The American Journal for Nurse Practitioners, 11*(4), 8-23.

Stanley, J. (2009). Reaching consensus on a regulatory model: What does this mean for APRNs? *The Journal for Nurse Practitioners, 5*(2), 99-104.

Styles, G., Schumann, M. J., Bickford, C., & White, K. M. (2008). Specialization and credentialing in nursing revisited. Silver Spring, MD: American Nurses Association. Retrieved from www.nursingworld.org/MainMenuCategories/ANAMarketplace/ANAPeriodicals/OJIN/TableofContents/vol132008/No2May08/ArticlePreviousTopic/EntryIntoPracticeUpdate.aspx.

CHAPTER 52

Global Nurse Migration

Barbara L. Nichols, Catherine R. Davis, and Donna R. Richardson

"Migration is one of the defining issues of the 21st century. It is now an essential, inevitable and potentially beneficial component of the economic and social life of every country and region."

—Brunson McKinley, Director General, International Organization for Migration

Migration within and between countries is commonplace and is expected to grow. The shortage of health care workers in developed countries drives migration, fuels aggressive recruitment, and is being temporarily resolved with migrant workers from developing countries. Since the domestic source of nurses in many countries is not keeping up with the increased demand, the gap will continue to be filled by foreign-educated nurses. This chapter discusses key nurse migration trends and challenges and their policy implications.

MIGRATION AND THE GLOBAL HEALTH CARE WORKFORCE

GENERAL TRENDS IN MIGRATION

Migration is the movement of people from one country to another (international or external migration) or from one region of a country to another (internal migration). In general, five main trends characterize migration in the twenty-first century:

1. The number of international migrants is increasing; it is estimated that 1 in 35 individuals, worldwide, is an international migrant (Kingma, 2006).
2. There has been growth in the migration of skilled and qualified workers (Organization for Economic Co-operation and Development, 2002), with female migrants accounting for an increasing proportion of all migrants.
3. Women are reported to be migrating without partners or families (Kingma, 2007).
4. Violence against health care workers and gender-based discrimination persist in many countries.
5. Migration affects both developed and developing countries.

Almost all countries are affected by migration in one way or another, but developing countries are disproportionately affected because of their much smaller workforces and greater health care needs. Some countries provide the world with needed goods and services and are considered source countries for migration. Other nations accept the goods and services provided and are considered receiving countries. The United States is predominantly a receiving country and a prime destination for international migration.

As of 2008, immigrants made up 12.5% (38 million) of the total U.S. population. Mexican-born immigrants accounted for 30.1% of all foreign-born individuals living in the U.S., followed by immigrants born in the Philippines (4.4%), India (4.3%), and China (3.6%). These four countries, combined with Vietnam, El Salvador, Korea, Cuba, Canada, and the Dominican Republic, made up 57.7% of all foreign-born individuals living in the U.S. in 2008 (Terrazas & Batalova, 2009). This pattern of Asian and Mexican immigration is quite different from the migration of Europeans in the previous century.

THE GLOBAL NURSE WORKFORCE

A number of "push" factors (reasons for leaving one's own country) and "pull" factors (reason for choosing a receiving country) motivate nurses to migrate. Some countries, despite their own domestic health care needs, cannot create enough jobs to employ the nurses they educate. Policies and restrictions related to pay and career structure, retention, recruitment, deployment, transfer, promotion, and the planning framework are other factors that "push" nurses to leave (Vujicic, Ohiri, & Sparkes, 2009).

Governmental policies on return migration and remittances also encourage nurses to seek employment in other countries. Return migration enables the source country to benefit from the skills acquired by the nurse while working in another country and thus provides an incentive for nurse migration. Remittance refers to the portion of an immigrant's income that returns to the source country in the form of either funds or goods. The World Bank estimates that global remittances reached $328 billion in 2008 (Orozco & Ferro, 2009). Nurses are more likely to be remitters than other migrants, remitting $8 billion to the Philippines and $5 billion to India in 2008. Remittances, which are the second most important source of external funding for developing countries (after direct investment), are generally used to provide financial support, decrease poverty, and improve education and health for families back home (Focus Migration, 2006).

Factors that "pull" nurses to developed countries include higher wages, improved living and working conditions, and opportunities for advancing their education and clinical skills. The continuing existence of gender-based discrimination in many cultures and countries, with nursing being undervalued as "women's work" relative to other professions, also encourages nurses to migrate. Table 52-1 presents the common push/pull factors that precipitate global nurse migration.

A migration-related issue that has received increasing attention is the effect of international nurse recruitment on local and global health care needs. When the U.S. nursing shortage exploded, so did the shortages in Canada, the United Kingdom (UK), and Australia. More troubling, many developing countries were experiencing nursing and physician shortages concomitantly with critical health challenges, such as HIV disease, infant mortality, and other public health problems. The developed countries encountered global criticism because they were accepting foreign-educated nurses from countries that needed nurses to meet their own health care needs. The question of how to balance the right of nurses to migrate for their own personal and professional reasons and the needs of people in both the source and receiving countries

TABLE 52-1 Common Push/Pull Factors That Precipitate Global Nurse Migration

Push Factors	Pull Factors
• Low salary	• Higher salaries
• Limited career opportunities	• Career opportunities
• Lack of professional respect/autonomy	• Professional autonomy
• Violence in the workplace	• Better way of life
• Poor retirement benefits and practices	• Families already in the receiving country
• Poor working conditions	• Better working conditions/adequate supplies and staffing
• Tradition of migration	• Better resourced health systems
• Rise of HIV/AIDS in the workplace*	• Provision of post-basic education
	• Political stability
	• Improved standard of living

*Particular to African and Caribbean countries.

is still unanswered. Some receiving countries, such as the UK, have issued agreements with source countries, such as South Africa, to limit their recruitment in that country. Others have provided scholarships and educational funding with the intent to replenish the source countries' supply of nurses. Return migration upgrades a country's nursing workforce.

TRENDS IN U.S. NURSE MIGRATION

The U.S. is one of the top receiving countries for migrating nurses. Foreign-educated nurses entering the U.S. workforce tend to be female, 30 to 35 years of age, and educated in baccalaureate programs. Generally, they have worked for 1 to 5 years in their home countries prior to migrating. When practicing in the U.S., the majority work in hospital settings (critical care and adult health), with long-term care being the second venue of choice (CGFNS, 2002).

Source countries that traditionally have provided nurses to the U.S. are the Philippines, Canada, and India. This pattern continues today and is augmented by emerging suppliers such as China, South Korea, sub-Saharan Africa, and the Caribbean. Foreign-educated nurses can be found in all areas of the country; however, five states receive the majority of migrating nurses (California, New York, Texas, Florida, and Illinois), though other states have begun seeing an increase—most notably Georgia and North Carolina.

In 1994, foreign-born nurses made up 9% of the U.S. workforce, but, by 2008, this percentage had increased to 16.3% (Buerhaus, Auerbach, & Staiger, 2009). It should be noted that "foreign-born" does not mean that the individual also was educated outside the U.S. Many foreign-born students enter the U.S. on a student visa to attend nursing school and then either return home or adjust their visa status to permanent and become part of the U.S. workforce. Initial findings from the 2008 National Sample Survey of Registered Nurses (NSSRN) indicate an increase in foreign-educated nurses in the workforce from 3.7% in 2004 to 5.6% in 2008, despite periods of retrogression implemented by the U.S. State Department (Health Resources and Services Administration [HRSA], 2010).

RETROGRESSION

Retrogression, the procedural delay in issuing visas when more visa applications have been received than visa slots exist, has limited the number of foreign-educated nurses who can obtain occupational visas to practice in the U.S. The Department of State determines when it is necessary to impose limits on the allocation of immigrant visas and to which countries retrogression will apply. Under retrogression, visa applications are not processed until the backlog is completed (Richardson & Davis, 2009). When retrogression was ordered in 2004, it applied only to China, India, and the Philippines and lasted for several months. The most recent retrogression (November 2006) was for all countries and continues as of 2010, causing a major decrease in the recruitment and visa certification of foreign-educated nurses (Richardson & Davis, 2009). A source country's economy may be dependent on how many of its citizens work overseas—a fact that fuels the push for changes in U.S. immigration and economic policies, which are needed to open the doors closed by retrogression and the downturn in the U.S. economy.

POLICY IMPLICATIONS FOR THE U.S. NURSING WORKFORCE

Imbalances in nurse staffing vary among nations, regions, states, levels of care, specialties, and organizations. The dynamics of supply and demand driven by an aging population, increasing demands for health care, and migration are out of balance with the growing global shortage. Nursing shortages are often a symptom of wider health system and societal elements. For sustainable solutions, it is not about just numbers of nurses but whether or not the health system enables nurses to use their skills effectively. Aiken and colleagues (2004) argued that "developed countries' growing dependence on foreign trained nurses is largely a symptom of failed policies and underinvestment in nursing."

Receiving countries have the following four major policy challenges:
1. Determining the relative contribution of foreign-educated nurses to their in-country nursing workforce
2. Assessing credentials and improving regulatory mechanisms for licensure/registration
3. Providing initial periods of supervised practice as well as language training, health system orientation, cultural orientation, and social support
4. Developing ethical policies regarding recruitment (Buchan, Parkin, & Sochalski, 2003)

The U.S. historically has viewed foreign-educated nurses as a "quick-fix option" to meet U.S. nursing shortages and escalating patient care demands. Although the U.S. has the world's largest nursing workforce, Buerhaus and colleagues (2009) predict that U.S. dependence on foreign nurses is going to be a reality for the foreseeable future, thus the previously mentioned policy challenges must be addressed.

DETERMINING THE RELATIVE CONTRIBUTION OF FOREIGN-EDUCATED NURSES

Similar to many countries, the U.S. needs to enhance, reorient, and integrate its workforce-planning capacity across occupations and disciplines to identify the workforce skills and the roles required to meet service needs. It also needs to improve day-to-day matching of nurse staffing with workload.

A systems perspective is required to achieve priority of roles and a better balance of registered nurses to other health professionals and support workers. Data on skill mix are limited, and studies need to be done to highlight the nature of effective utilization of nurse specialists and nurse practitioners in advanced roles for improving the effectiveness of skill mix across the continuum of nursing care. To ensure that the nursing care needs of the public are met, a broader

U.S. workforce policy is needed that balances foreign nurse recruitment and domestic needs. Table 52-2 presents a snapshot of the policy issues and strategic challenges that must be considered when migration policies are developed.

Keeping Track. Although foreign-educated nurses have been coming to the U.S. for over 50 years, there are no monitoring mechanisms in place to accurately report how many arrive, if and where they work (geographically and in what specialty), and how long they stay. The U.S. Citizenship and Immigration Service (USCIS) can tell us how many occupational visas they have issued, but neither by occupation nor by where the permanent visa holders are located. The only nurses the USCIS can accurately document are those on a temporary H-1C visa because it is limited to 500 per year. Trade NAFTA (TN) nurses, who also are on temporary status, are difficult to document because they may enter the U.S. on a daily basis if they are commuting from Canada to work in border states. This daily counting skews the tracking of the number of TN nurses.

Tracking by Nursing Organizations. Nursing organizations also are limited in their ability to document the number of foreign-educated nurses entering the U.S. The National Council of State Boards of Nursing (NCSBN) can provide data on the number of foreign-educated nurses taking the U.S. licensure examination, but this exam is given in regions around the world, and taking it does not ensure that the nurse is in or coming to the U.S.

CGFNS conducts a federal screening program called *VisaScreen®: Visa Credentials Assessment,* which is one of the requirements for an occupational visa; however not all nurses who complete the program will migrate in a given year. In addition, some nurses do not require an occupational visa, such as spouses or family of U.S. residents or citizens.

State boards of nursing also do not track the numbers of foreign-educated nurses. A few boards are beginning to collect aggregate data, but there is no universal data set. A major challenge for such data collection is that foreign-educated nurses may take one state's licensure exam to enter the U.S. but then apply for licensure by endorsement in a second state or even multiple states, depending on their work plans.

Monitoring Systems. The U.S. needs to establish a monitoring and tracking system for nurses who

TABLE 52-2   Policy Issues and Strategic Challenges That Must Be Considered When Migration Policies Are Developed

Policy Issue	Strategic Challenges
Demographics of workforce	Maldistribution of workers Aging nursing workforce Shrinking supply pool Variable retention Aging faculty Lack of prepared faculty
Poor or limited system planning for nursing workforce	Increasing RN supply Underfunding education programs for nurses Managing retention Improving recruitment Ameliorating effects of international recruitment/migration
Work/organizational environment	Opportunities for: • Career advancement • Continuing education • Professional development Reduction of occupational risks • Reducing violence in the workplace • Taking protective measures regarding HIV/AIDS Job satisfaction • Supportive supervision • Ability to use professional knowledge and skills Salary and wage structure Improving wage differentials between/among health professionals Workload/staffing Improving utilization and productivity of the health workforce
General governance and governmental administrative and bureaucratic policies	Human resource planning and management Managing the role of bilateral and multilateral development partners Lack of data and valid information Managing the change process Policy and health sector reform

have immigrated to work in response to the nursing shortage. Such a system is essential to determine whether or not the recruiting of foreign-educated nurses does in fact contribute to a decrease in the shortage—especially as employers continue to demand increased visas for nurses, and as governments and professions attempt to establish effective workforce development and nursing education policies and funding.

ASSESSING CREDENTIALS AND IMPROVING REGULATORY MECHANISMS FOR LICENSURE

The migration of nurses and other health professionals is not a new phenomenon, but one that is growing each year—fueled by such factors as in-country shortages of health professionals, the desire for a better way of life, and opportunity for personal and professional advancement. The immigration of foreign-educated nurses and other health professionals varies by profession and is regulated by law in the U.S.

U.S. Illegal Immigration Reform and Immigrant Responsibility Act. The 1996 Illegal Immigration Reform and Immigrant Responsibility Act (IIRIRA) resulted in significant changes to existing U.S. immigration laws. Although the IIRIRA was promoted as an illegal immigration bill, its provisions have had a serious impact on legal immigration as well (Whitehouse & Gale, 2009). Section 343 of the IIRIRA requires that all health professionals, except physicians, who come to the U.S. for the purpose of performing labor as health care workers on either a permanent or temporary basis must undergo a federal screening program before obtaining an occupational visa.

CGFNS was named in the legislation to conduct the screening program for all named health professions, including nurses (registered and practical), occupational therapists, medical laboratory technologists, medical laboratory technicians, physical therapists, physician assistants, speech-language pathologists, and audiologists. The regulations implementing the law became final in 2003.

VisaScreen®: Visa Credentials Assessment. The CGFNS program that meets Section 343 requirements is known as VisaScreen®. It includes an assessment of the health professional's education to ensure that it is comparable to that of a U.S. graduate in the same profession; verification that licenses are valid and unencumbered; demonstration of written and oral English language proficiency; and, in the case of registered nurses, verification that the nurse has passed a test of nursing knowledge, either the CGFNS Qualifying Exam® or the NCLEX-RN® examination. Once all of these elements are successfully completed, the applicant is awarded a VisaScreen® certificate that must be presented to a consular office or, in the case of adjustment of status, the Attorney General as part of the visa application.

Educational Credentials. The International Council of Nurses (ICN) has guidelines and advocates for educational standards for general nurses. Foreign-educated, first-level (Registered) nurses are generally diploma or baccalaureate prepared. However, the largest number of immigrant nurses is from the Philippines, a country that has required the baccalaureate for entry into nursing practice since the 1980s. Diploma programs are on the decline in the United Kingdom and India, where the country is phasing out diploma programs. Most provinces in Canada require that those entering nursing be prepared at the baccalaureate level. The U.S. will have to accelerate its conversion to the BSN entry level for registered nurses, or it will lag behind the global community in preparing nurses to meet global health care needs.

PROVIDING SUPERVISED PRACTICE, LANGUAGE TRAINING, HEALTH SYSTEM ORIENTATION, CULTURAL ORIENTATION, AND SOCIAL SUPPORT

With the increase in global nurse migration, clinical competency becomes critical as nurses transition to practice in receiving countries. The more similar the nurse's health care system is to that of the receiving country, the more closely matched are the nurse's clinical skills. Employers identify clinical proficiency as vital to a safe transition to practice in the U.S.—second only to English language proficiency (Davis & Kritek, 2005). However, for many foreign-educated nurses, clinical experiences in their home country do not prepare them for nursing practice in the U.S.

Receiving institutions should have policies in place that support formal transition programs that incorporate orientations tailored to the needs of the foreign-educated nurse and assign a preceptor for as long as needed. Because most errors are made within the first 6 months of practice (Davis & Kritek, 2005), preceptors should be assigned for as long as needed, but not less than 6 months. Preceptors not only provide clinical support for foreign-educated nurses, but also enable their integration into the workforce, promote social networking, and help to create positive practice environments.

Language. In the U.S., written and spoken language proficiency for those seeking an occupational visa is mandated by law. However, the portion of English language testing that many foreign-educated nurses find most challenging is spoken English. This raises concerns because so much of nursing practice requires good verbal communication skills—interacting with patients and their families, physicians, nursing colleagues, and other health professionals.

Receiving institutions need to create policies on the use of language and programs that enable mastery of the language of practice—not only the formal language but also the slang, idioms, and abbreviations. Foreign-educated nurses must attempt to use the formal language of the workplace—English in the case of the U.S.—rather than fall back on use of their native language, especially when working with colleagues from their own countries.

Acculturation. The acculturation of foreign-educated nurses to a new setting in a host or receiving country can take up to 12 months. During this time, the nurse goes through a number of stages. First there is initial excitement about working in a new environment. Then there is anxiety and a sense of isolation. In the next stage, the nurse feels a part of two cultures and explores his or her own beliefs and values about care as well as those of the institution. Finally, the nurse reaches the integration stage in which there is a renewed enthusiasm for work and a reconciliation of the differences between personal and institutional values.

Receiving institutions should adopt policies that ensure that foreign-educated nurses work in an environment that is free from oppression and that promotes integration of cultural competence into the daily practice of care. This might include an educational component that focuses on cultural awareness and increases staff knowledge of the most common cultures of their colleagues as well as their patients (Douglas et al., 2009).

DEVELOPING ETHICAL POLICIES REGARDING RECRUITMENT

In the 1970s, there were many reported instances of unethical recruitment practices and no international,

national, or industry oversight of the recruitment of nurses. The unethical practices included usurious fees for immigration services and travel, substandard housing, misrepresented charges, inequitable salaries and benefits, broken contracts, harassment, and threats of legal action and deportation.

CGFNS International was established in 1977 to create a program of credentials evaluation that not only ensured the competency of foreign-educated nurses but also was professionally ethical and responsible to both the foreign-educated nurses and the U.S. public. The need for such an entity was a novel and controversial idea at the time. Nevertheless, CGFNS was created at the behest of the U.S. Departments of State, Labor and Health, Education, and Welfare (HEW)—later known as the Department of Health and Human Services (DHHS)—and the Immigration and Naturalization Service (INS), later to be absorbed by the Department of Homeland Security (DHS).

Many of the unethical recruitment practices declined as the federal government and state boards of nursing began requiring education and licensure screening of foreign-educated nurses. Nevertheless, they have not disappeared entirely. As nursing shortages have increased and recruitment has become a lucrative business, such practices are recurring—often with new, inexperienced recruitment businesses located both in the U.S. and abroad.

In the 1989 Immigration Nursing Relief Act (INRA), which provided temporary visas (H-1A) for registered nurses, Congress included language for the protection of foreign-educated nurses who experienced discrimination in salaries, assignments, and benefits. It also imposed penalties and fines for employers who engaged in such practices. Although the legislation sunsetted in 1995, these protections are still in place and have been used to challenge unethical and illegal practices by health care employers.

Ethical recruitment practices have become a priority of the international and U.S. nursing communities, as well as human rights organizations. The World Health Organization (WHO) developed a Code of Practice on the International Recruitment of Health Care Personnel, which was adopted at the 63rd World Health Assembly in May 2010. The International Council on Nursing (ICN) issued a Code of Ethics for recruitment of nurses in 2007. National nursing organizations in the U.S. also have issued statements in support of ethical recruitment.

In 2008, the MacArthur Foundation funded the development of a U.S. Code of Ethics for Recruitment of Foreign-Educated Nurses that was issued in 2009 as a voluntary code. It was developed by an advisory council of stakeholders convened by AcademyHealth, a private sector health policy organization, and included representatives from unions, hospitals, nursing organizations, regulatory bodies, credentials evaluators, recruiters, staffing agencies, and immigration attorneys. The goal was to reduce the harm and increase the benefits of international nurse recruitment for source countries, receiving countries, U.S. patients, and migrant nurses. The council evolved into the Alliance for Ethical International Recruitment Practices. Subscribers to the Code will agree to abide by it. Nurses will be able to refer possible violations of the Code to the Alliance, which will assist in resolution of the infractions or refer them to advocacy or government bodies. This work is essential as it focuses on the actual practices of greatest concern— aggressive, predatory recruitment practices that are abusive to nurses seeking a better life for themselves and their families. Nursing leaders in the U.S. will need to proactively implement these guidelines and continue to monitor abuses that may emerge, and that could negatively impact the recruitment and retention of foreign-educated nurses.

All of these codes stress the need for informed consent and transparency to ensure that the nurse knows and understands the content of work contracts, requirements for immigration, and his or her rights and responsibilities.

SUMMARY

The impact of global nurse migration on developed and developing countries has fueled a worldwide nursing shortage. "The issues surrounding nursing shortages and global nurse migration are inextricably linked. Global nurse migration has become a major phenomenon impacting health service delivery in both developed and developing countries. The phenomenon has created a global labor market for health professionals and has fueled international recruitment. International migration and recruitment have become dominant features of the international health policy debate" (Nichols, 2007).

The loss of human resources through migration of professional health staff to developed countries usually results in a loss of capacity of health systems in developing countries to deliver health care equitably. Migration of health workers also undermines the ability of countries to meet global, regional, and national commitments, such as the health-related United Nations Millennium Development Goals (MDG). Data on the extent and impact of migration are often anecdotal and fail to shed light on the multiple interrelated causes and the multifaceted dynamics related to this complex phenomenon.

Without effective and sustained policy interventions, the global nursing shortage will persist, undermining global attempts to improve care outcomes and the health of all nations. In short, U.S. planning efforts should require the establishment of a national system that monitors the inflow of foreign nurses, their country of origin, the states and settings in which they work, and their impact on the nursing shortage.

For a list of related websites, please refer to your Evolve Resources at http://evolve.elsevier.com/Mason/policypolitics/

REFERENCES

Aiken, L., Buchan, J., Sochalski, J., Nichols, B., & Powell, M. (2004). Trends in international migration. *Health Affairs, 23*(3), 69-77.

Buchan, J., Parkin, T., & Sochalski, J. (2003). *International nurse mobility: Trends and policy implications.* Geneva: World Health Organization. Retrieved March 10, 2010, from http://whqlibdoc.who.int/hq/2003/WHO_EIP_OSD_2003.3.pdf.

Buerhaus, P. I., Auerbach, D. I., & Staiger, D. O. (2009). The recent surge in nurse employment: Causes and implications. Building a high-value nursing workforce. *Health Affairs Supplement, 28*(4), w657-w668.

CGFNS International. (2002). *Characteristics of foreign nurse graduates in the United States workforce.* Philadelphia: Author.

Davis, C. R., Kritek, P. B. (2005). Foreign nurses in the U.S. workforce. *Healthy work environments: Foreign nurse recruitment best practices.* Washington, D.C.: American Organization of Nurse Executives. Retrieved from www.aone.org/anoe/pdf/ForeignNurseRecruitmentBestPractices October2005.pdf.

Douglas, M. K., Pierce, J. U., Rosenkoetter, M., Callister, L. C., Hatter-Pollara, M., et al. (2009). Standards of practice for culturally competent nursing care: A request for comments. *Journal of Transcultural Nursing, 20*(3), 257-269.

Focus Migration. (2006). *Remittances: A bridge between migration and development.* Retrieved from www.focus-migration.de/Remittances_A_Brid.1200.0.html?&L=1.

Health Resources and Services Administration (HRSA). (2010). *The registered nurse population: Initial findings from the 2008 National Sample Survey of Registered Nurses.* Retrieved from http://bhpr.hrsa.gov/healthworkforce/rnsurvey/initialfindings2008.pdf.

Kingma, M. (2006). *Nurses on the move.* Ithaca, NY: Cornell University Press.

Kingma, M. (2007). Nurses on the move: A global overview. International Migration of Nurses [special issue]. *Health Services Research, 42*(3). June 2007, Part II, 1281-1298.

Nichols, B. (2007). *The impact of global nurse migration on health services delivery* (White Paper). Philadelphia: CGFNS International.

Organization for Economic Co-operation and Development. (2002). *International mobility of the highly skilled.* Paris: Author.

Orozco, M., & Ferro, A. (Eds.). (2009, August). Worldwide trends in international flows. *Migrant Remittances, 6*(2). Retrieved from www.microlinks.org/ev_en.php?ID=13069_201&ID2=DO_TOPIC.

Richardson, D. R., & Davis, C. R. (2009). Entry into the United States. In B. L. Nichols & C. R. Davis (Eds.), *The official guide for foreign-educated nurses: What you need to know about nursing and health care in the United States* (pp. 43-70). New York: Springer.

Terrazas, A., & Batalova, J. (2009, October 27). *Frequently requested statistics on immigrants and immigration to the United States,* Retrieved from www.migrationinformation.org/USfocus/print.cfm?ID=747.

Vujicic, M., Ohiri, K., & Sparkes, S. (2009). *Working in health: Financing and managing the public sector health workforce.* Washington, D.C.: World Bank.

Whitehouse, D., & Gale, D. (2009). Foreign-educated healthcare professionals in the United States healthcare system. In B. L. Nichols & C. R. Davis (Eds.), *The official guide for foreign-educated allied health professionals: What you need to know about health care and the health professions in the United States* (pp. 1-39). New York: Springer.

CHAPTER 53

Nurse Staffing Ratios: Policy Options

Joanne Spetz

"The problems of the world cannot possibly be solved by skeptics or cynics whose horizons are limited by the obvious realities."

—John F. Kennedy

The importance of nursing to the delivery of high-quality health care has been recognized since the inception of the practice of nursing. Various factors contribute to the quality of nursing care, including the expertise of nursing staff, availability of supportive personnel and other health professionals, good communication among the care team, and the nurse/patient ratio. The relative importance of each of these factors has been debated through the years, and it was not until the past decade that high-quality empirical research found consistent relationships between licensed nurse staffing and the quality of patient care (e.g., Needleman et al., 2002; Aiken et al., 2002; Lang et al., 2004; Kane et al., 2007; Unruh, 2008).

Concerns about the effects of changes in nurse staffing levels in the 1990s, combined with the increasing influence of nursing unions, resulted in the passage of California Assembly Bill (AB) 394 in 1999—the first comprehensive legislation in the United States to establish minimum staffing levels for registered nurses (RNs) and licensed vocational nurses (LVNs) working in hospitals. This bill required that the California Department of Health Services (DHS) establish the specific staffing ratios. These were announced in 2002 and implemented beginning in 2004. In May 2009, federal legislation was introduced in the Senate (S.1031) by Barbara Boxer (D-CA), largely based on California's regulations. Since then, other states and the federal government have considered, and are considering, their own regulations for nurse staffing in hospitals.

THE CONTEXT IN WHICH RATIOS WERE IMPLEMENTED

Throughout the late 1990s and early 2000s, there was substantial debate about changes that occurred in hospital staffing in the 1990s and the effects of such changes on the quality of care (Wunderlich, Sloan, & Davis, 1996; Aiken, Sochalski, & Anderson, 1996; Spetz, 1998; Unruh and Fottler, 2006). In some states, legislators and regulatory agencies considered staffing requirements to increase the numbers of nurses and other health care personnel working in hospitals and other settings. In 1996, California's DHS implemented regulations that require hospitals to use patient classification systems (PCSs) to measure the acuity of patients and determine nurse staffing needs for inpatient units on a shift-by-shift basis. These regulations augmented regulations implemented in the 1976-1977 fiscal year that required hospitals to staff a minimum of 1 licensed nurse per 2 patients in intensive and coronary care units.

The PCS requirements did not satisfy some nursing advocates, and the California Nurses Association (CNA) and the Service Employees International Union (SEIU) continued to press for fixed staffing ratios in both ballot propositions and legislation (Spetz, 2001). Nurse unions alleged that hospitals created PCSs to meet budget requirements rather than patient needs, and that compliance with PCSs was low (Spetz, et al., 2000). At the same time, there was widespread agreement that the fixed minimum staffing requirements that applied to intensive and coronary care units were successful in ensuring adequate nursing care.

As the 1990s ended, a shortage of RNs emerged, and concern about poor staffing in hospitals continued (Kilborn, 1999). It was in this environment that AB 394 was passed by the legislature. Previous Republican governors had vetoed similar legislation; union-friendly Democratic Governor Gray Davis signed AB 394 and satisfied the union efforts to pass minimum-ratio legislation. AB 394 charged the California DHS with determining specific unit-by-unit nurse/patient ratios (Table 53-1).

REGULATIONS

The DHS launched an extensive effort to determine the new minimum nurse staffing ratios. At the time, there was relatively little research that linked nurse staffing to the quality of patient care (Spetz et al., 2000; Kravitz et al., 2002); moreover, none of the published studies identified an ideal staffing ratio for hospitals (Lang et al., 2004). The DHS received recommendations about the ratios from stakeholders. The California Hospital Association (CHA) proposed a ratio of 1 licensed nurse per 10 patients in medical-surgical units and somewhat richer ratios in other units. The CNA recommended a ratio of 1 licensed nurse per 3 patients in medical-surgical units and richer ratios in other units. The SEIU recommended a ratio of 1 licensed nurse per 4 patients in medical-surgical units, and also made recommendations for staffing ratios for other health care workers. To help develop proposed ratios, the DHS commissioned a study by researchers at the University of California, Davis (Kravitz et al., 2002).

The proposed ratios were between those recommended by the CHA and the unions, with a 1:6 ratio in medical-surgical units starting January 1, 2004, and a 1:5 ratio in medical-surgical units commencing in January 2005. Other units have richer minimum-ratio requirements, as presented in Table 53-1. These minimum ratios do not replace the requirement that hospitals staff according to a PCS; if a hospital's PCS indicates that richer staffing is needed, the hospital should staff accordingly. However, the problems with the PCS requirements have not been remedied.

WHAT HAS HAPPENED AS A RESULT OF THE RATIOS?

The implementation of California's minimum nurse staffing ratio legislation has led to legal challenges and state government efforts to expand RN education. It also drove increases in hospital nurse staffing and

TABLE 53-1 California Minimum Licensed Nurse/Patient Ratios

Type of Unit	Ratio in 2004	Ratio in 2005	Ratio in 2008
Intensive or critical care	1:2	1:2	1:2
Neonatal intensive care	1:2	1:2	1:2
Operating room	1:1	1:1	1:1
Postanesthesia recovery	1:2	1:2	1:2
Labor and delivery	1:2	1:2	1:2
Antepartum	1:4	1:4	1:4
Postpartum couplets	1:4	1:4	1:4
Postpartum women only	1:6	1:6	1:6
Pediatrics	1:4	1:4	1:4
Emergency room	1:4	1:4	1:4
ICU patients in the ER	1:2	1:2	1:2
Trauma patients in the ER	1:1	1:1	1:1
Step-down	1:4	1:4	1:3
Telemetry	1:5	1:5	1:4
Medical-surgical	1:6	1:5	1:5
Other specialty care	1:5	1:5	1:4
Psychiatric	1:6	1:6	1:6

Sources: California Nurses Association. Retrieved from *www.calnurses. org/nursing-practice/ratios/ratios_index.html*; Spetz, J. (2004). California's minimum nurse-to-patient ratios: The first few months. *Journal of Nursing Administration, 34*(12), 571-578.

wages in California. Whether the ratios have improved patient safety is still up for debate.

LEGAL CHALLENGES

Two days before the ratios went into effect, the CHA filed a lawsuit arguing that the regulatory phrase "at all times" should not require that nursing coverage must comply any time a nurse leaves the work environment, such as during a break or restroom visit. The DHS contended that if the ratios were to have any meaning, they must be effective "at all times." The judge hearing the case agreed with the DHS in a May 2004 ruling (Berestein, 2004). The second major legal challenge to the ratio regulations came from Governor Arnold Schwarzenegger, who sought to delay the implementation of the stricter 1-licensed nurse to 5-patient ratio scheduled for January 2005. The DHS stated that the severe shortage of licensed nurses made it overly onerous for hospitals to meet stricter staffing requirements and therefore issued an emergency regulation suspending the change 2 months before it was to have occurred. The DHS also proposed changes to the regulations for emergency departments (Rapaport, 2004).

The CNA filed suit against the DHS in December 2004, alleging that the emergency order had illegally bypassed the legislature (LaMar, 2005). In early March, a Superior Court judge tentatively ruled that the DHS indeed had not followed the law when issuing the emergency regulation (Salladay & Chong, 2005). After attempts by the governor's administration to override and appeal the initial ruling, the judge's decision was finalized in May 2005 (Benson, 2005a; Benson, 2005b; Gledhill, 2005). The denial of the emergency order to delay the enrichment of the ratios forced hospitals to scramble to meet the new requirements.

EXPANSION OF NURSING EDUCATION

To assist hospitals in meeting the staffing ratio rules, both former Governor Davis and Governor Schwarzenegger dedicated funds to expanding nursing education and reducing attrition from nursing programs. The 2008 Annual Report reported that there had been a 54% increase in California RN graduates over the previous 4 years, and a 56% increase in nursing faculty (California Labor and Workforce Development Agency, 2009). In May 2009, it was announced that the Nurse Education Initiative would continue for a second round of 5-year grants, with an additional $60 million of Workforce Investment Act funds (Wasserman, 2009).

ENFORCEMENT ISSUES

The inspection and enforcement mechanisms of the DHS are relatively weak. The ability of the DHS to conduct inspections is hindered by ongoing state budget shortfalls. The DHS does not have the authority to impose fines or monetary penalties on hospitals that are found to violate the ratios, but instead requests and monitors plans submitted by hospitals to remedy the problem.

Other mechanisms exist to ensure that hospitals adhere to the ratios. First, government payers such as Medicare and Medi-Cal (the state Medicaid program) require that hospitals meet all state and federal regulations, and can deny payment to violators. Second, California's cap on malpractice awards does not apply in cases of negligence, and it is possible that a hospital could be determined negligent if it consistently did not adhere to minimum nurse staffing regulations

(Robertson, 2004). Third, unions draw public attention to hospitals that do not meet the staffing requirements, resulting in negative publicity for hospitals and increased scrutiny from DHS inspectors. Fourth, labor organizations that represent nurses, such as the CNA and the SEIU, have sought to incorporate staffing standards in their contract negotiations. Recent contractual agreements regarding nurse/patient ratios have come through standard contract negotiations (Gordon, 2005; Osterman, 2005).

ARE HOSPITALS MEETING THE RATIOS?

Studies of all California hospitals using annual hospital financial data submitted to the California Office of Statewide Health Planning and Development (OSHPD) have found that annual average numbers of RN productive hours and nurse staffing ratios in medical-surgical units increased markedly between 2001 and 2006 (Conway et al., 2008; Cook et al., 2010; Spetz et al., 2009). Most recently, Spetz and colleagues (2009) found that statewide average RN hours per patient day increased 16.2% from 1999 through 2006, to an average of 6.9 hours per patient day. Interviews conducted with hospital leaders by a research team at UCSF revealed that many chief nursing officers and other managers said they hired nurses in order to meet the ratios, and most noted that it is challenging to adhere to the ratios at all times, including during scheduled breaks (Chapman et al., 2009).

Analyses of aggregated data such as those collected by the California Nursing Outcomes Coalition (CalNOC) or OSHPD can indicate general trends in nurse staffing, but cannot determine whether or not specific hospitals are compliant with the staffing ratios. Quarterly or annual data provide only an average number of productive nursing hours over the time period, which does not capture monthly, daily, or hourly variation in nurse staffing or patient census. A hospital might appear to be compliant on average by staffing more richly than required during the day and violating the ratios every night. CalNOC data are further limited because not all hospitals are represented, while OSHPD data are limited by not providing unit-by-unit data. Moreover, the OSHPD staffing data are not limited to nurses who work directly with patients. Researchers and policymakers will need to survey hospitals directly to fully understand how hospital staffing has changed on a shift-by-shift, unit-by-unit basis as a result of the minimum nurse/patient ratios.

HAS THE MIX OF STAFF CHANGED?

There has been concern about the possibility that hospitals eliminated support staff positions because of the minimum licensed nurse staffing requirements (Spetz, 2001). Anecdotal evidence suggests that this occurred among some hospitals. In 2003, the SEIU filed a grievance against Stanford University Medical Center when that hospital issued layoff notices to 113 nursing aides in advance of the implementation of the ratios. The hospital planned to replace those positions with RNs. The SEIU charged that the elimination of the nursing aide positions was contrary to the spirit of the minimum ratios (Ostrov, 2003). In a study conducted by UCSF, some hospital leaders reported that they had laid off ancillary staff to use their personnel budgets to hire more RNs (Chapman et al., 2009). CalNOC analyses of staffing data suggest that the substitution of licensed nurses for unlicensed staff may be widespread; the increase in RN staffing was much larger than the overall staffing increase among their hospitals (Donaldson et al., 2005; Bolton et al., 2007).

HAVE HOSPITALS REDUCED SERVICES?

The California Hospital Association warned that strict minimum nurse/patient ratio requirements will force hospitals to reduce their services. To maintain the minimum ratios, hospitals might reschedule procedures, close selected units and beds, or shut their doors entirely. These fears seemed warranted when in January 2004, it was announced that Santa Teresita Hospital in Duarte, California, was closing its 39-bed inpatient department and emergency room because of its inability to meet the minimum ratios (Chavez, 2004). However, newspapers subsequently reported that nurses who had worked at the hospital said they were meeting the ratios without difficulty (Allen, 2004), and an analysis of financial data reported by the hospital to OSHPD revealed that the hospital had been suffering severe financial distress for several years before it closed (Spetz, 2004). Given this information, it seems unlikely that the ratios were the primary reason for the hospital's closure. Statewide, there have been few verified reports of the minimum nurse/patient ratios causing permanent closures of inpatient hospital units or beds. Whether there have

been permanent, important effects on health or access to care for Californians is unknown.

HAVE HOSPITALS SUFFERED FINANCIAL LOSSES?

In November 2004, the DHS argued that catastrophic financial losses that would result from implementing more stringent ratios in 2005 justified the issuance of an emergency order to delay ratios. However, there is no empiric evidence that staffing ratios have negatively impacted hospitals' financial status. Since 1999, hospitals have been financially buffeted by numerous factors, most notably changes in Medicare and Medicaid payment policy and requirements that hospital facilities meet seismic standards through retrofitting or new construction (Spetz et al., 2009). Average operating margins of California hospitals hovered between −2% and +2% from 1999 through 2006. Qualitative evidence published by the California HealthCare Foundation reported that hospital CEOs absorbed the costs of the ratios by reducing other budget areas, and some hospitals were able to obtain higher insurance reimbursement rates to cover additional staff expenses (Spetz et al., 2009). In an analysis of OSHPD hospital financial data, Cook and colleagues (2010) found no significant change in total annual labor costs for licensed nurses, total annual hospital costs, or hospital prices. Another study of California hospital data concluded that labor cost increases resulting from the nurse staffing ratios were not large enough to explain increases in hospital prices from 1999 through 2005 (Antwi, Gaynor, & Vogt, 2009).

ARE NURSES MORE SATISFIED?

Advocates of staffing ratio regulations link improved staffing to nurse satisfaction, and argue that greater nurse satisfaction will reduce nurse turnover and lead to better patient outcomes (Peter D. Hart Research Associates, 2003; Public Policy Associates, 2004; CNA, 2009). An analysis of nurse survey data collected for the California Board of Registered Nursing found that there were significant improvements in overall job satisfaction among hospital-employed RNs between 2004 and 2006 (Spetz, 2008). Nurse satisfaction also increased with respect to the adequacy of RN staff, time for patient education, benefits, and clerical support. However, these improvements in nurse satisfaction could not be directly linked to changes in nurse staffing at the hospital level or with regional changes in nurse staffing that may have resulted from the ratio regulations.

OTHER STATE AND FEDERAL PROPOSALS

The only Federal regulation that directly referred to nurse staffing levels in hospitals at this writing is the 42 Code of Federal Regulations (42CFR 482.23[b]), which requires hospitals that participate in Medicare to have "adequate numbers of licensed registered nurses, licensed practical (vocational) nurses, and other personnel to provide nursing care to all patients as needed" (American Nurses Association, 2009). In 2009, Senator Barbara Boxer (D-CA) introduced S 1031, and Representative Janice Schakowsky (D-IL) introduced H.R. 2273, both of which would require that hospitals implement nurse-to-patient staffing plans and meet minimum RN nurse-to-patient ratios for specified patient care units. Hospitals that treat Medicare and Medicaid patients would be required to meet these requirements, and supplementary funding would be made available through Medicare to finance the cost of the additional nursing staff. These bills were referred to committees after introduction, and had not been voted upon by those committees by the end of 2009.

Some states have pursued their own staffing regulations, in part because there is limited regulation at the federal level. State regulations generally take one or more of three approaches: a requirement that hospitals develop and implement nurse staffing plans with input from direct care nurses; requiring public disclosure of staffing levels; and/or establishment of fixed minimum staffing ratios. California is the only state to have implemented a law using this third strategy, although similar legislation has been proposed in other states, and is currently under consideration in Illinois, Michigan, Nevada, New York, and Pennsylvania. Most of these bills have been developed or supported by affiliates of National Nurses United, which is a national RN union spearheaded by the California Nurses Association.

Some states have opted to develop staffing regulations that offer hospitals more flexibility than do fixed minimum staffing ratios. Oregon, Texas, Nevada, Ohio, Rhode Island, Connecticut, Washington, and Illinois have signed into law requirements that hospitals implement and enforce a written nurse staffing policy. In most of these states, the staffing policy must be developed by a committee that includes staff nurses. For example, the laws for Oregon, Texas, Nevada, Washington, Illinois, and Connecticut require that the committee be composed of at least 50% direct care nurses. These laws often specify that staffing committees take into account patient acuity, physical configuration of the unit, and other factors when developing staffing plans. Rhode Island requires that hospitals submit a "core staffing plan" to the state department of health annually, with specific staffing for each patient care unit and each shift (American Nurses Association, 2009). In 2009, several states were considering regulations to require that hospitals establish staffing plans, including Florida, Pennsylvania, and Massachusetts.

The third, and least binding, approach to nurse staffing regulation is to mandate reporting of staffing ratios to the public or to a regulatory agency. In New York, for example, facilities must make available to the public information about nurse staffing and patient outcomes. Specific adverse events, such as medication errors and decubitus ulcers, are considered reportable information under this law. Other states with public reporting requirements are Vermont and Illinois. New Jersey's regulation mandates that hospitals post daily staffing information for each unit and shift, and also provide these data to state regulators, and in 2009 New York added a similar posting requirement to its regulations.

ISSUES THAT NEED TO BE ADDRESSED

Two issues central to the success of minimum nurse/patient ratios have not been addressed: Have the ratios improved the quality of patient care, and what was the total cost of the ratio regulations?

DID THE RATIOS IMPROVE THE QUALITY OF CARE?

Only a handful of published studies examine the effect of the minimum ratios on the quality of patient care. In the first paper published on this subject, the CalNOC analyzed rates of patient falls and hospital-acquired pressure ulcers between 2002 and 2004 in their sample of 68 hospitals and found that there was no statistically significant change that could be attributed to the ratios (Donaldson et al., 2005). A follow-up study of CalNOC data through 2006 confirmed these results, finding no improvement in rates of patient falls, prevalence of pressure ulcers, or prevalence of restraint use that could be associated with the implementation of staffing ratios (Bolton et al., 2007). Although these studies suggest that the ratios have not improved quality of care, there are several reasons these papers do not provide a definitive verdict on the ratios. First, as noted above, only a fraction of California hospitals was analyzed. Second, the outcomes examined might not be very sensitive to changes in licensed nurse staffing. Research studies that examine whether or not nurse staffing affects rates of hospital-acquired pressure ulcers and postoperative hip fractures (which would be caused by a patient fall) have produced mixed findings (Agency for Healthcare Research and Quality, 2005). Finally, these outcomes might be more sensitive to total staffing than to licensed nurse staffing. In this case, replacement of unlicensed staff with licensed nurses may have no net positive or negative effect.

Two recent studies echo the findings reported by the CalNOC researchers. Spetz and colleagues examined OSHPD patient discharge data for all non-federal, general acute care California hospitals from 1999 through 2006, and could not associate improvements in outcomes to the implementation of the ratios. The research team noted that many of the hospital leaders they interviewed expected that the staffing ratios would improve the quality of care, but few thought the ratios had met this expectation. In a more rigorous analysis of OSHPD data from 2001 to 2005, Cook and colleagues (2010) found no association between changes in nurse staffing and changes in pressure ulcer rates or failure to rescue a patient after a complication.

However, the newest study of the impact of the ratios on the work environment and quality of care finds improvements in nurse job satisfaction, burnout, and quality of care. Aiken and colleagues surveyed nearly 80,000 RNs in California, New Jersey, and Pennsylvania to learn their experiences with staffing, the work environment, and patient safety (Aiken et al., 2010). The survey data were linked to secondary data on patient outcomes collected by state government agencies. The researchers found that nurse workloads, measured as average patients per shift, were lower in California than in New Jersey and Pennsylvania, and that over 80% of California nurses reported that their assigned workloads were in compliance with the state's regulation. They indicated that improvements in their patient assignments had been achieved by there being more relief nurses to cover breaks, more nurses floating to other units, and greater use of supplemental and agency nurses. They also reported less use of LVNs, unlicensed personnel, and non-nursing support services, suggesting that hospitals compensated for RN staffing increases by reducing staff in other areas.

Aiken and colleagues (2010) also reported that nurses were more satisfied with their working conditions. Nurses in California were significantly more likely to report that their workload was reasonable, allowed them to spend adequate time with patients, and that they were able to take breaks during the workday. Nurses with lower workloads were significantly less likely to report that they received complaints from families, faced verbal abuse, were burned out, were dissatisfied, felt quality of care was poor, or were looking for new jobs. Perhaps most importantly, Aiken and colleagues found that across all three states, higher nurse staffing levels were associated with lower rates of 30-day inpatient mortality and failure-to-rescue. These relationships were stronger in California than in other states.

The study by Aiken and colleagues (2010) is limited by its use of cross-sectional data. Research based on a single year of data cannot identify the effect of *changes* in policy or practice on *changes* in patient outcomes. While the responses of nurses regarding the patient safety environment suggest that the lower workloads in California are associated with more positive nurse perceptions of patient safety, these perceptions may not lead to true improvements in patient outcomes. And, the analysis of patient outcomes was limited to two outcomes; while these are arguably among the most important, other outcomes should be assessed in the future.

There is a pressing need for more research on the effects of minimum ratios on patient care. Researchers should examine a variety of patient outcomes and sources of data, using various statistical methods. As Cook and colleagues (2010) note, it is not possible with secondary data to easily determine whether or not a hospital reallocated resources so they could increase nurse staffing at the expense of other quality-improving processes. It also is possible that changes in patient outcomes due to the staffing ratios will occur over a longer period of time, and thus empiric research will not measure improvements in outcomes for several more years. Further confounding the research on the quality impact of staffing ratios is the fact that many health systems and hospitals have established quality improvement programs in response to increased public attention to medical errors and patient outcomes. As of 2010, there has been no statewide analysis of the impact of these other quality-improvement programs and how their efforts may have complimented or detracted from the impact of nurse staffing ratios.

WHAT WAS THE COST OF THE RATIOS?

Any positive impact of minimum staffing ratios should be weighed against the costs of the ratios. At this time, those costs have not been accurately quantified. Numerous studies indicate that hospitals hired more licensed nurses to meet the ratios, and one study reported that nurse wages rose substantially in California (Mark et al., 2009). However, no research has tied these facts to overall increases in hospital costs or declines in hospital operating margins. A careful accounting of the extent to which increases in nurse staffing were necessitated by the ratios, and the cost of such increases, is necessary. Moreover, it is important to quantify the value of other investments hospitals might have made if they were not required to adhere to the staffing ratios. A hospital may have delayed implementation of a new infection-control system that would have reduced infection rates; this "opportunity cost" should be included as part of the overall cost of the staffing regulations.

WHAT NEXT?

Many states and the federal government are considering legislation to mandate minimum licensed nurse staffing ratios in hospitals (CNA, 2009). Even if these efforts fail, improvements in nurse staffing are likely to propagate across the United States. Recent research suggests that the ratio of cost per life saved associated with increasing nurse staffing is favorable as compared with many other health interventions (Rothberg et al., 2005), and thus hospitals are likely to turn toward improved nurse staffing as a way to meet quality goals at a reasonable price. However, even if more studies demonstrate that nurse staffing

is a cost-effective means to producing better health, researchers need to examine the effectiveness of a minimum staffing mandate. If California's regulation can be shown to have improved patient outcomes at an acceptable cost, it will be easy for other states to follow in California's footsteps.

For a list of related websites, please refer to your Evolve Resources at http://evolve.elsevier.com/Mason/policypolitics/

REFERENCES

Agency for Healthcare Research and Quality. (2005). *AHRQ quality indicators—Guide to patient safety indicators,* Version 2.1, Revision 3. AHRQ Publication No. 03-R203. Rockville, MD: Agency for Healthcare Research and Quality.

Aiken, L. H., Clarke, S. F., Sloane, D. M., Sochalski, J., & Silber, J. H. (2002). Hospital nurse staffing and patient mortality, nurse burnout, and job dissatisfaction. *Journal of the American Medical Association, 288*(16), 1987-1993.

Aiken, L. H., Sloane, D. M., Cimiotti, J. P., Clarke, S. P., Flynn, L., et al. (2010). Implications of the California nurse staffing mandate for other states. *Health Services Research, 45*(4), 904-921.

Aiken, L. H., Sochalski, J., & Anderson, G. F. (1996). Downsizing the hospital nursing workforce. *Health Affairs, 15*(4), 88-92.

Allen, M. (2004, January 10). Former Santa Teresita nurses speak out. *Pasadena Star-News,* A1.

American Nurses Association. (2009). Nationwide state legislative agenda, 2008-2009 reports: Nurse staffing plans and ratios. Retrieved from http://nursingworld.org/mainmenucategories/ANAPoliticalPower/State/StateLegislativeAgenda/StaffingPlansandRatios_1.aspx.

Antwi, Y. A., Gaynor, M., & Vogt, W. B. (2009, July). *A bargain at twice the price? California hospital prices in the new millennium.* National Bureau of Economic Research Working Paper 15134.

Benson, C. (2005a, June 8). Final ruling backs higher nurse ratio. *Sacramento Bee,* A5.

Benson, C. (2005b, March 15). Judge orders launch of nurse staffing rule. *Sacramento Bee,* A4.

Berestein, L. (2004, May 27). Industry group contends measure may hurt patients. *San Diego Union-Tribune,* C3.

Bolton, L. B., Aydin, C. E., Donaldson, N., Brown, D. S., Sandhu, M., et al. (2007). Mandated nurse staffing ratios in California: A comparison of staffing and nursing-sensitive outcomes pre- and post-regulation. *Policy, Politics, & Nursing Practice, 8*(4), 238-250.

California Labor and Workforce Development Agency. (2009). *California Nurse Education Initiative, annual report, 2008.* Sacramento, CA: California Labor and Workforce Development Agency.

California Nurses Association (CNA). (2009). *The ratio solution: CNA/NNOC's RN-to-patient ratios work—Better care, more nurses.* Oakland, CA: California Nurses Association. Retrieved August 10, 2009, from www.calnurses.org/assets/pdf/ratios/ratios_booklet.pdf

Chapman, S., Spetz, J., Kaiser, J., Seago, J. A., & Dower, C. (2009). How have mandated nurse staffing ratios impacted hospitals? Perspectives from California hospital leaders. *Journal of Healthcare Management, 54*(5), 321-336.

Chavez, S. (2004, January 9). Duarte hospital to close its ER. *Los Angeles Times,* B4.

Conway, P. H., Konetzka, R. T., Zhu, J., Volpp, K. G., & Sochalski, J. (2008). Nurse staffing ratios: Trends and policy implications for hospitalists and the safety net. *Journal of Hospital Medicine, 3*(3), 103-199.

Cook, A., Gaynor, M., Stephens Jr., M., & Taylor, L. (2010). *The effect of hospital nurse staffing on patient health outcomes: Evidence from California's minimum staffing regulation.* National Bureau of Economic Research Working Paper 16077. Cambridge, MA: National Bureau of Economic Research.

Donaldson, N., Bolton, L. B., Aydin, C., Brown, D., Elashoff, J., & Sandhu, M. (2005). Impact of California's licensed nurse-patient ratios on unit-level nurse staffing and patient outcomes. *Policy, Politics, & Nursing Practice, 6*(3), 1-12.

Gledhill, L. (2005, March 4). Governor loses to nurses in ruling He illegally blocked law that set staffing ratios, judge says. *San Francisco Chronicle,* A1.

Gordon, R. (2005, June 22). Nurses pact ready for vote: Plan would raise pay, offer higher signing bonus. *San Francisco Chronicle,* B4.

Kane R. L., Shamliyan T., Mueller C., Duval, S., & Wilt, T. J. (2007, March). *Nursing staffing and quality of patient care.* Rockville, MD: Agency for Healthcare Research and Quality.

Kilborn, P. T. (1999, March 23). Current nursing shortage more serious than those of the past. *New York Times,* A14.

Kravitz, R., Sauve, M. J., Hodge, M., Romano, P. S., Maher, M., et al. (2002). *Hospital nursing staff ratios and quality of care.* Davis, CA: University of California, Davis.

LaMar, A. (2005, January 19). Nurses protest delay of lower patient ratio, 1500 rally at Capitol to fight 3-year wait. *San Jose Mercury News,* B2.

Lang, T. A., Hodge, M., Olson, V., Romano, P. S., & Kravitz, R. L. (2004). Nurse-patient ratios: A systematic review on the effects of nurse staffing on patient, nurse employee, and hospital outcomes. *Journal of Nursing Administration, 34*(7-8), 326-337.

Mark, B.., Harless, D. W., & Spetz, J. (2009, February10). California's minimum-nurse-staffing legislation and nurses' wages. *Health Affairs, 28*(2), w326-w334.

Needleman, J., Buerhaus, P., Mattke, S., Stewart, M., & Zelevinsky, K. (2002). Nurse-staffing levels and the quality of care in hospitals. *New England Journal of Medicine, 346*(22), 1715-1722.

Osterman, R. (2005, July 13). Hospitals accept nursing ratios. *Sacramento Bee,* D1.

Ostrov, B. F. (2003, October 18). Stanford nursing levels studied. *San Jose Mercury News,* B3.

Peter D. Hart Research Associates. (2003, April). *Patient-to-nurse staffing ratios: Perspectives from hospital nurses.* Washington, D.C.: AFT Healthcare.

Public Policy Associates. (2004, June). *The business case for reducing patient-to-nurse staff ratios and eliminating mandatory overtime for nurses.* Lansing, MI: Michigan Nurses Association.

Rapaport, L. (2004, November 5). State eases nurse-staffing law until 2008—Hospital closings and delays in patient care prompt move. *Sacramento Bee,* A1.

Robertson, K. (2004). New nurse law fails to cause emergency. *Sacramento Business Journal, 21*(9), 1.

Rothberg, M. B., Abraham, I., Lindenauer, P. K., & Rose, D. N. (2005). Improving nurse-to-patient staffing ratios as a cost-effective safety intervention. *Medical Care, 43*(8), 785-791.

Salladay, R., & Chong, J.-R. (2005, March 4). Judge backs nurses over staffing. *Los Angeles Times,* B1.

Spetz, J. (1998). Hospital use of nursing personnel: Has there really been a decline? *Journal of Nursing Administration, 28*(3), 20-27.

Spetz, J. (2001). What should we expect from California's minimum nurse staffing legislation? *Journal of Nursing Administration, 31*(3), 132-140.

Spetz, J. (2004). California's minimum nurse-to-patient ratios: The first few months. *Journal of Nursing Administration, 34*(12), 571-578.

Spetz, J. (2008). Nurse satisfaction and the implementation of minimum nurse staffing regulations. *Policy, Politics, & Nursing Practice, 9*(1), 15-21.

Spetz, J., Chapman, S., Herrera, C., Kaiser, J., Seago, J. A., & Dower, C. (2009). *Assessing the impact of California's nurse staffing ratios on hospitals and patient care.* Oakland, CA: California HealthCare Foundation.

Spetz, J., Seago, J. A., Coffman, J., Rosenoff, E., & O'Neil, E. (2000). *Minimum nurse staffing ratios in California acute care hospitals.* San Francisco: California HealthCare Foundation.

Unruh L. (2008). Nurse staffing and patient, nurse, and financial outcomes. *American Journal of Nursing, 108*(1), 62-71.

Unruh, L., & Fottler, M. (2006). Patient turnover and nursing staff adequacy. *Health Services Research, 41*(2), 599-612.

Wasserman, J. (2009, May 23). $60 million targets state nursing shortage. *Sacramento Bee,* 6B.

Wunderlich, G. S., Sloan, F. A., & Davis, C. K. (Eds.). (1996). *Nursing staff in hospitals and nursing homes: Is it adequate?* Washington, D.C.: National Academies Press.

CHAPTER 54

TAKING ACTION
Aligning Care at the Bedside with the C-Suite

Linda Burnes Bolton and Margaret L. McClure

"Quality is the result of a carefully constructed cultural environment. It has to be the fabric of the organization, not part of the fabric."

—Phillip Crosby

All Americans should be afforded accessible care that is safe and of high quality. But what does this mean? We should be able to rely on our health care system to provide care for us that will not end up making us sicker. The 2001 Institute of Medicine (IOM) report, *Crossing the Quality Chasm: A New Health System for the 21st Century,* admonishes us to create a system that is safe, effective, patient-centered, timely, efficient, and equitable. To achieve these aims, the IOM report called for fundamental redesign of care systems. Getting there is not easy.

Nursing care is central to how better outcomes might be achieved. Inadequate nurse staffing has been linked to adverse outcomes, which increase the length of stay, sometimes significantly (Aiken, 2002). When the stay is lengthened, so is the cost. Five adverse events—medication errors, falls, urinary tract infections, pneumonia, and pressure ulcers—all associated with nursing care, were found to increase the cost of a hospital "case" by between $25 and $2384 (Pappas, 2008). The 2004 IOM report, *Keeping Patients Safe: Transforming the Work Environment of Nurses,* noted that "research is now beginning to document what physicians, patients, other health care providers, and nurses themselves have long known: how well we are cared for by nurses affects our health, and sometimes can be a matter of life or death" (IOM, 2004).

We must ensure that nurses are given the support they need to help prevent the enormous burden of medical errors and provide a patient-centered environment that is conducive to healing. Nurses must be empowered in their workplaces to proactively redesign work processes to achieve better clinical outcomes. To create this kind of active engagement, nurses must believe that their expertise is valued, know that they have a say in decisions, and be encouraged to lead and collaborate in quality improvement activities. By becoming an active participant in developing, implementing, and measuring the value of quality improvement activities, nurses have the opportunity to lead the way to better care. The following growing evidence shows that they can and will do so:

- Donahue (2009) saw a "consistent and sustained improvement in patient satisfaction scores" following the engagement of staff in a performance improvement effort.
- A nurse-led interdisciplinary team reduced falls among pulmonary rehabilitation outpatients by brainstorming ideas for improvement (Zant, 2009).
- Rutherford and colleagues (2009) found that ten facilities engaged in Transforming Care at the Bedside (TCAB) demonstrated improvements making care safer and more reliable and with better teamwork and staff vitality.

TCAB, a national program of the Robert Wood Johnson Foundation (RWJF) and the Institute for Healthcare Improvement (IHI) was designed in 2003 to engage and empower nurses and other front-line

417

BOX 54-1 RWJF Aligning Forces for Quality (AF4Q)

- An effort to improve "overall quality of health care in targeted communities, reduce racial and ethnic disparities and provide models for national reform" (Aligning Forces for Quality, 2009).
- AF4Q targets 15 communities nationwide that together cover 11% of the United States population.
- Multi-stakeholder leadership alliances of physicians, nurses, patients, consumers, purchasers, hospitals, health plans, and safety net providers work in each community to address AF4Q's focus areas of quality improvement, consumer engagement, and performance measurement and public reporting.

Source: *Aligning Forces for Quality*, 2009.

providers to: improve the quality and safety of patient care on medical-surgical units, increase the team vitality and retention of nurses, improve patient's and family members' experience of care, and improve the effectiveness of the health care team. Initial TCAB hospitals served as laboratories for innovation and change on medical-surgical units with a focus on improving patient care outcomes and the work environment for nurses and the health care team. TCAB nurses regularly proposed solutions that might address either team vitality, patient-centered care, a safety issue or eliminating system "waste." TCAB teams built knowledge and confidence in their redesign efforts by locally creating and testing new ideas, measuring outcomes, and implementing successful changes on their medical and surgical units.

A national learning community was created through site visits, teleconferences, and face-to-face meetings where collaborative learning thrived among front-line staff, midlevel managers, hospital executives, and nursing faculty. This community reinforced learning and became the force behind the significant replication of TCAB. TCAB continues through collaboratives led by the American Organization of Nurse Executives (AONE), through learning and innovation communities in IHI's IMPACT Network, and within RWJF's Aligning Forces for Quality initiative (Box 54-1). Hundreds of hospitals have now adopted TCAB as a way to deliver high-quality and safe patient care.

CASE STUDY

Cedars-Sinai Medical Center actively pursued participation in the launching and implementation of the TCAB initiative. The opportunity to partner with two of the most important organizations committed to improving health care—the RWJF and the IHI—was irresistible. Our missions are aligned, and our values are similar. It was a match that would benefit all three and lay the foundation for fundamental change in acute care.

BEGINNING

Cedars-Sinai was chosen to be one of the initial pilot organizations. It is one of several U.S. institutions that have achieved both Magnet and Leap Frog status. The operating premise was to select diverse institutions and determine if the application of an idealized design created by the IHI would be effective in different settings. The IHI Idealized Design Process is a collaborative among various institutions to design and implement comprehensive system redesign (Moen, 2002). Our acceptance of the invitation to participate was considered by our president, trustees, senior executives including the chief nursing officer (also known as the C-Suite for the CEO, COO, CFO, or CNO), nursing leadership, and staff. We had the opportunity to further our goals and values of *clinical excellence*, defined as quality and innovation; *service excellence* defined as extraordinary patient, employee, medical staff, community, and volunteer experiences; and *value* defined as the best processes at the right price, without waste.

We began by identifying two units and engaging the nursing director, manager, physician leader, education institution representative, patient representative, community service representative, and clinical leaders from across the organization.

FORMING AND STORMING

Cedars-Sinai had previously been engaged in a patient-focused care initiative led by the chief nursing officer. We had established solid liaisons with departments providing services to support the delivery of patient care and with physicians and education partners. We built on that foundation by calling together diverse voices to imagine the perfect work environment. We held a series of sessions to identify the "as-is states" of our environment, using a combination of

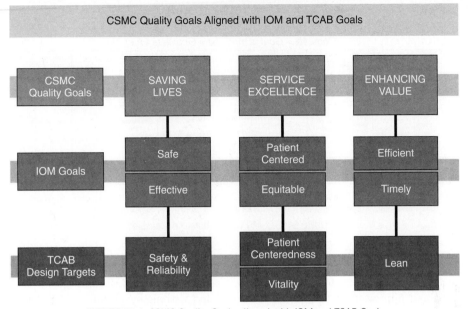

FIGURE 54-1 CSMC Quality Goals aligned with IOM and TCAB Goals.

the TCAB brainstorming techniques called *deep dives* and *snorkels,* as well as Technology Drill Down (TD2) strategies (Burnes Bolton, Gassert, & Cipriano, 2008) created by the American Academy Nursing. The TD2 process engages multiple stakeholders to describe their existing workflow practices, create a preferred state, and identify technology solutions to close the gap between the desired state and existing practices. Throughout the initial forming and storming period that lasted over 8 months, we had many opportunities to walk away, but we remained committed to the TCAB and institutional goals that were fully aligned, as shown in Figure 54-1.

IMAGINATION, INNOVATION, SPREAD, AND SUSTAINABILITY

Beginning in 2005, the initial 13 organizations moved from forming and storming to creating a community committed to imagining and creating innovative work environments. We launched multiple rapid-cycle tests of change that informed and shaped our experiences and resulted in a phenomenal explosion of unit-based performance improvement projects. Cedars-Sinai produced over 600 half-baked ideas that were tested and then adopted, adapted, abandoned, or implemented. Examples are as follows:

- We implemented hourly rounding, which decreased the number of patient falls. Subsequently, we spread the test of change across the organization.
- The use of orange slippers as a visual cue that the patient was at risk for falls didn't work, so we abandoned the test after three performance improvement cycles.
- We (as did other members of the innovation community) stole shamelessly 15 ideas from our community partners. "Steal shamelessly" is a tenet of TCAB to encourage spread of good ideas.
- We established structures within the organization to facilitate the implementation and spread of successful tests of change across the organization. We began with two surgical units. By 2006, we had spread TCAB to all 20 medical-surgical units, and by 2007 TCAB was embedded as an imaginative deliberative process carried out at the unit, department, and institutional level.

TCAB key steps are staff, patient, physician, and senior executive engagement; deployment of the idealized design model; measurement; and the use of data to obtain information that results in shared transformation of work environments. We worked with our education partners to embed the principles of TCAB in the undergraduate and graduate curricula for two universities.

The alignment of organizational and nursing priorities and targeted outcomes is critical. Throughout

QUALITY OUTCOME MEASURES
MONTH REPORTED: December 2009

	Saving Lives					Service Excellence				Enhancing Value		
CSMC Quality Goals	Saving Lives					Service Excellence				Enhancing Value		
TCAB	Safety and Reliability (updated monthly)					Vitality (updated quarterly)		Patient Centeredness		Lean (monthly)		
UNIT	Falls w/Injury per 1000 Pt Days	Hospital Acquired Pressure Ulcers (Stage III, IV & Unstageable) < 0	Med Errors (ADE) w/ Harm per 1000 Pt Days	BSI Prevention Bundle (Central Line Bundle) −100%	Code Blue per 1000 Pt Days (Non-ICU)	Voluntary Turnover (NQF) ≤4% Voluntary Controllable including FT, PT & No Benefit RNs Through Dec 2009	New Hire Turnover <4% Including FT, PT & No Benefit RNs Through Dec 2009	Rate Hospital 72% Updated Through Oct 09	Would Recommend 78% Updated Through Oct 09	Direct Patient Care Time Spent ≥70%	Toes Out/Toes In Total/Average times exclude EVS time <55 Min ED-Floor	Toes Out/Toes In Total/Average times exclude EVS time <55 Min ED-Floor
House-Wide Rollup	0	0	0.25	100.00%	0.84	2.90%	9.34%	68.1%	76.6%	70.45%	70	63

Code: ■ = Goal is met. □ = Goal is not met.

New Hire Turnover Rate - Numerator: All RNs hired and resigned within 12 rolling months. Denominator: All RNs hired within 12 rolling months.
Voluntary Turnover Rate - Numerator: All resigned RNs within 12 months for any of the TCAB (NQF) controllable reasons. Denominator: All RNs in the unit.

FIGURE 54-2 CSMC Quality Outcome Measures.

our participation with the RWJF and the IHI, we were willing partners in a commitment to create a model for engagement and improvement that would yield outcomes beyond the initial pilot. We created and distributed DVDs, papers, and PowerPoint presentations on how to engage, enrich, and evolve the nursing staff in the quest for excellence. We built upon our nursing strategic plan and the institution's quality and strategic plan to achieve our goals. The TCAB process became part of our overall operational plan (see Figure 54-1). We have achieved positive outcomes, as shown in Figure 54-2, and we are committed to spreading TCAB throughout the nation as part of the AONE TCAB community and the RWJF Aligning Forces initiatives.

SPREADING TCAB: THE AMERICAN ORGANIZATION OF NURSE EXECUTIVES

All hospitals are challenged to critically analyze their current methods of delivering care and services. What worked previously will not work in a future of fewer resources, greater patient chronicity, and extreme complexity. TCAB is a process that unites rapid-cycle redesign at the bedside with organizational vision and mission. The senior leadership must focus on creating viable business processes and programs to support key services and meet the expectation of staff, patients, and community. The senior goals are then translated at the bedside. For example, if safety metrics are board-level measures for quality, TCAB units incorporate the goals in their bedside redesign targets.

Decreasing nosocomial infections to zero is an institutional goal; TCAB unit goals—including 100% hand washing by all staff, use of wide sterile barriers for procedures, removing lines (peripheral, central, urinary) when no longer required—appear on the unit dashboard. There is a direct line between what happens at the bedside and what is reported in the board room.

The senior nursing team provides support and advocacy for the process by clearly outlining and articulating the vision and mission of TCAB. The TCAB process becomes a structure that supports shared decision-making at all levels. Staff learns that their participation is not optional; it is an essential component to success. There is consistent application of quality improvement that creates transformation experts. And, as these changes are introduced, the senior team serves as an advocate to move the changes through, remove barriers, and hardwire or institutionalize the successes.

AONE completed a two-and-a-half–year AONE/RWJF TCAB project with 67 hospitals, is working with the RWJF Aligning Forces for Quality Grant in 14 national communities, and has launched a national AONE TCAB learning community project. The greatest learning has been that TCAB transforms not only processes, but more importantly, culture. The culture of shared leadership and decision-making creates a foundation for doing the work with a shared vision and mission. TCAB is embedded into the formal shared governance structure and processes as a major spread technique. As staff learned how to conduct rapid-cycle tests of change, the Unit Practice Councils established goals for improvement based on the results. For example, staff set goals in the Unit Practice Councils to improve nurse retention and created a peer mentoring process to achieve desired institutional outcomes for the education, certification, and development of staff. This has signaled that TCAB is no longer a special project; it is the way that work will be done. Through our collaboration with the Robert Wood Johnson Foundation, we hope to engage hospitals throughout the nation to adopt TCAB processes and achieve a critical mass of facilities committed to improving the practice environment of nurses—a key strategy to keeping patients safe.

LESSONS LEARNED AND POLICY IMPLICATIONS

Transformation requires "all hands on board." It cannot be accomplished as a pure staff or executive model. Change must come by engaging both the clinicians with the knowledge about what needs to be done and those in positions with the power to enable change efficiently and effectively. The empowerment of nurses to bring up ideas, test them using the TCAB processes, and examine results to drive improvement occurred because they had the tools and support they needed from executives. Sustaining TCAB required the allocation of resources: time, funding and willingness of the C-suite to change. The commitment from institutional presidents and trustees was essential so that TCAB was not just a "flavor of the month" project (Lewis, 2009).

It is essential that nurses, physicians, and other direct care clinicians, educators, and patients be engaged to provide their recommendations on what works and doesn't work in the creation of a sustainable, efficient, effective, reliable, and equitable health care system. Those with resources to reform our system—elected officials at the local, state, and national levels; executives of insurance companies; pharmaceutical and medical device manufacturers; hospital associations; educators; quality and accrediting bodies; and consumers of health care—should examine the extraordinary outcomes that have emerged from TCAB. We established, launched, and spread an effective model for transformation of complex systems within America's hospitals. The idealized design applied on a larger scale has the potential to create the foundation for transformation of our health care system.

For a list of related websites, please refer to your Evolve Resources at http://evolve.elsevier.com/Mason/policypolitics/

REFERENCES

Aiken, L. (2002). Hospital nurse staffing and patient mortality, nurse burnout, and job dissatisfaction. *Journal of the American Medical Association, 288*(16), 1987-1993.

Burnes Bolton, L., Gassert, C. A., & Cipriano, P. F. (2008). Smart technology, enduring solutions. *Journal of Healthcare Information Management, 22*(4), 24-26.

Donahue, L. (2009). A pod design for nursing assignments. *American Journal of Nursing, 109*(11), 38-40.

Institute of Medicine. (2001). *Crossing the quality chasm: A new health system for the 21st century.* Washington D.C.: National Academies Press.

Institute of Medicine. (2004). *Keeping patients safe: Transforming the work environment of nurses.* Washington D.C.: National Academies Press.

Lewis, L. (2009) Commitment of the entire organization: Two CEO's reflect on TCAB. *American Journal of Nursing, 109*(11), 16.

Moen, R. D. (2002). *A guide for idealized design.* Cambridge, MA: Institute for Healthcare Improvement.

Pappas, S. H. (2008). The cost of nursing sensitive adverse events. *Journal of Nursing Administration, 38*(5), 230.

Robert Wood Johnson Foundation. (2009). Aligning Forces for Quality. Retrieved January 19, 2010, from www.forces4quality.org.

Rutherford, P., Moen, R., & Taylor, J. (2009). TCAB: The "how" and the "what." *American Journal of Nursing, 109*(11), 5-11.

Zant, W. (2009) Reducing falls among outpatients. *American Journal of Nursing, 109*(11), 41-42.

CHAPTER 55

TAKING ACTION
When a Hurricane Strikes: The Challenge of Crafting Workplace Policy

Janice M. McCoy and Susan McDonough Stackpoole

"The smart thing is to prepare for the unexpected."
—Chinese fortune cookie

At Cape Canaveral Hospital, the television announcers are relentless in their coverage of the approaching hurricane. The same message is heard from the TV in every patient's room: "Evacuate now!" The nursing staff hear the message, but they are focused on patient safety as their patients are loaded into waiting ambulances for the trip to their sister hospital in Melbourne, Florida, which is 35 miles to the south. The wind is increasing, as well as anxiety, as the staff hurry to finish, secure their areas, and evacuate to a safe location to wait out the approaching storm.

Hurricanes are a force of nature that challenges many states along the east and gulf coasts of the United States. Florida is especially vulnerable, and every community must be ready to respond quickly to protect its citizens and their property during violent weather. Cape Canaveral Hospital, one of three hospitals in Health First, Inc., is located 1 mile from the Atlantic Ocean in Cocoa Beach, Florida, and is under mandatory evacuation orders when a hurricane approaches from the east (Figure 55-1). Coordinating the evacuation process is a challenge, as patient safety and well-being are primary concerns. Time is a critical factor to ensure that the patients are relocated, the hospital is secured, and employees also have adequate time to prepare their homes and their families for evacuation. All of these things must be completed before the causeways are closed and travel to safety is no longer possible.

Multiple hurricane evacuations in recent years revealed problems at Cape Canaveral Hospital. The problems provided an opportunity to develop creative policy solutions. The policies were designed to address nursing staff expectations and responsibilities and to define the consequences of failure to adhere to these policies during hurricanes. The policy goal was to hold employees accountable for their job responsibilities, at a time when the community depends on them, without risking the safety of the employees and their families.

ANNUAL PREPARATION ACTIVITIES

Hurricane season begins June 1, but hospital planning and preparations begin every January. Health First, Inc. has a Hurricane Task Force that is composed of representatives from all of the Health First facilities. This interdisciplinary team meets to review the experiences from the previous year and to ensure that all of the policies address any issues that were identified. May is designated as Hurricane Preparedness Month, and all educational activities for staff and physicians are completed during the month.

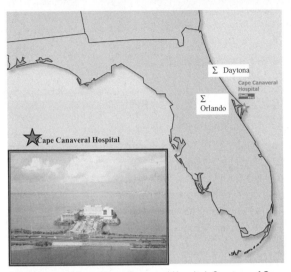

FIGURE 55-1 Map of Cape Canaveral Hospital. Courtesy of Cape Canaveral Hospital.

BEFORE THE STORM

Because of the nature of the preparation process, three planning phases have been defined: pre-storm, during storm, and post-storm. The pre-storm team includes all of the employees who are on duty at the time the evacuation is ordered. Hospital department evacuation plans have been developed that clearly define expectations of the employees. When this plan is activated, discharge or transfer orders for patients are obtained, patients and their health care records are prepared for transfer, and the nursing units are secured and closed down as the patients are discharged or transported to other facilities. Once the unit or department is closed, employees are allowed to leave. All staff members are expected to tell their directors where they will be during the storm and how they can be contacted.

DURING THE STORM

The "during storm" team is composed of the employees who are scheduled to work during the shifts when the hospital is closed. This may be only 1 day to 4 or more days, depending on the extent of the damage that occurs at the hospital. The expectation is that employees will report to work at another facility where patients have been transferred to assist the receiving hospital's staff with the extra workload. It is also expected that employees will report to the facility in advance of the storm to ensure that they are able to reach their destination safely. They are directed to bring enough food, clothes, and personal care items to last for several days.

AFTER THE STORM

The post-storm team includes employees who are able to return to the hospital as soon as the roads are passable to assess the damage and begin to prepare the facility to reopen. Certain departments arrive first, including security, administration, environmental services, food services, and plant operations, to begin the cleanup and ensure that the hospital is safe for staff and patients. Staff members involved in patient care are notified as soon as it is safe to return to reopen their units and begin the process of returning patients to the facility.

EMPLOYEE EXPECTATIONS

A brochure that is updated and distributed each year clearly explains the expectations for the employees, and meetings are held to review the information. Flyers entitled "Hurricane Preparedness Tips" are distributed monthly during hurricane season to all employees to reinforce the information in the brochure.

Health First developed a number of forms to clearly communicate the expectations for each individual employee, depending on his or her family situation.

The most important form is the employee "During Hurricane Exemption" form (Figure 55-2). This form is used by staff to request an exemption from working before, during, or after the storm. The eligible exemptions include the following:

- Providing care on a routine basis for an elderly immediate family member who does not qualify for a special needs shelter and for whom no other care provider is available
- Providing care on a routine basis for an immediate relative who is handicapped or has a chronic illness
- Providing sole care for a child under 2 years old
- Both parents of a child under 2 years old work for emergency service providers (e.g., hospital, law enforcement, fire and rescue) and are required to work during the storm simultaneously; the Health First employee is exempt

(Employee Directions: By June 1, send completed form to the Employment Manager and place a copy in your department Disaster Manual. Associates meeting any of the following exemptions must complete this form annually in May, and update as necessary throughout the hurricane season.)

Associate name: _____ Dept: _____

Facility: _____

I am requesting exemption from working at any Health First facility **during** a hurricane or other severe weather incident because I meet one of the following criteria:

☐ I provide care for an elderly immediate relative who cannot care for himself or herself on a routine basis. There are no other adult family members to provide this care. This person would not otherwise qualify for a special needs shelter.

☐ I provide care that cannot otherwise be delivered for an immediate relative who is handicapped or has a chronic illness.

☐ I am a sole caregiver with a child less than 2 years of age.

☐ When both parents of a child less than 2 years old, one of whom works for another emergency services employer (i.e., nursing, other hospital, law enforcement, fire and rescue, city employee), are required to work and have simultaneous roles during a storm, associate is exempt.

☐ When both parents of a child less than 2 years old work at Health First and normally would have simultaneous roles during a storm, one is exempt.

I certify that the above checked statement is true. I also understand that untrue statements may subject me to disciplinary action.

Associate signature: _____ Date: _____

Based on the above statement, I am in agreement that this associate be granted exemption from working during a hurricane or other severe weather incident.

Director's signature: _____ Date: _____

FIGURE 55-2 Cape Canaveral Hospital "During Hurricane Exemption" form.

- Both parents of a child under 2 years old work for the Health First Corporation and have simultaneous roles during a storm; one is exempt

The employee signs the exemption form, which must be approved by his or her direct supervisor and forwarded to the Employment Manager. The form is completed at the time of hiring and annually in May and is updated as necessary throughout the year.

CHILD CARE SERVICES

For employees who volunteer or are required to work during or after the storm, Health First provides childcare for children through age 20. Older children (over age 16) may be permitted to volunteer in the hospital in appropriate areas. A childcare enrollment form must be completed on hire and annually in May. If schools and daycare facilities are unable to open post-storm, working employees who have no other childcare options may bring their children to Health First–designated childcare facilities.

COMMUNICATION ISSUES

Health First uses numerous methods of communication to ensure that information is available to all employees throughout the entire disaster situation. Every employee is to provide contact information, including cell phone numbers or phone numbers where they can be reached if they are evacuating to another location. The corporation also sets up a hotline, which is updated on an ongoing basis and is accessible to all employees at any time. Announcements are also sent out via the media as appropriate.

It is important to use as many options as possible, because some may not be accessible as a result of power outages and overloaded phone lines.

PERSONAL IMPACT OF A STORM

One of the most difficult things to deal with is the stress on the employees who are trying to balance their personal needs with the job expectations. Health First encourages employees to make preparations at home at the beginning of the hurricane season so that supplies are available at a moment's notice. When a storm is approaching, personnel are expected to secure their property, make arrangements for their family members and pets, and pack the essentials that they will need during and after the storm. Depending on their previously agreed-on assignment, they will report to the appropriate facility to provide assistance during and after the storm.

Post-hurricane critiques are done on each hospital nursing unit, as well as hospital-wide, to identify areas for improvement of the disaster processes and to address the needs of the nurses and other staff members. A study by Cohan and Cole (2002) found that "There is robust evidence community-wide disasters lead to mental health problems." In addition, they identified that "posttraumatic stress disorder increases following natural disasters, including hurricanes" (Ironson et al., 1997). The hospital's pastoral services department provides opportunities for employees to attend counseling sessions. This enables employees to share their experiences and receive further care if needed. The Employee Assistance Program (EAP) is also available to all employees to assist with personal crises. Short-term counseling, identification of resources, and referrals for long-term services are included in the free sessions.

RECENT EXPERIENCE WITH DISASTER

Cape Canaveral Hospital was founded in 1963, and until 1995 had evacuated only once. Since 1996, with the improvement in storm predictions and warning systems, the accuracy of the information has improved considerably, resulting in a total of five evacuations since 1996. In the early evacuations, the policies and expectations were not clearly defined. Employees volunteered to assist as necessary, and the evacuation process was completed without incident. However, as the corporation grew to include three hospitals and other entities, it became increasingly important to more clearly define the responsibilities and expectations. During the evacuation in 1999 for Hurricane Floyd, approximately 100 associates failed to fulfill their obligations, and as a result 30 were terminated. Some personnel had evacuated to other states and were unable or unwilling to return for duty in a timely manner. Others simply abandoned their positions and quit. During the post-storm critique, it was apparent that the expectations were not clearly defined, and after careful review of individual circumstances, several employees were reinstated to their positions.

In 2004, four hurricanes struck the state of Florida, with three of them hitting the east coast of central Florida. Cape Canaveral Hospital was ordered to evacuate twice in 3 weeks which placed an incredible burden on the staff and available resources. Unfortunately, a number of employees had sustained significant damage to their homes and personal property during the first storm, which added to their stress in responding to the second. However, most employees provided the support needed to accomplish the task a second time.

Unfortunately, there were still a few employees who failed to meet their obligations and were terminated. It was a much better process than in 1999, because the policies were more clearly defined and communicated. Fellow employees also reinforced their obligations and expectations to their peers, and several made the statement when told that their co-workers were evacuating outside the immediate area, "You know you could lose your job if you do that, don't you?"

THE HURRICANE POLICIES

It became clear after the problems with the Hurricane Floyd evacuation in 1999 that Health First would benefit from improved policies to guide both employee and hospital actions and better define responsibilities. Policies that resulted include the following:

- *Hurricane and severe weather policy:* This clearly defines what is expected of each employee and employees' responsibilities in a hurricane.
- *Positive discipline and corrective action guide:* This includes "failure to report to work when scheduled

during a hurricane or other community crisis or disaster" in the list of violations that result in disciplinary action.

- *Department-specific plans:* These plans are guides for each hospital department for evacuation and staffing during a hurricane.

LESSONS LEARNED

CLEAR EXPECTATIONS ARE CRITICAL

The most important lesson learned from these disaster experiences was the need to clearly define organizational expectations in policies and communicate them to every employee. The employees' signatures on the forms indicate that they have reviewed and understand the information and agree to the expectations as defined. It is critical to inform employees that failure to meet their obligation may result in disciplinary action, up to and including termination, depending on the circumstances. After the 2004 hurricanes, an appeal process was also defined and implemented in which employees had a formal mechanism to tell their story and appeal their situation before executive leadership. The severity of infractions was defined, with corresponding disciplinary actions outlined, to ensure consistency across the entire system (Box 55-1). A detailed review was conducted to ensure that the follow-through was equal and consistent. Most of the original decisions were upheld after the appeal process. This was a critical factor for those employees who sacrificed their own needs to ensure that the needs of the patients and their fellow employees were met.

SAFE EVACUATION PLANS ARE NEEDED

Another lesson learned is that evacuation from coastal areas does not necessarily need to be far-away location to be safe. In the past, people were encouraged to move at least 2 hours away from the projected path of a storm, but experience has shown that this may be too far because of the huge traffic delays when trying to return home. As storms can be unpredictable in their direction and severity, it is now recommended that people remain as close to home as safely possible, as directed by local emergency authorities.

EMPLOYEE NEEDS

French, Sole, and Byers (2002), in a study on nurses' needs following Hurricane Floyd, found the primary

---

> **BOX 55-1** **Types of Disciplinary Action for Noncompliance with Hurricane Policies at Cape Canaveral Hospital**
>
> **Nondisciplinary action:** Miscommunication (includes instances of staff evacuating too far away and not being able to get back in time to meet their assignments so they arranged to "trade" with other staff, and instances when phone messages were left but the phones were out of service).
> - Hospital action: Written documentation and explanation to file.
>
> **Level 1**: Post-storm employees with extenuating circumstances (running out of gas, traffic backups, cleaning up from damage to their homes).
> - Hospital action: Nonpaid decision day (a day for the employees to consider their own desire to remain within the organization based on the expectations for them to continue in their roles).
>
> **Level 2**: Negligence on behalf of employee for defined storm responsibilities; effort made to return as soon as possible for post-storm duties.
> - Hospital action: 24- to 40-hour employee suspension; loss of annual team bonus for failure to support the team.
>
> **Level 3:** Flagrant disregard for responsibilities before, during, or after for one of the storms; either not scheduled or fulfilled scheduled shift before, during, or after second storm.
> - Hospital action: 40- to 80-hour suspension; loss of annual team bonus, for failure to support the team.
>
> **Level 4**: Flagrant disregard for responsibilities before, during, or after, for both storms; understood consequences as explained to and/or by their manager; no-call, no-show at any time.
> - Hospital action: Termination of employment.

---

concerns of nurses were family safety, pet care, and personal safety while at work. Secondary concerns were for basic needs, such as food, water, sleep, shelter, and rest. Health First recognized these employee concerns and addressed them. Before, during, and after the storms, they identified numerous ways to assist the employees to meet their personal needs. Cash advances were made available to assist with evacuation expenses (for hotels, gas, and food). Transportation between facilities was provided to ensure that staffing was adequate but that the

BOX 55-2 Health Care Worker Needs during Emergencies

- Security at work
- Training
- Shelter for self
- Health care
- Shelter for family
- Clarification of role
- Food
- Scheduled relief
- Compensation
- Security at home
- Stress debriefing
- Transportation
- Childcare, pet care, and elder care

From Martens, K. A., Hantsch, C. E., & Stake, C. E. (2003). Emergency preparedness survey: Personnel availability and support needs. *Annals of Emergency Medicine, 42*(4), S105.

It's about the aftermath, a lessening of a standard of living that is very disruptive to families" (Lapidario, 2005). Other issues that remain to be resolved include accommodations for employee family members and employee's pets that need a secure facility for shelter (Box 55-2).

Clearly defined policies, and communication of these policies to every employee of the organization, is essential to ensure that the needs of the hospital, its patients, and its employees are met in a fair and consistent manner. Health First implemented policy changes that clarified what was expected of the employees and the consequences that would occur if the policies were not followed. All of these efforts ensure adequate staffing during a disaster to meet the needs of hospitalized patients while also protecting the individual needs of the employees.

For a list of related websites, please refer to your Evolve Resources at http://evolve.elsevier.com/Mason/policypolitics/

employees did not have to drive their own vehicles during the storm. The action that was most appreciated was the roofing crew made available to provide temporary repairs to the homes of employees who suffered damage. This protected their property until permanent repairs could be made.

Counseling was offered to employees who had suffered losses and experienced anxiety as a result of the storms. According to the Florida Coalition Against Domestic Violence, "It's not the wind and the floods.

REFERENCES

Cohan, C. L., & Cole, S. W. (2002). Life course transitions and natural disaster: Marriage, birth, and divorce following Hurricane Hugo. *Journal of Family Psychology, 16*(1), 14-25.

French, E. D., Sole, M. L., & Byers, J. F. (2002). A comparison of nurses' needs/concerns and hospital disaster plans following Florida's Hurricane Floyd. *Journal of Emergency Nursing, 28*(2), 111-117.

Ironson, G., Wynings, C., Schneiderman, N., Baum, A., Rodriguez, M., et al. (1997). Posttraumatic stress symptoms, intrusive thoughts, loss, and immune function after Hurricane Andrew. *Psychosomatic Medicine, 59*(2), 128-141.

Lapidario, M. (2005, February 5). Domestic abuse rises after storms. *Daytona Beach News Journal*, 3C.

CHAPTER 56

Workplace Abuse in Nursing: Policy Strategies

Jane H. Barnsteiner

"Organizations learn and evolve through conscious, deliberate action. Deliberate action is ethical. When the time to act has come, it is unethical not to do something."

—David Thomas, ethicist

A culture of safety is necessary to achieve continuous and sustainable changes that promote patient safety and employee satisfaction in an organization. Bullying, harassment, and "disruptive behaviors" constitute workplace abuse and violate the principles of a culture of safety, endanger patients, and are a cause of employee dissatisfaction and turnover (The Joint Commission, 2008). Workplace abuse must be managed with a multifaceted approach that includes engaging top leadership, setting expectations, training and progressive discipline, and self-management.

Workplace abuse is an all too common experience in health care settings. More than 70% of physicians and nurses report that they have witnessed such disruptive behaviors (Rosenstein, 2002). Further, fewer than 10% of supervisors are reported to address issues of abuse in the workplace (AACN, 2005). A number of terms are used to describe workplace abuse and include disruptive behavior, bullying, and lateral violence. While the definition of each of these is slightly different, for the purposes of this chapter all are considered workplace abuse.

WHAT CONSTITUTES WORKPLACE ABUSE?

Workplace abuse is behavior that interferes with the ability of employees to provide safe and effective care, undermines the confidence of team members to effectively care for patients, and causes a concern for physical safety and/or undermines effective teamwork. Overt and passive activities meant to intimidate or disrupt care may be from peer to peer, physician to nurse, or supervisor to employee. While there is increasing concern related to abuse from patients and family members, this is not included as a focus of this chapter.

Workplace abuse may take a number of forms, including profane or disrespectful behavior; name calling; demeaning behavior; sexual comments or innuendos; racial or ethnic jokes; outbursts of anger; criticizing in front of patients or other staff; throwing objects; intimidation that suppresses input from other providers; and retaliation against clinicians who raise concerns about safety, conduct, or culture issues. It also includes a preceptor being visibly exasperated when asked a question by an orientee, gossip about co-workers, scapegoating, public verbal outbursts, refusal to answer questions or phone calls, intimidating body language, or physical violence.

Workplace abuse has a negative effect on the quality of patient care (Barnsteiner, Madigan, & Spray, 2001; Institute for Safe Medication Practices (ISMP), 2004; Johnson, 2009; Rosenstein & O'Daniel, 2005). This may result from a reluctance to ask questions related to patient care or workarounds because staff may avoid those known to be abusive. Examples include an RN not notifying an MD of a change in patient status, keeping silent about a safety concern rather than questioning a known disruptor, administering a medication despite serious unresolved safety concerns, or tolerating substandard care such as no hand washing or surgical site marking. It may affect work productivity by causing rework or delays in care. Public and private policies have been developed to reduce abuse among health care workers. These policies can and should be extended to the local work unit where the abuse takes place.

INCIDENCE

Reports vary on the incidence of workplace abuse. Rosenstein (2002) reported that 96% of nurses have witnessed workplace abuse. Diaz and McMillin (1991) reported that 64% of nurses have experienced disruptive behaviors, and 23% of nurses reported that something has been thrown at them. In a survey of nursing staff in a prominent children's hospital, 65% reported they had experienced verbal abuse by physicians in the past year, and 24% reported they had felt afraid while at work (Barnsteiner, Madigan, & Spray, 2001). Further, 97% of respondents in the survey stated that hospital leadership should be involved in solving issues of workplace abuse.

The American Association of Critical-Care Nurses collaborated on a large national survey that examined the challenges related to healthy work environments, one of which was workplace abuse (Maxfield, Grenny, McMillan, Patterson, & Switzler, 2005). Seventy-seven percent (77%) of respondents indicated that they work with someone who is condescending, insulting, or rude; 33% reported that they work with someone who is verbally abusive; and 52% work with clinicians who abuse their authority by pulling rank, bullying, and forcing their point of view on them. Only 2% of non-supervisors and 5% of supervisors confronted issues related to disrespect and abuse.

CAUSES

Various causes of workplace abuse have been postulated. Workplace abuse arises from individual and systemic factors (Johnson, 2009; The Joint Commission, 2008). There continues to be a steep power gradient among professionals, particularly between physicians and nurses. Fear of retaliation, lack of formal systems to report or address, and the high pressure and emotionality of the practice setting are contributing factors. Individuals who are abusive may be fatigued or immature, or may lack interpersonal or conflict-management skills. What is clear is that the behavior has been tolerated, and there has been a leadership indifference to workplace abuse in health care.

INDICATORS OF WORKPLACE ABUSE

Workplace abuse affects job satisfaction and retention. It is reported as the largest factor in job satisfaction for nurses. Rosenstein and O'Daniel (2005) reported that more than 30% of nurses knew at least one nurse who left because of workplace abuse. But we've known that abuse affects staff retention. In 1987, Cox reported that 18% of turnover could be attributed to workplace abuse.

A high rate of staff turnover is just one of a number of indicators that abuse is occurring in a workplace. Low ratings of overall job satisfaction—particularly of physician-nurse relationships, peer relationships, and relationships between staff and nurse managers—are all signs that workplace abuse may be a problem. The presence of cliques in a work area and reports of dueling units or shifts are also indicators (Alspach, 2008; Gilmore & Hamlin, 2003).

WORK ENVIRONMENT AND ERRORS

There have been numerous studies demonstrating the association between work environment and patient errors and the influence on job satisfaction and retention. In a study of more than 2000 health care professionals queried about workplace intimidation related to medication practices, 7% of respondents indicated that they were involved in a medication error during the past year in which intimidation played a role (ISMP, 2004). More than 45% of respondents in the ISMP survey indicated that past intimidating experiences caused them to not clarify medication orders or ask questions. Rosenstein and O'Daniel (2005) reported in a large survey of nurses that 17% of respondents were aware of a specific adverse event that occurred as a result of disruptive behavior.

There is an assumption that most health care workplace abuse is by physicians. A national sample survey of nurses who were victims of abuse said that intraprofessional abuse was commonplace (Vessey et al., 2009). Senior nurses, charge nurses, and nurse managers were identified as perpetrators of abuse. More than 50% of the respondents reported that they left their positions to take a new one after being abused. In a study of emergency nurses, 27% stated that they had experienced bullying in the previous 6 months, and there was a significant association of workplace abuse with intent to leave one's current position (Johnson, 2009; Rosenstein & O'Daniel, 2005).

COMMUNICATION AND HEALTHY WORK ENVIRONMENTS

Communication is a significant factor associated with workplace abuse. Rosenstein and O'Daniel (2008) reported that one in three nurses stated that they have difficulty speaking up when witnessing patient problems due to fear and intimidation. One common theme in the literature is the need to improve communication skills and for all health care workers to become skilled in negotiation and conflict resolution. Nurses need to become as proficient in communication skills as they are in clinical skills. When abuse is present, a dysfunctional cycle can evolve. Poor communication may lead to frustration and workplace abuse; conversely, workplace abuse leads to poor communication as staff wish to have as little contact as possible with an abuser. The Joint Commission analysis of sentinel events ranks poor communication the number-one factor following root cause analysis of events causing serious injury.

Facilitating teamwork and collaboration has been demonstrated to improve communication among health care providers. Components of teamwork include positive communication, intraprofessional and interprofessional collaboration, valuing each member of the health care team's contribution, active work to resolve conflict, and development of work-related shared vision and goals.

POLICY CONSIDERATIONS

There are numerous policies and practices that can be helpful in reducing workplace abuse. These policies can be categorized according to the following:
1. Education of health professions students
2. Standards from professional organizations
3. Policies from health care regulatory associations such as the Joint Commission and state and federal government
4. Individual institutional policies and practices
All policies and practices need to state clear expectations about acceptable behavior; training, coaching, and mentoring for those who struggle with the

policies; monitoring of the culture for violations; early intervention for even the mildest violations and progressive discipline for repeated violations; and systemic solutions to contributing causes. Clear expectations include a universal code of conduct that applies to everyone in the organization, including physicians, employees, and top leadership, and defines what teamwork, collaboration, and respect look like as well as unacceptable behaviors.

HEALTH PROFESSIONS EDUCATION

The Institute of Medicine (2000) spearheaded the movement to incorporate competencies needed by all health professionals, one of which is the ability to function effectively and collaborate on interprofessional teams. Leaders in the health professions have since moved to incorporate content related to communication, respectful behavior, and teamwork and collaboration into education programs. The American Association of Medical Colleges (2005) has defined standards and behaviors related to professionalism to be incorporated into prelicensure medical education. The Accreditation Council for Graduate Medical Education (2007) has established competencies related to professionalism to be incorporated into postgraduate programs.

Nursing has also defined standards related to developing professionals who have the knowledge, skills, and attitudes to work as member of a team and promote a healthy work environment. In the Essentials of Baccalaureate Education for Nursing, The American Association of Colleges of Nursing (AACN) (2008) has identified the knowledge, skills, and attitudes related to teamwork and collaboration. The AACN standards integrate the Quality and Safety Education in Nursing (QSEN) work that defined the prelicensure and graduate competencies for nursing related to the IOM components of quality health care (Cronenwett et al., 2007, Cronenwett et al., 2009).

PROFESSIONAL STANDARDS

Some nursing organizations have developed standards for healthy work environments that incorporate strategies to deal with workplace abuse. The American Organization of Nurse Executives (2005) standards related to professionalism are required to be met for certification as a nurse executive. The American Association of Critical-Care Nurses (2005) established standards for creating and sustaining healthy work environments.

REGULATORY APPROACHES

The Joint Commission, the major accreditation body for health care organizations, recognized the significant presence of workplace abuse in hospitals and published a Sentinel Event Alert in 2008, synthesizing research on workplace abuse and outlining steps organizations should take to stop workplace abuse (The Joint Commission, 2008). Additionally, the leadership standard (LD.03.01.01) has two performance elements that address behaviors that undermine a culture of safety and mandate the systems that organizations must put in place to facilitate a healthy work environment: The first is EP 4: The hospital/organization has a code of conduct that defines acceptable, disruptive, and inappropriate behaviors. The second is EP 5: Leaders create and implement a process for managing disruptive and inappropriate behaviors. Please visit the Joint Commission's website at *www.jointcommission.org/sentinelevents/sentineleventalert/sea_40.htm* to read the Sentinel Event Alert and view a list of recommendations for preventing and managing disruptive behavior in health care organizations.

The Occupational Safety and Health Act of 1970 was passed to ensure that all workers had safe and healthy working conditions. The Occupational Safety and Health Administration's (OSHA's) response to the problem of workplace violence has been to develop guidelines and recommendations for organizations implementing workplace violence prevention programs. In 1996, OSHA published Guidelines for Preventing Workplace Violence for Health Care and Social Service Workers. The guidelines are based on OSHA's voluntary generic Safety and Health Program Management Guidelines (OSHA, 2004).

There have been cases in which the courts have ruled that health care workers can sue workplace bullies for behavior that is not already covered under laws such as for assault. Employees must demonstrate that the behavior has resulted in them being unable to perform their responsibilities (Porto & Lauve, 2006; Klein, 2008).

INSTITUTIONAL APPROACHES

It is at the local level of the individual health care organization or unit where efforts to develop healthy work environments and stop workplace abuse are operationalized. To be successful, a multifaceted approach is required that incorporates both policies and practices. An executive team that wants to increase the level of respect in a workplace, eliminate abuse, and promote collaboration must develop policies to guide the organization. These often take the form of codes of conduct or directives. Policies, used alone, have limitations. Defining specific practices provides a complementary perspective to the policies. For example, when putting in place a "condition white" code, someone who is observing or experiencing abuse calls the code for supportive people to come and intervene. It is also the role of the executive team to identify system-level bottlenecks and constraints that prevent implementing and sustaining healthy work environments.

Employees may not experience their executive leadership as a reliable authority who is "just" and facilitates employees overcoming fear of reporting. Employees may fear that if they speak up, they will not be supported. They may experience a conflict between doing what is right for a patient or colleague and what is safe for them. If the leadership is committed to developing healthy work environments and eliminating workplace abuse, people in high-status positions cannot be exempt from the rules of conduct or from the disciplinary system. Oftentimes the medical staff has a separate organizing structure and is not held to the policies of the organization. It is necessary to harmonize and coordinate the disciplinary practices of the hospital and the medical staff. Organizations have a responsibility to provide a safe environment for all who work there. The Joint Commission (2008) recommends that organizations have a "zero tolerance" for intimidating or disruptive behaviors, and this needs to be defined in medical staff bylaws and organization policies and widely circulated throughout the organization so everyone is aware of it. Having a zero tolerance policy in effect may minimize frequency and the harmful effects of workplace abuse. A workplace abuse prevention program includes a reporting and documentation process and a prevention policy that includes strategies to be implemented system-wide when instances of abuse occur.

In addition to standards and policies, specific actions are needed to establish the policies and practices and for monitoring, including periodic organizational self-assessments to identify the issues and extent of workplace abuse. Educational programs are necessary to equip leaders and clinicians with good communication and conflict resolution skills and teach clinicians how to give direct feedback. TeamSTEPPS is an effective program to teach clinicians these skills. TeamSTEPPS is an evidence-based, government-sponsored program to improve teamwork and communication skills among health care workers. It incorporates the development of four skills; leadership, communication, situation monitoring, and mutual support. The program facilitates shared understanding and development of positive attitudes about teamwork. Please refer to *http:// teamstepps.ahrq.gov/* for more information.

WORK UNIT APPROACHES

Reducing anonymity; creating stable interprofessional teams; and using chain of command reporting mechanisms, interprofessional rounds, and 360-peer review[1] feedback methods are work unit approaches for reducing workplace abuse.

1. *Reduce anonymity.* Nurses often feel invisible to their colleagues, particularly physicians. They may not be addressed by name or receive eye contact. It is harder to treat someone disrespectfully when he or she is being addressed by name. Anonymity can be reduced by making it easy to see others' names and occupations. Face books, photo bulletin boards, and ID tags are ways of helping people put names to faces.

2. *Create stable interprofessional teams to promote healthy environments.* A significant stress in many organizations is the instability of clinical care teams. Frequent changes of residents and attending physicians hinder the relationship development that anchors teams and protects against disrespectful behavior. Stable, cohesive interprofessional teams provide the best patient care and are unlikely to behave unprofessionally toward

each other. A challenge for health care organizations is how to see the long-term benefits (greater patient satisfaction and staff retention and satisfaction) of stable interprofessional teams and appropriately compensate clinicians for this work.

3. *Eliminate the feeling that there's no support.* Often people who are being treated disrespectfully feel isolated, like there is no source of authority to appeal to and no available support. If the nurse has had an experience of verbal abuse from a physician colleague, she may hesitate to call about a patient condition. The nurse is balancing self-preservation with the interest of the patient. All staff needs education about the resources available. There should always be someone in the chain of command one can turn to for assistance. This may be a nursing supervisor or a physician director.

4. *Develop an understanding of other's roles and expertise.* It is not unusual for some professions such as nursing and physical therapy to feel devalued by physicians and not recognized for their expertise and contribution to patient care. Opportunities should be created for health care professionals to demonstrate what they do, what they have done, and what they have accomplished. Weekly interdisciplinary staff meetings co-chaired by physician and nurse leaders, short team huddles at the beginning of shifts, nurses presenting patients on interprofessional rounds, and task force membership strengthen interprofessional relationships and respect.

5. *Provide feedback on unprofessional behaviors.* Professionals may act unprofessionally partly because they do not manage their own stress and anxiety but also because they rarely get feedback on what their behavior means to others. 360-Feedback methods to survey the perceptions of staff, leadership, and physicians' professionalism from above and below facilitate individuals receiving feedback about how supportive or disruptive their behavior is viewed.

6. *Reduce fear of retaliation.* Twenty states currently have whistleblower laws that are intended to protect health care workers who speak out about situations that threaten the safety of patients and staff and from which they need protection (ANA, 2010). These laws are intended to prevent retaliation in the form of harassment, suspension, or firing for reporting these conditions.

[1]A "360 peer review" is an opportunity to obtain anonymous feedback and learn about one's strengths and areas for improvement from co-workers and supervisors. Formal feedback is usually requested via a survey from 5 to 10 peers and supervisors. Aggregated results are then provided to each person along with recommendations on behaviors to continue, those needing to be developed, and those needing to stop.

INDIVIDUAL APPROACHES

Individual clinicians have a responsibility to assess and develop their emotional maturity, collaboration skills, respectful negotiation, and effective and efficient communication. They need skills to discuss difficult topics with each other and the competence and confidence to confront anyone carrying out unsafe practices or abusing them or another colleague. They need to know how to tap into organizational resources. They need to learn how to remain approachable, even when stressed out. This includes treating team members with respect, pointing out mistakes in respectful and helpful ways, and responding to conflict by trying to work out the solutions.

A number of strategies can assist a clinician to develop these skills. The use of SBAR (Situation, Background, Assessment, and Recommendation) is a focused communication strategy for framing a critical conversation requiring a clinician's immediate attention and action. Cognitive rehearsal is an intervention strategy that teaches an individual a series of responses that allows them to respond differently to harmful interference or abuse (Griffin, 2004). For example, in the event of a verbal affront by a clinician, a response might be "The individuals I learn the most from are clear in their directions and feedback. Is there some way we can form this type of communication?" or "This is not the time or the place; please stop."

SUMMARY

Workplace abuse is a common occurrence in all health care settings. There continues to be a need to acknowledge the reality of the behavior and the negative impact it has on patient outcomes and employee job satisfaction and retention. A multipronged approach is needed to eliminate workplace abuse and promote development of healthy work environments. Policy and practice implications include: (1) incorporating components of teamwork and collaboration in health professions education; (2) continued development and dissemination of professional organization standards related to professionalism; (3) enforcement of health care regulatory policies related to elimination of workplace abuse; (4) development of institutional policies and practices to guide leaders and clinicians in developing healthy work environments and stopping workplace abuse; and (5) assuming personal responsibility for development of self-monitoring behavior.

For a list of related websites, please refer to your Evolve Resources at http://evolve.elsevier.com/Mason/policypolitics/

REFERENCES

Accreditation Council for Graduate Medical Education. (2007). *General competencies.* Chicago: ACGME. Retrieved from www.acgme.org/outcome/comp/GeneralCompetenciesStandards21307.pdf.

Alspach, G., (2008). Lateral hostility between critical care nurses: A survey report. *Critical Care Nurse, 28*(2), 1319.

American Association of Colleges of Nursing. (2008). *The essentials of baccalaureate education for professional nursing practice.* Washington, D.C.: Author.

American Association of Critical-Care Nurses. (2005). *AACN standards for establishing and sustaining healthy work environments: A journey to excellence.* Aliso Viejo, CA: American Association of Critical-Care Nurses.

American Association of Medical Colleges. (2005). Recommendations for clinical skills curricula for undergraduate medical education. Retrieved from https://services.aamc.org/publications/showfile.cfm?file=version56.pdf&prd_id=141&prv_id=165&pdf_id=56.

American Nurses Association. (2010). Whistleblower protection. *Nursing World.* Retrieved from www.nursingworld.org/MainMenuCategories/ANAPoliticalPower/State/StateLegislativeAgenda/Whistleblower_1.aspx.

American Organization of Nurse Executives (2005). Nurse executive competencies. *Nurse Leader, 3*(1), 15-22. Retrieved from www.nurseleader.com/article/PIIS1541461205000078/fulltext.

Barnsteiner, J., Madigan, C., & Spray, T. (2001). Instituting a disruptive conduct policy for medical staff. *AACN Clinical Issues, 12*(3), 378-382.

Cox, H. C. (1987). Verbal abuse in nursing: Report of a study. *Nursing Management, 18*(11), 47-50.

Cronenwett, L., Sherwood, G., Barnsteiner, J., Disch J., Johnson, J., et al. (2007). Quality and safety education for nurses. *Nursing Outlook, 55*(3),122-131.

Cronenwett, L., Sherwood, G., Pohl, J., Barnsteiner, J., Moore, S., et al. (2009). Quality and safety education for advanced practice nurses. *Nursing Outlook, 57*(6), 338-348.

Diaz, A., & McMillin, J. (1991). A definition and description of nurse abuse. *Western Journal of Nursing, 13*(1), 97-109.

Gilmore, D., & Hamlin, L. (2003). Bullying and harassment in perioperative settings. *British Journal of Perioperative Nursing, 13*(2), 79-85.

Griffin, M. (2004). Teaching cognitive rehearsal as a shield for lateral violence: An intervention for newly licensed nurses. *Journal of Continuing Education in Nursing, 35*(6), 257-263.

Institute of Medicine. (2000). *To err is human: Building a better health system.* Washington, D.C.: National Academy Press.

Institute for Safe Medication Practices. (2004). Survey on workplace intimidation. Retrieved from www.ismp.org/pressroom/pr20040331.pdf.

Johnson, S. L. (2009). International perspectives on workplace bullying among nurses: A review. *International Nursing Review, 56*(1), 34-40.

The Joint Commission. (2008). Behaviors that undermine a culture of safety. Sentinel Event Alert. Issue 40. Retrieved from www.jointcommission.org/SentinelEvents/SentinelEventAlert/sea_40.htm.

Klein, K. (2008). Employers can't ignore workplace bullies. *Bloomberg Business Week.* May 7. Retrieved from www.businessweek.com/smallbiz/content/may2008/sb2008057_530667.htm.

Maxfield, D., Grenny, J., McMillan, R., Patterson, K., & Switzler, A. (2005). Silence kills: The seven crucial conversations for healthcare. VitalSmarts Industry Watch.

Occupational Safety and Health Administration. (2004). *Guidelines for preventing workplace violence for health care & social service workers, OSHA*

3148-01R. Retrieved from www.osha.gov/Publications/OSHA3148/osha 3148.html.

Porto, G., & Lauve, R. (2006, July/August). Disruptive clinician behavior: A persistent threat to patient safety. *Patient Safety and Quality Healthcare.* Retrieved from www.psqh.com/julaug06/disruptive.html.

Rosenstein, A. (2002, July/August). The impact of nurse-physician relationships on nurse satisfaction and retention. *American Journal of Nursing, 102*(6), 26-34.

Rosenstein, A., & O'Daniel, M. (2005). Disruptive behavior and clinical outcomes: Perceptions of nurses and physicians. *American Journal of Nursing, 105*(1), 54-64.

Rosenstein, A., & O'Daniel, M. (2008). A survey of the impact of disruptive behaviors and communication defects on patient safety. *The Joint Commission Journal on Quality and Patient Safety, 34*(8), 464-471.

Thomas, D. (1993). *The ethics of choice: A quick guide.* Omaha, Nebraska.

Vessey, J. A., DeMarco, R. F., Gaffney, D. A., & Budin, W. C. (2009). Bullying of staff registered nurses in the workplace: A preliminary study for developing personal and organizational strategies for the transformation of hostile to healthy workplace environments. *Journal of Professional Nursing, 25*(5), 299-306.

CHAPTER 57

TAKING ACTION
Advocating for Nurses Injured in the Workplace

Anne Hudson

"If you ever think you're too small to be effective, you've never been in bed with a mosquito!"

—Wendy Lesko

When I was a nursing student, I learned to lift and move patients with techniques such as the under-axilla "drag lift," "bear hug," "pivot transfer," two-person "cradle lift," two-person "arm and leg lug," and others. I later learned that these techniques could be dangerous to the person performing them and were not approved for use in the United Kingdom.

One of my instructors warned about cumulative trauma back injury from lifting patients. She said, "Be careful with your back. Your job depends on your back." I dismissed this as impossible. Surely nurses would not lose their jobs because they were injured at work. I was unaware of the scope of back injuries in nurses or that manual lifting had been described as "deplorable … inefficient, dangerous to the nurses, and often painful and brutal to the patient" (Owen, 1999, p. 15). Patients can suffer pain, bruising, skin tears, abrasions, tube dislodgement, dislocations, fractures, and being dropped during attempts at manual lifting.

As an RN on medical/surgical, telemetry, and intermediate care units, I kept my patients pulled up in bed, turned frequently, and well-positioned, as well as lifting them to assist them to their walker, chair, and commode. In 2000, I suffered herniated lumbar discs and "cumulative trauma degenerative disc disease" from lifting patients. After spinal fusion surgery for placement of cadaver bone grafts and hardware, I had permanent lifting restrictions. I had to get an attorney and fight two court battles to prove that my spinal injury was from lifting patients in order to receive workers' compensation. I could not return to my position with lifting patients and was not selected for other nursing positions that did not require lifting. As a result, I was terminated. I became aware what happened to me was part of a larger problem, and I began educating myself. I was troubled by what I found. Though patient-lift equipment used by "lift teams" or nurses had proven since 1991 to prevent injury, nurses were still suffering severe injuries from performing manual patient lifting (Charney et al., 1991). I couldn't find any efforts to develop "safe patient handling" legislation.

My online research revealed nothing about "back-injured nurses." I contacted nursing schools, my state nursing association, and college and public librarians; still I found nothing. I contacted the American Nurses Association and learned that the preferred search term for the problem I was exploring was *patient handling*. Using this term, I found that 38% of nurses require time away from work during their career because of back injuries, and 12% leave nursing permanently due to back injuries, and that the Bureau of Labor Statistics (BLS) continually ranks nurses in the top 10 for work-related musculoskeletal disorders (MSDs) and reports that in 2007 nursing aides, orderlies, and attendants suffered the highest rate of MSDs, a rate of 252 cases per 10,000 workers, which is more than 7 times the national MSD average for all occupations (BLS, 2008).

I learned about cumulative trauma microfractures from lifting hazardous weights and about spinal injury to nurses from lifting patients. Because there are no pain receptors in the disc nucleus and vertebral endplates where microfractures typically begin, damage can occur over time without pain. Extensive damage may have already resulted in degenerative disc disease before severe pain announces extension of the injury from the center to nerves in the outer ring of the disc. By then, a career-ending or career-changing injury may have already occurred.

BECOMING A VOICE FOR BACK-INJURED NURSES

I discovered that the hospital had a "Back Injury Prevention Task Force" and requested to speak with the group. I presented research on safe lifting limits (35 pounds maximum for patient handling), spinal injury from patient lifting, preventing injuries with lift equipment, and how hospitals can save money through injury prevention techniques (Waters, 2007). I didn't receive an enthusiastic response. The group indicated that they were aware of what could be done to prevent injuries but had not tried to introduce workplace policies in the organization to prevent nurses from being injured.

My speaking out about preventing back injury began during a chance encounter with a patient lift equipment vendor who introduced me to William Charney, pioneer of "lift teams" and "no lift" policies. In 2001, Mr. Charney asked me to speak at a workshop in Portland, Oregon, on preventing back injuries with safe patient handling. I was glad to have the opportunity to discuss how nurses can be disabled by preventable injuries, issues related to loss of health insurance, and problems with employability.

Next, I spoke at the 3rd annual "Safe Patient Handling and Movement" Conference in Clearwater, Florida. By networking with new contacts, I went on to speak around the country at health and safety conferences, meetings of nursing organizations, hospitals, schools of nursing, workers' compensation training programs, and others. In 2005, I keynoted a conference for the Australian Nursing Federation (ANF) Victorian Branch "No Lifting Expo," the ANF Industrial Relations Organizers, and for the Injured Nurses Support Group (INSG).

In 2002, I published my first article about back injury issues in nursing. It was titled "Oh! My Aching Back!" In 2003, William Charney and I collaborated to co-edit a book titled *Back Injury Among Healthcare Workers: Causes, Solutions, and Impacts,* which was

about the epidemic of back injuries caused by dangerous manual patient-lifting practices. We addressed preventive technology and made a case for eliminating manual patient lifting. We included personal stories of back-injured nurses, revealing the lasting, devastating impacts of severe injury caused by physically lifting patients. Mr. Charney and I were the first voices in America since 2001 calling for state and national "safe patient handling-no manual lift" legislation. I contacted my local television station to increase public awareness of injuries caused by patient lifting. As a guest on a television news program, I had the opportunity to raise awareness about the problem. I continued to write about the problem, collaborated on peer-reviewed articles, and was invited to serve on the editorial board of the *Journal of Long-Term Effects of Medical Implants.* In 2007, my local newspaper published a full-page feature article about my efforts to address nurse injury from lifting patients. Despite all of these efforts to educate and raise awareness, action was still needed to address the problem.

ESTABLISHING THE WORK INJURED NURSES GROUP USA (WING USA)

I discovered that "no lifting" policies had been in place for years in the United Kingdom, Australia, and other countries, and that some nursing organizations provided support services for injured and ill nurses. There appeared to be no such assistance, information, or support in place for back-injured nurses in the United States. I contacted nurses who were involved in back injury protection efforts in other countries. My first international contacts were Maria Bryson, Royal College of Nursing Work Injured Nurses Group (RCN WING) Steward and Safety Representative in the UK, and Elizabeth Langford, Australian Nursing Federation (ANF) Victorian Branch, and Coordinator of Injured Nurses Support Group (INSG) in Melbourne. Inspired by my new friends who taught me about the services provided to injured nurses by RCN WING, and by ANF and INSG, I set out to work to develop similar services for U.S. nurses.

With the help of friends Teri Jennings and Marian Edmonds, we launched a website called "B.I.N. There—Back Injured Nurses," thus putting the phrase "back-injured nurses" into online search engines. In 2002, the name was changed to Work Injured Nurses'

Group USA (WING USA), and the website became *www.wingusa.org*. WING USA provides information about back injury in health care from manual patient lifting and serves as a meeting place for injured nurses from around the country. It is facilitated by a new effort for leaders in each state to provide injured nurses with a contact in their area for mutual support and encouragement, and for sharing experiences and information. Fifteen state leaders are currently active, and our goal is to identify one in each state. State leaders may also be involved in a variety of activities including group meetings, writing for publication, media outreach, speaking events, and political involvement for safe patient handling/no manual lift legislation. We hope that national nurse organizations will initiate broad programs to help injured nurses, particularly advocacy programs to help work-injured nurses remain employed.

Over 600 people receive WING USA's e-mail updates on legislation for safe patient handling. Recent legislative news posted at WING USA's website concerns the Coalition for Healthcare Worker and Patient Safety (CHAPS) visit to Capitol Hill to meet with U.S. Representatives and their staff in support of H.R. 2381, the Nurse and Health Care Worker Protection Act of 2009.

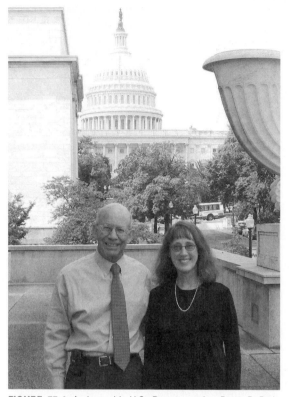

FIGURE 57-1 Author with U.S. Representative Peter DeFazio (D, OR) in Washington.

LEGISLATIVE EFFORTS TO ADVANCE SAFE PATIENT HANDLING

Since 2001, I have worked to advance legislation for "safe patient handling-no manual lift." This included working with labor unions, meeting with other back-injured nurses, meeting with legislators, and speaking out about the need for legislative efforts. I met with my U.S. Representative, Peter DeFazio (D-OR) (Figure 57-1) and his staff both in the district and in Washington. Congressman DeFazio became co-sponsor of H.R. 2381, the Nurse and Health Care Worker Protection Act of 2009. The legislation would mandate use of mechanical lift equipment for patients and residents nationally. A companion bill, S.B. 1788, was introduced in the Senate. At the time of this writing, both bills are in their respective committees.

We have made progress. Texas became the first state to require hospitals and nursing homes to implement a safe patient handling program. WING USA's website identifies state legislative initiatives pertaining to safe patient or resident handling. Laws in the three states of Ohio, New York, and Hawaii lend support to efforts for safe patient and/or resident handling. Laws in the seven states of Texas, Washington, Rhode Island, Maryland, Minnesota, New Jersey, and Illinois require development of safe patient handling policies, and/or implementation of safe patient handling programs, and/or use of mechanical patient lifting equipment, with variations in the scope and strength of requirements imposed by each state.

Most recently, I have joined the Coalition for Healthcare Worker and Patient Safety (CHAPS) to support passage of H.R. 2381/S.B. 1788—the Nurse and Health Care Worker Protection Act of 2009 (Figure 57-2). On July 23, 2009, ten members of CHAPS met with members of Congress and their staff, including U.S. Representative John Conyers (D-MI), author of H.R. 2381, which would mandate safe patient lift equipment and allow nurses and other health care workers to work without fear of being disabled and losing their positions due to back injury.

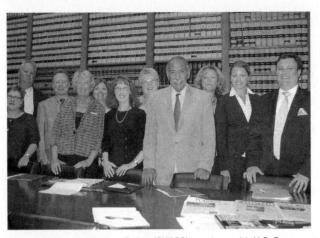

FIGURE 57-2 Coalition for Healthcare Worker and Patient Safety (CHAPS) members with U.S. Representative John Conyers, Jr. (D, MI) to support his sponsorship of H.R. 2381, the "Nurse and Health Care Worker Protection Act of 2009." *Photo left to right:* Sara Markle-Elder, UAN, AFL-CIO; Walter Frederickson, UAN, AFL-CIO; Bill Borwegen, SEIU; Susan Epstein, WING USA Connecticut State Leader; Donna Zankowski, AAOHN; Anne Hudson, founder, WING USA; Elizabeth Shogren, Minnesota Nurses Association; Congressman John Conyers; Marsha Medlin, founder, CHAPS; Erin Zrncic, senior nursing student, Indiana University of Pennsylvania; and Jay Witter, UAN, AFL-CIO.

At the time of this writing, no action has been taken on the bill.

THE FUTURE

I look forward to the day when (1) losing nurses to disabling injuries caused by the dangerous practice of manual patient lifting is recognized and addressed as a public health crisis; (2) legislation for safe patient handling protects all nurses and health care workers against life-altering injuries from lifting hazardous amounts of weight that are not permitted to be lifted by hand in other industries; (3) concern for the safety and well-being of nurses equals the concern for the patients in our care; and (4) nursing organizations assist back-injured nurses to remain employed so that nurses who have sacrificed their health and well-being in the care of others are no longer treated as disposable.

For a list of related websites, please refer to your Evolve Resources at http://evolve.elsevier.com/Mason/policypolitics/

REFERENCES

Bureau of Labor Statistics (BLS). (2008, December 1). *Jobs with most injuries and illnesses resulting in days away from work.* Retrieved from www.bls.gov/opub/ted/2008/dec/wk1/art01.htm.

Charney, W., & Hudson, A. (Eds.). (2004). *Back injury among healthcare workers: Causes, solutions, and impacts.* Boca Raton, FL: CRC Press.

Charney, W., Zimmerman, K., & Walara, E. (1991). The lifting team: A design method to reduce lost time back injury in nursing. *Journal of American Association of Occupational Health Nurses, 39*(5), 231-234.

Hudson, A. (2002). Oh! My aching back! *Revolution: The Journal for RNs and Patient Advocacy, 3*(5), 31. Retrieved from www.wingusa.org/aching.htm.

Owen, B. (1999). Decreasing the back injury problem in nursing personnel. *Surgical Services Management, 5*(7), 15-21.

Waters, T. (2007). When is it safe to manually lift a patient? *American Journal of Nursing, 107*(8), 53-58.

CHAPTER 58

TAKING ACTION
Influencing the Workplace by Serving on a Hospital's Board of Directors

Kristine M. Gebbie

"How wonderful it is that nobody need wait a single moment before starting to improve the world."

—Ann Frank

This discussion is focused on the governing body of the hospital: the board of trustees or board of directors. The reader should be able to identify key reasons for learning about the trustees of any place of employment and for considering seeking a seat on a board. The primary focus of this discussion is the board of a not-for-profit institution, whether established as a semi-public corporation to manage a public hospital or the board of a voluntary hospital, which includes those established by faith groups or concerned citizens. The basic structure is the same for advisory board of a public hospital or the board of a proprietary (for-profit) entity.

Trustees generally are individuals who are earning (or have earned) their livelihood elsewhere, who agree to serve for a number of hours per week or month participating in decision-making about a health care institution. The "pay" may be a chance to do good, to fulfill a sense of communitarian obligation, or, in a less positive perspective, to rub shoulders with people of social standing and money and gain public acclaim. The trustee as beneficent volunteer does not hold for all trustees, as those serving on the boards of proprietary hospitals or for-profit health institutions are compensated, often at a very generous level. The author's perspective is based on first-hand experience, having served for several years as director of a not-for profit, multistate social service agency, and currently serving as trustee of a not-for profit health care system with overlapping boards that includes a hospital, long-term care facility, community clinics, and a Medicaid insurance provider. In addition, during a period as state secretary of health, I served as one of the three voting members of a state authority providing funds for hospital construction.

WHY BE CONCERNED ABOUT TRUSTEES?

From the perspective of a busy nurse (or physical therapist, pharmacist, physician—any employee) rushing to complete what feels like a full day's work every hour of a hectic shift, nothing could be further from consciousness than questions such as "Who is the new trustee?" or "What did the board say about this month's quality dashboard?" or "How far down is our reserve fund depleted because of the market drop?" Yet the trustees establish policy, employ one critical staff member, and have final say on budget and staff appointments. A key question for anyone exploring a potential job should be, "What is my line of communication to and from the board of directors?" or "Who presents issues from this department to the trustees?" The response may well be, "No one ever asked that before!", but it never hurts to be first. The answer should include some reference to the organizational chart and the way in which senior staff bring reports up through the system, and it should convey decisions back out to all staff. For most nurses, the line is through the nursing hierarchy to the senior nursing executive, who reports to the Chief Executive Officer, who reports to the board.

In day-to-day matters, the trustees are invisible to almost everyone in a hospital. There may be a small office used by the Chair of the Board when in the building, with the secretary to the board in attendance. Or the board may simply be accommodated within the Chief Executive Officer's (CEO's) suite. Some members of the hospital leadership team (the CEO, the chief of the medical staff, perhaps one or two others such as the chief nursing officer) may sit with the board, either recognized in legal documents *ex officio* (with or without vote) or as a courtesy. The legal affairs office will be very aware of the board, given the number of official documents to be filed with state and federal agencies that require official board approval or signature. Professionals seeking privileges (e.g., physicians, nurse practitioners, nurse midwives, nurse anesthetists, physician assistants) may be aware of the delegated authority to grant privileges, as this approval is needed before any practice can begin.

The route to selection of a trustee or director is transparent in some institutions, but more often is an obscure process with at least as much "Who do you know?" as "What do you know?" In some places, the key question is "How much can you give?" Thirty years ago, I was present at a discussion of the failure of a particular health care organization to have a single nurse in a governing position, at which the debate-ending answer from the Chair of the Board was "We don't need nurses because the doctors on the board are all married to nurses." While this particular argument might well be hooted down in today's more sensitive age, it is certainly true that there are far more physicians than nurses serving on institutional boards. The reasons are multiple, and while partly sexist, they are definitely related to money. Physicians are more likely to have the income to purchase tables for 12 at annual fund-raisers, to be seen as critical to the bottom line if they admit many patients, and to move in social sets with the business executives and owners seen as essential to a successful board. It is the rare nurse that fits that description. Nurses are more likely to serve on a board when the charter or establishing document spells out some criteria such as neighborhood residence, or other category into which the nurse fits. While I might pride myself on bringing incredible expertise to the hospital board on which I sit, I must quickly acknowledge that I got onto the list of potential trustees because of a religious affiliation that must be held by a certain proportion of the board.

WHAT DO TRUSTEES DO?

A quick answer to the question of what trustees do is "They eat dinner and talk a lot," but this answer does not do justice to the critical role of trustees in shaping the mission of the hospital, assuring its finances, and achieving quality standards. The most visible activities of the Trustees are their routine and special meetings, whether of the full body or its committees. Staff members may also become aware of annual or more frequent fund-raising events such as gala dinners or auctions sponsored by the board. It is the content of the meetings, and the purposes to which the funds raised are directed that are the critical activities.

The mission and goals of the hospital may be stated in a general way in the articles of incorporation, as "for the purpose of providing hospital services to the people of the Northside," but it is the subsequent elaboration of the legal documents into a statement of mission and goals that should receive close attention. Whatever the stated mission, it should be visible or it is only rhetoric. Measures of successful match of action to mission include buildings (are they accessible to the population that is the target of services?), staffing (are the specialties matched to the goal?), and annual budgets (are funds going to areas designed to fix identified quality problems?). Mission statements in this context serve the same purpose they do in the general corporate world: broad statements of aspiration that may include references to the driving philanthropic or religious motivation for service. The mission is translated into goals and then into annual plans of operation and annual budgets not by the trustees in isolation, but by the executive staff of the organization, for subsequent approval by the board. Depending upon the operating style, one or more board committees may be consulted extensively before an annual budget is presented to the full board for action. The key individual in this process is the CEO, generally the only hiring decision made by the board. If the board has not selected a CEO who understands the mission of the institution and is capable of managing an organization toward achievement of the mission, the board has not been successful. And if the board does not allow the CEO the freedom to manage day-to-day operations without excessive second-guessing and interference, the board either does not understand its role, or has no confidence in the hiring decision it made.

Financial issues are central to the discussions of every board, whether it is the annual acceptance of an operating budget, a decision to incur debt to achieve a goal, or the understood obligation to contribute to capital projects through donations and fund-raising. Any stated objective that is not backed by resources is a hollow promise. A press release announcing "Northside Hospital, the place to come for cutting-edge cardiac care" will be meaningless if there is no cardiac catheterization laboratory, no capacity for angioplasty, and no cardiac surgery or rehabilitation. Each of these requires both equipment and a well-prepared staff. The capital investment in equipment or space may be the focus of an annual gala fund-raiser to which each trustee contributes. The ongoing service requires attention to the nursing and other professional staff, medical staff appointments, and such mundane matters as housekeeping and maintenance. Even a single week of "Sorry, we can't admit you today" caused by a shortage of staff and supplies can echo through the community and undo any good from the advertising campaign. Meeting this ongoing fiscal obligation usually begins with a finance committee of the board, meeting regularly with the CEO and chief financial officer, and reporting to the executive committee and eventually the full board.

The third major area of trustee responsibility and activity is in quality and regulatory compliance. No matter how secure the fiscal situation or how confident the board is in the CEO, no health care institution can function long without meeting at least minimal regulatory requirements, including such things as state laws requiring reports of unexpected patient deaths, federal payment requirements regarding accurate billing based on documented diagnosis, or The Joint Commission emergency preparedness standards. "Quality" has been a most elusive item to specify, quantify, and require. Media exposé of a hospital's failure to identify an incompetent physician, a fake nurse, or routinely unsterilized equipment happens all too often. It is the trustees who are ultimately responsible for any failure to assure both quality and compliance with regulations. This requires more than placidly accepting a quarterly report from the CEO and chief compliance officer that all reports are ready to be filed and all is well, followed by a unanimous voice vote of approval. A trustee committee that is treated as the equal of the finance committee should be charged with reviewing in depth both

routine practices and any major incidents that reflect a potential breach in quality and with proposing to the full board changes needed to maintain or improve quality. A member of the board who is a health professional may bring value added to this committee, through an ability to interpret terminology and issues to fellow trustees. The health professional on the quality committee is, however, in danger of becoming an apologist or defender of staff or procedures, failing to probe deeply enough or question history and habit.

NOTES ON BOARD SERVICE

This has been written as if all boards are actively engaged in their duties, asking critical questions at every meeting, reading all documents in advance, and keeping the leadership team on its toes. There are undoubtedly boards that do not meet this description: the board that is a rubber stamp on whatever is placed on the agenda by the CEO or the board chair. There are sufficient reports of institutions making egregious errors in staff appointments, in management of funds, or in serving patients in which it becomes clear that most members of the board, if not all, were paying no attention to their duties. And there are a few exemplary boards that are always on top of every issue, providing support to the CEO and leadership team while guiding them toward every more successful achievement of targets and goals. Most boards are in between, with directors or trustees taking time from earning their own living and caring for their families to serve their communities in multiple ways and to do their best to master the language of hospital governance, to follow the "dashboard" report each month, and to listen to presentations loaded with untranslated medical jargon.

Key to effective service on any board is allocation of sufficient time to do one's homework prior to any committee or board meeting. Failure to do so leads to the likelihood of accepting at face value every document presented in a crowded agenda, or failure to catch a quick slide over a potentially critical incident report. With reports read in advance, a board member comes into each meeting aware of the agenda, having routine matters separated from those critical items requiring attention, and ready to listen actively and interact strategically. This does not mean showing off an ability to identify every misplaced comma or spelling error; if those are found, handing a corrected copy to the secretary should suffice. Homework should lead to consistent priority setting, in which the attention of the board members is on those policy issues critical to achieving the mission of the institution, and not on day-to-day operations rightly delegated to the CEO and staff. For example, a report of a rising vacancy rate in nursing staff should not lead to questions about an individual resignation or hiring, but should stimulate questions about the work environment, actions to reduce turnover, relationship of active hiring to occupancy rate, and the experiences of comparable institutions in the area. A report on an untoward, unexpected event leading to a patient death (reportable to the board under some state laws) should not lead to extensive second-guessing of the specific care decisions, but an exploration of the quality control systems that were or were not in place, and action plans to avoid similar events in the future.

One of the dangers in any group that works together over time is the stereotyping of individual members or the assigning of standing roles, such as the "wet blanket," "CEO's cheerleader," or "technology-basher." Any one of these (or the many others) becomes a rut that can lead to the individual being ignored or even avoided by others. While the assignment to a specific committee and one's individual interests and skills will lead each board member to pay more or less attention to various items on the agenda or various aspects of the mission, no board member should become so categorized that the others have no need to attend to questions asked or comments entered into discussion. It is unfortunate that far too many nurses become stereotyped because they exclusively focus on issues of nursing contributions, the omission of nursing insights in reports, or the lack of nurses engaged in any particular aspect of hospital life. Nurses, whether they mean to be or not, are often identified as physician-bashers who are unable to acknowledge the essential partnership of these two key professions in the successful delivery of care. Even if (or especially if) the agenda seems far too concentrated on the fiscal at the expense of quality, or on immediate crises at the expense of long-term mission, it is essential to pay attention to all issues coming before the board. Members of other committees are going to take an issue far more seriously from a colleague who has exhibited wide-ranging attention to items on the agenda than to someone who only speaks up on a pet problem.

Finally, an institutional trustee from a health profession such as nursing can use his or her professional skills to advance the work of the board and model the positive impact of including the voice of nursing (or social work, pharmacy, dietetics) at all levels of decision-making. Assessing strengths and weaknesses, identifying potential supports, selecting goals that are achievable and remaining attentive to signs of new problems are all skills used in professional practice that can be transferred to the board room. A health professional can set an expectation that cultural competence and respect will permeate all activities of the institution. Questions about the evidence base for changing policy or adding a new therapeutic system should be second nature. Shaping questions or comments so that they are clear to listeners from differing backgrounds is essential. There may be other trustees who are considered key decision-makers because of their economic, social, or political standing in the community. There may be others who have years of philanthropic contributions to recommend them. Each trustee is chosen to fill a particular purpose, and has the power of having arrived at the table. Careful attention to each other trustee, and to each critical mission, fiscal, and quality decision can make the voice of any member important to the rest.

GETTING ON A BOARD

If you've never served on the board of trustees of a corporate entity or service organization, it is unlikely that you will be named to serve as a trustee of the largest health care system in your community. Start small, and start where you live. It is more likely that your first board appointment will be as an interested member of the service or catchment area of a community health center or ambulatory care network. Volunteer some time; help out at the fund-raiser if you can't afford to write a big check, let your interest in the overall success of the organization become known to neighbors and to the organization's leaders. Learn who the current directors are, and when you cross paths with one, let your interest in the organization be known by asking intelligent questions about current and future plans, with a positive tone. While whistle-blowers and loud complainers are sometimes brought onto a board as a co-opting move, it's not the best beginning. Each board membership opens the door to potential selection to the board of larger, more complex institutions. The same process applies: the nominating committee of the board is looking to select members who have a range of skills, work well with others, and are known to care about the community. The nurse who is known to be well-versed in current policy issues, able to communicate well with others, an enthusiastic supporter of institutions in the community, and known to local decision-makers would be a good candidate.

For a list of related websites, please refer to your Evolve Resources at http://evolve.elsevier.com/Mason/policypolitics/

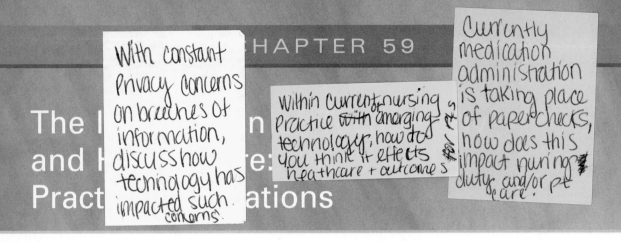

CHAPTER 59

The Impact of Technology and Health Reform: Practice Implications

Linda Burnes Bolton, Pamela F. Cipriano, and Carole Gassert

"Technology…is a queer thing. It brings you great gifts with one hand, and it stabs you in the back with the other."

—C.P. Snow

The dissemination and utilization of health information has been lauded as a key strategy in achieving the health reform goals of improved access to safe, reliable, efficient, and effective care for all and the elimination of waste, including unnecessary costs and overuse of services. In this chapter, we provide commentary on the demand for value-based health care,[1] the potential for technology to enhance nursing practice, and the role of nursing and its senior leaders in the acquisition and deployment of technology, including the opportunities to work with other clinicians to advocate for appropriate use of technology.

THE DEMAND FOR VALUE-BASED HEALTH CARE

One of the hallmarks of the twenty-first century is the explosion of technological devices and systems that touch every part of our lives. Nowhere is this more apparent than in health care. As a result, an enormous strain has been placed on the shoulders of those who make business decisions for health care organizations. Capital budgets are already at the breaking point, even though there is an amazing number of emerging technologies to consider purchasing (e.g., imaging, monitoring, communication devices, information management systems, pharmacological products, and implants)—all of which promise improved therapies, care delivery processes, and patient safety. Sorting these out can be quite time-consuming and often requires a level of knowledge that many executives simply do not possess. Moreover, consideration of this vast array is frequently complicated by the many disappointments that have accompanied the introduction of earlier versions of the technologies under consideration.

As a result, it has become increasingly important that each institution have its own means of confronting decisions related to technology, and that these questions always be addressed within a clear framework of policies and procedures. In fact, a helpful approach is one that represents a combination of evidence-based practice (something demanded of all clinicians but seldom expected of administrators) and informed consumer behavior. Value analysis and technology assessment are parts of the process, but the techniques to do this can be imprecise, and other business imperatives (e.g., maintaining a competitive edge and retaining physicians) may take precedence. Nonetheless, careful and deliberate consideration of technology purchases has become essential because of the magnitude of both the cost and potential impact, whether good or bad. In the future, robust comparative effectiveness research may shed more light on the effectiveness and efficiency of the most expensive technologies.

---

[1]Value-based health care entails attaining the greatest benefit for dollars spent, or improving outcomes for the same or reduced spending.

There is an urgency to understand the benefits of health care investments. In a 2009 Institute of Medicine report, "Value in Health Care: Accounting for Cost, Quality, Safety, Outcomes, and Innovation," health information technology was noted to be a prerequisite for attaining greater value in health care. The benefits were improved quality, ability to monitor outcomes, clinical decision support, collecting and developing evidence, tracking costs, streamlining paperwork, improving care coordination, and facilitating patient engagement. Although perspectives on the value of care differ for each stakeholder (i.e., the consumer, provider, and payer), the lack of uniform definition of value does not diminish the belief that outcomes can improve while reducing costs. Value-based payment approaches by payers such as Medicare link payment to performance in order to stimulate improvements in systems of care and, thus, better care coordination and reduction of unnecessary costs.

Use of technology is a key strategy for harnessing the power of data at the point of care and using these data for managing disease, identifying patient trends, and intervening on health problems earlier. Transforming technologies such as telehome care and telemonitoring are already showing reduced hospital admissions and lengths of stay, as well as decreased unplanned visits to health care providers. Devices that eliminate redundant nursing tasks can increase the nurse's time spent in direct care of patients, improving safety through direct observation and early interventions.

TECHNOLOGY ENHANCED NURSING PRACTICE

Health care organizations are making significant investments in technology to improve clinical care and slash error rates. Technology has been used extensively in the hospital for decades, but now it provides new capabilities for remote monitoring in homes, offering connectivity to portable devices such as cell phones and personal digital assistive devices. In this way, technology is becoming an effective tool for chronic disease management, prevention of hospitalization, and keeping people in their homes.

Nurses have begun to embrace the use of technology in all aspects of their practice. They perceive it as a means to improve the accuracy of care delivery,

reduce redundancy of activities such as data collection and documentation, reduce physical strain from moving patients, and improve workflow efficiencies. Nurses may also find that some technologies present barriers to efficient care if not developed to complement the nurse's workflow and human behavior. As a result, nurses may develop "workarounds" that circumvent the correct use of devices. Early bedside barcode medication administration scanners and complicated intravenous pumps with safety software required redesign and testing to ensure that nurses could use the technologies easily and efficiently.

THE EFFECT OF TECHNOLOGY ON NURSING PRACTICE: THE TD2 STUDY

In 2000, the Workforce Commission of the American Academy of Nursing (AAN) focused on ways to decrease the demand on registered nurses' time as a solution to the impending workforce shortage. Facing a different kind of shortage characterized by the aging population of nurses, a dwindling supply pipeline, an increase in demand for nurses, and a paucity of individuals prepared to fill the ranks of nursing faculty jobs, the Commission focused its attention on how the demands of patient care could be met in part by technology. It was thought that the growing availability of technology—devices, instruments, appliances, and information systems—offered important opportunities for reducing the demand on nurses' direct and non-direct care time. Likewise, technology was thought to have the potential for easing the physical burden of nurses' work through a variety of devices such as those used for moving patients. In short, the AAN Workforce Commission believed that innovative technology could be used to enhance patient care, improve efficiency, and make care safer for patient and provider.

To that end, the Commission convened an invitational conference in 2002 that was attended by nurses, physicians, pharmacists, health care provider organizations, government agencies, equipment suppliers, engineers, architects, futurists, and medical record system vendors to consider how technology might be deployed in an ideal care delivery system within the next decade. They proposed a redesigned future nursing work environment that effectively used technology to improve practice and patient care outcomes.

THE "TECHNOLOGY DRILL DOWN"

As a result of this invitational conference, the Workforce Commission, with funding from the Robert Wood Johnson Foundation, embarked on a project to develop a process for identifying potential technology solutions needed to support the redesign of practice environments in medical-surgical units of hospitals. A pilot study at three hospitals led to the design of the "Technology Drill Down" or "TD2" process whereby multidisciplinary participants described the current workflow for patient care activities, envisioned the ideal future state, identified gaps between the current and the ideal state, and proposed potential (real or imagined) technology solutions to close the gaps (American Academy of Nursing Drill Down, n.d.; Burnes Bolton, Gassert, & Cipriano, 2008) (Box 59-1).

With continued funding, the Workforce Commission conducted TD2s at 25 sites across the United States. More than 300 statements from the TD2 participants revealed 8 common workflow categories for which technology could provide improvements: admission, discharge, and transfer; care coordination; care delivery; communication; documentation, management of equipment and supplies, management of medication, and management of patient movement. The nurses and their colleagues also described process issues within these workflows with emphasis on concern for safety, including challenges related to documentation, access to information, inconsistency in process, workload, intrateam communication, clinical orders, systems integration, and data entry. The most creative work came from descriptions of almost 600 technology solutions that included information systems and a plethora of devices, hardware, and telecommunications tools, such as the following:

- Bedside computer system (hardware at point of care)
- Electronic medical record (clinical information system)
- CPOE (computerized provider order entry system)
- Tracking systems (supplies, equipment, patients, providers, staff)
- Robots
- RFID (radio frequency identification)
- PDA (personal digital assistant)
- MAR (medication administration record)
- Smart bed

BOX 59-1 The TD2 Process

The Technology Drill Down (TD2) process is a critical strategy to achieving the following goals:

- Identifying workflow processes that impede the delivery of safe, timely, and effective patient care
- Developing ideal workflows to improve care delivery quality
- Identifying the need for technology to address the gaps between current and ideal workflow processes
- Prioritizing the technology solutions for review and purchase

The TD2 process applies the following steps:

Step 1: Hospital system executives identify a medical/surgical unit that could benefit from a TD2.

Step 2: An internal TD2 facilitator is identified who uses the training materials from the American Academy of Nursing.

Step 3: Approximately 20 to 30 unit and interdepartmental representatives come together for 1½ days to map the gaps between current workflow and an idealized workflow and, most importantly, to identify potential technological applications that could close the gaps. (The TD2s engage not only RNs, assistive personnel, and unit clerks but also members of other departments whose work processes interface and are interrelated.)

Step 4: Group participants envision how the work would flow under ideal circumstances. As they talk, the facilitator uses a laptop computer to diagram the discussion, and the diagram appears on a screen for all participants to see. Participants then analyze and discuss their current environment, identifying how to bridge gaps between current state and ideal environment. Technologies to bridge gaps in processes are identified; participants identify specific requirements for new technologies and discuss how these technologies could reduce waste, add value to nurses' time, and create efficiencies in overall workflow and work processes.

Step 5: Hospital administrators, unit managers, and nursing staff use the information gathered to assist with making technology decisions.

The American Academy of Nursing website contains a detailed facilitator's guide to conducting a TD2, which is available at *www.aannet.org/i4a/pages/index.cfm?pageid=3318.*

- Smart pump
- WOW (wireless on wheels for mobile computing)

Above all, nurses expressed the need for a comprehensive electronic medical record coupled with order entry and point-of-care or bedside functionality that was handheld and voice-activated whenever possible. Four projected outcomes of the use of the suggested technology included eliminating non-valued work (e.g., redundant documentation), providing access to resources, accomplishing regulatory work, and creating an efficient use of space.

By far, the greatest redundancy was in documentation. Systems that reduce the demand for documentation of care, eliminate duplicate charting in multiple systems, and allow for auto-population of data through wireless transmission of data already entered, would provide the greatest relief. Similarly, using data in the system to accomplish charting, inventory control, and documentation for quality reporting was a plus. Access to resources is accomplished through tagging systems that reveal proximate locations of caregivers and supplies, two-way communication systems for immediate consultation with pharmacists, and systems with smart technology that provide decision support with real-time information. Capturing data in documentation that flows into needed regulatory reports relieves a burden of duplicate manual record keeping.

The TD2 results clearly demonstrated the complex environment and workflows of nursing care. The participants identified technology solutions and functional requirements for new or revised products that will improve workflow, effectiveness, and efficiency of nursing care. The benefits of implementing the results of a TD2 include improving the practice environment, retaining nurses, providing safer care, and increasing the time nurses spend in direct care of patients. An important insight from this work is the need to ensure that the perspectives of nurses and other front-line caregivers are incorporated into the design and implementation of systems and services in the patient care environment. Without this input, technology may be underutilized or misused, thereby reducing the inherent improvements in safety, quality, and efficiency that can be brought to bear by technology.

CONCLUSIONS FROM THE TD2 STUDY

The data from the TD2 study clearly indicated that nurses do not want to be passive consumers of technology. They want to be partners with the designers and producers of devices and systems in order to develop improved functionality and utility in care delivery. Nurses are disappointed with current technology and the all-too-frequent "workarounds" that

detract from their time with patients. TD2 participants expressed the importance of the need for vendors to "listen to the voice of the staff." Nurses know what technology works for them, what increases their workload, and what features will enhance safety and efficiency. They also voiced concern about non-compatible technologies and their potential to compromise safety. They asked that systems and devices be user-friendly, allow for rapid retrieval of data, and create efficiency at the point of care.

RECOMMENDATIONS FROM THE RESEARCH

Using the results of the TD2 study, nurses can make a strong business case that technology helps make care safer and more efficient. However, technology alone does not make care safe. Rather, it can optimize workflow and allow those delivering care to drive quality improvement (Murphy, 2009). Having a drug interaction alert appear at the point of care or being able to access another provider without experiencing a delay from an antiquated communication system drives better decision making, efficiency, and confidence on the part of the nurse.

The findings also support the use of technology to enhance the retention of nurses; this is directly related to the implementation of time-saving and step-saving devices, as well as systems that reduce the physical burden of work, while improving the safety and comfort of the work environment. The use of automated medication administration systems, mobile communication devices, moving and lifting equipment, automated tracking systems for timely delivery of supplies and equipment, and accurate automated patient identification systems enhance the nurse's use of time and energy. The voice of the nurse heard in the TD2 process supports current health policy proposals for health information systems standards for interoperability and data exchange, industry standards for communication, and safeguards for privacy and portability of health information.

PRIORITY SETTING FOR TECHNOLOGY ACQUISITION

There are always more requests for new technology purchases than can ever be accommodated. The recent recession has undoubtedly created a new view of priority setting/spending within all health care institutions in the U.S. Every proposal for acquiring new technology should be required to meet at least one of the following conditions:

- Solves an important institutional problem
- Increases patient safety
- Increases efficiency/cost savings
- Improves the patient experience/market share

Clearly these conditions are not mutually exclusive, and, in fact, it should be expected that most technological investments would have an impact on several, if not all, of the above. In addition, each should undergo rigorous cost/benefit analysis as a major component of the priority setting process.

It is important to mention that this vital work must involve the nurse executive as a key member of the team. Nursing is the core business of most health care delivery organizations; certainly this is true of inpatient facilities. Patients are admitted to hospitals because they are in need of *nursing* care, and they are discharged when the level of nursing care they require can be accommodated in other settings. It would seem peculiar, then, that there are instances in which the voice of nursing is not present in every step of the technology priority-setting process, a situation that can lead to disastrous results—for the institution, the staff, and the patients. Nurse leaders must help establish the value proposition for the acquisition of technology that enables the delivery of safe, efficient, and effective care (American Organization of Nurse Executives, 2007).

CHOOSING THE PRODUCTS

Once prioritized, the work of choosing the specific products must be undertaken in a rigorous, systematic manner. Unfortunately, there have been many instances in which the selection process is more often driven by the skill of the vendor's sales force than by the pursuit of evidence to support one decision over another. The latter should obviously become a formalized part of the organization's policy and procedures and should include *evidence* of the following:

- The involvement of knowledgeable end users in the design of the technology
- Adequate and thorough field trials
- High-level customer satisfaction at peer institutions

In instances in which major purchases are concerned, the above criteria should be supplemented with site visits to comparable facilities where the products are in use. Such visits should be made principally by the end-users who are expected to install and use the equipment or systems. In this way, the staff, along with the executives, will gain as thorough an understanding as possible of the advantages and the problems they may experience in adopting the particular technology under consideration.

Once purchased, the senior executives and the end-user staff need to adopt a very businesslike approach to the vendor or supplier. In other words, they need to demand that the product meets the institution's needs and performs in the manner promised. Too often, the staff find themselves trying to adapt to products that are not useful enough to them or, worse, that actually cause them additional work. This is where true executive leadership is most needed and where the pain of introducing new technology can be greatly reduced or eliminated altogether.

Much of this discussion has been aimed at the organizational level and the policies and procedures that should be in place inside each institution. At the larger policy level, however, there are improvements that are essential for health care executives to make through collective action with their colleagues and peers. Some efforts to achieve value-based care as it relates to technology can only be accomplished through collaboration with professional organizations (Department of Health and Human Services, n.d.).

SYNERGY WITH EMERGING HEALTH INFORMATION POLICY

Besides developing institutional policies for purchasing, deploying, and evaluating new technology, nurses need to be attentive to public policies around health information technology (HIT). This includes the electronic health record.

The American Recovery and Reinvestment Act of 2009 (ARRA) authorized the Centers for Medicare and Medicaid Services (CMS) to provide incentive reimbursement to eligible professionals and hospitals who demonstrate they are "meaningful users" of electronic health record technology

In December 2009, CMS and the Office of the National Coordinator (ONC) for Health Information Technology announced proposed regulations to define "meaningful use," as well as a set of standards, implementation specifications, and certification criteria for electronic health record technology. The HITECH Act set forth the expectation that adoption of an electronic health record was not an end goal, but rather, appropriate use of EHRs will improve health, enable better performance of our health care system, and achieve greater efficiency. The meaningful use of EHRs should achieve the following five goals recommended by the Health Information Technology Policy Committee, a federal advisory committee to the National Coordinator for HIT:

1. Improve quality, safety, and efficiency, and reduce health disparities.
2. Improve care coordination.
3. Engage patients and families.
4. Improve population and public health.
5. Ensure adequate privacy and security protections for personal health information.

The first two goals address the need for the health care team to be able to access and exchange comprehensive patient health data from all available sources. Nurses provided input into the rules to ensure inclusion of nurses as eligible providers, as well as identification of patient-centered documentation elements and critical data linked to improved decision-making and outcomes of care.

Following review of over 2000 comments, Health and Human Services Secretary Kathleen Sebelius issued final regulations in July 2010 addressing both meaningful use and certification standards. The regulations include incentives to be paid through the Medicare and Medicaid programs over 5 years, beginning in 2011, for the integration of HIT into clinical practices and health care organizations to enable them to move from measurement to constant improvement of health outcomes. If this expectation is not met, providers and hospitals will be subject to penalties or reductions in payments beginning in fiscal year 2015.

The regulations create a road map with two sets of requirements for hospitals and clinicians for Phase 1, covering 2011 and 2012. Using a certified EHR, eligible hospitals, including critical access hospitals, and providers, must meet a core set of measures (14 for hospitals and 15 for eligible providers) plus 5 selected from a menu of 10 additional measures for implementation over 2 years. Core elements include basic essential components of an EHR such as vital signs, demographics, active medications, allergies, problem lists, and clinical summaries. Each group will also report quality data, assure privacy and security of data, and achieve electronic prescribing for a portion of orders. The extent of implementation for each measure varies, such as percent of orders or transactions to show how one uses the EHR. Menu options range from drug-formulary checks to recording of advanced directives to sending preventive care reminders to patients.

Future rule making will address Stages 2 and 3, which are focused on capture and exchange of data related to coordination of care across transitions, greater access by patients to their health information, quality measurement, and research. Additionally, utilizing clinical decision support with improved access to comprehensive patient data is expected to demonstrate improvements in quality safety, efficiency, and population health outcomes.

These rules implementing provisions of the ARRA have broad effects on health care providers that will extend far into the future as EHR technology becomes the primary vehicle for measuring and evaluating quality outcomes. Nurses have participated in the debates about what constitutes "meaningful use" of technology and need to continue to do so. The American Academy of Nursing Workforce Commission recommendations from the TD2 study have been brought forward to the Office of the National Coordinator of HIT to inform discussions on developing policy and standards for information technology.

Nursing must seize the opportunity to be an influential participant so that it would not be uncommon to read headlines such as "National Nursing Leaders Join with Consumers and Physicians to Support New National Policy on (major health care issue)" or "Nursing Leads the Way in Controlling Costs While Improving the Coordination of Care" or "Nursing Leaders Asked to Help Craft New Healthcare Policy Initiative." We can do this. We have the knowledge and skills. We must mobilize our collective will to move forward our vision for a reformed health care delivery system that is enabled by the right technology and is co-designed by clinicians and those who would benefit from a technology-enhanced care delivery system.

For a list of related websites, please refer to your Evolve Resources at http://evolve.elsevier.com/Mason/policypolitics/

REFERENCES

American Academy of Nursing Technology Drill Down, 2004-2008. (n.d.). Retrieved from www.aannet.org/i4a/pages/index.cfm?pageid=3318.

American Organization of Nurse Executives. (2007). *Guiding principles for defining the role of the chief nurse executive in technology acquisition and implementation.* Retrieved from www.aone.org/aone/resource/PDF/AONE_GP_Technology_and_Acquisition_and_Implementation.pdf.

Burnes Bolton, L., Gassert, C. A., & Cipriano, P. (2008). Smart technology, enduring solutions, *Journal of Healthcare Information Management, 22*(4), 24-26.

Department of Health and Human Services, Centers for Medicare & Medicaid Services. (n.d.). CMS finalizes definition of meaningful use of certified electronic health records (EHR) technology. Retrieved from www.cms.gov/apps/media/press/factsheet.asp?Counter=3794&intNumPerPage=10&checkDate=&checkKey=&srchType=1&numDays=3500&srchOpt=0&srchData=&keywordType=All&chkNewsType=6&intPage=&showAll=&pYear=&year=&desc=&cboOrder=date.

Health Information Technology Policy Committee. (2009). Meaningful use objectives and measures: 2011-2013. Retrieved from http://healthit.hhs.gov/portal/server.pt/gateway/PTARGS_0_10741_888532_0_0_18/FINAL%20MU%20RECOMMENDATIONS%20TABLE.pdf.

Institute of Medicine. (2009). *Value in health care: Accounting for cost, quality, safety, outcomes, and innovation: Workshop summary.* Washington, D.C.: National Academies Press.

Murphy, J. (2009). Technology and nursing, a love/hate relationship. *Journal of Health Information Management, 23*(2), 9-11.

CHAPTER 60

The Influence of Magnet Recognition® on Organization and Workplace Policy

Karen Drenkard

"Excellent things are rare."

—Plato

UNCOVERING THE "FORCES OF MAGNETISM"

In the 1980s, a group of insightful nurse researchers used a unique approach to explore a nursing shortage phenomenon in United States hospitals. High RN turnover and vacancy rates were plaguing hospitals and health care organizations. Rather than study what was wrong with these organizations, the researchers chose to identify organizations in which things were going well and learn what was *right* with them. The American Academy of Nursing's (AAN) Task Force on Nursing Practice in Hospitals conducted a study of 163 hospitals to identify and describe variables that created environments that attracted and retained well-qualified nurses and promoted quality patient care. Forty-one of the 163 institutions were described as "magnet" hospitals because of their ability to attract and retain professional nurses. The characteristics that seemed to distinguish these "magnet" organizations from others became known as the "forces of magnetism."

ESTABLISHMENT OF THE MAGNET PROGRAM

In 1990, based on a recommendation of the American Nurses Association (ANA), the American Nurses Credentialing Center (ANCC) was established as a separately incorporated nonprofit organization through which the ANA offers credentialing programs and services. The initial proposal for the Magnet Hospital Recognition Program for Excellence in Nursing

Services was approved by the ANA Board of Directors in December 1990. The proposal indicated that the program would build upon the 1983 magnet hospital study conducted by the AAN. In 2002, the program name changed to the Magnet Recognition Program®. The program was based on the identified areas of research that were identified as the "forces of magnetism" that led to improved RN and patient outcomes in health care organizations. In 2008, the Commission on Magnet introduced a new vision and a new conceptual model that grouped the 14 forces of magnetism into 5 key components: (1) Transformational Leadership; (2) Structural Empowerment; (3) Exemplary Professional Practice; (4) New Knowledge, Innovations, and Improvements; and (5) Empirical Outcomes. These components are illustrated in Figure 60-1.

In 2010, there were over 370 U.S. hospitals and health care organizations that had achieved Magnet recognition, and 5 international organizations (in Australia, New Zealand, Lebanon, and Singapore). The Magnet Recognition® Program for hospitals influences workplace policy and the work environment for nurses—especially in acute care environments. This is reflected in the low RN turnover of 11.5% and vacancy rate of 3.6% at Magnet hospitals in the U.S. (ANCC, 2010).

This improvement in work environments is evidence-based. Research outcomes are correlating the impact of Magnet status on improved nurse outcomes and patient outcomes as well. Magnet hospitals have a history of positive nurse and work satisfaction linked to increased autonomy in practice, structural empowerment, participation in decision-making opportunities, and a positive work environment (Laschinger, Fingan, Shamian, & Wilk, 2004;

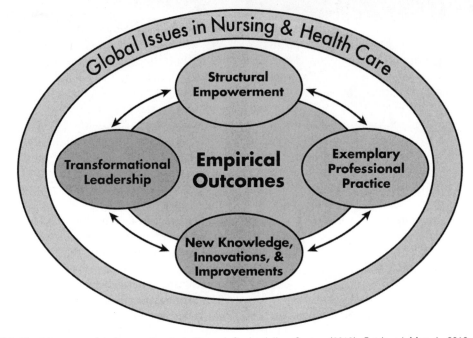

FIGURE 60-1 The Magnet model. Source: American Nurses' Credentialing Center. (2010). Retrieved May 4, 2010, from *www. nursecredentialing.com/Documents/Magnet/NewModelBrochure.aspx.*

Laschinger, Shamian, & Thomson, 2001; Rondeau & Wagar, 2006; Schmalenberg & Kramer, 2008; Smith, Tallman, & Kelley, 2006; Ulrich, Buerhaus, Donelan, Norman, & Dittus, 2007). A positive practice environment is increasingly linked to high quality care (Brooks, Titler, Ardery, & Herr, 2009; Titler et al., 2009; Vaughn et al., 2004). With the release of the 2008 Magnet model (see Figure 60-1) and corresponding manual, there is a requirement for Magnet organizations to have clinical, nurse satisfaction and patient satisfaction scores above the midpoint of the benchmark of the data set provided for review.

THE MAGNET APPLICATION PROCESS

Organizations pursuing Magnet designation work through a multistep process. Magnet designation is conferred for 4 years, and re-designation can be attained. The four phases of the Magnet application process include the following:

- Submitting an application, and conducting a self-assessment and gap analysis

- Submitting written documentation to demonstrate excellence in the nursing standards. This document is reviewed by knowledgeable and experienced appraisers, and if the standards of excellence are met, then the organization moves to the next phase.
- Participating in a site visit where the documents are verified, amplified, and clarified by interaction with direct patient care nurses.
- Final review and decision on the final credential by the Commission on Magnet.

The Magnet process is a rigorous one that often takes several years. Most health care organizations begin with an assessment of their current state based on the standards, called "sources of evidence" that are required to obtain Magnet recognition. Next, the organization applies and submits documentation. The documents must provide evidence to meet 88 standards across the five Magnet model components (leadership, structure, professional practice, new knowledge and innovation, and empirical outcomes). If a threshold of excellence is met through review of the documentation, a site visit is scheduled by appraisers to verify, amplify, and clarify the contents of the written documentation. The Magnet site visit is the organization's opportunity to demonstrate that the model components are fully developed, disseminated, and embedded in the culture of the organization (ANCC, 2008).

To achieve the Magnet credential, hospitals change processes and create policies to meet the required standards. The Magnet standards become a roadmap for nursing administrators to use to design structure and processes that support excellence in nursing care. The outcome requirements, added to the 2008 Magnet model, are incorporated into the expected Magnet documentation. Based on statistical analysis and scholarly review of the original Magnet requirements, the 2008 model was created to reflect the research and evidence that leads to positive nurse and patient outcomes.

ELIGIBILITY REQUIREMENTS

Eligibility requirements for Magnet recognition have driven change in hospitals. To apply for Magnet status, a hospital must have a chief nurse officer (CNO) who has a graduate degree and either a bachelor's or master's degree in the core science of nursing. As a result of this requirement, 100% of Magnet CNOs have graduate degrees. When turnover in chief nurses occurs, consideration of the education level of the CNO is a key concern in Magnet hospitals. As a result of the leadership requirements in the Magnet model, organizations develop programs and processes to develop leaders, as well as provide mechanisms for clinicians to be involved in decision-making. Shared governance structures are common in Magnet hospitals.

In another example of the influence of Magnet standards, Magnet organizations are required to describe and demonstrate the commitment of the health care organization to nurses' professional development, teaching and role development, community involvement, and recognition of nursing in the broader community. As a result of these requirements, programs and resources are allocated to improvement in the rates of RN to BSN graduates, certification rates, and new graduate orientation programs. All of these programs improve the workplace for nurses and, ultimately, patient care.

The Magnet model requires that organizations demonstrate outcomes. The outcome measures that are required include an evaluation of data that demonstrate top performance in nurse satisfaction, patient satisfaction, and clinical outcome measures of nursing-sensitive indicators. The standards also include requirements for workplace advocacy and addressing health disparities.

The requirements for demonstrating new knowledge, innovations, and improvements have encouraged research and evidence-based practice in hospitals. This is mostly due to the requirements that nurses at all levels evaluate and use published research findings in their practice. Examples of meeting these requirements include greater partnerships with universities and colleges to encourage faculty research in clinical areas, a focus on literature and evidence-based practice, and the completion of nursing research studies in clinical sites.

The Commission on Magnet is committed to continually raising standards as new research findings are generated. Similar to the policy process, the Magnet program is constantly being modified and improved based on evidence and research findings (Longest, 2006). In this way, the bar continues to be raised by the Commission on Magnet, and the emphasis on patient outcomes assures the relevance of the credential in the future.

For a list of related websites, please refer to your Evolve Resources at http://evolve.elsevier.com/Mason/policypolitics/

REFERENCES

American Nurses Credentialing Center. (ANCC). (2008). *Application manual, Magnet Recognition Program*. Silver Spring, MD: American Nurses Credentialing Center. Retrieved from nursecredentialing.org/Magnet/ProgramOverview/Magnet-Characteristics.aspx.

American Nurses Credentialing Center (ANCC). (2010). Magnet Program overview. Retrieved from nursecredentialing.org/Magnet/ProgramOverview/Magnet-Characteristics.aspx.

Brooks, J. M., Titler, M. G., Ardery, G., & Herr, K. (2009). Effect of evidence-based acute pain management practices on inpatient costs. *Health Services Research, 4*(1), 245-263.

Laschinger, H. K. S., Fingan, J. E., Shamian, J., & Wilk, P. (2004). A longitudinal analysis of the impact of workplace empowerment on work satisfaction. *Journal of Organizational Behavior, 25*(4), 527-545.

Laschinger, H., Shamian, J., & Thomson, D. (2001). Impact of Magnet hospital characteristics on nurses' perceptions of trust, burnout, quality of care, and work satisfaction. *Nursing Economics, 19*(5), 209-219.

Longest, B. (2006). *Health policymaking in the United States* (4th ed.). Chicago: Health Administration Press.

Rondeau, K. V., & Wagar, T. H. (2006). Nurse and resident satisfaction in magnet long-term care organizations: Do high involvement approaches matter? *Journal of Nursing Management, 14*(3), 244-250.

Schmalenberg, C., & Kramer, M. (2008). Essentials of a productive nurse work environment. *Nursing Research, 57*(1), 2-13.

Smith, H., Tallman, R., & Kelley, K. (2006). Magnet hospital characteristics and northern Canadian nurses' job satisfaction. *Canadian Journal of Nursing Leadership, 19*(3), 73-86.

Titler, M. G., Herr, K., Brooks, J. M., Xie, X. J., Ardery, G., et al. (2009). Translating research into practice intervention improves management of acute pain in older hip fracture patients. *Health Services Research, 44*(1), 264-287.

Ulrich, B. T., Buerhaus, P. I., Donelan, K., Norman, L., & Dittus, R. (2007). Magnet status and RN views of the work environment and nursing as a career. *Journal of Nursing Administration, 37*(5), 212-220.

Vaughn, T. E., McCoy, K. D., Beekman, S. E., Woolson, R. E., Torner, J. C., & Doebbeling, B. N. (2004). Factors promoting consistent adherence to safe needle precautions among hospital workers. *Infection Control and Hospital Epidemiology, 25*(7), 548-555.

CHAPTER 61

Collective Bargaining in Nursing

Judith Shindul-Rothschild

"Unions provide nurses with real power to protect their practice and their profession."
—Donna Kelly-Williams, RN, President of Massachusetts Nurses Association, March 2010

The number of registered nurses covered under collective bargaining agreements in the United States has been steadily rising since 2004 to 21.5% and is higher than for all U.S. workers (13.7%) and women in the workforce (12.9%) (U.S. Bureau of Labor Statistics, 2009) (Table 61-1). In 2008, approximately 17% of all U.S. hospital workers were covered by a union contract (U.S. Bureau of Labor Statistics, 2010). The three largest unions in the U.S. that represent registered nurses for collective bargaining are as follows:

- National Nurses United (NNU) is the largest union, representing over 150,000 registered nurses (Figure 61-1).
- Service Employees International Union (SEIU) represents 80,000 registered nurses.
- National Federation of Nurses (NFN) has 70,000 registered nurse members.

The NNU and SEIU are members of the AFL-CIO, while the NFN is associated with the American Nurses Association.

A BRIEF HISTORY OF COLLECTIVE BARGAINING IN NURSING

When the first nursing organizations were formed at the turn of the twentieth century, one of the central concerns was the exploitation of student nurses. After 6 months of coursework, it was common practice for student nurses to provide 3 years of unpaid labor working 12 to 16 hours a day. And yet surprisingly, in 1911, nursing organizations opposed the first labor legislation limiting the hours student nurses worked. Such contradictions would reappear throughout the history of collective bargaining in nursing.

Should nurses be aligned with the labor movement, or eschew any association with labor because it would diminish nursing's professional status? Would it be possible for one professional nursing organization to address professional advancement and workplace advocacy? While professional nursing organizations struggled with the philosophical view that any association with the labor movement would diminish nursing's aspirations to advance their professional status, rank-and-file nurses were participating in strikes in response to inhumane working conditions as early as the 1900s.

The original National Labor Relations Act (NLRA) enacted in 1935, mandated the right of hospital employees to collective bargaining. However, several actions, both by government and by nurses themselves, would hamper nurses' use of collective bargaining to improve their working lives. In 1947, the American Hospital Association persuaded Congress to include a clause in the Taft-Hartley Amendments to exempt private nonprofit hospitals from the National Labor Relations Act—a clause that remained in effect until 1974. Shortly thereafter, the membership of the American Nurses Association adopted a no-strike policy to quell fears that striking nurses would abandon their patients. In the face of these impediments, by the 1950s only 17 state nurses' associations had programs in place to represent registered nurses in collective bargaining activities.

Organized nursing's ambivalence toward the labor movement began to shift in the second half of the 1900s when low salaries and poor working conditions created persistent nursing shortages. By the 1960s, the

TABLE 61-1   Registered Nurse Employment in the U.S., Union Membership or Covered by Union Contracts, 1985-2008

Year	RN Employment	Union Members	Covered by Union Contracts	% Union Members	% Covered Union Contracts
2008	2,720,051	539,283	584,038	19.8	21.5
2007	2,577,560	499,763	555,657	19.4	21.6
2006	2,472,288	413,397	455,846	16.7	18.4
2005	2,402,429	398,447	450,247	16.6	18.7
2004	2,432,286	406,795	455,831	16.7	18.7
2003	2,425,429	410,727	471,936	16.9	19.5
2000	2,074,741	350,203	395,510	16.9	19.1
1995	1,949,020	300,931	360,766	15.4	18.5
1990	1,656,605	274,228	344,974	16.6	20.8
1985	1,421,280	222,138	285,128	15.6	20.1

Adapted from Hirsch, B. T., & Macpherson, D. A. (2010). V. Occupation: Union membership, coverage, density and employment by occupation, 2008-1985. *Union membership and coverage database from the current population survey.*

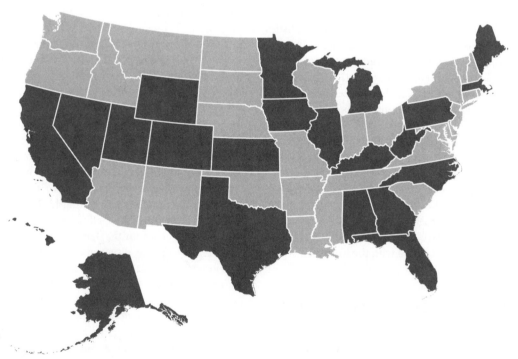

FIGURE 61-1 National Nurses United (NNU) Affiliated Member Organizations, 2009. Shaded states represent those with state nursing associations that are affiliate members of the National Nurses United. Note: RN members of the NNU are in all states. (Adapted with permission from *Building a National Nurses Union* by National Nurses United [December, 2009].)

civil rights movement and the women's liberation movement set the stage for nurses nationwide to embrace collective bargaining as a potent means to improve their professional and working lives. In the summer of 1966, registered nurses represented by the California Nurses Association (CNA) in 33 San Francisco hospitals submitted their resignations in response to the hospital association's failure to address nurses' deteriorating salaries. The unprecedented collective action by the CNA nurses forced hospital administrators to concede to the nurses' demands including a 40% pay increase. Emboldened by the success of the California nurses, registered nurses began to stage work stoppages throughout the United States.

By the time nurses arrived at the annual ANA convention in 1968, they came prepared to vote down ANA's 18-year-old no-strike policy. State associations soon followed the ANA's lead as they too abolished their policy of prohibiting strikes by nurses. Now, equipped with the necessary leverage to make collective bargaining effective, nurses quickly began to organize.

Registered nurses grew to support unions because of the measurable impact collective bargaining had on both salaries and working conditions. Early collective bargaining agreements addressed the traditional bread-and-butter issues of organized labor by establishing a 40-hour workweek, time and a half for overtime, paid vacation and sick leave, health insurance benefits, disability benefits, pensions, and salary increases. By 1969, nurses' salaries had surpassed the average income for female professionals and in response, vacancy rates in hospitals dropped for the first time into single digits (Aiken & Blendon, 1981). Labor economists uniformly concluded that collective bargaining was the major factor that forced hospitals to increase nurses' wages and drew thousands of nurses back into the labor force during critical shortages in the late 1960s and early 1970s (Yett, 1975; Feldstein, 1979).

Beginning in the early 1980s, pay equity and staffing agreements began to appear in collective bargaining agreements. To redress pay disparities between men and women, the Florida, Massachusetts, Pennsylvania, New York, and California Nursing Associations included comparable worth provisions—equal pay for performing work of comparable value, responsibility, and complexity—in all collective bargaining contracts. Language was negotiated in collective bargaining agreements requiring the participation of staff nurses in staffing decisions and the use of patient acuity systems to determine appropriate staffing levels. The California Nurses Association successfully lobbied for state regulations establishing RN-to-patient ratios in intensive care units. The professional and economic gains achieved by nurses in the 1980s through collective bargaining were often hard fought. In Massachusetts alone, nurses went on strike in eight hospitals to demand provisions in labor contracts that would improve the quality of patient care as well as wages (Wilson, Slatin, & O'Sullivan, 2006).

COLLECTIVE BARGAINING AND LEGISLATIVE INITIATIVES SINCE 2000

Nurses' professional and economic gains were again challenged beginning in 2000 by cost-cutting measures that threatened the welfare of nurses and their ability to provide safe patient care. Inadequate nurse staffing triggered a widespread practice of mandatory overtime in hospitals nationwide. Frustrated with the lack of responsiveness by hospital administrators and policymakers to unsafe staffing and inhumane working conditions, unions used their leverage in labor negotiations and in state legislatures to secure a series of reforms (Shindul-Rothschild, 1998) (Box 61-1).

Unions representing registered nurses sponsored legislation and negotiated contract language to establish safe staffing standards, whistle-blower protections for nurses who reported unsafe staffing conditions, and limits to mandatory overtime. In 2000, Massachusetts registered nurses at hospitals owned by Tenet Health Care would go on strike for 49 days over inadequate staffing and mandatory overtime. The late Senator Edward Kennedy (D-Massachusetts) interceded and negotiated landmark contract language to prohibit mandatory overtime that would serve as a model for nursing labor contracts nationwide (Massachusetts Nurses Association, 2003).

Unions representing nurses also successfully lobbied for state laws that would severely limit the practice of mandatory overtime for registered nurses. Minnesota Statute 181.275, enacted in 2002, prohibits an employer from taking action against a registered nurse who is mandated to work in excess of normal

BOX 61-1 National Nurses United RNs across the Nation Take Up the Fight

Key Components of Hospital Patient Protection Legislation

1. Legal recognition of the right of RNs to advocate for patients
2. Whistle-blower protection with substantive monetary fines
3. Unit-specific RN-to-patient ratios for acute-care hospitals
4. Restrictions on use of unlicensed assistive personnel
5. Patient classification system to determine additional staff, based on an acuity tool
6. Safe hospital care workplace standards
7. Strengthening emergency preparedness capacity with paid leave for volunteers

Key Components of Collective Bargaining Contracts

1. Establishing a secure retirement with guaranteed annual pensions
2. Professional practice committees—Staff RN-controlled committees with the authority to report unsafe practices and the power to make real changes
3. Mandatory overtime bans
4. Restrictions on unsafe floating
5. Enforceable staffing language
6. Technology protections to enhance, not replace, RNs' clinical judgment
7. Enhanced economic security in salary and benefits
8. Occupational health and safety protections, including contract language to prevent latex allergy and needlestick injuries, and language to address workplace violence and safe patient handling

Adapted from California Nurses Association/NNOC (2009). *The ratio solution*, pp. 12, 16.

TABLE 61-2 Registered Nurse-to-Patient Ratios in California (AB 394)

Specialty Unit	RNs	Patients
ER trauma	1	1
Operating room	1	1
Postanesthesia recovery	1	2
Intensive care/critical care	1	2
Neonatal intensive care	1	2
ICU patients in ER	1	2
Labor and delivery	1	2
Step-down	1	3
Antepartum	1	4
Postpartum couplets	1	4
Pediatrics	1	4
Emergency room	1	4
Telemetry	1	4
Other specialty	1	4
Medical/surgical	1	5
Postpartum women only	1	6
Psychiatric	1	6

Adapted from California Nurses Association/NNOC. (2009). *The ratio solution*, p. 8.

standards were fully implemented for all hospital units. During the phase-in period, the number of registered nurses increased by 11.2% on medical-surgical units and 4.8% on step-down units (Burnes Bolton et al., 2007). Job satisfaction of California registered nurses increased significantly with the greatest improvements in nurses' satisfaction with the adequacy of staff (Spetz, 2008). Improvement in nurses' satisfaction reversed the protracted trend of registered nurses leaving California, and the number of RNs with active licenses in California increased by more than 60,000 from the time the RN-to-patient ratio bill was first enacted until 2005 (Nelson, 2008) (see Chapter 53).

Studies have found associations between increased RN staffing and lower odds of hospital-related mortality and adverse patient events (Kane, Shamliyan, Mueller, Duval, & Wilt, 2007). In California, nurse-to-patient ratios have had the greatest improvement on patient outcomes in hospitals that began with the highest ratios (Sochalski, Konetzka, Zhu, & Volpp, 2008). The nurse staffing standards mandated in California are associated with significantly lower patient mortality, higher job satisfaction, and reports by both staff nurses and nurse administrators of improved quality of care (Table 61-2) (Aiken et al.,

working hours when the nurse clearly states that to do so would put patients at risk (Minnesota Nurses Association, 2007), and New York Labor Law 167 prohibits employers from mandating registered nurses to work overtime except in the event of an unforeseen emergency or other extraordinary circumstance such as a health care disaster (SEIU, 2010).

In 1999, the CNA became the first union in the nation to successfully lobby for an RN-to-patient ratio law, Assembly Bill 394. After an additional 9 years of bitter court battles between the CNA and the governor of California, the nurse-to-patient ratio

TABLE 61-3 Registered Nurse Mean Wages by Five Highest States and Nationally, 2003-2008

Year	MEAN WAGE RANK						#1 Mean Wage vs. U.S. Mean Wage
	#1	#2	#3	#4	#5		
2008	California $83,040	Massachusetts $79,390	Hawaii $77,950	Maryland $74,370	New York $73,160	United States $65,130	(22% higher) $17,910
2007	California $78,550	Massachusetts $74,940	Hawaii $74,200	New Jersey $70,900	Maryland $70,480	$62,480	(21% higher) $16,070
2006	California $75,130	Massachusetts $70,910	Hawaii $68,680	Maryland $68,370	New Jersey $66,600	$59,730	(21% higher) $15,400
2005	California $70,430	Maryland $67,330	Massachusetts $66,250	Hawaii $65,490	New Jersey $63,070	$56,880	(19% higher) $13,550
2004	California $66,920	Maryland $64,720	Massachusetts $62,490	Hawaii $60,920	New York $60,680	$54,210	(19% higher) $12,710
2003	California $62,270	Maryland $61,920	Hawaii $58,490	New York $57,900	Massachusetts $57,650	$51,230	(18% higher) $11,040

Adapted from *Occupational Employment and Wages, 29-1111 Registered Nurses* by the U.S. Bureau of Labor Statistics (2003-2008).

2010). The primary agenda of the newly formed NNU, which tripled in size in 2009, is to lead a highly visible, public campaign to enact RN-to-patient ratios across the U.S. Nurse staffing legislation is pending in at least 25 states (Conway, Konetzka, Zhu, Vopp, & Sochalski, 2008), and congressional legislation supported by the NNU to mandate RN-to-patient ratios has been introduced in the Senate (S. 1031) and in the House (H.R. 2273) in 2009 (see Chapter 53).

The recent success of collective bargaining, coupled with pervasive dissatisfaction among hospital nurses with their working conditions, is widely anticipated to lead to an expansion of unionization in the years ahead (Bureau of National Affairs, 2005, p. 1). Registered nurses who are union members have salaries on average that are 13% higher than their nonunion counterparts (Lovell, 2006). In Massachusetts, where 70% of hospital-employed nurses are represented by the Massachusetts Nurses Association (the highest union penetration in the country), nurses' salaries are 18% higher than the national average (Wilson, Slatin, & O'Sullivan, 2006; U.S. Bureau of Labor Statistics, 2003-2008) (Table 61-3). Although the value of RNs to improve patient outcomes has been proven through empirical research, hospital management continues to return to the tactics of de-skilling (substituting unlicensed personnel for RNs), casualization (substituting temporary RNs for full-time RNs), and speed-ups (increasing the number of patients assigned to

RNs) to achieve short-term savings. For growing numbers of registered nurses in the U.S., collective bargaining has become vital to upholding standards of professional nursing practice, economic security, and the quality of patient care.

For a list of related websites, please refer to your Evolve Resources at http://evolve.elsevier.com/Mason/policypolitics/

REFERENCES

Aiken, L. H., & Blendon, R. J. (1981, May). The national nurse shortage. *National Journal*, 948-953.

Aiken, L. H., Sloane, D. M., Cimiotti, J. P., Clarke, S. P., Flynn, L., et al. (2010). Implications of the California nurse staffing mandate for other states. *Health Services Research, 45*(4), 904-921.

Burnes Bolton, L., Aydin, C. E., Donaldson, N., Brown, D. S., Sandhu, M., Fridman, M., & Aronow, H. U. (2007). Mandated nurse staffing ratios in California: A comparison of staffing and nursing-sensitive outcomes pre- and postregulation. *Policy, Politics, & Nursing Practice, 8*(4), 238-250.

Bureau of National Affairs. (2005). *Union organizing in the health care industry: A BNA Plus special report*. Washington, D.C.: The Bureau of National Affairs.

California Nurses Association/NNOC. (2009). *The ratio solution*. Retrieved from www.calnurses.org/assets/pdf/ratios/ratios_booklet.pdf.

Conway, P. H., Konetzka, T., Zhu, J., Vopp, K. G., & Sochalski, J. (2008). Nurse staffing ratios: Trends and policy implications for hospitalists and the safety net. *Journal of Hospital Medicine, 3*(3), 193-199.

Feldstein, P. J. (1979). *Health Care Economics*. New York: Wiley.

Hirsch, B. T., & Macpherson, D. A. (2010). V. Occupation: Union membership, coverage, density and employment by occupation, 2008-1985. *Union membership and coverage database from the current population survey.* Retrieved from www.unionstats.com.

Kane, R. L., Shamliyan, T. A., Mueller, C., Duval, S., & Wilt, T. J. (2007). The association of registered nurse staffing levels and patient outcomes: Systematic review and meta-analysis. *Medical Care, 45*(12), 1195-1205.

Lovell, V. (2006). *Solving the nursing shortage through higher wages.* Washington, D.C.: Institute for Women's Policy Research. Retrieved from www.iwpr.org.

Massachusetts Nurses Association. (2003). MNA 1903-2003: A century of caring for the Commonwealth: Fact sheet and historical timeline. *The Massachusetts Nurse, 74*(3), 10-11. Retrieved from www.massnurses.org/files/file/News/newsletter/2003/April.pdf.

Minnesota Nurses Association. (2007). New law change: Mandatory overtime prevention law for state RNs. *Minnesota Nursing Accent, September/October,* 8-9.

National Nurses United. (December, 2009). *Building a national nurses union: The time is now!* Canton, MA: Massachusetts Nurses Association.

Nelson, R. (2008). California's Ratio Law four years later: Better staffing but no data on outcomes yet. *American Journal of Nursing, 108*(3), 25-26. Retrieved from www.nursingcenter.com.

Service Employees International Union (SEIU). (2010). *1199 Nurses won a ban on mandatory overtime: Now we need to enforce it.* New York: 1199SEIU. Retrieved from www.1199seiu.org/members/occupations/rn/mandatory_overtime.cfm.

Shindul-Rothschild, J. (1998). Nurses' day tribute: A nursing call to action. *American Journal of Nursing, 98*(5), 36.

Sochalski, J., Konetzka, R. T., Zhu, J., & Volpp, K. (2008). Will mandated minimum nurse staffing ratios lead to better patient outcomes? *Medical Care, 46*(6), 606-613.

Spetz, J. (2008). Nurse satisfaction and the implementation of minimum nurse staffing regulations. *Policy, Politics, & Nursing Practice, 9*(1), 15-21.

U.S. Bureau of Labor Statistics. (2010). *Career guide to industries (2010-2011 Ed.).* Washington, D.C.: U.S. Department of Labor. Retrieved from http://data.bls.gov/cgi-bin/print.pl/oco/cg/cgs035.htm.

U.S. Bureau of Labor Statistics. (2009). *Women in the labor force: A databook. September. Report 1018.* Washington, D.C.: U.S. Department of Labor. Retrieved from www.bls.gov/cps/wlf-databook2009.htm.

U.S. Bureau of Labor Statistics. (2003-2008). Occupational employment and wages, 29-1111 Registered Nurses. Retrieved from www.bls.gov/oes/current/oes291111.htm.

Wilson, B., Slatin, C., & O'Sullivan, M. (2006). Nurses respond to health care restructuring: The transformation of the Massachusetts Nurses Association. *Journal of Health & Social Policy, 21*(4), 51-72.

Yett, D. E. (1975). *An economic analysis of the nursing shortage.* Lexington, MA: Lexington Books.

CHAPTER 62

Workplace Advocacy

Dennis Sherrod, Wylecia Wiggs Harris, and Alfreda Harper-Harrison

"When people go to work, they shouldn't have to leave their hearts at home."

—Betty Bender

The CENTER for American Nurses (The Center), founded in 2003, was established to help nurses create healthy work environments through education and research. While other national nursing associations focus on national and state policy, the Center partners with organizations, state nurses associations, and individual registered nurses to develop resources, strategies, and tools to help nurses manage and influence evolving workplace issues.

WORKPLACE POLICY

Policy in the health care workplace establishes standards, identifies boundaries, and provides protections for employees, employers, and patients. Mutually determined, defined, and documented policy assists health care organizations to more efficiently and effectively provide quality patient outcomes. While much workplace policy is mandated from federal and state levels, helpful and meaningful policies shaping workplace culture, employee satisfaction, and positive patient outcomes are initiated and developed by passionate and expert health care professionals within the workplace itself.

THE CENTER FOR AMERICAN NURSES

The CENTER for American Nurses offers evidence-based solutions and powerful tools to equip nurses to navigate workplace challenges, optimize patient outcomes, and maximize career benefits. These tools, services, and strategies support nurses at all levels of experience who are striving to improve their practice

environments, meet their personal and professional goals, and promote excellence in patient care (Scott, 2008). Nurses face many challenges in the work environment such as increased workloads, fatigue, musculoskeletal injuries, difficult coworkers, and so on. The Center serves as a resource for nurses seeking to overcome these challenges and create work environments that support health care professionals as well as patients. For example, the Center offers an extensive program for nurses seeking to develop effective conflict engagement skills (CENTER for American Nurses, 2010). In addition, the Center provides resources to address lateral violence and bullying.

The Center monitors internal and external factors affecting the work environment through environmental scans and national surveys; provides leadership and vision in response to changing work environments; and develops and disseminates strategies to address personal and professional concerns that can initiate and shape workplace policy. For example, the Center hosts monthly webinars to explore issues such as becoming an exceptional charge nurse, defining respect, and surviving shift work. Recently, the Center partnered with the Women's Institute for a Secure Retirement (WISER) to create tools to help nurses increase their financial literacy.

Finally, the Center creates and disseminates position statements to guide the profession in specific areas that affect health care work environments. The Center's Zero Tolerance Policy addressing disruptive behaviors has been broadly recognized and used by facilities seeking to curb workplace violence.

To identify evolving workplace issues, the Center surveys the national nursing community and reviews the latest evidence-based research to develop fact sheets to educate nurses and provide solutions to identified concerns. Nurses may access the Center's information and services through individual memberships or through their state nurses association. Nursing associations and organizations whose primary purpose does not involve representation of its members for collective bargaining purposes are eligible for membership in the Center.

CURRENT WORKPLACE ADVOCACY POLICY ISSUES

MANDATORY OVERTIME

When overtime hours, particularly mandatory overtime, are required by organizations to provide adequate registered nurse staffing, nurses can be pushed beyond their capacity to work safely and to provide appropriate, quality care to patients. Extended work hours contribute to nurses' job dissatisfaction (Institute of Medicine, 2004; United States General Accounting Office, 2001). Additional shifts and hours are also reported to cause work-related illness and injuries (Christo & Pienaar, 2006; Cohen & Single, 2001) as well as health care errors (Institute of Medicine, 2004). The Center recommends that nurses develop workplace policies in collaboration with employers requiring no employee be forced to work overtime. In 2006, The Center adopted a position statement opposing mandatory overtime and outlining recommendations to decrease the physical and mental burdens such practices place on health care professionals (CENTER for American Nurses, 2006).

NURSE FATIGUE

It has been noted that fatigue impairs nurses' performance and increases the chance of making errors that affect health outcomes. It is not uncommon for nurses to work past the end of a scheduled shift. Those who work shifts lasting 12.5 hours or more have a 3 times greater risk for making errors (Rogers, Hwang, Scott, Aiken, & Dinges, 2004). To improve the work environment, the Center agrees with the recommendation made by the Institute of Medicine to prohibit mandatory or voluntary overtime in excess of 12 hours per 24-hour period and in excess of 60 hours per 7-day period (Institute of Medicine, 2004). Nurse fatigue is a controversial issue. Some support imposed limitations on work hours and shifts; others, particularly those who work overtime or have more than one job, believe they can self-regulate their work behaviors.

The Center has provided a number of publications on shifts, work hours, and nurse fatigue to inform nurses about personal safety and quality care. Examples include *Nurses and Fatigue* fact sheets and articles focusing on shifts and work hours posted on the Web and provided directly to state nurses association members for reprinting in their statewide publications. Future nurse fatigue workplace policies will need to balance the work interests of nurses and employers with the safety interests of patients.

MUSCULOSKELETAL INJURIES

Musculoskeletal injuries are common because of the need to lift, turn, and assist patients. Back, neck, and shoulder pain are the most common type and cost the industry an estimated 6 absentee days per nurse per year (Trinkoff, Lipscomb, Geiger-Brown, & Brady, 2002). The Center supports the American Nurses Association's (ANA) "Safe Patient Handling" campaign to encourage hospitals to provide lifting devices and lifting teams when transporting, lifting, and repositioning clients.

MATURE NURSES

The current nurse shortage is compounded by the large number of aging nurses. The average age of a nurse in the U.S. is estimated to be 47 years (HRSA Health Professions, 2010). Mature nurses work in environments that are often stressful, demanding, and lack retention incentives devised especially for older nurses. They are expected to mentor novice nurses and build healthy intergenerational collaborative work relationships. In addition, a majority lack the financial skills necessary to plan for retirement. The Center highlights workplace strategies designed to retain mature nurses, increase nurses' financial planning skills, and explore flexible staffing strategies that support the mature nurse.

WORKPLACE DESIGN

Workplace design profoundly affects nurses and patients in the health care environment. A well-planned facility design can improve the quality of care for patients, promote recruiting and retention of staff, and enhance operational efficiency and productivity (CENTER for American Nurses, 2007). The Center provides education about ergonomics, technology, and workplace design to promote the well-being and safety of health care workers and patients. Nurses are encouraged to participate as full partners in workplace design and redesign decisions (CENTER for American Nurses, 2007).

LATERAL VIOLENCE AND BULLYING IN THE WORKPLACE

Evidence validates that disruptive behaviors such as lateral violence and bullying negatively impact the health care work environment, the recruitment and retention of nurses, and the quality and safety of patient care (see Chapter 56). The Center has worked with other organizations to decrease such behavior.

INITIATING WORKPLACE POLICY

How can nurses influence workplace policy? First, nurses can stay informed by reading the literature in their area of practice and participating in webinars and discussion groups hosted by nursing organizations, such as the Center. It is important to respond quickly to federal or state policies that affect the workplace. The recent national impact of the H1N1 virus stimulated rapid revisions of workplace infection-control policies. If a policy is not supported by administration, build a strong, evidence-based case. Build support among colleagues. Seek information from the state nurses association or the Center. The Center's extensive resources in conflict engagement may be helpful. Involve other members of the health care team in developing workplace policy that provides a healthy work environment for quality patient care.

For a list of related websites, please refer to your Evolve Resources at http://evolve.elsevier.com/Mason/policypolitics/

REFERENCES

CENTER for American Nurses. (2006, June). *Opposition to mandatory overtime.* Retrieved from http://centerforamericannurses.com/associations/9102/files/Position%20StatementMandatory_Overtime.pdf.

CENTER for American Nurses. (2007, March). *Restructuring and redesigning nurses' work environments.* Retrieved from http://centerforamericannurses.com/associations/9102/files/Position%20StatementRestructuringRedesignNurse%20Work%20Environments.pdf.

CENTER for American Nurses. (2010). *Conflict engagement: Creating healthier work environments.* Retrieved from http://centerforamericannurses.com/displaycommon.cfm?an=1&subarticlenbr=235#Why_Conflict_Engagement.

Christo, B., & Pienaar, J. (2006). South Africa correctional official occupational stress: The role of psychological strengths. *Journal of Criminal Justice, 34*(1), 73-84.

Cohen, J., & Single, L. E. (2001). An examination of the perceived impact of flexible work arrangements on professional opportunities in public accounting. *Journal of Business Ethics, 32*(4), 317-319.

HRSA Health Professions. (2010). National sample survey of registered nurses. Retrieved from http://bhpr.hrsa.gov/healthworkforce/rnsurvey.

Institute of Medicine. (2004). *Keeping patients safe: Transforming the work environment of nurses.* Washington, D.C.: The National Academies Press.

Rogers, A. E., Hwang, W. T., Scott, L. D., Aiken, L. H., & Dinges, D. F. (2004). The working hours of hospital staff nurses and patient safety. *Health Affairs, 23*(4), 202-212.

Scott, D. (2008, June). The CENTER for American Nurses—Celebrating five years of workforce advocacy. *Nurses First, 1*(1). Retrieved from http://centerforamericannurses.com/associations/9102/Nurses%20First%206-08a.pdf?CFID=18577649&CFTOKEN=54450863&jsessionid=663093ac489e260f3b4e391a784233563517.

Trinkoff, A. M., Lipscomb, J. A., Geiger-Brown, J., & Brady, B. (2002). Musculoskeletal problems of the neck, shoulder, and back and functional consequences in nurses. *American Journal of Industrial Medicine, 41*(3), 170-178.

U.S. General Accounting Office. (July, 2001). Nursing workforce: Emerging nurse shortage due to multiple factors. GAO-01-944. Washington, D.C. Retrieved from www.gao.gov/new.items/d01944.pdf.

CHAPTER 63

Contemporary Issues in Government

Deborah B. Gardner and Amanda L. Ebner

"The bill I'm signing will set in motion reforms that generations of Americans have fought for and marched for and hungered to see."
—President Barack Obama, New York Times, March 23, 2010, before signing the Patient Protection and Affordable Care Act

On March 23, 2010, President Barack Obama signed into law H.R. 3590, the Patient Protection and Affordable Care Act (P.L. 111-148), and 7 days later he signed H.R. 4872, the Health Care and Education Reconciliation Act of 2010 (P.L. 111-152). This contentious yet long awaited legislation will fundamentally change the United States health care system. The reconciliation bill combined with the Senate-passed bill affects American health care in five notable ways.

First, the Act expands health care access for more Americans by preventing insurance companies from discrimination based on preexisting conditions (starting in 2014). Second, the bill also expands access by providing subsidies for American families earning up to $88,000 annually (for a family of four). Several non-profit advocacy organizations, including the Patient Advocate Foundation and Coverage for All, are already assisting families in securing coverage and prescription subsidies prior to the full reinstatement of the Act in 2014. Third, the Act extends prior policies, as dependent children will now remain insured under their parents' coverage until age 26. Next, access is increased as employers with more than 50 employees will be required to cover health care costs with steep per-employee fines for violations. Finally, the passage of the reconciliation bill adds new approaches with free preventive screenings to seniors on Medicare and closes the so-called "doughnut hole" in Part D prescription drug coverage by 2011. The combined legislation will extend coverage to an estimated 30 million uninsured Americans.

This legislation will require most Americans to have health insurance coverage and adds 16 million people to the Medicaid rolls. The law will cost the government about $938 billion over 10 years, according to the nonpartisan Congressional Budget Office, which has also estimated that it will reduce the federal deficit by $143 billion over a decade (Box 63-1). Indeed, the sheer scope and complexity of the nation's health care system as part of a larger political and global economic context make the implementation of this new health care legislation a most formidable endeavor. The 2076-page Affordable Care Act symbolizes the complexity of this reform effort.

Claims that health reform will fail continued as threats of repeal were voiced by Republican challengers even while President Obama was signing both Acts into law. And the public has heard these attacks on the reform loud and clear. According to a Gallup poll on health care reform taken a week after Obama signed the law, a solid majority of Americans think it will make both budget deficit and health care costs worse (Newport, 2010). Since key provisions don't begin until 2014, both skeptics and supporters will have plenty of time to assess the law, its prospects for success, and, of course, its forecasted cost.

This chapter focuses on the landmark legislation enacted by the 111th U.S. Congress to remedy this nation's broken health care system and the challenges reformers will face in implementing these policies. The history and current context that underscore this legislation will be described. The health care climate and institutional politics at the national and state levels of government are examined. The critical need to control health care costs, connect prevention with quality care and patient safety, integrate technology for improving health care coordination, contain the threat of bioterrorism, and combat the growing obesity epidemic will be explored. These are tangible

---

BOX 63-1 Understanding the Health Care Overhaul

From 2010 to 2019: The reconciliation bill combined with the Senate-passed bill will do the following:

- Spend $938 billion on expanding insurance coverage, including $464 billion in subsidies to help uninsured people buy coverage.
- Expand Medicaid coverage to 16 million additional people.
- Require many employers to offer coverage for their workers.
- Collect $69 billion in penalties from uninsured individuals and employers for non-coverage.
- Provide coverage through an insurance exchange to 24 million people.
- Reduce the number of uninsured by 32 million people, but leave 23 million (including illegal immigrants) not covered.
- Cut Medicare spending by $455 billion from currently-projected levels.
- Produce a net reduction in federal deficits of $143 billion.

Source: The Congressional Budget Office.

---

examples of issues that must be addressed in the redesign of a sustainable health care system that provides access to quality outcomes for all U.S. citizens regardless of income, race, or geographic location.

HISTORICAL PERSPECTIVE

Health care reform has been a holy grail of Democratic presidents. Truman, Johnson, Carter, and Clinton all set out to find consensus to provide every American with health insurance coverage, only to end up empty-handed. President Franklin D. Roosevelt hoped to include some kind of national health insurance program in Social Security in 1935. President Harry S. Truman proposed a national health care program with a multi-payer insurance fund. Since then, every Democratic president and several Republican presidents have wanted to provide affordable coverage to more Americans. President Bill Clinton offered the most ambitious proposal in 1993-1994

and suffered the most spectacular failure (Stolberg & Pear, 2010).

Despite these daunting precedents, the election of President Barack Obama was seen by most Democrats as a public mandate on health care reform. Its passage assures Obama a place in history as the American president who finally succeeded where others tried mightily and failed. One of the most significant differences between the Clinton reform efforts and those of 2009-2010 is that employers and corporations, alarmed at the soaring cost of health care, agreed that changes were necessary. Some of the same insurance companies, which helped defeat the Clinton plan, began 2009 by claiming that they accepted the need for change and wanted a seat at the negotiating table. As the bills developed, however, these powerful stakeholders became strong opponents of some Democratic proposals, especially one known as the "Public Option" to create a government-run insurance plan as an alternative to their offerings.

To give a sense of the contextual obstacles impeding the legislation's passage, the scale and quantity of problems confronting the country and President Franklin Roosevelt at the start of the Great Depression in 1929 are repeatedly evoked as the most comparable historic referent (Baker, 2009). "The Great Recession," prompted by overspeculation in finance and brought to light with the housing market collapse, demanded immediate and deliberate actions of risky unprecedented proportions early in the Obama presidency. Immediately after the president's election, critics argued that pressing priorities such as the U.S. economy, energy independence, global warming, and the Middle East needed attention more than health care reform. In addition to being confronted with major foreign policy decisions regarding the conflicts in Iraq and Afghanistan, on the domestic front, the administration's early months in office were indeed dominated by a single issue: the economy. In fact, the economy's relentless slide in late 2008 began reshaping the Obama team's agenda-setting. As president-elect, he was forced to contend with whether or not to bail out the financial system, and how to keep General Motors and Chrysler from going under (Stolberg & Pear, 2010). Because health care in this country is the most expensive in the world but not the strongest in health outcomes, 1 of every 6 dollars earned is spent on health care, and the current system has forced more than 1 million people into bankruptcy, the Obama administration argued that the biggest threat to the nation's economic balance sheet was the skyrocketing cost of health care (Gawande, 2009). To extend medical coverage to everyone was also a way to bring costs into control, thus health care reform was presented as an integral issue to economic stability.

President Obama's first major initiative incorporated the two inseparable issues in a stimulus package to pump money into a downward-spiraling economy. In February 2009, only 3 weeks after his inauguration, Congress passed the massive $787 billion American Recovery and Reinvestment Act (ARRA) in an effort to create jobs, stimulate economic activity, and increase transparency in government spending. Republicans derided the bill as unaffordable and excessive. Not a single Republican in the House voted for the package, and only three Republican senators did, narrowly avoiding a filibuster.

Under the aegis of economic recovery, the Act set aside more that $100 billion, enabling extensive provisions to address both immediate and long-term deficiencies in the health care infrastructure. For example, it helped an estimated 7 million unemployed Americans retain their health care coverage under COBRA and roughly 20 million Americans keep their Medicare coverage despite state budget shortfalls; allocated $1 billion toward prevention and wellness programming; and invested an immediate $24 billion for computerizing medical records to reduce costs and ensure patient privacy in records exchange (*www.Recovery. gov,* 2010). Furthermore, the Act provides funding for comparative effectiveness research, funds for the next generation of medical professionals, and invests in community health centers and health care technology for at-risk communities. Several states have already begun implementing strategies that mirror national health priorities, however, many of the states' reactions to federal reform have been neither uniform nor without contention.

THE ROCKY ROAD TO HEALTH INSURANCE REFORM: STATES REBEL

Despite the president's signature, the legislative work on the bill is not complete at the time of this writing, nor is the partisan clash over it. States have an extensive and complicated shared power relationship with the federal government in regulating various aspects of the health insurance market and in enacting health reforms. In general, the health insurance reform measures, covering both 2009 and 2010, seek to make or keep health insurance optional, and allow people to purchase any type of coverage they may choose. However, in response to federal health reform legislation, members of 39 state legislatures have proposed legislation to limit, alter, or oppose selected state or federal actions, primarily targeted at single-payer provisions and mandates that require purchase of insurance (Figure 63-1) (Cauchi, 2010).

Simply put, the individual mandate, passed by both chambers, requires people to buy health insurance or pay a financial penalty. Republicans argue that this is the government forcing people to buy a particular product. Democrats contend that the current system is forcing citizens out of health insurance or into few and expensive coverage options. Overall, Democrats designed this mandate to make reform more cost-effective by creating larger population pools that pay into the care of all risk levels. It is likely that the contours of this provision will be contentious and hotly debated in the judicial arena. Liberals argue that they have seriously reviewed the legalities of this mandate, and that the penalty is constitutional. Conservatives are advancing other constitutional arguments against reform plans including the regulation of insurance companies as the illegal seizure of private property. The pivotal argument here is that state law cannot nullify federal law. One strong source of congressional power is the General Welfare Clause, which provides the legislature with power to provide for the common defense and general welfare of the U.S. Jack Balkin, a constitutional law professor at Yale who wrote about the constitutionality of the individual mandate, argues that by insuring more people and preventing insurers from denying coverage because of preexisting conditions, the health reform bill serves the "general welfare" (Jost, 2010). While politicians and legal experts have expressed widely varying pro and con opinions on the validity of the approach, most experts see the purpose of these efforts as symbolic rather than legal, intended to send a message of political protest. Significantly, some analysts predict that partisan politics will delay and complicate implementation of health reform, as these legal collisions will be used as rallying points to

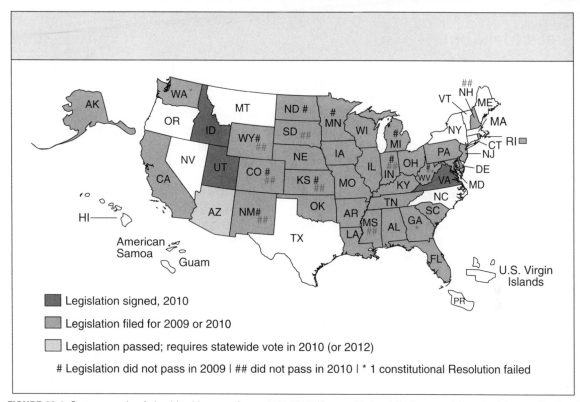

FIGURE 63-1 States opposing federal health care reforms, 2009-2012. (Source: National Conference of State Legislatures. Retrieved from *www.ncsl.org/?tabid=18906*.)

influence the 2010 congressional elections (Fletcher, 2010).

CONGRESSIONAL REFORM

In addition to the difficulty of dealing with a broken health care system, the months leading up to the health care reform vote revealed the legislative processes taking place in Congress to be in need of its own reform. While some argue that the fact that health reform legislation was passed refutes such a position, what is also apparent is that Democrats and Republicans currently vote against each other more regularly than at any time since Reconstruction. Two exemplars of legislative dysfunction during the health care debates were the misuse of the filibuster and the misrepresentation of reconciliation procedures.

Conventional wisdom acknowledges that the filibuster is most commonly used to obscure change and clarity in legislative discussion, if not paralyze it altogether. According to UCLA political scientist Barbara Sinclair, about 8% of major bills faced a filibuster in the 1960s, and in this decade it has risen to 70% (Klein, 2009). The second parody of deliberative democracy was the Republican battle against the use of reconciliation in the last days of the health reform legislation process. They argued that Democrats were using a procedural gimmick to "jam" the legislation through, and Democrats retorted by listing all the major bills the Republicans had passed via reconciliation when they were in the majority (such as the Medicare drug plan and both Bush tax cuts). The absence of bipartisanship and the use of the filibuster to obstruct progress rather than protect debate, has given any Congressperson the ability to hold a bill hostage to his or her demands. Some observers go so far as to argue that the continued misuse of the filibuster threatens successful governance overall (Klein, 2009). Certainly, the ability of the public to keep check on legislative decision-making has been undermined by these uncompromising, obfuscating practices.

THE BATTLE OVER PUBLIC OPINION

Efforts to make the legislation process transparent and intelligible for the public backfired in the thick of a contentious partisan background. Rarely have as many statistics been summoned, disputed, recorded, and maligned as during the months it has taken to pass the health care reform bill. Health care stirs powerful emotions, and the complexity of the subject, combined with round-the-clock politicized media coverage, makes it difficult for people to balance their emotional reactions with rational ones. Political observers note that as the public witnesses partisan polarization on an issue—with Democrats on one side and Republicans on the other—it receives a cue to harden its own opinions, which in turn reinforces the hardening of partisan political positions (Klein, 2010).

Political representatives used the debate over health care reform to accentuate differing ideologic approaches regarding the role of government. The role of government in this country has long been a deeply divisive issue. While across the citizenry, there is a shared belief that the role of government is to provide people the freedom necessary to pursue their own goals, in practice, outlining paths that carve a balance between individual rights and collective needs is fraught with political factionalism. Generally, conservative policies tend to emphasize the empowerment of the individual to solve problems rather than the government. In contrast, liberals see government action as necessary to achieve equal opportunity and tend to emphasize the role of the State in enacting and enforcing policies that empower individuals. Placing the role of the government somewhere in the middle, which is how the Obama administration describes its health care legislation, seemed to displease both liberals and conservatives. Amidst this ongoing context of zero-sum politicking in Congress, it is not surprising that while Americans vastly support the individual components of health reform they remain skeptical when asked about the hazy concept of "comprehensive reform."

During the congressional recess in August 2009, a wave of conservative protests almost ensured the death of health care reform. Opposition to the president's health care plans were likened on talk radio to something out of Hitler's Germany, lampooned by protesters at congressional town-hall-style meetings and vilified in television commercials (Begley, 2009). In response, President Obama confronted a critical Congress and a skeptical nation, decrying the "scare tactics" of his opponents and presenting a forceful case for a sweeping health care overhaul that had eluded Washington for generations. An instance of political machinations stifling discourse occurred during this same presentation when President Obama refuted claims that Democrats were proposing to provide health coverage to illegal immigrants, and Representative Joe Wilson of South Carolina yelled, "You lie!" Mr. Wilson apologized, but his outburst led to a 6-day national debate on civility and decorum, and the House formally rebuked him a week later. Not surprisingly, proponents of health care reform were shocked at the disparagement of the bill; however, its passage proved inevitable as the U.S. joins other nations in designing a more inclusive, universal model of health care.

FEDERAL IMPLEMENTATION OF HEALTH INSURANCE REFORM

The final health care bill targets three key operational sectors of health care: (1) insurance practice, (2) employer-based coverage mandates, and (3) subsidies for vulnerable populations. First-stage implementation of the new health care legislation began with the Department of Health and Human Services (DHHS) providing guidance through rule. Immediately after health reform was signed, HHS Secretary Kathleen Sebelius (USDHHS, 2010b) sent a letter to America's Health Insurance Plans (the trade association representing the plans) emphasizing the importance of compliance with the more immediately effective provisions in the health reform bill, specifically the "preexisting condition exclusion." She made it clear that rules to be established reinforce compliance with the requirements to ensure that children not be denied access to their parents' health insurance or denied treatment due to a preexisting condition.

To address the overlapping sectors of insurance practice and vulnerable populations, HHS has begun coordinating rapid implementation with state and insurance providers. Additional letters from Sebelius in April 2010 attempted to gather information on the number of states who would be interested in participating in the temporary high-risk pool program established by the new health insurance reform law (USDHHS, 2010b). States were given the option to provide coverage to the uninsured with preexisting conditions. The federal government will likely also offer a national pool. State-supported risk pools will phase out in 2014 when private insurance companies will be forced to sell policies to the "medically uninsurable" (Varney, 2010).

Currently, the high-risk pools in most states are largely viewed as a failure. Premiums and deductibles are wildly expensive, and the policies have spending caps that are frequently exceeded. For example, the California plan is capped at 7100 members and often has a waiting list. The new federal health care law sets aside $5 billion to fund new high-risk programs that are more affordable and open to more people. Deborah Chollet, a health insurance expert at the nonpartisan research firm Mathematica, says people who apply to the new programs will pay a standard rate, or the rate they would pay for a policy if they did not have a preexisting condition that previously excluded them from coverage (Varney, 2010). Although extending coverage to the previously uninsurable is perhaps the best-known section of the new health care legislation, significant changes are under way for conventional employer-based insurance programs as well.

HEALTH CARE WORKFORCE SHORTAGES AND REFORM RESOLUTIONS

The U.S. faces steep health care challenges as the "baby boom" generation enters retirement and as health care reform increases demand for services. America's health care professionals directly influence the cost and quality of health care through their diagnoses, orders, prescriptions, and treatments. Analysts are projecting a nationwide shortage of as many as 100,000 to 200,000 physicians and 250,000 public health professionals by 2020 (Dill & Salsberg, 2008), and 260,000 nurses by 2025 (Buerhaus, 2009a). Rural Americans and those living in other underserved areas across the country are especially vulnerable to health workforce shortages.

While the nursing shortage has been long-standing, Buerhaus (2009b) notes that although it is temporary, the recession has eased the shortage of hospital nurses, but large shortages are still expected in the next decade. The initial findings from the 2008 HRSA (USDHHS, 2010a) national survey of registered nurses released in 2010 also reports that the number of licensed registered nurses in the U.S. increased to a new high of 3.1 million between 2004 and 2008 reflecting a 5% increase. The ability to meet the country's demand for nurses remains a daunting goal. Over the past decade, numerous initiatives to recruit more nurses into the profession have been launched, and many are successful. While interest today in a nursing career is growing, with almost 50,000 qualified applicants turned away in 2008, this increase in demand reveals the complex problem of a low supply of nursing faculty as a primary barrier in the education pipeline for preparing the numbers and types of nurses so badly needed (AACN, 2009).

As policy efforts are developed to assure an adequate health care workforce, the question is whether the problem is a shortage of health professionals overall, or is it only with the distribution of certain types of health professionals in certain areas of need? The answer is both. Assessing, projecting, and planning health workforce needs is complicated, and no single entity in the U.S. is in charge of workforce planning (Derksen & Whelan, 2009). The absence of a cohesive approach to workforce shortages, training of health professionals across disciplines, and distribution of health professionals to areas of need must be addressed if health care reform policy is to be successfully implemented.

The federal government pays for health care workforce development through funding of two broad training categories. The first and largest payment comes from Medicare and Medicaid, which provide support for Graduate Medical Education (GME) by subsidizing hospital training through add-on payments. Teaching hospitals are reimbursed to train physicians in residency programs and for hospital-based nursing diploma education. Today with only 7% of nurses receiving their education in a hospital-based setting, nurses receive little benefit from this funding stream. Combining the last data available from 2007, approximately $12 billion was provided in GME subsidies (Derksen & Whelan, 2009). Medicare still pays about $150 million per year to these hospitals for nurses' training (Livsey, 2007).

The second and more modest funding component is provided through Health Resources and Services Administration (HRSA), an agency in the

Department of Health and Human Services that administers health workforce programs. With a 2010 budget of $7.2 billion, HRSA programs train health care professionals and place them where they are most needed. Grants support scholarship and loan repayment programs at colleges and universities to meet critical workforce shortages and promote diversity within the health professions.

Congress and the Obama administration began addressing workforce shortage issues by allocating $500 million to workforce development from the 2009 American Recovery and Reinvestment Act (ARRA). $200 million went to programs authorized by Titles VII (Health Professions) and VIII (Nurse Training) of the Public Health Service Act to expand training and educational opportunities. These sections of the Act include primary care medicine and dentistry programs, public health and preventive medicine programs, and scholarship and loan repayment programs. Of the $80 million awarded to date, about half has gone to students, health professionals, and faculty from minority and disadvantaged backgrounds. The other $300 million is being used to increase the capacity of the National Health Service Corps (NHSC). The NHSC, which is authorized through PHSA Title III, provides scholarships and loan repayment to health professionals who agree to work in areas with too few health professionals. It is worth noting that historically, for every federal dollar spent on HRSA's primary care, nursing, and dental workforce programs, teaching hospitals were paid $24 by Medicare and Medicaid to subsidize physician training. This reflects the severe funding inequities, as physician education and hospitals are strongly supported with GME funds, and nursing and other health professionals are minimally funded by comparison through HRSA dollars. The final Health Care Reform legislation includes important changes to this chronic issue as graduate nurse education and postgraduate experience demonstrations will be funded through Medicare funds (Kaiser Family Foundation, 2010).

The Patient Protection and Affordable Care Act (P.L.111-148) provides long-term strategies for improving health care workforce shortages. The first broad strategy authorizes the establishment of a multi-stakeholder Workforce Advisory Committee to develop a national workforce strategy. The second strategy entails an expansion of Medicaid to fiscally pay for health promotion and disease prevention as well as increases in Medicare payments for primary care physicians. Likewise, the laws and regulations that govern GME funding will expand from the strict hospital-based setting to the use of outpatient settings for residency training, and it will give priority to states with the largest rural and underserved areas as well as to primary care and surgery providers. Teaching Health Centers will be established that will be eligible for Medicare payments for operating primary care residency programs in 2010.

Another health reform workforce initiative includes support for the development of training programs that focus on primary care models such as medical homes, team management of chronic diseases, and those that integrate physical and mental health services. This initiative has a 5-year authorization. A complementary initiative provides training to family nurse practitioners who provide primary care in federally qualified health centers and nurse-managed clinics, again a 5-year authorization. Not only are these initiatives authorized for longer periods of time providing stronger program evaluation, they represent a realignment of federal incentives for improving our nation's health workforce capacity and quality. As the federal government has been looking at health reform from a national perspective, states have been struggling with the same issues locally.

STATE-LEVEL HEALTH REFORM

The number of uninsured people varies considerably from state to state, ranging from 2.7% of the population in Massachusetts, according to state government data, to 25.2% in Texas, according to a 2008 Kaiser report on state health facts. The number of uninsured increased during the recession as people lost jobs and employer-sponsored health insurance. Concerned about the problem of limited health insurance, states have taken a number of steps to expand access to coverage, including expanding public programs like Medicaid and CHIP, to cover additional children and adults.

States' fiscal concerns have slowed down their efforts to provide access to health insurance for the uninsured. In 2008, nearly half the states faced budget gaps, and by 2009 the number rose to two-thirds. The state budget situation is grim and getting worse with each new revenue revision. As of December 2008, at least 10 states have imposed and another 10 are considering across-the-board budget cuts. Six states (Maryland, New Hampshire, New York, South Carolina, Utah, and Vermont) have been forced to cut their Medicaid budgets. Currently, 30 states have proposed health care reform legislation they will consider alongside the federal reform legislation (National Conference of State Legislatures [NCSL], 2010a, 2010b).

The Commonwealth Fund Commission's report, the *2009 State Scorecard on U.S. Health System Performance* (2009), examines trends on state's progress toward achieving systems and models of health care that meet their residents' needs.

This report examines how states compare on 38 key indicators of health care access, quality, costs, and health outcomes. The findings of the report conclude that these indicators vary significantly depending on the state you live in. The scorecard findings reflect deteriorating coverage for adults and rising costs with broad geographic disparities and strong evidence of poorly coordinated care.

In 2009, Vermont, Hawaii, Iowa, Minnesota, Maine, and New Hampshire lead the nation as the top-ranked states in terms of performance. Patterns indicate that when public policies and state and local health care systems are aligned, individual states have the capacity to do much better. Vermont, Maine, and Massachusetts have enacted comprehensive reforms to expand coverage and put in place initiatives to improve population health and benchmark providers on quality. Minnesota is a leader in bringing public and private-sector stakeholders together in collaborative initiatives to improve the overall value of health care. Unfortunately, even these leading states face the problem of escalating health care costs (The Commonwealth Fund, 2009).

While other viable models are emerging at the state level, early attempts from Massachusetts and Vermont have received national attention and demonstrate the promise of innovative state reform efforts that are attempting to improve access while actively evaluating cost-effectiveness and quality changes.

HEALTH CARE QUALITY AND PATIENT SAFETY

The U.S. continues to spend more on health care than any other nation, yet numerous studies have found that there is no relationship between spending and the quality of care. The Institute of Medicine's Quality Initiative, launched in 1996, was a tipping point in collective learning about and acknowledging how poor the U.S. Health Care system was actually functioning. Documentation of the serious nature and high costs of hospital errors on human health and safety became a foundation for clinical practice reform (Institute of Medicine, 2001). Dougherty and Conway (2008) advocate a three-prong approach to transforming the quality of U.S. health care: translate scientific research into clinical practice, develop patient-specific evidence for effectiveness ("the right treatment for the right patient in the right way at the right time"), and make the policy changes necessary to improve population health (p. 2319).

While the value of decreasing error in caring for patients is supported by all health care professionals, the hidden and hierarchical culture in health care was one of fear, and to report error was to risk public "shame and blame." One legislative response to this critical issue in American health care was the passage of the 2005 Patient Safety and Quality Improvement Act. The Act established increased protection for reporting medical errors. As this culture shift supports the value for acknowledging errors and "near misses," and tools are developed to guide learning, a foundation is laid for a healthy inquiry into examining all clinical practice from a safety and quality point of view. Indeed, a paradigm shift from fear to accountability for medical professionals has certainly become a more consistent reality (Wachter & Pronovost, 2009). Health care quality has made significant headway as evidence-based practice has become an accepted standard for health care delivery and multiple institutions across the country guide the development for continual improvement. The Agency for Healthcare Research and Quality (AHRQ) a two-decade–old agency within HHS, was among the first to emphasize evidence-based practice. The AHRQ now provides 17 toolkits for multidisciplinary clinical professionals to address patient safety at the point of care in hospitals and outpatient settings, during consumer self-care, and for informal caregivers.

In terms of federal priorities in quality care, the Recovery and Reinvestment Act allocated $1.1 billion for comparative effectiveness research (CER), systematic research that compares different interventions and strategies to prevent, diagnose, treat, and monitor health conditions. Clinical effectiveness research is defined as a rigorous evaluation of the impact of different options that are available for treating a given medical condition for a particular set of patients. Such options are commonly drugs and surgery. Interest in CER has been spurred by ever-rising health care costs and the persistent nagging evidence of unexplained variations in clinical practice, which was first identified across large geographic regions in the Dartmouth Health Care Atlas and is now increasingly recognized in units as small as individual practices. However, there is controversy. Although some health professionals see such research as desired and even necessary given the current economic crisis and rise in health care spending, others fear a slippery slope leading to inflexible coverage decisions and even explicit rationing (Pentecost, 2009). This tension reflects the ongoing ambivalence regarding the changes that will be brought about through health care reform.

MEDICAL TECHNOLOGIES

While health care technology has had a pronounced effect on the growth in health spending, it has also yielded major improvements in quality and cost-effectiveness. Health care reform legislation will invest $24 billion for computerizing medical records. Audio-visual telemedicine using video-chat technology, which in recent years has replaced telephone-only formats, has already been credited with increased stroke evaluations in rural households; those using the technology report a 96% accuracy rate in diagnosis and treatment (Mayo Clinic, 2010). The benefits to making medical information electronic lie not only in improved treatment options but also in more immediate and convenient communication between clinicians, lowered costs of transferring and maintaining records, and minimized communication errors (Adams, 2010). The cost-reductive impact of telemedicine is felt across all major sectors of current health care spending and is particularly well-positioned to reduce expenditures in hospital and home care, which combined, represent 41 cents of every health care dollar (Hartman, Martin, McDonnell, Catlin; National Health Expenditure Accounts Team, 2009).

Older health care professionals, like many older Americans, are often slow or late adopters in the use of technology. The Health Information Technology for Economic and Clinical Health (HITECH) provisions within the Recovery Act of 2009 include physician penalties for non-adoption (lowered Medicare payments by 2015), yet economists estimate that the financial incentives offered to physicians in the $28 billion stimulus will far outweigh any potential non-compliance fees (Adams, 2010).

One continuing concern plaguing the speedy adoption of new health care technologies is privacy. However, ample privacy protections were written heavily into the 2008 medical records bill (H.R. 6357), which required the HHS Secretary to author an informed-consent agreement for all Americans whose data will eventually be digitalized (Armstrong & Nylen, 2008). Miller and Tucker (2009) found that in states where privacy regulations are at odds with the new federal medical records guidelines, aggregate electronic medical record (EMR) adoption by hospitals is reduced by 24%, a critically discouraging number given the minimal nationwide 25% EMR adoption goal of H.R. 6357. There are working models available to suggest the efficacy of an EMR/EHR program. Kaiser Permanente already has a linked electronic network of over 14,000 physicians that can access and share records, citing their "better management" practices as the basis for their claim that Kaiser patients have a 30% lower chance of dying from heart failure than members of the general population (Carey, 2008). Furthermore, the NIH Public Access Policy (revised in 2009), stating that the public has online open access to the results of all NIH-funded research via PubMed Central (PMC), sets a precedent for electronic and transparent transmission of health information that may loosen the tight grip of secrecy surrounding the availability, authority, and accessibility of health information in the U.S.

However, processes of communication, publication, and dissemination must continually be revisited to ensure that cutting-edge research and relevant results are reaching the at-risk populations most in need of clinical guidance. The battle between paper-based and electronic medical records may not be one of consent or even of funding, but rather one between the status quo and uncertainties of overhauling an institutionally entrenched records system. Recent information from the CDC suggests an increase in consumer use of the Internet to access health information and contact health care providers, signaling a

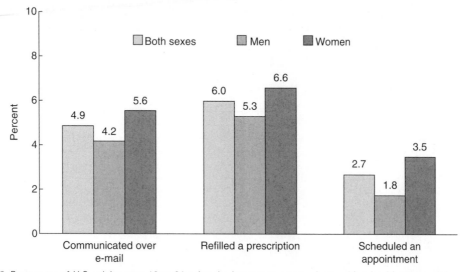

FIGURE 63-2 Percentage of U.S. adults ages 18 to 64 using the Internet to communicate with a health care provider, January-June 2009. (Source: Centers for Disease Control and Prevention [2009]. Retrieved from *www.cdc.gov/nchs/data/hestat/healthinfo2009/healthinfo2009.htm.*)

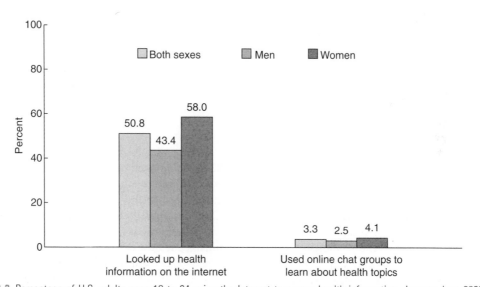

FIGURE 63-3 Percentage of U.S. adults ages 18 to 64 using the Internet to access health information, January-June 2009. (Source: Centers for Disease Control and Prevention [2009]. Retrieved from *www.cdc.gov/nchs/data/hestat/healthinfo2009/healthinfo2009.htm.*)

potential change in the norms of information access and distribution across the health care system (Figures 63-2 and 63-3).

Perhaps a more troubling issue for some bioethicists and critics of EMR are the developing national "biobanks" of medical information, in which genetic data is collected and analyzed for future disease prospects and susceptibilities. NIH is currently in the process of determining who will have access to large national databases of medical and genetic information and navigating the increasingly murky pool of private-interest database competitors such as Kaiser (Adams, 2010). As the value for technology continues to yield major improvements in quality and can be cost-effective, prevention has become a priority value as key to high quality and high cost savings.

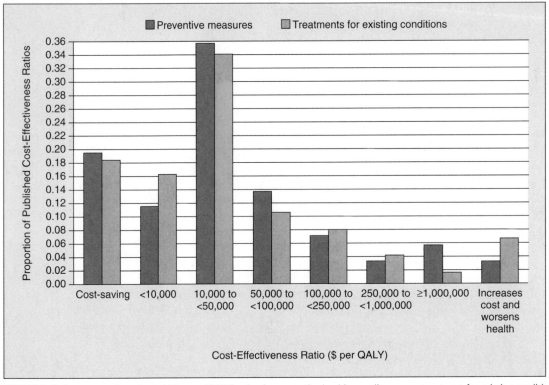

FIGURE 63-4 Dollars per quality-adjusted life-year (QALY) ratios for preventive health spending versus treatment for existing conditions. (Source: Cohen, J. T., Neumann, P. J., & Weinstein, M. C. [2008]. Does preventive care save money? Health economics and the presidential candidates. *New England Journal of Medicine, 358,* 661-663.)

PREVENTIVE HEALTH AND OBESITY

Nearly half of all cases of mortality in the U.S. are linked to social, environmental, and behavioral factors, including poor diet, sedentary lifestyle, substance use, and accidents. The relationship between these interacting spheres of risk and influence is dynamic and intentional and must be a stronger focus in national disease prevention and health promotion efforts. About 1 in 5 preventable deaths in the U.S. are attributable to tobacco use and high blood pressure, with obesity and physical inactivity responsible for another 1 in 10 (Danaei et al., 2009). With obesity and diabetes rates reaching unprecedented proportions, heart disease is on the rise, particularly among women, and comorbidities such as depression complicate the psychosocial experience of chronic disease; it is no surprise that public health discussions have recently returned to the power of prevention.

Studies suggest that as much as one third of the $2.1 trillion spent annually on health care does not actually improve health or prevent disease (Carey, 2008). Furthermore, De Lissovoy and colleagues (2009) estimated the surmountable costs to the U.S. economy of several chronic and acute medical conditions, concluding also that investment in preventive care and reorganization at several levels of the health care system would significantly reduce both direct and indirect costs (Figures 63-4 and 63-5).

Symptom-based and prevention-based health care are continually at odds, both in terms of resource allocation and evidence-based policy strategy. Whether health professionals should focus on controlling symptoms or preempting them is contested territory for policymakers and clinicians alike. The U.S. Preventive Services Task Force estimates that counseling adults to quit smoking, get screened for colorectal cancer, and get a flu shot could significantly reduce the 900,000 annual deaths categorized as

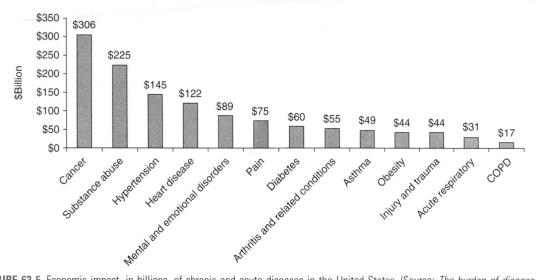

FIGURE 63-5 Economic impact, in billions, of chronic and acute diseases in the United States. (Source: *The burden of disease: The economic case for investment in quality improvement and medical progress—A literature review and synthesis*, Center for Health Economics and Science Policy, United BioSource, August 14, 2009.)

"preventable" at a net savings under current health care cost estimates (Cohen et al., 2008). Cost-effectiveness models examining the effects of preventive care measure outcomes in quality-adjusted life-years (QALY) consistently report positive results from relatively minor investments. Critics deriding prevention commonly misconceive that proponents think any intervention will cut costs and improve health; rather, the challenge facing health professionals today is identifying which resources must be deployed, through which delivery systems, and with what outcomes measures.

OBESITY-PREVENTION CARE WILL BE CRITICAL

Overweight and obesity prevalence are on the rise among all population sectors and all ages. According to two recent studies analyzing the biomedical samples of the 2007-2008 National Health and Nutrition Examination Survey (NHANES), 33.8% of adults and 16% of school-age children are obese (Gaziano 2010; Halfon, 2010). Few health problems afflict more people yet garner less clinical attention: one third of obese adults have never asked or been asked by their doctors about exercise (AHRQ, 2010). Comparatively, America's obesity rate is a full 6%

higher than the next most-obese nation (Mexico), with a rate nearly 10 times higher than those of Japan and South Korea (Organisation for Economic Co-operation and Development, 2009). The reality now is that Americans are more likely to be overweight than to pay their federal income tax (The Economist, 2010).

Many health care professionals liken the obesity epidemic to the tobacco crisis that plagued the latter half of the twentieth century. With expansive and expensive federal intervention, the proportion of U.S. adults who smoke fell from 42.4% in 1965 to less than 20% in 2007. Advocates claim that using similar strategies with comparable levels of federal and private funding will do the same for obesity prevalence over the next few decades (Englehard, Garson, & Dorn, 2009). These strategies include taxing "obesogenic" foods, simplifying nutritional information on food packaging, requiring restaurants to post nutrition information on menus, and limiting the amount of advertising for unhealthy or "junk" foods, and many of them have already been implemented at the state level (Englehard et al., 2009). Early efforts are making some inroads. Adult obesity rates have recently steadied, with no increase in obesity for American women from 1998 to 2008 and no increase for men from 2005 to 2008 (Gaziano, 2010).

Policy action regarding childhood obesity, a rate still on the rise, emerged in 2009 as a top priority for the Obama administration. The administration plans to reevaluate both the National School Lunch program as well as the Child Nutrition and WIC Reauthorization Act, with First Lady Michelle Obama launching her "Let's Move" initiative in 2009 to bring healthy foods to underserved areas, educate parents about healthy eating, serve healthier foods in schools, and increase physical activity among American youth (for more information, visit *letsmove.gov*). Furthermore, President Obama issued a memo on February 9, 2010, establishing an interagency Childhood Obesity Task Force set to "solve the problem of childhood obesity within a generation" (Obama, 2010).

Mirroring efforts to curb tobacco use in the 1980s and 1990s, public health efforts to address obesity include multilevel programs addressing individual behaviors, family and home environments, child care settings and schools, and worksites and medical communities. The proposed solutions vary in cost and scope; however, government subsidies for healthy foods; limits on advertising and distribution of unhealthy foods; and incentivizing healthy habits, recreational facilities, and community health infrastructures are paramount.

The necessity of partnerships between individual leadership, community activism, and government aid is evident; however, the political climate surrounding public health interventions is tumultuous. Kersh and Marone (2005) locate diseases like obesity alongside other contested health issues, such as tobacco use and the right to die, where the lines between public and private rights are blurred and the role of the courts and the government remains unclear. A recent study comparing public opinion about different anti-obesity initiatives suggests that 68% of Americans favor fresh food policies for public schools, 66% favor zoning laws requiring adequate recreational space in new developments, 37% support paid leave for exercise and employer-subsidized gym memberships, and less than 25% are in favor of graded insurance premiums based on weight status (Barry, Brescoll, Brownell, & Schlesinger, 2009). Nurses, physicians, and other health professionals must talk about obesity with patients in a way that is both clinically and personally relevant, while supporting initiatives to raise community awareness of the disease and its long-term effects.

BIOTERRORISM: THREATS AND PREPAREDNESS

Despite the predominance of competing health care issues including access to health care, rising pharmaceutical costs, insurance coverage, and Medicare expenditures, bioterrorism remains on the minds of policymakers and Americans alike. Following the attacks of September 11, 2001, *bioterrorism* became a priority on the national agenda with the first "Amerithrax" *(Bacillus anthracis)* scare. The scope and magnitude of a potential outbreak of chemical, biological, or nuclear aggression must, of course, be balanced with the immediate health care concerns listed earlier in the chapter in terms of resource allocation, preparedness efforts, staffing, and information dissemination.

In the U.S. the Centers for Disease Control and Prevention (CDC), the Department of Defense, the Federal Emergency Management Agency, the U.S. Public Health Service Commissioned Corps (PHS), and the Health Resources and Services Administration (HRSA) maintain comprehensive preparation plans in the event of a bioterrorist attack. For almost 25 years prior to the 2001 attacks, no large-scale investments had been made in the broader public health infrastructure. In response to perceived and actual threats, the federal government has since directed billions of dollars to shore up the nation's ability to prevent and respond to terrorist attacks, beginning with an infusion of, and continuing annual appropriations of over $40 billion. National security advocates emphasize the necessity of increased funding for a variety of medical countermeasures for potential bioterrorist attack. These measures, include those that detect, identify, prevent, or mitigate the health effects of biologic agents, were initially funded in a series of legislation from 2002 to 2006 (notably the Project Bioshield Act of 2004; Pandemic and All-Hazards Preparedness Act of 2006, and Bioterrorism Act of 2002) in an attempt to increase stockpiles and develop large-scale response plans in the case of bioterrorist activity (Maher & Lushniak, 2009). Liability concerns and access to unapproved countermeasures remain a threat to the success of bioterrorism initiatives.

President Obama's four-prong plan for biosecurity (i.e., prevent bioterrorist attacks with U.S. intelligence; build capacities to mitigate the consequences of bioterrorist attacks; accelerate the development of new medicines, vaccines, and production capabilities; and lead an international effort to diminish the impact of major infectious disease epidemics) suggests compliance with previous administrations' efforts in this area (O'Toole & Inglesby, 2009). Whether federal, state, and local preparedness efforts will be enough to combat the ever-changing technologies of bioterrorism is paramount; however, shifting social paradigms surrounding public health, weapons, and warfare also affect understandings of and responses to potential infectious attacks. As long as the public feels threatened by terrorist attacks, there will be urgent competition in public health priorities. The clear challenge is to avoid strengthening one focus at the expense of the other.

Presently, research agendas regarding bioterrorism are heavily subsidized by NIH and the CDC; however, experts believe that federal interests must be supplemented by private funding to effectively stockpile ample amounts of antidotes for potential infectious agents (Rubinson et al., 2005). In the event of a large-scale bioterrorist attack, clinical professionals must be prepared to dedicate local and regional planning time to bioterrorism preparedness from citizen to clinician, articulate reasonable expectations regarding the availability and use of federal aid, and develop a sound budget for the information technologies and legislative remedies necessary to administer large-scale emergency efforts.

Margaret Hamburg (1999), current commissioner of the Food and Drug Administration and former commissioner of health for the City of New York during the events of 9/11, believes "the public is key" in responding to public health emergencies, and emphasizes that "communication is vital" in "achieving a level of understanding that can form the foundation for sharing information and developing knowledge when a crisis occurs." A reassessment of public health infrastructures along with citizen education, health care professional planning, and adequate funding for bioterrorism preparedness initiatives are necessary to move toward a more comprehensive national security system. Nurses, often the first points of contact in disease surveillance and recognition, are poised to activate formal and informal networks in the case of a bioterrorist attack and mobilize community partnerships to help moderate the potential damages of such events (Akins, Williams, Silenas, & Edwards, 2005).

SUMMARY

Progress is uneven, but the general trend is clear; health care reform is moving forward and will change the U.S. health care system. The landmark legislation enacted by the 111th U.S. Congress will provide complex challenges for reformers in implementing these policies. While this initial health reform legislation may not go far enough for many, historically programs like Medicare and Medicaid, which passed with a limited payment structure, have improved over time. The combined health care legislation will extend coverage to an estimated 30 million uninsured Americans. Health reformers would argue that the bill is a start on cost control. Reinhardt (2010) suggests that if we want to have cost containment, it must be done rationally. More research is needed on bundling payments and comparative effectiveness. Effective quality and cost controls can occur as funding for healthcare workforce shortages is implemented and we see the results of health systems research improving care delivery. The scope of policy implementation will be extensive.

Nurses are important partners in shaping this new health care system. In reflecting on the journey that led to health care reform, we must appreciate how the interdependence of politics, global and local economics, past failures, diverse perspectives, shared values, and multiple avenues of communication shape the process and outcome. Policy change occurs through the influence of continual debate to find common ground and common goals. To lead in shaping a new health care delivery system, nurses need to *think both locally and globally.* Policy is more than politics, but politics are required. Therefore, our involvement is required. Connecting the interdependence of health care policy to other policy issues and understanding the interdependency within and across professions, as well as consumer perceptions, can open us to new possibilities and successes. Change is coming; rather than resisting it, we must embrace and influence it for the greater good.

For a list of related websites, please refer to your Evolve Resources at http://evolve.elsevier.com/Mason/policypolitics/

REFERENCES

Adams, R. (2010, February 1). IT plan called too much, too soon. *CQ Weekly*, 271.

Agency for Healthcare Research and Quality (AHRQ). (2010, April 13). Annual quality and disparities reports include data on rates of health care-associated infections, Obesity and Health Insurance (press release). Retrieved from www.ahrq.gov/news/press/pr2010/qrdr09pr.htm.

Akins, R. B., Williams, J. R., Silenas, R., & Edwards, J. C. (2005). The role of public health nurses in bioterrorism preparedness. *Disaster Management Response*, 3(4), 98-105.

American Association of Colleges of Nursing (AACN). (2009, September). *Fact sheet: Nursing shortage*. Retrieved from www.aacn.nche.edu/media/factsheets/nursingshortage.htm.

Armstrong, D., & Nylen, L. (2008, July 28). Measure aimed at increasing use of electronic health care records. *CQ Weekly*, 2063.

Baker, K. (2009, July). Barack Hoover Obama. *Harper's Magazine*, 319(1910), 9-37.

Barry, C. L., Brescoll, V. L., Brownell, K. D., & Schlesinger, M. (2009). Obesity metaphors: How beliefs about the causes of obesity affect support for public policy. *The Milbank Quarterly*, 87(1), 7-47.

Begley, S. (2009, August 15). *Attack! The truth about Obamacare*. Retrieved August 24, 2009, from www.newsweek.com/id/212131.

Buerhaus, P. I. (2009a). The recent survey in nurse employment: Causes and implications. *Health Affairs*, 28(4), w657-w668.

Buerhaus, P. I. (2009b, May/June). Massachusetts health care reform: Lessons for the nation? *Nursing Economics*. Retrieved from http://findarticles.com/p/articles/mi_m0FSW/is_3_27/ai_n31974421.

Carey, M. A. (2008, November 17). A battery of tests for health concepts. *CQ Weekly*, 3092.

Cauchi, R. (2010, April 13). *State legislation challenging certain health reforms, 2010*. Retrieved from www.ncsl.org/?tabid=18906.

Cohen, J. T., Neumann, P. J., & Weinstein, M. C. (2008). Does preventive care save money? Health economics and the presidential candidates. *New England Journal of Medicine*, 358, 661-663.

The Commonwealth Fund. (2009, October). Aiming higher: Results from a state scorecard on health system performance, 2009. The Commonwealth Fund Commission on a High Performance Health System.

Danaei, G., Ding, E. L., Mozaffarian, D., Taylor, B., Rehm, J., et al. (2009). The preventable causes of death in the United States: Comparative risk assessments of dietary, lifestyle, and metabolic risk factors. *PLoS Med*, 6(4), e1000058.

De Lissovoy, G., Pan, F., Siak, S., Hutchins, V., & Luce, B. (2009, August 14). *The burden of disease: The economic case for investment in quality improvement and medical progress*. Bethesda, MD: United BioSource.

Derksen, D. J., & Whelan, E. (2009, December). *Closing the health care workforce gap: Reforming federal health care workforce policies to meet the needs of the 21st century*. Washington, D.C.: Center for American Progress.

Dill, M. J., & Salsberg, E. (2008). The complexities of physician supply and demand. Washington Association of American Colleges Center for Workforce Studies, 2008. Retrieved from https://services.aamc.org/publications/index.cfm?fuseaction=Product.displayForm&prd_id=244.

Dougherty, D., & Conway, P. H. (2008). The "3Ts" road map to transform U.S. health care. *Journal of the American Medical Association*, 299(19), 2319-2321.

The Economist. (2010, January 21). The fat plateau (Web log message). Retrieved from www.economist.com/world/united-states/displaystory.cfm?story_id=15330562.

Englehard, C. L., Garson, A., & Dorn, S. (2009, July). *Reducing obesity: Policy strategies from the tobacco wars*. Washington, D.C.: Urban Institute.

Fletcher, P. (2010, April 7). *Florida says challenge to healthcare reform widens*. Retrieved from www.reuters.com/article/idUSTRE6363NL20100407?feedType=RSS&feedName=everything&virtualBrandChannel=11563.

Gaziano, J. M. (2010). Fifth phase of the epidemiologic transition. *Journal of the American Medical Association*, 303(3), 275-276.

Gawande, A. (2009, January 26). *Getting there from here: How should Obama reform health care?* Retrieved from www.newyorker.com/reporting/2009/01/26/090126fa_fact_gawande.

Halfon, N. (2010). Evolving notions of childhood chronic illness. *Journal of the American Medical Association*, 303(7), 665-666.

Hamburg, M. (1999). Addressing bioterrorist threats: Where do we go from here? *Emerging Infectious Diseases*, 5(4), 200.

Hartman, M., Martin, A., McDonnell, P., Catlin A.; National Health Expenditure Accounts Team. (2009). National health spending in 2007: Slower drug spending contributes to lowest rate of overall growth since 1998. *Health Affairs*, 28(1), 246-261.

Institute of Medicine. (2001). *Crossing the quality chasm: A new health system for the twenty-first century*. Washington D.C.: The National Academies Press.

Jost, T. S. (2010). Can the states nullify health care reform? *New England Journal of Medicine*, 362(10), 869-871.

Kaiser Family Foundation. (2010, April 8). Side-by-side comparison of major health care reform proposals. Retrieved April 15, 2010, from www.kff.org/healthreform/sidebyside.cfm.

Kersh, R., & Marone, J. A. (2005). Obesity, courts, and the new politics of public health. *Journal of Health Politics, Policy, and Law*, 30(5), 839-868.

Klein, E. (2009, December 26). The rise of the filibuster: An interview with Barbara Sinclair. *The Washington Post*. Retrieved from http://voices.washingtonpost.com/ezra-klein/2009/12/the_right_of_the_filibuster_an.html.

Klein, E. (2010, April 5). Welcome to smallville. *Newsweek*.

Livsey, K. R. (2007). Yesterday, today and tomorrow: Challenges in securing federal support for graduate nursing education. *Journal of Nursing Education*, 46(4), 176-183.

Maher, C., & Lushniak, B. D. (2009). Availability of medical countermeasures for bioterrorism events: U.S. legal and regulatory options. *Clinical Pharmacology & Therapeutics*, 85(6), 669-671.

Mayo Clinic. (2010, March 17). Telemedicine leads to better stroke evaluations in rural areas. Retrieved from www.mayoclinic.org/news2010-sct/5704.html.

Miller, A. R., & Tucker, C. (2009). Privacy protection and technology diffusion: The case of electronic medical records. *Management Science*, 55(7), 1077-1093.

National Conference of State Legislatures. (NCSL). (2010a, January). Access to health care: State legislation 2009. Retrieved from www.ncsl.org/Default.aspx?TabId=14516.

National Conference of State Legislatures. (NCSL). (2010b, April 14). Health reform is public law. Retrieved from www.ncsl.org/?tabid=17639.

Newport, F. (2010, March 30). *Americans remain concerned about costs of healthcare bill*. Retrieved from www.gallup.com/poll/127037/americans-remain-concerned-costs-healthcare-bill.aspx.

Obama, B. (2010, February 9). Memorandum for the heads of executive departments and agencies: Establishing a task force on childhood obesity. Retrieved from www.whitehouse.gov/the-press-office/presidential-memorandum-establishing-a-task-force-childhood-obesity.

Organisation for Economic Co-operation and Development. (2009, November). OECD health data 2009: Risk factors [Data file and code book]. Retrieved from www.oecd.org/document/16/0,2340,en_2649_34631_2085200_1_1_1_1,00.html.

O'Toole, T., & Inglesby, T. (2009). Biosecurity memos to the Obama administration. *Biosecurity and Bioterrorism: Biodefense Strategy, Practice, and Science*, 7(1), 25-28.

Pentecost, M. J. (2009, August). Comparative effectiveness research. *Journal of the American College of Radiology*, 6(8), 547-548.

Reinhardt, U. E. (2010, February 19). Once more, health care cost control. Retrieved from http://economix.blogs.nytimes.com/2010/02/19/once-more-health-care-cost-control.

Rubinson, L., Nuzzo, J. B., Talmor, D. S., O'Toole, T., Kramer, B. R., & Inglesby, T. V. (2005). Augmentation of hospital critical care capacity after bioterrorist acts of epidemics: Recommendations of the working group on emergency mass critical care. *Critical Care Medicine*, *33*(10), 2393-2403.

Stolberg, S. G., & Pear, R. (2010, March 24). Obama signs health care overhaul bill, with a flourish. *The New York Times*, A19.

U.S. Department of Health and Human Services (HHS). (2010a, March 17). *Initial findings: 2008 sample survey of registered nurses.* Retrieved from http://bhpr.hrsa.gov/healthworkforce/rnsurvey/initialfindings2008.pdf.

U.S. Department of Health and Human Services (HHS). (2010b, April 6). *Sebelius remarks: Health reform and you: How the new law will increase your health security.* Retrieved from www.hhs.gov/news/press/2010pres/04/20100406b.html.

Varney, S. (2010, April 15). New health law expands high-risk coverage. Retrieved from www.npr.org/templates/story/story.php?storyId=125600156.

Wachter, R. M., & Pronovost, P. J. (2009). Balancing "no blame" with accountability in patient safety. *New England Journal of Medicine*, *361*(14), 1401-1406.

www.Recovery.gov. (2010).

CHAPTER 64

How Government Works: What You Need to Know to Influence the Process

Karrie Cummings Hendrickson, Christine Ceccarelli, and Sally S. Cohen

"What government is the best? That which teaches us to govern ourselves."

—Wolfgang von Goethe

Nurses need to know how government works so that they can convince public officials to create policies that improve access to quality and affordable health care for all. This chapter provides an overview of the federal, state, and local levels of government, how each level works, and the relationships among them in a federalist system. Such information is essential to effect policy and bring nurses' unique perspective to those who make the final decisions—legislators, regulators, and staff who support them. Because budget policies underlie all health policy issues, this chapter also reviews the federal budget process and related state and local processes. All health programs require funding, and the budget process is the means by which the executive and legislative branches reconcile competing priorities and make budgetary decisions. In this chapter, we identify key access points for influencing policy at different levels and branches of government and throughout the federal budget process. We have used the issue of long-term care to demonstrate why nurses need to know how government works.

FEDERALISM: MULTIPLE LEVELS OF RESPONSIBILITY

The United States government is a federalist system. Simply stated, this means that the government consists of multiple levels, including both a centralized, national tier and at least one decentralized, subnational tier, and that power is shared among them. In the case of the United States, tiers include the federal, state, and local levels of government. Unlike a unitary state, a federalist system constitutionally divides sovereignty among the different governmental levels so that the policymakers at each level have final authority in some areas and can act efficiently and independently of each other. The U.S. Constitution divides governmental authority by prescribing the duties and responsibilities of the federal government and withholding both specified and unspecified powers for the states. The Tenth Amendment to the Constitution (also known as the State's Rights Amendment), ratified in 1791, helps to clarify how this authority is divided among the levels of government. It states, "The powers not delegated to the United States by the Constitution, nor prohibited by it to the States, are reserved to the States respectively, or to the people." This means that states have jurisdiction over issues that the Constitution does not explicitly grant to the federal government. This is a fundamental aspect of the Constitution; state policymakers often interpret their constitutional states' rights quite liberally.

Because the U.S. government is one of divided powers, citizens are accountable to three levels of authority. In a federalist system, the allocation of authority among the levels may vary over time, and successful state initiatives may eventually become national policy as part of the "marble cake federalism" of the U.S. (Nathan, 2006). Alternately, the federal government may participate in and influence local policy through government grants, sanctions, and federal mandates (federal requirements for state, local, or tribal governments to expend their own resources to achieve certain goals) (Hanson, 2004). Finally, many powers, such as taxation and law formation and enforcement, are shared equally among the levels of government and may be exercised in conjunction or independently. For more information on federalism and associated court cases, see the Rockefeller Institute website provided with the Web Resources on this book's Evolve website.

Because governmental powers and responsibilities laid out in the Constitution are imprecise and subject to interpretation, some controversy and conflict has occurred among all the levels of government, most particularly between federal and state authorities (Hanson, 2004). The U.S. Supreme Court, however, works to interpret the Constitution and maintain the balance of power among the levels of government (Hanson, 2004). It is important to understand the court's stand on federalism and states' rights when designing a federally administered program and planning its implementation. Court decisions may affect when, how, and by whom your program is implemented (see Chapter 7).

THE FEDERAL GOVERNMENT

The U.S. federal government is centered in Washington, D.C., and has 10 regional offices. These regional offices are instrumental in policy implementation and enhance access to federal officials for issues concerning health and well-being. Like the three levels of government, the three branches of the federal government represent a separation of powers and work as a series of checks and balances on one another. These branches require policymakers to work together to formulate policy that is acceptable to as many people as possible, and they are designed to prevent any individual or small group from making sweeping changes. For more information on the roles and powers of the federal government, see the U.S. Government's Official Web Portal website listed in Web Resources.

THE EXECUTIVE BRANCH

The role of the executive branch of the federal government is to implement laws and oversee their enforcement. The executive branch is made up of the Executive Office of the President (EOP); the Executive Cabinet; and many independent agencies, boards, committees, and commissions, the staffs of which

---

BOX 64-1 Obama Administration Offices and Agencies of the EOP

Council of Economic Advisors: *www.whitehouse.gov/administration/eop/cea*

Council on Environmental Quality: *www.whitehouse.gov/administration/eop/ceq*

The National Security Council: *www.whitehouse.gov/administration/eop/nsc*

Office of Administration: *www.whitehouse.gov/administration/eop/oa*

Office of Science & Technology Policy: *www.whitehouse.gov/administration/eop/ostp*

Office of Management and Budget: *www.whitehouse.gov/omb*

Office of the U.S. Trade Representative: *www.ustr.gov*

Office of National Drug Control Policy: *www.whitehousedrugpolicy.gov*

Office of the Vice President: *www.whitehouse.gov/about/vp-residence*

The White House Office

The Executive Residence

---

both advise the president and help to oversee the programs. Both the EOP and the Cabinet will be discussed here.

Executive Office of the President (EOP). The EOP consists of the president, the vice president, and related White House offices and agencies (Box 64-1) that develop and implement the policy and programs of the president. Of these offices, the Office of Management and Budget (OMB) is one of the most relevant to nursing. This office prepares the president's budget for presentation to Congress on the first Monday of every February. The budget reflects the president's national agenda and provides those seeking to influence policy a realistic picture of the likelihood of their project receiving funding. It also serves as a potential access point for policy change.

The president is the highest ranking elected federal official and serves as the head of the executive branch. The president also serves as the commander in chief of all U.S. military forces, and with the approval of the Senate, grants pardons, makes treaties, and appoints high-ranking officials such as Supreme Court justices and cabinet secretaries. One of the president's most notable domestic powers, however, is the veto, which effectively stops (or at least delays) a newly passed piece of legislation from becoming a law. This power is not to be taken lightly because, if the president invokes the veto, it can only be overridden by a two-thirds majority vote in both houses of Congress.

Of key importance to those hoping to influence policy are the powers of the president not defined in the Constitution, including the power to set the national agenda. This is sometimes referred to as "the power of the pulpit." Newly elected presidents bring their priority issues to the forefront of the American political agenda. Even though this may not result in policy change, it does open the door for discussion and debate of some issues and closes the door on others. For example, at the beginning of his presidency, President George W. Bush's proposals regarding Social Security, Medicare prescription drug coverage, and homeland security were high on the public and policy agendas. But the election of President Barack Obama in 2008 shifted emphasis away from those issues and onto discussions of revitalizing the domestic and worldwide economies, ending the war in Iraq, and providing universal health care. A savvy activist must be aware of policymakers' priorities and anticipate how changes in the political climate following an election may affect the politics of health policymaking.

White House staff are influential in setting national agendas and disseminating the president's priorities. These individuals are appointed by the president, but are not confirmed by Congress. Thus, they usually hold views similar to those of the president and are instrumental in White House decision-making. One can determine White House staff perspectives on health policy through newspaper and other media reports. For more information on the federal executive branch, see the U.S. Executive Branch websites listed in Web Resources.

The Cabinet. The Executive Cabinet is made up of the heads of 15 departments (see the President's Cabinet websites listed in Web Resources). After confirmation by Congress, cabinet members work with the president and oversee the enforcement and administration of federal law through regulation and the appropriation of funds. Although all cabinet departments may have jurisdiction over areas of interest to nurses, the ones most relevant to nursing practice are discussed next.

The Department of Health and Human Services (HHS). According to their website

---

> **BOX 64-2 The 11 Agencies Included in the Department of Health and Human Services**
>
> Centers for Medicare and Medicaid Services:
> www.cms.hhs.gov
> Centers for Disease Control and Prevention: www.cdc.gov
> Food and Drug Administration: www.fda.gov
> Indian Health Service: www.ihs.gov
> Administration for Children and Families: www.acf.hhs.gov
> Administration on Aging: www.aoa.gov
> Agency on Toxic Substances and Disease:
> www.atsdr.cdc.gov
> Health Resources and Services Administration:
> www.hrsa.gov
> Office of the Inspector General: www.oig.hhs.gov
> Substance Abuse and Mental Health Service
> Administration: www.samhsa.gov
> National Institutes of Health: www.nih.gov
> Agency for Healthcare Research and Quality:
> www.ahrq.gov

(www.hhs.gov), the HHS is "the United States government's principal agency for protecting the health of all Americans and providing essential human services, especially for those who are least able to help themselves." To accomplish this mission, HHS incorporates the Office of the Secretary as well as 11 agencies (Box 64-2) that oversee more than 300 programs such as Head Start, Vaccines for Children, Medicare, and Medicaid. HHS is responsible for the distribution of the second largest portion of federal budget. New programs or changes to existing programs advocated by health professionals will likely be overseen by HHS. Therefore, it is vital to understand its structure and functions. For more information on HHS, see the websites listed in Web Resources.

The Social Security Administration (SSA). Economic security for most retired workers age 65 or older in the U.S. is guaranteed through Social Security, funded through payroll contributions. The SSA also provides monthly benefits to permanently disabled workers who have contributed to the program, as well as Supplemental Security Income (SSI) payments to needy elderly, blind, and disabled individuals. Participation in the program also enables elderly and disabled individuals to qualify for Medicare health coverage, currently administered by CMS (see Chapter 37). For more information about the

SSA and its benefits, see the website listed in Web Resources.

The Department of Defense (DOD). U.S. military spending makes up the largest portion of the federal budget, and a large part of that money goes to health care. The DOD provides care to all active duty military personnel, retirees, National Guard and Reserve members, and their families, approximately 9.4 million people stationed throughout the world (DOD, 2009). The military employs over 35,000 nurses, runs 63 military hospitals, oversees 413 medical and dental clinics, and provides funding for nursing research. For more information on the DOD and TRICARE, its health maintenance organization, see the DOD website in Web Resources. (See also Chapter 19.)

The Department of Veterans Affairs. Through the Veterans Health Administration, the Department of Veterans Affairs oversees programs to provide health care and other services to U.S. military veterans and their families. In 2008, approximately 5.5 million people received care at a VA facility (U.S. Department of Veterans Affairs, 2008). The Veteran's Administration also manages the largest medical, nursing, and health professions training program in the U.S. Over 90,000 health professionals receive training in VA medical centers annually (U.S. Department of Veterans Affairs, 2009). (See also Chapter 20.)

The U.S. Department of Education. The Department of Education, along with the Health Resources and Services Administration of the Department of Health and Human Services, provides billions of dollars in grants and loans for students to attend college and professional schools, including schools of nursing. This is highly relevant to nurses, particularly in times of nursing shortage, because the department works with hospitals and other government agencies to provide incentives such as loan repayment programs, which attract nurses to the most underserved areas (U.S. Health Resources and Services Administration [HRSA], 2009). In February 2009, President Barack Obama signed the American Recovery and Reinvestment Act, part of which expanded federal funds available for the loan repayment for nurses (HRSA, 2009).

Regulatory Functions of the Executive Branch of Government. The executive branch of the federal government is responsible for implementing laws enacted by Congress. This task falls to staff of the relevant departments and agencies, often with input from the agencies under the EOP. Once a law is enacted, the federal agency staff develops regulations for implementation of the relevant program, which specify definitions, authority, eligibility, benefits, and standards. This step is necessary because while the laws passed by Congress express the legislators' intentions, they do not spell out the details of the new program (Smith, Greenblatt, Buntin, & Clark, 2005).

The regulations (or rules) are published in the *Federal Register,* giving interested individuals and organizations a limited opportunity to review and comment. This is an important access point for nurses interested in shaping health policy. Agency staff reviews all of the comments and then issues final regulations in the *Federal Register*. These regulations govern how agencies and individuals in states and localities are to implement the law. For more information on regulatory functions of the federal government and the *Federal Register*, see the *Federal Register* website in Web Resources.

THE LEGISLATIVE BRANCH

The legislative branch of the federal government consists of the Congress, which is divided into two chambers—the Senate and the House of Representatives. Members of Congress are elected by their constituents. The Senate, with two members from each state, has 100 seats. The House of Representatives has 435 voting seats and 6 non-voting seats, with each state's number of representatives based on its population size. The number of members in each state's delegation may change every 10 years based on the results of the national decennial census. Members of the Senate and House are elected for 6-year terms and 2-year terms, respectively.

The primary role of the legislative branch is the formulation of laws for recommendation to the president. The process of creating such laws can be long and arduous, and is thoroughly discussed in Chapter 65. It is key to note, however, that once a new topic or bill is introduced into a congressional chamber, it is often assigned to one of the committees or subcommittees for further discussion and hearings. In 2009, the Senate had 16 standing committees and 4 select committees, while the House of Representatives had 20 standing committees and 2 select committees. Select committees do not have the legislative jurisdiction of standing committees, but facilitate agenda

TABLE 64-1 Standing Committees of the U.S. Senate with Jurisdiction over Health Policy Issues

Committee	Jurisdiction
Agriculture, Nutrition, and Forestry *http://agriculture.senate.gov*	Agricultural economics and research Food Stamp programs Human nutrition School nutrition programs
Appropriations *http://appropriations.senate.gov*	Appropriation of revenue
Armed Services *http://armed-services.senate.gov*	Issues relating to national (common) defense
Banking, Housing, and Urban Development *http://banking.senate.gov/public*	Construction of Nursing Homes Public and Private Housing
Budget *http://budget.senate.gov*	Congress's annual budget plan
Commerce, Science, and Transportation *http://commerce.senate.gov/public*	Science, engineering, and technology research and development and policy
Energy and Natural Resources *http://energy.senate.gov/public*	Emergency preparedness Nuclear waste policy
Environment and Public Works *http://epw.senate.gov/public*	Air pollution and environmental policy Solid waste disposal and recycling
Finance *http://finance.senate.gov*	Public moneys and customs Health programs under Social Security Act Health programs financed by a specific tax or trust fund
Government Affairs *www.whitehouse.gov/omb/mgmt-gpra_gprptm*	Census and collection of statistics Studying the efficiency of government departments Evaluating the effects of enacted laws National security
Health, Education, Labor, and Pensions *http://help.senate.gov*	Aging Biomedical research and development Domestic activities of the Red Cross Individuals with disabilities Public health Student loans Wages and hours of labor
Indian Affairs *http://indian.senate.gov/public*	Indian Health Service
Veteran's Affairs *http://veterans.senate.gov*	Life insurance for members of the armed forces Veteran's hospitals and medical care

setting by focusing on specific issue areas. Between them, the House and Senate share four joint committees. The committee stage is a critical step for the nurse activist to recognize because it provides one of the primary points of entry into the policy arena. The assignment of a bill to a committee signals to those who care about the issue that it is time to act. Although this point of entry is not without roadblocks, measures can be taken to help keep the issue salient. Successful entry requires that the policy advocate be knowledgeable about the committee with jurisdiction, its members, and their priorities. It also requires that they be prepared with both a primary and backup policy plan, be willing and able to educate committee members and their staff, and be capable of providing persuasive testimony before committee members. For a complete list of committees and their health-related jurisdictions, see Tables 64-1 and 64-2. A complete listing and other information is also available on the department websites listed in Web Resources. By

TABLE 64-2 **Standing Committees of the U.S. House of Representatives with Jurisdiction over Health Policy Issue**

Committee	Jurisdiction
Agriculture http://agriculture.house.gov/index.shtml	Human nutrition and home economics WIC and Food Stamps Rural development Bioterrorism
Appropriations http://appropriations.house.gov	Appropriation of revenue
Armed Services http://armedservices.house.gov	Common defense National security Benefits of members of the armed forces (including health care) Scientific research and development is support of the armed services
Budget http://budget.house.gov	Budget Resolutions and budget process
Education and Labor http://edlabor.house.gov	Child labor Head Start and other early childhood education Child abuse prevention and adoption Food programs for schools Education and labor generally Worker's compensation
Energy and Commerce http://energycommerce.house.gov	Biomedical research and development Health and health facilities (except health care supported by payroll deductions) Public health and quarantine
Financial Services http://financialservices.house.gov/jurisdiction.html	Public and assisted housing
Homeland Security http://homeland.house.gov	National security Science and technology preparedness
Natural Resources http://resourcescommittee.house.gov	Water and power Indian affairs
Science and Technology http://science.house.gov	Environmental research National Science Foundation Science Scholarships
Veteran's Affairs http://veterans.house.gov	Veteran's hospitals, medical care, and treatment
Ways and Means http://waysandmeans.house.gov	Customs Tax exempt foundations National Social Security Health programs under the Social Security Act and those financed by a specific tax

following the link to each committee, one can obtain information about committee and subcommittee membership, complete jurisdiction, hearings, recent bills, and other timely health policy information. The status of all federal bills can be obtained at one of the most important websites for congressional information: http://thomas.loc.gov/. Finally, it is also important to recognize that the members of congressional staffs are accessible via phone and the Internet. Nurses should be familiar with not only representatives from their home state but also other legislators who either support their issue or sit on a committee with jurisdiction over it.

Congressional Caucuses are another way that congressional members provide a forum for issues or legislative agendas. Caucuses generally exist in the

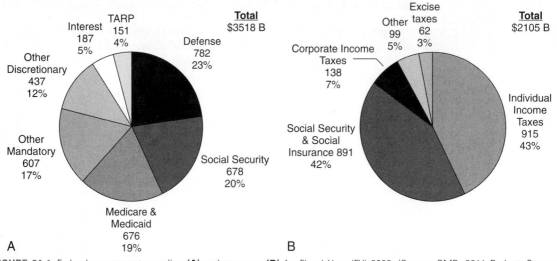

FIGURE 64-1 Federal government spending **(A)** and revenues **(B)** for Fiscal Year (FY) 2009. (Source: OMB, 2011 Budget, Summary Table S-3.)

House of Representatives and can consist of both representatives and senators interested in diverse topics including individual disease conditions and health professions. The 111th Congressional Nursing Caucus is co-chaired by Lois Capps, RN (D-CA) and Steven LaTourette (R-OH). Nurses interested in a specific area of health care can identify whether a caucus exists for that area and its congressional members by visiting *www.house.gov.*

THE FEDERAL BUDGET

Anyone involved with national health policymaking follows the federal budget process closely. The federal budget is the end result of collaboration between the executive and legislative branches. The executive branch sets the national agenda as outlined in the presidential budget, and the legislative branch, with the help of the Congressional Budget Office (CBO), reevaluates the budget and divides and allocates the available monies among the programs seeking funding.

Policy advocates need to be very familiar with the federal budget process because it sets the structure and timeline for important policy work. Its appropriation process provides key access points for nurses to educate staff members and provide testimony. The federal government's fiscal year runs from October 1 through September 30. For example, the fiscal year 2011 runs from Oct 1, 2010 to September 30, 2011.

The budget process officially begins each year in early February when, after months of analysis by the OMB, the president officially presents his budget to Congress.

The House and Senate budget committees work with the CBO to create budget resolutions for their respective chambers. According to congressional rules, these are supposed to be passed during March, but due to conflicts over budget priorities, consensus is not always easily reached. Once passed, a conference committee composed of both senators and representatives works to resolve the differences between the two budget resolutions and combine them into a single resolution that should pass both houses by April 15, but again, may be delayed. Once passed, the final budget resolution lacks the power of law, but is important as a blueprint for subsequent budget legislation.

After passage of the resolution, the next steps are enacting budget reconciliation legislation and enacting appropriation bills. A reconciliation bill is a piece of legislation that reconciles the amount of money coming into the government (taxes) with the amount of money the government is spending. (See Chapter 65 for more information on authorization and appropriations.) Figure 64-1 depicts some of the data used to calculate the reconciliation each year and shows how tax revenues compare with government spending. An appropriations bill is a piece of legislation that

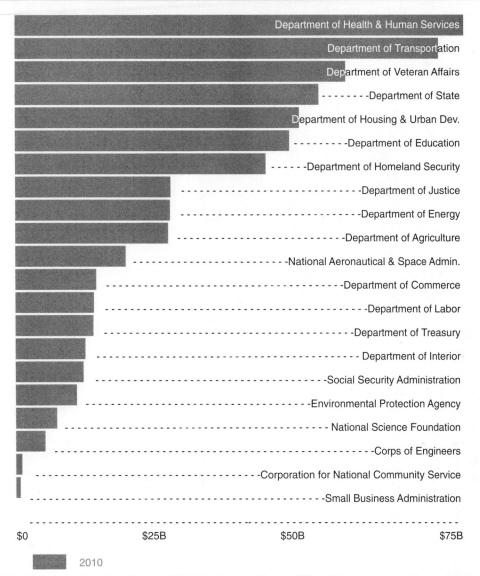

FIGURE 64-2 Allocations in President Obama's 2010 federal budget. (Source: Office of Management and Budget, Washington, DC.)

prescribes how much money will go to each program named in the federal budget. Figure 64-2 depicts early appropriations for President Obama's 2010 Budget.

Both reconciliation and appropriation deliberations entail hearings and opportunities for nurses to present testimonies as the legislators try to determine how best to allocate the funds for the upcoming fiscal year. Many programs such as Social Security and Medicaid receive *nondiscretionary* funds as laid out by their authorizing legislation. These programs are *entitlements*, meaning Congress is required to fund all

individuals and programs that are eligible under law. The only way entitlement funding can be decreased is by changing eligibility or diminishing services through revisions in law. Such highly contentious discussions may be part of reconciliation or budget deliberations in an effort to reduce federal spending.

Other programs, however, such as the National Institutes of Health and AIDS funding, are *discretionary* in nature, meaning that their funding is determined annually under the *appropriations* process. Figure 64-3 depicts discretionary spending and major

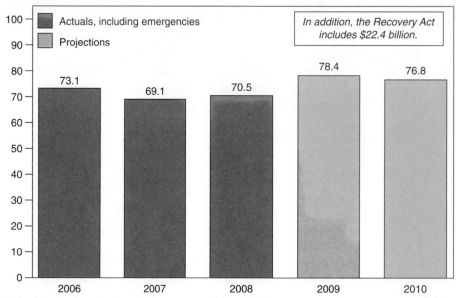

Discretionary budget authority in billions of dollars

FIGURE 64-3 Federal health spending: discretionary budget authority in billions of dollars. (Source: Department of Health and Human Services.)

BOX 64-3 Major Department of Health and Human Services Expenditures

- $81.3 billion requested to support the HHS mission
- $2.5 billion to enable health centers to provide affordable high-quality primary and preventive services to underserved populations including the uninsured
- $32.1 billion for the National Institute of Health; $6 billion of this is allocated for cancer research
- $25.5 billion in additional Medicaid assistance to help states maintain their Medicaid programs
- 4.4 billion for the Indian Health Services
- $4.0 billion for the FDA
- $10 million for the federal employee wellness program
- $169 million for the National Health Services Corps to install providers in underprivileged areas

Source: *FY 2011 Fact Sheet,* OMB Home. Retrieved from *www.whitehouse.gov/omb/factsheet_department_health/iati.*

BOX 64-4 Glossary for the Federal Budget Process

Reconciliation Bill: A piece of legislation that balances the amount of money coming into the federal government (taxes) with the amount of money the government intends to spend in the coming year.

Appropriations Bill: A piece of legislation that prescribes how much money will go to each program named in the federal budget.

Entitlement (Mandatory) Spending: Money for programs that, by law, Congress must fund in full each year. Example: Medicare

Discretionary Spending: Money for programs, the funding for which is debated annually during the appropriations process.

---

expenditures of HHS. (Also refer to Box 64-3.) Representatives of the constituent organizations involved with these programs must, with the help of advocates, provide testimony and lobby to request annual funding from the government. (For useful budget terminology, see Box 64-4.)

The Senate and House Committees on Appropriations. The role of the appropriations committees is described in the U.S. Constitution, which states that before the federal government may spend any money, it must be reviewed by Congress and appropriated "by law." This power is sometimes referred to as the "power of the purse." Appropriations bills must be enacted by September 30 for the ensuing fiscal year, which begins on October 1. Failure to do so may result in a government shutdown. The appropriations access point is important because Congress has money ready to spend and is weighing its options as to how best to spend it. Successful testimony at this point can result in money being dispersed to your program.

In sum, reconciliation and appropriations are important aspects of the budget process. Excellent information and a citizen's guide to the federal budget are available at the Center on Budget and Policy Priorities and the Government Printing Office websites listed in Web Resources.

STATE GOVERNMENTS

Each state government has its own constitution, which, similar to that of the federal constitution, defines the roles of each of the three branches of government (legislative, executive, and judicial) at the state level. Each state's constitution is unique and is based on the state's history, population, philosophy, and geography. State constitutions and individual state laws cannot, however, conflict with federal law or with the U.S. Constitution. Links to the websites of each state along with full text of the constitutions of all 50 states can be found at the websites listed in Web Resources.

Although there is much variation in the structure and day-to-day functioning of different state governments, there are enough similarities for comparison. Only the basics of the state executive and legislative branches will be discussed here. For complete information on your home state, visit your state government's website.

EXECUTIVE BRANCH

Similar to the president at the federal level is the governor at the state level. All but six states also have lieutenant governors, whose roles are comparable to that of the vice president. The powers of these officials vary widely among the states, but they all have some common duties—the preparation of the state budget for presentation to the legislature and management of the approved budget. Also, like the president, the governors have the power to veto or approve state-level legislation along with the power to make appointments to influential positions such as the state board of health. Most states also have lieutenant

governors who often have a leadership position in the legislature.

The governor's veto power, however, is slightly different from that of the president. Known as the "line item veto," it allows the governor to cross out or delete sections of a bill before signing it into law. This is helpful for combating "riders," legislators' favorite programs, which may be attached to bills. President Bill Clinton sought a line item veto on the federal level, but it was ultimately struck down by the Supreme Court. An attempt by President George W. Bush to enact an alternate way for the president to exert pressure on Congress to rescind portions of legislation was also unsuccessful. Therefore, the president must still sign a bill in total or veto it.

Regulatory Function of State Governments

Translating Laws into Regulations. Together, the 50 states employ about 5 million people in state agencies who work to translate the intentions of state legislatures, outlined in new laws, into sets of rules and regulations, which define how those intentions will become reality (Smith et al., 2005). The crafting of regulation language is a process as important as the law itself, since it determines how it will be implemented. Once a set of rules is approved, within 30 days, it has the force of law and becomes a part of the state's administrative code. Thus, laws and regulations work together to determine how public policy is implemented (Donovan, Mooney, & Smith, 2009).

The leaders of state agencies also work to influence policy. Many are elected officials, who attempt to keep campaign promises through the rules and regulations outlined in the agency (Smith et al., 2005). The regulatory role of the executive branch makes it a prime target for the nurse activist. Creating and maintaining relationships with both appointed and elected officials helps to ensure that once your bill is enacted, its implementation matches the law's intent and your original vision. Agency personnel responsible for writing new regulations often benefit from the input of practicing health professionals, especially in specialty practice areas. Nursing input in these situations can be critically important to ensure that rules governing professional practice are realistic and meet patient needs adequately.

Regulation of Health Professionals. One of the most visible roles of the state executive branch with respect to health care is the licensing and regulation of professionals, including nurses (see Chapter 66).

Each state sets both the educational and testing requirements for licensure and limits the scope of nursing practice through the state's nurse practice act. Even though some states have entered into compacts allowing nurses to practice in multiple states, the practice regulations continue to vary widely among states, particularly with regard to the scope of advanced nursing practice. Questions or disputes related to interpretation of state regulations are typically referred to the state's office of the Attorney General. Complete information on the regulations in your area, a list of states in the licensure compact, and links to all 50 state boards of nursing are available on the website of the National Council of State Boards of Nursing (see Web Resources). Familiarity with state licensing boards, as well as with state agencies such as departments of public health or social services, can be very beneficial to nurses in their quest to influence policy. These agencies also serve as consultants on issues pertaining to health care to both executive and legislative branches of government. Working with staff of these agencies can help enhance your policy efforts.

LEGISLATIVE BRANCH

All 50 states have state legislatures with roles similar to that of the U.S. Congress. These groups create and pass new laws and serve as a check and balance to the executive branch by evaluating the governor's budget and appointments. Beyond this basic structure, some aspects of the state legislatures may differ. One state, Nebraska, has a legislature with a single house, whereas the other 49 states have bicameral (two-house) legislatures. While most state legislatures meet every year, five states have legislatures that meet only every other year: Montana, Nevada, North Dakota, Oregon, and Texas. Just as at the federal level, it is important to get to know not only the representatives from your home district but also those who support your issue, as well as members of committees with jurisdiction over your area of interest.

LOCAL GOVERNMENT

There are many types of local governments in the U.S. including entities such as counties, cities, towns, villages, and school districts. Local governments often have elected executive leaders. They may be referred to as mayors, in a county, city, or town, or as superintendents in school districts. The legislative branch at the local level is often composed of an elected council or board, which works to create the laws governing the locality. These laws, of course, cannot conflict with state or national laws.

While the structure and function of local-level governments vary even more widely than the governments at the state level, they serve as vital links between the local citizens and the state and nation (Donovan et al., 2009). Federal health policy can influence local health initiatives through transfer of billions of dollars in grant money to local entities, which disperse funds to community health agencies. These grants are often accompanied by defined health goals such as improved child immunization (Metzenbaum, 2008). Alternately, due to rising health care costs of municipal employees and retirees, local governments often elect to institute their own health care reforms without waiting for federal or state initiatives. These programs can take the form of health screenings, wellness programs, and public education (Barkin, 2007; Wagner, 2010).

As local government responsibility for the health care of citizens has increased, it offers nurses increasingly accessible opportunities to influence policy. Getting to know, understand, and maintain a relationship with local officials is often much more feasible than it is with officials at the state or federal levels. In addition, addressing issues and testing proposals at the local level will allow evaluation and improvement before moving to the state or federal level.

The nurse's strategies for influence at the local level are the same as those at the state and national levels, with one possible exception. Because of the nature of localities, policy advocates and policymakers may also be neighbors, friends, or colleagues. Such informal relationships must be carefully balanced, but they may also aid the policy advocate in gaining access to influence change. For more information on local governments, see the state and local government websites in Web Resources.

TARGET THE APPROPRIATE LEVEL OF GOVERNMENT

The principle of divided powers is a cornerstone of our government in terms of both the levels (federal, state, and local) and the branches (executive, legislative, and judicial). The founding fathers saw this system of checks and balances as key to preventing the accumulation of power by any one group and thereby helping to maintain a democratic nation. Although this organizational structure may present challenges to nurses aiming to influence policy, it is important to understand which issues fall under the jurisdiction of each level of government and the tasks that are shared responsibilities among the levels.

When it comes to the health and health care of U.S. citizens, the preamble to the Constitution addresses the government's responsibility by stating that one of the government's purposes is to "promote the general welfare." At the time of the writing in 1787, the term *welfare* referred to the health, happiness, prosperity, and well-being of the people and should not be confused with the social programs it may be associated with today (Mount, 2010). Since that time, each level of government has addressed its responsibilities in different ways.

Today, the federal government is broadly responsible for many health policies regarding the organization, financing, and delivery of health care. More specifically, federal issues typically include programs enacted by Congress and the president, such as Medicare, Medicaid, and Veterans Affairs, as well as the administration of programs that fall under federal jurisdiction including NIH, the CDC, the FDA, and the DHHS.

At the state level, governments protect the public and affect the delivery of health care through licensing of health care professionals, regulating health insurance coverage, and developing long-term care policy (Reinhard, 2002). Local governments oversee the provision of health care through administration and funding of safety-net programs and public hospitals and, more broadly, by addressing the public's general health by providing public education, waste management, fire and police protection, and public health initiatives (Donovan et al., 2009).

Because the process of promoting the general welfare at the national level has not always been easy, over time, the powers associated with the implementation of programs have shifted from the federal level to the state and local governments, a process called *devolution*. Each state and locality implements federal programs, such as those funded by block grants and those that are shared federal-state responsibilities (e.g., Medicaid), in very different ways. Despite the

fact that this may or may not result in better outcomes for the program, it definitely creates challenges for the nurse activist trying to understand the policies that affect patient care. Remember that the system is murky, and any particular issue may require attention at all three levels of government. Federal laws often provide funding and overarching direction, states are often the lead funding agencies under block grants or matching federal-state programs, and local agencies may receive funding from state or federal authorities to administer programs. Each level of government also operates programs that are independent of the others.

Many health care initiatives fall to multiple levels of government for both funding and administration. For example, covering the uninsured falls under all three domains, depending on the proposal under debate. Medicaid, which provides insurance for the poorest Americans, is administered by federal and state authorities. Similarly, many education programs, although administered by local education agencies, entail some federal involvement. Laws such as the Elementary and Secondary Education Act (reauthorized as the No Child Left Behind Act in 2001) are federal initiatives with grants to states, which in turn allocate funds to local agencies. The full text for all laws is available on the Internet at *http://thomas. loc.gov*.

Some public health issues, such as emergency preparedness, which is overseen by the Department of Homeland Security and executed by the Federal Emergency Management Agency (FEMA), also involve all three levels of government. Implementation of disaster response and security of mass transit has become primarily a local responsibility, resting with local public health, hospital, and crime enforcement authorities. The federal and state governments, however, retain a great deal of administrative control as well as responsibility for security of air traffic.

PULLING IT ALL TOGETHER: COVERING LONG-TERM CARE

This example will demonstrate how an issue can span multiple levels (federal, state, and local) of government, with each level developing and implementing policy to reach the best workable solution for the public welfare. Meeting the long-term care (LTC) needs of elderly and disabled Americans is too complex and costly for one government level. This issue is addressed primarily through a federal/state partnership, with each state deciding the combination of LTC services available and the eligibility criteria required for persons to access them. According to the Centers for Medicare and Medicaid Services, the U.S. spent $51.7 billion in Medicaid LTC expenditures in 2006 (Klees, Wolfe, & Curtis, 2009). The responsibility for this cost is shared between the federal government and the states, occupying an increasingly larger share of state Medicaid budgets.

Millions of elderly and disabled Americans currently require help with activities of daily living to ensure their safety and health, and this population is expected to grow rapidly. According to the AARP Policy Institute, the population 65 or older is projected to grow by 89% from 2007 to 2030, more than four times faster than the general population (AARP Public Policy Institute, 2009). Most help is given by family and friends, but when this is not available, personal resources are usually used to pay for needed care. Medicaid is the safety net program available to Americans when they exhaust personal resources to pay for their LTC needs. For more information on the scope of the problem of long-term care coverage in the U.S., see the websites on long-term care listed in Web Resources. (Also see Chapter 24.)

Federal Medicaid funds available to states to help cover LTC costs are supplemented by matching state funds, and states must conform to federal rules and regulations including the right of every eligible beneficiary to benefit from the program. However, each state develops its own policies governing Medicaid eligibility, benefits provided, and reimbursement levels. This enables states to respond appropriately to the needs of its citizens as well as the limits of its budget. Because institutional care must be a covered Medicaid LTC service, all those eligible to receive services can be cared for in a nursing home. Local governments participate by ensuring that these facilities meet all local fire and safety requirements.

The majority of Americans wish to remain in their homes as long as they can, receiving "in-home" LTC services if possible. To accommodate public preference and reduce institutional Medicaid costs, many states have sought Medicaid "waivers" from the federal government in order to offer alternate home and community LTC services. Recent federal Real Choice System Change grants are also available to assist states address barriers to provision of more home- and community-based long-term care. Thus, both federal and state LTC policy continues to evolve, responding to public demand for changes in services as well as the need to control escalating costs. Nurses can help to advocate for choice in patients' LTC settings by lobbying state legislators to pass enabling legislation and testifying at public hearings on these issues. States and localities assist elderly and disabled persons in additional ways, recognizing that their resources may be limited. These efforts indirectly help defray LTC costs and can include reductions in property taxes, grants to cover energy costs, and sliding-scale fees for home care services.

SUMMARY

To influence many health policies that span levels of government, it is important for nurses to understand federalism and how it has shaped implementation of myriad public health programs. Targeting actions to influence legislators and other government officials on a piece of legislation may require a multilevel approach. Such an approach, however, reflects the realities of the U.S. federalist structure. The nurse interested in improving long-term care choices—or any other health policy issue—needs to know how the government works in order to know how to plan appropriate strategies.

For a list of related websites, please refer to your Evolve Resources at http://evolve.elsevier.com/Mason/policypolitics/

REFERENCES

AARP Public Policy Institute. (2009, June). *Fact sheet: Providing more long-term support and services at home: Why it's critical for health reform.* Retrieved from http://assets.aarp.org/rgcenter/health/fs_hcbs_hcr.pdf.

Barkin, R. (2007). Scaling back: Locals target bloated health care costs with programs to shape up employees. *American City & County, 122*(5), 32-34.

Department of Defense (DOD). (2009). *TRICARE: Your Military Health Plan.* Retrieved from www.tricare.mil/mybenefit/ProfileFilter.do;jsessionid=KLwVX5clTzNh380Mp4kmGbMHPBcT2xmpryT2pJwX2nljn2tchwm2!620604795?puri=%2Fhome%2Foverview%2FWhatIsTRICARE.

Donovan, T., Mooney, C. Z., & Smith, D. A. (2009). *State and local politics. Institutions and reform.* Belmont, CA: Cengage Learning Wadsworth.

Hanson, R. L. (2004). Intergovernmental relations. In V. Gray & R. L. Hanson (Eds.), *Politics in the American states: A comparative analysis* (pp. 31-60). Washington D.C.: CQ Press.

Klees, B. S., Wolfe, C. J., & Curtis, C. A. (2009, November 1). Brief summaries of Medicare & Medicaid. Retrieved from www.cms.hhs.gov/MedicareMedicaidStatSupp/downloads/2009BriefSummaries.pdf.

Metzenbaum, S. H. (2008). From oversight to insight: Federal agencies as learning leaders in the information age. In T. J. Conlan & P. L. Posner (Eds.),

Intergovernmental management for the twenty-first century (pp. 209-242). Washington D.C.: The Brookings Institution.

Mount, S. (2010, January 24). The U.S. Constitution online. Retrieved July 4, 2005, from www.usconstitution.net/glossary.html.

Nathan, R. P. (2006, September). Updating theories of American federalism. Presented at the Annual Meeting of the American Political Science Association, Philadelphia. Retrieved from www.rockinst.org/pdf/federalism/2006-09-02-updating_theories_of_american_federalism.pdf.

Reinhard, S. C. (2002). State government: 50 paths to policy. In D. J. Mason, J. K. Leavitt, & M. W. Chaffee (Eds.), *Policy and politics in nursing and health care.* (4th ed., pp. 491-497). St. Louis: Saunders.

Smith, K. B., Greenblatt, A., Buntin, J., & Clark, C. S. (2005). *Governing states and localities.* Washington, D.C.: CQ Press.

U.S. Department of Veterans Affairs. (2008). *Facts about the Department of Veterans Affairs.* Retrieved from www1.va.gov/vetdata/docs/Pamphlet_2-1-08.pdf.

U.S. Department of Veterans Affairs. (2009). *Fact sheet: Department of Veterans Affairs.* Retrieved from www1.va.gov/opa/fact/docs/vafacts.pdf.

U.S. Health Resources and Services Administration (HRSA). (2009). Grants. Retrieved from www.hrsa.gov/grants/default.htm.

Wagner, D. M. (2010). Local government leaders initiate health care reforms. *Public Management, 92*(1), 11-12.

CHAPTER 65

An Overview of Legislation and Regulation

Nancy Ridenour and Yvonne Santa Anna

"Law is order, and good law is good order."

—Aristotle

INFLUENCING THE LEGISLATIVE PROCESS

Public policy formation in the United States often appears to be indecisive and slow, and it can be difficult for the casual observer to distinguish the subtleties of the process. These nuances require that the observer select a conceptual model of policymaking to assist in understanding the specifics of the policy-making process—that is, why a particular proposal is enacted or defeated. Chapter 6 set forth several models for policy analysis. These can clarify how an issue is placed on the formal agenda for authoritative decision-making. Nurses who understand this process can better influence the development of sound health policies for their patients, their patients' families, and the profession of nursing.

This chapter will describe the path by which a bill becomes a federal or state law in the U.S., with primary emphasis on federal processes. The legislative path differs only slightly between the federal and state levels and from state to state.

INTRODUCTION OF A BILL

Only a member of the U.S. Congress (or of a state legislature) can introduce bills, though the idea for a bill can come from anyone, including constituents. A legislator can introduce any one of several types of bills and resolutions by simply giving the bill to the clerk of the house or, in Congress, placing the bill in a box called the *hopper* (Congressional Quarterly, 2008). In the U.S. Senate, a senator can postpone the introduction of another senator's bill by 1 day by

voicing an objection. Legislation is often introduced simultaneously in the Senate and the House of Representatives as a pair of companion bills.

A member of Congress or state legislator who understands the legislative process in depth can contribute more to either the passage or defeat of a bill than one who is an expert only on its substance. However, the numerous players involved (the executive branch, the legislature, constituents, and special interest groups) and the complexity of the legislative process make it far easier to defeat a bill than to pass one.

Every bill introduced in Congress faces a 2-year deadline; it must pass into law by then or die by default. Box 65-1 provides an overview of the various types of bills that can be introduced by members of Congress. Legislators introduce bills for a variety of reasons: to declare a position on an issue, as a favor to a constituent or a special interest group, to obtain publicity, or for political self-preservation. Some legislators, having introduced a bill, claim that they have acted to solve the problem that motivated it but do not continue to work toward enactment of the measure, blaming a committee or other members of the legislature if no further action is taken. Passage of a bill requires that at critical points in the policymaking process "a problem is recognized, a solution is available, the political climate makes the time right for a change, and the constraints do not prohibit action" (Kingdon, 1984, p. 93). Although meeting these conditions helps a bill to rise on the decision agenda, nothing can guarantee enactment.

INFLUENCING THE INTRODUCTION OF A BILL

Nurses can influence the introduction of bills as constituents and as members of professional associations

---

BOX 65-1 Types of Bills in the U.S. Congress

Bill: This is used for most legislation, whether general, public, or private (i.e., initiated by non-congressional sources). The bill number is prefixed with HR in the House and S in the Senate.

Joint resolution: This is subject to the same procedures as bills, with the exception of any joint resolution proposing an amendment to the Constitution. The latter must be approved by two thirds of both chambers, whereupon it is sent directly to the Administrator of General Services for submission to the states for ratification, rather than to the president. There is little difference between a bill and a joint resolution, and often the two forms are used interchangeably. One difference in form is that a joint resolution may include a preamble preceding the resolving clause. Statutes that have been initiated as bills have later been amended by a joint resolution and vice versa. The bill number is prefixed with HJ Res in the House and SJ Res in the Senate.

Concurrent resolution: This is used for matters affecting the operations of both houses. The bill number is prefixed with H Con Res in the House and S Con Res in the Senate.

Resolution: This is used when a matter concerns the operation of either chamber alone; adopted only by the chamber in which it originates. The bill number is prefixed with H Res in the House and S Res in the Senate.

From Congressional Quarterly. (2008). *Guide to current American government.* Washington, D.C.: Congressional Quarterly.

---

that lobby Congress. They can call attention to problems in funding health care, such as the need for expanded services for uninsured children, the need for long-term care coverage under Medicare, or the need to increase reimbursement for nursing services. Legislators like to work with organized groups that have strong positions on a bill, such as the American Nurses Association, American Association of Colleges of Nursing (AACN), American Association of Nurse Anesthetists, National Organization of Nurse Practitioner Faculties, or the state nurses associations.

Frequently, associations are asked to assist in drafting legislation and in lobbying members of the legislature. Coalitions of interested organizations are created to present a united front, a clear message, and a strong constituency to persuade legislators to support a particular bill (see Chapter 86). Enactment, if achieved at all, may take several legislative sessions.

Identifying the appropriate sponsor to introduce a bill is critical to its success. In selecting a primary bill sponsor, it is best to ask a member of a committee that has jurisdiction over the issue you wish to have addressed. For example, in the U.S. Senate, the Finance Committee has jurisdiction over the Medicare program and decides which Medicare-related legislation is sent to the full Senate for a vote. Legislation that would address changes in direct reimbursement of nurse practitioners (NPs) or nurse anesthetists under Medicare would be less likely to be tabled (i.e., never acted upon) if a member of the Senate Finance Committee was a primary sponsor of the measure.

COMMITTEE ACTION

Committees are centers of policymaking at both federal and state levels. It is in committee that conflicting points of view are discussed and legislation is often refined and amended. Successful committee consideration of bills requires organization, consensus building, and time; only about 15% of all bills referred to committees are reported out for House and Senate consideration.

The Senate and House have separate committees with distinct rules and procedures. Committee procedure provides the means for members of the legislature to sift through an otherwise overwhelming number of bills, proposals, and complex issues. Within the respective guidelines of each chamber, committees adopt their own rules to address their organizational and procedural issues. Generally, committees operate independently of each other and of their respective parent chambers (Schneider, 2008).

There are three types of committees at the federal level: standing, select, and joint. A standing committee has permanent jurisdiction over bills and issues in its content area. Some standing committees set authorizing funding levels, and others set appropriating funding levels for proposed laws. This two-step authorizing-appropriating process is designed to concentrate the policymaking decisions within the authorizing committee and decisions about precise funding levels within the appropriations committees.

A select committee cannot report out a bill and is often created by the leadership to address a special problem or concern. A joint committee consists of members of both the House and Senate. One type of a joint committee is the conference committee, in which members of each chamber and party work together to address differences in their respective bills.

In congressional committees, leadership and authority is centered in the chair of the committee. The chair, always a member of the majority party, decides the committee's agenda, conducts its meetings, and controls the funds distributed by the chamber to the committee (Schneider, 2007). The senior minority party member of the committee is called the *ranking minority member* (or *ranking member*). The committee's subcommittees also have chairs and ranking members. Often, but not always, the ranking member assists the chair with some of the responsibilities of the committee or subcommittee. The committee chair usually refers a bill to the subcommittees for initial consideration, but only the full committee can report out a bill to the floor (Schneider, 2007). For example, the House Ways and Means Committee refers most Medicare bills to the House Ways and Means Subcommittee on Health. If the subcommittee wishes to take action on the bill, it usually will schedule at least one hearing to discuss the substance of the proposed legislation.

In very unusual circumstances, a few bills will bypass the committee process. This can only happen if the leadership of the majority consents. For example, according to a U.S. House Select Committee on Aging Fact Sheet, "Since the Roosevelt era, major pieces of social legislation, including civil rights reforms and labor reforms, such as the wage and hours bill, were forced to bypass committees of jurisdiction because the committees refused or delayed in allowing the House to consider them" (Pepper & Roybal, 1988, p. 1). In the end, however, committees and subcommittees usually select the bills they want to consider and ignore the rest. Committees thus perform a gate-keeping function by selecting from the thousands of measures introduced in each session those that meet their party's leadership priorities and that they consider to merit floor debate.

Consideration of bills whose content overlaps the jurisdictions of different committees falls to the leader of the chamber to decide. Health care issues, for example, can cut across the jurisdiction of more than one committee. When this occurs in the House, upon advice from the Parliamentarian, the Speaker of the House will base his or her referral decision on the chamber's rules and precedents for subject matter jurisdiction and identify the appropriate primary committee and other committees for the bill's referral (Schneider, 2007). The Parliamentarians in both chambers have a key role in advising the member of Congress presiding over a bill on the floor. While a member is free to take or ignore the Parliamentarian's advice, few have the knowledge of the chamber's procedures to preside on their own. The primary committee has primary responsibility for guiding the referred measure to final passage. Referrals to more than one committee can have a positive effect by providing opportunities for greater public discussion of the issue and multiple points of access for special interest groups, but this can also greatly slow down the legislative process (Davidson, Oleszek, & Lee, 2007).

A committee can handle a bill in any of the following ways (Congressional Quarterly, 2009):

- Approve a bill with or without amendments.
- Rewrite or revise the bill, and report it out to the full House or Senate.
- Report it unfavorably (i.e., allow the bill to be considered by the full House or Senate, but with a recommendation that it be rejected).
- Take no action, which kills the bill.

AUTHORIZATION AND APPROPRIATION PROCESS

To understand the legislative process and to analyze individual pieces of legislation, it is important to know the distinction between authorizing legislation and appropriating legislation. Because a considerable amount of congressional activity is concerned with decisions related to spending money, and because much of this activity has a direct effect on health care and nursing programs, it is especially important for nurses to be familiar with the authorization-appropriation process. Programs and agencies such as the Nurse Education Act, Scholarships for Disadvantaged Students, the National Health Service Corps, the National Institute of Nursing Research, the National Institutes of Health, and the Agency for Health Care Policy and Research are all subject to the authorization-appropriation process.

Before any of these programs can receive or spend money from the U.S. Treasury, a two-step process must occur. First, an authorization bill allowing an agency or program to come into being or to continue to exist must be passed. The authorization bill is the substantive bill that establishes the purpose of, and guidelines for, the program and usually sets limits on the amount that can be spent. It gives a federal agency or program the legal authority to operate. Authorizing legislation does not, however, provide the actual dollars for a program or enable an agency to spend funds in the future. Renewal or modification of existing authorization is called *reauthorization* (see Chapter 64).

Second, an appropriation bill must be passed. The appropriation bill enables an agency or program to make spending commitments and to actually spend money. In almost all cases, an appropriation bill for an activity is not supposed to be passed until the authorization for that activity is enacted. That is, no money can be spent on a program unless it first has been authorized to exist. Conversely, if a program has been authorized but no money is provided (appropriated) for its implementation, that program cannot be carried out (Schick, 2007).

The authorization-appropriation process is determined by congressional rules that, like most congressional rules, can be waived, circumvented, or ignored on occasion. For example, failure to enact an authorization does not necessarily prevent the appropriations committee from acting. If an expired program—for example, the Nursing Education Act—is deemed likely to be reauthorized, it may receive funds. These must be spent in accordance with the expired authorizing language.

Today, much of the federal government is funded through the annual enactment of 13 general appropriations bills. Whether agencies receive all the money they request depends, in part, on the recommendations of the authorizing and appropriating committees. Each chamber has authorizing and appropriating committees, and these have differing responsibilities. For federal nursing education and research activities, the authorizing committees are the Senate Health, Education, Labor, and Pensions Committee and the House Energy and Commerce Committee. The appropriating committee for federal nursing education and research programs are the Senate and House appropriations committees and their subcommittees on Labor, Health and Human Services, Education, and Related Agencies (Figure 65-1).

COMMITTEE PROCEDURES

Committee consideration of a measure usually consists of three standard steps: hearings, markups, and reports.

Hearings. Hearings can be legislative, oversight, or investigative; each of these types of hearing may be either public or closed (Schneider, 2007). When the committee leadership decides to proceed with a measure, it will usually conduct hearings to receive testimony in support of a measure. From these hearings the committee will gather information and views, identify problems, gauge support for and opposition to the bill, and build a public record of committee action that addresses the measure (Schneider, 2007). Although most hearings are held in Washington, D.C., field hearings in the members' respective states are also held.

Most witnesses are invited to testify before the committee by the chair, who is a member of the majority party and who sets the agenda for the hearing proceedings. The ranking minority member may have an opportunity to request a witness, but it is up to the discretion of the chair to agree to the selection of the witness. Written testimony can also be submitted to the committee by persons who do not have the opportunity to speak their position on a measure in person.

Nurses can influence the policymaking process by testifying at bill hearings. Frequently, committees prefer to deal with large, organized groups that have a position on an issue rather than with private individuals. Professional nursing organizations testify on behalf of their members. Congressional hearings are listed in the official House and Senate websites at *www.house.gov* and *www.senate.gov*. C-SPAN provides live and recorded coverage of hearings at *www.c-span.org*.

Constituents can influence the committee process by meeting with and writing to members of the committee. Concerns expressed by constituents are given serious consideration.

Lobbyists often meet with all members of the committee to express their client's position on a measure. Professional associations often activate a grassroots network of members, asking them to contact the committee members to request co-sponsorship of, or opposition to, the measure.

The hearing process at the state level is similar, as is the importance of an organized approach to presenting testimony. When several representatives of nursing plan to testify on a bill, it is more efficient and effective for them to coordinate their testimony, raising different aspects of an issue rather than repeating the same points. It is also important for various nursing representatives to emphasize those issues

HOW A BILL BECOMES A LAW

The Federal Level

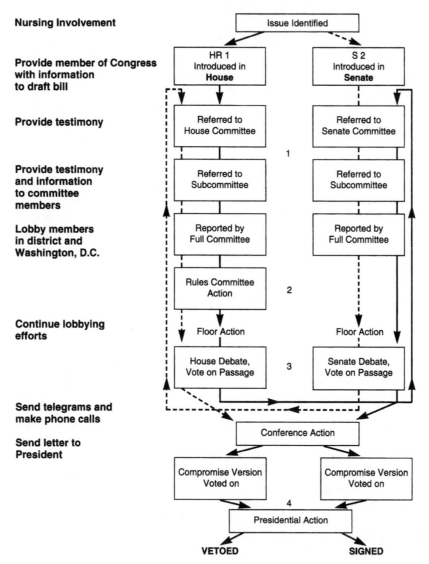

Nursing Involvement

Provide member of Congress with information to draft bill

Provide testimony

Provide testimony and information to committee members

Lobby members in district and Washington, D.C.

Continue lobbying efforts

Send telegrams and make phone calls

Send letter to President

1, A bill goes to full committee first, then to special subcommittees for hearings, debate, revisions, and approval. The same process occurs when it goes to full committee. It either dies in committee or proceeds to the next step.

2, Only the House has a Rules Committee to set the "rule" for floor action and conditions for debate and amendments. In the Senate, the leadership schedules action.

3, The bill is debated, amended, and passed or defeated. If passed, it goes to other chamber and follows the same path. If each chamber passes a similar bill, both versions go to conference.

4, The President may sign the bill into law, allow it to become law without his signature, or veto it and return it to Congress. To override the veto, both houses must approve the bill by a $^2/_3$ majority vote.

FIGURE 65-1 How a bill becomes a law.

where there is agreement; a unified message can strengthen the impression of a powerful coalition. And a hearing room packed with a supportive audience makes a powerful statement to legislators about support for an issue.

Markups. When legislative hearings are concluded, a subcommittee decides whether to attempt to report a measure. If the chair decides to proceed with the measure, she or he will generally choose to continue with the legislative process to "mark up" the bill. A markup is the committee meeting where a measure is modified through amendments to clean up problems or errors within the measure (Schneider, 2007). A quorum of one third of the committee is required in both chambers to hold a markup session (Schneider, 2007). A markup session can weaken or strengthen a measure. Pressure from outside interest groups is often intense at this stage. Under congressional "sunshine rules," markups are conducted in public, except on national-security or related issues.

After conducting hearings and markups, a subcommittee sends its recommendation to the full committee, which may conduct its own hearings and markups, ratify the subcommittee's decision, take no action, or return the bill to the subcommittee for further study.

Reports. The rules of both the Senate and the House dictate that a committee report accompany each bill to the floor. The report, written by committee staff, describes the intent of legislation (i.e., its purpose and scope). It explains any amendments to the bill, and any changes made to current law by the bill; estimates the cost of the bill to the government; sets out documentation for the bill's legislative intent; and often contains dissenting views on the measure from the minority-party committee members.

A committee's description of the legislative intent of the bill is extremely important, especially for the government agency that will implement and enforce the law. Sometimes the report contains explicit instructions on how the agency should interpret the law in regulations, or the report may be written without great detail. Sometimes an agency will interpret the law narrowly, particularly if it is written vaguely. For example, when certified nurse midwives received reimbursement authority under the Medicare program, the agency chose to reimburse them only for gynecologic services, not for all the services covered by Medicare, which they are legally able to provide. This was a narrow interpretation of the law and was not the intent of Congress.

The committee report is also important because it offers those interested in the bill an opportunity to promote or protect their interests. Committee staffs frequently include the report language suggested by special interest groups if it is congruent with the bill.

FLOOR ACTION IN THE HOUSE AND SENATE

After a bill is reported out of committee, it can be placed on a calendar of chamber business and scheduled for floor action by the leadership of the majority party (Schneider, 2007). If the bill is not controversial, it may be dealt with expeditiously. Otherwise, it is placed on the chamber's calendar for future consideration. Both the rules governing the calendar on which a bill is placed and the subsequent floor procedures differ between the House and Senate and among state chambers. Box 65-2 compares the House and Senate procedures for scheduling and raising measures.

The influence of the committee chair and ranking member of the committee that reports out a measure is maintained throughout the floor proceedings. They continue to manage the measure by "planning parliamentary strategy, controlling time for debate, responding to questions from colleagues, warding off unwanted amendments, and building coalitions in favor of their positions" (Schneider, 2007, p. 6). Box 65-3 compares House and Senate rules for floor consideration of a measure. In the House, the Committee on Rules governs proceedings on the floor; there is no such committee in the Senate.

When a bill moves to the floor, special interest groups continue to lobby its opponents, its proponents, and particularly undecided legislators, attempting to influence the outcome of the vote. This process is usually begun after the introduction of the bill, when lobbyists meet with the members of the referring committee to gather support for the measure, and continues until the bill is signed into law. When a bill moves to the floor, constituents are activated to contact the members of the legislature from their own districts. Members listen attentively to their constituents, and so lobbying should continue until the moment of the vote, especially lobbying of undecided members. Lobbyists are known to wait outside the cloakroom in the "lobby" to catch the attention of members as they move in and out of the chambers.

BOX 65-2 Scheduling and Raising Measures in the U.S. House and U.S. Senate

House

Four calendars (Union, House, Private, Discharge)

Special days for raising measures*

Scheduling by speaker and majority party leadership in consultation with selected representatives

No practice of "holds"

Powerful role for Rules Committee

Special rules (approved by majority vote) govern floor consideration of most major legislation

Non-controversial measures usually approved under suspension of the rules procedure

Difficult to circumvent committee consideration of measures

Senate

Two calendars (Legislative and Executive)

No special days

Scheduling by majority party leadership in broad consultation with minority party leaders and interested senators

Individual senators can place "holds" on the raising measure, within limits

No committee with role equivalent to that of House Rules Committee

Complex unanimous consent agreements (approved by unanimous consent) govern floor consideration of major measures

Non-controversial measures approved by unanimous consent procedure

Easier to circumvent committee consideration of measures

Adapted from Schneider, J. (2008). *House and Senate rules of procedures: A comparison* (Congressional Research Service order code RL30945, CRS-6). Washington, D.C.: CRS.

*There are special days for calling up bills under the suspension of the rules and Calendar Wednesday procedures, for raising measures from the Private Calendar, and for bringing up legislation involving the District of Columbia.

BOX 65-3 Floor Procedures of the U.S. House and the U.S. Senate

House

Presiding officer has considerable discretion in recognizing members

Rulings of presiding officer seldom challenged

Debate time always restricted

Debate ends by majority vote in the House and in the Committee of the Whole (i.e., the membership of the House)

Most major measures considered in Committee of the Whole

Number and type of amendments often limited by special rule; bills amended by section or title

Germaneness of amendments required (unless requirement is waived by special rule)

Quorum calls usually permitted only in connection with record votes

Votes recorded by electronic device; electronic vote can be requested only after voice or division vote is completed

House routinely adjourns at end of each legislative day

Senate

Presiding officer has little discretion in recognizing senators

Rulings of presiding officer frequently challenged

Unlimited debate;* individual senators can filibuster

Super-majority vote required to invoke cloture; up to 30 hours of postcloture debate allowed[†]

No Committee of the Whole

Unlimited amendments; bills generally open to amendment at any point

Germaneness of amendments not generally required

Quorum calls in order almost any time; often used for purposes of deliberate delay

No electronic voting system; roll-call votes can be requested almost any time

Senate often recesses instead of adjourning; legislative days can continue for several calendar days

---

Adapted from Schneider, J. (2008). *House and Senate rules of procedures: A comparison (Congressional Research Service order code RL30945, CRS-6)*. Washington, DC: Congressional Research Service.

*Except when complex unanimous consent agreements or rule-making provisions in statutes impose time restrictions.

[†]Adoption of the motion to table by majority vote also ends Senate debate. Use of this motion, however, is generally reserved for cases when the Senate is prepared to reject the pending bill.

A vote on the bill is taken after the debate and amendment process is completed. There are three methods of voting: (1) voice vote, which calls for members to answer yea or nay (victory is judged by ear); (2) division vote, which requires a head count of those favoring and those opposing an amendment; and (3) recorded teller vote, which records each legislator's name and position taken on the vote.

Recorded votes are the most valuable to lobbyists and constituents because they document how the member voted—helpful information in determining whether or not to continue support for a legislator and as a predictor of a legislator's future stands on issues.

CONFERENCE ACTION

Before a bill can be sent to the executive branch for consideration, identical bills must be passed in both chambers. Frequently, the bills originally considered by the House and Senate chambers are not identical, so members of each chamber must meet to resolve the differences. This is often where much of the hard bargaining and compromising takes place in the passage of legislation. The leaders of each chamber appoint conferees, usually senior members of the committees with jurisdiction over the bill, to meet with the conferees of the other chamber.

A joint conference offers another opportunity for groups and individuals to persuade members to support various positions on controversial aspects of the bill. Frequently, there is controversy over the amount of money allocated to a federal program. For example, House and Senate funding authorizations for nursing education programs can differ by tens of millions of dollars. Generally, supporters of a program would lobby for the version of the bill authorizing the largest amount of funding for it.

When agreement is reached on the controversial provisions of the measure, a conference report is written explaining the differences considered in resolving the issue. Both chambers must then approve the conference version of the bill for the bill to become law.

SENATE ROLE IN THE CONFIRMATION PROCESS

The role of the Senate in the confirmation process is defined in the U.S. Constitution. Article II, Section 2 states that the president "shall nominate, and by and with the Advice and Consent of the Senate, shall appoint high government officials" (Tong, 2008). The Senate gives its advice and consent to presidential appointments, to Supreme Court nominees, and to other high-level positions in the cabinet departments and independent agencies of the government. The Senate also confirms appointments of members of regulatory commissions, ambassadors, federal judges, U.S. attorneys, and U.S. marshals. Appointees named to be Supreme Court Justices and Cabinet secretaries receive close scrutiny by the full Senate and Senate committees.

There are several steps in the confirmation process. First, the president submits a nomination in writing and forwards it to the Senate. The nomination is read on the floor of the Senate and is given a number. Second, the Senate Parliamentarian, acting on behalf of the presiding officer, refers each nomination to the committee or committees of jurisdiction. Confirmation hearings, generally open to the public, can be held, but they are not held on all nominations. Supreme Court nominees and senior administration officials or controversial nominees are given the closest scrutiny in hearings. Senators can use the committee hearings as a forum to advance their own policy and political agenda, to determine or challenge the administration's positions on policy issues, and to receive commitments from a nominee. The committee has the option to report the nomination favorable, unfavorable, or without recommendation, or take no action at all. If the committee moves to report the nomination, it is filed with the Senate's executive clerk, who assigns a calendar number and places the nomination on the Executive Calendar.

The third step in the confirmation process involves floor consideration of the nomination. During this step, the Senate will meet in an executive session to consider the nomination. Nominations are subject to unlimited debate, subject to cloture being invoked (which requires 60 votes). The Senate has three options in its advice and consent role: confirm, reject, or take no action on the nomination. Confirmation requires a simple majority vote. Once the Senate has acted on a nomination, the Secretary of the Senate transmits the results of the nomination to the White House. In some instances, one or more senators can place a hold on a nomination, which can delay or prevent the nomination from reaching the floor for further action. Senate rules require any pending nominations to be returned to the president when the Senate is in recess for more than 30 days or adjourns between sessions. Presidents have made court appointments without the Senate's consent, when the Senate was in recess. These court "recess appointments" are temporary in nature, with the nominee's term expiring at the end of the Senate's next session.

EXECUTIVE ACTION

After both chambers have passed identical versions of a bill, it is ready to go to the executive branch. The executive (president or governor) has the power to sign a bill into law, veto it, or return it to the legislature with no signature and a message stating his or her objections. If no further action is taken, the bill dies; or, the legislature may decide to call for another floor vote to overturn the executive's veto. A two-thirds vote is required to override an executive veto in Congress and in many states. Under the U.S. Constitution, a bill becomes law if the president does not sign it within 10 days of the time she or he receives it, provided Congress is in session. Presidents occasionally permit enactment of legislation in this manner when they want to make a political statement of disapproval of the legislation but do not believe that their objections warrant a veto. If Congress adjourns before the 10-day period expires, the unsigned bill does not become law. In this case, the bill has been defeated by the pocket veto (Congressional Quarterly, 2009).

REGULATORY PROCESS

As important as it is to become skilled at influencing the legislative process, it is equally important to influence the regulatory process (see Chapter 64). Regulations have a direct impact on a nurse's work and professional life. As changes in health care financing and delivery structures are driving changes in the current health care provider licensing system, many states are considering changes in the regulation of nursing, from amending the Nurse Practice Act to accomplishing a major overhaul of the entire licensing system. Many of these changes will take place in the regulatory arena within a nurse's state. Other health care–related regulations that can have an impact on nursing practice may also take place within the federal domain.

Though some regulations may be developed or amended without legislation, other regulations are created by the details of new or amended laws. The development of such regulations takes months and sometimes years. It is this important step—the development of regulations—that may be overlooked by organized groups and individuals working to influence policy and the political process (Figure 65-2).

One of the largest federal agencies having primary responsibility for health care programs is the Department of Health and Human Services (HHS). The Centers for Medicare and Medicaid Services (CMS) is the administrative agency in HHS that directs the Medicare and Medicaid programs. A major role of government regulation is to interpret the laws. The laws that Congress and state legislatures pass rarely contain enough explicit language to closely guide their implementation. It is the responsibility of the administrative agencies to promulgate the rules and regulations that fill in the details of those laws. The health policy positions of the executive or legislative branch of government will determine the laws that are passed, but once enacted, laws and their accompanying regulations will shape the way health policy is translated into programs and services.

Regulations specify definitions, authority, eligibility, benefits, and standards. Their development is shaped not only by the law but by the ongoing involvement and input of professional associations, providers, third-party payers, consumers, and other special interest groups (Box 65-4).

The administrative agencies, usually part of the executive branch of government, may enact, enforce, and adjudicate their own rules and regulations, thus assuming (in this context) the functions of all three branches of government (legislative, executive, and judicial). For example, some administrative agencies can sit in judgment of previously enforced agency regulations that are now in dispute and judge whether to uphold or overturn them. Agencies are created through legislation that broadly defines their structure and function. They must develop their own regulations that set policy to govern the behavior of agency officials and regulated parties; spell out their procedural requirements, such as rules governing notices of intent, comment periods, and hearings; and develop enforcement procedures. For example, the Food and Drug Administration sets and monitors standards for foods and tests drugs for purity, safety, and effectiveness, while the Environmental Protection Agency, among other activities, controls health risks from water-borne microbes in drinking water through the development and implementation of regulations.

The promulgation of regulations is guided by certain rules. Key among these, at the federal level, is the requirement that the agency responsible for implementing a law publish a draft of any proposed

THE REGULATORY PROCESS

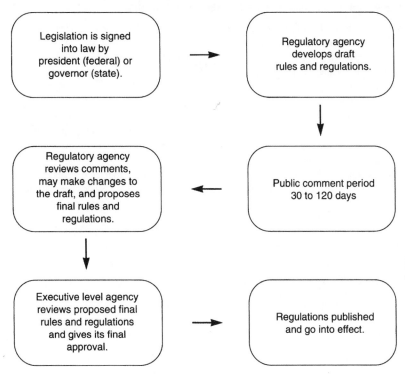

FIGURE 65-2 The regulatory process.

regulation or set of regulations in the Federal Register. The Federal Register is the official daily publication for administrative regulations, including rules, proposed rules, and notices of federal agencies and organizations, as well as executive orders and other presidential documents. The publication of proposed regulations offers an opportunity for interested parties to react to the draft before it becomes final. Commenting on draft regulations is one of the most important points of involvement in the entire legislative process (Longest, 1997). States follow similar procedures.

A REGULATORY EXAMPLE: THE AMERICAN ASSOCIATION OF COLLEGES OF NURSING AND EDUCATION REQUIREMENTS FOR NURSE PRACTITIONERS AND CLINICAL NURSE SPECIALISTS

The following example illustrates the impact of nurse practitioners, clinical nurse specialists, professional associations, and consumers have had on the regulatory process as it relates to Medicare and Medicaid

reimbursement. The history of reimbursement for advanced practice nurses involves several points where coalition building and lobbying Congress lead to incremental changes in the reimbursement of advanced practice nurses (Figure 65-3).

The initial Medicare laws were promulgated in 1965. At that time, nurse practitioners were not well established as providers; therefore traditionally regulatory language does not include advanced practice nurses in the definition of physician. In order to include advanced practice nurses, each section of CMS regulations needs to be changed to include other providers such as nurse practitioners and clinical specialists. Such changes require significant effort on the part of nurses to overcome opposition (see Chapter 69).

Prior to the Balanced Budget Act (Balanced Budget Act [BBA], 1997), NPs and CNSs were paid for services only when provided in a rural setting, in nursing facilities, or in some cases when assisting in surgery (MedPAC, 2002). The BBA (Balanced Budget Act) of 1997 removed restrictions on the geographic areas

BOX 65-4 How to Influence Legislative and Regulatory Processes

- Become informed about the public policy and health policy issues that are currently under consideration at the local, state, and federal levels of government.
- Become acquainted with the elected officials that represent you at the local, state, and federal levels of government. Communicate with them regularly to share your expertise and perspective on health care and nursing issues.
- Call, write, or send a fax or e-mail message to your legislator, stating briefly the position you wish him or her to take on a particular issue. Always remember to mention that you are a registered nurse and that you live and vote in the legislator's district.
- Request that legislation be introduced or a regulatory change made. Offer your expertise to assist in developing new legislation or in modifying existing legislation and rules.
- Become active in your professional association and work to activate a strong grassroots network of members who are prepared to contact their elected representatives on key health care issues.
- Attend a public hearing on a bill or regulation to show support for an issue, or actually testify yourself.
- Build your own political resume by becoming active in local politics in your area.
- Volunteer to work on the campaigns of candidates who are knowledgeable and supportive of nursing's perspective on health care issues.
- Seek appointment to a government task force or commission to have the opportunity to make legislative, regulatory, and public policy changes.
- Seek election to public office or employment in an administrative or executive agency.
- Explore opportunities to be involved with the policy and legislative process through internships, fellowships, and volunteer experiences at the local, state, and federal levels.

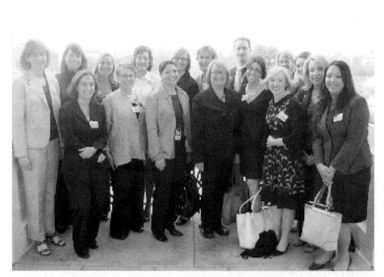

FIGURE 65-3 Nursing policy and organizational leaders on the Capitol balcony, September 30, 2008. Nancy Ridenor, first row, center. They met to work on the document "Commitment to Quality Health Care Reform: A Consensus Statement from the Nursing Community." Photo published with permission of Nancy Ridenor.

and settings in which NPs, CNSs, and PAs could be reimbursed and raised limits on Medicare payment levels to 85% of the physician fee schedule. As the states changed their laws to require advanced practice nurses to have masters degrees, CMS rules attempted to keep pace. Since 2003, nurses applying for a Medicare number for the first time are required to have the masters degree to be eligible for Medicare Part B coverage of services (Federal Register, 1999).

The development of the doctor of nursing practice (DNP) required a revision of CMS regulations. A provider could obtain the DNP without earning the masters in nursing. Without a revision of the regulations, those with the DNP without the masters degree would not be eligible for Medicare reimbursement. AACN took the lead in negotiating with CMS to discuss the need to update CMS requirements to include the emerging DNP. CMS responded by proposing rules to encompass the DNP recognizing the need to revise the regulation (Federal Register, 2008a). The comments in response to the proposed regulation are summarized in the Federal Register (2008b).

For a list of related websites, please refer to your Evolve Resources at http://evolve.elsevier.com/Mason/policypolitics/

REFERENCES

Balanced Budget Act (BBA). (1997). *Increased Medicare reimbursement for nurse practitioners and clinical nurse specialists, Section 4511.* Retrieved from http://frwebgate.access.gpo.gov/cgi-bin/getdoc.cgi?dbname=105_cong_bills&docid=f:h2015enr.txt.pdf.

Centers for Medicare and Medicaid Services (CMS). (2009). *E-rulemaking overview.* Retrieved from http://cms.hhs.gov/eRulemaking.

Congressional Quarterly. (2008). *Guide to current American government.* Washington, D.C.: *Congressional Quarterly.*

Congressional Quarterly. (2009). *Congress 101: The legislative process.* Washington, D.C.: Congressional Quarterly. Retrieved from http://corporate.cq.com/wmspage.cfm?parm1=231.

Davidson, R. H., Oleszek, W. J., & Lee, F. E. (2007). *Congress and its members.* (11th ed.). Washington, D.C.: Congressional Quarterly.

Federal Register. (1999, July 22). Department of Health and Human Services. Centers for Medicare and Medicaid Services. Nurse practitioner qualifications. *Federal Register, 64*(140), 39625-39626. Retrieved from www.gpoaccess.gov/fr/advanced.html.

Federal Register. (2008a, July 7). Department of Health and Human Services, Centers for Medicare and Medicaid Services. Educational requirements for nurse practitioners and clinical nurse specialists. *Federal Register, 73*(130), 38576. Washington, D.C.: U.S. Government Printing Office. Retrieved from http://edocket.access.gpo./2008/pdf/E8-14949.pdf.

Federal Register. (2008b, November 19). Department of Health and Human Services. Center for Medicare and Medicaid Services. Educational requirements for nurse practitioners and clinical nurse specialists. *Federal Register, 73*(224), 69853-69854. Retrieved from www.gpoaccess.gov/fr/advanced.html.

Kingdon, J. (1984). *Agendas, alternatives, and public policy.* Boston: Little, Brown.

Longest, B. B., Jr. (1997). *Seeking strategic advantage through health policy analysis.* Chicago: Health Administration Press.

MedPAC. (2002). Medicare payment to advance practice nurses and physician assistants. Retrieved from www.medpac.gov/publications/congressional_reports/jun02_NonPhysPay.pdf.

Pepper, C., & Roybal, E. (1988). *H.R. 3436 Fact Sheet: Financing and cost controls.* Washington, D.C.: U.S. House of Representatives Select Committee on Aging.

Schneider, J. (2007). *The committee system in the U.S. Congress (Congressional Research Service order code RS20794).* Washington, D.C.: Congressional Research Service.

Schneider, J. (2008). *House and Senate rules of procedure: A comparison (Congressional Research Service order code RL30945, CRS-6).* Washington, D.C.: Congressional Research Service.

Schick, A. (2007). *The federal budget: Politics, policy, process.* (3rd ed.). Washington, D.C.: Brookings Institution.

Tong, L. (2008). *Senate confirmation process: A brief overview (Congressional Research Service order code RS20986).* Washington, D.C.: Congressional Research Service.

CHAPTER 66

Nursing Licensure and Regulation

Edie Brous

"[T]he liberty component of the Fourteenth Amendment's Due Process Clause includes some generalized due process right to choose one's field of private employment, but a right which is nevertheless subject to reasonable government regulation."

—United States Supreme Court, *Conn v. Gabbert,* 526 U.S. 286, 291(1999)

The application process for nursing educational programs has become progressively more competitive. The accepted student must then meet the stringent academic rigors of a challenging curriculum, followed by successful completion of state board examinations before being initially licensed to practice. The extensive ordeals in reaching the qualifications for licensure have led some to believe they have earned the right to practice professional nursing. The practice of nursing, however, is not an unqualified *right*. It is also a *privilege,* and privileges must be preserved. To maintain one's license in good standing and continue practicing, nurses must understand that *rights* are always accompanied by *responsibilities*.

This chapter will provide an overview of the regulatory processes, both those that are internal to nursing and those that impose obligations from outside the profession. While external regulatory schemes impact all health care providers, it is the internal process of self-regulation that greatly influences nursing practice and defines nursing as an autonomous profession.

HISTORICAL PERSPECTIVE

Prior to 1903, nursing regulation in the United States was limited to lists or registries of those who had been trained as nurses. In 1903, North Carolina created the first board of nursing (BON) and enacted a Nurse Practice Act (NPA). Within 20 years, this had been followed by all other states. As nursing boards

developed standards to define nursing practice and prevent unqualified persons from practicing, licensure became mandatory and each state developed an examination process toward that end (Damgaard et al., 2000). Members of each state BON met collectively with members of the American Nurses Association (ANA) Council on State Boards of Nursing. This gave way to the National Council of State Boards of Nursing (NCSBN) in 1978. Today there are 60 constituent member boards (including all 50 states and some U.S. territories). Educational requirements have been standardized and modernized, as has the examination process (NCSBN, 2009b). The NCSBN has published a model NPA and interfaces with the International Council of Nurses (ICN). The NCSBN and ICN have issued independent and joint position papers.

The scope of nursing practice has greatly expanded but remains state-specific at all levels of practice. Advanced practice nursing, as with RN, LPN/LVN, or nursing attendant practice, remains within the regulatory purview of each state or territory. The composition and authority of each board, the methodology for addressing complaints, the definition of professional misconduct, and the qualifications for remaining in good standing are examples of state-specific regulation. For this reason, nurses at all levels of practice must understand and abide by the NPAs of each state in which they practice.

THE PURPOSE OF PROFESSIONAL REGULATION

The government has an obligation to protect its most vulnerable citizens. This social contract with the public is the reason nursing is a regulated profession. Those who are sick, infirm, young, elderly, disabled, or in any manner unable to advocate for themselves may be endangered by unqualified practitioners.

Nursing regulation provides public accountability. A member of the lay public may not have the ability to recognize and protect himself or herself from incompetent providers. Government oversight of licensed nurses by a body of nursing experts is intended to keep patients safe by ensuring competence.

SOURCES OF REGULATION

NURSING BOARDS

The initial qualifications for licensure, continuing educational requirements, disciplinary procedures, complaint resolution processes, professional misconduct or unprofessional conduct definitions, mandatory reporting requirements, and specific scopes of practice are determined at the state level. Some states have separate licensing boards for registered nurses and licensed practical or vocational nurses, while other states have unified boards for regulating all nurses. BONs are given their authority through state laws or administrative procedure acts.

HEALTH AND HUMAN SERVICES

As stated on the HHS website, "[T]he Department of Health and Human Services (HHS) is the United States government's principal agency for protecting the health of all Americans and providing essential human services, especially for those who are least able to help themselves" (HHS, 2009). Through various administrative agencies, HHS regulates issues such as civil rights, privacy, food and drug safety, the Medicaid and Medicare programs, health care fraud, medical research, technology standards, and tribal matters. It serves as the umbrella organization for such agencies as the Centers for Medicare and Medicaid (CMS), the Food and Drug Administration (FDA), the Centers for Disease Control and Prevention (CDC), and the Office for Civil Rights (OCR), among others. The integrity of all HHS programs is protected by the Office of the Inspector General (OIG) through audits and exclusion lists, as discussed in the following paragraphs.

CENTERS FOR MEDICARE & MEDICAID SERVICES

Medicare and Medicaid are government health insurance programs for qualifying individuals. Medicare is a federally-administered program available to persons 65 or older, persons under 65 with certain disabilities, and persons of all ages with end-stage renal disease. Medicaid is a state-administered program available to low-income individuals and families meeting federal and state eligibility criteria. Health care providers must be compliant with regulations and criteria called "Conditions of Participations" (CoPs) and "Conditions for Coverage" (CfC) to be eligible for Medicare or Medicaid reimbursement. The OIG may place a provider on a "List of Excluded Individuals/Entities." The exclusion program is designed to protect the health and welfare of the nation's older adults and poor individuals by preventing certain providers from participating in the Medicaid or Medicare programs. Nurses placed on the exclusion list may not be employed by any employers receiving state or federal funding.

THE JOINT COMMISSION

Compliance with the Medicare and Medicaid CoPs may be demonstrated with Joint Commission accreditation (United States Code, 2009). The CMS will "deem" an organization as meeting certification requirements by virtue of having met The Joint Commission's standards. Those standards include nursing performance elements such as policies and procedures, safety initiatives, reporting mechanisms, communication systems, sentinel events, quality improvement practices, staffing effectiveness, credentialing, and other performance indicators. The goal of The Joint Commission survey and accreditation process is to improve patient outcomes through improved performance.

FEDERAL, STATE, AND LOCAL LAW

Public health codes are laws enacted to promote community health and safety. They address emergency preparedness, communicable diseases, environmental controls, utilization of health care facilities, staff credentials and competency, policies and procedures, sanitation, housing, childhood nutrition, mental health issues, food safety, and many other elements related to nursing care. Public health laws exist at the local, state, and federal level and may be enforced by civil or criminal penalties.

ORGANIZATIONAL POLICY

Nurses are responsible to be familiar with their employer's policies and procedures and to adhere to them. An organization's protocols may be used to establish the practice standards to which the nurse will be held. They exist to provide standardization and consistency. Failure to abide by an institution's rules may endanger patients and expose the nurse and the employer to liability.

LICENSURE BOARD RESPONSIBILITIES

PROTECT THE PUBLIC

The primary function of a BON is protection of the health, safety, and welfare of the public and maintenance of the public's trust in the profession by ensuring that those individuals who engage in the conduct described in the Nurse Practice Act are properly trained and licensed. The state in which an applicant seeks licensure (by reciprocity or endorsement) must confirm that the applicant is, in fact, a licensee in good standing in another jurisdiction. To confirm that this is the case, state boards will perform licensure verification. Approximately 38 states participate in NURSYS®, an online process for providing immediate verification information to the requesting board.

ISSUE AND RENEW LICENSES

An initial professional license issued by a nursing board is valid for the licensee's lifetime, but the licensee must periodically register that license to continue practicing. The licensee must meet the board's registration requirements to be issued a registration certificate. Such requirements typically include continuing education, clinical practice, the absence of a criminal record, and continued good moral character. The cyclical process of reregistering a license is commonly referred to as a *renewal process*.

To comply with their legislative mandate to protect the public, BONs define the required elements of nursing education. Graduation from a school that is accredited in one state may not meet the requirements for licensure in another state.

INVESTIGATION AND PROSECUTION OF COMPLAINTS

BONs are statutorily mandated to investigate all complaints against health care providers covered by the state's NPA. Some cases may be resolved through informal procedures, while others require formal hearings. Licensees against whom a complaint has been lodged should be advised of the allegations and of their rights. Although nurses may represent themselves, it is strongly advised that they seek legal counsel when responding to Board inquiries, even when the allegations appear baseless.

LICENSURE REQUIREMENTS

EXAMINATION

A candidate for entry into nursing practice as an RN or LPN/LVN must apply for licensure to a board of nursing and receive an Authorization To Test (ATT). He or she then may be allowed to schedule an appointment to take the National Council Licensure Exam (NCLEX-RN or NCLEX-PN). Successful completion of the examination is required to be granted an initial licensure.

ENDORSEMENT

A nurse currently licensed in one jurisdiction may be granted a license in another jurisdiction without retaking the NCLEX upon meeting certain conditions. Typically the requirements include graduation from an accredited program, English proficiency, clinical practice experience or a refresher course, and good moral character. Additionally, the nurse may be required to explain criminal activity or disciplinary actions in the home state. Interstate compact agreements may also allow multistate licensure (MSL).

NURSING LICENSURE COMPACT

A multistate compact, referred to by the NCSBN as a "mutual recognition model," allows RNs or LPN/LVNs to work across state lines in certain circumstances. Nurses residing in compact member states known as *residency* or *home states* may practice in other compact member states known as *remote states*. Nursing practice must be compliant with the NPA and the nursing licensure compact administrative rules of each state. Nurses must remain within the specific scope of practice in the state in which they are practicing (the state in which the patient is located). Home states and remote states communicate through a coordinated database, and both may take disciplinary action against a licensee when indicated. A separate licensure compact for advanced practice nurses has not been implemented, but three states (Texas,

Iowa, and Utah) have passed laws authorizing their participation (NCSBN, 2010).

NURSE PRACTICE ACTS

The state regulation of nursing occurs within the context of statutory mandates. Sets of laws enacted to protect the public specify the scope of practice for nursing attendants, LPN/LVNs, RNs, and APNs; outline the authority of the Board; define professional misconduct; and detail the investigation and disciplinary processes for resolving complaints.

SCOPE OF PRACTICE

The scope of practice for all levels of nursing has evolved and expanded considerably since the first NPA was enacted. Medical societies frequently react to advancements in nursing practice by challenging BON authority to define expanded roles, particularly regarding advanced practice roles. Medical societies have made arguments that advanced nursing practice encroaches upon the practice of medicine, specifically regarding NPs, Nurse Midwives, and Clinical Nurse Specialists. The American Medical Association (AMA), for example, has proposed or adopted resolutions opposing the creation of a board of midwifery and proposing greater physician oversight of midwifery practice (AMA, Resolution 204, 2008), requiring Doctors of Nursing Practice to function under the supervision and authority of physicians (AMA, Resolution 214, 2008) and "protecting" the terms *doctor, resident,* and *residency* by restricting their use to physicians, dentists, and podiatrists (AMA, Resolution 232, 2008). Such actions by the AMA consistently oppose the independent practice of other practitioners and declare the need for physician supervision and authority over all other providers. In 2005, the AMAs Resolution 814 even suggested that physicians should usurp the legislatively-granted authority of other licensing boards. Nursing organizations, such as the American Nurses Association (ANA), view these efforts as a divisive attempt to restrict the practice of other providers and presume authority over all professions. The use of terms such as "limited licensure health care provider," "mid-level professional," or "non-physician" reflects the AMA's anachronistic view of all health care providers as physician extenders (American Academy of Nurse Practitioners [AANP], 2006) and inaccurately suggests that nursing boards do not keep patients safe.

ADVISORY OPINIONS AND PRACTICE ALERTS

Many nursing boards release opinions regarding scope of practice, professional misconduct definitions, or delegation questions to clarify the board's position on certain matters. These advisory opinions may be released independently or in conjunction with other organizations. Practice alerts may also be released advising the nursing community and the public at large of rule changes or urgent issues. Nurses should go to their BON's website periodically to monitor such communications.

THE SOURCE OF LICENSING BOARD AUTHORITY

Nursing is regulated at the state level. Laws referred to as "Administrative Procedure Acts" or "Civil Procedure Codes" vary by state and determine the structure and authority of the BON. In some states, the BON is an independent agency, while in other states the BON operates under a larger state agency. Typically the BONs that are consolidated under larger umbrella agencies are functionaries of the Secretary of State, the Department of Health, the Division of Consumer Affairs, Education Departments, or other regulatory and licensing agencies. In yet other states, BONs are hybrid organizations, functioning as institutions that are partially independent and partially affiliated with other agencies. Rules and regulations for nursing practice may also be found in public health and general business laws. The court system generally supports the exclusive authority of the BON but will consider conflicts between employment practices and BON directions.

Courts may also hear conflicts between the BON and other agencies, as exemplified in *K.C. et al. v. Jack O'Connell, et al.* (American Nurses Association, et al., 2008). The American Diabetes Association (ADA) and the parents of several diabetic students brought a class-action lawsuit claiming that the California Department of Education (CDE) violated the educational rights of diabetic students. In the absence of adequate numbers of school nurses, the parents claimed they had to remove their children from the school or leave their jobs to administer insulin. The CDE settled with the parents and issued a "Legal Advisory on the Rights of Students with Diabetes in California's K-12 Public Schools" in which local education agencies were required to train non-licensed volunteers to administer insulin.

The ANA, the California Nurses Association (CNA), and the California School Nurses Association (CSNA) challenged this legal advisory in court, arguing that the directive could not be followed as it violated the California NPA (ANA, 2008). The NPA specifically restricted medication administration to licensed nurses. While the matter was pending, the California Board of Registered Nursing issued a public statement (CBRN, 2007) in which nurses were advised to adhere to the NPA and practice in accordance with the Board's standards.

The American Diabetes Association (ADA) intervened in the lawsuit, arguing that federal disability laws entitled diabetic students to insulin administration as a component of their educational rights. As such, in the absence of sufficient school nurses, schools were required to train unlicensed employees in insulin administration. The court ruled that the CDE legal advisory was unenforceable, as the CDE had exceeded its authority. The opinion stated that the CDE's legal advisory conflicted with state law because the NPA clearly defined the administration of medications as nursing practice. Although the decision should imply that school funding decisions must include adequate nursing staffing, the case has been appealed. Legislation and public hearings are being conducted regarding the issue. Many BONs are considering this issue in home care as well as school settings.

DISCIPLINARY OFFENSES

BONs investigate all complaints they receive. While gross negligence and unsafe practice are obvious sources of disciplinary action, many actions not directly related to patient care may fall within the definition of professional misconduct and result in disciplinary action. Failure to advise the BON of name or address changes, failure to repay student loans, failure to pay child support, driving under the influence, failure to file or pay taxes, dishonesty in licensure or job applications, falsified or deficient documentation and record-keeping, improper delegation, diversion of controlled substances, or criminal convictions are some examples of actions that may result in BON disciplinary action.

COMPLAINT RESOLUTION

The BON may offer the nurse an opportunity to settle the matter informally, rather than conducting a full hearing. A settlement called a Consent Order may be reached in which the nurse stipulates to certain findings and agrees to discipline that has been negotiated. Informal settlement conferences offer the advantage of lower legal costs and more rapid resolution of the complaint. The nurse may elect to attend a formal hearing rather than agree to a Consent Order if the settlement agreement offers a disciplinary action the nurse considers too harsh. A formal hearing may also be preferred when the disciplinary action of a proposed Consent Order would trigger an OIG exclusion.

DISCIPLINARY ACTIONS

The BON may close the file if its investigation finds no violations. The complainant will be advised that the investigation is complete and the matter is resolved. No action is taken against the nurse. The BON may find violations that can be addressed by issuing a letter of reprimand, but no other action. Letters of reprimand may be publicly posted as disciplinary actions. Nurses may also be fined, and/or ordered to attend corrective education.

For more serious practice or ethical issues, the BON may impose practice restrictions and place the nurse on probation. During the probationary period, the nurse may be required to submit periodic employer reports, demonstrate attendance in an impaired provider program, and comply with other terms. Licenses may also be suspended. The period of suspension may be actual suspension, during which time the nurse is not permitted to work, or stayed (temporarily set aside) during which time the nurse is permitted to work while remaining on probation.

The most severe penalty, revocation, is reserved for cases in which the BON believes the nurse presents a serious danger to the public and cannot be rehabilitated to safely practice. A revocation permanently terminates a person's license, prohibiting practice and the use of nursing titles. The individual may no longer represent himself or herself as a nurse. The BON may entertain a petition for reinstatement after revocation in certain cases where the individual can demonstrate rehabilitation and competence. Mandatory waiting periods may be imposed before requests for restoration will be entertained, and formal restoration hearings may be required.

When faced with formal disciplinary hearings, some nurses may agree to voluntarily surrender their nursing licenses. In doing so, the nurse must understand that the forfeiture of the license is permanent. Such surrender still constitutes a disciplinary action tantamount to revocation. The surrender process, sometimes referred to as "Discipline by Consent," is an application that the BON may or may not accept. Temporary surrenders may be negotiated for nurses who agree to enter professional assistance programs for impaired providers. Entry into such programs may provide immunity from further disciplinary action if the licensee meets all other required criteria.

Non-punitive peer assistance programs may provide an alternative to discipline but have not been uniformly adopted by all jurisdictions. Those states and territories that have adopted such alternative to discipline programs may require the absence of patient harm for nurses to qualify for participation. The ANA endorses these programs, stating, in part, that, "alternative approaches have been demonstrated to be at least as effective in protecting the public safety as more antiquated punitive methods. The ANA has resolved to work with these few states to pursue the legislative and regulatory modifications necessary to implement an 'alternative to discipline' model for impaired nurses" (ANA, 2010).

Alternatives to discipline programs may address impairment from mental illness as well as from chemical addiction. The use of a medical model, as opposed to a punitive model in addressing mental illness and/ or chemical addiction is preferable because it is more consistent with the board's stated goal of protecting the public. Additionally, such diversion programs allow the nurse to be rehabilitated and support reporting systems. Nurses working in states without such programs should become active in lobbying for their adoption. Some states have an additional category of license surrender called "Voluntary Relinquishment." This is a form of surrender unrelated to disciplinary action, in which the licensee is retiring, moving out of state, or for other reasons choosing not to practice nursing in the state.

Appealing board decisions is a difficult, expensive, and frequently unsuccessful process. All internal administrative steps must be completed before seeking redress in the courts. The court will only reverse BON decisions under narrow circumstances. The licensee appealing a BON decision must prove that the BON has violated the constitution or the law, has exceeded its authority under the statute, that it took actions that were an abuse of discretion or arbitrary and capricious, or that the actions taken by the BON were unsupported by the evidence.

COLLATERAL IMPACT

The emotional, financial, legal, and professional impact of BON disciplinary action can be profound. Evidence of board disciplinary action may be admissible in medical malpractice lawsuits, or in criminal prosecution. OIG exclusions and data bank listings may render a nurse unable to work, even when holding a license in good standing. Subsequent licensure in another profession or jurisdiction may be difficult or impossible to obtain. Reputation damage is very difficult to overcome. The emotional distress can be considerable, even disabling. Long after the BON has resolved the complaint, the licensee may continue to experience sequelae.

REGULATION'S SHORTCOMINGS

Although professional licensing boards are entrusted with keeping the public safe, there is no evidence basis that the current regulatory system for BONs is effective in improving nursing practice. Some BON practices may, in fact, be antithetical to patient safety goals. Punitive cultures undermine patient safety by deterring essential error-reporting. BONs that fail to distinguish between intentional misconduct and inevitable human error perpetuate an ineffective response to adverse events by blaming the end user, or direct provider for the error. This *sharp-end* focus fails to account for the dangerous systems in which nurses practice and compromises the error-analysis process necessary to prevent recurrence. As opposed to *latent-error* focus, which does positively impact patient safety, such *active-error* focus has a paradoxical and perverse effect on patient safety initiatives.

The level of penalty imposed may be determined by the level of injury to the patient, which is both inequitable and counterproductive. Outcome-oriented discipline results in inconsistency from one licensee to another for the same infraction. Safety experts recommend evaluating processes, not outcomes. The public is not kept safe by imposing a harsher penalty on a nurse because the patient was injured. The nurse whose patient is not injured by the identical error may be a less cautious provider and actually pose a greater risk to patients but receives a lighter penalty with this approach.

Lengthy suspensions create rusty practice skills. The technical competence and knowledge required for safe practice are not enhanced by removing a clinician from the workforce. Practice deficiencies are not corrected by levying fines or publishing disciplinary actions on the Internet. Without addressing the underlying root causes and contributing factors of nursing errors, they will persist and endanger patients.

Public safety cannot be attained in the absence of nursing advocacy. Patients cannot be kept safe unless their providers are adequately supported. BON advisory opinions are often unavailable or inadequate. Statements such as, "Nurses should work collaboratively with their employers" or "Until the matter is resolved nurses are advised to use their best judgment" offer no direction to the practitioner faced with questionable work situations. While the NCSBN could provide an enormous amount of guidance, much of the Council's published materials are restricted to board members and unavailable to the practicing nurse. Many NPAs use generic language when addressing "professional misconduct" or "unprofessional conduct" and do not provide definitions to guide practice or educate a nurse regarding potential violations.

The defense of a licensee may be compromised when the BON has information which the licensee is unable to access. Privacy and confidentiality provisions of the administrative statutes are sometimes written or interpreted in such a manner as to prevent even the target of the investigation from obtaining all evidentiary materials. The discovery rights to which a criminal or civil defendant would be entitled may not be afforded to licensees in an administrative action.

Disciplinary actions taken against licensees can destroy reputations and careers. As such, there should be an adequate appeal mechanism. Courts tend to defer to the expertise of the BON and uphold BON decisions. This deference is based upon a rationale that the BON's unique nursing expertise distinguishes it as the most qualified body to render decisions. Disciplinary hearings in some states, however, may be conducted by non-nurse administrative personnel with absolutely no expertise in nursing.

The collateral impact of disciplinary action may be ultimately more destructive than the actual disciplinary action itself, even serving as a constructive revocation. Onerous practice restrictions compromise employment opportunities. A temporary suspension may be all that is required for OIG exclusion. The inability to practice for several years may make an eventual return to practice logistically impossible, regardless of licensure status. This undermines efforts to rehabilitate motivated professionals. Such constructive revocations contribute to the nursing shortage by accelerating the exodus of providers from the workforce. The consequent reductions in staffing levels endanger, rather than protect patients.

Board members may not be selected by members of the nursing profession. They are frequently appointed by the governor or some other state selection method. As such, appointees may be selected more by political motivations than qualifications the regulated community would find essential. BONs are bureaucratic structures, many of whom are underfunded and understaffed. Levels of efficiency vary. Due process rights in agencies differ substantially from due process rights in a court of law. The "right to a speedy trial" in the criminal system, as well as the standards and goals that move civil suits forward on mandated schedules, do not exist in the administrative setting. The investigative and hearing process can take months or years from initial complaint to final resolution. This lengthy process is traumatizing even to those nurses who are ultimately vindicated.

Most people understand the need for legal representation to protect their freedom and physical possessions in criminal or civil lawsuits, yet many nurses try to represent themselves with the BON. A professional license is also a valuable asset that requires zealous protection and skilled advocacy. Some BONs make telephone calls to licensees. In these circumstances, nurses may unknowingly make statements against their interest. Nurses may also sign agreements with the BON not understanding the long-term collateral impact of doing so. BONs do not always advise licensees that they can and should seek legal representation at all stages of the process.

SUMMARY

It is critical that nurses read and understand their NPAs. Although all nurses make human mistakes, they should not unexpectedly find themselves defending their license for failure to educate themselves regarding the rules. Nurses must study and adhere to their state's continuing education requirements, scope of practice, definitions of professional misconduct, reporting requirements, and standards of practice. Nebulous areas of practice should be identified to the BON, and advisory opinions should be requested. Clinical practice can only be evidence-based if nurses belong to professional organizations and regularly read the literature. Physical limitations must be respected to reduce the clinical error associated with sleep-deprivation impairment. If contacted by telephone, nurses should advise the BON that they wish to speak with counsel before making any statements or signing any papers. All nurses should independently maintain professional liability insurance rather than relying on employer coverage. Personal policies may provide the coverage for disciplinary actions and licensure defense that employer policies do not. A professional license is a valuable asset that may be considered a property right. It is not a right that can be taken for granted, however, and nurses can only protect their licenses by fully understanding the responsibilities that accompany them.

For a list of related websites, please refer to your Evolve Resources at http://evolve.elsevier.com/Mason/policypolitics/

REFERENCES

American Academy of Nurse Practitioners (AANP). (2006, June 1; updated 2006, August 26). Health professionals urge cooperative care; Oppose SOPP & AMA Resolution 814. Retrieved from www.apta.org/AM/Template.cfm?Section=Home&TEMPLATE=/CM/ContentDisplay.cfm&CONTENTID=31550.

American Medical Association House of Delegates. (2005, September 21). Resolution 814: Limited Licensure Health Care Provider Training and Certification Standards. Retrieved from www.aaom.info/ama814.pdf.

American Medical Association House of Delegates. (2008, April 28). Resolution 204: Midwifery Scope of Practice and Licensure. Retrieved from www.ama-assn.org/ama1/pub/upload/mm/471/204.doc.

American Medical Association House of Delegates. (2008, April 30). Resolution 232 (formerly 303): Protection of the terms "Doctor" "Resident" and "Residency." Retrieved from www.amaassn.org/ama1/pub/upload/mm/471/annotatedb.doc.

American Medical Association House of Delegates. (2008, May 7). Resolution 214: Doctor of Nursing Practice. Retrieved from www.ama-assn.org/ama1/pub/upload/mm/471/214.doc.

American Nurses Association. (2010). Impaired Nurse Resource Center. Retrieved from www.nursingworld.org/MainMenuCategories/ThePracticeofProfessionalNursing/workplace/ImpairedNurse.aspx.

American Nurses Association, et al. v. Jack O'Connell, State Superintendent of Public Instruction, et al., California Superior Court, Judge Lloyd Connelly, No. 07AS04631, Judgment dated December 29, 2008.

Damgaard, G., Hohman, M., & Karpiuk, K. (2000, September 8). History of Nursing Regulation. Retrieved from http://doh.sd.gov/boards/nursing/Documents/WhitePaperHistory2000.pdf.

Hughes v. Freeman Health System, 283 S.W.3d 797 (Mo. App. S.D., 2009).

The Joint Commission. (2009). Retrieved from www.jointcommission.org.

National Council of State Boards of Nursing. (2010). APRN Compact. Retrieved from www.ncsbn.org/917.htm.

National Council of State Boards of Nursing. (2009a). Complaints. Retrieved from www.ncsbn.org/181.htm.

National Council of State Boards of Nursing. (2009b). History. Retrieved from www.ncsbn.org/181.htm.

United States Code. (2009). Title 42, Chapter 7, Subchapter XVIII, Part E, § 1395(bb), Effect of Accreditation. Retrieved from www.law.cornell.edu/uscode/42/1395bb.html.

United States Department of Health and Human Services. (2009). Retrieved from www.hhs.gov/about.

CHAPTER 67

Regulating Industrial Chemicals to Protect the Environment and Human Health

Charlotte Brody

"Only within the moment of time represented by the present century has one species—man—acquired significant power to alter the nature of his world."

—Rachel Carson

The problem of environmental contaminants has a long history in the United States. In 1785, the lawmakers of Massachusetts added a preamble to explain the purpose of the new law they were putting into place:

> *Whereas some evilly disposed persons, from motives of avarice and filthy lucre, have been induced to sell diseased, corrupted, contagious or unwholesome provisions, to the great nuisance of public health and peace. (Swann, 2001)*

The Massachusetts Act Against Selling Unwholesome Provisions is one of the first examples of a law aimed at protecting the health of the American public from contaminated products and the "avarice-motivated" people who sell them.

In 1906, the United States Congress passed the Food and Drug Act. In 100 years since, consumers have come to expect that the federal government's laws and enforcement mechanisms provide the scientific inspections that are beyond our reach as ordinary consumers. The public believes that, given the existence of the FDA and the Consumer Product Safety Commission, the products we use every day have gone through rigorous safety and efficacy testing and official review of these tests before they can be sold. The FDA does require extensive animal and human studies that are scrutinized by institutional review boards before being conducted (Meadows, 2002). But recent

headlines have shown that this process isn't enough to fully protect the public from unnecessarily dangerous prescription drugs. Lurking below the headlines is the larger story of industrial chemicals that work like drugs but are put on the market without any FDA-like approval or labeling requirements.

HISTORY OF CHEMICALS CAUSING DISEASE AND THE LACK OF REGULATION

Mercury provides one example of how long science has recognized that chemicals can harm health. Galen, born in 129 AD, described mercury as "a cold poison." In 1860, Transactions of the Medical Society of New Jersey published a clinical description of "mecurialism" among workers who used mercury to make fur hats (Hightower, 2004). The Mad Hatter in Lewis Carroll's 1865 classic Alice in Wonderland exhibited the most visible of these symptoms of "tremor, psychic disturbances such as irritability, timidity, irascibility and difficulty in getting along with people, headaches, drowsiness, gastrointestinal disturbances, sore mouth, insomnia and weakness."

Our early knowledge about the hazards of mercury and other chemicals was mostly ignored as the twentieth-century economy built itself on the use of thousands of chemicals. These chemicals were introduced into the marketplace without any government-required premarket studies of possible health effects. Only when people in certain occupations with certain exposures started developing certain diseases did the health professions and the public learn of a chemical's danger. In the 1920s, the press covered the story of the 11 men who died and the 149 more who were poisoned by the tetraethyl lead being added to gasoline (Rosner & Markowitz, 2002). In 1928, a medical journal published the first finding of benzene-related leukemia, and reports of lung cancer associated with asbestos exposure started showing up in the medical literature in the 1930s and 1940s (Gee et al., 2001). In 1970, animal studies were published that showed that exposure to vinyl chloride, the basic component of vinyl or PVC, resulted in angiosarcoma, a cancer of the blood vessels in the brain or liver at half the exposure level that workers were being told was safe (Rosner & Markowitz, 2002).

These stories of workers, exposure, and disease share a plotline. First, the studies showing harm are ignored. Then they are disputed, usually by the industry that employs the affected workers. When those positions are overwhelmingly challenged by the scientific evidence and political will, the argument shifts to how much exposure to that chemical is necessary before workers start getting a specific disease. Instead of focusing on finding safer alternative materials or processes that would eliminate the exposure problem, scientists and policymakers review the animal and human studies on exposure to a certain industrial chemical, decide the amount of exposure that the studies show will cause a health problem, add a safety factor, and set a limit for exposure.

This policy option, most often called *risk assessment,* is used to set limits on exposure not only to substances present in factories but also to chemicals added to personal care products; contaminants in drinking water; toxic contaminants in food; outdoor air pollution from vehicles, factories, and power plants; and indoor air pollution from building materials and furnishings. Risk assessment is based on the following assumptions:

- That we have the information we need to make good decisions
- That most chemicals are benign
- That although chemicals may cause harm when workers are overdosed, there is a safe level for even the most dangerous chemicals
- That exposure to the less-benign chemicals will result in unique disease that can be tied to the exposure to a single chemical
- That it is morally acceptable to wait and see what disease manifests itself in exposed workers and,

since Love Canal, exposed communities before taking action.

The Toxic Substances Control Act of 1976, or TSCA (pronounced "toska"), enshrines this set of assumptions. TSCA finds all chemicals in use before 1976 to be safe unless the government can prove that their use poses "an unreasonable risk." More than 99% of the volume of chemicals on the market today is part of the TSCA inventory list of "innocent until proven guilty" chemicals. There are additional requirements for new chemicals under TSCA. This higher standard for chemicals created after 1976 has limited innovation by promoting the continued use of chemicals that were grandfathered in at a lower standard (Tickner, Geiser, & Coffin, 2005).

Drugs must be shown to be safe, but chemicals must be shown to be guilty. Federal law requires rigorous reviews of the animal and human data by the FDA before a drug can be commercially sold, but the U.S. Environmental Protection Agency (EPA) has to gather the evidence to prove that a chemical "will present an unreasonable risk," that the regulation it proposes to reduce the risk to "an acceptable level" is the least burdensome to industry, and that the benefit of the regulation outweighs the cost to industry.

The numbers reveal the level of protection that results from these two very different regulatory methodologies:

- According to the Tufts Center for the Study of Drug Development, about 1 in 5 drugs that enter clinical testing ultimately is approved by the FDA (Meadows, 2002).
- According to the U.S. Government Accountability Office (GAO) June 2005 report, of the 60,000 chemicals on the TSCA inventory, the EPA has successfully restricted 5.

A coarse mathematic comparison yields this statistic: 80% of new drugs never get to market, but only 0.008% of TSCA-listed chemicals have been restricted by government action.

EMERGING FIELD OF ENVIRONMENTAL HEALTH

Chemicals work very much like pharmaceutical drugs. Specifically, for both:

- The size of the patient matters, especially when the patient is still in utero.
- The unique sensitivities of the patient matter.

- Interactions, synergies, and cumulative effects matter.

SIZE MATTERS

Prescribing the correct dose, depending on the size and age of the patient, is a standard part of the practice of medicine. If a drug is considered safe for children, the appropriate dose is much smaller than the adult amount. And many drugs that are approved for adult use are restricted for pregnant women because of the potential impact on the developing child.

An exposure to chemicals from a product or a food, or from air, water, or soil pollution, takes place without modification in dose. So when a 6-foot man eats mercury-contaminated tuna with his newly pregnant wife, the mercury in the fish may not harm either adult but can profoundly affect the brain and nervous system development of a fetus. When human populations have been poisoned by mercury in environmental accidents, exposed pregnant women who reported few or no symptoms have given birth to children who had severe brain and nervous system damage (National Research Council Commission on Life Sciences, 2000).

SENSITIVITY MATTERS

Asking a patient if he or she is allergic to any food or drug is essential to the delivery of any health service. And warning of side effects, even if they are unlikely to occur in most patients receiving a particular medication or treatment, is routine. Just as with drugs, some people can be harmed by chemical exposures that do not seem to affect other people. Studies suggest that genetic differences are at least partly responsible for these differences. A 2004 study of women in Connecticut, for example, showed that women with a particular variation of a gene that helps metabolize toxic substances have a greater risk for breast cancer if they are exposed to PCBs (Zhang et al., 2004).

INTERACTIONS MATTER

Why do we ask patients about the medications they are currently taking? One important answer is so we don't prescribe another medication that might create a dangerous drug interaction. Studies are suggesting that interactions, synergies, and cumulative effects also take place between chemicals. In 1997, Lancet published a study by Rothman and colleagues that shows that people exposed to the Epstein-Barr virus and PCBs had a higher risk of non-Hodgkin's lymphoma than people exposed to only one risk factor.

Cumulative effects can also make tiny doses add up to harm. Rajapakse, Silva, and Kortenkamp (2002) are among the scientists who have noted how chemicals that work like estrogens can mix with natural hormones in the body and double the effect of natural estrogen. What's safe one at a time isn't so safe in combination (e.g., a patient who takes three cold medicines in one swallow and experiences undesirable results).

REGULATING CHEMICALS LIKE WE'RE SUPPOSED TO REGULATE DRUGS

As the emerging field of environmental health teaches us that chemicals work like drugs, we can also be learning from the history of drug regulation about how we might regulate chemicals.

- Use carefully constructed animal studies to predict human effects.
- Heed early warnings. When good science shows that a chemical is causing harm to animals or humans, mandate the move to safer substitutes.
- Build good policies on good data and the government's ability to act on the findings.

An important difference between chemicals and drugs makes the recognition of animal studies particularly important: Because chemical exposures in humans do not cure disease or alleviate pain, it is not ethical for society to engage in the types of human studies that we use for pharmaceuticals. Studies have repeatedly demonstrated, for example, that the male reproductive system of laboratory animals can be harmed by exposure to the phthalate DEHP in utero or before puberty (Center for the Evaluation of Risks to Human Reproduction, 2005). Other studies have shown that male infants receiving treatment in a neonatal intensive care unit (NICU) can be exposed to DEHP in PVC medical devices at levels higher than those that cause harm in animal studies (Green et al., 2005). Is it ethically appropriate to purposefully expose baby boys in NICUs to DEHP and then follow them to adulthood to determine if the animal studies accurately predict that their reproductive capacities are harmed?

After Vioxx and Bextra, two pain-relieving prescription drugs, were pulled off the market over an

8-month period in 2004 and 2005, the FDA's top officials acknowledged that their Adverse Event Reporting System (AERS) was flawed and called together experts to determine how to improve the system (*American Journal of Health-System Pharmacy*, 2005). The AERS process and its flaws underscore the importance of taking action based on the timely recognition of a problem by well-resourced, independent reviewers who are fed information from a broad and diverse group of trained observers and who are protected from inappropriate industry influence. Because most chemicals are on the market without any government review or permission, public policy that requires premarket and postmarket health testing of chemicals and that adequately collects and acts on adverse chemical events are even more important. This improved FDA-like approach would replace the failed EPA TSCA system, which has led to federal action only a handful of times.

ABSENCE OF INFORMATION IS NOT THE SAME AS ABSENCE OF HARM

When the Canadian government legislated a comprehensive review of chemicals in commerce in 1999, the resulting findings showed that the government had no toxicity data for more than 90% of chemicals. We are in the dark about the toxic effects of most chemicals. Public and corporate policy should be based on knowing that what we cannot see can still hurt us.

NUMBER AND QUALITY OF THE STRESSORS ON THE PATIENT MATTER

Not every person who is exposed to a virus will get sick. The strength of the immune system, access to health care services, family support, the existence of other disease, age, weight, alcohol or tobacco use, mental state, and other risk factors can all make a difference. Studies of human blood and urine by the U.S. Centers for Disease Control and Prevention (CDC), the Environmental Working Group, and Commonweal have demonstrated that every person has a body burden of toxic chemicals. But for communities bordering polluting industries, for children growing up in neighborhoods full of diesel engine fumes, for farm workers working in fields sprayed with toxic pesticides, the impacts of toxic chemicals can be much worse. In 1991, recognition of this disparity or environmental racism led to a national conference: the First National People of Color Environmental Justice Leadership Summit. The summit defined environmental justice as the antidote to environmental racism and created the Principles of Environmental Justice based on the shared recognition that social justice issues such as race, class, income status, and political power were inextricably linked to environmental justice issues such as the proximity of polluting industries and hazardous waste sites.

ANY STRESSORS YOU CAN REMOVE MATTER

In Lisbeth B. Schorr's 1988 book *Within Our Reach—Breaking the Cycle of Disadvantage,* she describes the stressors or risk factors for "rotten outcomes" for America's disadvantaged children and the elements of successful programs to prevent those rotten outcomes. Schorr explains that "it takes multiple and interacting risk factors to produce damaging outcomes. Lasting damage occurs when the elements of a child's environment—at home, at school, in the neighborhood—multiply each other's destructive effect." But just as the adding on of risk factors can multiply harm, their removal can divide the negative impact.

The implication is clear: The prevention of rotten outcomes is not a matter of all or nothing. It will be of value if we can eliminate one risk factor or two, even if others remain. By distinguishing between those factors we can do something about and those we cannot, the problem becomes less intractable. There are many environmental health factors we can do something about. From transforming our personal habits to transforming global chemicals policy, we can make the problem of chemicals less intractable.

CHANGING POLICIES

Some cities have taken their cues from the environmental health work of hospitals and have banned the sale of mercury-containing thermometers. Other municipalities have made it illegal to use lawn pesticides for cosmetic purposes. San Francisco and other Bay Area governments have passed the precautionary principle ordinances that require their purchasing departments to select products and services that minimize negative impacts to human health and the environment, driving manufacturers to engage in research and development toward the production of more innovative alternative products. The District of Columbia passed an ordinance forbidding the rail shipment of toxic chemicals through the heart of that city.

Many communities have also adopted environmentally preferable purchasing policies that encourage public expenditure on products that are more protective of public health.

In Maine, Washington, Minnesota, Connecticut, and many other states, new laws are being passed that phase out the use and the production processes that produce certain toxic chemicals. As their predecessors did more than 100 years ago, state legislators are trying to protect their constituents in the absence of federal law. But just like 100 years ago, we need a federal solution.

The European Union has created a modern chemicals policy for their continent. The new law, called *REACH* (Registration, Evaluation, Authorisation and Restriction of Chemicals), requires chemical companies that sell to the European market to either provide health studies that show that a chemical is safe or take the chemical off the market. This "no data, no market" approach to chemicals is what we need in the U.S. to move us toward a chemical regulation system like the drug-approval system of the FDA. Coupled with an adverse event reporting and action program that recalls chemicals from the market that are strongly linked to disease, the U.S. could begin to heal the harm created by the use of chemicals. Furthermore, if these chemical policy reform efforts are linked with the reduction of other stressors like racism, inadequate housing, unsafe working conditions, and limited access to health care services, we will have affirmed the aspirations of the 1785 Massachusetts legislature in reducing a "great nuisance of public health and peace."

For a list of related websites, please refer to your Evolve Resources at http://evolve.elsevier.com/Mason/policypolitics/

REFERENCES

American Journal of Health-System Pharmacy. (2005). *FDA's adverse-event surveillance needs improvement, advisers say.* Retrieved from www.ajhp.org/cgi/content/full/62/13/1336.

Center for the Evaluation of Risks to Human Reproduction. (2005). Draft NTP-CERHR expert panel update on the reproductive and developmental toxicity of di(2-ethylhexyl) phthalate. Retrieved from http://cerhr.niehs.nih.gov/news/dehp/DEHP-Update-Report-08-08-05.pdf.

Gee, D., Vaz, S. G., Harremoes, P., MacGarvin, M., Stirling, A., et al. (2001). Late lessons from early warnings: The precautionary principle, 1896-2000. Retrieved from http://reports.eea.eu.int/environmental_issue_report_2001_22/en.

Green, R., Hauser, R., Calafat, A. M., Weuve, J., Schettler, T., et al. (2005). Use of di(2-ethylhexyl) phthalate-containing medical products and urinary levels of mono(2-ethylhexyl) phthalate in neonatal intensive care unit infants. Retrieved from http://ehp.niehs.nih.gov/docs/2005/7932/abstract.html.

Hightower, J. (2004). Environmental health, mercury and human health: A case study in science and politics. *San Francisco Medicine, 77*(4). Retrieved from www.sfms.org/sfm/sfm404e.htm.

Meadows, M. (2002). The FDA's drug review process: Ensuring drugs are safe and effective. Retrieved from www.fda.gov/fdac/features/2002/402_drug.html.

National Research Council Commission on Life Sciences. (2000). Toxicological effects of methylmercury. Retrieved from www.nap.edu/books/0309071402/html/R1.html.

Rajapakse, N., Silva, E., & Kortenkamp, A. (2002) Combining xenoestrogens at levels below individual no-observed-effect concentrations dramatically enhances steroid hormone action. *Environmental Health Perspectives, 110*(9), 917-921.

Rosner, D., & Markowitz, G. (2002). Industry challenges to the principle of prevention in public health: The precautionary principle in historical perspective. Retrieved from www.publichealthreports.org/userfiles/117_6/117501.pdf.

Rothman, N., Cantor, K. P., Blair, A., Bush, D., Brock, J. W., et al. (1997, July 26). A nested case-control study of non-Hodgkin lymphoma and serum organochlorine residues. *Lancet, 350*(9073), 240-244.

Schorr, L. (1988). *Within our reach: Breaking the cycle of disadvantage.* New York: Anchor Press.

Swann, J. P. (2001). *History of the FDA.* Retrieved from www.fda.gov/oc/history/historyoffda/default.htm.

Tickner, J. A., Geiser, K., & Coffin, M. (2005). The U.S. experience in promoting sustainable chemistry. Retrieved from www.springerlink.com/app/home/contribution.asp?wasp=52a196a5053d4a739a8b2b4896f11a2a&referrer=parent&backto=issue,10,11;journal,3,4;linkingpublicationresults,1:112851,1.

U.S. Government Accountability Office (GAO). (2005). Report to congressional requesters, chemical regulation: Options exist to improve EPA's ability to assess health risks and manage its chemical review. Retrieved from www.gao.gov/new.items/d05458.pdf.

Zhang, Y., Wise, J. P., Holford, T. R., Xie, H., Boyle, P., et al. (2004). Serum polychlorinated biphenyls, cytochrome P-450 1A1 polymorphisms and risk of breast cancer in Connecticut women. *American Journal of Epidemiology, 160*(12), 1177-1183.

CHAPTER 68

Lobbying Policymakers: Individual and Collective Strategies

Ellen-Marie Whelan and Michael P. Woody[1]

"The greater the obstacle, the more glory in overcoming it."

—Molière

The word *lobbying* often generates negative connotations. However, the word *lobbyist* may come from the early days of the United States government when constituents with interests in legislation or policy would wait outside the doors of the U.S. House or Senate chambers—in the lobby—to approach their legislators as they entered or exited. The idea of a citizen government may seem far removed from today's polarized political environment. Still, with the right combination of dedication, strategy, and persistence, individual citizens can and do have access to and accountability from elected officials—and you don't have to be a paid lobbyist to make a difference.

Many citizens also lobby Congress, as well as state and local officials. Nurses have some significant advantages when it comes to working to influence an elected official. They are ranked first in trustworthiness in the Gallup Organization's most recent poll on honesty and ethics in professions (Saad, 2008) and in each Gallup poll ranking since nursing was added in 1999, except for one year (in 2001, firefighters were rated number 1 after their heroic acts during the September 11 terrorist attacks). Nursing is 3.1 million individuals strong, composing the largest group of health care professionals in the U.S. The combination of credibility and numbers is important to legislators.

[1]This chapter is revised from earlier versions authored by Melinda Mercer Ray, Shelagh Roberts, Mary Foley, and Catherine Dodd.

LOBBYISTS, ADVOCATES, AND THE POLICYMAKING PROCESS

Lobbying is a form of advocacy. Both paid, professional lobbyists and unpaid advocates may "lobby" a specific issue with the intention of influencing policymakers. However, the Internal Revenue Service (IRS) makes a clear distinction between lobbying and advocacy. The IRS defines a lobbyist as "A person who represents the concerns or special interests of a particular group or organization in meetings with lawmakers" (2010). Most have experience in some aspect of the political or policy process, often as former elected officials or their staff, and have practical expertise in the legislative process or a specific policy area. Professional lobbyists are employed by trade associations (such as the American Nurses Association), law firms, companies, public interest groups, and non-profit agencies. There are certain limits, though, on the lobbying activities of non-profit agencies as determined by the IRS.

LOBBYIST OR ADVOCATE?

Citizen advocates, on the other hand, are not paid and spend most of their time doing something else. While both lobbyists and advocates may "lobby" Congress, there is an important legal distinction between the two. For example, at the federal level, in 2007, Congress passed new registration requirements for "registered" lobbyists. If an individual spends more than 20% of his or her time on lobbying activities, then he or she is required to register with Congress, report what he or she is working on, and report political contributions above a certain limit. States have requirements also.

Lobbying has become a politically charged word in recent years, with professional lobbyists often being blamed for policy failures, corruption in the political process, and symbols of what is wrong with Washington D.C. Anti-lobbyist sentiment was a prominent part of President Barack Obama's campaign narrative, but has been central to the political dialogue for years. Politicians often decry "special interests" and purport to favor the "public interest" even though the terms are subjective. Indeed, the Jack Abrahmoff scandal and other high-profile cases help solidify the view of "lobbyist as a villain" in the public's mind. However, anti-lobbyist rhetoric undermines the profession's legitimate place in the policy process and denigrates the essential work lobbyists and advocates do to communicate policy ideas to Congress and the executive branch. In reality, legislation—the regulation of human activity—can be blindingly complicated. Members of Congress and state legislators write the laws, presidents and governors execute the laws, but all have precious little experience with every aspect of the complex society they are elected to govern. Providing information to elected officials is essential to the coherence of policymaking through law and regulation, its function in the real world, on professions and on real people. Without lobbying, policy would have more unintended consequences than it already does.

WHY LOBBY?

The most common reason people get involved with lobbying is because they see something that needs to be fixed. Nurses may see issues in their workplace that affect patients and coworkers that stimulate the desire to find a solution. Another reason is to offer expertise on policy proposals being considered by Congress or state legislators. For example, if Congress wants to alter the way nurse anesthetists are reimbursed under Medicare, there may be unintended consequences for the profession. A knowledgeable nurse or nursing group could explain the benefits and potential harm of policy alternatives. Unless a nurse represents their professional association as a paid lobbyist or serves as an appointed or elected representative, they often lobby due to their beliefs and values.

STEPS IN EFFECTIVE LOBBYING

RESEARCH

The first step in the lobbying process is to find out as much as you can about your area of interest or the issue that concerns you. Become a kind of detective. Uncover the legislative history, stakeholders, important elected officials, and policy particulars of bills related to your issue of interest. Your job is to learn as much as you can about the issue so that you can decide what your best lobbying approach will be.

Nearly all professional nursing associations, health care associations, and think tanks post political position statements on their websites. Many have legislative affairs sections that display sample letters or issue briefs to help you frame your arguments in favor of, or in opposition to, a particular bill or policy. For additional guidance, or if you have an expertise to offer, contact someone in the federal or state government affairs department. Most government agencies make detailed documents, including bill texts and summaries, federal agency reports and studies, and countless sources of federal data available online. The Library of Congress's website *(www.thomas.loc.gov)* offers complete listings of bills that can be searched by subject, key word, co-sponsor, date of introduction, and bill title or number. In addition, every state has a webpage with detailed information regarding elected officials and legislative activity. While the states' websites vary in the degree of detail they provide, almost every one includes the names of, and contact information for, state senators and representatives, as well as a search function to identify your legislator according to zip code or city name. These searches will identify bills on your issue of interest in great detail and can help you gain knowledge of the legislative histories behind a given subject. Tracking a bill is also very important, as the legislative process is, by design, one of compromise. Knowing where a bill is in the process, and what has changed or remained the same, will enable you to speak accurately about your support for, or opposition to, a bill at the right time.

IDENTIFYING SUPPORTERS

First, identify members of Congress or state legislatures who have been leaders on the particular issue. For example, if you search a site using the key word *breastfeeding,* you can identify legislators with a long history of introducing or co-sponsoring breastfeeding legislation. When approaching the legislator for support, you will be able to build on his or her previous knowledge and initiatives to craft a workable legislative strategy. Once you identify the issue that you want to lobby on, and you have educated yourself as to its legislative history and the current status of bills related to it, the next step is to determine (1) whom you need to contact to bring about change and (2) the best mode of communication to accomplish that change.

CONTACTING POLICYMAKERS

At the federal level, your primary contacts are the congressional staff members in the offices of your representatives and senators. They work with other congressional offices and interest groups to craft provisions in legislation. Your first step at the federal level is to identify the person in your legislator's office who is responsible for your issue. Nursing and health-related issues will likely be the "legislative assistant" who works on health care policy. Sometimes, though, responsibility for health care issues can be divided among several staff people, particularly if the member of Congress serves on a committee that has jurisdiction over health. Therefore, it is best to obtain specific information about who covers your particular issue of interest, not just who covers health care issues. Usually, the easiest way to identify the correct person on your issue is to telephone your member's Capitol Hill office and ask for the name of the individual who handles that issue. Once you have identified the proper staff member, you should address all correspondence or requests for meetings to that person.

Types of Congressional Staff. At the federal level, there are two types of staff who work on policy: those in the members' personal offices and those who work at the committee level. Some members of Congress are leaders on an issue because they have a personal or constituent-related connection to it, whereas others serve on committees that have jurisdiction over significant health care matters, such as the committees that oversee federal health programs or appropriations. Although there also are district offices for both representatives and senators in the members' home states, these offices generally handle constituent services rather than policymaking responsibilities.

However, this might be a good place to start if your issue has strong implications for your state or district.

Political staff often experience high turnover rates, so you should confirm that the contact information you have is current, particularly if you are relying on a published directory. Staff usually rely on experts in the field to help them understand the background of certain legislative issues. A staff member would need input from experts who actually work in nursing in order to get a firm grasp on what might be short-term and long-term strategies to recruit and retain nurses. Registered nurses and professional nursing organizations have the insight and the credibility to explain the complexities of the educational needs, overtime requirements, harried work environments, or the implications of an aging nursing workforce.

At both state and federal levels, it is important to recognize the critical role the staff plays in crafting legislation and helping to determine legislative priorities for the member of Congress for whom they work. With the broad range of issues that members of Congress must address, they rely on staff to brief them on issues. Members also look to staff to craft legislation and make recommendations about what issues to champion. It is unrealistic to expect a meeting with a member of Congress in most circumstances, and you can accomplish a great deal by meeting with a staff member who will be involved in writing legislative language. Additional avenues of access may result from your participation in an association or coalition that has broad appeal to the member.

Building Relationships. Opportunities to build personal relationships are often easier at the local and state levels than at the federal level, for the simple reason that there are more occasions for networking and building personal relationships with policymakers where you both live. In your community, you can invite an official or his or her staff to meetings of your professional organization, or you can invite the policymaker to address the group at a meeting or luncheon. You should also regularly attend local and state meetings or committee hearings on issues in the home district. Additional opportunities for networking and visibility occur when you volunteer to serve on a task force in your community, take part in a political campaign, become involved in the political party structure, or run for office yourself. Through the informal exchanges with legislators and policymakers these activities provide, you can build the foundations for lasting relationships.

HOW SHOULD YOU LOBBY?

PERSONAL VISITS

Face-to-face lobbying is generally perceived as the most effective strategy. If you have arranged a personal visit with a legislative assistant or other staff member, or with a member of Congress or state or local official, you can apply many of the same guidelines for crafting your message that you would employ in letter writing. Know the current status of legislation; keep the visit brief, as time is usually short; keep your points succinct and germane to the topic; illustrate your expertise or concern with personal examples; and identify your practice setting. Finally, don't forget to ask for a specific action or request to close the meeting. This is your "ask" and the reason for the visit. For example, "We hope we can count on you to vote next Wednesday to increase funding for nursing education." Box 68-1 contains tips for effective visits to policymakers.

It is recommended that you provide a one-page fact sheet to staff in advance of the meeting, and have a copy available to leave with whomever you meet as well. For example, if you are demonstrating the need for increased funding for nursing scholarships, you could provide a graphic representation—a chart or table—that illustrates the low rate of increase for nursing scholarships since they were initiated, particularly compared with grants or scholarships for other health professions. Make sure your name and contact information is on this document. Any resource that provides data or illustrates points in the form of easily digestible tidbits ("talking points") can be useful to the staff member when he or she briefs the elected official, writes speeches, or drafts press materials. Be sure to bring business cards to distribute.

TELEPHONE CALLS

Telephone calls are not ideal for introducing yourself to a legislative assistant. It is better to write a letter or make a personal introduction at an appropriate forum, such as a legislative briefing, to make the initial point of contact. After a letter has been received, it is perfectly acceptable to call the legislative assistant to whom you have written in order to confirm that the

---

BOX 68-1 Tips for Effective Lobbying

Prepare for the Visit
- Make an appointment with the policymaker or his or her staff member.
- Determine which issue(s) you want to discuss (not more than three).
- Research the issue(s). Learn about your legislators' records on these and related health issues.
- Become familiar with the opposition's views and arguments on the issue(s).
- Prepare materials such as copies of position papers, and a memo or fact sheet summarizing your main concerns.
- Work with other members of a coalition.
- Confirm the appointment the morning of or day before the meeting.
- Arrive on time and be patient.

Conduct the Visit
- Identify yourself as a member of your nursing or health care group.
- Thank the person you are meeting with for previous support.
- State your position or that of the coalition you are representing.
- Support your position with facts, but also use personal stories when possible.
- Ask the legislator or staff to clarify their position on the issue.
- Ask the legislator to take a specific action such as sponsoring a bill, or voting for or against a pending measure.
- Say "I don't know" if you don't know the answer to a question, and offer to get an answer.
- Thank the person who met with you.

Follow-up after the Visit
- E-mail or call legislators and staff to thank them for their time; remind them of anything they agreed to do, and send additional information you agreed to provide.
- Share the results of your meetings with your organization.
- Find out when the legislators will be in your home district hosting town hall meetings or forums, and organize a group to attend.
- Maintain communication with legislators and their staff through letters, telephone calls, and visits.

Adapted from the American Nurses Association. (2010). *Hill basics: Lobbying.* Retrieved from *www.nursingworld.org/Main MenuCategories/ANAPoliticalPower/Federal/ToolKit/Lobbying. aspx.*

letter was received or to ask if he or she would like any further information. Telephone calls are, of course, expected if you are actively working with a legislative assistant or other staff member on a particular piece of legislation or if you have an ongoing relationship with that person. Placing numerous telephone calls to someone with whom you have no established relationship, however, can identify you as a nuisance. With written communication, the person can respond according to his or her own timetable, whereas a phone call is sometimes an interruption.

A pitfall of communicating by telephone is that there is no written record of a telephone call. Additionally, when you communicate with staff via telephone, you have no way of guaranteeing that either your message or your personal information (e.g., your name, telephone number, or address) is recorded correctly. And even if they are recorded correctly, you have no assurance that they will be forwarded to the correct person. A telephone call may be worthwhile simply to express your support for, or opposition to, a legislative issue that is currently on the floor of the House or Senate for debate and will be coming up for a vote. Most congressional offices keep a running tally of yes or no votes from constituents who call the office during a contentious debate. Telephone calls can also be a good means of obtaining brief information or following up with someone with whom you have already established a relationship. Always follow up with a personal thank-you note or e-mail acknowledging the call.

LETTER-WRITING

Written communication to Congress has changed dramatically over the past decade after the anthrax attack in 2001, where letters containing anthrax spores were mailed to several news media offices and two U.S. Senators. Since that time, all mail delivered to Congress must go through an irradiation process. This process creates new compounds, which results in a different look, feel, and even smell. In many cases, it ruins the mail rendering it virtually unreadable. Because of this, electronic correspondences have become the norm for communicating with Congress. Though "letters" are still a critical way of communicating with Congress, they should be put into the body of an e-mail when possible.

When you write a letter to a member of Congress or a state or local official, there are some general guidelines to follow. First, direct your letter according to the legislator's responsibility. For example, do not write a letter regarding problems with your state's nurse practice act to a federal legislator, who has no authority on that issue. As an individual, your correspondence will be considered only if you write to the elected official who represents you. If you have a reputation as an expert or you have a personal relationship with an elected official, your letter may have impact. Personal letters still carry more weight than form letters, petitions, e-mails, or phone calls. If the elected official has a history of support of the issue, it is always important to start each communication with a thank-you and an acknowledgement of his or her support.

A further clarification of who to write pertains to an issue you may want to influence at the committee level, but your elected official is not on that committee. At the federal level, if your member of Congress is not on the committee, you can still communicate your opinion by addressing your letter to the chair of the committee at the committee address (not at the chair's congressional personal office address). Committee information, such as chair names, committee members, and committee address, is available on the Internet. State practices may vary, so again, check with your local guidelines. In crafting the message of your letter, identify yourself as a nurse, particularly if the legislation has anything to do with health care. Include hospital or other practice setting information as well as professional credentials, and make sure to include a return address, telephone number, and e-mail address if appropriate. See Box 68-2 for an example of a letter to a policymaker.

Include information about how proposed legislation would influence your personal experiences, or provide personal anecdotes that demonstrate your firsthand knowledge of, and experience with, a certain issue. State clearly what your position is, what your major concern about the proposal is, and whether you want the official to support, or oppose, the proposal. Again, tracking the legislation throughout the process will require that you include relevant committee or hearing information and bill numbers in your correspondence. Keep your letter brief and to the point.

E-MAIL

For many members of Congress and their staffs, e-mail is a preferred means of communication. E-mail correspondence has the following advantages:

- *Directness.* The information is sent directly to the person you identify.
- *Timeliness.* Correspondence is immediate, in most cases.
- *Flexibility.* Legislative staff can open e-mail in their own time frame, unlike telephone calls, which are often unscheduled interruptions.
- *Attachments.* Important articles, reports, or other information that support your ideas can be attached with e-mail.

BOX 68-2 Sample Letter to a Policymaker

Mary Breckenridge, RN
2500 Market Street, Suite 100
San Francisco, CA 94109

The Honorable Jackie Smith
California State Assembly
State Capitol
Sacramento, CA 95814

Dear Assemblywoman Smith:

I am a certified nurse-midwife and a member of the California Nurse-Midwives Association. I am writing to urge your support for Senator Jones' bill, S.B. 255, which will replace the words physician "supervision" in the language of our Nursing Practice Act with the more accurate words physician "collaboration," thereby defining the relationship between physician and nurse-midwife in accordance with the Joint Statement of Practice Relations Between Obstetricians and Gynecologists and Certified Nurse-Midwives. The bill will also allow hospitals to consider granting staff privileges to certified nurse-midwives, thereby expanding access to low-cost, effective, safe care to women who wish to use our services.

I am a graduate of UCSF School of Nursing and practiced as a registered nurse in Maternal and Child Nursing prior to returning to school to become a certified nurse-midwife. I have practiced nurse-midwifery for the past 10 years and can vouch for the fact that the relationship I enjoy with my referring obstetricians is collaborative and supportive. In most instances, they never see my patients, nor are they required to do so, although under current law they are required to sign off on the charts related to those patients. They, and I, see this as an unnecessary step that bears no relationship to patient care or safety. Barriers such as this supervisory requirement add additional expense and may delay access to care by requiring signoff of charts prior to initiation of essential care. I urge you to support S.B. 255, and I would appreciate knowing your position on the bill.

Sincerely,
Mary Breckenridge, RN

When sending e-mail, remember to include your name, address, telephone number, and e-mail address. Observe the usual rules for written correspondence. E-mail is clearly a valuable tool if you are actively working with other organizations or with congressional staff on documents that need to be shared, such as when you are drafting legislation.

PROVIDING HEARING TESTIMONY

Providing testimony at a government hearing is an important way to go "on the record" about an issue on behalf of an organization or as a constituent. Hearings are increasingly designed by committee staff to highlight an issue, but they are not, in fact, where most of the key information is shared or decisions are made. As an individual, or on behalf of an association, you may request to testify on a particular issue. It is more likely that your coalition or organization will receive a call from a legislative office requesting that testimony be given from your group. Federal testimony is accepted in two forms for most committees: as oral remarks (those who are asked to testify) or as written testimony. Written testimony can be provided to the committee by the witness as a supplement to the oral remarks, or it can be provided by any association or individual choosing to submit it for the record. This testimony, including the transcript of the hearing, will eventually be compiled and published as a permanent record of the hearing.

Although there is limited opportunity to testify at hearings, it is important that you know how to prepare and conduct yourself in the event that you do testify. All committees and their subcommittees have a format they use to conduct the hearing; formats differ not only from state to federal committees but also from one committee to the next. Generally, there is a time limit placed on the length of an individual's remarks. You will use this time to present your position on the legislation or issue in an interesting and informative way. Some committees use a green-yellow-red light system to keep the witnesses on time. It is important that you follow the rules and conclude your comments when the red light comes on or your time has elapsed. Frequently, this is not your last word on the subject, as the committee will often engage in a question-and-answer period with a witness following the presentation of testimony.

A senior legislator chairs committee hearings. The hearing is called to order, and then the chair often begins with remarks. Following the chair's remarks, any other legislators on the committee that choose to provide opening remarks will be given the opportunity to do so. Do not be surprised if the elected officials come and go during the meeting. The staff is always present and, in fact, will be responsible for the key messages you bring, and they will also rely on the written materials. The hearing then turns to the panel(s) of witnesses for their comments on the legislation or issue being considered at the hearing.

If you are asked to testify, it is important that you learn all you can about the politics and the issue before your testimony. This is where association representatives are invaluable. Typically, they will be the ones who call and ask if you would be willing to testify. If you receive the call from them, rely on them for the drafting of remarks, briefing on the issue and the politics, rules of the hearing, and other matters. Request that they attend the hearing with you and support you through the process. If you receive a request directly from a legislator's office, you may choose to call your association representative to see if he or she is willing to provide support for your testimony. Review your remarks; practice them before friends, family, and colleagues—even a mirror. Make sure you personalize your testimony and use phrases that are comfortable for you. Identify some of the questions you might be asked, and think through your responses. See Box 68-3 for a list of books with additional information about lobbying.

COLLECTIVE STRATEGIES

Although the potential power of the individual nurse-constituent is great, the power base grows when nurses come together with a unified voice to advocate for change. Nursing groups can be influential with policymakers at all levels of government—from local boards to Congress. Elected officials often welcome opportunities to address the core constituencies in their districts to show that they care about the issues back home, and the possibility of good coverage in local newspapers can also be an incentive to those representatives with an eye toward re-election. Local nursing groups can sponsor legislative luncheons or celebrate National Nursing Week by inviting a policymaker to either join them at a meeting or address the group. Groups can award legislators with annual "leadership" or "advocate" recognition. Such

---

BOX 68-3 Books on Lobbying

- Donald deKieffer. (2007). *The Citizen's Guide to Lobbying Congress.* Chicago Review Press.
- Deanna Gelak. (2008). *Lobbying and Advocacy: Winning Strategies, Resources, Recommendations, Ethics and Ongoing Compliance for Lobbyists and Washington Advocates.* The CapitolNet.
- Stephanie Vance. (2009). *Citizens in Action: A Guide to Lobbying and Influencing Government.* Columbia Books.
- Jack Maskell. (2009). *Lobbyist Registration and Compliance Handbook: The Honest Leadership and Open Government Act of 2007 and the Lobbying Disclosure Act Guide, House … and Lobbying Regulations for Nonprofits.* The CapitolNet.
- Frank Baumgartner, Jeffrey Berry, Marie Hojnacki, David Kimball, & Beth Leech. (2009). *Lobbying and Policy Change: Who Wins, Who Loses, and Why.* University of Chicago Press.
- Brian Adams. (2007). *Citizen Lobbyists: Local Efforts to Influence Public Policy.* Temple University Press.

---

grassroots activities are excellent ways to increase awareness of nursing issues and to make sure that nurses are represented when health care policy is being developed. The other model for grassroots action works in a reverse organizational pattern. Many national nursing organizations have local or statewide chapters. The headquarters of an association might be in Washington, D.C., while the local chapters, sections, or branches can be spread out nationwide. This model is effective because the local or regional branch of the organization has the name recognition, resources, and prestige of the national association on their side as they pursue activities at the local level. In this way, local chapters enjoy the added strategic benefit of integrating their grassroots activities with the overall strategic lobbying goals of the national organization. The local group can then look to the national organization for position papers, copies of testimony, briefing documents, or other data on a given issue for use at the local level. Coordination of activities at the local and national levels of the same organizations is critical to ensure that all representatives of the umbrella organizations are spreading consistent messages and positions with policymakers and to avoid any conflicts that might undermine the overall lobbying strategy.

In terms of collective lobbying strategies, one of the most common, and increasingly most effective, options for bringing about change is to create or join a coalition. As the number of interest groups has increased, with almost every niche group having its own association or group, it has become more important to reach consensus and refine priorities with groups that share your interests before approaching federal policymakers with priorities or legislative remedies. Coalitions simplify the workload of legislators and their staff by saving them time. A meeting with one coalition representing 25 groups will take much less time than 25 meetings with representatives from each group. In fact, coalition expert Kevin Hula (1995) states that because of increasing demands on time, "Groups are pressured to work out their differences before approaching Congress, rather than requiring Congress to sort out a seemingly infinite number of differences among groups" (p. 243).

For a list of related websites, please refer to your Evolve Resources at http://evolve.elsevier.com/Mason/policypolitics/

REFERENCES

Hula, K. (1995). Rounding up the usual suspects: Forging interest group coalitions in Washington. In A. J. Cigler & B. A. Loomis (Eds.), *Interest group politics* (4th ed.). Washington, D.C.: Congressional Quarterly.

Internal Revenue Service. (2010). Glossary. Retrieved from www.irs.gov/app/understandingTaxes/student/glossary.jsp#L.

Saad, L. (2008). *Nurses shine, bankers slump in ethics ratings: Annual honesty and ethics poll rates nurses best of 21 professions.* Retrieved from www.gallup.com/poll/112264/nurses-shine-while-bankers-slump-ethics-ratings.aspx.

CHAPTER 69

TAKING ACTION
An Insider's View of Lobbying

Betty R. Dickson

"There are two things you don't want to see being made—sausage and legislation."

—Attributed to Otto von Bismark

"So, what do you do?" is a question I am frequently asked. To which I reply, "I am a lobbyist." The looks that follow are either scornful, surprised, quizzical, astonished, or thoughtful. I wonder if the questioner associates all lobbyists with those who have been involved with high-profile scandals. Most likely the question is a reflection of not knowing what I do and a curiosity about the job.

The reality is that few people know what *really* happens in the halls and offices of government. To be a successful lobbyist includes attending plenty of committee meetings, knowing the bill-writing process, watching and understanding political maneuvering, sitting through innumerable working meals and receptions, developing different friendships, watching and working in elections, and imparting reams of information. While nurses are excellent caregivers and the backbone of our health care system, few understand the influence that laws and regulations have on their practice; fewer are skilled at the long process of creating positive outcomes. My role as a lobbyist parallels advice from my mother: "Don't cross the street without looking both ways." In other words, "don't approach a legislative body without a professional lobbyist, one who knows the ins and outs of the system."

I watch hundreds of schoolchildren, parents, teachers, and single-issue citizens converge on the Mississippi state capitol during the annual three-month legislative session. I watch as they wander the halls of what is probably one of the most beautiful capitol buildings in the United States. They come to observe, speak out about their issue, be recognized from the visitor gallery, and tour the magnificent capitol building. Then they go home.

For 20-plus years, I have mentored nursing students and practicing nurses as they come to observe and be publicly recognized by legislators in the chambers. A few have spent the entire day with me, following closely as I attend committee meetings, listen to testimony and debates, and conduct personal visits with legislators. They leave with a new respect for the role of a lobbyist and the importance of having someone represent nursing during the legislative session.

There's an old cliché—There are two things one ought not to watch: making sausage and observing the legislative process. Watching the lack of/or uninspiring debate, or the grandstanding by legislators can be strange to the novice. Most of those who look behind the scenes or witness the process in depth are fascinated. Some even become "hooked" and come back again.

With these one-day visits, visitors miss stories like the Bilbo statue, a bronze, life-size rendering of one of Mississippi's most notorious racist governors who also served in the U.S. Senate. It once stood in a prominent place in the capitol, and as more and more African Americans were elected to the legislature, the statue began to be moved around. Today it has been relegated to one of the conference rooms—an insignificant place on the first floor of the capitol. Many of the older lobbyists know the significance of Bilbo's positioning today—a tribute to how far Mississippi has come and a testimony to the rise in power and influence of African-American legislators.

Visitors may not appreciate the excitement of watching a plan for legislation come to fruition—all the time, effort, and expertise negotiating that made it possible. As a result, they may not appreciate why a profession, business, or organization needs representation by a lobbyist.

GETTING STARTED

I started working as a lobbyist (Figure 69-1) in 1989 when I began a long journey learning the ropes of lobbying in a small state, rich with tradition and history—some bad, some notorious. In 1988, I became executive director of the Mississippi Nurses Association (MNA) and began my career as a lobbyist. Thankfully, my background as a journalist and newspaper editor, and my experience in government and public relations was a perfect combination for the responsibility of lobbying.

Throughout the years, the MNA has had 95% of its legislation passed, some of which includes the following:

- Securing significant annual funding for nursing education
- Obtaining additional pay for school nurses who become certified
- Increasing the number of school nurses
- Creating a $12,000 per year stipend for nurses to obtain a master's or doctoral degree if they teach in a school of nursing
- Securing inclusion of nurse practitioners in most health care networks, and getting reimbursed at the same rate as physicians
- Obtaining controlled substance authority for nurse practitioners
- Establishing the Office of Nursing Workforce

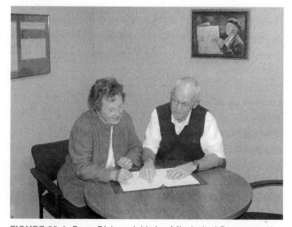

FIGURE 69-1 Betty Dickson lobbying Mississippi Representative Cecil Brown.

I worked for a group of nursing leaders in the MNA who understood the value of using the political arena to protect and advance the profession.

POLITICAL STRATEGIES

GETTING NURSES ON EVERY HEALTH-RELATED STATE AGENCY

My lobbying career got off to a big start. Innocently, I took the MNA leadership seriously when they told me their major objective was to have nurses at the seat of every table where health care decisions were made. During my first year at the MNA, our lobbyist was a nurse-attorney. During Desert Storm, the nurse/lobbyist went to work full-time for a law firm to fill a vacancy created by an attorney/guardsman who was called to active duty. I became the MNA's only lobbyist.

But while she was still working, we developed a strategy to access every code section in the law for every health care agency. We planned to try and amend the law to mandate that a nurse be on every governing board of any health-related agency, including the Department of Education. Although the legislation would define my career and reputation, I was totally unaware of the enormous opposition to "touching" any regulatory board's composition. That first legislative session turned out to be one of getting acquainted with division and department heads, getting a comprehensive education about government agencies, and getting a ton of teasing from other lobbyists who thought this was a pretty gutsy move for a newcomer.

Of course, the bill had little chance of passage, but once we searched the Mississippi code, drafted the bill's language, asked a legislator to introduce the bill, and attempted to get a committee hearing on the bill, I learned the legislative process from the bottom up. To this day, those agency heads who are still around ask me at the beginning of each session if I have any surprises up my sleeve. It's good to keep them guessing. As a result of that initiative and even without passage of the bill, the Department of Mental Health and the Department of Health, to this day, have a registered nurse on the Boards, including one who served as chair. As nurses serve on various boards, their value increases. Today nurses serve on numerous boards and committees in state government. Every time a piece of legislation comes forward in the Mississippi legislature, I am there as a lobbyist to ensure the insertion of the words *nurse, school nurse,* and *nurse practitioner* where appropriate in health-related legislation and regulation.

NUMBERS CONNOTE STRENGTH

Lobbying is about counting. I can count, nursing leadership can count, and legislators especially know the value of numbers. We use the strength of numbers to influence legislators. In the early 1990s, there were over 40,000 RNs and licensed practical nurses (LPNs) practicing in Mississippi, and we had to establish a mechanism to bring representatives from all those nurses together. We created the MNA's Nursing Organizations Liaison Committee (NOLC) to bring 25 nursing organizations together to plan and agree on a legislative agenda. Representatives from each group worked collaboratively on a statewide nursing summit that 700 to 800 RNs and students attend annually. We invited key legislators to join us, and they could count the numbers for themselves. It was through this coalition that nursing began to be recognized as a significant force at the state capitol. That same coalition continues to work today in a collaborative effort to maintain a strong legislative presence.

LONG-TERM STRATEGIES FOR LONG-TERM SOLUTIONS: TACKLING THE NURSING SHORTAGE

When the NOLC was formed, I told the group, "MNA is furnishing the lobbying for all of you. There's a way for you to participate and to provide support for this effort" and they have. This group was involved in passing the law creating the Office of Nursing Workforce (ONW). My role as a lobbyist is to ensure that this office is adequately funded. The nursing shortage has been a major focus of the group. We developed long-range legislative plans. The first step was to retain nursing faculty, and the best way to do so was to provide faculty with a competitive salary. In 2007, we worked with the legislature to obtain a $6000 pay raise for all nursing faculty in the state. In 2008, the second installment of the pay raise was enacted; nursing faculty received their second raise of $6000. Many of those considering retiring changed their minds, while others decided to become teachers. In 2008, the next step was to add one additional faculty in all schools of nursing. That too was successfully enacted.

In 2008, I lobbied to fund a study about simulation labs and how they could increase enrollment. The legislature appropriated $75,000 for this initiative. In 2009, they funded the next step, allocating $500,000 to the Office of Nursing Workforce to coordinate where, when, and how to implement a simulation lab program.

A million here, a million there, and the next thing you know is that Mississippi has invested millions of dollars to resolve the nursing shortage. As a result, faculty numbers have stabilized and enrollment has increased.

CALL IN THE NURSES

It helps to have a successful political action committee behind you (which the MNA has), and it helps to have a plan to "call in the nurses" when the need arises. I know that legislators really fear having large droves of citizens come to the capitol—whether it's truckers, physicians, loggers, hair braiders … or nurses. I remember one issue in the early 1990s when an attempt was made to establish medication technicians in nursing homes. Nurses were strongly opposed to this new provider whose only requirement was a high school education and a few weeks of training. The vice chair of the House of Representatives Public Health and Welfare Committee was assigned the bill and scheduled a public hearing. MNA arranged for over 100 nurses, in uniform, to attend the hearing. When the committee chair couldn't get everyone in the regular conference room on the first floor because there were so many nurses, he moved us to a larger room on the second floor. It became apparent that the second room was too small, so he moved us to an even larger room back again on the first floor. Imagine 100 nurses marching to a room on the first floor, and then marching upstairs to another room, then down the stairs to the room on the opposite end of the hall. It created a lot of excitement, lots of stares, and lots of curiosity. It also established several points about the nursing community: We are well organized, there are a lot of us, and we will make plenty of calls to our legislators.

When the chair finally got the hearing under way, the nurses were breathing pretty heavily; but when testimony began, the breathing became a little more pronounced. And when one of the opponents, during testimony, said something disparaging about nurses, all 100 gasped in unison. It even scared me, and I was on their side. Needless to say, the chair ended the hearing without a vote on the bill. Mississippi still does not have medication technicians.

BE IN THE RIGHT PLACE AT THE RIGHT TIME

Successful lobbying often depends on being in the right place at the right time. Once a state senator called me to review an immunization bill he wanted to introduce. After reading through the bill, I told him that I thought we were already doing what he wanted to do with the legislation. His reply was that he wanted an immunization bill! I told him I would get back with a suggestion. I was the MNA's representative on the Mississippi State Health Department's Immunization Task Force, so I called the chief of staff at the health department, a nurse. She suggested that we convince him to introduce a bill for a statewide immunization registry, one of the goals of the task force. I did. He loved the idea. He introduced a bill, and we worked very hard for passage. Today there is a statewide registry for tracking immunization. The result is that Mississippi has one of the highest immunization rates in this country.

The same nurse and I were in the capitol during a legislative session when we were called by the chair of the Public Health and Welfare committee, who wanted to implement a school-based clinic pilot for the state. We were given the assignment to come up with language for an amendment to an education bill that would authorize the pilot project. She grabbed an envelope, and we crafted the language on the back. Reading it over carefully, we went back into the meeting where she handed the chair the envelope and he passed it to the bill writer. It became law.

PUTTING FROGS IN A WHEELBARROW: USE HUMOR AS A TOOL

Sometimes humor can disarm even the most stoic adversary. After we were successful in getting the bill passed to create the Office of Nursing Workforce (ONW) through the House and the Senate and then back to the House for final approval, a community college president appeared at the weekly committee meeting and told the chair that the community colleges were opposed to our bill. We were completely blown away by this opposition at the final hour. The chair gave us one day to work out the problem.

Luckily, the community college presidents were meeting the next day, so I arranged an audience with them by convincing an old friend, who was a president, to get a group of us on the agenda. Several of us appeared the next day but were getting nowhere. The head of the community college board kept saying we didn't need the ONW. We tried to reason with him: "We have no accurate data on nursing in Mississippi; we need better communication between the schools of nursing and hospital nursing administration; we need to develop workforce strategies." Nothing was working with the all-male audience. Finally, I placed both hands on the table and asked: "Mr. Chairman, have you ever tried to put frogs in a wheelbarrow?" A slight smile appeared on his face. "Where are you going with this?" he asked. I explained, "We have been trying to get these folks working together. First, we get the community college nursing programs in the wheelbarrow. Then we turn around and try to pick up the baccalaureate programs and put them in the wheelbarrow. Then we try to get hospital administration in the wheelbarrow. Then we turn around, and the other two have jumped out. We need a way to get them all in the wheelbarrow at the same time." They all laughed and, with further discussion, agreed to support our bill.

USE YOUR BEST ASSETS

When Mississippi's first Republican governor since reconstruction, Kirk Fordice, created the state's Health Care Commission, I was appointed to represent nursing. When it came time for nursing to make a presentation on nursing's role in health care and how we could improve the status of health care in Mississippi, MNA chose three outstanding leaders to make our case. The first was a diminutive, perky nurse president of MNA who could spit out data in rapid fire delivery; the second was our impressive Board of Nursing executive director, whose ability to think on her feet and whose sense of humor was incredible; and finally, a tall blond dean of a school of nursing and former Alabama Maid of Cotton, whose intelligence was only exceeded by her good looks. When the nurses finished their presentation and walked back to their chairs, the president of the hospital association whispered to me, "You don't play fair!" As a result of our unfair play, the commission recommended, and the legislature passed, legislation to increase funding to three existing nurse practitioner programs and to add two new programs—all to increase the numbers of NPs so that rural Mississippi could experience better health care coverage.

USE PROVEN STRATEGIES

Learning from past experiences was important when nurse practitioners asked MNA to help with regulations about signing forms that, by law, required a physician signature. Once again, we did a code search of the rules and found every law requiring a physician signature and drafted a bill to change the language to say "or nurse practitioner" (see Chapter 65). The process was the same as the one we used to get nurses on state agency boards; finding a simple word or phrase that could be added to an existing law—and thus expand NP practice. It involved numerous forms, one of which was an authorization for handicapped parking. The addition of "nurse practitioner" affected many agencies, thus creating a lot of attention. We explained that the NP was the provider and that the physician was not always on site. In order to get a physician signature, the patient had to schedule an appointment with the physician, thus creating additional cost and additional paperwork. The bill passed, and the result was that all agencies affected changed all their forms to include NP signatures.

BE PATIENT; DO NOT GIVE UP

My job as a lobbyist has been to shepherd legislation to expand NP practice. In the early 1980s, there were only a handful of NPs practicing in the state. In the early 1990s, there were about 400. By 2009, there were almost 2000, not including Certified Registered Nurse Anesthetists (CRNAs). Eventually, some NPs opened their own practices. This was perceived as a threat by the Mississippi State Board of Medical Licensure (MSBML) and the Mississippi Medical Association (MMA). Under the old law, the Board of Nursing (BON) was required to "jointly promulgate" any regulation affecting the NP. The MNA was successful in getting a law passed in 1994 that required the BOML to also "jointly promulgate" any regulations affecting NPs. This meant that both boards had to "jointly promulgate." This set up a scenario in which we spent fifteen years arguing back and forth between the two professions whenever any regulatory changes were suggested by one of the boards. We were able to gain ground by introducing bill after bill to remove the restrictions, and, through legislative

support, we actually forced the BOML to compromise on many of the restrictions. But keeping the regulatory process effective and timely was impossible, much like walking through molasses. It took 2 to 3 years to get anything done.

When the NPs approached the MNA regarding prescriptive authority for controlled substances, we went to the BOML asking for an opportunity to jointly promulgate regulations to make it happen. They refused to work with us. We went to the legislature and asked for a bill to give the NPs controlled substance prescriptive authority. We also told the legislators that it could be done through the regulatory process, but the BOML would not cooperate. The chairman of Public Health and Welfare called all stakeholders to his office and gave strong directions for the two parties to work together through the regulatory process, or else he would look at a change in the law. It took another year, but regulations were passed to give controlled substance prescriptive authority.

In 2009, the MNA went back to the legislature with a bill to completely remove joint promulgation of rules. Once again, the Public Health Chairman forced the parties to work together, and, after many negotiations, all parties came to agreement and the bill became law on July 1, 2010. Now the Board of Nursing could regulate NPs without joint promulgation with the BOML. But it took 20 years!

What made the difference? First was the fatigue factor; after all those years, key legislators were tired of trying to resolve issues between the BON and the BOML. Secondly, there was a vast increase in the number of NPs. More and more legislative families were using NPs as their primary provider. Many had daughters and sons who were NPs. And MNA pounded the legislators with the outcome data about NP practice. Thirdly, we figured out some fancy political maneuvering. When the BOML opposed our legislation, we suggested that we take the regulations under which the NPs had been successfully practicing for years and move them into legislation. This was a strategy I had considered for 20 years. It actually was suggested by a physician who supported NPs and encouraged us to consider legislation instead of regulation. The legislators thought the logic was sound, because NPs were already practicing successfully under the regulations and moving them into legislation did not change any of their practices. Today, NPs continue to work in a "collaborative" arrangement with physicians.

The efficiency of eliminating joint promulgation has greatly shortened the promulgation of rules. For example, practice guidelines for NP hospitalists and NPs in pain management were developed quickly but thoroughly. The process is simple: Bring together interested NPs, look at national guidelines, study the research, create appropriate practice guidelines, present them to the BON, seek public and medical input, and present final proposals to the BON. Instead of taking 2 years, as it would under joint promulgation, it took from 1 to 3 months to implement. This new painless, seamless, timely process would not have been possible without years of work by a seasoned lobbyist.

THERE REALLY IS A NEED FOR LOBBYISTS

There are no secret ingredients to lobbying. Legislators, especially in states where staff are limited, depend on lobbyists to provide information about issues, to muster support for pet projects, and to help with their campaigns. There is so much legislation that can affect nursing practice. From issues like Medicaid to the State Department of Health, from the nursing shortage to mandatory overtime, there must be nursing representation in state and federal policy arenas. Box 69-1 provides an example of how nurses can use lobbying to provide patient care. It requires expertise in the intricacies of the legislative and regulatory process, in knowing the implications of suggested legislation or regulation, knowing who is your ally and who is your obstacle, developing trust among policymakers and other stakeholders, and knowing when the "right" people are in the "right" places to implement change. It requires seeing the process like a puzzle or poker game: "Know when to hold and when to fold." It helps to be creative and look at surprise approaches to problems. Lobbyists keep their fingers on the pulse of health care legislation and regulations. They are skilled communicators, who know when to call out the nurses. Organizational success in policy arenas is often directly related to the effectiveness of the lobbying effort. Unless nurses do this as a full-time job, they rarely have the time to

---

BOX 69-1 **Nurses Taking Care of Patients through Effective Lobbying**

In the summer of 2008, a nurse practitioner from Pelahatchie, Mississippi, lost her mother for several hours. An Alzheimer's patient, she was with her husband who left her seated in a store mall while he went to get the car. When he returned, she was gone.

The search that began involved her daughter working with the Ridgeland Police, Jackson Police, and several television stations as she frantically tried to find her mother. What ensued was a horrible 13-hour hunt that ended with good news. Her mother was located at Cabot Lodge Hotel in Jackson at 2:30 AM. During the 13 hours, the family initiated every move: furnishing her picture to local television stations, working with several police departments, calling all area hospitals, calling hotels—all of which led to the good ending.

The nurse practitioner, seeing a need to develop a plan for others who had elderly parents with dementia, turned to the Mississippi Nurses Association.

Several geriatric nurse members of the MNA came together to work on the issue. At the MNA convention in October 2009, a resolution was passed to pursue legislation to set up a Silver Alert system in Mississippi, which was similar to the Amber Alert for children. Members rallied around this issue, worked closely with the MNA lobbyist, helped draft legislation, and convinced two powerful legislators to sponsor bills in each house. The MNA worked with the Department of Public Safety to craft the language; enlisted support from the Alzheimer's Association, the AARP, and nursing home associations; came to the Capitol to testify; and worked diligently to pursue what they saw as a real need for elderly patients with dementia.

On the day of testimony before the House Judiciary B Committee, the MNA lobbyist received a message from an NP on her cell phone that an elderly woman had been reported missing in Meridian, Mississippi, and was later found dead in a nearby creek. The message was relayed to the chairman, who spoke eloquently on the need for this bill and the timely message he had just received.

This legislation passed the House and Senate and was signed by the governor. It went into effect in July 2010.

---

assume the lobbying function. My advice to nursing: Don't be caught without one.

For a list of related websites, please refer to your Evolve Resources at http://evolve.elsevier.com/Mason/policypolitics/

CHAPTER 70

Political Appointments

Judith K. Leavitt and Mary W. Chaffee

"Ask not what your country can do for you. Ask what you can do for your country."

—John F. Kennedy

The wheels of the United States government, as well as state governments, are powered by three groups of employees: those who are elected to office, those who are career employees, and those who are appointed to serve. Each offers an opportunity to influence public policy, but the path to an appointment differs from the others. To attain a political appointment, nurses should be familiar with how the appointment process works, what is needed to be a viable candidate for an appointment, and how to prepare for the process.

WHAT DOES IT TAKE TO BE A POLITICAL APPOINTEE?

Richard Nathan (2009), an authority on political appointments states:

> *The politics of getting appointed and then being in the public service are intense. One appeal of appointive office is that, unlike elective offices, most people in these jobs are not constantly caught up in political fundraising and campaigning. Still, one cannot succeed in government without being political. A thick skin, the courage to take a stand, and the quickness of wit to defend it are essential qualities for appointive public service. It is exhilarating at the top, but it can also be nerve-racking too. Successful appointed leaders need a keen intuitive feel for the constant bargaining that the American political process requires. Most appointees are qualified and willing to serve when asked. (p. 11)*

Then why seek a political appointment and the resulting political pressures? Nathan (2009) identified the following reasons why individuals seek political appointments:

1. Public service can produce a gratifying sense of accomplishment.
2. Public service can lead to recognition and prestige.
3. Successful leadership in public service can enhance the chances of landing a well-paid job after exiting government service.

There is a large demand for appointees. Nathan (2009) estimates that 400,000 individuals serve in appointed positions in the federal, state, and local governments. In addition to recognizing their extensive numbers, Nathan tips his hat to their influence: These (appointed) officials ... "do the heavy lifting of policymaking and management inside America's governments and play a significant role as change agents in the nation's political system. Yet books about American government tend to ignore them and focus instead on elected office holders" (p. 10). David Lewis, a political scientist at Vanderbilt University, examined 600 government programs and the 234 managers that ran them (Lewis, 2008). He found that the political appointees were better educated and had excellent records before their appointments. It was the career employees who were better at getting the work done through strategic planning, program design, and financial oversight (Vedantam, 2008). Yet the political appointees may bring fresh ideas, enthusiasm, and a closer connection with the public to the government workplace.

GETTING READY

Once you decide you are interested in a political appointment, how do you get started? Determine where your interests and experience lie. Is there something you wish to change or a service you desire in your community or state? Do you have the expertise

---

BOX 70-1 Government Political Appointment Resources

State Government

Contact the offices of individual secretaries of state, or check their websites for appointment opportunities at the state level. For example, search online for "California Secretary of State." Employment sites and professional organizations update postings for appointment opportunities on a regular basis.

Federal Government

The federal government provides many public resources. One of the most important is the official *Plum Book*. Every 4 years, just after the presidential election, Congress publishes U.S. Government Policy and Supporting Positions, more commonly known as the *Plum Book*. (The *Plum Book* is so called because of the color of the book.) At the end of the 110th Congress, the *Plum Book* catalogued over 7000 federal civil service positions in the legislative and executive branches of the U.S. government that are potentially available for noncompetitive appointment. The electronic version of the *Plum Book* is actually located at the Government Printing Office's website at *www.gpoaccess.gov/plumbook/.*

BOX 70-2 Non-Government Political Appointment Resources

- The National Women's Political Caucus (NWPC) *(www.nwpc.org)*. The NWPC is a grassroots membership organization that assists in the identification, recruiting, training, and support of women for elected and appointed office at all levels of government. The NWPC is also the chair of the Coalition for Women's Appointment, a 60-member organization that assists women who seek presidential and gubernatorial appointments.
- The National Council of Women's Organizations (NCWO) *(www.womensorganizations.org)*. The NCWO is an organizing council of over 200 women's organizations representing more than 10 million members. Their goal is to advocate change on many issues of importance to women, including equal employment opportunity, economic equity, media equality, education, job training, women's health, and reproductive health, as well as the specific concerns of mid-life and older women, girls and young women, women of color, business and professional women, homemakers, and retired women.
- The Brookings Institution *(www.brookings.edu)*. The Brookings Institution provides information for those interested in pursuing a presidential nomination. They have done a number of studies about the appointment process and making government processes more effective.
- The Rutgers Center for American Women and Politics (CAWP) *(www.cawp.rutgers.edu)*. The CAWP is a unit of the Eagleton Institute of Politics at Rutgers University, the state university of New Jersey. It is nationally recognized as the leading source of scholarly research and current data about American women's political participation. It is an excellent source for learning about campaigns, elections, and appointments.

---

to be competitive for a federal appointment? Is your ultimate goal to seek political office? Will serving in a political or public role enhance future advancement in your career? See Boxes 70-1 and 70-2 for some useful resources.

IDENTIFY OPPORTUNITIES

How does a nurse determine where the opportunities are? The types of political appointments run the gamut. For instance, a position on a state board of health affords an opportunity to develop policy, whereas an appointment to an election commission is a mechanism for carrying out state law. Most state nurses associations, specialty organizations, and other professional organizations offer appointment information. At the state level, the state nurses' association should be able to assist in finding positions as well as guide nominees through the process. Organizations such as the ANA and the American Organization of Nurse Executives (AONE) offer help at the federal level. Other sources include nonpartisan organizations such as the League of Women Voters. State and federal health-related coalitions may support nurses

for particular positions, and political parties may offer support in some cases. For example, MassGAP is a bipartisan coalition of Massachusetts women's groups that works to increase the number of women appointed by the governor to senior-level cabinet positions, as agency heads and to state selected authorities and commissions (MassGAP, 2010).

Nurses can seek appointment at many levels, and the appointment doesn't necessarily have to be focused on health or health care. At the community level, nurses could serve on county health boards, task forces on redevelopment, or a local recreation committee to address policies that expand walking paths and bike trails. Community and county appointments could include the zoning commission, planning commission, hospital boards, boards of education, or councils on aging or economic development. State appointments could be as a public university trustee, a department head, or to a state board or commission. Federal opportunities exist in all federal agencies—both in Washington D.C. as well as in regional offices around the nation (Box 70-3).

MAKING A DECISION TO SEEK AN APPOINTMENT

Seeking a political appointment, at any level, is not a decision to be taken lightly. Consider some of the following questions to determine whether or not this path is right for you. Some questions will be more important if you are considering a full-time federal assignment rather than a part-time community role (Box 70-4).

PLAN YOUR STRATEGY

When you've identified the appointment you are interested in, the next step is being nominated. Determine the process used for nomination, and identify who will make the appointment. Having the support of more than one organization strengthens your chance for nomination. A number of factors should be considered when a plan is developed.

THE VETTING PROCESS

The scrutiny of an appointee's past is called the *vetting* process and serves as a quality check prior to appointment. Vetting involves the review of financial history, personal history and relationships, tax records, business transactions and ventures, family history, and other personal credentials. Vetting can also involve the process of preparing a candidate for the nomination hearing process. Vetting can result in the withdrawal of a nomination when unfavorable information is uncovered. Recall the circumstances surrounding the 2009 vetting of former Senator Tom Daschle, nominated by President Obama to serve as Secretary of Health and Human Services. Daschle was forced to withdraw following a revelation of unpaid taxes from consulting fees and unreported gifts of a car

---

BOX 70-3 Finding Opportunities to Serve in an Appointed Status

Although health and health care services appointments may be attractive to nurses, there are many types of appointments, not directly related to health, where nursing expertise can benefit constituents. These include the following:

- *Commerce and economic development.* Tourism and industrial development appointments could benefit from nursing expertise. A nurse's knowledge of the health care system could provide industries considering relocation with valuable information about what they can expect for their employees' health care. In many states, health care is one of the top three industries.
- *Conservation.* Environmental issues affect the health care of every community. For example, a nurse could provide expertise regarding hazardous waste, the value of clean water systems, or preserving green space.
- *Corrections.* Nurses' expert health care knowledge could play a valuable role in policy decisions regarding the health care and education of incarcerated persons. Nurse practitioners provide much of the health care in many of today's correctional facilities (both public and private).
- *Education.* Nurses could offer valuable insight on policy decisions regarding school-based health care services and health curricula. A nurse's knowledge of budgeting and cost-effective management could assist in the budget process.
- *Health and human services.* A wide variety of appointments exist at the local, state, and federal levels.
- *Higher education.* Policy decisions are made by state agencies and boards that have authority over colleges and universities.
- *Licensure and regulatory boards.* State boards of health determine policy regarding the health of the public, including drinking water, restaurant inspections, and health care provider licensure. State boards of nursing regulate the practice of nursing and offer the opportunity to nurses to serve on their governing boards. Some state boards of medicine make decisions regarding the practice of nurse practitioners and may have seats available for a nurse appointee.
- *Public safety.* Nurses can bring important perspectives to agencies and boards involved in public safety related to domestic violence, gun laws, and motor vehicle safety.
- *Transportation.* Nurses have seen firsthand the effect of motor vehicle accidents and can be valuable partners in improving safety through political appointments on transportation and highway safety organizations.

BOX 70-4 **Questions to Consider When Seeking a Political Appointment**

If you're considering a political appointment, ask yourself these questions:

- Can you take time away from your job or your family to meet the demands of the position?
- How often will meetings be held? What will your time obligation be? Is this a full-time position or a group that meets occasionally?
- Will your employer support you? Will you have family support?
- Will your employer provide the time for you to serve, or will you be required to take vacation time?
- Why do you want to serve in this position? Can you articulate why you are qualified?
- What are the strengths and weaknesses you would bring to the position?
- What is your connection to your community? Do you know your neighbors? Have you served in volunteer organizations? Having a solid base of support from your neighbors, your friends, and your fellow volunteers in local organizations will enhance your chances of success.
- Where do you fit in the political spectrum? Are you registered to vote as a Democrat, Republican, or Independent? Party affiliation provides important linkages to support from individuals and groups.
- How will your education, background, and experience serve you in the desired appointment? Candidates should be able

to identify aspects of each that will qualify them for the position.

- How are your health and your family's financial situation? Careful analysis should be given to each.
- Who makes the appointment? Is it the governor, the lieutenant governor, or the Speaker of the House of Representatives?
- Are there educational or geographic requirements? In Mississippi, the Nurse Practice Act requires a baccalaureate degree as the basic qualification for one board of nursing position and an associate degree as the basic qualification for another. One position is designated for an advanced practice nurse, and another is designated for a nurse educator. Some appointments require certain credentials (e.g., being a physician or a nurse).
- Which stakeholders care about who gets this position? Do you have influence with them? Are there other nominees under consideration?
- Is there a match between your qualifications and the requirements of the position? Carefully review local, state, or federal laws applicable to the appointment.
- Do you have a chance of getting the position? What connections do you have with individuals and organizations that will make the decision?

---

and driver services. Bernard Kerik, nominated by President George Bush, abruptly withdrew his name from nomination for Secretary of Homeland Security when multiple issues were uncovered during his vetting. At the state level, scrutiny is less intense but still will include a thorough review of a candidate's personal and public life.

POLITICAL PARTY AFFILIATION

Political party affiliation is an important factor in securing support for a political appointment. Most appointments are made as rewards for loyal support. The support could be as simple as volunteering in a local or state party office, organizing a fund-raising event for your party, writing letters, or making contributions to a candidate or the party. It can also involve becoming recognized for expertise in the appointment domain. For example, Virginia Trotter Betts identified her political affiliation as key to her appointment as Senior Advisor on Nursing and Policy

to the Secretary and Assistant Secretary of Health of the U.S. Department of Health and Human Services (HHS) under President Bill Clinton. She credited a long-standing relationship with the Clinton-Gore administration after the American Nurses Association (ANA) became the first health care group to endorse the candidates in 1992. Betts had been a Robert Woods Johnson fellow in the office of then-Senator Al Gore. When he ran for vice president, she worked on his campaign. After her federal appointment, Betts was appointed by Tennessee Governor Phil Bredesen as Commissioner of Mental Health and Developmental Disabilities because of her federal experience and her expertise in mental health.

GETTING SUPPORT

Dr. Mary Wakefield was appointed by President Barack Obama as Administrator of the Health Resources and Service Administration (HRSA) in HHS. She is former chief of staff to two North Dakota senators and an appointee to several federal health care commissions. She advises that expertise alone might get you a position, but frequently it requires becoming known to the decision-makers. She emphasizes the need to have the support of nursing as well as other major organizations and influential individuals that can advocate for you. The more broad-based support you have, the better your chances of being noticed. Wakefield says that to successfully obtain an appointment, you must have a two-pronged approach: You need to have the expertise required by the position and a network of relationships built over time with policymakers. Wakefield highlights the importance of making it easy for people to help you. She recommends that nurses not just ask someone to write a letter of support, but that the potential nominee write the letter and provide it to the person providing the recommendation or that person's staff. If you desire, a phone call can be made on your behalf; provide the person making the call with a brief memo about your qualifications and why you would make a great candidate (Chaffee, 2000).

USING THE POWER OF NETWORKS

Few people have the clout or power to be appointed without broad support. The executive responsible for making the appointment wants to be certain that the appointee is respected and approved by many constituents. For nurses, this means mobilizing groups or individuals outside of nursing. These can be other policymakers, such as members of Congress, if one is seeking a federal position. At the state level, it might mean other health professionals, such as physicians, social workers, or the hospital association, as well as consumer groups such as the AARP.

Patricia Montoya was a federal political appointee in the Clinton administration serving as Commissioner to the Administration on Children, Youth and Families. At the state level, she was appointed by Governor Bill Richardson of New Mexico as Secretary of Health and Human Services. Montoya reports that she was appointed to both positions because she had both experience and expertise and a well-developed political network. Montoya worked on the campaigns of President Clinton and Governor Richardson and worked with Governor Richardson on his nurse advisory group when he served as a member of Congress. Several influential individuals who were familiar with her qualifications advanced her name as a nominee. Montoya says that she has always mixed practice and politics in her career and credits her work with the ANA for advancing her political education (Montoya, 2007).

CONFIRMATION OR INTERVIEW?

Depending on the type of appointment you desire, you may need to participate in confirmation hearings or interviews. It is vital to be familiar with the position and the organizational hierarchy in which it falls, as well as current issues facing the organization. Such interviews can be intense and require careful preparation.

When preparing for either a hearing or interview, consider the following questions:

- What do I need to bring?
- Who will be conducting the hearing or interview?
- What questions will I be asked?
- Will I have the opportunity to ask questions?
- Should I have representation or sponsorship at the confirmation hearing?

Be honest about personal and family finances, anything in the past that could be damaging, public records, or media reports. Be prepared to respond to questions; it helps to practice for the interview with someone who can be tough and give honest feedback.

COMPENSATION

Federal appointments follow published compensation schedules. State appointees may have compensation set by statute. Potential appointees should request information in advance of an appointment about compensation—both direct compensation and reimbursement for expenses incurred before accepting an appointment. Pay alone generally does not motivate appointees; some high-level appointees may actually receive less compensation than they could receive in the private sector.

AFTER THE APPOINTMENT

RELATIONSHIPS WITH SUPPORTERS

Once you've passed the background checks, survived the interviews, and have been appointed to a position, there is nothing more important than thanking all those who supported your appointment. Send letters of appreciation to recognize the efforts of others in helping you attain your appointment.

Once you are appointed, consider whom it is your duty to serve. If yours is a public appointment, your allegiance must be to your constituents. If it is to a health care organization's board of directors, your responsibility is to the patients and community. It is important that you retain your autonomy if the appointment is of a regulatory nature. If an association or other group was instrumental in your nomination and subsequent appointment, maintain open communication to keep them informed and to listen to their concerns. If your appointment is to represent a specific group on a task force or other group, close communication is necessary to convey the viewpoints of those you represent.

EXPERIENCES OF NURSE APPOINTEES

DR. SHIRLEY CHATER

Federal appointee Dr. Shirley Chater served as U.S. Commissioner of the Social Security Administration during the Clinton administration from 1993-1997. Dr. Chater's appointment was unusual because she did not seek it. Rather, it evolved from her leadership, her health care knowledge, and her experiences with the former governor of Texas. Her appointment was supported and promoted by her former colleagues and the American Nurses Association. It is a story of unexpected opportunity that resulted in the most senior appointment of a nurse in the Clinton administration.

Prior to her federal appointment, Chater was President of Texas Woman's University. For the previous 17 years, she held joint faculty appointments at the University of California, San Francisco and the University of California, Berkeley, and for five years she served as Vice Chancellor for Academic Affairs at the University of California, San Francisco. She became known to President Clinton in several ways. The first was through lobbying efforts with ANA, and the second was through chairing a major commission on health reform in Texas. This led to then–Texas Governor Ann Richards urging President Clinton to appoint Chater to a senior position. Chater was then selected by Dr. Donna Shalala, Secretary of HHS, to serve as administrator of the Social Security Administration (SSA) which at the time was in HHS.

Chater's background as a nurse and an administrator was crucial to the work she did. After her first year as SSA administrator, SSA was made an independent agency. It gave Chater an opportunity to attend presidential cabinet meetings and be involved in policy decisions in many areas. It also gave her the opportunity to change the SSA culture and business practices to that of an agency that put customers first—reminiscent of the focus of nursing. She indicated that influencing and implementing policies that affected clients was the most rewarding part of the position.

Chater's advice for others seeking a high-level appointment in government is that one must have a strategy developed with supporters whose voice and influence will be strong and persistent. It helps to have appropriate education and experience. And one must be prepared for the vetting process, which can be long and difficult. When asked if it was worth it, Chater said unequivocally yes, it provided the experience of a lifetime (personal communication, December 2009).

MARILYN TAVENNER

Marilyn Tavenner served as Virginia Secretary of Health and Human Services from 2006 to 2009. In 2010, President Barack Obama appointed her as Principal Deputy Administrator for the Centers for Medicare and Medicaid Services (CMS), an agency within HHS. As second in command of CMS, Tavenner oversees more than 4400 employees; an annual budget that exceeds $670 billion; and the provision of health care benefits to roughly 98 million people enrolled in Medicare, Medicaid, and the Children's Health Insurance Program (CHIP). She started her career as a staff nurse, moved to chief nursing officer, and eventually moved to chief executive officer (CEO) of two hospitals in the Hospital Corporation of American (HCA) system in Virginia. She then moved to a more senior position in HCA, as Group President of Outpatient Services in their corporate office in Tennessee. During that time, she served as chair of the Virginia Hospital Association and was a member of the Board of Trustees of the American Hospital Association.

Tavenner became acquainted with Tim Kaine prior to his election as Virginia's governor. As a hospital CEO, she worked on projects with Mr. Kaine as well as serving as head of his campaign's policy working group. After his election, she called to congratulate him, and he asked her to interview for a position in his administration. It was the broad support of groups she had worked with that moved her nomination forward. These included the Virginia Nurses Association, the Virginia Hospital Association, the Virginia Medical Association, the American Organization of Nurse Executives, insurance firms, long-term care organizations, and other nursing groups close to the governor. That network was glad to rally support when she asked for help.

Once appointed to the state position, she went to work reorganizing the agency and creating one of the first state health reform commissions during a time of extreme budget challenges. Tavenner was able to create nursing positions in many agencies, including creating a department of health professions headed by a nurse. She established a health workforce center that instituted nursing scholarships for graduate education and resulted in a major increase in nursing faculty in the state. It also resulted in a 50% increase in nursing school enrollment. In addition, she expanded medical school enrollment to meet the projected shortfall of physicians.

Ms. Tavenner's advice for others seeking an appointment is threefold:

- Get involved in your community, and develop a broad network of support.
- Get involved in political campaigns and party organizations, and in developing policy platforms.
- Give financial contributions to candidates whom you support (J. K. Leavitt, personal communication, December 5, 2009).

RITA WRAY

Rita Wray, Deputy Executive Director of the Mississippi Department of Finance and Administration, got her start through a neighbor's invitation to a County Republican Women's Club meeting. She was drawn to the party because she agreed with the values that the party espoused: personal responsibility, free markets, low taxes, and fiscal conservatism. Wray was a nurse executive with a consulting business focused on regulatory compliance, risk management, corporate communication, and professional practice issues. She was also active in leadership positions with the American Nurses Association, the Susan G. Komen Breast Cancer Foundation, and National Coalition of 100 Black Women, Inc. But her political connections, made through running for a seat in the Mississippi legislature (unsuccessfully) and working for the successful election of Governor Haley Barbour, made her

a candidate for an appointment when Barbour was elected. In 2008, she became the sixteenth president of the Mississippi Federation of Republican Women (MFRW) and the first African American.

Wray credits her selection for the political appointment as the result of her business acumen, her work with the party, her leadership ability, her interpersonal and communication skills, in addition to her race and gender. She advises others to use the steps of the nursing process: Assess strengths and abilities, develop a plan to demonstrate how those match the ones needed for the appointment, implement the plan, and evaluate outcomes. Above all, she recommends, use the power of connections (J. K. Leavitt, personal communication, March 2010).

SUMMARY

When Dr. Catherine Dodd, a nurse from California, was interviewed by former Secretary of HHS Donna Shalala for an appointment as a regional director, Shalala commented that she had appointed three nurses to federal positions. Shalala's respect for nurses was clear in her appraisal, according to Dodd. Shalala stated, "Nurses understand health care issues, they can talk to anybody and they come prepared to work—they can hit the ground running." Entering public life as an appointee is a noble and challenging endeavor that nurses who wish to make a difference should consider.

For a list of related websites, please refer to your Evolve Resources at http://evolve.elsevier.com/Mason/policypolitics/

REFERENCES

Chaffee, M. W. (2000). In the health policy spotlight: An interview with Dr. Mary Wakefield. *Policy, Politics & Nursing Practice, 1*(1), 53-59.

Lewis, D. (2008). *The politics of presidential appointments: Political control and bureaucratic performance.* Princeton: Princeton University Press.

MassGAP. (2010). *MassGAP: Moving women ahead in Massachusetts.* Retrieved from www.massgap.org.

Montoya, P. (2007). *Making the most of political appointments: My life as a federal and state official.* In Mason, D., Leavitt, J., Chaffee, M. Policy and Politics in Nursing and Health Care (5th ed.). (pp. 699-702). St Louis: Elsevier.

Nathan, R. P. (2009). *Handbook for appointed officials in America's governments.* Retrieved from www.rockinst.org/pdf/government_reform/2009-handbook_for_appointed_officials_in_america%27s_governments.pdf.

Vedantam, S. (2008, November). Who are the better managers—Political appointees or career bureaucrats? Retrieved from www.washingtonpost.com/wp-dyn/content/article/2008/11/23/AR2008112302485.html?sub=AR.

CHAPTER 71

TAKING ACTION
Influencing Policy as a Member of the San Francisco Health Commission

Catherine M. Waters

"In every community, there is work to be done. In every nation, there are wounds to heal. In every heart, there is the power to do it."

—Marianne Williamson

I was appointed as a Commissioner to the San Francisco Health Commission by the Mayor of San Francisco, Gavin Newsom, in 2008. I replaced a nurse, Dr. Catherine Dodd, who had 1 year left in her term when she was appointed as the Mayor's Deputy Chief of Staff for Health (Figure 71-1). Commissioner Dodd recommended me to the Mayor's Office to complete her term. I was told that other candidates, mostly physicians, were being considered also for the position. In the span of two weeks, I was notified by the Mayor's Office that I had been appointed, and I was sworn in at City Hall the following week. I am certain that the synergy of various nursing connections and networks was an influential factor in my appointment.

After completing my 1-year term, I was reappointed by the Mayor in 2009 to a 4-year term. The reappointment required that I testify before the city's Board of Supervisors for approval. In my televised testimony, the Board of Supervisors queried me about my commitment to the citizens of San Francisco and whether or not my views were independent of the Mayor's views. I emphasized that the Health Commission is an independent, autonomous body that provides health advice to the Mayor on behalf of the residents of San Francisco.

In addition to my service on the full Health Commission, I am a member of the Joint Conference Committee that oversees San Francisco General Hospital and Trauma Center, a member of the Community and Public Health Joint Conference Committee that oversees community programs and public health prevention activities, and a liaison to the San Francisco Health Plan, the program that provides health access to low- and middle-income San Francisco residents.

APPLYING MY NURSING BACKGROUND IN COMMISSION ACTIVITIES

I bring expertise to my work as a public servant from my background as a doctorally-prepared registered nurse, a university faculty member, a nurse scientist, and a citizen. My community-based participatory research and teaching, which focuses on health-promoting lifestyle interventions in collaboration with public and private community partnerships, informs my policy work and decision-making on the Health Commission. Making decisions and having debate about the multifaceted issues that come before the Health Commission requires the application of diplomacy, democracy, politics, and the art and science of nursing. During my tenure, the primary focus of the Health Commission has been on deciding where spending reductions have to be made within the Department of Public Health. Diplomacy and democracy are about differences, which are bound to diverge when different viewpoints and demands are expressed freely between competing interest groups or individuals for limited funds and resources.

The Health Commission hears arguments from disparate sides; I listen with diligence and in earnest

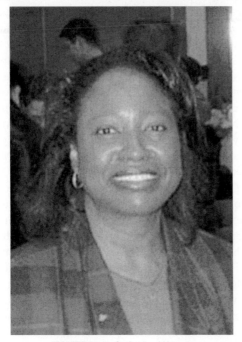

FIGURE 71-1 Catherine Waters.

central principle of public health nursing is to achieve the greatest good for the greatest number of people by working with the population as a whole and as an equal partner (Levin et al., 2008). Adhering to this code of ethics requires being guided by a moral compass and philosophical and ethical values in order to help people live more healthful lives in the context of mutual respect, fairness, and justice.

I believe I have a moral obligation and duty to do the greatest good for the greatest number of people and engage in actions that cause the least harm to the fewest number of people. During this economic downturn, some people would question my use of morality and dismiss it as naïve, but morality has a place in policymaking and decision-making, especially when it involves the safety of the public's health. Ideology may not be a prudent course of action during this time, but making sure that every person has a fair chance for a healthy life and an equal opportunity for quality health care is not about ideology; it is about the inherent and inalienable right to life, liberty, and the pursuit of happiness, which is not possible without good health. As a society, we have little to gain and everything to lose under a disparate health care system.

from a nursing perspective. How do I prioritize and decide which programs that serve as the safety net for vulnerable populations take precedence over other programs that serve vulnerable populations? As a nurse, how do I in good conscious vote for the reduction and elimination of programs that I know may prove to be detrimental to the public's health, particularly to populations who are the most vulnerable, but often, who have no voice, no power, and no leadership? I try to give voice to these stakeholders who often cannot speak for themselves. There is no magical formula to determine budget cuts that are difficult, painful, inevitable, and indispensable. I use principles of public health nursing, my professional expertise for the past 15 years, to guide me in policymaking and decision-making. Prior to public health nursing, my expertise was in oncology nursing.

Public health nursing contributes to population-focused health through effective partnerships with communities and populations to identify specific public health needs and concerns, address those issues at multiple levels, and use the political process to assure healthy communities via an ecological approach (American Nurses Association, 2007). The

OVERVIEW OF THE SAN FRANCISCO HEALTH COMMISSION

As the governing and policymaking body of the Department of Public Health, the San Francisco Health Commission (referred to as the Health Commission), is mandated by the City and County Charter to manage and control the City and County hospitals, to monitor and regulate emergency medical services, and to oversee all matters pertaining to the preservation, promotion, and protection of the lives and the physical, mental, and environmental health of San Francisco residents (Health Commission, 2008).

THE COMMISSION'S SCOPE OF WORK

The Commission considers issues including approval of the budget of the San Francisco Department of Public Health; estimates of revenues and expenditures; budget modifications; fund transfers and reappropriations; accepting and expending grants and receipt of gifts; entering contractual agreements; and reviewing proposed rates, fees, and other similar charges. The Health Commission also considers policy matters relating to health needs of the public, including program additions, deletions, or modifications and the closing and building of hospitals in San Francisco. All declarations of policy are made in the form of a resolution, and if approved, the Health Commission forwards the resolution to the Mayor for submission to the Board of Supervisors.

INFRASTRUCTURE

The Health Commission is composed of seven members from diverse backgrounds and is led by a president and vice president. Health Commissioners are appointed by the Mayor and approved by the Board of Supervisors and serve 4-year terms. The Health Commission conducts all of its business in a public forum; however, it may meet in closed session. Members of the public are encouraged to attend the meetings and address the Health Commission. Public comments are heard prior to the vote on action items. Four Joint Conference Committees compose the Health Commission. One reviews financial reports of and approves contracting services for the Department of Public Health. Another provides oversight for the Department of Public Health programs and its city-wide contractors that deliver services on behalf of the Department of Public Health. The remaining two committees provide oversight of health care delivery services for the City and County of San Francisco's two hospitals, Laguna Honda Hospital and Rehabilitation Center and San Francisco General Hospital and Trauma Center. In addition to the Joint Conference Committees, the President of the Health Commission appoints one Commissioner to be a liaison to three governing bodies needing Health Commission representation.

DIFFICULT DECISIONS

Some of the issues that I've been involved in have been challenging. I had to consider whether to vote to eliminate services (that would prevent ophthalmologic problems for persons with diabetes, reduce clinical hours during the week and eliminate a weekend day of clinical services for persons seeking urgent

care, and eliminate integrated behavioral and medical services for persons living with the human immunodeficiency virus and acquired immunodeficiency syndrome) in order to budget for mandated cost-of-living allowances for health care personnel. These health services programs were implemented to prevent complications, such as blindness, emergency department overuse, and stigmatization, in these populations. Why would we dismantle services that were designed to save lives, improve quality of life, and decrease health care costs?

The Health Commission cannot spend money that it does not have. However, I feel an obligation to advocate for the public to do the greatest good for the greatest number of people and cause the least harm to the fewest number of people. The Health Commission's budget principles dictate that it will develop a budget to maximize revenues; minimize the impact on vulnerable populations—those with the lowest income, severest illness, disproportionate health disparities, and are homeless; and preserve its core functions (i.e., primary care, emergency care, and protection of the public's health through education and infectious disease control). Using these budget principles, I voted in favor of a wait-and-see approach to see how the overall budget would unfold before approving cuts in services that might harm the most vulnerable populations. In waiting for a thorough assessment of the fiscal impact of decisions to reduce and eliminate services, it reflects my belief that the balance sheet should reflect the Department of Public Health and its partners' values, not the other way around.

THE BALANCE OF POWER

The balance of power in San Francisco's local government is similar to the balance of power in the United States federal government. The Health Commission falls under the executive branch because its members are appointed by the mayor. The powers and duties of the Health Commission are in accordance with the City and County Charter. The Board of Supervisors composes the legislative branch and approves the appointments made by the mayor. Serving as the judicial branch, the San Francisco City Attorney Office provides legal services to the mayor, Board of Supervisors, and Health Commission. The Health Commission recommends programs to be funded, eliminated, or reduced; the Board of Supervisors determines expenditures for those programs; the mayor considers implementation of the expenditures recommended by the Board of Supervisors; and the City Attorney's Office provides advice about the legality of expenditures.

THE PUBLIC'S TRUST IN NURSES AND WHAT IT MEANS

According to the 2008 *USA Today*/Gallup poll, rating the honesty and ethics of workers in 21 different professions, for the seventh straight year, nurses are the most trustworthy, honest, and ethical of health care professionals (Saad, 2008). The public values and trusts nurses—a trust that is an honor that brings with it responsibility and commitment to serve the public. I believe it is my moral obligation and duty to ensure the delivery of services to assure the welfare of the public, to be honest in delivering information, to develop trusting partnerships, and to recognize the status of people who are inextricably bound to their social context. With this responsibility comes internal vigilance and being a part of the decision-making process in a discriminate and participatory manner. It is a *fata morgana*, a mirage, to believe budget cuts will not have a negative impact on the health of vulnerable people. In a decent, democratic society, there are certain obligations that are not subject to trade-offs or negotiations. Health care is one of those obligations.

I believe nurses know better than anyone where the system works and where it does not work, and they know how to improve quality of care and serve clients more effectively and efficiently. Despite it being difficult to prioritize resources among people who are all at-risk, I have learned to articulate my viewpoint, defend my position, face controversy, build a consensus, and debate issues of vital importance with diplomacy. Admittedly, this can sometimes be a slow and fragile process, especially if the process is conducted democratically and diplomatically.

SUMMARY

All of the Health Commissioners do not always agree, but we engage and dialogue to find common ground with each other, the Department of Public Health and its partners, and the public to develop a common agenda and vision. The debate can and should be nuanced, principled, and spirited. Arguing over ideas is different from suppressing, changing, or ignoring opinions. Transparency and inclusiveness of decision-making and negotiation, action in the face of uncertainty, and accountability are fundamental to the success and maintenance of democracy in public health.

There are many health needs in San Francisco, but there are limited funds and resources available to address them. We cannot do everything that would be desirable to eliminate health disparities. This is the time to set priorities and consider inescapable trade-offs and opportunity costs with creative and innovative practices. This is an appropriate time to rethink how the Department of Public Health does business—moving from a model of "more quantity of services" to "quality of care and value of services" with more focus on outcomes. Difficult decisions must be made because of the fiscal reality.

For a list of related websites, please refer to your Evolve Resources at http://evolve.elsevier.com/Mason/policypolitics/

REFERENCES

American Nurses Association. (2007). *Public health nursing: Scope and standards of practice.* Washington, D.C.: Author.

Health Commission. (2008). *Rules and regulations.* San Francisco: Author.

Levin, P. F., Cary, A. H., Kulbok, P., Leffers, J., Molle, M., & Polivka, B. J. (2008). Association of Community Health Nursing Educators. Graduate education for advanced practice public health nursing: At the crossroads. *Public Health Nursing, 25*(2), 176-193.

Saad, L. (November 24, 2008). Nurses shine, bankers slump in ethics ratings. Annual honesty and ethics poll rates nurses best of 21 professions. Gallup. Retrieved from www.gallup.com/poll/112264/Nurses-Shine-While-Bankers-Slump-Ethics-Ratings.aspx#2.

CHAPTER 72

Nursing and the Courts

David M. Keepnews and Virginia Trotter Betts

"Power concedes nothing without a demand. It never did and it never will."

—Frederick Douglass

The courts are an important source of health policy. Their deliberations and decisions hold significant implications for nurses and the patients, communities, and populations they serve. Many nurses and other health professionals (like most nonlawyers) may think of legal and judicial processes as arcane, highly technical, even frightening, and better left to legal experts to address and understand. But nurses should not regard the legal system as the exclusive domain of lawyers and judges any more than they regard the legislative process as belonging only to lobbyists and legislators. In fact, anyone who seeks to understand policy needs at least a basic knowledge not just of the impact of court decisions, but also how advocates respond to and even influence the outcomes of those decisions.

This chapter provides an overview of the legal and judicial system and the role of the courts in shaping policy. It is not a comprehensive overview; rather, it aims to provide the reader with a general understanding of this area and its critical importance for nursing.

THE JUDICIAL SYSTEM: A BRIEF OVERVIEW

The United States has two major, parallel court systems: federal and state. The federal courts have jurisdiction over matters that involve federal law (generally, those that pertain to the U.S. Constitution, federal statutes and/or the actions of federal agencies). Federal courts can also hear complaints that arise between parties in different states if a sufficient monetary amount (currently a minimum of $75,000) is in dispute. The trial courts for the federal system (the entry point for most federal cases) are called district courts; there are 94 federal district courts located throughout the U.S. and its territories. Federal courts of appeal, also referred to as Circuit Courts, are organized into 11 geographic circuits plus the District of Columbia Circuit Court and the Federal Circuit Court (Want, 2009). The U.S. Supreme Court is the federal court of last resort—there is no higher court to which its decisions can be appealed.

Each state has its own court system. State courts generally rule on issues arising under the state's constitution and laws. (State courts may also hear some claims that arise under federal law or the U.S. Constitution.) Generally, state court systems include trial-level and appellate courts, with a high court as the court of last resort. (The high court is known as the Supreme Court in most states, but not all; in New York State, for example, it is known as the Court of Appeal.) Often, trial courts are further subdivided on the basis of subject matter, an amount in dispute or a type of remedy. (Thus, states may have a family court, probate court, municipal court, mental health court, and so on.) On certain matters, decisions of a state Supreme Court may be appealed directly to the U.S. Supreme Court.

JUDICIAL REVIEW

In *Marbury v. Madison* (1803), the U.S. Supreme Court first asserted its power to declare a law null and void if it is found to violate the Constitution. This concept of judicial review has evolved into one of the courts' most important powers because it grants them significant influence over government action. Another important doctrine, *stare decisis* ("let the decision stand"), set the course for judicial precedents by adhering to previous findings in cases with substantially comparable facts and situations. Thus, courts grant deference to their own prior rulings. Courts are not completely bound by precedent, and they sometimes overrule their prior decisions, but they are expected to depart from precedent based on compelling and clearly articulated reasons.

The scope of the Supreme Court's influence on American life expanded greatly in the years after the Civil War when the Fourteenth Amendment to the Constitution, ratified in 1868, limited states' abilities to restrict the rights of their citizens, including the right to due process and the equal protection of the law. This amendment made many state laws susceptible to challenge in the federal courts, particularly as the Supreme Court ruled that the Fourteenth Amendment had the effect of making most of the rights in the Bill of Rights (e.g., the right of free speech under the First Amendment) applicable to the states.

THE CONTEXT FOR COURT DECISIONS: THE CONSTITUTION AND THE BRANCHES OF GOVERNMENT

The U.S. Constitution sets out the basic structure of the federal government. State constitutions do the same for each state government. A key element of this structure is a system of checks and balances between the three branches of government: the legislative branch (Congress, state legislatures, local legislative bodies), the executive branch (the president, governors, and the government agencies they administer), and the judicial branch (the federal and state courts). Within this structure, each branch carries out specific functions, but no branch is completely autonomous. For example, Congress passes legislation, but the president can either sign or veto it, and Congress can override a presidential veto by a two-thirds majority. Federal executive agencies such as the U.S. Department of Health and Human Services are accountable to the President, but their budgets depend on actions by Congress. The federal courts act independently of the President and Congress, but judges are nominated by the President subject to confirmation by the U.S. Senate.

The Constitution is our fundamental source of law. All government action must be consistent with it. This is true of the U.S. Constitution (which applies to the actions of the federal and state governments) and

each state constitution (which apply to the actions of each respective state).

The U.S. Constitution is the legal source of the rights and freedoms that Americans enjoy. While much of the Constitution is concerned with the structure and functions of the federal government, the first ten amendments to the Constitution—known as the Bill of Rights—define the basic rights of all people in the U.S. including freedom of speech; freedom of assembly; freedom of religion; freedom from unlawful searches and seizures; protection against being deprived of life, liberty, or property without due process; and others. In the U.S., the rights outlined by the Bill of Rights are defined primarily as limitations on government's power to restrict or deny them. Thus, for example, the First Amendment reads as follows:

Congress shall make no law respecting an establishment of religion, or prohibiting the free exercise thereof; or abridging the freedom of speech, or of the press; or the right of the people peaceably to assemble, and to petition the Government for a redress of grievances.

(While the Bill of Rights specifically focuses on the federal government, the Fourteenth Amendment—as noted earlier—has had the effect of applying most of these rights to actions by state governments as well.)

Because the Bill of Rights applies to government action, it does not directly limit the behavior of private individuals (including employers). Other laws may apply to actions by employers and individuals—for example, whistleblower laws that protect employees' rights to report unethical or illegal conduct.

Laws passed by Congress must be consistent with the U.S. Constitution. Any laws passed by a state legislature must be consistent with the U.S. Constitution and the state constitution. Laws or ordinances passed by a local legislative body (such as a City Council) must be consistent with the federal and state constitutions and any other legal documents that set out the structure and functions of local government (such as a city charter).

Rules or regulations issued by the executive branch (administrative agencies) must be consistent with the Constitution. There must also generally be some statutory (legislative) source of authority for them to act. For example, the U.S. Secretary of Health and Human

Services is authorized by federal law to issue rules and regulations to carry out the functions of her department, including the administration of the Medicare program (42 U.S.C. Sections 1302 and 1395 [2008]); this is the basis for that agency to adopt regulations spelling out Conditions of Participation that hospitals and other health care organizations must meet in order to participate in the Medicare and Medicaid programs (42 CFR Chapter IV, Subchapter G, 2004.) The federal Administrative Procedure Act (5 U.S.C., Chapter 5 [2009]) and parallel state laws also spell out the procedures that government agencies must follow in issuing regulations—for example, how much notice must be provided to the public and how members of the public can provide comments on proposed regulations. The actions of an executive agency may be challenged on the basis that it has allegedly acted without legal authority or fails to comply with procedural requirements.

For example, in *Spine Diagnostics Center of Baton Rouge, Inc. v. Louisiana State Board of Nursing* (2008), a Louisiana appellate court considered a challenge to a Board of Nursing Advisory Opinion that interventional pain management is within the scope of practice of Certified Registered Nurse Anesthetists (CRNAs). The court upheld a trial court finding that this Advisory Opinion constituted a "rule" (regulation) expanding the CRNA scope of practice into an area in which they had not traditionally practiced. The court agreed that interventional pain management is "solely the practice of medicine." Since this "rule" expanding (according to the court) CRNAs' scope of practice had not been issued in accordance with the state's Administrative Procedures Act (including advance notice and an opportunity for public comment), it was found to be an improper attempt at rule making. The state Supreme Court subsequently declined to hear an appeal of the decision thus allowing it to stand.

Two other examples, both pertaining to nurse staffing ratios in California, also help to illustrate the court's power to review agency actions. In 1999, California enacted Assembly Bill (AB) 394, which requires hospitals to abide by mandatory nurse staffing ratios. AB 394 directed the California Department of Health Services (CDHS) to issue regulations implementing the ratios. When the CDHS issued its ratios regulations in 2002, they included a proviso that the ratios be in effect "at all times." The state hospital

association argued that this requirement was too rigid—that applying it during meal and bathroom breaks would be costly and impractical. They sued the CDHS, seeking to have that provision overturned. A California Superior Court ruled against them, finding that the "at all times" language accurately reflected the intent of AB 394 and that eliminating it would render the law "meaningless" (Egelko, 2004).

Another section in the regulations initially set requirements for nurse staffing on medical-surgical units at 6 patients per licensed nurses (6:1), but included a change to a required 5:1 staffing ratio, scheduled to go into effect on January 1, 2005. At the behest of a newly elected governor, the CDHS issued emergency regulations to delay implementation of the 5:1 ratio until January 1, 2008. California law allows a state agency to issue emergency regulations (which are not subject to requirements for advance notice and public comment) "if the emergency situation clearly poses such an immediate, serious harm that delaying action to allow public comment would be inconsistent with the public interest" (California Government Code Section 11346.1).

The California Nurses Association, a major proponent of mandatory nurse staffing ratios, sued to stop the emergency regulations (and thus to stop delay in implementation of the more stringent staffing ratios). A Superior Court judge granted their request, finding that the CDHS had failed to follow required procedures for changing state regulations and that it had not demonstrated that the delay was needed for the immediate preservation of public health and safety (*California Nurses Association v. Schwarzenegger et al.,* 2005). The planned 1:5 ratio for medical-surgical units was implemented; an appeal of the judge's decision was later dropped (Martin, 2005).

IMPACT LITIGATION: ESTABLISHING RIGHTS

Over the decades, advocates have had a strong tradition of using the courts strategically to establish, affirm, or clarify rights. Litigation that is pursued with a goal of achieving a broad social affect that sets a significant precedent or benefits a class of people is often referred to as *impact litigation*. Impact litigation "is most commonly understood to mean litigation that is expected to have far-reaching results" (Churchill, 2009).

A major example of impact litigation is *Brown v. Board of Education,* the 1954 case in which the U.S. Supreme Court struck down school segregation and mandated that states begin a process of desegregating their public schools. The Court unanimously found that segregated public school education constituted a state policy of inferior education—that "separate educational facilities are inherently unequal"—and that it thus violated the Equal Protection Clause of the Fourteenth Amendment to the U.S. Constitution. This case had been pursued by civil rights advocates who sought to use the courts as a vehicle for vindicating their rights as promised by the U.S. Constitution.

Another prominent example of using the courts to forge social policy is *Roe v. Wade* (1973) in which the U.S. Supreme Court found that women had a right to choose abortion without unreasonable state restrictions. The Court made its ruling on the basis of its interpretation of various amendments to the Constitution that taken together conferred a right of privacy that included self-determination in seeking a medical procedure to terminate pregnancy. Although *Roe v. Wade* has been modified and narrowed in some respects by subsequent Supreme Court decisions, the basic right of a woman to choose abortion to terminate an unwanted pregnancy as established by the Court in 1973 has remained intact and continues as current reproductive health policy.

Litigation has also helped to establish and advance tobacco policy (Parmet, 1999). Through both individual lawsuits and class actions, advocates have sought to hold the tobacco industry accountable for illnesses and deaths caused by tobacco use. These legal efforts have also helped publicize important, previously undisclosed information about the tobacco industry and its practices and about the serious health effects of tobacco use, adding ammunition to both legal and political efforts to limit access to and use of tobacco. In 1998, 46 states settled a lawsuit against U.S. tobacco manufacturers, agreeing on payments to states of over $250 billion, as well as restricting advertising and marketing of tobacco products (Wilson, J., 1999). This multistate settlement helped to spur increased social and political support for numerous public health–oriented anti-tobacco efforts. In 2009, Congress passed—and President Obama signed—the Family Smoking Prevention and Tobacco Control Act giving the Food and Drug Administration authority

to regulate tobacco and further restricting tobacco advertising. Tobacco companies challenged this new law in court. In January 2010, a federal court struck down some of the bill's provisions, but upheld key provisions, including FDA regulation and some advertising restrictions (Wilson, D., 2010; *Commonwealth Brands Inc. v. U.S.,* 2010).

INTERPRETING AND ENFORCING EXISTING LEGISLATION

EXPANDING LEGAL RIGHTS THROUGH LITIGATION

Laws passed at the federal or state level often create rights or remedies that can be legally enforced through the courts. The Americans with Disabilities Act (ADA) provides for equal treatment for disabled Americans and bars discrimination in a number of areas including employment and public accommodations. For example, a person with a disability who is able to perform the essential aspects of a job with reasonable accommodation cannot be fired or denied a promotion on the basis of her or his disability. While the ADA applies principles of equality and fair play that are basic to American law and public life, it also created specific, enforceable rights.

In *Olmstead v. L.C.,* (1999), the Supreme Court found that states are required to place persons with mental disabilities in community settings rather than in institutions when the State's treatment professionals have determined that community placement is appropriate, the transfer from institutional care to a less restrictive setting is not opposed by the affected individual, and the placement can be reasonably accommodated, taking into account the resources available to the State and the needs of others with mental disabilities.

ENFORCING LEGAL AND REGULATORY REQUIREMENTS

The courts are often used as a means to seek enforcement of existing regulatory requirements. Nursing organizations sometimes turn to the courts to challenge practices they believe violate state nurse practice acts. For example, the American Nurses Association (ANA), ANA/California, and the California School Nurses Organization sued the California Department of Education (CDE) challenging a CDE directive authorizing insulin injection in public schools by unlicensed personnel. The CDE had issued this directive in connection with its settlement of a suit by parents of diabetic students who, the parents had charged, were being denied needed care by the lack of school personnel qualified to administer insulin (CDE, 2007). The nursing groups challenged this practice as a violation of California's Nursing Practice Act and questioned the authority of the CDE to issue a directive on nursing practice. The trial court issued an order stopping the CDE directive; (*American Nurses Association California v. Connell*, 2008); that order was subsequently stayed (essentially, put on hold) pending appeal.

ANTITRUST LAWS

Federal and state antitrust laws are designed to protect consumers by prohibiting anticompetitive business practices. These laws have their roots in the end of the nineteenth century when large and powerful businesses combined into alliances and colluded on prices, distribution, and other practices. Such collusion effectively eliminated competition among these businesses and blocked newer companies from entering the market. Such practices operated to the detriment of the consumer. Antitrust protections have been a legal area to which nurses and others have sometimes looked for relief from practices that block their full participation in the health care marketplace.

Traditionally, health professionals were largely free from antitrust scrutiny under an exemption for "learned professions." In 1975, the U.S. Supreme Court essentially eliminated that exemption (*Goldfarb v. Virginia State Bar*, 1975). Over the past 3 decades, antitrust laws have become significant to the health care industry. Beginning in the 1990s, merger activity among hospitals, insurance companies, and health systems brought attention from antitrust enforcement agencies.

Although federal antitrust laws are enforced through two federal agencies, the Federal Trade Commission (FTC) and the Antitrust Division of the Department of Justice (DOJ), private parties can also bring antitrust suits directly in federal court. In June 2006, class action antitrust suits were filed on behalf of nurses in Detroit, San Antonio, Albany, Chicago, and Memphis. (Class action suits seek to vindicate the rights of an entire class of individuals who share a common interest giving rise to the suit and who seek a common outcome.) These suits alleged that hospitals and health systems in each of those metropolitan areas had secretly shared nurses' pay and planned raises, agreeing not to compete with each other on compensation. This collusion between erstwhile competitors, the suits alleged, violated federal antitrust laws (Evans, 2007; Miles, 2007). Some hospitals opted to settle without going to trial. An Albany, New York, health system reached a $1.25 million settlement (Greenhouse, 2009); a Detroit health system agreed to a $13.6 million settlement (Greene, 2009).

Professional associations can also be subject to antitrust scrutiny. For example, in a prominent case, the U.S. Supreme Court found that an agreement by a county medical society to establish maximum fees for medical procedures constituted illegal price-fixing (*Arizona v. Maricopa County Medical Society*, 1982). In *Wilk v. American Medical Association* (1990), the AMA was found to have violated antitrust laws for anticompetitive activities aimed toward chiropractors. The AMA had advised that physicians were guilty of unethical conduct if they referred patients to chiropractors or accepted referrals from them, since one of the AMA's ethical principles barred cooperation with "unscientific practitioners." A group of chiropractors filed suit against the AMA and prevailed in the Seventh Circuit Court of Appeals, which found that this was part of an attempt to conduct an illegal group boycott of the chiropractic profession.

CRIMINAL COURTS

Many of the court decisions that have an impact on health policy and nursing practice are civil actions. In some prominent instances, however, actions in criminal courts have posed significant policy implications for nursing as well. For example, while negligent acts or commissions that lead to patient injury or death are usually addressed in civil suits by the injured party (or his or her family), on occasion they have led to criminal prosecution. In 2006, a Wisconsin nurse faced criminal charges for negligence leading to the tragic death of a teenage mother in labor. She was charged with Neglect of a Patient Causing Great Bodily Harm—a felony. This case drew national attention because of concern that criminalizing medical errors was over reaching and excessive and that emphasizing individual blame rather than systems-level accountability for errors and their prevention could actually impede efforts to improve patient safety. The Wisconsin nurse eventually accepted a plea bargain, agreeing to plead "no contest" to two misdemeanor charges and accepting 2 years' probation and restrictions on her work hours; in addition, the Wisconsin Board of Nursing suspended her license for 9 months (Treleven, 2006).

In 2006, 10 nurses simultaneously resigned their positions at a Long Island nursing home. These nurses were among a larger group—all of them recruited from the Philippines—working in facilities owned by the Sentosa Care nursing home chain. These nurses had complained that many of the promises made to them when they were first hired regarding wages, working, and living conditions had been broken. The nurses, fearing retaliation by their employer, resigned with minimal notice. The facility, whose patients included ventilator-dependent children, covered their shifts with other nurses. After receiving a complaint from the nursing home, the state's board of nursing found no basis to proceed with a patient abandonment complaint. An investigation by the state Department of Health later yielded a conclusion that no patients had been put at risk. Nonetheless, the local county District Attorney filed criminal charges against the nurses, indicting them for conspiracy and for putting children and disabled patients at risk.

The case raised significant concerns not only about mistreatment of immigrant nurses but about the rights of all nurses (Keepnews, 2009). Nursing organizations, including the ANA, the New York State Nurses Association, and the Philippine Nurses Association of America, supported the nurses' call for charges to be dropped. The trial court judge refused to drop the charges. However, the nurses filed an appeal of this decision. A state appellate court issued an order that the trial be stopped. The court found that "criminalizing [the nurses'] resignations" would have the effect of unjustifiably "abridging the nurses' Thirteenth Amendment rights"—referring to that Constitutional amendment's prohibition on involuntary servitude (*Matter of Vinluan v. Doyle*, 2009).

INFLUENCING AND RESPONDING TO COURT DECISIONS

Judges are supposed to rule based on facts and law, not according to public or political pressure. There are established channels for advocates to seek to persuade judges through written and oral argument, presentation of witnesses, and other evidence. In a strict sense, this precludes attempts by non-parties to a case to lobby for or influence the outcome of judicial proceedings.

However, in reality, several factors may influence the outcome of court decisions. In a very general sense, judges often take changing social attitudes and standards into account in their rulings. Judges also differ in their own judicial philosophy. The views of federal judicial appointees and their judicial record may influence a president's decision to nominate someone to the district or appellate courts and to the Supreme Court. (Past judicial rulings may also be a factor in the Senate's ultimate decision whether or not to confirm a nominee.) Thus, supporting one or another candidate for president is, in a general but important sense, one way of seeking to influence the courts' decision-making on major issues. The appointee frequently matters. (However, it should be noted that judges' opinions and attitudes often shift over time and cannot always be reliably predicted. Justice Harry Blackmun, often characterized as a liberal Court member, and who wrote the majority opinion in *Roe v. Wade*, had been nominated to the Supreme Court by President Nixon.)

INFLUENCING THE COURTS: AMICUS CURIAE BRIEFS

A more direct route for influencing courts' decisions is through filing amicus curiae ("friend of the court") briefs. Amicus briefs provide an important tool for advocacy groups to make their views known on a case with broad implications, even when they are not parties to that case. When (with the court's permission) groups and/or individuals file an amicus brief, they bring their perspectives, data, and beliefs about the issues before the court in order to influence how the court should rule.

Examples of cases in which nursing organizations have filed amicus briefs include the following:

- *Lark v. Montgomery Hospice* (2008). ANA, the Maryland Nurses Association, the American College of Nurse-Midwives, and the Public Justice Center filed an amicus brief in Maryland's high court in support of a nurse who had accused her employer of violating that state's health care whistleblower law.

- *Spine Diagnostics Center of Baton Rouge, Inc. v. Louisiana State Board of Nursing* (2008). The ANA, the Louisiana State Nurses Association, and the Louisiana Alliance of Nursing Organizations jointly filed an amicus brief with a Louisiana appellate court in support of a state board of nursing advisory opinion that interventional pain management is within the scope of practice of Certified Registered Nurse Anesthetists. The American Association of Nurse Practitioners, the Louisiana Association of Nurse Practitioners, and the National Council of State Boards of Nursing each also filed an amicus brief in this case.
- *Olmstead v. L.C.* (1999). The American Psychiatric Nurses Association joined several other organizations in an amicus brief before the U.S. Supreme Court to support the right of disabled persons to receive care in non-institutional settings.
- *Sullivan v. Edward Hospital* (2004). The American Association of Nurse Attorneys (TAANA) filed an amicus brief with the Illinois Supreme Court arguing that only nurses are qualified to provide expert testimony on nurses' standard of care.
- *Matter of Vinluan v. Doyle* (2009). ANA and NYSNA filed an amicus brief urging a New York State appellate court to stop the criminal trial against 10 Filipino nurses who had resigned their positions at a Long Island, New York, nursing home.
- *Commonwealth Brands Inc. v. U.S.* (2010). The Oncology Nursing Society joined with 10 other organizations in support of FDA regulation of tobacco manufacturing, sales, and advertising.

RESPONDING TO COURT DECISIONS

Appealing an Unfavorable Decision. When faced with an unsatisfactory court ruling, interest groups potentially have several options. The first is to appeal the decision to a higher court. Generally, there must be grounds to appeal beyond just not being satisfied with the outcome. For example, the losing party may argue that the court made an error in how it applied the law, or in refusing to consider relevant evidence. There is no guarantee that an appellate or higher court will agree to hear an appeal.

"Repudiating" the Court. When a court's decision is based on its interpretation of a law, another option is to change the law in order to (explicitly or implicitly) repudiate the court's interpretation. Accomplishing this requires a political strategy to win the support of sufficient numbers of members of Congress or state legislators.

For example, in *Ledbetter v. Goodyear Tire & Rubber Co., Inc.* (2007), the U.S. Supreme Court interpreted the equal-pay provisions of Title VII of the Civil Rights Act of 1964 as meaning that a violation occurs only at the time that a biased pay scale is instituted, not each time workers are paid unequally as a result of that policy. This had the effect of limiting an employee's ability to file a discrimination claim— even if an employee only actually learned of this unequal pay policy some time after it had been implemented. In response, Congress passed and President Obama signed the Lilly Ledbetter Fair Pay Act of 2009.

Revising the Law. Another response to a court decision invalidating a law may be to enact a law that has similar goals but is tailored to avoid the problems the court found. For example, in 2007, the New York City Board of Health adopted a regulation requiring some restaurants to visibly post nutritional information for its menu items. (Specifically, the regulation applied this requirement to restaurants that were already posting this information voluntarily.) The New York State Restaurant Association sued in federal court to stop this regulation. A district court judge ruled against the city finding that the law was pre-empted by a federal law, the Nutrition Labeling and Education Act of 1990 (NLEA), Pub. L. No. 101-535, 104 Stat. 2535 (1990). The Board of Health then adopted a revised requirement—now codified as New York City Health Code Section 81.50—requiring nutritional posting by all restaurants that are part of a chain with at least 15 outlets nationwide.

The restaurant association challenged this revised Health Code requirement, charging that it was pre-empted by federal law and that it violated the First Amendment (by requiring restaurants to "speak" a message with which they might not agree). This time, however, the same federal judge ruled in the city's favor and upheld the city's nutritional posting requirement (Barron, 2008). This decision was subsequently upheld by the Second Circuit Court of Appeals.

Pursuing Multiple Strategies. Sometimes multiple strategies are pursued to respond to an unfavorable court ruling. One example concerns the issue of when nurses can be considered supervisors under the National Labor Relations Act (NLRA). The NLRA provides employees with a number of protections including the right to engage in concerted action regarding wages, hours, and working conditions, to organize unions, and to bargain collectively with their employers. Some employers have argued that nurses, because they sometimes direct the work of other employees, are "supervisors" and are therefore not covered by the act. In *NLRB v. Health Care and Retirement Corp.* (1994), the Supreme Court invalidated the rationale that the National Labor Relations Board (NLRB) had previously used to find that nurses were not supervisors. (The NLRB had found that nurses direct the work of other staff, such as licensed practical nurses and nursing assistants, in the interests of patient care, and not "in the interests of the employer.")

The decision understandably caused a great deal of concern among nurses because it potentially jeopardized the collective bargaining rights of many registered nurses (RNs). The ANA and nurses' unions worked to mitigate its impact. They opposed employers' attempts to exclude charge nurses from collective bargaining units and supported subsequent NLRB decisions that directing the work of others in providing patient care does not make RNs ineligible for collective bargaining.

In 2001, the U.S. Supreme Court revisited the issue of nurses as supervisors in *NLRB v. Kentucky River Community Care*. This decision rejected the NLRB's argument that, in directing the work of others, nurses do not exercise "independent judgment" as used in the NLRA to (in part) define "supervisors." In 2007, the NLRB applied the Court's reasoning in a trilogy of decisions (Oakwood Healthcare, Inc.; Golden Crest Healthcare Center, and Croft Metals, Inc.). These cases cemented concerns among nursing organizations, unions, and other supporters of employees' rights regarding nurses (particularly charge nurses)—as well as lead workers in other industries—being excluded from the NLRA's protections. In response, those organizations have supported passage of the Re-empowerment of Skilled and Professional Employees and Construction Tradeworkers (RESPECT) Act, which would amend the NLRA to tighten the definition of supervisor. (At the time of this writing, the RESPECT Act has not been passed.)

However, this situation also points to the importance of the political context for shaping the legal environment. Just as the president nominates federal judges, he or she also nominates members of the NLRB (subject, as with judicial nominations, to Senate confirmation). The NLRB decisions ruling against broadly classifying nurses (or charge nurses) as supervisors were issued during the Clinton administration; the Kentucky River NLRB decisions were issued during the George W. Bush administration. As of this writing, President Obama's NLRB nominees have yet to be confirmed by the Senate, but the outcome of issues addressed by the Bush-era NLRB may likely be different if and when the NLRB revisits them.

Amending the Constitution. Another potential means of responding to an unsatisfactory court decision—particularly if the decision is based on an interpretation of the Constitution—is to amend the Constitution. In most cases, this is much easier said than done. Generally, amending the U.S. Constitution requires approval by not only a $\frac{2}{3}$ majority of both houses of Congress but also by $\frac{3}{4}$ of the states.

Amending state constitutions, however, is often a different story. States differ in their procedures for amending their state's constitution. One example that has captured national attention has occurred in California. In 2008, the California Supreme Court ruled that denying same-sex couples the right to marry was a violation of the equal protection clause of the California State Constitution (*In re Marriage Cases*, 2008). Opponents of same-sex marriage gathered enough signatures to place Proposition 8, a state Constitutional amendment, on the ballot. That amendment, which California voters narrowly approved in November 2008, declared that only marriage between a man and a woman is valid or recognized in California, thereby repudiating the court's interpretation by changing the constitution. (A federal district court subsequently ruled that Proposition 8 violates the U.S. Constitution [*Perry v. Schwarzenegger*, 2010]; an appeal of that ruling is pending as of the time of this writing.) A similar scenario—a popular vote amending the state constitution in order to overturn a state Supreme Court decision allowing same-sex marriage—took place in Maine in 2009 (Goodnough, 2009). Nationally, the issue of same-sex marriage continues to play out in courts, state legislatures, and public opinion.

PROMOTING NURSING'S POLICY AGENDA

Health care practice and health policy continue to change rapidly in often chaotic and unpredictable ways. Nursing needs to utilize a full range of effective strategies to achieve its policy goals. Nursing organizations—and all nurses who seek to understand and change policy—should be familiar with sources of policy at all levels of government. Successful policy strategies must include being knowledgeable about the role of the courts in health policy and being prepared to respond to and, when possible, seek to influence the outcome of court decisions.

For a list of related websites, please refer to your Evolve Resources at http://evolve.elsevier.com/Mason/policypolitics/

REFERENCES

American Nurses Association California v. Connell, California Superior Court, Case No. 07AS04631. (2008).

Americans with Disabilities Act of 1990, P.L. 101-336, 42 U.S.C. § 12101 et. seq.

Arizona v. Maricopa County Medical Society, 457 U.S. 332 (1982).

Barron, J. (2008). "Restaurants Must Post Calories, Judge Affirms." *New York Times*, April 17, 2008. Retrieved from www.nytimes.com/2008/04/17/nyregion/17calorie.html.

Brown v. Board of Education, 347 U.S. 483 (1954).

California Department of Education (CDE). (2007), "Children with diabetes win assurance of legally required services at school." Retrieved from www.cde.ca.gov/nr/ne/yr07/yr07rel97.asp.

California Nurses Association v. Schwarzenegger et al., California Superior Court for Sacramento, Case No. 04CS01725 (2005).

Churchill, S. (2009). Making employment civil rights real. Amicus (Harvard Civil Rights-Civil Liberties Law Review online supplement). Retrieved from http://harvardcrcl.org/amicus/2009/10/22/employment-civil-rights.

Commonwealth Brands Inc. v. U.S., 2010 U.S. Dist. LEXIS 6316, USDC W.D.Ky (2010).

Egelko, B. (2004). "Judge upholds nurse rules/Hospitals must continue to maintain staffing ratios at all times" *San Francisco Chronicle*, May 27, 2004. Retrieved from http://articles.sfgate.com/2004-05-27/business/17427543_1_california-nurses-association-nursing-shortage-ratios.

Evans, M. (2007). Nurses' wage war. Modern Healthcare, December 17, 2007. Retrieved from www.modernhealthcare.com/article/20071217/REG/71213005.

Goldfarb v. Virginia State Bar, 420 U.S. 905 (1975).

Goodnough, A. (2009). "A Setback in Maine for Gay Marriage, but Medical Marijuana Law Expands." *New York Times*, November 4, 2009. Retrieved from www.nytimes.com/2009/11/05/us/politics/05maine.html.

Greene, J. (2009). "St. John Health agrees to $13.6 million settlement with nurses." *Crains Detroit Business*, March 30, 2009. Retrieved from www.crainsdetroit.com/article/20090330/FREE/903309950.

Greenhouse (2009). "Settlement in nurses' antitrust suit." *New York Times*, March 9, 2009. Retrieved February 9, 2010, from www.nytimes.com/2009/03/10/nyregion/10settle.html?_r=3

In re Marriage Cases (2008). 43 Cal.4th 757.

Keepnews, D. M. (2009). Welcome news in the Sentosa nurses case. *Policy, Politics, & Nursing Practice, 10*(1), 4-5.

Lark v. Montgomery Hospice, 414 Md. 215 (2008).

Ledbetter v. Goodyear Tire & Rubber Co., Inc. 127 S, Ct. 2162, 550 US 618, 167 L. Ed, 2d 982 — Supreme Court (2007).

Marbury v. Madison, 5 U.S. 137 (1803).

Martin, M. (2005). "Governor drops fight with nurses on staffing." *San Francisco Chronicle*, November 12, 2005. Retrieved from http://articles.sfgate.com/2005-11-12/news/17397694_1_nurse-to-patient-california-nurses-association-rose-ann-demoro.

Matter of Vinluan v. Doyle. (2009). 2009 NY Slip Op. 219. New York State Supreme Court, Appellate Division, Second Department (January 13, 2009). Retrieved from www.courts.state.ny.us/courts/ad2/calendar/webcal/decisions/2009/D20723.pdf.

Medicare Conditions of Participation, 42 CFR Chapter IV, Subchapter G (2004).

Miles, J. (2007). The nursing shortage, wage information sharing among competing hospitals, and the antitrust laws: The nurse wages antitrust litigation. *Houston Journal of Health Law & Policy, 7*, 305-378.

NLRB v. Health Care and Retirement Corp, 511 U.S. 571 (1994).

NLRB v. Kentucky River Community Care, 532 U.S. 706 (2001).

Olmstead v. L.C., 527 U.S. 581 (1999).

Parmet, W. (1999). Tobacco, HIV and the courts: The role of affirmative litigation in the formation of health policy. *Houston Law Review, 36*, 1663.

Perry v. Schwarzenegger, 591 F.3d 1147 (2010)

Roe v. Wade, 410 U.S. 113 (1973).

Spine Diagnostics Center of Baton Rouge, Inc. v. Louisiana State Board of Nursing, Louisiana Court of Appeal (First Circuit). No. 2008 CA 0813, December 23, 2008.

Sullivan v. Edward Hospital, 806 NE 645 (Ill. 2004).

Treleven, E. (2006). "'I'd give my life to bring her back'; Nurse gets probation in pregnant teen's death." *Wisconsin State Journal*, p. A1, December 16, 2006.

Want, R. (Ed.). (2009). *Federal-state court directory*. New York: Want Publishing.

Wilk v. American Medical Association, 895 F. 2d 352 (7th Cir. 1990; cert. denied, 498 US 982) (1990).

Wilson, D. (2010). "Judge Lifts Some Tobacco Ad Limits." *New York Times*, January 5, 2010. Retrieved from www.nytimes.com/2010/01/06/business/media/06smoke.html.

Wilson, J. J. (1999). Summary of the Attorneys General Tobacco Settlement Agreement. Retrieved from http://academic.udayton.edu/health/syllabi/tobacco/summary.htm.

CHAPTER 73

The American Voter and the Electoral Process

Karen O'Connor and Jon L. Weakley

"Suffrage is the pivotal right."

—Susan B. Anthony

American democracy requires elected officials in the legislative and executive branch to create public policy. Legislation is created in legislatures and Congress and signed into law by the president or governor. Consequently, it is critical who those legislators and chief executives are because they determine whose interests are represented in the policy arena.

Citizens exercise a key political act when they vote for candidates who support particular policy positions. In the United States, opportunities to vote abound. Elections range from local party officials to those for the U.S. President and members of Congress. Thus, the 3.1 million nurses in the U.S. have significant potential to affect health policy through the ballot as well as having clear policy preferences to articulate to legislators. As the 2009-2010 debates about health care revealed, it is crucial to have elected officials who support the interests of the health care community.

Yet U.S. voter turnout for elections remains low compared to other industrialized nations, perhaps due to the sheer number of elections and lack of clarity of issues in this country. Examining and understanding basic election law, voting behavior, how campaigns work, and how to lobby optimizes the potential for nurses and voters more generally to affect the policy process.

VOTING LAW: GETTING THE VOTERS TO THE POLLS

The Framers of the U.S. Constitution initially granted voting rights to all property-owning, white men. But,

as our notion of equality expanded, so did voting opportunities for additional groups. States are granted the right to establish voter standards unless outlawed by amendment or by U.S. Supreme Court decisions. Over time, the Constitution was amended to grant suffrage first to free men regardless of "race, color … [or] previous condition of servitude," (Fifteenth Amendment, 1870), then women (Nineteenth Amendment, 1920), and, most recently, those age 18 and older (Twenty-Sixth Amendment, 1971). Currently, there are attempts in many states to re-enfranchise the more than 5 million convicted felons who are barred from voting. The U.S. Constitution prohibits poll taxes (Twenty-Fourth Amendment, 1964), which were passed largely by Southern lawmakers with the intent to disenfranchise largely poor African Americans.

Federal legislation has also eliminated literacy tests and property ownership as qualifications to vote. The Voting Rights Act of 1965 was enacted with support from President Lyndon B. Johnson. The Act targeted all of the southern states and others with high concentrations of minority voters—particularly African Americans—whose voter turnout lagged behind their percentage of the voting-age population. Recognizing that voter repression and intimidation was happening, the Act streamlined many state election procedures by introducing national standards (and compliance measures) designed to promote electoral equality. Where necessary, it also authorized the U.S. Attorney General to replace local voting registrars with federal registrars, and procedures to register voters were standardized in specific states. The immediate consequence was to enfranchise large blocks of African-American voters, particularly in the South. It also caused formerly conservative Democrats to join the Republican Party.

Voter registration of minorities and the poor continued to lag behind that of white voters until the early 1990s. Grassroots civil rights and good government organizations around the country pushed for voter registration reform, citing much higher registration and turnout rates in other nations. In many locales, registration was difficult. Prior to passage of the National Voter Registration Act of 1993 (known hereafter as the "Motor Voter law"), modes of registration varied widely from state to state, from the ease at shopping malls and post offices to more difficult access in isolated board of elections offices, removed from public transportation. Behind the push for the Motor Voter law was the argument that increased accessibility of voting registration would increase voter turnout. When President Bill Clinton signed the Motor Voter law, voter registration sites were expanded specifically to include social services and motor vehicle registry offices, hence the appellation. While the Motor Voter law was effective in increasing registration dramatically, its effects on actual turnout were less notable (Brown & Wedecking, 2006).

A CALL FOR REFORM

In 2000, the hotly disputed presidential election between Vice President Al Gore and Texas Governor George W. Bush produced a massive albeit brief public outcry for reforms of voting methods. Across the nation, especially in Florida, voting technology was revealed to be outdated, malfunctioning, or still inaccessible for certain voters, especially African Americans and Hispanic people who repeatedly found their names wrongfully purged from lists of eligible voters. With visions of hanging chads dancing in their heads, members of Congress passed the Help America Vote Act (HAVA) in 2002. It provided federal funding to states and localities to replace old voting technologies. It also mandated that at least one voting device at each precinct be accessible to voters with disabilities. The act also allows voters whose names do not appear on registration lists to vote with provisional ballots, which can later be verified, and if proven legal, counted. This measure allows all citizens who are properly registered to have their votes counted. Although these reforms sought to expand not only the number of Americans registered to vote but also the percentage of those voting, overall turnout increased only moderately after HAVA's passage.

Still, many new technologies sought to streamline the voting process as well as improve its ease and accuracy. The efforts were not without controversy. For example, many voters argued that some digitized ballots that leave no paper trail for verification could be manipulated easily or sabotaged. Steps have been taken to ameliorate these concerns, but the reforms have been gradual and have not yet yielded immediate, tamper-free, accurate results across localities and states (Renner, 2008). Congress has considered a variety of bills to modify current HAVA verification standards, such as requiring all states to have voter-verifiable paper audit trails, but these efforts have failed and have lost their sense of immediacy as the tainted 2000 election faded from memory and was replaced by concerns about the economy, health care, and two wars.

Unless a requirement is specified in the Constitution or by federal law, states have the power to define and change election laws. Despite the Voting Rights Act of 1965, the Motor Voter law, and HAVA, voting laws still vary considerably from state to state. All states allow some sort of early or absentee voting with mail-in ballots if individuals are unable to vote in their designated precincts on Election Day.

Modes of voting are different from jurisdiction to jurisdiction. Oregon residents, for example, vote by mail-in ballot only, making voting booths obsolete. As of 2009, nine states allow same-day voter registration, and several states do not require any voter registration at all. In the 2004 and 2008 general elections, many states opened polling places days or even weeks prior to Election Day in a process called *early voting*; in these states, a significant number of voters opted to vote early. In 2008, early voters who identified as Democrats outnumbered those who identified as Republicans, reversing the earlier trend of Republican dominance in early voting states (Wolf, 2008). HAVA provided a greater range of options and times to register and to vote. Hence, voting is among the simplest ways for nurses to influence public policy since longs shifts on Election Day no longer means that the only opportunity to vote is missed.

VOTING BEHAVIOR

Research on voting behavior seeks primarily to explain two phenomena: voter turnout (that is, what factors contribute to an individual's decision to vote or not to vote) and voter choice (once the decision to vote has been made, what leads voters to choose one candidate over another).

VOTER TURNOUT

Turnout is the proportion of the voting-age public that votes. Those eligible to vote include all citizens of the U.S. who are age 18 or older. States regulate voting eligibility in a number of ways, from preventing felons from voting to having strict single-day, limited voting hours.

Turnout is especially important in American elections because most candidates are elected in winner-take-all systems, where an election's outcome can be influenced by a single voter. (A few states still require candidates to receive 50 + 1% of the vote; without it, runoff elections are necessary.)

In spite of the reforms, the U.S. continues to lag well behind many other constitutional democracies in terms of voter turnout. Many industrialized societies report that upwards of 90% of all eligible voters do so. In contrast, only about 63% of eligible voters went to the polls in the 2008 presidential election. Even though pundits and academics alike were expecting historic turnout in light of then-Senator Barack Obama's (D-IL) voter mobilization efforts and apparent energizing of young voters, only modest gains in overall voter turnout were recorded (Gans, 2008). Turnout is of great concern, especially if non-voting is seen as a sign of political alienation, dissatisfaction with the status quo, anger at negative campaigns, and/or voter cynicism.

Why such low voter turnout rates? According to one 2008 Census Bureau study, 18% of Americans say that school or work conflicts made them too busy to vote. Approximately 15% cite illness or personal emergencies in explaining why they did not vote. Other explanations include apathy, being out of town, not knowing or not liking the candidates, registration problems, or shear forgetfulness. A breakdown of turnout rates by demographic categories reveals dramatically different turnout rates among different groups (Table 73-1). According to the table, turnout was lowest among the Asian/Pacific Islander population and highest among White, Non-Hispanic people. Turnout rates increase with age, and a higher percentage of women than men voted in the 2008 presidential election.

TABLE 73-1 Voter Turnout and Vote Choice by Age, Race/Ethnicity, and Gender, 2008 Presidential Election

	TURNOUT		VOTE CHOICE	
	Number (in Thousands)	Percent Registered	Obama	McCain
Age				
18 to 24 years	12,515	48.5	66	32
25 to 44 years	42,366	60.0	58	40
45 to 64 years	50,743	69.2	50	49
65 years and older	25,520	70.3	45	53
Race/Ethnicity				
White, Non-Hispanic	100,042	66.1	43	55
African American	16,133	64.7	95	4
Asian/Pacific Islander	3357	47.6	61	35
Hispanic	9745	49.9	67	31
Gender				
Man	60,729	61.5	49	48
Woman	70,415	65.7	56	43

Source: U.S. Census Bureau, Retrieved from *www.census.gov/Press-Release/www/releases/archives/voting/013885.html.*

PATTERNS IN VOTER CHOICE

Getting voters to the polls and providing fair and dependable mechanisms is one issue; how people vote is another. Deep divisions exist within the electorate across different social and demographic factors. Understanding the habits of American voters is important as nurses seek allies for their policy agendas.

Factors known to influence voter turnout include political party, religion, race and ethnicity, gender, and age. From the earliest days of our democracy, most political power has been vested in two political parties. Although some third parties are powerful at the local level, no third-party candidate has won a presidential election. Political scientists have long sought to discover why people vote the way they do. Research reveals that several demographic characteristics correlate with voting behavior.

Political Party. Party identification is the most powerful predictor of voting behavior. Quite obviously, self-described Democrats tend to vote for Democratic candidates, and self-described Republicans often vote for Republican candidates. Although intense partisanship has increased over the last electoral cycles, many voters now identify as Independents, in addition to those who register for either party. Voting for candidates from other parties, especially in state presidential primaries where Independents may choose a party at the poll or the state allows voters of either party to vote in the primary of another, can affect electoral outcomes drastically. Independents who make up as much as one-third of the voters in a general election are a focus of partisan candidates trying to sway them to "their" side (O'Connor & Sabato, 2009).

Religion. Since the 1980s, religion has become the second most common predictor of voting. Religious groups also vote in distinct patterns. Fundamentalist or Evangelical Christians are most likely to vote for conservative, Republican candidates and have become a major source of former Governor of Alaska, Sarah Palin's support. Jewish voters are also a politically cohesive group; the vast majority align with Democrats and have done so for decades. In 2008, for example, 77% of all Jewish American voters cast their ballots for Senator Barack Obama in the general election (Haaretz Service and News Agencies, 2008).

Catholics are a somewhat politically cohesive group. For years, they tended to be Democrats. However many support Republican candidates when issues of gay rights or abortion are major issues in an election. The Roman Catholic Church, as much as evangelical churches, often makes voter recommendations largely based on candidates' positions on abortion. The Church hierarchy has threatened high profile legislators such as House Speaker Nancy Pelosi and 2004 Democratic presidential candidate, John Kerry. Rep. Patrick Kennedy (D-RI) even cited pressure from the Church as one of the reasons he chose not to seek reelection in 2010. In 2008, 54% of the Catholic voters chose Barack Obama for President in the general election in spite of his pro-choice views (O'Connor & Sabato, 2009).

Race and Ethnicity. Democrats have long enjoyed the support of the African-American community. Single, African-American women are the most supportive of Democratic Party candidates. In the 2008 presidential election, 95% of African Americans voted for Barack Obama, while only 4% supported John McCain. Typically, African Americans vote at lower rates than white Americans, but in 2008, Obama successfully mobilized young African-American voters to the point that they voted at higher rates than any other group in 18- to 24-year-olds (Edwards, 2009). Turnout of other minority groups also increased in the 2008 presidential election.

While African Americans tend to have consistent voting patterns, other racial groups are less consistent. The 2000 Census revealed that the U.S. Hispanic community is slightly larger in size than the African-American community; thus, Hispanics have the potential to wield enormous political power. In California, Texas, Florida, Illinois, and New York, five key electoral states, Hispanic voters have emerged as powerful allies for candidates seeking office, and, no doubt, were among the major reasons for President Barack Obama's selection of the self proclaimed "wise Latina woman," Judge Sonia Sotomayor, to be his first appointment to the U.S. Supreme Court. Hispanics[1] tend to align with the Democratic Party except for those of Cuban descent, who overwhelmingly vote for Republicans. In 2008, approximately 49% of Hispanic voters cast their ballots for Barack Obama. Asian/ Pacific Islanders are even more heterogeneous than their racial/ethnic counterparts. In 2008, for example, Chinese Americans and American Indians generally supported Senator Barack Obama, while Vietnamese Americans tended to support Senator John McCain's candidacy (NAAS, 2008). Citizens who identify as Asian/Pacific Islanders are diverse in terms of political leanings, so generalizing for this broad minority group can be misleading. As noted above, though, other races and ethnicities have more consistent voting patterns, as Table 73-1 illustrates.

Gender. In general, women are more Democratic than white men. Unmarried women are even more likely to vote for a Democrat than married, white women who face cross demographic pressures. The Democratic Party tends to support more liberal policies of concern to women, such as health care, contraceptive and reproductive rights, and equal pay. Women also are more likely than men to align with the Democratic Party's positions on social welfare and

---

[1]The author acknowledges the controversy over the proper terminology of this group, ranging from *Hispanic* to *Latino* and/ or other terms; the term *Hispanic* is that which is used in the U.S. Census and is thus used in this work.

military issues (Box-Steffensmeier et al., 2004). In every election since 1980, women have supported Democratic candidates, especially at the presidential level, at statistically significant higher rates than men. Furthermore, women are far more likely to support female candidates than are men. Studies on representation suggest that women and minority groups tend to vote for candidates who match their demographic characteristics because they believe that the candidates can understand their life experiences and will thus promote policies that are friendly to them.

Age. Age has long been associated with party identification, as most voters develop their partisan affiliations based on formative political experiences growing up. For example, many voters who were young during the Reagan years identify with the Republican Party. Today, generally the very youngest and very oldest voters tend to prefer the Democratic Party, while middle-aged voters disproportionately favor the Republican Party (O'Connor and Sabato, 2009). The Democratic Party's more liberal positions on social issues tend to resonate with today's moderate but socially progressive adults. The nation's oldest voters, who tend to focus on Social Security and Medicare, tend to favor the Democratic Party's consistent support for these programs and are generally skeptical of privatization plans often supported by Republicans. Middle-aged voters, often at the height of their careers and consequently at the height of their earning potential, tend to favor the low taxes championed by Republicans (Flanigan and Zingale, 2006).

ANSWERING TO THE CONSTITUENCY

Does it make a difference if the members of Congress come from or are members of a particular group? Are they bound to vote the way their constituents expect them to vote even if they favor another policy? Years ago, British political theorist Edmund Burke and members of Parliament posited that the answers to these questions depend on a person's philosophy of representation. It can be argued that a representative is a trustee who listens to the opinions of constituents and then can be trusted to use his or her own best judgment to make final decisions. In contrast, those who believe in delegate representation contend that representatives should vote exactly how their constituents would, regardless of the representatives' own

views. Clearly, these two modes of representation are not exclusive, nor do representatives subscribe to one view entirely. Therefore, a third theory exists: legislators act as politicos, alternately donning the hat of trustees or delegates, depending on the issue or the environment (O'Connor and Sabato, 2009).

Of course, how representatives view their roles does not completely explain whether it makes a difference if a representative is young or old; male or female; African American, Hispanic, or Caucasian; or gay or straight. Can a man, for example, represent interests of women as well as women can?

VOTING DISTRICTS

According to the Constitution, the U.S. Senate is composed of 100 senators—two from each state, and two shadow senators who have non-voting status from the District of Columbia. Representation in the U.S. House of Representatives is based on the population of each of the states. There are 435 seats in the House of Representatives (plus 5 non-voting delegates representing the District of Columbia, the U.S. Virgin Islands, Guam, American Samoa, and the Northern Mariana Islands, and a resident commissioner representing Puerto Rico). The Congress determines the number of seats in the House, and each state is apportioned seats based on a census taken decennially by U.S. constitutional mandate. How those seats are allotted within the states is up to the states and is a process referred to as redistricting. Redistricting involves the state legislators, who want to optimize the majority party's political power. When legislators redraw district lines, they often engage in a practice called gerrymandering—drawing lines most advantageous to their political party. This is called "packing." Or, they may break up the districts of prominent representatives of the opposite party, called "cracking," which weakens the chances of a member of the opposition from winning in the redrawn district.

In the last few decades, northern and Mid-Atlantic states have lost congressional seats to the South and West, particularly California, which has one-seventh of the members of Congress. With growth and contraction has come an additional challenge: meeting the mandates of the Voting Rights Act of 1965, which requires that districts could not be cracked to minimize representation of minorities. Thus, state lawmakers have ended up drawing oddly shaped districts to achieve their goals. While insisting that districts facilitate the election of minorities, the U.S. Supreme Court has ruled that racially gerrymandered districts do not serve a compelling government interest and are thus unconstitutional (O'Connor and Sabato, 2009).

Redistricting is an extremely contentious process that has tremendous potential to affect the outcome of elections and the types of lawmakers elected. Many states hold hearings as new district maps are drawn, providing citizens and groups of citizens—such as nurses—input into a process that is so critical to the outcome of public policy.

INVOLVEMENT IN CAMPAIGNS

CHOOSING "YOUR" CANDIDATE

Political parties and women's groups are important resources for finding candidates. Recruiting candidates requires that they are knowledgeable about the electoral process and can tap into resources of time, money, and volunteers to execute a successful campaign. A new Women's Campaign Forum (WCF) program, She Should Run, allows friends to be formally invited to consider a run for office at all governmental levels.

What traits do interest groups look for in a candidate? What issues are key to support? Researching candidates via the Internet is an effective way to determine which candidate is likely to support issues of concern to nurses and patients. Interest groups provide invaluable information on most national and many state candidates. (See Chapters 74 and 81.)

Tracking who gives money to a particular candidate is an indication of how a candidate might vote. Interest groups may also publish materials such as voting guides or score cards to guide potential voters toward or away from candidates.

The websites of candidates and political parties usually define their policy positions. Consider the questions in Box 73-1 as you make a decision about which candidates to support. Information from reputable media sources can prove helpful. The national and local chapters of the League of Women Voters can be an important resource.

CAMPAIGNING

An opportunity for nurses to get their voices heard is by participating in political campaigns as a group.

BOX 73-1 Questions to Ask When Considering Candidates

1. What kinds of experiences would the candidate bring to office?
2. Are the candidate's political skills and knowledge sufficient and respected by his or her peers?
3. If the candidate is an incumbent (already holding the office and seeking reelection) or held another office previously, what is his or her voting record in terms of nursing or comparable policies?
4. Has the candidate established positions on issues pertaining to health care and nursing policy, and, if so, what are they?
5. What positions of leadership could enable this candidate to be more effective if elected?
6. Is the candidate's campaign well-organized and relatively straightforward in its message?
7. Can the candidate raise money well and keep an organized and transparent budget?
8. Can the candidate actually be elected by the population at large? Is his or her name recognizable by the general public?
9. What does public opinion indicate about the potential of this candidate to be victorious?
10. Who supports this candidate's campaign, both through fund-raising and endorsements?
11. How has the media covered the candidate?
12. Is there any damaging evidence—whether it be a policy stance or personal shortcoming—that would be exploited by opposition or would prevent you or the general public from voting for the candidate?

Adapted from Dato, C. (2006). *The American voter and electoral politics.*

Nurses have participated in political workshops offered by numerous national women's groups, unions, and the American Nurses Association. Nurses have unique skills that enable them to be both consultants on policy as well as organizers, negotiators, and communicators on behalf of candidates they support. Even making small monetary donations or distributing campaign materials can make an impact on the outcome of elections.

Of course, nurses can seek elective office, and they often do. Service on town councils, school or advisory boards, as well as in state legislators and Congress are essential in increasing the visibility of nurses as political actors.

GETTING THE "BEST" CANDIDATE

Women's rights groups have been vital to the political success of nurses, especially since most nurses are women. All three nurses in the House were supported by EMILY's List. EMILY'S List was founded in 1985 to support pro-choice Democratic women candidates. Now one of the largest and most influential political action committees (PACs), it dwarfs all other women's PACs in size of contributions to candidates. It bundles contributions for endorsed candidates and provides candidate training, consultants, and get-out-the-vote efforts to increase the number of women in Congress as well as create more public awareness of important issues and those candidates' stances on issues.

PACs are the fund-raising arm of organizations. While organizations and their PACs can endorse candidates under the initial provisions of the Bipartisan Campaign Reform Act (as it was interpreted in 2008), only PACs could donate a set amount of money to candidates in both primary and general elections. But, in 2010, the U.S. Supreme Court ruled that the provision providing limits on spending was unconstitutional, violating freedom of speech. Thus, there are now no limits on how much organizations can spend to support candidates in national elections. Nurses and others must be aware of these changes when dealing with campaign contributions, since the larger health insurance industry has more money than nurses or physicians to spend on elections.

CAMPAIGN FINANCE LAW

Campaign finance laws were created in the 1970s amid public concerns about transparency in campaign spending. While the original 1971 Federal Election Campaign Act (FECA) was largely ineffective and vague, amendments to FECA in 1974 had more ambitious goals, including the following:

- Contribution limits for individuals, interest groups, and political parties in national elections
- Spending limits for individuals, interest groups, political parties, and candidates in national elections
- Mandatory disclosure of campaign contributions and spending
- Establishment of a non-partisan Federal Election Commission to oversee and enforce campaign laws

PACs were established to channel money to candidates, but since these spending limits were put in place, nearly 4000 PACs have been established (Francia, Joe, & Wilcox, 2008). The stringent spending requirements were loosened after the Supreme Court's ruling in *Buckley* v. *Valeo* in 1976, which found that spending money was a right of free speech. Only if presidential candidates waived their First Amendment rights by accepting public funds, could they be subjected to campaign spending limits. Every presidential candidate who was eligible for public funding accepted it and waived their free speech rights until Barack Obama in 2008. His decision not to accept public financing allowed him unlimited fund-raising power. He was still subject to contribution limits, but he had no limits on how much he could spend, so he was able to raise and spend over $750 million, while John McCain was limited to his public allotment of $84 million.

During the 1990s, the problem of soft money—unreported and unlimited but legal contributions to political organizations but not candidates—illustrated loopholes within FECA, leading to the passage of the Bipartisan Campaign Reform Act of 2002 (also known as the BCRA or the McCain-Feingold Act in honor of its sponsors). This law banned large soft money contributions and enacted limits on campaign advertising, timing, and spending. Since the Supreme Court ruled its spending provisions unconstitutional, the 2010 national elections are the first test with no spending limits.

TYPES OF ELECTIONS

There are three types of elections: primary, general, and presidential.

PRIMARY ELECTIONS

In the primary election, voters decide which candidate will represent the party in the general election. In some states, there are *closed primaries,* meaning only a party's registered voters may cast a ballot to determine the candidate for the general election. In contrast, *open primaries* allow independents and members of other parties to participate. Closed primaries are generally considered healthier for the two-party system because they prevent members of one party from influencing the elections of another party. In some states, if none of the candidates in the primary secures a majority of votes, a runoff primary occurs, where the top two candidates vie in a second contest for at least 50% plus one of the votes.

GENERAL ELECTIONS

Once candidates from the primary election are decided, each state holds its general election. (States often hold elections for state and local office on off- and odd-numbered years.) In general elections, voters decide which candidates from opposite parties will hold elective public office. Many local elections, especially for judges, are non-partisan.

PRESIDENTIAL ELECTIONS: A SPECIAL CASE

In all elections except for the presidential election, people vote directly for the candidate. In the case of presidential elections, voters actually vote for electors instead of the candidates themselves. Electors are representatives from each state who convene at the Electoral College to elect a president. While the Electoral College itself has been a contentious issue recently, the Electoral College remains intact.

THE MORNING AFTER: KEEPING CONNECTED TO POLITICIANS

After a candidate wins the election, it is vital to advance one's interests even if the person who won was not the preferred candidate. Just as their roles in campaigns are crucial, nurses can continue to act as champions of policy and sources of information to influence the politicians while in office. Nurses can join the staff or volunteer for the elected official and be involved with policy issues more directly. In whatever way possible, nurses must develop relationships with policymakers if they expect to influence policy.

For a list of related websites, please refer to your Evolve Resources at http://evolve.elsevier.com/Mason/policypolitics/

REFERENCES

Box-Steffensmeier, J., De Boef, S., & Tse-min, L. (2004). The dynamics of the partisan gender gap. *The American Political Science Review, 98*(3), 515-528.

Brown, R. D., & Wedecking, J. (2006). People who have their tickets but do not use them. *American Politics Research, 34*(4), 479-504.

Edwards, T. (2009, July 20). Voter turnout increases by 5 million in 2008 presidential election, U.S. Census Bureau reports (Press Release). Retrieved from www.census.gov/Press-Release/www/releases/archives/voting/013995.html.

Flanigan, W., & Zingale, N. (2006). *Political behavior of the American electorate* (11th ed.). Washington, D.C.: CQ Press.

Francia, P., Joe, W., & Wilcox, C. (2008). Campaign finance reform—Present and future. In R. J. Semiatin (Ed.), *Campaigns on the cutting edge* (pp. 156-174). Washington, D.C.: CQ Press.

Gans, C. (2008, November 6). *Much-hyped turnout record fails to materialize: Convenience voting fails to boost balloting.* (Press Release). Retrieved from www1.media.american.edu/electionexperts/election_turnout_08.pdf.

Haaretz Service and News Agencies. (2008, November 5). Barack Obama wins 77 percent of the Jewish Vote, exit polls show. Retrieved from www.haaretz.com/news/barack-obama-wins-77-percent-of-jewish-vote-exit-polls-show-1.256651.

NAAS (2008, October 6). *Comprehensive new survey shows Asian Americans could play key role in outcome of presidential election.* (Press Release). Retrieved from www.naasurvey.com/assets/NAAS-DC-pr.pdf.

O'Connor, K., & Sabato, L. (2009). *American government, roots and reform (2009 ed.).* New York: Longman.

Renner, T. (2008). Election administration—Trends in the twenty-first century. In R. J. Semiatin (Ed.), *Campaigns on the cutting edge.* (pp. 175-193). Washington, D.C.: CQ Press.

U.S. Census Bureau. (2008). Current population survey, November 2008. Retrieved from www.census.gov/hhes/www/socdemo/voting/publications/p20/2008/tables.html.

Wolf, R. (2008, October 22). Dems get big boost in early voting; Trend is a reversal of pattern favoring GOP. *USA Today*, p. A1.

CHAPTER 74

TAKING ACTION
Anatomy of a Political Campaign

Greer Glazer and Charles Alexandre

"A campaign is about defining who you are—your vision and your opponent's vision."

—Donna Brazile

Is it hard to imagine why anyone would stand in the rain or snow from 6:00 AM to 6:00 PM on Election Day handing out information about a political candidate. How about someone driving a candidate to eight events in one long 14-hour day covering 250 miles? People work on political campaigns for a variety of reasons, and understanding their motivation is critical to building a strong volunteer program.

WHY PEOPLE WORK ON CAMPAIGNS

People's motivations for working on campaigns fall into four general categories: (1) belief in an issue or a candidate, (2) network building, (3) party loyalty, and (4) personal payback.

BELIEF IN AN ISSUE OR CANDIDATE

Some people work for a candidate because they feel strongly about issues they support and champion or conversely want to defeat the opponent because of where he or she stands on the issues. For example, Democratic presidential candidate Barack Obama preached a message of change that resonated with voters. The 2008 presidential election resulted in higher voter turnout than had been seen in many years (61.7% of eligible voters as compared to 60.1% in 2004 and 54.2% in 2000) (McDonald, n.d.). Obama's message clearly resonated with minority voters with 96% of African Americans and 67% of Hispanics supporting him over John McCain, the Republican candidate. Obama garnered the support

of 70% of unmarried women and 56% of women overall. Obama also beat Senator McCain among voters under age 30 by a margin of 34%. Interestingly, since the election of Jimmy Carter in 1976, no Democrat has had the support of more than 38% of white men until 2008, when Obama took 41% of the white male vote (U.S. News Staff, 2008).

NETWORK BUILDING

Some people are drawn to campaigns to build their own social network. Getting these volunteers involved in social activities will keep them involved in campaign activities.

PARTY LOYALTY

Some people work for the candidate because they are loyal to the political party. Candidates target close races in which they believe an infusion of financial and human resources can change the outcome of the election. Party loyalists will travel to different states to work on campaigns in which they can make a difference in the election. In 2008, nurses traveled to a variety of states to attend rallies and events to support presidential candidates and help their candidate gain visibility to garner press coverage.

PAYBACK

Tangible paybacks include paid work for the campaign, course credit for students, and, if the candidate is elected, appointment to staff, appointment to key commissions or boards or other political appointments, and support for specific legislation. Greer Glazer worked on Ohio Congressman Eric Fingerhut's campaign by coordinating house parties in one city in his district and was appointed to his 19th Congressional District Healthcare Advisory Committee. Intangible benefits may include recognition for the work and a desire to contribute to the democratic process.

Understanding why people work on campaigns enables the campaign to successfully recruit volunteers. However, understanding why people work on campaigns does not necessarily help to retain them. You must also be aware of why people stop working on campaigns.

WHY PEOPLE STOP WORKING ON CAMPAIGNS

The major reason why people stop working on campaigns is that their roles and campaign activities are not aligned with their motivation for working on the campaign. It would not make sense to ask someone who is pro-choice to work on the campaign of a candidate who is anti-choice. Even if the activities match the campaign worker's motivation, people leave campaigns because they lose interest, aren't given enough positive feedback and recognition, don't feel part of the larger whole, lose faith that the candidate can win the election, feel that the work is boring, have competing outside interests such as family and work obligations, and are not enjoying themselves. What are campaign activities that either engage or disengage campaign workers?

THE INTERNET AND THE 2008 ELECTION CAMPAIGN

The Pew Research Center (2004) declared the Internet an essential part of American Politics. Four years later, the 2008 Pew Internet & American Life Project (Pew Research Center, 2009) reported that 55% of the adult population in the United States went online to take part in or get news about the 2008 election campaign (Box 74-1). This marked the first time "more than half the voting-age population used the Internet to connect to the political process during an election cycle" (Pew Research Center, 2009, p. 3).

Edsall (2008) described the growth in the significance of the Internet as causing an upheaval in U.S. politics by "creating (1) innovative ways to reach voters; (2) a radically changed news system; (3) an unprecedented flood of small donors; and (4) newly empowered interest groups on the left and the right." (p. 1). In 2007, for the first time, some presidential candidates began their campaigns by announcing

---

BOX 74-1 Internet Use by Politically Engaged Individuals during the 2008 Presidential Campaign

- 42% of all Internet users went online to learn about a candidate's position on an issue or to check a candidate's voting record.
- 45% of all Internet users watched political videos.
- 17% of all Internet users went online for customized political news (signing up for e-mail alerts or RSS feeds).
- 33% of all Internet users shared campaign information by forwarding political commentary, audio files, videos, or photographs.
- 18% of all Internet users posted questions or comments where others could read them.
- 9% of all Internet users contributed money to candidates online.
- 6% of all Internet users signed up to volunteer for a campaign.
- 26% of all Internet users who voted in 2008 went online for help with voting (to find polling places, get information about early or absentee voting, or check the status of their voter registration).

Adapted from Pew Research Center. (2009). *The Internet's role in Campaign 2008.* Pew Internet and American Life Project.

---

their candidacy on the Internet. Most notably Hillary Clinton stated her intention to run by announcing the formation of a presidential exploratory committee over the Internet using a video in her living room in Chappaqua, New York (Edsall, 2008).

Supporters of both major candidates used the Internet during the 2008 campaign, although supporters of McCain were more likely to use the Internet than Obama supporters (83% vs. 76%). This is not surprising because higher levels of income and education, which describe Republican and non-Republican supporters of McCain, are indicators of Internet use. Overall, supporters of candidate Obama participated in a wider range of online political activities than their Republican counterparts. For example, Obama supporters were more likely to post comments about the campaign online, go online to volunteer for the campaign, and to donate money to the candidate (Pew Research Center, 2009).

Who were the online political users of the 2008 election campaign? Not surprisingly, of all voting age adults using the Internet, young adults under age 30 have the highest level of Internet use, although adults in all age groups are political users of the Internet. For example, 74% of 18- to 24-year-olds were active politically online during the 2008 campaign, as were 71% of 25- to 34-year-olds, 65% of 30- to 49-year-olds, 57% of 50- to 64-year-olds, and 22% of adults age 65 years and older. Demographically (gender, race, and geography), political Internet users are similar in makeup to the adult population as a whole, though the political Internet user tends to have higher levels of income and education than the total U.S. population.

SOCIAL NETWORKING WEBSITES

New phenomena not readily available during the 2004 election campaign but used extensively during the 2008 campaign were social networking websites (e.g., MySpace and Facebook) and video-sharing websites (e.g., YouTube). The Pew Research Center (2008) reported that 27% of adults under age 30, including 37% of those age 18 to 24, reported getting election campaign information from social networking websites. Recognizing the significance of such websites, the Obama campaign hired Facebook co-founder Chris Hughes to help develop the Obama campaign website. Using the social networking site model, the Obama website encouraged visitors to connect with others in their neighborhoods, volunteer for the campaign, make contributions, and keep up with the latest campaign news. The Obama campaign set up accounts on multiple social websites including Facebook, MySpace, MyBatanga, MyGente, AsianAve, and Twitter (Terhune, 2008). Use of these social websites helped Obama gain the edge in the youth vote that helped him clinch the Democratic nomination (Journalism professor discusses use of internet in elections, 2008).

CAMPAIGN ACTIVITIES

Campaign activities can be divided into basic-level campaign activities and advanced-level campaign activities. Basic campaign activities include organizing phone banks and literature drops, office work, poll watching, organizing house parties, driving candidates, fund-raising, serving as a health policy advisor, organizing voter registration, and providing Internet communication about a candidate. Advanced-level campaign activities and roles usually require full-time involvement and include the campaign manager, finance director, political director, operations director, communications director, and new-media or Internet director.

BASIC-LEVEL CAMPAIGN ACTIVITIES

Basic-level campaign activities are easily undertaken by nurses because they are used to working on teams and in groups, have good communication skills, and are well organized. There are some issues that need to be considered before volunteering. First, are you doing this for your personal benefit or for an organization's benefit?

Although there are no limitations on your involvement in a campaign as a private individual, in some cases it may be inappropriate for you to work on a political campaign as a representative of a particular organization. Some organizations are prohibited from engaging in political activity or candidate endorsements based on federal election law and their tax status (see Chapter 80). Political involvement on behalf of that organization may cause problems for the organization as well as the campaign. Be sure that your participation in a campaign is approved by the organization that you represent.

Once you have the green light, don't be shy about making sure the campaign is aware of your affiliation. If you want an organization to get credit for your participation, you need to identify yourself as a representative of that organization. It would be best to have a group of individuals from your organization take responsibility for a specific campaign activity or project. The American Nurses Association organizes Campaign Activity Night (CAN) in the fall of each national election year. During that night, nurses nationwide are asked to work on campaigns. At the state level, nurses in Ohio formed the Ohio Nurses Democratic Caucus, an affiliate of the Ohio Democratic Party, to promote candidates and issues important to them. The caucus has a mission based on informing nurses about health care priorities of the Democratic Party and to inform the Party about issues important to nurses (Ohio Nurses Democratic Caucus, n.d.).

The second issue to consider is how much time you have to volunteer. Campaigns count on their volunteers, and if you sign up to do something, it is important that you follow through. Obviously the more time and involvement you have, the greater will be the payback. For those who have more time, decide whether you want to be involved in many activities or stay focused on one activity. Keep in mind that it is easier to quantify one's contribution and get credit for the work when you can be identified as filling a specific role such as driver, house party coordinator, or heath policy advisor.

The last issue to consider is when to get involved in the campaign. If possible, it is best to get involved early in the campaign. Candidates remember their early supporters. It is easier to carve out your niche when there are fewer people involved in the early stages of the campaign.

TYPES OF CAMPAIGN ACTIVITIES

Phone Banks. Phone banks are frequently used to contact voters for voter identification, to communicate the candidate's message, to determine support or nonsupport of a specific candidate or issue, and to ensure turnout on Election Day. They are also used to recruit volunteers, raise money, and ensure turnout at campaign events. Nurses are usually experienced at phone banking because of their excellent communication skills.

Literature Drops. Volunteers often go door to door to drop off campaign literature. Leafleting is a form of literature distribution that is limited to public places. Literature drops and leafleting are low-impact voter contacts with low cost and little ability to target voters. Other low-impact activities include buttons and bumper stickers, lawn signs, billboards, and human billboards. High-impact voter contact activities include: door-to-door canvassing, house parties, special events, and get-out-the-vote activities.

Door-to-Door Canvassing. Door-to-door canvassing is a traditional type of voter contact in which the volunteer knocks on the door and speaks with the voter. Your goal may be to share the candidate's message or to determine the voting preference of the residents of the house.

House Parties. House parties are given by a volunteer in a targeted area where neighbors, friends, and colleagues are invited to the volunteer's house to meet the candidate. Greer Glazer served as house party coordinator for Lee Fisher during his campaign for Ohio State Senate. When Fisher was elected State Senator, Greer served in an advisory capacity on nursing and health issues. He subsequently ran for

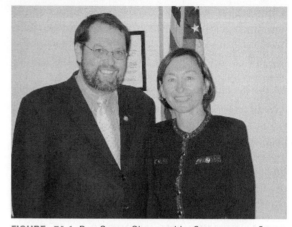

FIGURE 74-1 Dr. Greer Glazer with Congressman Steven LaTourette (R-OH) at the AACN Congressional Reception.

and was elected to the office of Ohio Attorney General. At the time of this writing, Fisher is Ohio Lieutenant Governor and a candidate for the U.S. Senate. The relationship that had been developed by working on all of his campaigns was very helpful when Greer was able to have access to discuss Medicaid payments for advanced practice nurses.

Created Events. Created events are the best way to create the environment for the candidate's message and to target it to a specific group (Figure 74-1). Senator Sherrod Brown of Ohio (D-OH) routinely holds such events. These include meetings with nurses to discuss health care issues, meetings with senior citizens to discuss prescription drug coverage, or town hall meetings to discuss larger policy issues such as social security. Every detail is planned in advance. Nurses participated in a variety of created events during the 2008 presidential campaign. For example, Barack Obama participated in an event sponsored by the Service Employees International Union (SEIU) spending a day with a home health care nurse in California (SEIU, 2007). Later in the campaign, President Obama again spent time with a nurse at Barnes-Jewish Hospital in St. Louis (Rhee, 2008). The campaign used these events to elaborate on the candidate's position and to provide visual images, using the public's trust in nurses, to enhance support for his candidacy.

Timing for media events can be created by the campaign or dictated by opportunities that arise to highlight a candidate's position. Examples of events created by the campaign might include staging a worker rally, holding a press conference in front of a hospital to discuss the need for enhanced medical insurance for children, or interviewing senior citizens about Medicare. For added exposure, clips from rallies or interviews might also be posted as a video on the candidate's website.

Unplanned media opportunities use news events to highlight a candidate's position with regard to a current event. It can provide an opportunity to differentiate the candidate from the opposition candidate or to highlight one's leadership. For example, as the national economy spiraled downward near the end of the 2008 campaign, McCain attempted to make a bold statement by suspending his campaign, flying to Washington, and working with Congress to develop an economic recovery plan. In contrast, Obama continued campaigning, choosing to stay out of Washington to not overshadow the work of Congress. When no recovery plan was forthcoming, McCain's perceived lack of leadership with respect to the economy likely hurt his chances for election. Media coverage of such events creates powerful messages for the public.

Political Action Committees. In addition to candidate media events, supportive organizations and individuals may use their own resources to generate media coverage for a particular issue. Political action committees (PACs) are groups that are organized to engage in political activity, though they are not endorsed by a particular candidate or political party (Law Library, n.d.). PACs may be sponsored by businesses, labor unions, or special-interest groups for the purpose of raising and spending money to support or denounce legislative initiatives. For example, Emily's List *(www.emilyslist.org)* is a PAC that supports pro-choice women running for governor or Congress. The American Nurses Association's (ANA's) political action committee, ANA-PAC, has actively taken out newspaper ads, made radio spots, and purchased political paraphernalia to advocate for nurse-friendly candidates.

Get-out-the-Vote Activities. The candidate can have the most campaign funds, best message, and most efficient operation, but if the campaign is unable to get supporters out to vote on Election Day, the candidate will not win. Phone banks are used to get out the vote. The same messages can be e-mailed to listserves of supporters. Door-to-door canvassing is also effective in getting out the vote. Campaigns have poll workers who track supporters voting and report back to the campaign so that nonvoters can be contacted.

ADVANCED-LEVEL CAMPAIGN ACTIVITIES

The *campaign manager* has overall responsibility for the strategic and technical decisions of the entire campaign and creates the campaign and business plans. The campaign manager sets the tone to motivate staff and volunteers, who work long hours for little or no payment. For example, the 2008 election illustrates that strategic use of the Internet should be an integral part of any campaign. The Internet is most effective when it is integrated into the entire organization. Internet-based tools must focus on bringing interested people together offline ("Joe Rospars Discusses Online Outreach in Political Campaigns," 2009). For example, the Obama campaign provided opportunities on virtually every webpage for supporters to sign up for house parties, local rallies, and other campaign-related activities.

The *finance director* has overall responsibility for campaign finances. This individual manages fundraising and oversees a finance committee and fundraising events, and how the money is spent. This is the person who determines, with the political director and the communications director, how much to spend on media, special events, travel, staff, and so on. The 2004 elections proved that fund-raising via the Internet must be a critical component of the campaign. During the 2004 election, Democrat Howard Dean pioneered the use of Internet-based campaign donations amassing a database of 600,000 supporters. Although he lost the presidential nomination, he changed the playing field by reaching out to average Americans on the Internet and using credit card links to generate huge sums of money from many small donors (Edsall, 2008; Terhune, 2008). By the 2008 election cycle, all candidates used the Internet to enhance fund-raising for their campaigns. No one was more effective than the Obama campaign raising nearly $750 million while establishing a database of 13 million donors (Brooks, 2009).

The *political director* has overall responsibility for campaign strategy to determine how to position the candidate as the person to win. A major responsibility is developing an opposition strategy. In the 2008 election, the Internet not only became an effective medium for fund-raising, but it also provided extensive constituent outreach that resulted in a very large online constituency. The Obama campaign did an outstanding job of recruiting and developing an online constituency by having people register on the campaign's website; sending routine e-mail messages with consistent and compelling messages; creating online polls, surveys, and discussions (blogs); asking those visiting the website to forward messages to friends and relatives (viral marketing); and creating urgency. Importantly, every contact from the Obama campaign included a request for a campaign donation with an active credit card link.

The *communications director* has overall responsibility for the campaign theme. A campaign message is the basis for a successful communication plan. Joe Rospars, former new media director for the Obama 2008 presidential campaign, defined the prerequisite for a successful campaign as "a candidate and a message that resonates with people and a staff of dedicated people that believe in the candidate and the message in order for it to work" (Joe Rospars discusses online outreach in political campaigns, 2009, p. 9). Rospars went on to state that "building of networks among the supporters within the context of your organization and the campaign where people can step up and become owners of the campaign and owners of the organization and recognized the collective power to come together in small groups, and also in a big way, together create change" (p. 10).

Planning the message involves research about the voters: Who are the most and least likely to vote for your candidate, and who are most persuadable? What are the issues that are important to them, and what positions taken by a candidate would influence them to vote or not vote for the candidate? When will the voter likely make a decision about who she or he will vote for? Where do the voters live? Why do they support, do not support, or are undecided about the candidate?

Throughout a campaign, candidates seek as much control as possible over how much they and their opponents are perceived by the media and the electorate. Communications directors carefully craft messages about their candidate as well as about the opponent, often based on research and polling. The goal is to ensure that their campaign defines the candidate and, the greatest extent possible, the opponent on their own terms. In 2008, 24% of Americans reported that they viewed something about the

election campaign in an online video. Among adults under age 30, 41% reported viewing at least one political online video. The rise of YouTube and other similar websites has been both a help and a hindrance to candidates. On the positive side, these websites allow the candidate's campaign to post videos that define the message about an issue. For some candidates, these websites may also work against them (Pew Research Center, 2008). For example, videos of some controversial sermons of Barack Obama's pastor, Jeremiah Wright, became the focal point of the Democratic campaign for a period of time, distracting the candidate from his planned campaign message. In this case, videos posted on the Internet forced the Obama campaign off message, spending valuable time denouncing the content of the sermons rather than defining his campaign message.

Web-base political websites also became important players in the coverage of the 2008 election campaign. Sites like the Huffington Post, Salon, Politico, and the National Review Online have created a culture of immediacy with respect to the political process. No longer do campaign communication directors plan their political events or news conferences around the predictable schedule of the national network news and newspapers. Partisan and non-partisan websites alike are constantly searching for the next new policy statement from a candidate's campaign to be immediately analyzed and criticized on the Internet long before the traditional media are able to respond (Edsall, 2008).

The Internet proved to be an essential communication tool for developing and executing candidates' messages in the 2008 campaign. For the first time, more than half (55%) of the U.S. adult population went online to participate in the electoral process (Pew Research Center, 2009). The new media (Internet) director, having overall responsibility for the development and implementation of all website content for the campaign, became a key figure on the campaign team.

Involvement in political campaigns provides nurses a wonderful opportunity for influencing candidates about health issues, for meeting people, and for bringing a nursing perspective to the political process.

For a list of related websites, please refer to your Evolve Resources at http://evolve.elsevier.com/Mason/policypolitics/

REFERENCES

Brooks, M. A. (2009). *Challenges ahead for new White House Web team.* Retrieved from www.america.gov/st/usg-english/2009/January/20090123153511hmnietsua0.1627008.html.

Edsall. T. B. (2008). *The new media and U.S. politics.* Retrieved from www.america.gov/st/freepress-english/2008/April/20080513173442WrybakcuH0.1571619.html.

Joe Rospars discusses online outreach in political campaigns. (2009). Retrieved from www.america.gov/st/washfile-english/2009/March/20090331113206xjsnommis0.5156214.html.

Journalism professor discusses use of Internet in elections. (2008). Retrieved from www.america.gov/st/washfile-english/2008/November/20081103154651ptellivremos8.393496e-02.html.

Law Library. (n.d.) *Political action committee—Further readings.* Retrieved from http://law.jrank.org/pages/9252/Political-action-Committee.html.

McDonald, M. (n.d.). *United States election project.* Retrieved from http://elections.gmu.edu/voter_turnout.htm.

Ohio Nurses Democratic Caucus. (n.d.). Mission statement. Retrieved from http://ohdemnurses.org/about/mission-statement.

Pew Research Center. (2004). *The Internet and campaign.* Pew Internet and American Life Project. Retrieved from www.pewinternet.org/Reports/2005/The-Internet-and-Campaign-2004.aspx.

Pew Research Center. (2008). *Social networking and online videos take off: Internet's broader role in campaign 2008.* Pew Internet and American Life Project. Retrieved from www.people-press.org/report/384.

Pew Research Center. (2009). *The Internet's role in Campaign 2008.* Pew Internet and American Life Project. Retrieved from www.pewinternet.org/Reports/2009/6-The-Internes-Role-in-Campaign-2008.aspx.

Rhee, F. (2008). *Obama does "work day" with nurse.* Retrieved from www.boston.com/news/politics/politicalintelligence/2008/06/obama_does_work.html.

Service Employees International Union (SEIU). (2007). Barack Obama walks in the shoes of Alameda County homecare worker. Retrieved from www.seiu1021.org/Barack_Obama_Walks_in_the_Shoes_of_Alameda_County_Homecare_Worker.aspx.

Terhune, L. (2008). *Internet revolutionizes campaign fundraising.* Retrieved from www.america.gov/st/elections08-english/2008/July/20080710130812mlenuhret0.6269953.html.

U.S. News Staff. (2008). 5 Voting demographics where Barack Obama made headlines. Retrieved from http://politics.usnews.com/opinion/articles/2008/11/06/5-voting-demographics-where-barack-obama-made-headlines.html.

CHAPTER 75

TAKING ACTION
Nurses for Obama: My Advocacy and Experience on the Campaign Trail

Pamela J. Johnson

"In the face of impossible odds, people who love their country can change it."

—Barack Obama, from his February 10, 2007, presidential announcement

I grew up in Mississippi in the late 1960s and early 1970s during the civil rights and women's rights movements. My interest in advocacy and political activism was born in those volatile and challenging years. I saw my mother's efforts in the civil rights movement, which also influenced me. My mother, Nellie Johnson, went from paying poll taxes to becoming the first female and first African-American election commissioner in Tunica County, Mississippi. When 18-year-olds got the right to vote, no one I knew was more excited than I was. I cast my first vote for President in 1972.

MEETING STATE SENATOR BARACK OBAMA

I attended nursing school at the University of Wisconsin at Milwaukee and eventually moved to Chicago, Illinois, to work as a home health nurse. I first met then–Illinois State Senator Barack Obama in 2000. The Democrats had won a majority vote in the Illinois State Senate, and the Senate president, Emil Jones, Jr., had appointed Mr. Obama as Chair of the Illinois Senate Health and Human Services Committee. At the time, I was serving as chair of the Health Policy Committee of my local National Black Nurses Association chapter. I invited Mr. Obama to address our members at a monthly meeting. At this meeting, I realized I was in the presence of a truly special public servant.

We were impressed with how Senator Obama explained his ideas for improving the health care system in Illinois, his views on the numerous problems that the state was facing as well as how they could be fixed, and his ability to explain complex issues. Later in his career, during the presidential campaign, Barack Obama would be criticized for being "too professorial." But our nursing group appreciated how he educated us. When Mr. Obama left our meeting, he challenged the nurses who had attended to hold him accountable for following through on his promises to work to improve the health care system in Illinois.

Prior to the Democrats gaining control of the Illinois State Senate in 2001, Mr. Obama was one of few Democrats to get legislation passed. He earned my respect by demonstrating excellent negotiating skills, reaching out and involving those who disagreed with him, and having the willingness to compromise with Republicans.

Mr. Obama served three terms in the Illinois Senate from 1997 to 2004. While serving, he was involved with health care and social issues that were important to me. He sponsored, co-sponsored, or supported legislative initiatives including expansion of the State Child Health Insurance Program (S-CHIP), which made Illinois the only state at that time to cover all children from birth to 19 years old; the Hospital Report Card Act, which made it possible for consumers to learn how their hospitals fared on key quality measures; ethics legislation related to campaign finance reform; expansion of the state Earned Income Tax Credit to assist low-income working people; legislation to curb racial profiling during traffic stops; and legislation to overhaul the state's death penalty laws. Mr. Obama co-sponsored the Abandoned Newborn Baby Act which allowed mothers of newborns to bring their unwanted babies to any fire or police station, hospital, or other safe havens without fear of prosecution. The National Black Nurses Association provided input and testimony at the hearings on the health care legislation. I testified before the Senate Judiciary Committee in support of the Abandoned Newborn Baby Act. It was passed by the legislature and signed into law in 2001 by former Governor George Ryan.

MY WORK ON MR. OBAMA'S CAMPAIGN FOR U.S. SENATE

I, and others in Illinois, recognized that Senator Obama had a bright future. I was not surprised when he announced in 2003 that he was going to run for the United States Senate seat being vacated by Peter Fitzgerald. We also recognized that Mr. Obama's U.S. Senate campaign would have to overcome major obstacles. Mr. Obama had little name recognition outside of Illinois, he had no money (senate campaigns cost millions of dollars), he had a funny-sounding name, and he was a liberal who was against the war in Iraq. Early in the Democratic primary, Mr. Obama was not the clear favorite.

FUNDRAISING FOR THE SENATE CAMPAIGN

To help raise the critical "early money" for Mr. Obama's Senate campaign, I turned to my personal address book. I called every single person in the book whose phone number was current—even those who I had not seen or heard from in years! I worked to convince my friends, colleagues, and family members to support Mr. Obama in the Senate race and to work for his election victory (Figure 75-1). Fortunately, I have a large network of family and friends across the country who I viewed as potential supporters. I went through my file of business cards and contacted many people, including members of professional organizations such as the Cook County Physicians Association, the Chicago Medical Society, and the Cook County Bar Association. I networked with fellow church members and members of the Chicago

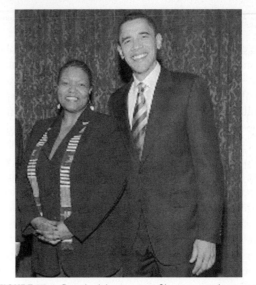

FIGURE 75-1 Pamela Johnson at an Obama campaign event.

Chapter of the National Black Nurses Association. Basically, anyone I had met in my entire adult life got to listen to my Obama-for-Senate pitch. My friends and colleagues from outside of Illinois were not exempt. I encouraged them to support Mr. Obama because he had the potential to become only the fifth African American to serve in the U.S. Senate. I held an "Obama for Senate" fund-raiser at my home early in the campaign. Family members, friends, professional colleagues, and members of the Chicago Chapter of the National Black Nurses Association attended. Many attendees had never contributed to a political campaign before. We were able to speak briefly with candidate Obama and hear his views on the issues before he was whisked off to the next campaign event. This event in my home raised several thousand dollars of seed money and helped me reach the fund-raising goal of $3000 that I had pledged to meet. I asked people who could not attend to send contributions so I could submit them to the campaign treasurer. By doing this, I felt that there was a greater chance people would follow through on their pledges to provide contributions and that I would be able to document the total amount of contributions I was acquiring. About 20 to 30 people attended these events.

CANDIDATE'S FORUMS

As chair of the Chicago Chapter of the National Black Nurses Association's Health Policy Committee, one of my responsibilities was to inform members about health and social issues legislation at the local, state, and national levels. We held the forums only during the primaries because in the most solidly "blue" (or Democratic) city in one of the most solidly "blue" states, it was a given that whomever won the Democratic primary would win the general election. To ensure a successful forum, we sent out letters of invitation and contacted other professional organizations and solicited them to be co-sponsors. We were so excited the day of the forum to have Barack Obama and the other candidates discuss their views on the issues and take questions from the audience.

VOLUNTEERING FOR THE CAMPAIGN

I volunteered for the Obama Senate campaign by working on phone-banks, sending out letters and flyers, attending rallies (and getting fired up with other supporters!), doing door-to-door canvassing, and talking with many people about why I supported Mr. Obama. On March 16, 2004, Barack Obama won the Illinois Senate primary, winning nearly 53% of the vote. We celebrated that night, but we knew we had a general election to win in November. So the next morning, it was back to work.

MR. OBAMA'S DEMOCRATIC NATIONAL CONVENTION SPEECH—A TURNING POINT

On July 27, 2004, Barack Obama delivered the keynote address at the Democratic National Convention and gained national attention. I was riveted to my television as Mr. Obama delivered the address. I cried, cheered, high-fived, and, finally, silently reflected as he stated, "We are not red states or blue states, but we were the United States of America," and discussed his book, *The Audacity of Hope*. I was inspired by what I felt was the speech of a great leader. When I got to work the next day, Senator Obama's speech was the topic of many conversations, and I first heard talk that he should run for president.

When Mr. Obama won the seat in the U.S. Senate in November 2004, he beat his Republican opponent, Alan Keyes, by 76%. Volunteering for Obama in the general election campaign was fun and challenging, and it allowed me to use many of the nursing skills I acquired over the years, including organizational skills, written and oral communication skills, and research and problem-solving skills. Seeing Senator-elect Barack Obama, his wife Michelle, and their daughters on stage at the victory party at the Chicago Hyatt Hotel made all the hard work worthwhile. As he thanked his supporters and outlined his plans for his Senate tenure, I could not help but think, "He's not going to stop at the U.S. Senate."

"YES WE CAN"

On a cold day in February 2007, Senator Obama announced that he was going to run for the presidency. I knew this would be difficult. I thought Hillary Clinton would be a formidable opponent, and I had concerns about racial attitudes in America. In my final analysis, I put aside my doubts and fears and fell back to a position that makes all the difference in Chicago politics: loyalty. When Senator Obama formed his presidential exploratory committee, I was among the early supporters and used my contacts from the last race to raise funds. I traveled as a campaign volunteer to Indiana, Wisconsin, and Pennsylvania. Senator Obama ran a disciplined, highly organized, honorable campaign for which I was proud to have been a volunteer. We were rewarded for our hard work with a victory on an unseasonably warm November 4, 2008, night that President-elect Obama called "our time, our moment." He was speaking to us, the new generation of leaders and activists, at Grant Park in Chicago. We were ecstatic that he was now the president-elect and would be inaugurated in January 2009 as the 44th President of the U.S.

A CHALLENGE FOR NURSES—YES WE CAN

Dr. Martin Luther King, Jr. said, "Everybody can be great, because everybody can serve." As the largest group of health care professionals and the group consistently rated as one of the most trusted by Americans, nurses have a tremendous opportunity as well as an obligation to "get off the bench and get in the game" (to use a sports metaphor). Politics affects all that we do, and there are ways for everyone to be involved. We can make a difference. Are you going to make a difference or remain on the bench and complain when your team loses?

For a list of related websites, please refer to your Evolve Resources at http://evolve.elsevier.com/Mason/policypolitics/

CHAPTER 76

Is There a Nurse in the House? The Nurses in the United States Congress

Mary W. Chaffee

"I have seen in the Halls of Congress more idealism, more humanness, more compassion, more profiles of courage than in any other institution that I have ever known."

—Hubert H. Humphrey

The U.S. Congress is a democratically-chosen body elected at regular intervals to represent the interest of each state's citizens. The Congress consists of 535 members—435 in the House of Representatives and 100 in the Senate. The 111th Congress of the United States, elected in November 2008, included 2 state troopers, a retired U.S. Navy vice admiral, 4 ministers, 3 organic farmers, an FBI agent, a television reporter, 16 physicians, an astronaut, 2 bank tellers, 38 mayors, a waitress, a meat cutter, a former first lady of the U.S. and 2 former state first ladies, a riverboat captain, a volunteer fireman, an auctioneer, an NFL football player, a mountain guide…and 3 nurses (Congressional Research Service, 2008). The first U.S. Congress met in 1789. In 1992, 203 years later, Eddie Bernice Johnson became the first nurse elected to serve in the U.S. Congress. Johnson (D-TX-30) has been joined by Lois Capps (D-CA-23) and Carolyn McCarthy (D-NY-4). Four more nurses were elected in the 2010 midterm election and will serve in the 112th Congress. The new nurse-members are Renee Ellmers (R-NC), a former critical care nurse; Diane Black (R-TN), a former emergency nurse; Ann Marie Buerkle (R-NY), a former school nurse; and Karen Bass (D-CA), a former nurse and physician assistant.

Though elected to represent their constituents, Congress as a whole does not always reflect the population characteristics of the nation (Heineman, Peterson, & Rasmussen, 1995). For example, 51% of the 2000 U.S. population was female (U.S. Census Bureau, 2005). However, only 17.7% of the 111th Congress was female (Congressional Research Service, 2008).

THE NURSES IN CONGRESS

The three nurses who served in the 111th Congress arrived at their positions through extremely different paths. One replaced a spouse who died while serving in Congress, another ran for office after the incumbent refused to take a stand on gun control following an act of gun violence that killed her husband, and the third ran for Congress after serving in her statehouse. Though their backgrounds are different, their records demonstrate consistent commitment to improving health and social policy. All serve in the House of Representatives; no nurse has yet served in the Senate. Table 76-1 describes the three nurses who served in the 111th Congress.

THE HONORABLE EDDIE BERNICE JOHNSON

Congresswoman Eddie Bernice Johnson's political career began with the urging of friends after she had worked as a nurse for 15 years. She campaigned for, and won, a seat in the Texas House of Representatives. President Jimmy Carter appointed her to serve as the Department of Health, Education and Welfare Regional Director in 1977. Following elected service in the Texas State Senate, she was elected to the U.S. House of Representatives in 1992 (Johnson, 2007).

TABLE 76-1 About the Nurses in the 111th U.S. Congress*

	Congresswoman Eddie Bernice Johnson	Congresswoman Carolyn McCarthy	Congresswoman Lois Capps
Represents	Texas' 30th (Dallas County/City)	New York's 4th (Long Island)	California's 23rd (Southern California)
Education	• BS Nursing, Texas Christian University • MS Public Administration, Southern Methodist University	• LPN, Glen Cove (NY) Nursing School	• BS Nursing, Pacific Lutheran University • MA Religion, Yale University • MA Education, University of California, Santa Barbara
Nursing experience	• Dallas Veteran's Administration Hospital	• 30 years as an ICU and home health nurse	• Director, Santa Barbara County Teenage Pregnancy and Parenting Project • Instructor, Early Childhood Education, Santa Barbara City College • Nurse Manager, Yale New Haven Hospital
Elected to Congress	1992	1996	1998
Number of terms served	9	7	6
Congressional Committee assignments	Committee on Science and Technology • Subcommittee on Energy and Environment • Subcommittee on Research and Science Education Committee on Transportation and Infrastructure • Subcommittee on Aviation • Subcommittee on Railroads, Pipelines, and Hazardous Materials • Subcommittee on Water Resources and Environment (Chairwoman)	Committee on Education and Labor • Subcommittee on Healthy Families and Communities (Chairwoman) • Subcommittee on Health, Employment, Labor, and Pensions Committee on Financial Services • Subcommittee on Capital Markets, Insurance, and Government Sponsored Enterprises • Subcommittee on Financial Institutions and Consumer Credit	Committee on Energy and Commerce • Subcommittee on Energy and Environment • Subcommittee on Health (Vice Chair) Committee on Natural Resources • Subcommittee on Insular Affairs, Oceans and Wildlife • Subcommittee on National Parks, Forests, and Public Lands

*Four more nurses were elected to serve in the 112th Congress.

A lifetime member of the National Black Nurses Association, Johnson has been recognized by a number of organizations for her efforts in the areas of health care, science, and transportation (Figure 76-1). She serves now as a Senior Democratic Deputy Whip, Chair of the Texas Democratic Delegation, and Chair of the Congressional Black Caucus in the 107th Congress. Johnson has advocated for reauthorization of the Children's Health Insurance Program and support for family members of patients with Alzheimer's disease, and she introduced legislation that would help unemployed manufacturing workers be retrained for the health care workforce (About Eddie Bernice Johnson, 2009). Johnson has worked with The Century Council, a not-for-profit group funded by the distilling industry, to caution teens about the dangers of underage drinking, and driving while intoxicated (Harakal, 2009). In 2008, she was honored by the Society of Women Engineers with their first-ever President's Award for her work in promoting diversity and inclusion as a legislator and as co-chair of the House Diversity and Innovation caucus (Society of Women Engineers, 2009).

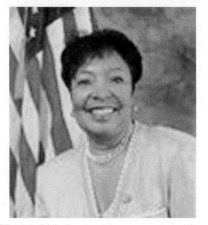

FIGURE 76-1 Eddie Bernice Johnson, member of Congress.

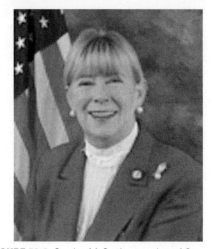

FIGURE 76-2 Carolyn McCarthy, member of Congress.

THE HONORABLE CAROLYN MCCARTHY

Carolyn McCarthy's story demonstrates how life can turn on a dime. In 1996, she was a New York wife, mother, and nurse. Shortly after, her life story was made into a television movie, she appeared on Oprah, and she addressed the Democratic National Convention (McCarthy, 2007). McCarthy's life changed course on December 7, 1996, when her husband Dennis and son Kevin were shot by a gunman aboard the Long Island Railroad. Her husband died, and her son faced a difficult recovery from his wounds. When shortly after the shootings her congressman, Representative Daniel Frisa, voted to repeal the assault weapons ban, her anger led to her run against him (McCarthy, 2007). *The New York Times* called her "The Long Island Everywoman, forced into the limelight by a flash of violence, who reluctantly capitalized on her own celebrity to take on and defeat one of the most daunting political machines in the nation" (Barry, 1996).

Though recognized for her legislative efforts focused on gun violence, Congresswoman McCarthy is not a one-trick pony (Figure 76-2). *The New York Times* endorsed her reelection in 2004 noting, "If Carolyn McCarthy were only a one-issue representative, it would still be difficult to discount the amazing influence she has had in her four terms in the fight for gun control. But Ms. McCarthy, who became a Democrat and won the congressional seat after her husband was killed and her son wounded by a gunman on a commuter train, has taken on much more. A novice when she first entered the world of politics, Ms. McCarthy has grown into a strong and forceful representative for the region and an important voice on issues like health care and education" (*The New York Times*, 2004).

Much of her legislative focus has remained on controlling gun violence, and she has found some success. In 2008, President George W. Bush signed into law McCarthy's bill, the National Instant Criminal Background Check System (NICS) Improvement Amendments Act. The bill provides grants to states to upgrade information and identification technologies for firearms eligibility. She has supported efforts to reform the U.S. health system and joined President Obama for a White House summit on health reform in July 2009 (Congresswoman Carolyn McCarthy Biography, 2009). She played a significant role in developing legislative solutions to the nursing shortage, including as co-sponsor of the Nurse Reinvestment Act signed into law in 2002 (GovTrack. US, 2009).

THE HONORABLE LOIS CAPPS

After practicing nursing for 30 years, Lois Capps accompanied her husband, Walter Capps, from California to Washington D.C. when he was elected

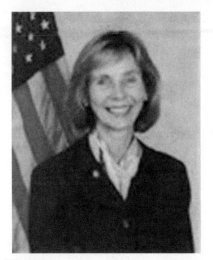

FIGURE 76-3 Lois Capps, member of Congress.

as a member of Congress in 1996. Nine months later he died following a heart attack, and Capps was approached about filling his seat. Though she questioned what she could offer to the community, Ms. Capps agreed. Congresswoman Capps reports that many of her legislative priorities are derived from her experience as a nurse (Capps, 2007).

Congresswoman Capps has encouraged other nurses to consider running for elective office and points out that she was 60 years old when she was first elected to Congress (Figure 76-3). Capps believes that nurses' voices should be heard in the policymaking process (Capps, 2007).

EVALUATING THE WORK OF THE NURSES SERVING IN CONGRESS

Many individuals and groups offer opinions on the performance of members of Congress. Overall approval ratings are calculated by numerous organizations. PollingReport.com compiles approval ratings from many of them (PollingReport.com, 2009). These, of course, offer only aggregated views of how Congress as a whole is doing—not how individual members are viewed. Citizens offer qualitative evaluations of individual members by speaking out, blogging, protesting, and bestowing awards. One measure of the individual member is his or her reelection success. None of the three nurses in the 111th

Congress was beaten in a reelection bid. Altogether, they have been reelected 19 times.

POWER RANKINGS

Roll Call, a Capitol Hill newspaper, analyzes the relative power of each member of Congress. The assessments of power are based on a member's ability to acquire earmarks, positional power (committee assignments), legislative activity, and indirect influence. In 2009, McCarthy was rated the 62nd most powerful member in the House of Representatives, Capps was ranked 65th, and Johnson was ranked 264th (*Roll Call,* 2009).

POLITICAL PERSPECTIVE

National Journal ranks lawmakers on how they vote relative to each other on a conservative-to-liberal scale. The ratings are based on votes in three areas: economic issues, social issues, and foreign policy (*National Journal,* 2009). Table 76-2 demonstrates the most recent *National Journal's* ratings of the three nurses in Congress.

PolitiFact.com, a Pulitzer Prize–winning organization, evaluates the veracity of lawmakers on its "Truth-o-Meter" (PolitiFact.com, 2009). A search of PolitiFact did not uncover any findings regarding statements by the nurses in Congress.

INTEREST GROUP RATINGS

Some interest groups grade, rate, or rank members of Congress on issues of interest to the group. For example, the Cato Institute, a supporter of free markets, evaluates the support that members of Congress provide for open trade. Their searchable online database permits users to examine the level of support that members of Congress have provided for free trade (Cato Institute, 2009). The National Rifle Association grades members on their support for the 2nd Amendment (the right to bear arms). Their grades are available on their "Political Victory Fund" website—but the information is available to members only (National Rifle Association, 2009). One would expect that McCarthy's grade is less than an A.

CAMPAIGN FINANCING

The Center for Responsive Politics, formed in 1982, is a non-partisan watchdog group whose mission is to

TABLE 76-2 National Journal's Ratings of the Nurses in the 111th U.S. Congress (2007)

	LIBERAL RATINGS			CONSERVATIVE RATINGS			COMPOSITE SCORE Liberal	COMPOSITE SCORE Conservative
	E	S	F	E	S	F		
Eddie Bernice Johnson	60	92	77	40	0	23	77.7	22.3
Carolyn McCarthy	67	77	78	31	23	22	74.3	25.7
Lois Capps	82	92	94	0	0	4	94	6

How to read these ratings: A score of 82 on economic issues, for example, means that the representative was more liberal than 82% of her House colleagues on key economic votes in 2007. The designations E, S, and F refer to the "economic" and "social" and "foreign" policy votes used to determine overall ratings (*National Journal*, 2009).

TABLE 76-3 Nurses in the 111th Congress: 2008 Election Cycle Fund-Raising

	Congresswoman Eddie Bernice Johnson	Congresswoman Carolyn McCarthy	Congresswoman Lois Capps
Raised	$527,856	$1,336,619	$1,054,974
Spent	$459,462	$1,520,492	$957,695
Debt	$83,395	$0	$0

Source: Center for Responsive Politics (*www.OpenSecrets.org*).

TABLE 76-4 Contributions to Nurses in the 111th Congress by Geography

	Congresswoman Eddie Bernice Johnson	Congresswoman Carolyn McCarthy	Congresswoman Lois Capps
In-state	$146,265 (80%)	$228,561 (64%)	$363,559 (92%)
Out of state	$36,946 (20%)	$127,070 (36%)	$33,250 (8%)
No state	$0	$0	$0

Source: Center for Responsive Politics (*www.OpenSecrets.org*).

"inform, empower, and advocate" (Center for Responsive Politics, 2009). The organization is an independent non-profit that manages an extensive online database that tracks money in politics. The group's website, *www.OpenSecrets.org*, provides access to extensive data about politicians: where their contributions come from and how they spend money. Table 76-3 demonstrates overall fund-raising and expenditures of each nurse in Congress during the 2008 congressional election cycle. McCarthy had the largest campaign war chest of the three nurses and acquired over one-third of her contributions from outside her state (Table 76-4). Capps, in comparison, received only 8% of her campaign funds from outside of California, her home state.

SOURCES OF CAMPAIGN FUNDS

The Center for Responsive Politics (2009) reports that Lois Capps manages to beat opponents, even when they outspend her. The bulk of her funds come from constituents in Santa Barbara, California, and she has great support from the nursing community. Nurses have donated more to her than any other member of Congress except former Senator Hillary Clinton. Health professionals are her second largest industry donors (Table 76-5). McCarthy and Capps receive significant support from the health professions, and all three are well-supported by lawyers and law firms.

Johnson received nearly two-thirds of her 2008 campaign funds from PACs, while McCarthy and

TABLE 76-5 Top 5 Contributors to Nurses in the 111th Congress (2008 Election Cycle)

	Congresswoman Eddie Bernice Johnson	Congresswoman Carolyn McCarthy	Congresswoman Lois Capps
Top 5 contributors	American Association for Justice ($10,000)	PMA Group ($23,000)	American Association for Justice ($10,000)
	Credit Union National Association ($10,000)	Plumbers and Pipefitters ($12,000)	American Bankers Association ($10,000)
	International Brotherhood of Electrical Workers ($10,000)	Air Line Pilots Association ($10,000)	American College of Radiology ($10,000)
	Laborers Union ($10,000)	American Association of Oral and Maxillofacial Surgeons ($10,000)	American Nurses Association ($10,000)
	National Association of Realtors ($10,000)	American Bankers Association ($10,000)	International Brotherhood of Electrical Workers ($10,000)
Top 5 industry contributors	Transportation unions ($44,500)	Health professions ($110,310)	Health professions ($164,350)
	Real estate ($38,500)	Securities/investments ($61,400)	Retired ($78,550)
	Lawyers/law firms ($38,250)	Retired ($50,550)	Democratic/liberal ($48,150)
	Railroads ($33,200)	Lawyers/law firms ($47,450)	TV/movie/music ($38,550)
	Construction ($32,300)	Builders Trade unions ($44,500)	Lawyers/law firms ($34,960)

Source: Center for Responsive Politics (www.OpenSecrets.org).

TABLE 76-6 Nurses in the 111th Congress: Sources of Campaign Funds (2008)

	Congresswoman Eddie Bernice Johnson	Congresswoman Carolyn McCarthy	Congresswoman Lois Capps
Individual contributions	$194,660 (37%)	$798,640 (60%)	$559,982 (53%)
PAC contributions	$333,196 (63%)	$524,571 (39%)	$489,139 (46%)
Candidate self-financing	0	0	$0
Other	0	$13,408 (1%)	$5853 (1%)

Source: Center for Responsive Politics (www.OpenSecrets.org).

Capps received the majority of their funds from individuals (Table 76-6).

Compared with their colleagues in the House, the nurses in Congress sponsored and co-sponsored significantly more bills than their average colleagues in the 110th Congress. Johnson sponsored 57 bills, earning her a ranking of 21st out of 451; McCarthy sponsored 62 bills, ranking her 14th out of 451; and Capps sponsored 26 bills, ranking her 147th out of 451 (Table 76-7).

EARMARKS

Earmarks are funds provided by Congress that are awarded for a specific project or program, usually in a Member's home district or state. In 2008, McCarthy sponsored or co-sponsored the most earmarks of the three nurses (28 earmarks valued at

$31,342,214), earning her a ranking of 185th among her peers. Capps sponsored the fewest earmarks of the nurses and earned a ranking of 321st among her peers (Table 76-8).

The effectiveness of members of Congress, including the three nurses who serve their constituents there, cannot be determined with only one measure. A full analysis may cause the reader to recall the old story of three sightless men touching different parts of an elephant and describing the animal. Each measure adds something to the analysis—and many measures are focused only on what is of use to the analyst.

For a list of related websites, please refer to your Evolve Resources at http://evolve.elsevier.com/Mason/policypolitics/

TABLE 76-7 Nurses in Congress: Legislative Activity in the 110th Congress

	Congresswoman Eddie Bernice Johnson	Congresswoman Carolyn McCarthy	Congresswoman Lois Capps
Number of bills sponsored	57	62	26
Ranking among 451 members	21st	14th	147th
Number of bills co-sponsored	300	200	100
Ranking among 451 members	48th	109th	236th

Source: Center for Responsive Politics (www.OpenSecrets.org).

TABLE 76-8 Nurses in the 111th Congress: Earmark Activity (Fiscal Year 2008)

	Congresswoman Eddie Bernice Johnson	Congresswoman Carolyn McCarthy	Congresswoman Lois Capps
Number of earmarks sponsored or co-sponsored	11	28	19
Value of earmarks	$17,266,500	$31,342,214	$11,618,000
Ranking (of 451 members)	254th	185th	321st

Source: Center for Responsive Politics (www.OpenSecrets.org).

REFERENCES

About Eddie Bernice Johnson. (2009). Congresswoman Eddie Bernice Johnson website. Retrieved from http://ebjohnson.house.gov.

Barry, D. (1996, November 7). L.I. widow's story: Next stop, Washington. *The New York Times.* Retrieved from www.nytimes.com/1996/11/07/us/li-widow-s-story-next-stop-washington.html?scp=72&sq=.

Capps, L. (2007). A Nurse in Congress. In D. Mason, J. Leavitt, & M. Chaffee (Eds.), *Policy and Politics in Nursing and Health Care* (5th ed., pp. 723-725). St. Louis: Elsevier.

Cato Institute. (2009). Free trade, free markets: Rating Congress. Retrieved from www.freetrade.org/congress.

Center for Responsive Politics. (2009). About us. Retrieved from www.opensecrets.org/about/index.php.

Congressional Research Service. (2008). Membership of the 111th Congress: A profile. Retrieved from www.senate.gov/CRSReports/crs-publish.cfm?pid=%260BL)PL%3B%3D%0A.

Congresswoman Carolyn McCarthy biography. (2009). Retrieved from http://carolynmccarthy.house.gov/index.cfm?sectionid=223&sectiontree=4,223.

GovTrack.US. (2009). H.R. 3487: The Nurse Reinvestment Act. Retrieved from www.govtrack.us/congress/bill.xpd?bill=h107-3487.

Harakal, M. (2009). Congresswoman Eddie Bernice Johnson (TX-30) welcomes Brandon Silveria to encourage teens to make the right choice during prom and graduation season. Retrieved from www.centurycouncil.org.

Heineman, R., Peterson, S., & Rasmussen, T. (1995). *American government.* (2nd ed.). New York: McGraw-Hill.

Johnson, E. (2007). My path to Congress. In D. Mason, J. Leavitt, & M. Chaffee (Eds.), *Policy and politics in nursing and health care* (5th ed., pp. 729-730). St. Louis: Elsevier.

McCarthy, C. (2007). I believed I could make a difference. In D. Mason, J. Leavitt, & M. Chaffee (Eds.), *Policy and politics in nursing and health care* (5th ed., pp. 726-728). St. Louis: Elsevier.

National Journal. (2009). National Journal's 2007 vote ratings. Retrieved from www.nationaljournal.com/voteratings.

National Rifle Association. (2009). Political victory fund candidate grades and endorsements. Retrieved from www.nrapvf.org/Elections/Default.aspx.

The New York Times. (2004, October 24). For Congress on Long Island. *New York Times.*

PolitiFact.com. (2009). The Truth-o-meter: Separating fact from fiction. Retrieved from www.politifact.com/truth-o-meter.

PollingReport.com. (2009). Congress job rating. Retrieved from www.pollingreport.com/CongJob.htm.

Roll Call. (2009). Power rankings. Retrieved from www.congress.org/congressorg/power_rankings/overall.tt#house.

Society of Women Engineers. (2009). *The Society of Women Engineers honors Congresswoman Johnson with President's Award.* Retrieved from http://societyofwomenengineers.swe.org.

U.S. Census Bureau. (2005). We the people: Women and men in the United States. Retrieved from www.census.gov/prod/2005pubs/censr-20.pdf.

CHAPTER 77

TAKING ACTION
Nurse, Educator, and Legislator: My Journey to the Delaware General Assembly

Bethany Hall-Long

"I have come to the conclusion that politics are too serious a matter to be left to the politicians."
—General Charles de Gaulle

MY POLITICAL ROOTS

I am a nurse, and I became the first health care professional elected into the Delaware General Assembly as well as the first Registered Nurse elected. The roots of my public service began in a farming community where I volunteered to help others in my church and with neighborhood organizations. At the age of 12, I was a candy-striper in a local hospital and continued my civic work during my teen years. When I entered college, I joined a political party. Though my parents were not politically active, my great-grandfather was a member of the Delaware House of Representatives in the 1920s, and I am a descendent of Delaware's 16th governor.

My interest in politics began while working with underserved residents while completing my master's degree in community health nursing in the late 1980s. I used an earlier edition of this book in my graduate program and vividly recall reading the chapters about becoming involved in politics. I began working with my local city government, the League of Women Voters, and a federal health clinic that served the homeless. Before these experiences, I had thought that public policy was "remote" to nursing and somewhat "dry." These experiences changed my perspective.

VOLUNTEERING AND CAMPAIGNING

I went on to volunteer with nonprofit and civic organizations, join professional associations, and complete my doctoral degree in nursing administration and public policy. During this time, I served as a United States Senate Fellow and as a U.S. Department of Health and Human Services policy analyst for the Secretary's Commission on Nursing. These experiences exposed me to national policy work, federal officials, leaders in the nation's health associations, and international researchers. I became actively involved with veteran's organizations since my husband was active duty military. I also became a volunteer on political campaigns and with the Democratic Party. I had excellent mentors to assist me with both my nursing and my political career paths. All of these experiences helped me understand the policy process and the importance of building relationships.

I began my work in politics to make a difference in the lives of many citizens who lack life's necessary resources. As a public health nurse, I had an interest in improving the services available to vulnerable populations. I continue to work to advance issues important to the residents I represent. These include health care, the environment, land preservation, education, and economic development.

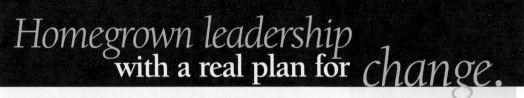

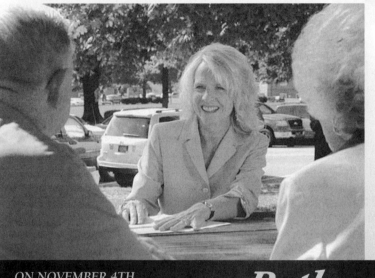

Homegrown leadership **with a real plan for** *change.*

Born and raised on a Delaware farm, Bethany Hall-Long's roots run deep in our state. As a nurse, a UD professor and a mother, Bethany understands the challenges facing Delaware's families. As our next State Senator, Bethany has a plan to improve the lives of Delaware's citizens – and the experience with proven results to make it happen.

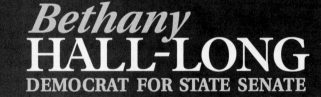

ON NOVEMBER 4TH, give Delaware's families a strong voice in the State Senate.

www.hall-longforsenate.com

Bethany **HALL-LONG**
DEMOCRAT FOR STATE SENATE

Paid for by the Committee to Re-Elect Bethany Hall-Long

FIGURE 77-1 Dr. Hall-Long's campaign literature identifies her as a nurse and educator.

THERE'S A REASON IT'S CALLED "RUNNING" FOR OFFICE

A number of factors influenced my decision to run for public office in 2000, including my desire to make a significant contribution to the public's health. As a university faculty member, I assigned students to various public health and health policy assignments. In these experiences, I witnessed the need for expert health knowledge in the Delaware General Assembly. The time was ripe within the political party and within my district to run for the Delaware legislature. I ran for office for the first time in 2000 and lost by a mere 1%. I had run against a long-term, male incumbent and learned some important political lessons. In 2002, political redistricting left a vacant seat and I ran again. This time, I won in a tough election against the president of the local school board. After serving 6 years in the House, I campaigned for, and won, a State Senate race in 2008 (Figure 77-1).

A DAY IN THE LIFE OF A NURSE-LEGISLATOR

No two days in politics are alike. Each elected official's experiences and perceptions are linked to his or her beliefs, the district's beliefs, the state's legislative rules, and any external economic or social pressures. In

Delaware, serving as a legislator is a part-time job. Delaware's bicameral legislative session is a total of 45 days per year. Session convenes each January, and the legislature must pass the budget bill and recess by July 1. We meet three days a week—Tuesday, Wednesday, and Thursday. I spend the other days on constituent work, meetings, speeches, and continuing my other job as a nursing faculty member. Between July and January, my days are filled with at least 8 to 12 hours of meetings, community work, and, in election years, with campaign activities. On occasion, there are Special Sessions in the fall when the Senate convenes.

Much of a state legislator's time is spent on the capital and operating budgets of the state, as well as handling Senate confirmations. These activities need to be completed by the end of the state's fiscal year: July 1. My most important role is to represent my constituents at committee meetings, at public hearings, on task forces, and as a sponsor or co-sponsor of relevant bills. My district is both rural and suburban and has numerous policy needs: smart growth, transportation, education, health care, and economic development.

I juggle caring for my family, legislative work, and nursing education. I'm up at 5 AM to exercise, and then I have breakfast meetings with constituents or campaign committee members. Following the meetings, I usually put on my other "hat" and spend time with my nursing students. I return phone calls in my car as I head into the state capital. When I arrive in my office, I'm greeted with phone messages, e-mail, and the pressing issues of the day. I share one staff member with two other officials. Session begins around 2 PM when we enter caucus for 30 to 45 minutes to discuss the legislative agenda and bills to be voted upon. One day a week, there are committee hearings. In the afternoon, I squeeze in more phone calls, RSVPs, research with the lawyers, and then head back to the floor for votes.

After each legislative day, there are usually receptions sponsored by interest groups. These provide time for lobbyists and members to review issues and concerns and highlight state funding efforts or programs. Typically, I attend several civic or association meetings each evening after the session in my district (I balance these with my son's sporting and school events.). These meetings are important for gathering community input, staying current on issues, and letting my constituents know that I am concerned about their issues. It all takes a lot of time, energy, and a few cups of coffee.

WHAT I'VE BEEN ABLE TO ACCOMPLISH AS A NURSE-LEGISLATOR

I have sponsored or co-sponsored a range of legislation as a member of the House and Senate: Health, Education, Transportation, Veteran's, Agriculture, Natural Resources and the Environment, Homeland Security, Community and County Affairs, and Insurance committees. As the only health care professional in the Delaware General Assembly, I have been the prime sponsor of some important health bills and on task forces such as the Governor's Cancer Council and the Health Fund Advisory (Master Tobacco Settlement Committee). I have worked on public health and environmental policies. These policy issues have included occupational health, cancer, minority health, dental care access, health professions, environmental justice, chronic illness, mercury removal from the environment, school health, early childhood education, prescription assistance, and end-of-life care decisions. I have found that having a nursing background is extremely valuable in influencing a wide variety of policy issues.

I've worked very closely with the farmers in my district—I was raised on a farm, and know how vital farming is. I was pleased to sponsor, as my first piece of legislation, the farmland preservation license tag. In addition, I have sponsored land use legislation that helps with county, municipal, and state communication. One percent of the U.S. population consumes more than 25% of all health care expenditures, and 5% of the population accounts for more than 50% of the total expenditure (U.S. Department of Health and Human Services, 2004). Chronic illness is a major issue for Delaware, as it is for the nation. I sponsored legislation to establish a blue ribbon task force to analyze the problem of chronic illness in Delaware and develop policy recommendations. The task force identified strategies including disease standards of care for health professions, improved communication between insurers and providers, outreach to the at-risk, and the use of a disease management approach with Medicaid patients and in the business community.

I was the prime House sponsor of legislation creating a cancer consortium for Delaware. This group has completed a comprehensive assessment and plans to tackle our high cancer mortality rates. I am pleased to say that the cancer incidence and cancer rates have dropped since the creation of this body. The state has implemented the consortium's many recommendations, including establishing a free treatment program for cancer patients who lack insurance, adding statewide caseworkers, and creating screening programs. Recently, I was pleased to update the state's Indoor Tanning Laws to prohibit children under age 14 years from using tanning beds and for those age 14 to 18 years to require parental consent.

HIV infection rates in Delaware are among the highest in the nation. I co-sponsored needle exchange legislation several years back, and it has shown a positive impact on HIV infection rates. I was pleased to sponsor the legislation to create a state Office of Health and Safety for public programs. All these examples of sponsored legislation involve a team effort with other officials, individuals, lobbyists, and organizations or advocates.

TIPS FOR INFLUENCING ELECTED OFFICIALS' HEALTH POLICY DECISIONS

What have I learned as a legislator that can help other nurses who are seeking to influence policy? You must communicate well to influence policy, and nurses are naturally gifted communicators and problem solvers. In a study of nurse leaders in federal politics, I found that the political strategies used most frequently by nursing organizations are direct contacts, grassroots efforts, and coalition formation (Hall-Long, 1995).

Nurses should not be intimidated by needing to call, write, or visit their elected officials. It is important when meeting with elected officials that you are prepared. Have a one-page fact sheet to leave behind (not a binder of information), and be prepared to summarize your issue and offer solutions in less than 5 minutes.

If nurses don't speak up on health care issues, who will? Physicians? Hospital associations? Insurers? If nurses don't speak up, legislators will only hear from other groups. You've heard the expression, "It's not whether you win or lose but how you play the game." Well, in politics, how you play the game can determine whether you win or lose an issue. Increasing your influence by working in a group or coalition is an extremely effective strategy.

IS IT WORTH IT?

Life as an elected official has been better than I could have imagined. Though it has taken some time away from my family and my scholarship, it has been worthwhile. I encourage other nurses to consider how they might serve—including running for elected office.

For a list of related websites, please refer to your Evolve Resources at http://evolve.elsevier.com/Mason/policypolitics/

REFERENCES

Hall-Long, B. (1995). Nursing education at political crossroads. *Journal of Professional Nursing, 11*(3), 139-146.

U.S. Department of Health and Human Services (DHHS). (2004). *The burden of chronic diseases and their risk factors: National and state perspectives 2004.* Washington, D.C.: DHHS.

CHAPTER 78

TAKING ACTION
Into the Rabbit Hole: My Journey to Service on a City Council

Holly Edwards

"Service is what life is all about."
—Marian Wright Edelman

Nursing was a career change for me. I had a degree in psychology and a master's degree in education and was working in a homeless shelter. When I began studying nursing at Hampton University, I was a bit older than my classmates. I had to work as well. It was tough. Between semesters, I would read *Alice in Wonderland,* a childhood favorite and a great way for me to escape. Even as an adult, I admired Alice's boldness when she just jumped into the rabbit hole. Little did I know that entering local politics was going to be my own "rabbit hole" experience.

I moved to Charlottesville, Virginia, because of an employment-scholarship program offered by the University of Virginia Health Sciences Center. When I moved there in 1991, I intended to stay for 18 months and then return to my home in Washington, D.C. That's not what happened.

WORKING AS A NOVICE

As a new graduate, I struggled to organize my patient care. It took awhile for me to find my voice as a nurse. With the help of really great mentors and spending nights reading Patricia Benner's *From Novice to Expert,* I was able to climb the clinical ladder. I reached a point where I could balance my clinical work at the hospital with volunteer service in the community. I became the first president of the Black Nurse's Association of Charlottesville, Virginia. I also became involved with creating a network of parish nurses in a chapter of the Health Ministries Association.

I became aware of many social issues while at the University of Virginia. The University's Board of Visitors issued a resolution that acknowledged the role of the university in slavery (University of Virginia Board of Visitors, 2007), and I was deeply affected by this. As I learned about health disparities in the African-American community and the importance of advocacy for the disenfranchised, I knew I wanted to learn more about the Charlottesville community. I wanted to contribute, and I became a health fair waiting to happen! Health education and outreach were ways I could create trust and build a bridge to link people to health services. I volunteered and served on boards including Charlottesville City Schools' School Health Advisory Board, Prevention and Treatment Committee, Quality Community Council, the Shelter For Help in Emergency, HIV/AIDS Services Group, and the University of Virginia Health System, Department of Chaplaincy Services and Pastoral Education, Professional Consultation Committee. I worked hard to learn about the community, but it was while I cared for an elderly woman that I learned a special lesson.

A LESSON ABOUT THE POWER OF POLICY

While I was working on a general medicine unit, an elderly African-American woman was admitted for evaluation of confusion. It was discovered she had a urinary tract infection. She was given antibiotics and improved dramatically. When I assessed her, I asked her what day it was and other routine questions. She answered them appropriately. But she gazed through the window the entire time I questioned her. When I asked her what was she looking at, she said, "My house." When I looked out the window to follow her gaze, I saw a parking lot and railroad tracks. I documented my assessment that she was improving but was still confused.

Years later, I found out that the land obtained for the hospital where I had cared for the elderly woman had been an African-American neighborhood. City policy had guided the rezoning of the neighborhood in order to build the hospital. This experience made me realize the powerful impact policy has on human lives. I became curious about the impact of government policies and their effects on the community. I wondered if decision-makers took into consideration the policies that affect the day-to-day lives of people.

TWIN MIRACLES

As I worked to become engaged in the Charlottesville community, I became engaged myself. I was married in 1993, and in 1995 I gave birth to twins. Several years later, something happened that I didn't expect to happen: I was pregnant again—with twins (Figure 78-1). Being pregnant makes you do a lot of thinking. Being pregnant and on bed rest because you are 45 years old and expecting a second set of twins was more than just a contemplative exercise for me. The reality of raising children in a complex world was overwhelming. During this time, I found that bed rest during pregnancy is really spiritual boot camp.

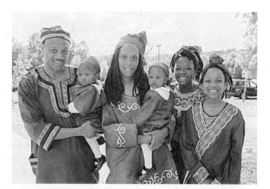

FIGURE 78-1 Councilwoman Holly Edwards and her family. (Photo credit: Lester Frye.)

SHIFTING DIRECTION

After my second set of twins was born, I decided to leave night shift work at the hospital. I took a position as Program Coordinator for Charlottesville's Public Housing Association of Residents (PHAR). PHAR is a citywide association for public housing residents. In this role, I was able to plan and implement the Intern Leadership Development Program for Public Housing Residents. My philosophy of "meeting people where they are" framed how I would plan programs and support the interns so they would be successful. I watched the interns struggle and grow. I pushed them to go to the next level in their lives. I realized that if I was really going to "walk the talk: of what I was teaching, I had to do the same. For me, it meant another level of civic engagement—and that meant running for city council.

The first part of my journey to the city council was to hold a press conference to announce my candidacy. I chose to do it at Crescent Halls, a public housing site for older adults and the disabled. It was the right place to demonstrate my commitment to housing, and it highlighted my values. My family surrounded me as I made my speech. My platform would be focused on issues in education, housing, and health care.

I told the audience, "I believe that my journey to this moment is a natural consequence of the events and my involvement in the community since I arrived in Charlottesville 16 years ago … one by one I have taken people to the food bank, provided transportation to doctor appointments, made arrangements to get prescriptions filled, encouraged people to maintain a steady job. I have, one by one, connected resources so rent can get paid, served food for the homeless, coordinated health fairs, held hands, wiped tears, and maintained my motto of "meeting people where they are." But now it's time for me to go upstream to explore the systemic issues that foster the struggle to find an affordable place to live. It's time to go upstream to find out how sustainable jobs can be created, and it's time to go upstream to promote the health and wellness for all of the citizens of Charlottesville. As a parish nurse, I learned the importance of a holistic approach to care emphasizing the relationship between mind, body, and spirit. It's that same approach to care that I will apply to the issues to which I am concerned … It's time for me to go upstream. There is a time for everything, and

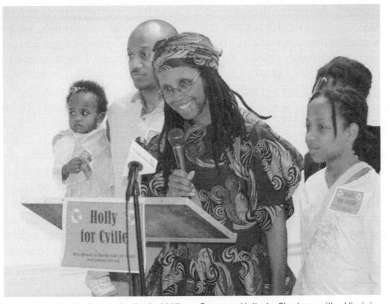

FIGURE 78-2 Holly Edwards and her family on April 12, 2007, at Crescent Halls in Charlottesville, Virginia, as she announces her candidacy for Charlottesville City Council. (Photo credit: George Loper.)

everything on earth has its special season. This is my season, and I invite you to join me in my journey and I ask for your support at the Democratic Nominating Convention on June second" (Figure 78-2).

THE CAMPAIGN GOES FORWARD

A number of publications covered my announcement, and they all clearly identified me as a nurse (Charlottesville Tomorrow News Center, 2007). Being a nurse provided a unique framework for my campaign. It was centered in how I could be a person voters would trust. After the announcement of my candidacy, the work of creating name recognition began in earnest. I made telephone calls, knocked on doors, and encouraged my friends to have house parties so I could meet their neighbors. And this was just to rally support for me at the Democratic primary. The only time I took a break in campaigning was following the tragic shootings at Virginia Tech.

My website provided an opportunity for people to get to know me. The following homepage welcome message described how many nurses have taken on leadership roles in Charlottesville:

We have a long tradition in Charlottesville of nurses stepping up to play active roles in the public life of this community. I think of our former Mayors, Nancy O'Brien, and Charles Barbour, the late Grace Tinsley, my friend David Simmons—all of them were trained as healers and caregivers, and all of them have made enormous contributions to the health and vitality of our city. It would be a great honor for me to follow in their footsteps as I pursue this journey. (Hollyforcville.org, 2007)

ON TO THE ELECTION

I received the nomination! I was on my way as a candidate in the upcoming November 3, 2007, election. Campaigning now included participating in neighborhood forums. That meant I had to be well-versed on the city's issues. I spent a lot of time studying the city budget, meeting with leaders in the community, and getting a clear understanding of the city council and the city manager form of government.

When I spoke to groups, I emphasized that a healthy city not only includes the citizens making responsible choices but also the city's environment. A parent can't send a child outside to play if there are safety concerns in a neighborhood. I was concerned about the city's aging infrastructure. And I found ways to remind people about making healthy lifestyle choices. The theme for the Democratic ticket was "Building Better Communities." I was able to use my nursing experience in many parts of the campaign. At the last candidate forum before the election, I stated the following:

I bring understanding that roads are important, but it's also important to build roads of social equity. I think it is important to plant trees, but it is also important to plant seeds of hope. I bring understanding of a balanced budget, but it's also important to have citizens that lead balanced healthy lives.

On election night, I listened to the election results on the radio at home with my family. I'll never forget the look on my father's face when the final results came in and it was clear that I had won.

SERVICE ON THE CITY COUNCIL

Since my election, I have initiated the dialogue on race utilizing the Study Circle Model to develop not only an opportunity to listen to sensitive issues but also develop an action plan. I established a health summit, now held annually, to address health issues that impact the community. I've worked to address a true health priority: the African-American infant mortality rate in Charlottesville.

An area in which I really stretched was to address the tension that surrounded our community water supply plan. The future of our water supply is the most important public health, safety, and sanitation issue for the entire community. It was decided that to best serve the constituents, an elected official would become a member of the Rivanna Water and Sewer Authority Board. I am the first to serve on that board.

The future will bring continued work on affordable housing, improving the graduation rate, access to quality health care, and workforce development. Workforce development will have as a priority the importance of workplace skills and job placement for people completing jail terms and returning to the community. In addition, I will have a defined leadership role on Council as I, on January 4, 2010, accepted the nomination of vice-mayor for the Council. One highlight of my service was seeing Charlottesville build a relationship with a sister city in Africa. In 2009, the city council voted to have Winneba, Ghana, become Charlottesville's sister city. My nursing background has been helpful to me as an elected official.

Everything turns into a care plan including the need to evaluate the plan to make sure it is effective. I also have a holistic approach to issues that creates a new way of framing them so we can focus on what we have in common. You might think nursing was a career change *for* me, but actually the career changed me. Nursing is a calling, and I heard the shout loud and clear.

For a list of related websites, please refer to your Evolve Resources at http://evolve.elsevier.com/Mason/policypolitics/

REFERENCES

Charlottesville Tomorrow News Center. (2007). Edwards announces bid for City Council. Retrieved from cvilletomorrow.typepad.com/charlottesville_tomorrow_/2007/04/edwards.html.

Hollyforcville.org. (2007). Holly Edwards for City Council. Retrieved from http://hollyforcville.blogspot.com.

University of Virginia Board of Visitors. (2007). University of Virginia's Board of Visitors passes resolution expressing regret for use of slaves. *UVA Today*. Retrieved from www.virginia.edu/uvatoday/newsRelease.php?id=1933.

CHAPTER 79

TAKING ACTION
Truth or Dare: One Nurse's Political Campaign

Barbara B. Hatfield and Brenda C. Isaac

"All serious daring starts from within."
—Harriet Beecher Stowe

My dream had always been to be a wife, mother, and nurse. Never in my wildest dreams did I envision a career in politics. Having graduated from a hospital-based diploma program, I was content to raise my family and work as a staff nurse in Charleston, West Virginia. As I became more experienced in my career, I began to be increasingly frustrated by the lack of power that nurses have in health care decisions. My colleagues and I saw the problems on a daily basis but felt powerless to make needed changes. Living and working in the capital city, we constantly heard about the activities of the West Virginia legislature. The legislative meeting schedules were printed daily in the local newspapers.

After one particularly discouraging day, some of the nurses on my unit suggested that we sit in on a Health Committee meeting at the House of Delegates. Working full time and raising our families didn't leave much time for outside activities, but one day after work we decided to go and listen for ourselves. In the 1980s, nurses still wore white uniforms. Because we hadn't had time to change, we were immediately recognized as nurses. To our amazement, no one serving on the Health Committee had any health care experience. In a moment of levity, I commented to my friends that if these guys could get elected, I probably could, too. At least I would understand what they were discussing. We all laughed because, of course, I had no intention of ever running for office.

My offhand comments, intended to be funny, were taken quite seriously by two of my colleagues. They decided that one of them would be my campaign manager and the other my public relations chairperson. I still had no intention of actually running but agreed to go with them to a workshop entitled "How to Get Women and Minorities Elected to Office," which was sponsored by the National Organization for Women. After attending the workshop and reading the book that they provided, I was more convinced than ever that my running for office was a futile cause. I promptly forgot about my threat.

My friends, however, didn't forget and began to spread the word. Before I knew it, I was being contacted by other nurses who wanted to help with my campaign for the House of Delegates. To pay the filing fee, they had collected $33 by asking 33 nurses for a dollar each. I called a meeting at my house, and 15 nurses showed up, excited and ready to go. All of us realized that the power that we wanted and needed was in the political arena. Suddenly, I found myself on a roller coaster, and I couldn't get off.

In my House of Delegates district at this time there were 12 vacant seats. The 12 top vote getters from the Democratic Party ran against the 12 from the Republican Party in the general election. Our first challenge was to make it through the primary. Thirty-four other candidates were running, many of whom were seasoned politicians. Our first big obstacle was money, or the lack of it. None of my backers had money, and I certainly had no personal wealth. We began by collecting small donations of $15 to $25 from individual nurses. The nurses that donated were charged to collect from other nurses. The campaign manual suggested going after endorsements from groups and organizations. I received support from the West Virginia Nurses Association and the West Virginia

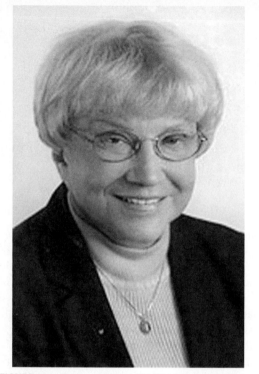

FIGURE 79-1 Barbara Hatfield, RN, West Virginia legislator.

Association of School Nurses, which were small but very politically active; the teachers' associations; the Hospital Association; and the Medical Association. The last two groups endorsed me because I was a nurse but never expected me to win and dropped their support after my first election. They never quite understood that my first loyalty was, and still is, with nurses and their patients rather than with doctors and hospital administrators.

My campaign "staff" consisted of volunteer nurses who took pictures, researched key issues, designed brochures and flyers, and formed phone banks. We found out that if you aren't one of the "good ole boys," you get very little help or advice from the party. There was no money to buy mailing lists, so we had to be creative. For 2 months, we went to the Voter's Registration Office every night after work, looked at every voter's card in the targeted precincts of my district, and got the names and addresses of the voters who had voted in the last three elections. From these, we developed mailing and walking lists.

The guide instructed us to do three mail-outs. We had the money to do one. There was only one way to get our literature out. The volunteer nurses formed teams and walked from house to house, knocking on doors and leaving brochures. To our delight, we discovered that everybody loves nurses and enjoys talking to them. Two weeks later, I covered those same precincts to introduce myself.

Through all of these efforts, I became known as the "nurse" candidate. This helped to pull me out of the pack of 35 candidates. To get free publicity, we stood on street corners and along the highways, often in uniform, holding signs with slogans like "Elect a Nurse" and "Every House and Senate needs a Nurse." By now, my volunteer nurses and their friends were so excited and encouraged that my biggest fear was letting them down, so I never stopped. Although I tried not to think about it, deep down I still didn't think we stood a chance of winning.

The night of the primary election, I didn't plan a party because I couldn't face the nurses if I lost. My close friends, who had worked so hard, sat with me as the first returns came in. In disbelief, we listened as my name began to be mentioned in the top 12. At the end of the evening, I was not only one of the 12 winners but had come in third. The nurses had won a big one! Suddenly reality set in. We looked at each other and exclaimed, "We have to do this all over again for the general election," which was less than 6 months away.

After a month's rest, we did it all over again, and once again were victorious in the general election. When the elation faded, I realized that I didn't have a clue what to do next. The campaign manual had instructed me how to win but didn't say anything about how to be a good legislator. I quickly discovered that my past training had prepared me well. As a nurse, I had been playing politics throughout my hospital career.

With name recognition and a positive voting record, I have continued to win elections. We still struggle to raise money, and I still depend heavily on the dedicated nurses and other friends who volunteer to help me. The grassroots campaign is still an effective way to win, although, with the growing importance of the media, candidates must raise more money than ever. Those of us without large corporate donations have to rely on small donations from a lot of people. Fortunately, over the years we have broadened our base to include social workers, teachers, labor unions, and others who fight for the "little guys." The nurses, however, are always my mainstay.

During each campaign, I have, in addition to the volunteers, a few nurses who stay close to me. They are always there to provide support when I get discouraged and give me strength when I want to quit. As the battles get tough, they keep me focused on our real objective—making life better for the people of West Virginia.

I am currently serving my seventeenth year in the West Virginia House of Delegates. The elections still aren't easy, but, with 16 years of name recognition and a record that I am proud of, the money flows a little more smoothly and the races are becoming manageable. Through lots of hard work and a positive change in House leadership, I am now vice chairperson of the Health and Human Resources Committee that once had no health professionals as members. As health care becomes a primary issue for the state, I am frequently consulted by other legislators, committee chairs, and even the governor. Through legislation, I created a Behavioral Health Commission that is working to improve mental health care statewide, and I serve on the Commission. I have been able to take a major role in health care reform for the state and have championed several bills that have had direct, positive impact for nurses and their clients, such as the prohibition of mandatory overtime for nurses and funding for additional school nurses to care for our children.

Since I was first elected, my office has been a refuge for nurses and other health care workers who come to the Capitol to be heard. Now, however, my visitors include those representing hospitals, business, labor, and industry. I never tire of finding new ways to serve the people of West Virginia. I am known throughout the legislature as the "nurse in the House," and I wear that label with pride. Maybe someday soon I will be known as "one of a number of nurses in the legislature." When that day comes, I will know that I have truly accomplished my dream.

For a list of related websites, please refer to your Evolve Resources at http://evolve.elsevier.com/Mason/policypolitics/

CHAPTER 80

Political Activity: Different Rules for Government-Employed Nurses

Tracy A. Malone and Mary W. Chaffee

"Government of the people, by the people, for the people, shall not perish from the Earth."

—Abraham Lincoln

The 2008 presidential election was historic in many ways. The election was the first in which an African American was elected to the presidency, and the first time the Republican Party nominated a woman for vice president. With the highest voter turnout in at least 40 years, more Americans were mobilized than ever before to be politically active. But some were called to task for their efforts to influence the process:

- A senior administrator at the Department of Veterans Affairs Medical Center in Georgia is alleged to have sent over 30 e-mails directed toward the success or failure of political parties or candidates in the 2008 presidential election. Several e-mails asked the recipient to take further action such as forwarding the e-mail to even more recipients or voting online. The administrative officer's official title and agency information was included in the majority of the e-mails. The United States Office of Special Counsel is seeking removal of the administrator.
- Three federal employees are being investigated for unlawful political activities for allegedly sending an e-mail falsely accusing then-candidate Barack Obama of being a "radical Muslim." All three forwarded the erroneous chain e-mail from their government e-mail accounts.

U.S. citizens celebrate many freedoms—speaking out on radio call-in shows, participating in public demonstrations, and campaigning for political candidates. It seems to be a paradox, then, that the U.S. government restricts the type of political activity in which government-employed nurses, as well as other employees, may participate. This policy may appear to be a restriction of political freedom and the right to free speech, but the limits serve as a means of protecting government employees from coercion. Nearly 60,000 nurses nationwide are subject to these restrictions.

Two major regulations affect the political behavior of government-employed nurses. First, the Hatch Act limits the political activity of civilian nurses serving in a variety of government agencies, including the Veterans Administration, the Department of State, the U.S. Public Health Service, and the civil service system. Second, a Department of Defense regulation limits the political activity of nurses who serve on active duty in the U.S. Army, Navy, and Air Force.

Using the Internet for partisan political communication has caused some government employees to wind up in trouble. John Mitchell, Communications Director for the Office of Special Counsel (OSC) has cautioned federal employees about using the Internet. Quick access to the Internet from work "makes it easier for people to make a mistake." He also added "Now people can step into trouble very easily just by forwarding a message that someone else sent to them." (Federaltimes.com, 2008).

THE HATCH ACT

The Act to Prevent Pernicious Political Activities, more commonly known as the Hatch Act, was passed in 1939. The Hatch Act restricts the political activity of executive branch employees of the federal government, the District of Columbia (DC) government, and certain state and local agencies. Because the original Hatch Act was extremely restrictive, multiple attempts have been made to amend the legislation and loosen restrictions. In 1993, Congress passed legislation that substantially amended the Hatch Act, allowing most federal and DC employees to engage in many types of political activity. Although these amendments did not change the provisions applying to state and local employees, they do allow most federal and DC government employees to take part in political management or in political campaigns. The Office of Personnel Management (OPM) published the translation of the amendment into specific regulations in the *Federal Register* on July 5, 1996. Nurses employed by the federal government in any status (i.e., full-time, part-time, permanent, temporary) are subject to restrictions on political activity. Nurses covered by the Hatch Act include federal employees, DC employees, employees of state or local agencies funded by the federal government, and commissioned officers in the U.S. Public Health Service (American Nurses Association [ANA], 1992).

WHY WAS THE HATCH ACT PASSED?

The political activity of government employees is restricted to protect employees from coercion by corrupt politicians and political organizations. In the 1930s, a Senate panel discovered that certain federal employees had been coerced to support specific political candidates in order to keep their jobs. Senator Carl Hatch of New Mexico introduced legislation that was enacted in 1939 to end this practice. Senator Hatch also feared the development of a national political machine made up of federal employees following the directions of their employers. In addition, the Hatch Act maintains the political neutrality of government offices.

WHAT IS POLITICAL ACTIVITY?

Political activity is defined as any activity that is directed toward the success or failure of a political party, candidate for partisan political office, or partisan political group. For nurses covered by the Hatch Act, a wider range of political activities is now permitted because of Hatch Act reform, with the following specific restrictions:

Nurses covered by the Hatch Act *may:*
- Register and vote as they choose and assist in voter registration drives
- Express opinions about candidates and issues
- Participate in campaigns in which none of the candidates represent a political party
- Contribute money to political organizations
- Attend political fund-raising functions, political rallies, and meetings
- Join and be active members of a political party or club
- Sign nominating petitions
- Campaign for or against referendum questions, constitutional amendments, or municipal ordinances
- Campaign for or against candidates in partisan (political party–affiliated) elections
- Be candidates for public office in nonpartisan elections
- Make campaign speeches for candidates in partisan elections, as long as the speech does not contain an appeal for political contributions
- Distribute campaign literature in partisan elections
- Help organize a fund-raising event, as long as they do not solicit or accept political contributions
- Display a partisan bumper sticker on a private automobile used occasionally for official business
- Contribute to a political action committee through a payroll deduction plan

Nurses covered by the Hatch Act *may not:*
- Solicit or receive political contributions from the general public
- Coerce other employees into making a political contribution
- Become personally identified with a fund-raising activity
- Participate, even anonymously, in phone-bank solicitations for political contributions or solicit political contributions in campaign speeches
- Display partisan buttons, posters, or similar items on federal premises, on duty, or in uniform
- Participate in partisan political activity while on duty, when wearing an official uniform, using a government vehicle or in a government office
- Sign a campaign letter that solicits political contributions
- Use official authority or influence to interfere with an election
- Solicit or discourage political activity of anyone with business before their agency

- Be candidates for public office in a partisan election
- Wear political buttons on duty

Although Hatch Act reform has resulted in greater opportunity for political participation, handling political contributions remains off limits. Personally accepting, soliciting, or receiving political contributions is not permitted under current regulations.

HATCH ACT ENFORCEMENT

The U.S. Office of Special Counsel (OSC) is an independent federal agency charged with enforcing the Hatch Act and several other federal laws. Headquartered in Washington, D.C., the OSC investigates and, when warranted, prosecutes violations before the Merit Systems Protection Board. The OSC serves a dual role under the Hatch Act. Its mission includes preventing Hatch Act violations through the use of advisory opinions, and enforcing and prosecuting violations of the act when they do occur. Each year the OSC issues approximately 2000 advisory opinions, enabling individuals to determine whether and how they are covered by the act and whether their contemplated activities are permitted under the act. The OSC also enforces compliance with the act, receiving and investigating complaints alleging Hatch Act violations (OSC, 2009).

The OSC reports increased requests for advisory opinions on political activity during presidential election periods. During the 2008 election period, the OSC saw a considerable increase in both the number of complaints—the highest on record—and the seriousness of Hatch Act violations by federal employees (OSC, 2009). With a rise in political advocacy by federal employees, there are more possibilities for violations. An online poll of federal employees regarding their compliance with the Hatch Act was conducted by the *Federal Times* on November 5, 2008, the day after the presidential election. Fifteen percent of those who responded reported that they saw frequent violations of the Hatch Act in the workplace.

Today the most common way federal employees run afoul of the Hatch Act is through misuse of e-mail. When a federal employee sends an e-mail that advocates support or opposition of a partisan candidate running for office and does so from a government computer, in a government building, or while on duty in a federal job, he or she violates the Hatch

Act. Most state employee violations involve members who were unclear as to their ability to run for public office while serving in state government.

With the wave of new political appointees that entered government service as a result of the 2008 presidential election, the OSC stepped up efforts to get the message out that federal employees, political and career, must use the many opportunities available to them to learn about Hatch Act regulations. Although the OSC will prosecute violations of the Hatch Act, it views its primary role as helping federal employees avoid such violations in the first place.

PENALTIES FOR HATCH ACT VIOLATIONS

Federal employees who violate the Hatch Act may be punished by removal or a minimum 30-day suspension without pay. Violations of the Hatch Act applicable to state and local employees are punishable by removal or by forfeiture, by the employer, of an amount equal to up to 2 years of the charged employee's salary. In matters not sufficiently serious to warrant prosecution, the OSC will issue a warning letter to the employee.

DEPARTMENT OF DEFENSE REGULATIONS ON POLITICAL ACTIVITY

Restrictions similar to those in the Hatch Act regulate the political behavior of the nurses in the U.S. Army, Navy, and Air Force, including those in the National Guard and/or in Reserve status. The "spirit and intent" of Department of Defense Directive 1344.10 (Department of Defense, 2008) prohibits any activity that may be viewed as associating the Defense Department with a partisan political cause or candidate. The following restrictions apply:

Nurses in the armed forces *may*:

- Register, vote, and express their personal opinions on political candidates and issues, but not as representatives of the uniformed services
- Encourage other military members to vote, without attempting to influence or interfere with the outcome of an election
- Contribute money to political organizations, parties, or committees favoring a particular candidate

- Attend partisan and nonpartisan political meetings or rallies as spectators when not in uniform or on duty
- Join a political club, and attend meetings when not in uniform
- Serve as nonpartisan election officials, if they are not in uniform, if it does not interfere with military duties and approval is provided by the commanding officer
- Sign a petition for legislative action or for placing a candidate's name on a ballot, but in the service member's personal capacity
- Make personal visits to legislators, but not in uniform or as official representatives of their branch of service
- Write a letter to the editor of a newspaper or other periodical expressing personal views on public issues or political candidates
- Display a political bumper sticker on a private vehicle
- If an officer, seek and hold nonpartisan civil office on an independent school board that is located on a military reservation

Nurses in the armed forces *may not*:

- Use their official authority to influence or interfere with an election
- Solicit votes for a particular candidate or issue
- Require or solicit political contributions from others
- Participate in partisan political management, campaigns, or conventions
- Write or publish partisan articles that solicit votes for or against a party or candidate
- Participate in partisan radio or television shows
- Distribute partisan political literature or participate in partisan political parades
- Display large political signs, banners, or posters on a private vehicle
- Use contemptuous words against the president; the vice president; Congress; the secretaries of defense or transportation or the military departments; or the governors or legislators of any state or territory where the service member is on duty
- Engage in fund-raising activities for partisan political causes on military property or in federal offices

- Attend partisan political events as official representatives of the uniformed services
- Campaign for or hold elective civil office in the federal government, or the government of a state, a territory, DC, or any political division in those areas
- Nurses serving in the military are encouraged to obtain an official opinion from a military lawyer if they are unsure about participating in a specific political activity.

American nurses have created new horizons in policy and politics by becoming increasingly sophisticated in their political knowledge and by becoming actively involved in influencing health care in many environments. Many have translated professional nursing skills into effective political skills. Government-employed nurses should have their voices heard, as all other nurses have the opportunity to do, and participate actively in the political process. However, it is critical that they be aware of and abide by the laws and regulations designed to offer them a nonpartisan workplace and protection from coercion. Although the availability of information and educational materials on political activity and government employment is abundant, it is the nurse's responsibility to review and understand the provisions of the Hatch Act and Department of Defense regulations to avoid any unnecessary violations or misuse of their key positions in the U.S. government.

For a list of related websites, please refer to your Evolve Resources at http://evolve.elsevier.com/Mason/policypolitics/

REFERENCES

American Nurses Association (ANA). (1992). The political nurse: Your rights under the Hatch Act. *Capital Update, 10*(1), 4-5.

Department of Defense. (2008). DoD Directive 1344.10, Political activities by members of the armed forces. Retrieved from www.dtic.mil/whs/directives/corres/pdf/134410p.pdf.

Federaltimes.com. (2008). What to know about Hatch Act. Retrieved from www.federaltimes.com/index.php.

U.S. Office of Special Counsel (OSC). (2009). U.S. Office of Special Counsel Fiscal Year 2008 Report to Congress. Washington D.C.: U.S. Office of Special Counsel.

CHAPTER 81

Interest Groups in Health Care Policy and Politics

Joanne Rains Warner

"Politics isn't about big money or power games; it's about the improvement of people's lives."

—Paul Wellstone

A month before Barack Obama's inauguration, health care interest groups had formed coalitions in order to urge the president-elect "to follow through on your campaign promise and commit to making healthcare and financial security reform a priority in the first 100 days of your administration." This urgent plea signaled new possibilities of societal willingness to reform health ("Interest Groups," 2008). Fast-forward 8 months when the health care reform efforts had intensified and President Obama was chiding special interest groups for "fighting to block his healthcare overhaul." His strategy to engage special interests early and substantively was clearly a lesson learned from the failed reform efforts under President Bill Clinton (Espo, 2009). In the final analysis, the health reform efforts that history will record for President Obama will involve the robust influence of interest groups vociferously defending their stake and preferences in the structure and financing of the health care system.

Interest groups play a significant role in health care reform and any other issue. However, they are a paradox within our governing system. We need and value them; at the same time, they annoy and distract us. We embrace them as empowering opportunities for citizen involvement, and we resent their influence and perception of buying elections and votes. The love-hate ambivalence is born, in part, by the way a notion crafted in 1787 has translated into the technological, Washington-centric, mass communication political era of the twenty-first century. Democracy within the individualistic American society presents inherent tensions that are both our genius and our burden.

An interest group is a collection of people who pursue their common interests by influencing political processes. They are also known as *factions, special interests, pressure groups,* or *organized interests.* The original definition depicted them as "united and actuated by some common impulse of passion, or of interest, adverse to the rights of other citizens, or to the permanent and aggregate interests of the community" (Madison, 1787, paragraph 2). The mere act of organizing presupposes "some kind of political bias because organization is itself a mobilization of bias in preparation for action" (Schattschneider, 1960/2005, p. 279). Today, political arenas at the federal, state, and local levels experience the activity of organized groups who influence elections, votes, societal opinion, and the policy process itself.

This chapter gives context to the duality of distrust and appreciation for interest groups while also portraying them as a significant feature of our governing system. It traces the historical roots and development of interest groups, describes their functions and methods, and concludes that they embody the good, the bad, and the ugly of governance effectiveness. It also describes the contemporary terrain of health care interest groups, as well as a discernment framework for interest group involvement.

DEVELOPMENT OF INTEREST GROUPS

James Madison's *The Federalist No. 10* (1787) is part of his treatise on the preferred structure of a republic. He proposes that rather than removing the causes of factions, the best wisdom is to control the effects of interest groups. To do otherwise is to undermine liberty. The legitimate roots of interest-group organizing are therefore traced to the framers of the Constitution and the birth of the American version of democracy. Several decades later, the French philosopher and politician Alexis de Tocqueville traveled and observed this country from an outsider's perspective. His *Democracy in America* (1835) endures as a classic description of our inclination to form associations for common purpose and to create a vibrant political structure independent of the state (de Tocqueville, 1835/2000).

The impetus to organize exists not only within the American people but also within the structure of our political system. The separation of powers and responsibilities in the federal system provides multiple points for exerting pressure on the policy process. Groups can influence outcomes through elections, work within each legislative chamber, executive branch pressure, and in the regulatory and implementation process at any level of government (Skocpol, 2003). This diffusion of power presents many opportunities for persuasion.

Historically, groups formed around interests such as abolition of slavery and prohibition of alcohol. At the turn of the twentieth century, the federal government and the associated bureaucracy blossomed, as did the presence of interest groups based in Washington. Business-oriented groups formed during the Progressive Legislative Era (early 1900s) and the New Deal Era (1930s). The social activism of the 1960s generated more groups focused on civil rights, the environment, and specific economic and humanitarian causes (Ness, 2000).

As the power and money of these groups grew, Congress acted to rein in their influence and limit direct contributions to candidates. However, the reforms that grew from the Watergate scandal of the 1970s inadvertently enhanced their power and diminished the leverage of political parties by promoting the formation of political action committees (PACs). Through PACs, the pooled money of many became more influential than that of a single donor. The Bipartisan Campaign Reform Act of 2002, also known as the McCain-Feingold Act, revised the Federal Election Campaign Act of 1971 to control "soft money" contributions—funds funneled through political parties to candidates or causes—and the funding of electioneering issues ads (Federal Election Commission, 2009a). Today, PACs who receive soft money have profound influence that society would like to curb but politicians seem to find advantageous. The politician's resistance to change is also supported by a 1976 Supreme Court ruling *(Buckley v. Valeo)* that equated (unlimited) financial contributions as a constitutionally-protected form of free speech. For good or ill, money of special interests continues to grease our electoral, bureaucratic, and political wheels (Ness, 2000).

From the perspective of this historical development, several kinds of interest groups in existence today are evident: the older trade unions and business associations that protect and advance their economic interests, and the groups that tap the energy of newer social movements or contemporary issues (Fiorina, Peterson, Johnson, & Mayer, 2009). Within the latter group, there are consumer-focused interest groups that provide information and are especially active in the current health care reform debate. Examples include the U.S. Public Interest Research Groups (USPIRGs) who aspire to be the "advocate for the public interest" when special interest lobbyists threaten to dominate the dialogue, silence the voice of common citizens, and impede reform on issues of health, economy, and democracy (U.S. Public Interest Research Groups, 2009); Essential Action (a component of Essential Information), which provides information and wage campaigns on topics that are not visible in the mass media or on political agendas, including access to medicines and the global effort to reduce tobacco use (Essential Information, 2009); and the Center for Science in the Public Interest (CSPI), whose consumer advocacy in health and nutrition involve novel research, equipping citizens and policymakers with useful information, and ensuring that science and technology serve the public good (CSPI, 2009). These examples demonstrate the enduring nature of interest groups juxtaposed an evolving list of groups and issues.

When is a special interest group not what it appears? Astute citizens and policymakers need to be aware of "front groups" whose public persona is that of an unbiased, independent group but whose funds and agendas are from an industry or political party. Recent examples relate to health concerns. The Center for Consumer Freedom, whose message of individual choice is a front group for the restaurant, alcohol, and tobacco industries, opposes public health messages of science, health advocates, and environmental groups calling them a "growing fraternity of food cops, health care enforcers, anti-meat activists, and meddling bureaucrats who 'know what's best for you'" (Source Watch, 2009). Contributions Watch is a public relations front group masquerading as a public interest campaign reform group; their agenda is to smear and discredit their political enemies, and their funding has been revealed as entirely from the tobacco-and-food conglomerate Philip Morris (Stauber & Rampton, 2004). The popular "Get Government Off Our Back" (GGOOB) campaign was also exposed as a tobacco industry front group that rallied diverse groups to oppose policy. Analysis of GGOOB suggests that knowing a group's history and funding can limit the harmful effects of misrepresentation and highlights how ideologic arguments can diminish the power of solid science and research findings in policymaking (Apolionio & Bero, 2007). The presence of front groups calls each information consumer—citizen and policymaker—to a vigilance about the bias and intention of groups who advocate and provide information.

FUNCTIONS AND METHODS OF INFLUENCE

How do interest groups function within our complicated governance system? What operating methods can they use to advance their causes, and how do they determine which to use? Their methods include lobbying, grassroots mobilization, influencing elections, shaping public opinion, direct action, and litigation.

LOBBYING

Lobbying involves the direct influence of public officials and ultimately an influence on their decisions or legislation. Wolpe (1990) presented a concise description of lobbying as "the political management of information" (p. 9) because it involves educating, shaping opinions, and offering research, data, and analyses. Lobbyists also often assist in bill drafting and revision. By hiring full-time Washington- or state-based lobbyists, groups have a more enduring presence in the legislative processes; this also allows ongoing relationships between staff, officials, and lobbyists to become the foundation of influence. Lobbyists become adept at the nuances of the legislative process and provide nimble responses.

The number of federal lobbyists increased from 10,661 in 1998 to 14,838 in 2008, and the total lobbying spending costs during the same period increased from $1.44 billion to $3.30 billion (Center for Responsive Politics, 2009a). Of the top 20 lobbying industries in 2009, 5 are related to health causes: pharmaceutical/health products, insurance, hospitals/nursing homes, health professionals, and health services/HMOs, in order of size (Center for Responsive Politics, 2009b). Lobbying is thus a substantial business.

GRASSROOTS MOBILIZATION

Grassroots mobilization involves indirectly influencing officials through constituency contact. More decentralized politics and expanded options in technology and communication make grassroots involvement effective and popular. Pseudo-grassroots efforts that mobilize technology more than citizens are mockingly called *astroturf lobbying;* another version is *grass-tops lobbying,* when a prominent personality is used to champion an issue through ads or letters. Most interest groups employ some version of grassroots mobilization.

Grassroots lobbying is effective for several reasons. It signals to officials that an issue is significant enough to prompt citizen action. It indicates that citizens can be mobilized to support this issue (which might also be true for the official's next election!). Lastly, it strengthens the communication and accountability between the legislator and the citizens; both realize the other is following their activities (Bergan, 2009).

ELECTORAL INFLUENCE

Electoral influence can be considered the "primary prevention" of policymaking because it is important activity that precedes policy work. It determines who is elected to the policymaking table in the first place to debate and shape future policies (Warner, 2002). Successful electoral campaigns need three resources: time, money, and people; interest groups can provide the last two. PACs are the primary vehicles for raising and donating money to the elections of individuals determined to match the interests and values of the group. Just as interest groups provide a collective voice, PACs provide the collective financial support. For example, the American Nurses Association (ANA) formed the ANA-PAC in 1974 to support candidates for federal office who match the ANA agenda and values, with the ultimate intent of improving the health care system (ANA, 2009). Through campaign reform efforts in 2002, the influence of PACs has been contained. PACs can only give $5000 per election (primary, general, or special) and $15,000 annually to a national party, while individuals can give up to $4800 per year to each candidate who runs in both a primary and general election (Federal Election Commission, 2009b).

SHAPING PUBLIC OPINION

Shaping public opinion overlaps with electoral influence and grassroots mobilization; it involves issue advocacy and public persuasion, similar to campaigning for an issue. Think of it as an infomercial that sells an issue or as direct mail tactics that use paper or technology to blanket an area with a perspective. Think of the ways the impression of societal consensus or preference could, in turn, persuade policymakers as they vote and create policy. Most of these initiatives cost money, but occasionally groups obtain "free" media coverage in the form of news coverage.

Interest groups can also employ *direct action* to accomplish their goals with visibility and drama. Examples include peaceful demonstrations, boycotts, marches, riots, or violent acts. Groups representing social causes and contemporary issues employ direct action more often than professional or trade groups. Media coverage for these events is a desired strategy to reach larger audiences.

LITIGATION

Lastly, *litigation* provides another method to shape governance toward the goals of the group. The *Brown v. Board of Education of Topeka, Kansas* is a classic example of years of strategic effort culminating in a significant judicial ruling changing the landscape of society. The National Association for the Advancement of Colored People (NAACP) was the interest group championing social justice and the elimination of racial discrimination who organized 200 plaintiffs in 5 states to bring cases of racial segregation and discrimination in schools to the Supreme Court. Rippling beyond application to education, this ruling affected racial discrimination throughout society, and it inspired interest groups to pursue their proposed change through the court system (Brown Foundation for Educational Equity, Excellence and Research, 2004).

Given the menu of methods discussed in this chapter, how do interest groups create their action plans? Victor (2001) suggested that they make three decisions. First, they determine whether their efforts are individual or orchestrated in coalition with other groups. Coalition work provides the advantages of pooled resources within a complex process, but it involves coordination, negotiation, and potential compromise. Second, they consider at which stage of the legislative process to focus their efforts (e.g., societal agenda setting, committee, full chamber, or regulatory process). Finally, a choice of tactics is necessary. This choice hinges on the group's resources, various contextual characteristics (for example, which political party is in control), and whether there is more concern for legislative detail or general ideologic posturing (Fiorina et al., 2009).

Each interest group, therefore, develops a distinct identity that originates in its choices, resources, and purpose. This discussion of function and method illustrates that their influence within the governance process, whether nuanced or bold, can span the entire process and can range from superficial to substantial.

Related to the scope of influence of interest groups is the question of their effectiveness. The critique ranges from the good to the bad and the ugly. Many maintain that they successfully enhance our democratic processes with varied inputs. Those who defend the value and influence of groups maintain that they "fulfill some of America's earliest and most enduring political ideals" (Ness, 2000, p. xx [preface]), as argued by James Madison. In doing so, they prevent violence and tyranny in society by engaging citizens in social change through other means. In theory, groups represent our pluralistic and transparent mode of government. In practice, scholars believe that their influence is often cancelled out by the opposing groups lobbying, media, or actions (Fiorina et al., 2009).

The bad and the ugly of their influence were termed *demosclerosis* or the clogged vessels of our governmental body and subsequent policy gridlock. This acknowledges that the maximum well-being of the country cannot be achieved through the collective concerns of special interests, and that we grind into inaction with too much attention to special groups vying for their own advantage (Rauch, 1994). Quadagno (2005) presents a bold, relevant example of demosclerosis by concluding that health care reform has been thwarted by special interests over the years and that these groups are the "primary impediment to national health insurance" (p. 207). Even as the anti-reform coalition has changed over the years from primarily physicians to insurers, its goal of inertia and status quo has prevailed over the reformers' efforts.

LANDSCAPE OF CONTEMPORARY HEALTH CARE INTEREST GROUPS

A *Pittsburg Post-Gazette* editorial warned President-Elect Obama against health care reform early in his presidency because "the field is a rat's nest of entrenched interests" (*Pittsburgh Post-Gazette,* 2008, p. 2). This unsavory reference underscores the complex, historic, and dominant nature of health care interests. Who are these players, what money is involved, and what is nursing's place and relative effectiveness in the context of federal lobbying groups?

The Center for Responsive Politics (a non-partisan, non-profit research group that tracks money in politics) includes five categories in the health industry sector: health professionals, health services/health maintenance organizations, hospitals/nursing homes, pharmaceuticals/health products, and miscellaneous health concerns. Funds from interest groups are predominantly spent on lobbying and on campaign contributions, and the health industry is heavily involved in both. The health sector ranked first in money spent in 2008 lobbying: $485 million and 3562 lobbyists reported (Center for Responsive Politics, 2008). And, as noted earlier in the chapter, among the list of Top 20 lobbying industries in 2009, 5 relate to health care. In the 2008 federal election, 127 health-related PACs contributed over $49 million to influence elections. Significant influence and money are also organized through health interest groups (Center for Responsive Politics, 2008).

The list of stakeholders concerned with health care reform also includes those outside the health industry (e.g., insurance corporations, labor unions, chambers of commerce, and a host of business and consumer groups such as the American Association of Retired Persons). In fact, from an ecological perspective, few topics do not eventually trace back to health and the human potential it impacts.

TABLE 81-1 Health Professionals' PAC and Individual Contributions to Campaigns

Election Cycle	Total Contributions	% to Democrats	% to Republicans
2008	$95,072,269	52	47
2006	$54,822,896	37	62
2004	$72,240,908	37	63
2002	$42,349,265	38	62
2000	$47,473,952	41	58
1998	$31,443,750	41	59
1996	$37,737,154	36	64
1994	$30,404,022	45	54
1992	$27,865,967	50	49
1990	$15,251,544	49	51
Total	$467,742,215	43	56

Adapted from Center for Responsive Politics. (2009). Health professionals: Long-term contribution trends. Retrieved from *www.opensecrets.org/industries/indus.php?ind=H01.*

Table 81-1 presents trended amounts of campaign contributions made by health professionals from 1990 to 2008. This includes both PACs of health professionals and individual contributions. It demonstrates dramatic increases in campaign contributions and variation in the partisan allocations, usually related to which party is in power. Clearly, health professionals are engaged in electoral politics.

Nursing has experience and success with collective involvement in campaigns. The American Nurses Association (ANA) has provided a collective voice and presence in Washington from 1974 to the present. Their goal is the "improvement of the healthcare system in the United States" by contributing to candidates who support the ANA policy agendas (ANA, 2009, p. 1). Decisions to endorse candidates are made by the Board of Trustees. It is important for ANA members to realize that endorsement decisions are based on agreement with ANA's policy stands and not on the party of the candidate. In the 2008 cycle, 86% of the contributions went to Democrats and 14% to Republicans. Of the health industry PACs that contributed to federal candidates in the 2008 election cycle, five were nursing groups. Their contributions are listed in Table 81-2.

Trended data provide interesting information about the choices that nurses make for their collective electoral influence. The ANA-PAC raised and spent over $1 million in one election cycle (1994) and has

TABLE 81-2 **2008 Nursing PAC Contributions to Federal Candidates**

Nursing Political Action Committee	Amount Contributed
American Association of Nurse Anesthetists	$860,574
American Nurses Association	$562,466
American College of Nurse Midwives	$28,500
American Academy of Nurse Practitioners	$17,500
American College of Nurse Practitioners	$3500

Adapted from Center for Responsive Politics. (2008). PACS health: PAC contributions to federal candidates. Retrieved from *www.opensecrets.org/pacs/sector.php?cycle=2008&txt=H01*.

not reached that amount since. The amount of funds spent by the ANA-PAC in the last three presidential campaigns cycles (2008, 2004, and 2000) averaged $856,000. Contrast this to trended data about the American Association of Nurse Anesthetists whose PAC has exceeded $1 million in every election cycle from 1998 through 2008, with a record high of $1.6 million in 2008 (Center for Responsive Politics, 2009c, 2009d). A simplistic assumption is that nurses donate closer to their specialty, yet the fuller explanation is likely more complex and not yet explained.

When the campaign dust settles and policy-making continues, lobbyists base their advocacy on the values and positions of the group. The ANA, for example, has a long history of supporting universal access to health care, including advocacy for Medicare and Medicaid in the 1960s and its landmark *Nursing's Agenda for Healthcare Reform* in 1991. The 2008 *Health System Reform Agenda* presents the perspective needed within the current national reform debate. Emphasized are affordable health care for all, community-based primary care, and the four pillars of an excellent system: access, quality, cost, and workforce (ANA, 2008).

With ready access to information about campaign funds and donor lists, one would think that correlations could be readily drawn between dollars and votes. Sites like the Center for Responsive Politics *(www.OpenSecrets.org)* present the whole range of congressional bills and their summary, status, and list of supporters and opponents. Click yet deeper, and you will find the committee membership with their

campaign contributions. Political scholars, however, argue against simplistic analyses that would disregard the myriad of other factors that determine whether a bill progresses or passes (Victor, 2001).

The landscape, therefore, for health care reform in 2009 is populated with many interest groups, some in the health industry and many with a vested interest in the cost, outcomes, and structure of the reform efforts. Significant money goes into elections and lobbying. Nursing's involvement is evident in both areas, and while it may not be ranked in the most powerful (i.e., most wealthy) organizations, its currency in the policy arena is trust, integrity, and a reputation for championing quality safe care for all within an equitable and accessible system.

ASSESSING VALUE AND CONSIDERING INVOLVEMENT

Most life choices involve a "what's-in-it-for-me?" appraisal. In addition to that routine discernment, the robust ambivalence and distrust surrounding interest groups heightens the need for evaluation criteria. How can nurses and other health care providers assess the qualities of an interest group? Where should they allocate their finite resources of time, energy, money, and reputation? What merits their involvement?

Table 81-3 portrays queries that provide a framework for discernment as nurses assess an interest group and determine whether or how they will become involved. The framework also provides language and justification for decisions. This intentional approach matches the spirit, though not the rigor, of the scientific evidence-based nature of our profession. The nine queries are not listed by priority, as the weight of their importance will differ with various interest groups.

Nurses can engage in the discernment and defend their involvement in terms of the nine guiding principles, which may prove more thoughtful than replicating the behaviors of our parents or following the crowd with little or no personal intention.

SUMMARY

In a democracy and within an era of informatics, technology, and mass communication, special interest groups are an integral aspect of the governing process. They are sanctioned by our Constitution, valued as a

TABLE 81-3 **Framework for Assessing Interest Groups**

Factor	Questions to Assess the Factor in an Interest Group
Efficiency	What portion of the group's budget supports advocacy, education, or the social interest represented, compared to the portion that supports the group's infrastructure, overhead, or administration?
Effectiveness	What is the track record of accomplishments related to education, awareness, legislation, or cultural change? What outcomes can be credited to the group, either individually or in coalition?
Values	Do the values of the group align with your personal, political, and professional values? Do your beliefs match the values that inspire the group's work? Does this work stir some passion in you?
Tactics	Do you support the methods used by the group? Do the tactics match your preferred approach to social change, including options such as violence, protesting, nonviolent resistance, media campaigns, or organized action?
Visibility and responsiveness	Does the group have the level of public visibility that you prefer? Do they employ the level of outreach to their members that you prefer? Do they communicate clearly and consistently with the constituency?
Social norms	Does the group match your local culture and the social norms of the people with whom you associate? Would your involvement in this group change the way people perceive you personally or professionally? Does that perception matter to you?
Perception	What is your perception of the leaders and key stakeholders of the interest group? Does that perception matter to you?
Costs	What would involvement require of you? Are there dues or voluntary financial commitments? Can you contribute the amount of time required? Will they ask to use your name, title, or reputation, and will any unintended implications involve professional cost? Does your employer prohibit or discourage involvement with this group?
Benefits	What's in it for you? Will you obtain any profit, professional advantage, or membership benefits? Do you value the social benefit of association? Are you willing to be involved for altruistic intentions? Are you willing to be involved if the benefits go to others, for example, an underrepresented population, the environment, or a cause beyond your immediate life?

vehicle for citizen participation, and also despised as an underhanded and unequal wielding of influence through money. Despite societal ambivalence, they are likely here to stay. Perhaps the best approach is to cleverly frame them. Republican strategist Mary Matalin whimsically noted, "They're stakeholders when they're with you, and they're interest groups when they're against you" (Espo, 2009, p. 8). Or perhaps the best advice is to intentionally discern our own involvement, know how the rules are played, and use the power of interest groups to further the causes and values we treasure.

For a list of related websites, please refer to your Evolve Resources at http://evolve.elsevier.com/Mason/policypolitics/

REFERENCES

American Nurses Association. (2008). ANA's health system reform agenda. Retrieved from www.nursingworld.org/HSRA08.

American Nurses Association. (2009). ANA-PAC. Retrieved from www.nursingworld.org/MainMenuCategories/ANAPoliticalPower/ANAPAC.aspx.

Apolionio, D. E., & Bero, L. A. (2007). The creation of industry front groups: The tobacco industry and "Get Government Off Our Back". *American Journal of Public Health*, *97*(3). Retrieved from http://ajph.aphapublications.org/cgi/reprint/AJPH.2005.081117v1.

Bergan, D. E. (2009). Does grassroots lobbying work? A field experiment measuring the effects of an e-mail lobbying campaign on legislative behavior. *American Politics Research*, *37*(2), 327-352.

Brown Foundation for Educational Equity, Excellence and Research. (2004, April 11). *Brown v. Board of Education*: About the case. Retrieved from http://brownvboard.org/summary.

Center for Responsive Politics. (2008) Influence and Lobbying: Health. Retrieved from www.opensecrets.org/industries/indus.php?ind=H.

Center for Responsive Politics. (2009a). Lobbying database. Retrieved from www.opensecrets.org/lobbyists/index.php.

Center for Responsive Politics. (2009b). Lobbying: Top industries. Retrieved from www.opensecrets.org/lobby/top.php?indexType=i.

Center for Responsive Politics. (2009c). PACs: American Association of Nurse Anesthetists. Retrieved from www.opensecrets.org/pacs/lookup2.php?strID=C00173153.

Center for Responsive Politics. (2009d). PACs: American Nurses Association. Retrieved from www.opensecrets.org/pacs/lookup2.php?cycle=2008&strlD=C00017525.

Center for Science in the Public Interest. (2009). Mission. Retrieved from www.cspinet.org/about/mission.html.

de Tocqueville, A. (1835/2000). *Democracy in America* (H. C. Mansfield & D. Winthrop, Trans.). Chicago: University of Chicago Press.

Espo, D. (2009, August 19). *"Special interests" on both sides in health fight.* The Associated Press. Retrieved from www.google.com/hostednews/ap/article/ALeqM5jqi0vd508ygGwuXhWnP0tMBDigkQD9A65H8O0.

Essential Information. (2009). Essential Action. Retrieved from www.essentialaction.org.

Federal Election Commission. (2009a). Bipartisan campaign reform act. Retrieved from www.fec.gov/pages/bcra/bcra_update.shtml.

Federal Election Commission. (2009b). Contribution limits for (2009-2010). Retrieved from www.fec.gov/info/contriblimits0910.pdf.

Fiorina, M. P., Peterson, P. E., Johnson, B., & Mayer, W. G. (2009). *The new American Democracy* (6th ed.). San Francisco: Pearson.

Interest groups ask president-elect Obama to address healthcare reform, other issues. (2008, December 18). *Medical News Today.* Retrieved from www.medicalnewstoday.com/articles/133477.php.

Madison, J. (1787, November 22). The Federalist No. 10: The utility of the union as a safeguard against domestic faction and insurrection. *Daily Advertiser.* Retrieved from www.constitution.org/fed/federa10.htm.

Ness, I. (2000). *Encyclopedia of interest groups and lobbyists in the United States* (vol. 1). New York: Sharpe Reference.

Pittsburgh Post-Gazette. (2008, December 17). Road to reform: Daschle is well positioned to revamp health care [Editorial]. *Pittsburgh Post-Gazette.* Retrieved from www.post-gazette.com/pg/08352/935535-192.stm#ixzz00z09rLM1.

Quadagno, J. (2005). *One nation uninsured: Why the U.S. has no national health insurance.* New York: Oxford University Press.

Rauch, J. (1994). *Demosclerosis: The silent killer of American government.* New York: Random House.

Schattschneider, E. E. (1960/2005). The scope and bias of the pressure system. In G. M. Scott (Ed.), *Choices: An American government reader* (pp. 276-280). Boston: Pearson. (Reprinted from *The semisovereign people: A realist's view of democracy in America,* by E. E. Schattschneider, 1960, Austin, TX: Holt, Rinehart & Winston.)

Skocpol, T. (2003). *Diminished democracy: From membership to management in American civil life.* Norman, OK: Oklahoma University Press.

Source Watch. (2009). Center for Consumer Freedom. Retrieved from www.sourcewatch.org/index.php?title=Center_for_Consumer_Freedom.

Stauber, J., & Rampton, S. (2004). Wolves in sheep's clothing: "Special-interest watchdog" exposed as tobacco industry front group. *Full Frontal Scrutiny.* Retrieved from www.frontgroups.org/node/310.

U.S. Public Interest Research Groups. (U.S. PIRGs). (2009). Mission statement. Retrieved from www.uspirg.org/about-us/mission.

Victor, J. N. (2001). The challenges of evaluating interest group influence in Congress: A study of the 106th House Resources Committee. Paper presented at the 2001 Midwest Political Science Association Meetings, Chicago, IL.

Warner, J. R. (2002). Campaign management: Policy's primary prevention strategy. In D. J. Mason, J. K. Leavitt, & M. W. Chaffee (Eds.), *Policy and politics in nursing and health care* (ed. 4, pp. 579-583). Philadelphia: W.B. Saunders.

Wolpe, B. C. (1990). *Lobbying Congress: How the system works.* Washington, D.C.: Congressional Quarterly.

CHAPTER 82

Current Issues in Nursing Associations

Linda J. Shinn

"Associations are the hidden glue of our society and economy. Like the mortar that holds the bricks of a building in place, associations go largely unnoticed, yet they do much to hold the entire structure together."

—Jim Collins (ASAE, 2006)

Associations are groups of people who have joined together to pursue a common purpose or goal. For registered nurses, nursing associations have worked to achieve policies to ensure that nurses have fair pay; hours of work that approximate the rest of the labor force; opportunities to practice according to their preparation; prescriptive authority; a safe workplace; and a patient load that does not outstrip their capacities. Each of these achievements has been hard won and benefits all nurses without regard to their membership in a professional nursing organization. However, all of these accomplishments came through the work of organizations.

While continuing to work on behalf of the profession, nursing associations are confronting issues such as dwindling resources (including money and manpower); competition between and among all groups that speak for nursing; integration of cultures and generations; and the need to do ever better and to do more with less.

The issues can broadly be characterized as challenges in membership, leadership, and advocacy.

NURSING'S PROFESSIONAL ORGANIZATIONS

While the American Nurses Association (ANA) has generally been known as the organization that represents the profession across all education, practice, and demographic spectrums, a number of organizations focused on specialties and subspecialties in nursing practice have formed over the years. For example, the American Association of Nurse Anesthetists was organized in 1931 followed by the Association of Collegiate Schools of Nursing in 1932 and the Association of Operating Room Nurses in 1949. Other organizations focused on ethnicity, demographics, and scholarship have also emerged, such as the National Association of Hispanic Nurses; the National Council of State Boards of Nursing; and Sigma Theta Tau. Many of these organizations advocate for nurses and nursing in their particular area of interest. Most also advocate for patients. For example, through its chapters, the National Black Nurses Association (NBNA) has tackled the issue of obesity by providing screening and education to local communities (NBNA, 2008).

It is estimated that there are over 100 nursing associations organized in specialty practice areas or other spheres of interest. Many of these organizations establish standards of practice; offer certification programs; provide continuing education opportunities; publish professional journals; and lobby lawmakers and regulators on matters of public policy. A number of the organizations compete with each other for the time, talent, and dues money of nurses. There is often rivalry among organizations as to who will represent the profession in the halls of Congress, before state legislatures, or in the media. It is interesting to note that the ANA now states that it "represents the interests of the profession," though historically it claimed it represented the profession of nursing (ANA, 2010). The inability of the nursing profession to speak with "one voice" is an age-old predicament for the profession.

There is evidence that nursing organizations realize that collaboration rather than competition among

BOX 82-1 Alliance Member Organizations

- Academy of Medical-Surgical Nurses
- Academy of Neonatal Nursing, LLC
- Air & Surface Transport Nurses Association
- American Academy of Ambulatory Care Nursing
- American Academy of Nurse Practitioners
- American Association of Colleges of Nursing
- American Association of Critical-Care Nurses
- American Association of Heart Failure Nurses
- American Association of Legal Nurse Consultants
- American Association of Neuroscience Nurses
- American Association of Nurse Anesthetists
- American Association of Occupational Health Nurses
- American College of Nurse Practitioners
- American Holistic Nurses' Association
- American Medical Informatics Association
- American Nephrology Nurses' Association
- American Nurses Association
- American Organization of Nurse Executives
- American Pediatric Surgical Nurses Association
- American Psychiatric Nurses Association
- American Society for Pain Management Nursing
- American Society of PeriAnesthesia Nurses
- American Society of Plastic Surgical Nurses
- Association for Radiologic and Imaging Nursing
- Association of Black Nursing Faculty, Inc.
- Association of Nurses in AIDS Care
- Association of Pediatric Hematology/Oncology Nurses (APHON)
- Association of periOperative Registered Nurses
- Association of Rehabilitation Nurses
- Association of Women's Health, Obstetric and Neonatal Nurses

- Commission on Graduates of Foreign Nursing Schools
- Dermatology Nurses' Association
- Developmental Disabilities Nurses Association
- Emergency Nurses Association
- Hospice and Palliative Nurses Association
- Infusion Nurses Society
- International Association of Forensic Nurses
- International Nurses Society on Addictions
- NATCO, The Organization for Transplant Professionals
- National Association of Neonatal Nurses
- National Association of Nurse Massage Therapists
- National Association of Orthopaedic Nurses
- National Association of Pediatric Nurse Practitioners
- National Association of School Nurses
- National Council of State Boards of Nursing
- National Gerontological Nursing Association
- National League for Nursing
- National Nursing Staff Development Organization
- National Student Nurses' Association, Inc.
- Nutrition Support Nurses Practice Section of A.S.P.E.N.
- Oncology Nursing Society
- Pediatric Endocrinology Nursing Society
- Preventative Cardiovascular Nurses Association
- Rheumatology Nurses Society
- Sigma Theta Tau, International: Honor Society of Nursing
- Society of Gastroenterology Nurses and Associates, Inc.
- Society of Otorhinolaryngology and Head-Neck Nurses
- Society of Pediatric Nurses
- Society of Trauma Nurses
- Society of Urologic Nurses and Associates
- Wound Ostomy & Continence Nurses Society

Source: *www.nursing-alliance.org/content.cfm/id/members*, May 20, 2010.

organizations and across specialties will advance the profession. For example, the ANA has increasingly taken on the role of convener or partner with other nursing organizations for several initiatives including a study of the Economic Value of Nursing (ANA, 2008a) and an Assessment of Safety, Quality and Effectiveness of Care Provided by Advanced Practice Nurses (ANA, 2008b). The American Organization of Nurse Executives (AONE) and the American Association of Critical Care Nurses (AACN) collaborated in the publication of *The Nurse Manager Inventory Tool* and the provision of nurse manager certification.

Sixty nursing organizations representing over 700,000 nurses have joined the Nursing Organiza-

tions Alliance (The Alliance, 2010) (Box 82-1). The Alliance was created to replace the National Federation of Specialty Nursing Organizations and the Nursing Organization Liaison Forum in an effort to bring all nursing organizations under one roof to "...promote a strong voice and cohesive action to address issues of concern to the nursing community" (The Alliance, 2001). This initiative to bring nursing organizations together under one banner appears to be in conflict with the ANA, as the ANA allows for organizations representing the interests of nurses to affiliate with it (ANA, 2008c). Conversely, the Alliance's "Guiding Principles" state that "The Alliance does not have delegated authority to speak for nursing or any member organization" (The Alliance, 2001). Such policies and practices make it difficult for the Alliance to speak with a strong voice or to take cohesive action, the purpose for which it was founded.

The Nurse in Washington Internship (NIWI) is held annually under the auspices of the Alliance to prepare participants to influence health policy. The NIWI has been successful in introducing attendees to the "Washington scene" including policymakers and colleagues from other nursing organizations. For many, it is their first experience lobbying their members of Congress. However, there has been concern about the lack of follow-up to ensure that participants are mentored and stay engaged in shaping health policy after participating in the program.

There are mixed views about the value of the Alliance. Some view the Alliance as weak because all nursing organizations are not members, such as the American Association of Nurse Attorneys or the American Academy of Nursing. Others point to the fact that the Alliance has no delegated authority to speak for nursing or any member of the Alliance. Instead groups join the Alliance because it serves as a forum to develop business and personal relationships and to learn about each other's work enriching the profession.

Is there a need for professional organizations? "Why do we need so many nursing organizations?" Historically, organizations are formed around a particular issue. Some are formalized with bylaws, officers, dues and staff, such as the National Nursing Staff Development Organization (NNSDO). Others, such as the International Academy of Nursing Editors (INANE) convene but have no formal structure. Some organizations have dissolved over the years, such as the National Association of Colored Nurse Graduates, and others have arisen to take their place, such as the National Black Nurses Association. However, if history is any guide, organizations will continue to be formed. Some will grow and prosper; others will languish or die, and as the nature of nursing practice and health care policy changes, so will organizations.

Nursing groups continue to debate whether or not organizations should be homogenous (i.e., for registered nurses only) or heterogeneous (i.e., including licensed practical nurses, technicians, physicians, or other health care personnel). Having individuals with different credentials and expertise increases membership that can enable added resources; yet it can also result in an organization that is unable to meet the needs of a diverse constituency with divergent goals. In addition, nursing influence in a heterogeneous organization can be diminished. Focusing on core mission and business can be challenging. Hard economic times nudge groups to look beyond their mission, often for new revenue sources, or to engage in issues that might be tangential to their mission, however the expansion can bring in more members, customers, and money. Tough economic times result in decreased membership and decreased participation in an organization's programs often when the need for mobilization is most crucial. In 2010, conference attendance across nursing organizations was down 30% to 40%.

MEMBERSHIP

From the 250-member Rheumatology Nurses Society (RNS) (RNS, personal communication, March 20, 2009) to the 180,000-member American Nurses Association (ANA, 2010), nursing organizations represent a small percentage of the nation's 3.1 million registered nurses. Despite exhortations to nurses to join associations to advance the welfare of the profession, protect its practice, or work on behalf of patients, there are many reasons that nurses do not connect to professional organizations. Those that do not belong fail to recognize that every registered nurse benefits from the work of professional organizations, whether a member or not. This fact is a powerful persuader against "joining up" and one not easily overcome.

Earlier generations of nurses joined associations for altruistic reasons. Today, the decision to join is much more "What's in it for me?" Nurses often do not understand how much associations do in public policy and what the benefits are to all. Although public policy is already expensive and time-consuming for organizations, much more effort is needed in helping nurses understand how this improves practice and income. Nurses often respond with "Nobody asked me" when asked why they have not joined a nursing association. Perhaps all of organized nursing should embark upon a campaign to help stamp out "Nobody asked me!"

Informal conversations with nurses reveal that those who join associations do so for two primary reasons: networking and information. A formidable competitor today is the Internet. The Internet provides access to limitless information, and sites such as LinkedIn, Twitter, and Facebook supply ample networking opportunities. Nursing organizations are rising to today's challenges in a variety of ways. The American Nephrology Nurses Association (ANNA) is considering offering its journal articles through podcasts. The Oncology Nursing Society (ONS) offered its Institute of Learning on site and virtually in 2009. The ANA has Facebook and LinkedIn community groups for information sharing. Also, the Internet permits associations to bring people together instantaneously for opinions and votes on issues. The ANA has used its Nursing World website to conduct an online poll related to its Safe Staffing Saves Lives Campaign. Over 15,000 respondents weighed in on staff shortages (ANA, 2009).

Membership retention is another issue for nursing organizations. Association membership marketing experts report that a member who joins and remains in membership for 3 years is most likely to keep the membership for a career lifetime. Whether dues are paid by an individual or employer, membership dues are often the first items cut in tough economic times. In a recent survey regarding the recession, 14.1% of association members from across 77 professional and trade associations said they would drop their membership regardless of who pays (Junker, 2009).

Nursing organizations also struggle with diversity. While these groups have worked hard to diversify membership across racial, ethnic, and gender lines with modest success, generational issues are now a central issue. "Baby boomers" (born between the mid 1940s and 1960s) and their parents, the silent generation (born between the mid 1930s and 1940s), have been loyal association supporters. Generation X (born between the mid 1960s and 1970s) has not joined associations in droves. Generation Y (those born between the late 1970s and late 1990s) is perceived to be more involved in and connected to others not only through the Internet but through the community volunteer experience required during their secondary education. The challenge is to get young people to join and older people to remain (Shinn, 2009).

Formidable competitors, including not-for-profit and for-profit groups that provide goods and services traditionally provided by professional organizations, increase the competition for membership in existing organizations.

ADVOCACY

Nursing organizations have long advocated for causes or interests through lobbying Congress and state legislatures; developing and advancing public policy positions; creating political action committees; appearing before federal or state agencies and courts of law; collaborating with other groups on matters of mutual concern; setting standards of practice; establishing a code of ethics; and establishing credentialing mechanisms. This work is time-consuming, expensive, and resource-intensive. It is often supported by member dues or contributions. Lean times and dwindling association membership threaten these efforts. While there are many national nursing organizations that lobby Congress, there are few at the state and local levels. The result is that other stronger groups can have more influence. Physician groups, pharmaceutical organizations, hospital associations, and other provider groups can be counted on to fill any vacuum created by the lack of a strong voice for nursing at state and local levels.

One of the most controversial advocacy activities in the profession has been collective bargaining. The ANA was certified by the National Labor Relations Board as a labor union in 1949. Shortly, several state nurses associations began to represent nurses in the employment setting to influence policy related to wages, hours, and working conditions. In 2008, "nearly 20% of the 2.7 million RNs in the nation were unionized" (Carlson, 2009).

While some nurses have valued representation in the employment setting, others have found it foreign, labeling it unprofessional. And many nurses have debated whether or not it is possible for a professional association to pursue a policy of being a multipurpose association, attentive to issues such as standards of practice, research, ethics, and education as well as wages, hours, and working conditions. Within ANA, there has been a continuous debate over the amount of resources going to collective bargaining activities. State nurses associations that represent nurses for collective bargaining have historically had larger memberships and contributed more dues to the ANA. Some of these groups have wanted a larger portion of their ANA dues to be invested in union work.

The United American Nurses (UAN) was founded in 1999 within the ANA "by activist nurses...who believed in the creation of a powerful, national, independent and unified voice for union nurses." The UAN affiliated with the AFL-CIO in 2001. While the UAN was founded within the ANA, disagreement between the organizations over allocation of resources, sovereignty of state labor relations programs, the multipurpose nature of the ANA, and the locus of decision making resulted in the ANA and the UAN parting company. Subsequently, the UAN, the California Nurses Association, and the Massachusetts Nurses Association joined together to create the National Nurses Union (NNU) in late 2009 (Union Democracy Review, 2009). The group is affiliated with the AFL-CIO and has recently entered into an agreement with the Service Employees International Union (SEIU) in which the NNU will organize nurses while the SEIU organizes other types of health care workers. It is expected that the NNU will have about 125,000 members (Carlson, 2009) (see Chapter 61). Early in 2009, the National Federation of Nurses (NFN) was formed by several state nurses associations that broke away from the UAN wishing to remain allied with the ANA and the tenets of a multipurpose association. It is estimated that these state associations represent about 70,000 registered nurses. The NFN's focus is a "labor agenda that supports and advances the economic and general welfare, workplace conditions, and practice of registered nurses through collective bargaining and shared decision making" (NFN, 2009). The NFN has elected a leadership team and will open a headquarters office and employ a chief staff executive. The NFN is not affiliated with the AFL-CIO or the SEIU. The NNU will be a formidable competitor for the NFN. Such diverse groups as the Teamsters, Brotherhood of Decorators and Paperhangers, American Federation of Teachers, and American Federation of State, County and Municipal Employees represent smaller numbers of nurses.

When the UAN was founded, several nurses' associations that did not engage in collective bargaining believed that the ANA needed to invest in resources to influence the working conditions of nurses who did not choose to be unionized. They believed that the ANA's union label was hampering their membership recruitment efforts and hindering their ability to work with other state-based groups such as hospital associations and regulatory agencies.

In an effort to respond to states that did not engage in collective bargaining, the ANA created the Center for American Nurses (CAN) to focus on work place issues. The CAN's mission is creating healthy work environments through advocacy, education, and research (see Chapter 62). Although the center was created under the auspices of ANA and is located in the same office building, it is incorporated as a separate entity with a separate board of directors and distinct programmatic efforts, and has become more independent of ANA.

Advocacy for and by nurses also occurs in nonnursing organizations. For example, nurses have served as leaders in many national and consumer organizations, including the AARP, the American Society of Association Executives (ASAE), home care organizations (see Chapter 25), and groups such as the American Heart Association. They have contributed their knowledge, skills, and expertise to carrying out the missions of these organizations helping to shape their policies and practices.

LEADERSHIP

Volunteer leaders committed to the purpose and programs of the organization lead nursing associations through governing boards and committees. Leaders may be elected or appointed to office and come from diverse practice, educational, experiential, and demographic backgrounds. Volunteers are the life-blood of organizations and provide countless hours in advancing the mission.

As a result, current issues in organizational leadership include succession planning, that is, the identification, development, and engagement of future leaders. There is concern about a future leadership crisis as veteran nurses retire or become disabled and younger nurses find other causes to volunteer for. It is only recently that associations have paid attention to talent management, as volunteers are in short supply because of work demands, family commitments, and economic constraints.

Many groups report the recycling of leaders, particularly at the local organizational level. The tendency to recycle leaders can be attributed, in part, to an unwillingness to take a chance on a potential star or the belief that "you must pay your dues like I did" prior to mounting the leadership ladder. In addition, those who aspire to leadership roles often report that there are social, issue-related groups that are more worthy of the investment of time and energy.

Volunteering rates among young adults increased dramatically between 1974 and 2006 (Corporation for National and Community Service, 2008). This may augur well for associations in the future, although current and future generations will want something meaningful to do when volunteering their time and will expect that what they do will make a difference in their lives and the lives of others. Likewise, work-life balance has become a mantra for Generation Y, and associations are viewed as work.

Yet more organizations are paying attention to grooming future leaders. For example, the Oncology Nursing Society (ONS) has created a leadership academy devoted to the development, grooming, and mentoring of leaders. The ONS reports a 20% increase in volunteering for leadership positions in the last few years and attributes this increase to the academy (A. Stengel, personal communication, March 3, 2008). Organizations are trying to match their volunteer opportunities to the interests of Generation X and Generation Y. For example, the Society for Human Resource Management has chosen a member of Generation Y to head up its Green initiative (Brost, 2009).

Some organizations are experimenting with "virtual" volunteering to populate leadership ladders. Volunteering off site in cyberspace permits people to contribute their time without leaving their home communities or taking time away from work and certainly appeals to younger generations used to working online. Micro volunteering is also becoming popular, permitting people to do small, bite-sized jobs without making a long-term time commitment. Associations are also bringing people together for more time-limited, specific tasks. For example, one organization is experimenting with a leadership cabinet convening aspiring leaders to advise senior leaders and act as a conduit for young member interests.

Organizations with a compelling purpose and engaged in meaningful work are organizations that have no shortage of volunteer leaders. Habitat for Humanity is a high-profile community activity for which many volunteer. Nursing organizations have to determine what members have a passion for and then figure out how to match the jobs that need to be done to the interests of those in their ranks.

In the author's experience, nursing associations that involve nurses in community service work such as blood pressure screening, vaccination campaigns, or diabetes detection find ample enthusiastic workers. It may be time for nursing organizations to create a kind of "nursing habitat for humanity" as a way to get nurses invested in the association experience and to stimulate membership and leadership.

SUMMARY

The issues in contemporary organizations are complex. As the world becomes more complex and diverse, groups will be confronted with more and more challenges. While technology enables nurses to gather more information, communicate with more people in more places, and practice in more sophisticated settings with an array of new tools and strategies, there is still a desire among people for good, old-fashioned human contact—in practice and social settings. Nursing organizations provide the milieu for such contact.

It is still not clear who really speaks for nursing. This is perhaps the most troubling issue confronting the profession. With innumerable organizations trying to get the attention of employers, policymakers, and the public on behalf of nurses to advance a particular case or cause, no one group emerges as the single, strong, authoritative voice. A cacophony of disparate voices does the profession no good. It allows those outside the profession to fill the void by speaking for nursing. It dilutes the policy initiatives the profession undertakes on behalf of its members and the people for whom it cares. Hopefully the profession will begin to address the problem in a way that strengthens the profession and enables nursing to have a premier place in influencing health care.

For a list of related websites, please refer to your Evolve Resources at http://evolve.elsevier.com/Mason/policypolitics/

REFERENCES

The Alliance. (2001). Retrieved from www.nursing-alliance.org.

The Alliance. (2010). Retrieved from www.nursing-alliance.org/content.cfm/id/members.

American Nurses Association. (2008a). ANA on behalf of the larger nursing community announces the release of a first of its kind study on the economic value of nursing. Retrieved from www.nursingworld.org/mediaresources/pressreleases.

American Nurses Association. (2008b). Assessment of safety, quality and effectiveness of care provided by advanced practice nurses. Retrieved from www.nursingworld.org/mediaresources/pressreleases.

American Nurses Association. (2008c). *Bylaws as amended June 27, 2008.* Silver Spring, MD: Author.

American Nurses Association. (2009). Safe staffing saves lives campaign. Retrieved from www.nursingworld.org/Quick-Poll/Poll-Results.

American Nurses Association. (2010). About ANA. Retrieved from www.nursingworld.org/FunctionalMenuCategories/AboutANA.aspx.

American Society of Association Executives. (2006). *7 Measurers of success: What remarkable associations do that others don't*. Washington, DC: Author.

Brost, K. (2009, August-September). The Gen Y factor secrets to attracting and engaging "new age" attendees. *Association Conventions and Facilities, 2*(4), 16-20.

Carlson, J. (2009). Laboring to unite. In *Modern Healthcare News.Com*. (November 16). Retrieved from www.modernhealthcare.com/apps/pbcs.dll/article?AID=/20091116/REG/911139998.

Corporation for National and Community Service, Office of Research and Policy Development. (2008). Volunteering in America: Research highlights. Retrieved from www.volunteeringinamerica.gov/assets/resources/VIA_Brief_FINAL.pdf.

Junker, L. (2009, September). So, is it over yet? *Associations Now, 5*(10), 12.

National Black Nurses Association. (2008). NBNA Obesity Initiative. Retrieved from www.nbna.org/index.php?option=com_content&view=article&id=81&Itemid=119.

National Federation of Nurses. (2009). Our Constitution. Retrieved from http://www.nfn.org/about/constitution.

Shinn, L. (2009). *American Nephrology Nurses Association trends and considerations: Planning for the future: A report*. Unpublished report.

Union Democracy Review. (2009). Three major nurses unions unite in AFL-CIO. Retrieved from www.uniondemocracy.org/UDR/183Three_major_nurses_unions_unite_in_AFLCIO.htm.

CHAPTER 83

Professional Nursing Associations: Meeting Needs of Nurses and the Profession

Pamela J. Haylock

"Great organizations demand a high level of commitment by the people involved."

—Bill Gates

The landmark *Woodhull Study on Nursing and the Media* (Sigma Theta Tau International, 1998), published over a decade ago, identified inaccurate portrayals of nurses and nursing in the media as especially problematic if the profession is to be actively represented in policymaking at all levels, ranging from institutional to federal policymaking circles. Recommendations of the report centered on the invisibility of nursing and, subsequently, the absence of a recognized nursing voice. Nearly a decade later, Buresh and Gordon (2006), authors of *From Silence to Voice,* asserted that the public does not understand nurses and the significance of nursing work; further, nurses' reluctance to talk about their work is potentially catastrophic for nursing. The continued misunderstanding of nursing by the public and those with influence renders nursing vulnerable to limited support and resources for education and practice (Buresh & Gordon, 2006).

A 2009 Gallup survey reveals findings similar to those of the *Woodhull Study*—that opinion leaders do not perceive nurses as important decision-makers or revenue generators, even as nurses are trusted sources of information, second only to physicians (Robert Wood Johnson Foundation [RWJF], 2010). The 2009 findings reveal that nurses are expected to have the least amount of influence on future health care reform compared to other stakeholders, including patients and physicians. A major barrier to nurses' abilities to influence policy development and management of health systems and services is the perception that nursing does not have a single voice in speaking on national issues (RWJF, 2010). Getting to that single voice requires high levels of commitment by nurses to the profession and to their professional organizations.

Professional nursing associations offer members opportunities to engage in discussions and advance solutions for issues of quality, access, and costs of care (Ridenour & Trautman, 2009) and at the same time, advance the profession. Active and engaged members influence the direction of their associations, as well as the ways in which nursing and nursing care are considered, defined, taught, and delivered. Members can be involved in establishing organizational priorities, including research; the organization's advocacy priorities; and efforts to establish and advance nursing care through development of guidelines, standards, and education that reinforce consistent evidence-based practice. It is at these levels of involvement that members can influence the future of the nursing profession (Lambert & Lambert, 2005).

EVOLUTION OF NURSING ORGANIZATIONS

Nursing organizations emerged in the late nineteenth and early twentieth centuries as nursing became a social force. The first nurses' organization, the Royal British Nurses' Association, was founded in 1887. In North America, nursing groups initially appeared as alumnae associations focused on nursing schools and alumnae groups. Need for a broader focus became apparent along with the recognition of the importance of nursing influence (Dolan, Fitzpatrick, & Herrmann, 1983). A meeting of superintendents of nurse training schools was held at the 1893 Chicago World's Fair, resulting in the formation of the American Society of Superintendents of Training Schools (ASSTS). ASSTS became the National League of Nursing Education, and later, the National League for Nursing. In 1896, 10 alumnae associations merged to become the Nurses' Associated Alumnae of the United States and Canada. The group's name changed in 1899 to the Nurses' Associated Alumnae (NAA) of the United States. The American Nurses Association (ANA) was formed in 1911 as the successor to the NAA. State nurses associations were organized in 1901 to enhance nurses' influence in state legislative initiatives for the registration of nurses and to control nursing practice, including improving employment conditions, limiting duty hours, and advocating hospital employment of greater numbers of graduate nurses (Reverby, 1987).

The International Council of Nurses (ICN), founded in 1899, is the oldest international association of professional women (Dolan, Fitzpatrick, & Herrmann, 1983). Membership in the ICN was initially offered to self-governing national nurses associations, a requirement designed to encourage formation of associations in every country, thereby elevating nursing standards globally. Today, the ICN membership is a federation of national nurses associations representing the nursing profession in over 128 nations, with a mission "to represent nursing worldwide, advancing the profession and influencing health policy" (ICN, 2010).

Between 1950 and 1980, changes in nursing practice resulted in a transition from pupil nurse-provided care in hospitals to hospital-employed nurses, and related changes in nursing education (Lynaugh, 2008). The Nurse Training Act of 1964 (NTA), a component of President Lyndon Johnson's Great Society initiative, reflected the centrality of nurses and nursing to America's health agenda. Nurse traineeships supported the development of masters degree programs, and nurses were encouraged to enroll through availability of tuition and stipends. The NTA was a catalyst for the development of many specialty nursing organizations in the 1970s.

NURSING ORGANIZATIONS AND TODAY'S NURSES

Working together, association staff, volunteer leaders, and members can find and optimize the match between the motivation of current and potential members to join and volunteer, the creation of meaningful volunteer opportunities, and member benefits (Sadler, 2003) and organizations' needs to benefit the profession and society.

There are over 120 nursing specialty associations in the U.S. (Guide to Nursing Organizations, 2010). Additional associations have international and multidisciplinary membership, and still others represent ethnic groups, specialties, and specific interests of nurses. Participation in discipline-based and multidisciplinary associations is a philosophically-based responsibility nurses can choose to accept as a way of fulfilling a commitment to society, advancing nursing, and affording an interface between nursing, other professional disciplines, and society (Felton & Van Slyck, 2008). Some nursing leaders assert that membership in a "unified professional organization is a privilege and a requirement for the advancement of the profession" (Carson & Dinkel, 2008). The *Code of Ethics for Nurses* (ANA, 2001) section 9, articulates the following complementary roles of professional associations and association members:

The profession of nursing, as represented by associations and their members, is responsible for articulating nursing values, for maintaining the integrity of the profession and its practice, and for shaping social policy. (p. 24)

Regardless of their focus, nursing associations facilitate and accomplish the work of the profession by a variety of means, typically described in mission statements, bylaws, and charters of committees and other working groups. The existence of so many diverse nursing organizations has advantages and disadvantages for the profession. On one hand, the diversity and large number of organizations would seem to indicate that there is an organization to fit most if not all of nurses' needs and interests. Conversely, the diversity and large number of organizations creates competition for members, resources, media attention, and, in general, it complicates, dilutes, and weakens the efforts of the profession to speak with a single and forceful voice.

Mission statements define organizational purpose—its reason to exist (Nanus, 1992). Current mission statements and organizational visions and goals are usually offered on home or "about us" pages of organizations' websites. The ANA mission is "Nurses advancing our profession to improve health for all" (ANA, 2010a). The mission of the American Nephrology Nurses Association is "to advance nephrology nursing practice and positively influence outcomes for individuals with kidney disease through advocacy, scholarship, and excellence" (ANNA, 2010). The Oncology Nursing Society (ONS) mission is "to promote excellence in oncology nursing and quality cancer care" (ONS, 2010). Each mission statement stipulates the "work" of the profession in slightly different ways but shares intentions to advance the profession and practice and, thus, to enhance individual, group, or community health-related outcomes.

THE RELATIONSHIP OF ASSOCIATIONS AND THEIR MEMBERS

Nursing associations need members, and nurses need associations. Benefits flow both ways—from the association to its members, and from members back to the association. Despite changes in health care and nursing, and differences and similarities in generational cohorts of nurses, altruistic motives and the desire to make a difference in peoples' lives continue to lead people to choose nursing as a career path (Sadler, 2003; Price, 2008). Volunteer activities offer avenues through which an individual member can contribute to his or her profession and to make a difference (Stengel, Gobel, & Itano, 2009; Sadovich, 2005; Sadler, 2003).

MEMBER BENEFITS

Traditional benefits of organizational involvement are unique blends of products and services that define the value of membership, including the following (Smith et al., 2008):

- Information and knowledge collection and dissemination
- Networking and engagement
- Advocacy
- Volunteer opportunities

- Chapter or component benefits (local, regional, and special interest networking and project participation)

Findings from a study of members' decisions to join and volunteer conducted by the American Society of Association Executives revealed personal benefits that are important to members holding governance and committee roles, general members, and nonmembers (Inzeo, 2009). Governance and committee members value networking and leadership opportunities highest, whereas general members rate access to the most up-to-date information in the field highest. Networking opportunities ranked second among general members.

Nurses appreciate traditional membership benefits and also value the benefits specific to nursing. Professional association membership offers nurses a broader perspective of nursing (the trends and concerns of the profession); connections to peers, mentors, and leaders; and support for collaborative action among nurses (Frank, 2005). A 2007 survey of ONS members found that members place a high value on educational resources (e.g., publications, conferences, and Web-based offerings), networking opportunities provided by involvement in chapters, special interest groups, project teams, and giving and receiving mentoring (ONS, 2007).

EDUCATIONAL RESOURCES

New knowledge is essential to competent nursing practice, and specialty associations play vital roles in providing members with ongoing learning resources and opportunities. Typically, nurses join professional organizations for continuing education, to be updated on professional issues, and for networking opportunities. Educational offerings become increasingly important to nurse members as nurses' employers institute cuts in nursing education budgets. Creative application of electronic communications and forums including social networking and Internet-based courses are increasingly available from nursing associations.

CAREER ADVANCEMENT

Joining and volunteering for a professional nursing association provides opportunities to find or get promoted to a preferred role, and to develop the skills to become a recognized leader in one's chosen field. Members who choose involvement beyond paying dues and receiving preset member benefits can observe, learn, and differentiate between leadership and management—observing colleagues who are effective (or not) in moving professional and personal agendas forward, and learning from colleagues' successes and disappointments. Mentoring opportunities and relationships that occur as a result of association activities can affect one's personal and professional development and career directions.

ANTIDOTE TO COMPASSION STRESS AND FATIGUE

While not articulated in literature, benefits attributed to organizational engagement may well contribute to career satisfaction among nurses. Societal expectations that nurses provide continual and compassionate care—even in the face of physical and emotional exhaustion, constant exposure to suffering, intense emotional experiences, limited budgets, diminished staffing levels, administrative demands, and workplace communication issues (a few of the challenges nurses face)—can undermine career satisfaction among nurses, setting the stage for burnout, compassion stress, and compassion fatigue (Maslach, 1976; Maslach & Leiter, 1998; Medland, Howard-Ruben, & Whitaker, 2004). Nurses who participate in association conferences or who use association-sponsored networking tools report feeling professionally supported and invigorated as an outcome of these collegial interactions (Sadovich, 2005).

PROFESSIONAL SATISFACTION

Professional satisfaction is vital, and active organizational engagement can provide varied and valuable sources of satisfaction. A survey of ONS members, for example, found the following four major satisfaction factors (Stengel, Gobel, & Itano, 2009):

- Opportunities to meet, work, and socialize with colleagues in the field
- The feeling that you are giving back to the profession
- An opportunity to work with others toward a common goal
- The ability to apply existing skills

LEADERSHIP DEVELOPMENT

Professional associations provide members opportunities to develop and fine-tune leadership skills that are critical for nurses who aspire to any level of influence within and outside of their professional organizations. Participation in development of programs, products, and services offers members experience in group process, meeting facilitation, consensus-building, negotiating, communications, and other essential leadership skills that will be useful throughout a lifetime—inside and aside from nursing.

WHERE AND WHEN TO VOLUNTEER

CHOOSING WHICH ORGANIZATION TO JOIN

It is unlikely that any single nursing association will address a member's array of professional needs and interests (Carson & Dinkel, 2008). Many nurses are members of several associations, with each association representing an individual's interests, professional affiliation, and practice specialty. A nurse whose goal is to be involved in general professional issues might find value in joining and actively engaging in an organization like the American Nurses Association. Someone interested in international nursing issues is advised to look into pathways to contribute to one of the international associations. Clinical practice issues are more likely to be addressed within specialty organizations or organizations that focus on particular roles, for example, the Academy of Medical-Surgical Medical Nurses, the National Association of Clinical Nurse Specialists, and the American Organization of Nurse Executives.

Membership in an organization that promotes interdisciplinary and interorganizational collaboration can be an added benefit of organizational membership. Organizations whose members represent multiple disciplines connected to a specialty area—for example, organizations that include nurses, physicians, researchers, social workers, industry, and administrators—expand the context of the issues being considered.

Collaboration among the ANA, its affiliates, and specialty nursing associations is one way in which nursing could speak with one voice, and in a voice with sufficient volume to achieve greater influence in health policy. The ANA addresses economic and general welfare of nurses, develops clinical standards, lobbies lawmakers, and attempts to speak to the needs of all nurses. State association affiliates have historically been effective lobbying forces for improved working conditions for nurses and better care for consumers (Rhodes, 2008).

The ANA currently lists fewer than 200,000 registered nurse members, including members of state nursing associations, members of ANA constituent associations, and individual affiliate members (ANA, 2010b). Even though ANA membership currently represents approximately 6% of the over 3 million registered nurses in the U.S., the ANA identifies itself as the voice of nursing and is recognized as such by federal and many state governments. Beginning in the 1980s and continuing through the first decade of the twenty-first century, the ANA has experienced continued disaffiliations and decreasing membership. Areas of discontent include questions around the ANA's success in representing the interests of staff nurses, and state associations' disappointment in the efforts of the United American Nurses (UAN), the ANA's collective bargaining organ (ANA/CA, 2010), causing numerous state nurses associations to disaffiliate from the ANA. In 2006, the ANA announced its decision to discontinue its affiliation with the *American Journal of Nursing (AJN)*. The split, identified as a business decision, ended the century-old relationship between the *AJN* and the ANA (Fitzpatrick, 2006; Mason, 2006), and the *AJN's* inclusion as an ANA-member benefit. The continuing drop in ANA membership threatens its ability to retain its claim to represent American nurses and, likewise, any claim to be a strong and unified voice of American nursing. Without an effective coalition to represent professional nursing, the profession will have less than optimal influence in health policy.

WHEN TO JOIN AND HOW TO VOLUNTEER

When to join and volunteer in a professional nursing association is an individual decision. Carefully assessing organizational structure, understanding the organization's purpose, and one's potential for rewarding engagement can guide a nurse in deciding which nursing associations are likely to match his or her professional and personal needs. Prospective members should get a complete understanding of an organization's mission, goals, priorities, and political agenda; structure; support resources; and an individual member's potential to be involved and be heard. Attending a local or national meeting, observing the levels of collegial exchange, and speaking with current members are useful ways to get a complete picture of an organization.

Organizational Structure. It is important to have a thorough understanding of an association's organizational structure and processes—why it exists, what it purports to do, how it runs, and who runs it—as well as informal norms and expectations. Formal structure is determined by the organization's mission statement and bylaws, which are, in turn, operationalized by governing policies and processes. The mission statement, bylaws, and policies are published documents that are accessible not only to potential and current members but also to the general public. Processes, including step-by-step procedural directions, are generally made available to members on request. The subtle, implied, yet important, norms and expectations are discernible through formal and informal networking, collegial discussion, and astute observation.

Bylaws. Bylaws, the organizational "rule book," govern internal affairs and identify who has power and how that power works. Bylaws outline the purpose of the organization; membership criteria; financial and legal procedures; the number of board meetings; how the governing board operates; and the size, number, selection, and tenure of board members (Tesdahl, 2003). The significance of bylaw changes is reflected in the formality of the process. It is often important that proposed bylaw changes be reviewed by legal counsel and a parliamentarian before being submitted to the governing board. Rationale and arguments for and against the proposed changes are usually required components of the proposal, and sponsors are identified when the change is put to a vote of the organization's members.

Governance Policies. The organization's values and perspectives are blended into policy that codifies what staff can or cannot do and also the governing board's process and relationships (Carver, 1997). John Carver, a theorist and consultant on governance design, suggests that organizational effectiveness is supported by board policies that fall into four groups: (1) the desired "ends"—the reason the organization exists; (2) executive limitations, or the unacceptable means of achieving the ends; (3) governance process; and (4) board-staff linkages (Carver & Carver, 2006).

Processes and Procedures. Step-by-step "how-to" directions are offered in organizational policy and procedure manuals. The most common processes available to general members who wish to influence organizational direction or agendas, aside from bylaw amendments, include the following:

- Drafting and presenting organizational resolutions and position statements
- Suggesting organizationally branded projects, products, and services
- Introducing issues for consideration by the governing board
- Presenting issues for discussion in forums offered during general business and "town hall" or open meeting agendas

Resolutions are statements that reflect the organizational mission and goals and are proposed for endorsement and action by members. Resolutions are used to inform members or other designated constituencies about an issue and to show support (or lack of support) for programs or legislative initiatives. Members who submit resolutions are usually required to follow a formalized process that includes meeting established deadlines and using a designated format. Resolutions that meet established criteria are then put before the organization's voting body.

Position statements or simply *positions,* are documents that are issued under the auspices of the governing board, to articulate the organization's official stance on issues relevant to its mission. They are intended as instruments of change: to promote a common understanding and a collective response to issues of importance to organizational constituencies. The need for an organizational stance may be identified and suggested by general members and/or members in formal leadership roles. General members communicate this need via formal and informal member-leadership channels. Position statements are released only after the governing board gives final approval. Most nursing organizations post position statements on their websites so that their perspective is accessible to all constituents and to reach a broad audience.

Projects, products, and services that are consistent with an organizational mission offer important and meaningful opportunities for involvement and participation of members and are a critical factor in promoting members' commitment to the organization. Shepherding an idea from conception to completion, and successful dissemination is probably one of the most rewarding aspects of membership. When the final product is perceived as valuable, it reflects well on the organization. This level of work is generally assigned to committees, working groups, teams, and task forces composed of appointed expert members. Through such involvement, nurses get to exercise creativity, use their skills and knowledge, and be part of a collaborative effort with inherent opportunities to be mentored or to mentor others, to be exposed to new ideas and new ways of doing things, and to achieve success in a potentially complex process.

VOLUNTEERING

Volunteering to be part of a working group whose charge reflects a member's interests and expertise is a common route to gaining exposure and the credibility necessary to be influential enough to effect change. Most projects, products, and services mirror the creators, offering members the chance to influence policy in subtle ways. For example, work on a patient education tool provides the nurse member with the opportunity to convey ideas she or he believes are important directly to the patient population and, ultimately, to effect changes in nursing practice. Organizational publications provide numerous ways to affect organizational direction. Serving as a manuscript reviewer, a contributing editor, or as an editorial board member for publications allows members to participate in shaping organizational publications, another avenue for influence within and outside of the organization.

Although simply paying membership dues does benefit an organization, the real value of membership most often comes as a result of meaningful volunteer activities. Finding the right fit between one's professional needs; personal aspirations; and the mission, form, and function of the organization is central to individual members' abilities to be satisfied by what the organization offers. Elements that contribute to member satisfaction include the combined effects of social networking; the availability of programs and services that meet the needs of current, new, and the next generation of nurses; and acknowledging members' needs to balance their lives with the demands of career, work, and involvement in organizational activities (Wright, 2009).

Finding meaningful volunteer opportunities within an association involves additional fact-finding by the member. Assessing the match accurately requires learning about the terms of volunteer roles, anticipated workload, meeting schedule, and the identified "deliverable" associated with the volunteer effort. Thorough assessment and deliberate decision-making can make the difference between an exercise in frustration and an enriching volunteer experience.

Committee, Task Force, and Other Volunteer Roles. Nursing organizations traditionally use committee structures that focus on functional areas in the organization. Membership commitments are typically at least a full year, sometimes more. Regardless of the name given to working groups—whether "committees," "teams," or "task forces"—committee work is usually essential to an organization's ability to survive and thrive. They allow the association board to focus on "the big picture and critical decisions" (Lawrence & Flynn, 2006, p. 84). Standard nursing association committees and working groups include those that focus on recruiting and retaining members, nomination and election processes, educational efforts, clinical practice issues, research priorities, annual conferences, and health policy or government relations. Any and all association committees and working groups, by virtue of the quality and outcomes of efforts undertaken, can influence the direction of the organization and health policy.

Political Action Committees. Some nursing associations elect to create political action committees (PACs). It is illegal for incorporated nonprofit organizations to use funds to support candidates for federal elections, but association-related PACs are allowed to solicit funds and make contributions to candidates for federal office. Most association-related PACs adopt bylaws and governing boards separate from the affiliated association, providing opportunities for nurse members to focus entirely on issues of political influence. Since they were legitimized in 1971, PACs have become effective in channeling members' contributions to candidates who are sympathetic with organizational aims (Jacobs, 2007).

Trend analyses indicate that members want to volunteer, but increasingly prefer to participate in time-limited projects. For example, task forces are usually project-specific, have a specific deliverable with tangible results, and disband when the project is completed. Organizations that use task forces or advisory groups within their structures offer volunteers choices from among diverse and meaningful projects and a variety of time commitments. Increasing the number and variety of volunteer opportunities increases the breadth of interest areas and volunteer opportunities, but also requires interaction with and oversight by staff to assure that assigned tasks are being completed. In these situations, concerns sometimes arise among members about shifts from staff-managed to staff-controlled models. Association leaders, staff, and members must work together to identify volunteer member needs and develop a variety of meaningful volunteer opportunities to address those needs.

Governance Roles. Governance roles relate to the elected leadership roles in the association: president, vice-president, and/or president-elect, secretary, treasurer, and other members of the board of directors. These roles are usually filled by long-term experienced members and require commitments lasting several years. Criteria and qualifications for these volunteer roles will differ slightly within various associations and are defined in organizational bylaws or policies.

GETTING WHERE YOU WANT TO BE IN AN ASSOCIATION

Application and selection processes for working groups vary widely among nursing organizations, but this procedural information is easy to find. Successful previous volunteer roles, authored submissions, "letters to the editor" in organizational publications, and visibility in other organizational endeavors provide ways to attract the attention of those responsible for making appointments. Increasingly, association leaders are using formal application processes, providing mechanisms that increase the pool of potential volunteers beyond a small and connected inner circle. Although nurses are reluctant to appear boastful, it is essential that a members' experience and the skills that she or he brings to the group are clearly delineated and highlighted in the application to draw attention during applicant selection processes. Public speaking and writing skills are especially valued in nursing associations.

Once an appointment is secured, performing at or above expectations is essential. Group members need to understand group norms that establish a new member's standing as a valued colleague. As a member joins a new group, a brief self-introduction is a helpful way to identify the newcomer's interest in this group's work and the attributes he or she brings to the group. Task force and team leaders, governance and committee chairpersons value knowledge of members' areas of interest, expertise, and skills and areas in which members would welcome mentoring or would be able to serve as a mentor.

SUMMARY

Nursing associations around the world advocate, in one way or another, advancing the nursing profession and excellence in nursing practice and specialty settings, and they share a common cause of promoting health and well-being of the populations being served. Early in their careers, nurses look for ways to make meaningful contributions—to make a difference in the care of individual patients. Often they look to professional associations for ongoing information, education, collegial networking, and other resources to support career development. Opportunities to expand a nurse's level of influence beyond one-to-one direct care are the essence of the value of association involvement for nurses. The contributions of committed volunteers are essential for nursing associations to optimally influence the health and well-being of the individuals and communities being served. Association involvement offers nurses many opportunities to learn, practice, and polish the leadership skills that will maximize their influence in associations, work, community, and other policy development settings, and to support the next generations of nurse leaders who will continue the vital work of the nursing profession.

For a list of related websites, please refer to your Evolve Resources at http://evolve.elsevier.com/Mason/policypolitics/

REFERENCES

Guide to nursing organizations. (2010). *Lippincott's 2010 nursing career directory, 110*, 28-31.

American Nephrology Nurses' Association. (2010). The Association: Mission statement. Retrieved from www.annanurse.org/cgi-bin/WebObjects/ANNANurse.woa/wa/viewSection?s_id=1073744048&ss_id=536873278.

American Nurses Association. (2001). *Code of ethics for nurses with interpretive statements*. Washington, D.C.: American Nurses Association.

American Nurses Association. (2010a). Mission statement. Retrieved from www.nursingworld.org/about/mission1.htm.

American Nurses Association. (2010b). ANA FAQ. Retrieved from www.nursingworld.org/FunctionalMenuCategories/FAQs.aspx#member.

American Nurses Association/California. (2010). What are the differences between ANA\C and CAN Organizations? Retrieved from www.anacalifornia.com/Differences%20Between%20CNA%20and%20ANA%20.doc.

Buresh, B., & Gordon, S. (2006). *From silence to voice: What nurses know and must communicate to the public* (2nd ed.). Ithaca: Cornell University Press.

Carson, E., & Dinkel, S. (2008). Point counter-point: Are nursing associations such as ANA relevant to today's NP needs? *Journal for Nurse Practitioners, 4*(7), 526-527.

Carver, J. (1997). *Boards that make a difference* (2nd ed.). San Francisco: Jossey-Bass.

Carver, J., & Carver, M. (2006). Carver's policy governance model in nonprofit organizations. Retrieved May 18, 2010, from www.carvergovernance.com/pg-np.htm.

Dolan, J. A., Fitzpatrick, M. L., & Herrmann E. K. (1983). *Nursing in society: A historical perspective* (15th ed.). Philadelphia: W.B. Saunders.

Felton, G., & Van Slyck, A. A. (2008). Self-examination: Giving, membership, and worth. (Opinion). *Nursing Outlook, 56*(4), 191-193.

Fitzpatrick, J. J. (2006). A statement by nurse editors in response to the American Nurses Association's decision to discontinue its affiliation with the *American Journal of Nursing*. [Editorial]. *Applied Nursing Research, 19*(4), 173-176.

Frank, K. (2005, July). Benefits of professional nursing organization membership. *AORN Journal*. Retrieved from http://findarticles.com/p/articles/mi_m0FSL/is_1_82/ai_n15394456.

International Council of Nurses. (2010). About ICN. Retrieved from www.icn.ch/about/about-icn.

Inzeo, C. (2009). Making the decision to join and volunteer. *The Journal of Association Leadership, 4*(4), 74-90.

Jacobs, J. A. (2007). *Association law handbook: A practical guide for associations, societies, and charities*. Washington, D.C.: American Society for Association Executives and The Center for Association Leadership.

Lambert, V. A., & Lambert, C. E. (2005). Professionalism: The role of regulatory bodies and nursing organizations. In: J. Daly, et al. (Eds.), *Professional nursing: Concepts, issues and challenges* (pp. 245-256). New York: Springer.

Lawrence, B., & Flynn, O. (2006). *The nonprofit policy sampler* (2nd ed.). Washington, D.C.: BoardSource.

Lynaugh, J. E. (2008). Nursing the great society: The impact of the Nurse Training Act of 1964. *Nursing History Review, 16*, 13-28.

Maslach, C. (1976). Burned-out. *Human Behavior, 5*(16).

Maslach, C., & Leiter, M. (1998). *The truth about burnout: How organizations cause personal stress and what to do about it*. San Francisco: Jossey-Bass.

Mason, D. (2006). The ANA and AJN: A 107-year relationship ends. *American Journal of Nursing, 106*(9), 10-11.

Medland, J., Howard-Ruben, J., & Whitaker, E. (2004). Fostering psychosocial wellness in oncology nurses: Addressing burnout and social support in the workplace. *Oncology Nursing Forum, 31*(1), 47-54.

Nanus, B. (1992). *Visionary leadership: Creating a compelling sense of direction for your organization*. San Francisco: Jossey-Bass.

Oncology Nursing Society. (2007). Oncology Nursing Society environmental scan: A basis for strategic planning. Author. Retrieved from http://onsopcontent.ons.org/CorporateReports/environmental.shtml.

Oncology Nursing Society. (2010). Mission statement. Retrieved from www.ons.org.

Price, S. L. (2008). Becoming a nurse: A meta-study of early professional socialization and career choice in nursing. *Journal of Advanced Nursing, 65*(1), 11-19.

Reverby, S. M. (1987). *Ordered to care: The dilemma of American nursing, 1850-1945*. Cambridge, UK: Cambridge University Press.

Rhodes, J. (2008). Point counter-point: Are nursing associations such as ANA relevant to today's NP needs? *Journal for Nurse Practitioners, 4*(7), 526-527.

Ridenour, N., & Trautman, D. (2009). A primer for nurses on advancing health reform policy. *Journal of Professional Nursing, 25*(6), 358-362.

Robert Wood Johnson Foundation. (2010). *Nursing leadership from bedside to boardroom*. Princeton, N.J.: Robert Wood Johnson Foundation. Retrieved from www.rwjf.org.

Sadler, J. J. (2003). Who wants to be a nurse: Motivation of the new generation. *Journal of Professional Nursing, 19*(3), 173-175.

Sadovich, J. M. (2005). Work excitement in nursing: An examination of the relationship between work excitement and burnout. *Nursing Economic$, 23*(2), 91-96.

Sigma Theta Tau International. (1998). *The Woodhull Study on nursing and the media: Health care's invisible partner.* Indianapolis: Sigma Theta Tau, International.

Smith, B. G., Haas, J., Turner, M. M., Grant M. N., Cleaver S., et al. (2008). Member value proposition. ASAE Membership Associapedia Idea Swap. Retrieved from www.asaecenter.org/wiki/indix.cfm?debug=false&page=Member%20Value%20Proposition.

Stengel, A., Gobel, B., & Itano, J. (2009). Decision to volunteer. Proceedings of the Oncology Nursing Society's 34th Annual Congress. April 30 to May 3, 2009. San Antonio, TX.

Tesdahl, D. B. (2003). *The nonprofit board's guide to bylaws: Creating a framework for effective governance.* Washington, D.C.: BoardSource.

Wright, L. D. (2009). Nursing professional associations are struggling for members: Nursing associations of the past should not be the nursing associations of the future. *Nursing Law and Order,* Nov 12, 2009. Retrieved from www.nursing-jurist.com.

CHAPTER 84

TAKING ACTION
The Center to Champion Nursing in America: Mobilizing Consumers and Other Stakeholders

Brenda Cleary and Susan C. Reinhard

"The mission of the Center to Champion Nursing is to assure every American has access to a highly skilled nurse when and where they need one."

—Center to Champion Nursing in America

The Center to Champion Nursing in America (CCNA) was launched in 2007. Robert Wood Johnson Foundation (RWJF) officials approached AARP's leaders to discuss a potential collaborative effort among the RWJF, the AARP, and the AARP Foundation. The intent was to bring the consumer voice from a national powerful consumer organization to help galvanize broad-based support for sustainable solutions to seemingly intractable challenges (e.g., the nurse and nurse faculty shortage, and health care delivery). The center would offer substantial potential for the AARP to bring attention to evidence-based nursing models, the contributions of advanced practice nurses, and the need to prepare nurses with the skills needed for the twenty-first century.

At the time of the CCNA's inception, the AARP had three nurses on its board of directors and had just hired a nurse to lead its public policy think tank: the AARP Public Policy Institute. The timing was ripe to create a new center that could imagine new partnerships with nurses and other stakeholders who care about how people of all ages access high-quality, affordable health care. As a nonprofit, non-partisan membership organization of about 40 million members, the AARP is dedicated to leading positive social change through research/information,

advocacy, and service—consistent with its message: *"AARP...The Power to Make it Better."*

The mission of the center is to assure that every American has access to a highly skilled nurse when and where they need one. The goals include the following:

- Increase education capacity to prepare more RNs with skills needed in the twenty-first century.
- Increase the number and diversity of nurses remaining in the profession to serve twenty-first century health care needs.
- Remove barriers that limit nurses' ability to provide the health care consumers need.
- Increase the influence of nurses in high levels of health care, policy, business, and community decision-making.

THE CENTER TO CHAMPION NURSING IN AMERICA AS A CONSUMER-DRIVEN FORCE FOR CHANGE

The CCNA leverages internal influence within the AARP in order to champion nursing solutions as part of changing how the nation delivers health care. For example, the AARP Board of Directors and its National Policy Council consider major strategic initiatives, which successfully promoted transitional care as one of its six major priorities in the health care reform law. The AARP, in collaboration with national nursing organizations, also successfully supported

Medicare funding for graduate nursing education as part of health care reform. Through its policy and government relations divisions, the CCNA's issues are considered in the larger context of consumer priorities. Since the nursing center has a full-time senior legislative representative funded and positioned in AARP's Government Relations and Advocacy department, priority nursing issues such as increased funding for educational capacity get daily attention. The AARP also contracts the services of a well-known and respected expert consultant in nursing and health care policy at the federal level. Working closely with the nursing community, advocacy staff who focus on nursing issues have made significant progress in advancing policies that provide historically high funding for nursing education, with a focus on graduate preparation to increase the numbers of faculty and Advanced Practice Registered Nurses (APRNs).

The AARP is a large, complex organization, with a vast communications network. To facilitate the integration of messaging related to nursing, the center's Manager of Communications and Outreach is also part of the Integrated Communications division at the AARP. She works closely with CCNA's Information and Publications Manager to promote the flow of frequent and timely Web-based communications. The CCNA serves as a clearinghouse for nursing information through a web-based repository of information (issues and evidence-based solutions) for public reference.

Doctorally-prepared nurses serve as the center's Chief Strategist, Director, and Strategic Policy Advisor. The Strategic Policy Advisor supports the evidence base for both policy analysis and Web-based resources. The center also assists AARP State Offices in addressing nursing issues at the state level, with the primary contact being a Senior Manager for Operations and Integration hired internally through the AARP.

The center leverages external influence in several ways, including the Champion Nursing Council, the Champion Nursing Coalition, and Champion Nursing Teams in 30 states. The center also convenes hill briefings, roundtables, forums, and summits.

The Champion Nursing Council is an advisory group made up of the four organizations of the Tri-Council (American Association of Colleges of Nursing, American Organization of Nurse Executives, American Nurses Association, and the National League for Nursing), along with other major nursing

organizations with workforce planning and policy interests. The Champion Nursing Coalition represents the voices of consumers, purchasers, health care delivery systems and providers. Its purpose is to raise awareness about nurses' roles in health care reform and achieve permanent solutions to the looming crisis of inadequate numbers of nurses with the right skill sets.

Champion Nursing State Teams represented 18 lead states selected in 2008 with 12 teams added in 2009. The work was initiated through two national summits on expanding nursing education capacity that CCNA sponsored in partnership with the RWJF, the U.S. Department of Labor's Employment and Training Administration, and the U.S. Department of Health and Human Services Health Resources and Services Administration. The CCNA provides ongoing technical assistance (TA) in expanding capacity that relies upon and utilizes the recognized best practices and expertise of the original state teams to help advance and enhance the efforts of newer states. Recently, TA has focused on two learning communities of states already committed to either broadly implementing nursing education redesign or to expanding the use of technology to enhance nursing education. Site visits in 2009 included one to Oregon, featuring the Oregon Consortium for Nursing Education model (Tanner, Gubrud-Howe, & Shores, 2008), and the other to the Smart Hospital Regional Simulation Center at the University of Texas–Arlington. The learning communities also connect via an extranet accessed through the CCNA website. State team leaders reconvened in Washington in 2010. Among states with 2008 and 2009 comparative enrollment data in pre-licensure nursing education programs preparing registered nurses, 71% increased enrollments statewide, despite significant budget cuts.

In 2009, a Capitol Hill briefing was held on nurses' roles in health care reform and targeted to Hill staff from key committees: Senate Finance; Senate Health, Education, Labor and Pensions; House Ways and Means; and House Energy and Commerce: Health Subcommittee. The briefing was followed later in the year by an AARP/CCNA Solutions Forum, in collaboration with *Health Affairs* and the RWJF. The solutions forum allowed the CCNA and the AARP to extend the message that the goals of health care reform and economic recovery would not be met unless we build, empower, and deploy a twenty-first century health care workforce. A richly-skilled and effectively integrated nursing workforce offers an essential tool for achieving high-quality health care. The AARP helped to raise the consumer voice around critical needs for more primary and preventive care, chronic care management and care coordination, and transitional care that are core elements of a more effective and efficient health care delivery system, in which nurses play a large role. The forum highlighted five *Health Affairs* papers on addressing nursing workforce issues as part of health care reform that were released at the event.

EVOLVING STRATEGIC PRIORITIES

The CCNA has the following strategic priorities that continue to evolve in response to changes in the environment, particularly health care reform:

- Increase our nation's education capacity to prepare more RNs with the skills needed in the twenty-first century, through faculty development, increasing resources for graduate nursing education, education redesign, and strategic partnerships such as community colleges and universities working together to prepare a highly educated nursing workforce.
- Improve the numbers and diversity of the nursing workforce entering and remaining in the profession. The center's current strategic focus areas are on retention of older nurses and reducing turnover among new RNs entering the workforce.
- Enhance nursing practice and access to care by understanding barriers to advanced practice at the state level as well as federal barriers limiting APRNs from meeting consumer health care needs. RNs, as a whole, will need to delegate more tasks while maintaining oversight of the plan of care, especially in home- and community-based settings. Recently, the AARP Board of Directors approved adding new language to the *AARP Policy Book,* which guides AARP policy initiatives at both the state and federal level. The language proposes that current state nurse practice acts and accompanying rules should be interpreted or amended where necessary to allow APRNs to practice as fully and independently as defined by their education and certification.
- Strengthen nursing leadership by working with our Champion Nursing State Teams and AARP State

Offices, to increase the contributions nurses make on high-level decision-making bodies in various entities such as health care delivery systems, higher education, member associations, community organizations, and state and federal government.

LESSONS LEARNED

The early history of the CCNA and what we have been able to achieve in a relatively short period of time has involved both driving and restraining forces, although fortunately driving forces have mostly prevailed. It takes strategic effort on the part of many to integrate a new entity with a relatively singular focus in a large, powerful, and complex organization like AARP. The natural affinity between nurses and consumers seems obvious. However, it requires special attention to reaching out to consumers, helping them to understand the myriad of ways that nurses contribute to health and health care, and also careful attention to crafting messages to which consumers can relate.

It also takes strategic effort to gain the trust and acceptance of the nursing community and its diverse array of organizations. We have worked hard to earn the respect and trust of nursing organizations and to be perceived as a value-added, consumer-driven force for change as we collaborate to advance the profession's work in enhancing the quality, access, and affordability of health care. This same scenario applies to other stakeholders as well.

Finally, it requires new levels of thinking to analyze nursing solutions in a health care reform environment. Positioning CCNA within the AARP Public Policy Institute has proven to be a very important driver of success in terms of the think tank and policy analysis elements of our work. The many kinds of support provided by the AARP Foundation as well as our funder, the RWJF, have been drivers to creating an environment in which this young center can thrive.

For a list of related websites, please refer to your Evolve Resources at http://evolve.elsevier.com/Mason/policypolitics/

REFERENCE

Tanner, C. A., Gubrud-Howe, P., & Shores, L. (2008). The Oregon Consortium for Nursing Education: A response to the nursing shortage. *Policy, Politics, & Nursing Practice, 9*(3), 203-209.

CHAPTER 85

TAKING ACTION
The Raise the Voice Campaign: Nurse-Led Innovations Changing Public Policy

Diana J. Mason and Elizabeth Parry

"Innovation distinguishes between a leader and a follower."

—Steve Jobs

Nurses have long been innovators to ensure that people get the health care they need. Florence Nightingale changed a military hospital to improve soldiers' chances of survival during the Crimean War. Lillian Wald started public health nursing, school nursing, and the Visiting Nurse Service of New York to ensure that poor immigrants living on Manhattan's Lower East Side had access to care. Today, nurses continue this tradition of serving underserved and vulnerable populations through innovative interventions and models of care.

In 2006, the American Academy of Nursing (AAN) launched the *Raise the Voice* campaign to identify and promote nurse-led innovations that fill in the gaps in a health care system that emphasizes high-tech, acute care at the expense of services that focus on health promotion and wellness, chronic care management, and care coordination. The brainchild of then–AAN board members Joanne Disch, PhD, RN, FAAN, and Karlene Kerfoot, PhD, RN, FAAN, the project has been funded by AAN, a Robert Wood Johnson Foundation grant, and support from various organizations. Many of these organizations are represented on a National Advisory Committee that was chaired first by University of Miami President Donna Shalala, PhD, and then-Governor Ed Rendell, (D-PA). By 2010, the *Raise the Voice* initiative had identified over

40 "Edge Runners"—innovators who have designed nurse-led models of care with strong clinical and financial outcomes. Many have been unable to garner the attention and political support needed to disseminate their models. This chapter highlights several innovations developed by AAN Edge Runners to illustrate their scope, challenges, and policy implications, as well as how *Raise the Voice* has been able to support their spread. More information on the campaign and additional Edge Runners can be found at *www.aannet.org/raisethevoice*.

INNOVATIONS AND POLICY

ADDRESSING SOCIAL DETERMINANTS OF HEALTH: CHICAGO PARENT PROGRAM

Deborah Gross, PhD, RN, FAAN, recognized that child abuse often stems from parents who are unschooled in effective approaches to responding to problems with their children's behaviors and may be reluctant to adopt approaches that are inconsistent with their cultural beliefs and norms. Gross developed a culturally-specific parenting program in collaboration with an advisory group of African-American and Hispanic parents from various socio-economic backgrounds. Tested in seven Chicago daycare programs with funding from the National Institute of Nursing Research, this 12-week program uses videotaped scenarios to prompt discussion about parenting challenges and how to best deal with them.

In a comparative study, parents who completed the program demonstrated more effective and appropriate approaches to dealing with their children's behavioral problems, and their children demonstrated lower rates of these problems (Gross, Garvey, Julion, & Fogg, 2007; American Academy of Nursing, n.d.). The cost of the program is a modest $300 per child and provides a return on investment of more than 900%. The Mayo Clinic and Chicago Head Start have adopted the model.

KEEPING PEOPLE IN THEIR COMMUNITIES: LIVING INDEPENDENTLY FOR ELDERS

This University of Pennsylvania School of Nursing innovation aims to keep older adults out of nursing homes and at a lower cost than institutionalized care. Living Independently for Elders (LIFE) is a Program of All-Inclusive Care for the Elderly (PACE) supported by Medicare and Medicaid as a capitated benefit; LIFE is the only PACE program operated by a school of nursing. An adult day center is the focal point of the program, where older adults come to socialize, receive primary care from an interdisciplinary team led by nurse practitioners, and obtain other health and social services to remain healthy and as independent as possible. The program reduced common adverse occurrences of declining health among older adults, including falls, unnecessary medications, emergency room use, hospitalizations, and nursing home placement. LIFE has accomplished this at a cost that is less than what would be necessary for institutional care (Sullivan-Marx, Bradway, & Barnsteiner, 2010; Kane, Homyak, Bershadsky, & Flood, 2006).

THE IMPORTANCE OF OUTCOME DATA: THE NURSE-FAMILY PARTNERSHIP

Harriet Kitzman, PhD, RN, FAAN, in collaboration with David Olds, PhD, developed the Nurse-Family Partnership program to help high-risk mothers give their children a better start in life through home visitations by nurses prenatally and for the first two years of the child's life. The nurse works with mothers and their families to live healthier lives and make educated decisions about their own and their children's futures. Through the Nurse-Family Partnership, nurses' work to help parents in targeted communities give their children a better start and help improve health outcomes throughout the child's life.

Kitzman and Olds understood the importance of conducting carefully constructed studies to examine short-term and long-term maternal and child outcomes, as well as financial outcomes. Among other outcomes, these studies document across three communities (Elmira, New York; Memphis; and Denver) that the model reduces the rate of unintended repeat pregnancies, child abuse, and arrest by age 15 years; and it increases the likelihood that the mother will complete high school or a GED. The Rand Corporation found that the program had the highest return on investment among all home-visiting and child welfare programs evaluated, with an average return on investment of up to $5.70 per dollar spent (Karoly, Killburn, & Cannon, 2005).

These data provided compelling evidence for spreading the model. In 2010, the Nurse-Family Partnership was serving families in more than 375 counties in 29 states across the nation, with the goal of making the program available to all low-income, first-time families. The Obama Administration has included in its proposed budgets to expand the program, although there is no requirement that the visitors be nurses, despite evidence that nurses produce the best outcomes (Karoly et al, 2005). In fact, when studies of programs that use non-nurse visitors are added to systematic reviews of home visitation programs for at-risk women and their children—as was done in two Cochrane Collaboration Reviews—the evidence was inconclusive. Olds challenged these Cochrane Reviews, arguing that they mixed the Nurse-Family Partnership model with other programs that did not use nurses or have the same rigor; the Cochrane Collaboration agreed and withdrew the reviews (Bennett et al., 2008).

Not all nurse innovators have the kind of outcome data that policymakers want and need to justify new programs and funding. While an anecdote indicating success can make an important point, it is essential to have the data to back up the assertion. For example, it is powerful to say that "more children have received the necessary vaccinations before the school year started," but it is important to support the statement with statistics. After hearing such a claim, the first logical question a policymaker or a member of the media will ask is: "How much is more? How many more children were completely vaccinated before the first day of school? What did it cost? Did it save money?"

REMOVING BARRIERS TO DIFFUSING INNOVATIONS: THE ELEVENTH STREET FAMILY HEALTH SERVICES

The Eleventh Street Family Health Services of Drexel University was founded by Patricia Gerrity, PhD, RN, FAAN, who also leads this nurse-managed health center in North Philadelphia. Eleventh Street uses a transdisciplinary model of care, providing clients with access to the expertise of whichever health care providers are needed. Although Eleventh Street relies upon teams of a nurse and social worker, clients have access to other health professionals. It has served low-income, mostly African-American community members who have lacked insurance or were dissatisfied with care elsewhere. Eleventh Street also focuses on aggregate-level interventions to address common chronic health problems such as obesity, diabetes, and hypertension. It uses cooking classes to teach good nutrition or groups for addressing violence. Eleventh Street has improved clients' diabetes management, control of hypertension, and the prevalence of low-birth-weight babies (American Academy of Nursing, n.d.).

There are over 200 nurse-managed health centers in the United States that vary in focus and level of sophistication. Some, like Eleventh Street, are federally qualified health centers and serve as "medical" or health homes for the clients they serve. In 2010, 11 nurse-managed centers in Pennsylvania applied to the National Committee on Quality Assurance (NCQA) for medical home status, which would make them eligible for additional payments for care coordination. The NCQA congratulated them on meeting all but one of the criteria for medical home designation—they were not led by physicians. As a result, the NCQA would not award them the designation.

The AAN and the National Nursing Centers Consortium have shared this story whenever and wherever possible as an example of the unnecessary barriers that impede access to affordable, high-quality care. With support for infrastructure development (including health information technology capacity) and removing barriers to fair payment for services, nurse-managed centers could be ramped up to help the nation build its network of community health centers that are needed to meet the escalating need for primary care services.

DEFINING THE "POLICY ASK": THE TRANSITIONAL CARE MODEL

In 2004, 1 of every 5 Medicare patients was rehospitalized within 30 days of discharge; 67% of those with medical conditions were hospitalized or died within a year. The cost of such rehospitalizations to Medicare was estimated at $17.4 billion (Jencks, Williams & Coleman, 2009). Mary Naylor, PhD, RN, FAAN, developed an effective way to break this cycle through helping elderly patients and their families make the transition from hospital to home and improve their ability to manage chronic illnesses that can exacerbate and lead to hospitalization. Naylor's evidence-based model of transitional care was developed with funding from the National Institute of Nursing Research. It uses advanced practice nurses to work with patients and family caregivers during hospitalization and for up to 90 days postdischarge.

The Transitional Care Model has repeatedly shown longer intervals before rehospitalizations and fewer rehospitalizations overall, when compared to traditional methods of discharge planning and follow-up. Following a 4-year trial with a group of elderly patients hospitalized with heart failure, the APN Care Model cut hospitalization costs by more than $500,000, compared with a group receiving standard care—for an average savings of approximately $5000 per Medicare patient (Naylor et al., 2004).

When a program expands beyond the initial population it was designed to serve, it demonstrates its durability and adaptability—two components that are necessary for diffusing innovations in care. Because Naylor had such strong clinical and financial outcome data, she was able to interest others in replicating and adapting the model, including Aetna and Kaiser Permanente. But how could it be available as a benefit paid for by Medicare? The AARP saw the potential of the model to improve the health of its members and worked with Naylor to define the "policy ask" to take to Congress. As a result, in 2009, Representatives Earl Blumenauer (D-OR) and Charles Boustany (R-LA) introduced H.R. 2773, the Medicare Transitional Care Act, which would create a new benefit under Medicare to coordinate care throughout acute episodes of illness, develop a streamlined plan of care to prevent future hospitalizations, and prepare the beneficiary and family caregivers to implement the care plan. Subsequently, transitional care demonstration projects were included in the Affordable Care Act of 2010. The support of the AARP, a powerful consumer organization, was instrumental in defining the "policy ask," moving forward this next phase in testing and spreading transitional care.

MAKING THE INVISIBLE VISIBLE

Even when nurses have solid data to back up their innovations, it is still hard to get policymakers and the media to listen to the story. And though nurses are one of the most trusted professions, they are often not viewed as researchers, entrepreneurs, or business experts. Nurses must work harder to demonstrate that they are and can develop a health care solution, run a program, collect data, and, most importantly, improve health outcomes.

Nurses must think of different angles for the story. Providing timely and accessible care is an important part of the story, but it is not the only part. For example, making the business case can resonate with many different audiences. A personal story from a person served by the innovation can be a powerful hook to gain the attention of journalists and policymakers.

The American Academy of Nursing has used nurses' leadership and trusted voice to educate members of Congress, the media, and various thought leaders that nurse-led innovations should be studied, replicated when possible, and scaled-up when applicable. In 2009, Governor Ed Rendell and Donna Shalala, PhD, participated in an AAN webcast that discussed, among other things, the steps the governor had taken in Pennsylvania to remove barriers to nurse-managed centers and access to advanced practice nurses. In addition, the AAN produced a video on the campaign that highlights the Eleventh Street Family Health Service and other Edge Runners, with commentary from Dr. Shalala and Riza Lavizzo-Mourey, MD, MBA, the president of the Robert Wood Johnson Foundation. Both are available on the Academy website.

The *Raise the Voice* campaign has also led to broader recognition that nurses have solutions for our ailing health care system and must participate in the policy discussions about how to reform health care.

This has been accomplished through letters to the editor, interviews with the media, testimony before Congress, planned events for policymakers and journalists that showcase Edge Runner work, and working with partners, including consumer organizations, to convey the message that nurse-designed models of care are producing positive clinical and financial outcomes. The Academy has also facilitated meetings with advanced practice nursing organizations to discuss strategies for removing barriers to advanced practice nurses and have sought to make the good work and expertise of these organizations visible. And while more can and will be accomplished, the *Raise the Voice* campaign has had tremendous success in making policymakers and the general public aware that nurses can improve health care delivery.

This is a particularly important time for making nurses' work and voices heard. Multiple commissions are required under the Affordable Care Act of 2010 to support and evaluate demonstration and pilot projects to test ways to improve the quality and cost of care. The Act includes opportunities to test transitional care, home visitation programs for high-risk mothers, and nurse-managed centers. Nurses' education and expertise offer a unique perspective to the challenges that patients, families, and communities face in accessing affordable, coordinated, and effective care. Nurses must make the case that no single group of professionals or politicians will solve these complex health care problems alone. Any hearing, debate, demonstration project, or discussion about ways to reform health care that do not include significant input from nurses will fail to draw on critical insight and innovative solutions from the nation's largest health care profession—and will ultimately be unsuccessful.

Raise the Voice has begun the important conversation about how nurses' innovative solutions can transform health care delivery. The American Academy of Nursing has identified Edge Runners who demonstrate how nurses are already taking action to improve health care in their communities. *Raise the Voice* has and will continue to offer alternative ideas about how to promote the health of the nation.

For a list of related websites, please refer to your Evolve Resources at http://evolve.elsevier.com/Mason/policypolitics/

REFERENCES

American Academy of Nursing. (n.d.). *Raise the Voice campaign: Edge runners.* Retrieved from www.aannet.org/edgerunners.

Bennett, C., Macdonald, G., Dennis, J. A., Coren, E., Patterson, J., et al. (2008). Home-based support for disadvantaged adult mothers. *Cochrane Database of Systematic Reviews, Issue 1.* Art. No.: CD003759. Retrieved from www.mrw.interscience.wiley.com/cochrane/clsysrev/articles/CD003759/frame.html.

Gross, D., Garvey, C., Julion, W., & Fogg, L. (2007). Preventive parent training with low-income, ethnic minority families of preschoolers. In J. M. Briesmeister & C. E. Schaefer (Eds.), *Handbook of parent training: Helping parents prevent and solve problem behaviors* (3rd ed., pp. 5-24). Hoboken, NJ: John Wiley & Sons.

Jencks, S. F., Williams, M., & Coleman, E. (2009). Rehospitalizations among patients in the Medicare fee-for-service program. *New England Journal of Medicine, 360*(14), 1418-1428.

Kane, R.L., Homyak, P., Bershadsky, B., & Flood, S. (2006). Variations on a theme called PACE. *Journal of Gerontology, Series A: Biological Sciences and Medical Sciences, 61*(7), 689-693.

Karoly, L., Killburn, M. R., & Cannon, J. (2005). *Early childhood interventions: Proven results, future promise.* Arlington, VA: RAND Corporation. Retrieved from www.rand.org/pubs/monographs/2005/RAND_MG341.pdf.

Naylor, M., Brooten, D., Campbell, D., Maislin, G., McCauley, K., & Schwartz, J. S. (2004). Transitional care of older adults hospitalized with heart failure: A randomized, controlled trial. *Journal of the American Geriatrics Society, 52*, 675-684.

Sullivan-Marx, E.M., Bradway, C., & Barnsteiner, J. (2010). Innovative collaborations: a case study for academic owned nursing practice. *Journal of Nursing Scholarship, 42*(1), 50-57.

CHAPTER 86

Coalitions: A Powerful Political Strategy

Rebecca (Rice) Bowers-Lanier

"When spider webs unite, they can tie up a lion."
—Ethiopian proverb

Federal health care reform catalyzed the formation of coalitions whose aims were in support of or in opposition to all or some of the proposals. Because of the complexities of health care reform, virtually no patient, provider, financing, medical device, pharmaceutical company, or other health industry group was left untouched by reform. Many formed coalitions as a strategy to influence their positions. The power of coalitions lies in their ability to bring people together from diverse perspectives around clearly defined purposes to achieve common goals. Strength lies in numbers—in working together and in strategizing for success.

In this chapter, we will compare two coalitions for health reform—one at the national level and one at the state level. The National Coalition on Health Care (National Coalition) formed in 1990. It includes over 70 national organizations ranging from the AARP through the U.S. Conference of Catholic Bishops (one nursing organization belongs—the American College of Nurse Midwives) (National Coalition on Health Care, 2010). Its purpose is to advocate for health reform that ensures access to health care for all, cost management, and quality and safety.

In 2009, the state-level coalition formed but disbanded within weeks. It was created to represent the interests of stakeholders opposing a legislative initiative aimed at insuring more Virginians through stripped-down, low-cost insurance policies. If passed, the plans would have eliminated such benefits as well-baby examinations, immunizations, diabetic test strips, hospice care, and mental health coverage. Within a day, lobbyists representing the imperiled mandated benefit groups, for individual and group plans, galvanized into a coalition (Mandate-Lite Coalition) to oppose the bill.

What factors contribute to success or failure of coalitions? How do we go about forming and maintaining coalitions? What are the ingredients? How do we know when or whether coalitions achieve their goals? This chapter details the ingredients for successful coalition building, maintenance, and success. The ingredients work in small sizes for local and regional coalitions and are equally effective in creating and sustaining larger coalitions at the local, state, national, and international levels.

BIRTH AND LIFE CYCLE OF COALITIONS

In simplest terms, a coalition is a group of individuals and/or organizations with a common interest that agree to work together toward a mutually defined goal (Berkowitz & Wolff, 2000). Spangler (2003) defines coalitions as temporary alliances of groups in order to achieve a common purpose or to engage in joint activity. Coalitions are means to achieving goals that individual members cannot easily achieve by themselves. Because of the numbers of members or groups involved, the formation of a coalition can shift the balance of power in a challenging situation. Even people who are less powerful and resourced can form coalitions that can be successful against opponents with more resources and status (Spangler, 2003).

Coalitions arise out of challenges or opportunities, and the key for all coalitions is to maintain their effectiveness until they achieve their goals. For some coalitions, the work may be completed within a matter of weeks, such as with the Mandate-Lite Coalition;

others, like the National Coalition, persist for years to address a continuing problem.

BUILDING AND MAINTAINING A COALITION: THE PRIMER

ESSENTIAL INGREDIENTS

To build and maintain an effective coalition requires four ingredients: leadership, membership, resources, and serendipity. First and foremost is leadership. Coalitions cannot exist without outstanding leadership. Leaders may exist a priori or may emerge early from the membership of the coalition, but without leaders, coalitions will falter and fade away.

Two types of leaders are critical to coalition work: inspirational and organizational. An inspiring leader uses personal strengths and power to constructively and ethically influence others to an endpoint or goal. She or he motivates others to participate and meet their obligations. The leader balances a personal inner drive to move forward while assisting coalition members to solve problems and make decisions, knowing when to steer forward, when to idle, and when to back up, if necessary (Bleich, 2007; Siek & Hague, 1992). An organized leader possesses the skills to keep members on track between meetings, ensures that communication methods are in place, and follows through on coalition assignments. Inspiration and organization may coexist in one person; but frequently two leaders are needed to serve the coalition.

As important as leaders are, they are no more important than the coalition members, without whom the coalition would not exist. Members increase the productivity of the coalition. But they also increase the potential for conflict. Members increase the visibility of the coalition, because they represent diverse constituencies and networks. Members must commit to the goals of the coalition. The extent to which members value belonging to the coalition will help, in part, to gauge their commitment and willingness to work for the groups goals. Membership should be beneficial for the coalition and the individual (Berkowitz & Wolff, 2000; Rabinowitz, 2010).

Coalitions need adequate resources to accomplish their work. Resources are the tools for the leaders and members to accomplish the coalitions' goals. They include money and in-kind donations from members and others, such as support for developing marketing materials, purchasing supplies, putting on educational sessions, and developing and maintaining websites and social media.

Finally, an essential ingredient for coalition success is serendipity—the happy occurrence of an opportunity not specifically sought—so long as coalition members take advantage of the serendipitous event or opportunity. Successful coalitions use resources at hand, devise innovative ways to sustain their work, seize opportunities that come along unexpectedly, and are willing to take risks. In order to effectively use serendipity, leaders and members must obligate themselves to conduct continual environmental scans, such as tracking current events, connecting with many different kinds of people, and spending time thinking creatively.

The National Coalition and the Mandate-Lite Coalition illustrate these ingredients. The leadership of each is strikingly different yet successful. A staff of 14 leads and manages the work of the National Coalition. The Board of Directors is led by a president with years of experience in working in non-profit organizations devoted to civil and human rights. The staff consists of lawyers, public relations specialists, and policy consultants. This coalition's leadership, therefore, consists of both inspiring and organizational leaders. The Mandate-Lite Coalition, on the other hand, congealed quickly with two lobbyists assuming informal leadership positions. Both shared roles in organization and inspiration, but in this case, organization was more critical than inspiration, because members were inspired to oppose the insurance bill. Most important in this case was to define the work, assign members to complete it, report frequently on progress, and find legislators to support them. The two informal leaders consulted with one another frequently and kept the coalition's work on track.

Membership in the two coalitions is very different. As indicated, the National Coalition has over 70 organizational members, and the Mandate-Lite Coalition consisted of lobbyists representing many of the insurance mandates and the people potentially affected by the loss of mandates (e.g., children's health, poverty law, social justice economists, hospice, hemophilia, cancer, and mental health). In the latter case, members joined out of the desire to assure that their particular mandates would not be stripped in the bill; all realized that their effectiveness would be better served by working together than separately.

The third ingredient, resources, highlights the differences in the funding for the two coalitions. In addition to the National Coalition's 501(c)(3) tax-exempt status, it has an action fund with a 501(c)(4) tax-exempt status, which enables that arm to lobby for the coalition's aims. Anyone can donate to the action fund, and the National Coalition encourages donations. These funds are not tax deductible, since they are used for lobbying purposes. The Mandate-Lite Coalition, on the other hand, had no fiscal resources. Volunteers provided the work, including a position statement (from the social justice economists), amendment language for the bill to create a requirement for an annual report of effectiveness (from the poverty law center member), and the strategy for getting the amendment introduced (from a former state senator who lobbied for one of the member groups).

Finally, the ingredient of serendipity can best be illustrated by the Mandate-Lite Coalition, which formed and achieved its work around a number of serendipitous happenings. One member tagged the bill and brought it to the attention of other stakeholders. The social justice advocates were asked to participate, and they found evidence of similar bills' ineffectiveness in other states. In addition, they performed an economic analysis and distributed it to each member of the legislative committee hearing the bill. All coalition members agreed to texting each other when they found out new information. While many of these occurrences were unplanned from the beginning of the coalition's work, all members took advantage of their potential and utilized each in conducting the work of the coalition. No chance happening was allowed to pass without someone analyzing its usefulness to achieve the coalition's goals.

COALITION STRUCTURE

Structure refers to the organization of the coalition, and it defines the procedures by which the coalition operates. The structure serves the members, not the other way around. It also includes how members are accepted, how leadership is chosen, how decisions are made, and how differences are mediated. Effective coalitions operate using group process, meaning that they go through a life cycle that involves "norming and storming" (creating group behavioral norms and

settling disagreements) before establishing group processes. Having a structure helps provide a framework for the processing that must take place in order for the coalition to be active and successful.

Coalition structure, while necessary, is dynamic, depending upon the resources and the cause. Some coalitions are highly structured, with formal committees, task forces, or work groups, and communication mechanisms; others are more loosely structured, with shared leadership and work done by ad hoc groups. Moreover, the structure may change over time, depending on the lifespan and work of the coalition. Highly structured coalitions may be necessary if the coalition work is complex and multifaceted, involving more than one goal. Committees and/or task forces may be established around the goals.

Coalition structure should make provisions for governance. This is especially true if the size exceeds 15 people. Beyond this number, the group becomes too large for effective, efficient decision-making. The governance committee should, at the very least, include all committee and work group chairs to facilitate communication. The committee should represent the diversity of the members (Smith & Bell, 1992).

No matter what coalitions call themselves or how they structure themselves, an important factor to achieving goals is to engage appropriate support systems. Someone must agree to do a task, and that someone should have the means to get the task done. The work may be done by volunteers, as it is in many coalitions. However, there may be consequences to all-volunteer efforts. Often, paid staff can deliver on the tasks and move the coalition along more effectively, especially when the work is complex and multifaceted.

DECISION-MAKING

Decision-making is a source of great concern, usually at the beginning of a coalition's life. Because members represent different constituencies and perspectives, they will often not trust one another. Everyone wants to protect his or her own interests. As the coalition decides on its mission and goals, it also has to figure out how it will make its decisions. Most often, decisions are made without voting by consensus; members simply agree or disagree. However, when decisions are close, coalition members should step back and discuss the situation again. When one is operating on consensus, the coalition members must come to a decision with which all are comfortable. What frequently happens is that alternative solutions are offered until one is made to which all can agree. Consensus building is by nature time-consuming, but it fosters involvement and buy-in from all the coalition members, and coming to consensus requires leadership skill and finesse (Berkowitz & Wolff, 2000).

MEETINGS

Coalitions must meet; otherwise, the work doesn't get done. People come to coalition meetings for at least two reasons—to get work done and to make social connections. The meetings must combine both, in just the right combination, to keep people coming back.

The interval between meetings and the time of meetings is very important. The time interval should be long enough for members to accomplish their assignments. Meetings should consist ideally of presenting alternatives for action and making decisions. If the interval between meetings is too long, little interim work will get done, as the human response is to wait until right before a meeting to complete an assignment. The leader should confirm with members the amount of time each will need to get the work accomplished in the interim and then schedule the next meeting accordingly.

The content of the meeting should be focused on problem solving and decision-making. There should be a sense among members that work is being done and decisions made; otherwise, results-oriented members will soon stop attending meetings. A good meeting has energy. If the meeting is primarily conducted to exchange information, some members will see this as a waste of their time, and they may drop out. Alternatives such as e-mail and electronic bulletin boards exist for disseminating information. Consequently, coalition leaders and members should regularly assess the content of the meetings to see what works and what doesn't and to make necessary adjustments.

PROMOTING THE COALITION

What good is a coalition if no one knows it exists? Coalitions are formed to advance a common agenda, and communication is the vehicle with which that agenda is advanced. Early on in the coalition's life, members must develop and implement a communications plan aimed at getting the coalition's message out to the broader community of interest. The plan should include branding (i.e., logo and tag line), ways to reach intended audiences (i.e., website and social marketing venues, such as Facebook and Twitter), and assigning individuals to keep the communication up-to-date and vibrant.

FUNDING

Coalition work takes money. Some coalitions, like the Mandate-Lite Coalition, run on little or no money, using the time and talent of their members. These coalitions may be unable to sustain their work over the long haul because of lack of resources. Generally speaking, coalitions will need to look for additional funds to stay solvent and accomplish their work. How much money is needed depends on several factors. First are the mission and aims of the coalition. Second, the strategic plan will define the resources needed; then members can decide how to best obtain the funds. Third, members should develop a fund-raising plan that includes tailoring the message to prospective funding sources, assigning people to make the contacts, communicating the mission and aims of the coalition, and seeking funding.

PITFALLS AND CHALLENGES

Coalitions usually start out with a flurry of excitement and activity. Leadership plays a critical role in sustaining the excitement and guiding the activity. Nevertheless, coalition work is difficult and complex, with lots of challenges. Following are some common pitfalls and challenges, with suggestions for overcoming them.

FAILURE TO GET THE RIGHT PEOPLE TO PARTICIPATE

Coalitions should attract those who are most interested in seeing that the work gets done, and these members will commit to participating in the coalition. At regular intervals, coalitions should assess who is "at the table" and who is not. The following two common membership errors exist: First is the error of exclusion of an entire group of stakeholders. In examining the purpose of the coalition, members should ask themselves these questions: "Who have we excluded?" "Whose expertise do we need?" "Who may work to derail the coalition's work if not invited to become a member?"

The second error in coalition membership is not achieving buy-in from major players, like the "800-pound gorillas." Coalition members should identify these individuals/organizations and seek their buy-in. For example, a nursing coalition that does not include the major leaders or associations may have difficulty advancing its agenda.

CULTURAL AND LANGUAGE DIFFERENCES AMONG COALITION MEMBERS

Because coalition members represent different perspectives on the goals and mission of the coalition, all must learn the meaning of significant words used by coalition members. Sometimes simple words carry completely different connotations, such as the word *time* for nurse administrators (who operate day-to-day) and nurse educators (who operate by semesters). Coalition leaders and members must continually be attuned to words that have different connotations, and they should agree on a common definition (if possible) or agree to understand the differences in the meaning of words.

PERSISTENT DISTRUST AMONG COALITION MEMBERS

Distrust is perhaps one of the thorniest challenges that coalition leaders face, because much of the success of coalitions comes from the ongoing interaction among members that allays misperceptions and builds trust. When members become disengaged from coalition work, their absence can derail progress, especially if they fail to keep their own constituencies informed. Another source of distrust emanates from long-standing perceived inequalities among members, such as active membership of licensed practical nurses or certified nursing assistants in a nursing coalition. To overcome distrust, leaders and members must work diligently on including these potentially disenfranchised members. In the end, people must feel valued and treasured for all their participation and contributions to the enterprise.

CONTROL FREAKS AND PROTECTING TURF

The tendency to control and protect turf can happen at the individual member level and at the coalition level. At the individual level, there are those in whom coalition success breeds a new brand of person—one who knows "the truth" and is always willing to share it. These individuals need to be gathered back into the fold and made to feel that their ideas are worthy, but at the same time, they must understand that they do not possess all the answers to the work at hand. At the coalition level, successful coalitions may easily rest on past achievement and ignore the need for retooling for ongoing challenges. Hence, competing coalitions may form, leading to turf protection and dysfunctional competing coalitions.

POOR HANDLING OF DIFFERENT PERSPECTIVES

By their very nature, coalitions consist of individuals representing constituencies with differing perspectives on issues. For example, hospital associations are concerned with adequate reimbursement from insurers; quality, safety, and risk management; surpassing their current market edge; and maintaining an adequate nursing workforce to preserve patient safety and quality of care. Nurses associations' primary advocacy concerns are about the practice of registered nurses, including staffing and standards and ethics of nursing practice. Consequently, the perspectives of hospitals and nursing associations frequently differ over practice issues such as mandatory overtime and staffing ratios. Both types of organizations are concerned with quality and safety of care, thus working together can be most effective in creating solutions. Coalition leaders and members have an obligation to recognize points of contention and determine how they will be handled—by consensus, compromise, or agreeing to avoid the conflict if it is not essential to the work of the coalition (Siek & Hague, 1992).

FAILURE TO ACT

Coalitions begin with fire in their bellies. Unfortunately, going from words to action is sometimes more difficult than members had originally thought. Some coalitions formulate and reformulate action plans ad infinitum without getting to the action piece. However, action is the coalition's currency. Without action, there will be no resources to support the work. At least two factors contribute to failure to act. One is lack of leadership, and the other is the inability for the coalition to coalesce around solutions. To resolve the leadership issue, new leaders will have to emerge. Resolving the consensus issue requires a regrouping and reexamination of the purposes of the coalition and an analysis of whether or not any consensus can be achieved.

LOSING BALANCE

Coalition leaders and members wear out. Managing, leading, and working in coalitions drain energy. All members are entitled to personal lives and must know that they do not have to keep their coalition jobs for life. Each person must assess his or her readiness to step aside and support the leadership and membership activities of new recruits. Therefore, coalitions should set in place a means for leadership succession planning at regular intervals.

POLITICAL WORK OF COALITIONS

Should coalitions speak out on issues that matter to them? Should nursing coalitions speak out for nursing? Of course they should. But advocacy work has its downsides and upsides.

REASONS NOT TO ADVOCATE

When coalitions advocate for certain positions, they run into opposition from stakeholders who diverge from those positions. The further coalitions go out on the limb, the more people line up to saw off the limb. In fact, coalitions stand to lose their financial support if they go too far. In addition, there are legal restrictions on advocacy by tax-exempt groups in lobbying, so coalitions may be forced to pull back if they become too forcefully active. Therefore, coalitions should choose their battles carefully, making certain that they are willing to accept the consequences of winning or losing (Bowers-Lanier, 2010).

REASONS TO ADVOCATE

Nursing and other health care coalitions that are established to advocate for particular legislative or policy initiatives will be successful if the initiatives are enacted into law or become established policies. When that happens, the coalition will have met its goal, and it may disband. Alternatively, it may envision another goal and begin work toward accomplishing that.

HOW TO ADVOCATE WITH GRACE

The solution, of course, is to proceed with care. By its very nature, advocacy involves risk. Coalition members should work out their differences and carefully select the words they will use when advocating for positions. Coalition members should agree in advance on the advocacy approaches they will take

TABLE 86-1 Coalition Formative Evaluation

Evaluation Type	Questions to Be Answered
Formative	Questions to be asked at a regular basis (by meeting, monthly, quarterly at maximum) <ul><li>Membership<ul><li>Are the right member organizations at the table?</li><li>Who is missing?</li><li>Are all equal players?</li><li>Why or why not?</li></ul></li><li>Coalition work<ul><li>How is it being accomplished?</li><li>Is there a better way to do the work?</li><li>What is it?</li><li>How would we know?</li></ul></li><li>What are the barriers and facilitators to goal achievement?</li><li>Is the work plan on schedule?<ul><li>How can the barriers be minimized?</li><li>How can the facilitators be maximized?</li></ul></li></ul>
Summative	Semi-annually or annually: Goal achievement <ul><li>Have the goals been achieved?<ul><li>Why or why not?</li><li>What strategies should be changed?</li></ul></li><li>Are the goals still relevant to the mission of the coalitions? Why or why not?</li><li>Has the coalition achieved its stated goal? Should it be disbanded? Why or why not?</li><li>Is there additional work to be done and the will to do it?</li></ul>

that will not jeopardize their legal status as well as disenfranchise funders and members.

EVALUATING COALITION EFFECTIVENESS

Coalitions should evaluate their effectiveness on a regular basis. Evaluation helps to keep members on track, determine strengths and areas for improvement, and in the final analysis, determine whether the coalitions' goals are met or if further work is needed. Evaluation should be both formative (assessing the progress of the coalition on a continual and regular basis such as after each meeting) and summative (assessing the status of coalition deliverables after a defined period of time such as annually) and should occur at regular intervals. Stakeholders create coalitions to bring diverse groups of people together around a common cause. Table 86-1 lists the questions governing formative and summative coalition evaluation.

Coalition work can be extremely exciting and fulfilling. By bringing together individuals who represent varying perspectives, coalitions can achieve their goals through active involvement of these diverse members and their constituencies. Leaders must emerge or be selected who are passionate about the cause and who can simultaneously attend to detail and create an organized structure for the coalition work. Coalitions must meet regularly and take action on their decisions. In the end, coalitions must determine how and when to advocate for their mission and evaluate their effectiveness in order to stay viable.

For a list of related websites, please refer to your Evolve Resources at http://evolve.elsevier.com/Mason/policypolitics/

REFERENCES

Berkowitz, B., & Wolff, T. (2000). *The spirit of the coalition*. Washington, D.C.: American Public Health Association.

Bleich, M. (2007). Managing and leading. In P. Yoder-Wise (Ed.), *Leading and managing in nursing* (4th ed., pp. 2-20). St. Louis: Mosby.

Bowers-Lanier, R., (2010). Advocacy in the public arena. In K. A. Polifko (Ed.), *The practice environment of nursing* (pp. 565-592). Clifton Park, NY: Delmar Cengage Learning.

National Coalition on Health Care. (2010). Retrieved from http://nchc.org.

Rabinowitz, P. (2010). Coalition building I: Starting a coalition. In Wolff, T., *Community tool box*. Retrieved from http://ctb.ku.edu/en/tablecontents/section_1057.htm.

Siek, G., & Hague, C. E. (1992). Building coalitions: Turf issues. Retrieved from http://wch.uhs.wisc.edu/docs/PDF-Pubs/TurfIssues-12.pdf.

Smith, P., & Bell, C. H. (1992). Building coalitions: Structure. Retrieved from http://wch.uhs.wisc.edu/docs/PDF-Pubs/Structure-11.pdf.

Spangler, B. (2003). Coalition building. In G. Burgess & H. Burgess (Eds.), *Beyond intractability*. Retrieved from www.beyondintractability.org/essay/coalition_building.

CHAPTER 87

TAKING ACTION
A Rough Road in Texas: Advanced Practice Nurses Build a Strong Coalition

Lynda Woolbert

"You will never change anything by talking to your-selves. Stop complaining to other APNs and start edu-cating people who can help fix the problem."

—Kathy Hutto

ALL IS NOT ROSY IN TEXAS

All advanced practice nursing legislation introduced in Texas from 1979 to 1985 was defeated. Texas advanced practice nurses (APNs) finally got physician-delegated prescriptive authority in 1989. This passed only with stipulations that APNs work sites that serve certain medically underserved popula-tions and because Texas would have lost federal funds if it hadn't passed (Texas Nurses Association, 2009).

Four women changed the political balance of power for Texas APNs. Elaine Brightwater, a certified nurse midwife (CNM); Carol Cody and Zo DeMarchi, both women's health nurse practitioners (WHNPs); and Ira Gunn, a certified registered nurse anesthetist (CRNA), advocated at the Texas State Capitol for their respective advanced practice nursing (APN) organi-zations. They recognized the need to hire a lobbyist to focus on APN issues and to have a policy group directly accountable to their organizations. The nurses knew legislation that was good for nurse practitioners (NPs) and clinical nurse specialists (CNSs) sometimes undermined the practices of CNMs and CRNAs, so this new group had to balance the needs and interests of the four APN roles.

THE COALITION FOR NURSES IN ADVANCED PRACTICE IS BORN

In 1991, the four APNs met with a few others to devise a plan to obtain funding and support from their orga-nization's boards and members. They desired to form a coalition of APN organizations and hire a lobbyist. By November 1991, these goals were accomplished. By 1992, the Coalition for Nurses in Advanced Practice (the CNAP or the Coalition) had officers, and it was incorporated and designated as a 501(c)(6) organiza-tion. The CNAP was, and remains, a coalition of Texas APN organizations. The group's primary purpose is to advocate for APNs at the Texas legisla-ture and with Texas regulatory agencies. The CNAP has no individual members and is accountable to its member organization's boards. Each board deter-mines how much it contributes and names represen-tatives to attend CNAP meetings.

THE COALITION'S OPERATING PROCEDURES

The CNAP operates on consensus. If a decision has the potential to harm any group of APNs, the Coali-tion does not pursue it without specific approval by the group that might be harmed. It is a "one for all and all for one" philosophy set forth in the operat-ing principles adopted in February 1992 (CNAP, 1992). These principles have never been amended

---

BOX 87-1 **The Coalition for Nurses in Advanced Practice: Objectives**

1. Expand prescriptive authority.
2. Ensure clinical privileging with due process.
3. Increase third-party reimbursement.

---

and serve to keep the CNAP true to its roots. The structure is nimble and produces swift decisions when needed.

The consensus model is a key to the CNAP's continued existence and success. The leaders who established the CNAP knew that power must be balanced among the four APN groups. CNAP representatives need to have a good understanding of each other's practices to make wise policy decisions. To that end, the initial CNAP representatives educated the lobbyist and each other about each APN role's history, legal framework for practice, and resulting practice barriers, as well as the history and structure of each member organization.

THE COALITION'S OBJECTIVES

Kathy Hutto, the Coalition's principal lobbyist, led the transition from talk to action. She said, "It's been important to learn about your practices and the barriers you work around to take care of your patients. Now it's time to figure out what to do about it. You need to identify three goals to focus our efforts." Three broad objectives were defined that remain the core of the CNAP's legislative and regulatory work today (Box 87-1). The three-pronged approach serves APNs well. In years when the Coalition cannot make progress in one area, representatives focus on one or both of the others. Kathy Hutto gave CNAP representatives another valuable insight regarding taking action: "You will never change anything by talking to yourselves. Stop complaining to other APNs and start educating people who can help fix the problem."

ACTION LEADS TO ACCOMPLISHMENT

In 1992, the Texas Medicaid program reimbursed only four types of APNs. CNMs were reimbursed at 65% of the physician's fee, and CRNAs, FNPs, and PNPs were reimbursed at 70% of the physician's level. APNs wanted to expand Medicaid coverage to include all types of NPs and CNSs and increase the reimbursement rate to 100% for all categories of APNs. The Texas Medical Association opposed those changes. At the time, the Texas Department of Human Services Board approved the types of Medicaid providers and their reimbursement rates. Most of the Human Services Board members were not familiar with advanced nursing practice. APNs were selected to testify at a hearing on the matter, and Kathy Hutto, the lobbyist, helped them prepare testimony. Critical work occurred before the hearing. CNAP members educated board members, while Kathy Hutto and others met with Texas Medicaid staff. Supportive board members were asked to discuss the issue with other members and were encouraged to ask questions that reinforced information favorable to APNs. The CNAP left the Human Services Board hearing with a substantial win that day. All APN categories would be reimbursed at 85% of the physician's fee.

THE COALITION'S CHALLENGES

FUNDING

Any organization that retains lobbyists requires a healthy revenue stream. The CNAP does not have that. The Coalition values the participation of essential APN stakeholders over money, and minimum dues to join are only $500. Member organizations contribute in proportion to their membership and ability. The CNAP relies on contributions from individual APNs; those represent about half of the Coalition's income.

NEGOTIATING BOUNDARIES WITH ESTABLISHED ORGANIZATIONS

The CNAP negotiates relationships with a number of organizations. When it was established, it intruded on the Texas Nurses Association's "turf." A mediator helped the parties develop a good working relationship. The Coalition must actively maintain relationships with its member organizations. The CNAP bears the responsibility for delivering unique services and consistently articulating the value of its services to member organizations so they continue to recognize the Coalition's value.

TABLE 87-1 Number of Texas Advanced Practice Nurses and Physicians and Their Affiliated Lobbyists

| Provider Group | NUMBER IN TEXAS (2009) | |
	Providers	Lobbyists[c]
APNs (All)	10,801 (unduplicated)[a]	8
CRNAs	2,298[a]	
CNMs	287[a]	
CNSs	1,293[a]	
NPs	6,923[a]	
Physicians	47,759[b]	49

Sources: [a]Numbers of APNs are from "Currently Licensed Texas RNs Recognized as Advanced Practice Nurses by Country and Recognition Group," by Texas Board of Nursing, September 1, 2009. Retrieved from *www.bon.state.tx.us/about/stats/09-apn.pdf.*
[b]Number of physicians is from "Physicians In and Out of State," by the Texas Medical Board, September 2009. Retrieved from *www.tmb.state.tx.us/agency/statistics/demo/docs/d2009/0909/inout.php.*
[c]Lobbyist data is from "Lobby Lists & Reports," by Texas Ethics Commission, 2009. Retrieved from *www.ethics.state.tx.us/dfs/loblists.htm.*

THE OPPOSITION

The biggest challenge the CNAP faces is also the reason it exists. The Texas Medical Association (TMA) has 43,000 members (Texas Medical Association, 2009). Through its county medical societies, TMA has a network of physicians that keep legislators informed about medicine's issues. In 2009, TMA had 27 lobbyists, and an additional 22 lobbyists represented other medical associations (Texas Ethics Commission, 2009). In contrast, CNAP member organizations had about 6000 individual members and 8 lobbyists (Table 87-1).

BUILDING INFLUENCE WITH LIMITED RESOURCES

When the CNAP was established, most Texas state policymakers had never heard of APNs. This has changed dramatically due to CNAP's efforts to include APNs in legislation and rule making where appropriate. CNAP's strategy to influence policy with limited resources used these guidelines:

DEFINE WHAT IS WANTED

Kathy Hutto's direction to define three goals exemplifies the principle of identifying and succinctly articulating the group's goals.

USE GRASSROOTS STRATEGIES FOR STATEWIDE SUCCESS

There is one way to overcome overwhelming odds in politics: effective constituents. APN constituents who create positive relationships with legislators, through work in campaigns and with regular contact, are at the top of the influence pyramid with that legislator. The work of educating and motivating APNs to develop relationships with legislators is ongoing. The CNAP asks APNs to give their fair share. They are asked to make seven contacts with their legislators in each 2-year election cycle.

HIRE THE RIGHT LOBBYIST

The CNAP's founders interviewed Kathy Hutto after getting recommendations from lobbyists, legislators, and their staff. Kathy represents a variety of businesses and associations and maintains a portfolio of 10 to 15 clients. The Coalition benefits from her legislative expertise and the power she generates by lobbying for other clients that are much larger and have more PAC money than the Coalition.

FIND AN AFFORDABLE WAY TO BE A VISIBLE PART OF A POLITICAL ACTION COMMITTEE

The CNAP never formed its own political action committee (PAC) because of complex ethics rules and reporting requirements. Instead, the Coalition became a sponsoring organization of the RN PAC. In return, for sharing administrative expenses and adding to the contributor base, the RN PAC gave APNs recognition by changing its name to the Texas RN/APN PAC.

FOCUS ON REGULATION AS MUCH AS LEGISLATION

During legislative sessions, in addition to advocating for APN legislation, the CNAP also tracks at least 300 bills and asks for amendments to include RNs or APNs whenever appropriate (usually 20 to 25 bills per session). On average, about 7 bills pass each session that contain amendments sought by CNAP lobbyists. The CNAP also monitors the *Texas Register,* the weekly publication that includes all proposed and adopted state agency rules. The Coalition comments on proposed rules to include APNs whenever appropriate. At least three or four times a year, state agencies amend rules based on the CNAP's comments. State agencies ask the Coalition to attend stakeholder meetings, and APNs have the opportunity to shape the language in draft rules.

SUMMARY

The CNAP was born from frustration with the status quo and a vision for a better future for APNs and their patients. The Coalition was the first statewide advanced practice nursing coalition of its kind. Today, it remains the driving force for legislative and regulatory change for APNs in Texas. The CNAP exists because strong opposition creates a shared need for APN organizations to band together to achieve goals. The Coalition provides governmental expertise, concentrates power for all APN groups, and provides important services for member organizations. To stay viable, the CNAP always balances member's interests

and clearly communicates the value it brings to individual APNs and APN organizations throughout Texas.

For a list of related websites, please refer to your Evolve Resources at http://evolve.elsevier.com/Mason/policypolitics/

REFERENCES

Coalition for Nurses in Advanced Practice [CNAP]. (1992). Operating principles. Retrieved from www.cnaptexas.org/displaycommon.cfm?an=1&subarticle nbr=8.
Texas Ethics Commission. (2009). Search lobbyist clients. Retrieved from http://webdev.ethics.state.tx.us/search/lobby_search.cfm#Clients.
Texas Medical Association. (2009). Your voice, your vision, your TMA. Retrieved from www.texmed.org/Template.aspx?id=88.
Texas Nurses Association. (2009). History of Texas Nursing Practice Act. Retrieved from www.texasnurses.org/displaycommon.cfm?an=1&subartic lenbr=156.

CHAPTER 88

TAKING ACTION
The National Coalition for Lesbian, Gay, Bisexual, and Transgender Health

Scott Weber, Rebecca Fox, and David Haltiwanger

"The good we secure for ourselves is precarious and uncertain until it is secured for all of us and incorporated into our common life."

—Jane Addams

Health disparities have been noted in a number of ethnic and racial minority groups in the United States. It is now recognized that lesbian, gay, bisexual, and transgender (LGBT) individuals may experience the same type of poorer health and health outcomes. As with other groups, this is partly explained by differences in access to health care, lack of knowledge regarding the health issues of the LGBT community, and, sometimes, overt discrimination. The National Coalition for LGBT Health (the Coalition) was established to respond to a lack of focus in clinical care and research on sexual orientation and gender identity minorities—and their health needs. In addition, there was a perceived need for an organization to engage in public policy advocacy for the LGBT populations. Research literature and clinical case studies were demonstrating variations in health behavior as well as disparities in access to care among these groups (Harris Interactive, 2008). The HIV/AIDS crisis, which inordinately affects younger gay men, helped to bring a focus to the health of sexual minorities. Research has begun to demonstrate significantly higher risks for sexually transmitted infections, substance use, partner violence and abuse, and some cancers in LGBT populations (Hidalgo, Peterson & Woodman, 1985; Marmot & Wilkinson, 1999; Diamant, Wold, & Spritzer, 2000; Dean, et al., 2000; Ellis, Bradford, & Honnold, 2001; Linde, 2003; Bradford, 2005; Makadon, 2006; Makadon, Mayer, Potter, & Goldhammer, 2008). More recent research is examining disparities in senior care as well as parenting identity development and family planning among LGBT adolescents and young adults.

THE COALITION'S HISTORY

The Coalition, headquartered in Washington, D.C., was formed on October 14, 2000, when a group of community health advocates from across the U.S. convened in the nation's capital to discuss the need for including LGBT health issues in the federal government's *Healthy People 2010* objectives. At that meeting, we recognized that a coordinating structure was needed to advance our interests at the White House, as well as in the U.S. Department of Health and Human Services, Congress, and elsewhere. Many of the participants at that first meeting knew each other from conferences put on by the National Lesbian and Gay Health Association, an organization that had ceased to exist due to organizational problems. Learning from that group's demise, the leaders of the Coalition committed to a primary focus on advocacy, especially LGBT health advocacy within the federal government. We were committed to running a lean operation—beginning with a single full-time employee. In the beginning, the Coalition used donated office space at an LGBT community health center. In 2005, we moved into our own office space,

637

BOX 88-1 **Long-Range Goals of the National Coalition for Lesbian, Gay, Bisexual, and Transgender Health**

1. Increase knowledge regarding LGBT populations' health status, access to and utilization of health care, and other health-related information.
2. Increase LGBT participation in the formation of public- and private-sector policy regarding health and related issues.
3. Increase availability of, access to, and quality of physical, mental, and behavioral health and related services for the LGBT population.
4. Increase professional and cultural competencies of providers and others engaged in health and social service delivery to the LGBT population.
5. Eliminate disparities in health outcomes of LGBT populations and the community including differences that occur by gender, race/ethnicity, education or income, disability, nationality, geographic location, age, sexual orientation, gender identity, or presentation.

---

became incorporated, and successfully pursued obtaining 501(c)(3) non-profit status.

By obtaining grants from foundations, we've increased our resources and expanded our staff. With more personnel, we now have the ability to carry out policy analysis and to take the lead in federal advocacy in pursuit of the Coalition's agenda. The coalition's work is focused on five areas: (1) research, (2) policy, (3) programs and services, (4) professional and cultural competency, and (5) diversity of the national LGBT community (Box 88-1).

MEMBERS, AFFILIATES, AND STAFF MEMBERS

The Coalition has 65 organizational members and 50 individuals. The organizations include national LGBT and HIV/AIDS groups, community health centers, community centers, and departments of health. Individual members tend to be researchers or activists concerned with LGBT health. The Coalition works with these groups in different ways. For example, the Coalition works with national LGBT organizations to increase their focus on health as a social justice issue. For local groups without an advocacy arm, the Coalition connects them into federal policy and advocacy work.

Increasing numbers of nurses are involved in the work of the Coalition through participation in research projects; participation in policy advocacy work at federal, state, and local levels; service on the board of directors and other committee work; and personal or organizational memberships.

THE COALITION'S ACCOMPLISHMENTS

The Coalition works on multiple levels within Congress, the Administration, federal Agencies, and the LGBT community and its allies. This work has included such issues as *Healthy People 2010* and *Healthy People 2020*, working with the Substance Abuse and Mental Health Services Administration (SAMHSA), health care reform, and LGBT data collection.

THE COALITION'S OBJECTIVES IN HEALTHY PEOPLE 2010

Healthy People 2010 was the catalyst for the formation of the Coalition. *Healthy People* provides science-based, 10-year national objectives for promoting health and preventing disease (U.S. Department of Health and Human Services, 2009). We believed it was vital that LGBT health objectives be included in this program, which is viewed as a blueprint for improving the Nation's health (Box 88-2).

The Coalition succeeded in maintaining LGBT health objectives in *Healthy People 2010*. Advocacy strategies included regular contact with the leadership of the *Healthy People 2010* agencies responsible for the maintenance and evaluation of *Healthy People 2010's* impact. We participated in meetings with the U.S. Surgeon General and staff from the U.S. Department of Health and Human Services, Office of Disease Prevention and Health Promotion.

HEALTHY PEOPLE 2020

Healthy People 2020 is the federal government's plan for the road ahead. The Coalition has had a great deal of success around *Healthy People 2020*. We sent five press releases to LGBT-specific press outlets and obtained media coverage in Atlanta's LGBT newspaper, *Southern Voice*. The Coalition rallied members to participate in public forums organized by the Department of Health and Human Services *Healthy People 2020*. The organization created six documents to aid

BOX 88-2 Guiding Principles for Lesbian, Gay, Bisexual, and Transgender Inclusion in Healthcare Reform

Healthcare access must be assured to all persons regardless of sexual orientation, gender identity, gender, gender expression, or disorder of sex differentiation/intersex.

Healthcare services access and payment coverage must include a full range of legal reproductive health services, including family planning and pregnancy termination services, regardless of ability of patients to pay for these services.

The organization of the U.S. healthcare system must include a robust public insurance option that can effectively complete with private insurers to reduce costs, improve access to care, and maintain or improve care quality.

Opportunities and funding for health research must include programs that include a focus on health disparities of LGBT adults and adolescents.

Opportunities and funding for education and training of clinical care providers, including nurses, physicians, dentists, behavioral health specialists, and other health professionals, must include a focus on sensitivity toward and cultural competence of services to LGBT adults and adolescents.

Federal, state, and local data reporting and analysis systems must include key clinical and financial information elements that are relevant to LGBT adults and adolescents, including collecting and aggregate analyzing data regarding sexual orientation, gender identity, and relationship recognition status of all patients.

Healthcare services for Americans who are sexual orientation or gender identity minorities must preserve the confidentiality, privacy, and dignity of all LGBT patients.

Military personnel seeking medical care in military hospitals must be able to be open, honest, and complete about their sexual orientation or gender identity when seeking services and not fear risking discharge from the military services.

Source: Scott Weber, December 2009.

our members' work, including fact sheets, press releases, and talking point briefs. This work had a clear impact on the development of *Healthy People 2020*. LGBT health concerns were the second most frequently discussed topic at the *Healthy People* public forums. This prominence, in conjunction with testimony from the Coalition's Executive Director, led the HHS Secretary's Advisory Committee overseeing the development of *Healthy People 2020* to include sexual orientation as a key factor in America's health disparities. The Coalition also focused on increasing the amount of data collection on LGBT health and health disparities. The Coalition has advocated for the inclusion of standard LGBT demographic items on several federal health surveys, such as the National Health Interview Survey (NHIS).

WORK WITH THE PRESIDENTIAL TRANSITION TEAM

The Coalition met many times with then–President-elect Barack Obama's Presidential Transition Team (PTT) in late 2008 and early 2009. The Coalition hosted and coordinated the first-ever meeting with a PTT focused solely on LGBT health concerns. In addition, the PTT invited the Coalition to participate in conference calls on LGBT and HIV/AIDS issues. The Coalition was the only organization to speak at these meetings on the needs of transgender individuals. The Coalition was the only LGBT group invited to participate in PTT meetings focused on women's health and minority health that included the president-elect's top domestic policy staff. At each of these meetings, the Coalition presented its *Guiding Principles for LGBT Inclusion in Healthcare Reform*. This document lays out a comprehensive policy outline for ensuring the inclusion of LGBT concerns at all levels of the health care reform process. These meetings have continued with Coalition participation in meetings on health disparities, data collection, and health care reform.

LESBIAN, GAY, BISEXUAL, AND TRANSGENDER CULTURAL COMPETENCY CURRICULUM

The Coalition has worked as the lead organization to advocate for and develop a curriculum produced by the Substance Abuse and Mental Health Service Administration (SAMHSA). SAMHSA is an agency of the U.S. Department of Health and Human Services (HHS) that focuses on the lives of people with or at risk for mental health and substance abuse disorders. This curriculum enables providers of substance abuse and treatment services to train staff to become culturally competent when working with the LGBT community. The lack of LGBT-sensitive and -competent treatment providers is a critical problem given the widespread nature of this issue within the LGBT community. It is important for clinicians and researchers to understand the definitions of key terms as well as identified privacy and access concerns. Many LGBT individuals prefer to obtain care and services from providers who already have some awareness, sensitivity, and science-based knowledge of health concerns of the community. In the case of medical care of transgender individuals, relatively few physicians and other clinicians are well trained in this highly developed and specialized area of medicine. Without the work of the Coalition, this curriculum would not have been created to address the LGBT community's needs.

RAISING AWARENESS

In 2003, the Coalition launched the First Annual LGBT Health Awareness Week via an online and media campaign addressing health issues of cancer, domestic violence, smoking, mental health, HPV, hepatitis immunization, nutrition and weight, and sexual health. The Coalition has since produced this every year as a tool to educate members of the LGBT community and those who provide health care to them.

The Coalition continues to grow and flourish. The organization marked its tenth anniversary in 2010 by continuing extensive outreach to grow its membership base and expand its policy reach, and continuing to bridge the gap between the LGBT movement and health advocacy. The Coalition remains committed to its core vision of improving the health and well-being of lesbian, gay, bisexual, and transgender individuals and communities. It will achieve its vision through public education, coalition building, and advocacy efforts that focus on research, policy, education, and training. The Coalition remains dedicated to the concept that its ability to effect change will be determined by our bringing together the rich diversity of the LGBT community at a national level—across gender/gender identity, race/ethnicity, disability, education, income, age, and geography.

For a list of related websites, please refer to your Evolve Resources at http://evolve.elsevier.com/Mason/policypolitics/

REFERENCES

Bradford, J. (2005). *Lesbian health in the U.S.: Our foundation and our future.* Gay and Lesbian Health Association.

Dean, L., Meyer, I. H., Robinson, K., Sell, R. L., Sember, R., et al. (2000). Lesbian, gay, bisexual and transgender health findings and concerns. *Journal of the Gay and Lesbian Medical Association, 4*(3), 102-151.

Diamant, A. L., Wold, C., Spritzer, K., & Gelberg, L. (2000). Health behaviors, health status, and access to and use of health care: A population-based study of lesbian, bisexual, and heterosexual women. *Archives of Family Medicine, 9*(10), 1043-1051.

Ellis, J. M., Bradford, J. B., & Honnold, J. (2001). Identification and description of lesbians living in households reporting same-sex partnerships using micro-data samples. Paper presented at the National Lesbian Health Research Conference, San Francisco.

Harris Interactive, "Nearly one in four gay and lesbian adults lack health insurance," May 19, 2008, Retrieved from http://reuters.com/article/pressRelease/idUS141734+19-May-2008+BW20080519.

Hidalgo, H., Peterson, T. I., & Woodman, N. J. (Eds.). (1985). *Lesbian and gay issues: A resource manual for social workers.* National Association of Social Workers.

Linde, R., The Fenway Institute & the GLBT Health Access Project. (2003). *Gay, lesbian, bisexual and transgender health access training project participant resource manual.* Boston: The GLBT Health Access Project.

Makadon, H. J. (2006). Improving healthcare for the lesbian and gay communities. *New England Journal of Medicine, 354*(9), 895-897.

Makadon, H. J., Mayer, K. H., Potter, J., & Goldhammer, H. (Eds.). (2008). *Fenway guide to lesbian, gay, bisexual and transgender health.* Philadelphia: American College of Physicians.

Marmot, M. & Wilkinson, R. (1999). *Social determinants of health.* New York: Oxford University Press.

U.S. Department of Health and Human Services. (2009). Healthy people. Retrieved from www.healthypeople.gov/HP2020.

CHAPTER 89

TAKING ACTION
The Virginia Nursing Kitchen Cabinet

Judith B. Collins and Rebecca (Rice) Bowers-Lanier

"The activist is not the man who says the river is dirty. The activist is the man who cleans up the river."

—Ross Perot

In the mid-1990s, Virginia nurse leaders began a journey toward speaking with one voice for nurses and nursing in the public policy arena. This chapter chronicles the journey focusing on the development and growth of the "Nurses' Kitchen Cabinet," a loosely organized group of nurse leaders committed to a common nursing policy agenda during the 2005 gubernatorial campaign. We also discuss the ensuring influence of nursing in gubernatorial health policy reflected over a 4-year administration. Finally, we discuss the important factors contributing toward the success of the Kitchen Cabinet and lessons learned for the future.

THE CONTEXT

Our journey began with nurse leaders' commitment to working together in the policy arena. We had already strengthened the Virginia Nurses Association's commitment to working with all nurses and nursing organizations; formed the Legislative Coalition of Virginia Nurses (LCVN); broadened the membership in the Nurses' PAC (N-PAC, the political action committee for nurses in the state); and established a tax-exempt public-private partnership, the Virginia Partnership for Nursing (VPN), to develop and implement nursing workforce development activities.

By 2005, the LCVN, the VPN, and the N-PAC still had not attained a "tipping point" in advancing public policies supporting the profession despite their successes in bringing nurses together around legislative activity, launching statewide campaigns for nurse education and recruitment, and contributing to campaigns. Our goal was to make certain that the gubernatorial candidates knew nursing's platform and included nurses in health policy decisions in the executive branch. To accomplish this, Virginia nurses created the Kitchen Cabinet.

The mission of the Kitchen Cabinet was to educate the candidates about the nursing shortage, propose solutions, influence political campaigns, and change public policy. The members were volunteer nurse opinion leaders who were passionate about the mission and able to be dynamic and agile as the process unfolded. All nursing stakeholders were at the table—practice, education, associations, regulators, and policy influencers. The methods required the Kitchen Cabinet to separate policy development from electoral politics for action. Thus, though members differed on political persuasion, the Cabinet developed a common policy platform.

THE POLICY DEVELOPMENT

The Kitchen Cabinet agreed on a plan to work together to develop a consensus, nonpartisan policy platform (Box 89-1). The process of policy development entailed hearing from and acting on the requests from the VPN, which includes all stakeholders in nursing practice, and the state's educational programs.

The first request, from the VPN, focused on creating a center for nursing workforce development. The Commonwealth had no ongoing systematic process for collecting and analyzing data about the supply and demand for nurses. Without adequate data, workforce planning had been based on national and anecdotal workforce data. In 2000, we had successfully lobbied for a one-time appropriation to study the nursing workforce; the report was completed in 2001. It served as a catalyst for subsequent work on nursing education, particularly at the associate degree level. But the data collection and analysis were not sustained subsequently.

The second request centered on obtaining funds to support an increase in educational capacity. We used three data sources to support this request: national supply and demand projections estimated at the state level; National League for Nursing and American Association of Colleges of Nursing data on the aging faculty with impending plans for about 50% of faculty to retire within the next decade; and increasing demands for nursing education slots throughout the Commonwealth. Using the data available about the nursing workforce in Virginia, we were able to devise the following simple sound-bite message used by all:
- "By 2020, 20,000 nurses short."
- "1 in 3 Virginians will be without a nurse."

BOX 89-1 **Virginia Nurses' Kitchen Cabinet Policy Platform for the 2005 Gubernatorial Campaign**

- A commitment to nursing workforce development with the creation of a statewide center for nursing
- A commitment from the Commonwealth to increase the educational capacity of the state's schools of nursing

---

THE POLITICS IN ACTION

Having created the policy platform, we were ready to move on to the political action plan. First, we paired and embedded nurse liaisons with each of three gubernatorial candidates. We created "Nurses for Kaine" (D) (Figure 89-1), "Nurses for Kilgore" (R), and "Nurses for Potts" (I). Second, each of the nurse liaison groups met with the candidates or the campaigns early to deliver our message about nurses, nursing, and patient care. We all agreed to hold at least one fund-raiser for the candidates and be available to work for each campaign. We all enlisted other nurses to become part of the grassroots work. And finally, N-PAC contributions were hand-delivered to each of the campaigns. Our decision to contribute to each campaign was based on past experience and pragmatism. In a previous gubernatorial campaign, our N-PAC had endorsed the losing candidate. In Virginia, memories are long, and that decision may have been a factor in nursing's lack of visibility and influence during that governor's tenure. For pragmatic reasons (and because many PACs contribute to all campaigns), we decided to contribute equally to all three campaigns. In this case, hedging our bets paid off in the long run.

THE IMPACT

As it turned out, we met with huge success in our inaugural launch of the Kitchen Cabinet. Timothy M. Kaine was elected governor, and he appointed two

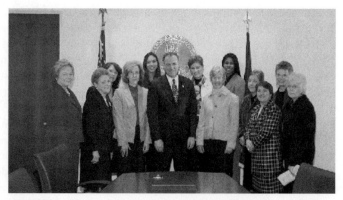

FIGURE 89-1 Governor Timothy M. Kaine with the Nurses Kitchen Cabinet.

Kitchen Cabinet nurses to his health policy transition team. Both of these nurses then received gubernatorial appointments in the administration—one serving as the first nurse to head the Department of Health Professions (the umbrella health professions regulatory agency), and the other as Chair of the Virginia Council on the Status of Women.

The governor also appointed other nurses in his administration and fostered the implementation of one of the long-term goals of the nursing community: He appointed nurses to key positions. Marilyn Tavenner was appointed to be Secretary of Health and Human Resources, which was a cabinet-level position. Her success in this role came to the attention of the Obama administration, and she was appointed Principal Deputy Administrator of the U.S. Centers for Medicare and Medicaid in 2010. In 2006, the governor also appointed nurses to serve on his Health Reform Commission (HRC) and on Commission workgroups.

In addition to ensuring the presence of nurses in the executive branch and on gubernatorial-appointed councils and commissions, we were incredibly successful in advancing our policy agenda. The primary overarching health workforce recommendation of the governor's HRC was that the Commonwealth should invest in a health workforce data center. Though nursing's request and dream was a nursing workforce center, through the art of negotiation and compromise, we recognized the need for data on all health professions and thus supported this concept. The Health Professions Workforce Data Center (the Center) is now a reality, housed within the Department of Health Professions. Its initial focus has been on the nursing profession, followed closely by medicine. In 2009, the Center issued its first report on the supply of nurses and the status of nursing education. Its next venture for nursing will be to analyze the supply of nurse practitioners.

Our second policy platform request, to increase the educational capacity and faculty salaries in schools of nursing, was realized in 2007. The governor submitted a budget request for a 10% increase in nurse faculty salary at all public colleges and universities.

> **BOX 89-2 Golden Nuggets of Lessons Learned by the Virginia Nurses Kitchen Cabinet**
>
> - Start early and act strategically by assuring that action steps are consistent with achieving Cabinet goals.
> - Speak in a unified voice on the planks of the policy platform for nursing.
> - Educate the candidates on the policy "asks," and remind them often through a consistent nursing presence in the campaign.
> - Cast a wide net for action, and include nurses from all service and education sectors.
> - Involve nurses as grassroots advocates for the campaigns to contribute financially, display yard signs, make phone calls, and so forth.
> - Trust one another to deliver the nursing message for the greater good.
> - Keep the message focused on the nurse's role in patient care and outcomes.
> - Have fun, and celebrate all successes!

This request has been sustained despite the state's difficult economic realities.

Through all of these years, Virginia nurses have grown in the ability to work collectively and collaboratively to achieve an agreed-upon set of common nursing policy goals. We also realize that our Kitchen Cabinet approach needs ongoing nurturing and rejuvenation with each election cycle. For the Kitchen Cabinet leaders, this process takes energy and commitment to advance the profession in a political environment. We have learned several critical lessons, including the importance of speaking with one voice, enhancing grassroots support, educating and supporting all candidates, and the art of negotiation and compromise. These "golden nuggets" of lessons learned in policy development and policies in action are included in Box 89-2. We encourage you to form a Kitchen Cabinet in your state to bring nurses together for policy development and political action—the potential outcomes are exciting!

For a list of related websites, please refer to your Evolve Resources at http://evolve.elsevier.com/Mason/policypolitics/

CHAPTER 90

The Politics of the Pharmaceutical Industry

Doug Olsen

"There's a better way to do it…find it."

—Thomas Edison

Prescription medications have been a mainstay of modern medical therapy since the 1920s, starting with insulin for diabetes and followed by the development of vaccinations for prevention and antibiotics. This trend accelerated in the 1950s, with the development of drugs to treat chronic and incipient conditions, hypertension, heart disease, type II diabetes, psychiatric disorders, and cancer. Ten years ago, when physicians were surveyed about the most important innovations in medical treatment since 1976, 11 of the top 20 were medications (Fuchs & Sox, 2001). Today, 46.5% of Americans take at least one prescription drug (National Center for Health Statistics [NCHS], 2009), and 71% of all outpatient visits result in a prescription (Cherry et al., 2008).

This demand fuels a large, profitable industry with $192 billion in sales and $36 billion in profits in 2002 (Fortune 500, 2003). Health care was 15.3% of the GDP in 2006, with 10% ($672 per person) of total health expenditures going for prescription drugs (Centers for Medicare & Medicaid Services [CMS], 2008). There was a 171% increase in overall prescribing in the outpatient setting from 1995-1996 to 2004-2005, with the increase being over 500% for some types of drugs (Figure 90-1) (NCHS, 2009).

Demand combined with large sums of money in the pharmaceutical industry translates into political clout. According to Public Citizen's Congress Watch in 2002, the industry spent $91.4 million in lobbying with 675 individual lobbyists. Also in 2002, the industry spent $17.6 million on advertising during the legislative process to create Medicare Part D.

The United States pharmaceutical industry emphasizes the money it spends on research and development. Estimated at $58.8 billion in 2007, it is the most visible figure in the Pharmaceutical Research and Manufacturers of America (PhRMA) *2008 Annual Report* (2008a). However, critics claim that research funded by the National Institutes of Health (NIH) and buyouts of drugs in-testing from small entrepreneurial efforts make up an increasing proportion of development funds, and that actual basic research by the large pharmaceuticals is shrinking (Angell, 2004). While the industry trumpets research and development funding, it combines marketing and administration costs, making it difficult to obtain reliable figures for marketing. The total marketing budget for the industry was estimated at $29.9 billion in 2005, up from $11.4 billion in 1997 (Donohue, Cevasco, & Rosenthal, 2007).

These numbers reveal an American industry driven by market forces to maximize return on investment. Some industry analysts express concern that overemphasis on "low-hanging fruit" in the form of me-too drugs (drugs with similar effects to available medications) and increasing market share by advertising have deemphasized basic research, resulting in less innovation (Public Citizen's Congress Watch, 2002).

VALUES CONFLICT

The industry is designed to produce profits, and like the manufacture of most other commodities in the United States, the manufacture of medications is shaped by market forces. However, medications, essential to health care, are also held to be a public good. The dual private-enterprise/public-good nature of drug manufacturing helps explain some of the industry's controversial aspects including industry-funded education and advertising campaigns aimed at clinicians and directly to patients. Reinhardt (2001)

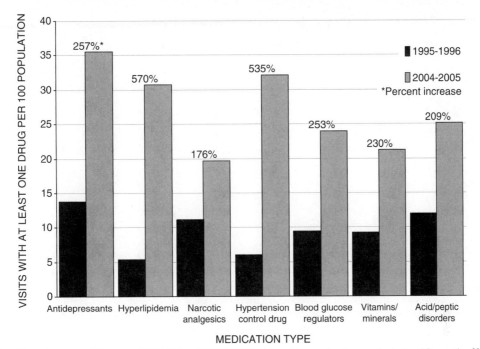

FIGURE 90-1 Outpatient prescribing from 1995-1996 to 2004-2005. (Data from Centers for Disease Control and Prevention [CDC]. [2009]. National Center for Health Statistics health, 2008 with chartbook. Hyattsville, MD. Retrieved from *www.cdc.gov/nchs/data/hus/hus08.pdf.*)

states, "On some occasions, lawmakers and the general public seem to expect pharmaceutical firms to behave as if they were community owned, nonprofit entities. At the same time, the firms' owners ... always expect the firms to use their market power and political muscle to maximize the owners' wealth" (p. 137).

A free enterprise system that lacks the ability to patent new items discourages innovation because inventions that can be freely copied confer little economic inventive for developing novel products (Taylor, 2007). The industry puts the expense of bringing a new drug to market at $1.3 billion (PhRMA, 2008c). So, to offset development expenses and encourage innovation, new medications are patented with exclusive marketing rights for 7 years (PhRMA, 2008c). This creates an incentive to deliver new drugs to market, while striving for rapid clinical acceptance. Financial assessments of a pharmaceutical company always include the "pipeline" or the drugs in development. Companies are often on a boom-bust cycle, with profits soaring when a new drug emerges and falling when the pipeline dries up (Ekelund & Persson, 2003).

The ceaseless search for blockbuster drugs results in drug development focused on those classes of medication producing large profits. The three top sellers are antidepressants, drugs for acid reflux, and statins for cholesterol reduction. Drug development based on potential profit will differ from development based on dispassionate assessment of public need. The Orphan Drug Act of 1983, providing financial incentives to develop treatments for rare diseases, is an example of an attempt to mitigate the effect of the industry's dual nature on development of new drugs.

Drug companies increase profits in two ways, bringing new medications to market and increasing the market for existing medications. Firms increase market share by advertising to prescribers and the public, as well as promotion activities that include sponsorship of clinical education and assistance to patient advocacy groups. One of the chief promotion methods to clinicians, called *detailing*, combines education-like activity with traditional advertising. In detailing, a company representative provides clinicians with educational materials, free samples, meals, and "reminder" items, including mugs, pens, or toys.

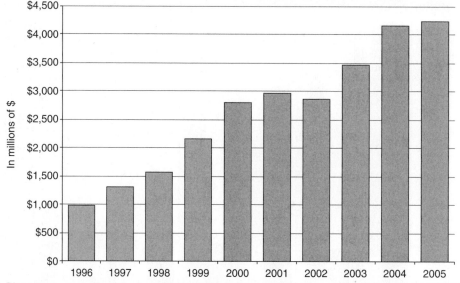

FIGURE 90-2 Direct-to-consumer advertising from 1996-2005. (From Donohue, J. M., Cevasco, M., & Rosenthal, M. B. [2007]. A decade of direct-to-consumer advertising of prescription drugs. *New England Journal of Medicine, 357*[7], 673-681.)

In 2005, an estimated $6.8 billion dollars, or 22% of promotion spending, went to detailing. In addition, $18.4 billion, 58% of promotion spending, went to free drug samples (Donohue, Cevasco, & Rosenthal, 2007).

DIRECT TO CONSUMER MARKETING

Direct to Consumer (DTC) advertising began in earnest in 1997, 6 months after David Kessler, who opposed easing regulations to allow more DTC, left his post as commissioner of the U.S. Food and Drug Administration (FDA). At that time, it was made easier to comply with the regulatory requirement that DTC broadcast advertising contain a "major statement" of the drug's risks, and "adequate provision" for consumers to obtain full information about the drug. These conditions are now satisfied with a risk statement and referral to concurrent print ads, websites, or toll-free telephone numbers (Bradford, Kleit, Nietert, & Ornstein, 2005). Industry spending on DTC advertising is estimated to have increased from $579 million in 1996 to $3.8 billion in 2004 (Bradford et al., 2005) (Figure 90-2). Profit spurred the growth of DTC marketing, and it is estimated that money spent on DTC advertising produces a fourfold return

in sales (Rosenthal, Berndt, Donohue, Epstein, & Frank, 2003).

The heated debate about DTC advertising highlights the ambivalence over medications as both public good and lucrative product. Both sides in the debate frame arguments in terms of DTC's effect on public health, passing over profitability as a rationale for favoring DTC advertising. Ethical and policy reasons favoring DTC advertising include increased public awareness of treatment options and enhanced ability for informed choices by consumers. One argument against DTC advertising is that the information disseminated by the ads is biased—designed to build profit and not simply a dispassionate account of risks, benefits, and alternatives essential to informed choice.

Research shows that while awareness is increased, the information received by the public through advertising is problematic. A series of FDA surveys (Aikin, Swasy, & Braman, 2004) indicates that the public and physicians view DTC advertising as raising awareness of treatment options and stimulating clinical discussion, but also note that the ads tend to overemphasize benefits. Woloshin, Schwartz, and Welch (2004) found that consumers, when given effectiveness data, perceived drugs as less beneficial than when given the qualitative data typical of most drug advertising.

Wilkes, Bell, & Kravitz (2000) reported that 43% of consumers believed that only completely safe drugs could be advertised, and 21% believed that advertising was restricted to extremely effective drugs.

The industry largely confines advertising to a few classes of drugs that generate the greatest profit rather than focus on distributing information on the basis of public need (Donohue, Cevasco, & Rosenthal, 2007). The drug with the most DTC spending treats heartburn, and a sleep aid ranks second (Donohue, Cevasco, & Rosenthal, 2007). There are also indications that prescribing patterns are influenced in ways inconsistent with health priorities. Weissman and colleagues (2003) found that 25% of patients who asked clinicians about an advertised drug received a new diagnosis; erectile dysfunction was the most common new diagnosis.

Another concern about DTC marketing is disease mongering, that is, promoting exaggerated perceptions of the seriousness of known disorders or even inventing new diseases to open new markets and improve sales. Conditions offered as examples include female sexual dysfunction, erectile dysfunction, acid reflux, insomnia, and allergies (Applbaum, 2006).

CONFLICT OF INTEREST

The large quantity of money spent promoting drugs to clinicians raises conflict-of-interest concerns that arise from the industry's dual nature. The public wants treatment to be based solely on a clinical assessment of the patient's best interests, not on personal or monetary considerations tied to specific medications, but industry promotion is designed to sell particular drugs in service of the company's primary goal of profitability.

EDUCATION

Drug companies are a major sponsor of medical continuing education. Between 1998 and 2003, commercial sponsorship of continuing medical education went from $302 million to $971 million (Steinbrook, 2005). Industry marketing has become so integral to clinical education that PhRMA (2008c) claims, "Restricting pharmaceutical marketing would likely significantly reduce the dissemination of information about new treatments..." In a report in the *New England Journal of Medicine,* Steinbrook (2008)

concluded, "Continuing medical education has become so heavily dependent on support from pharmaceutical and medical device companies that the medical profession may have lost control over its own continuing education." In 2008, the Association of American Medical Colleges (AAMC) identified the conflict between medical treatment as a social good and medical treatment as a commodity. In their report "Industry Funding of Medical Education," the AAMC states "these conflicts can have a corrosive effect on three core principles of medical professionalism: autonomy, objectivity, and altruism" (AAMC, 2008, p. 4).

Both the American Nurses Association through the American Nurses Credentialing Center (ANCC) and the American Medical Association (AMA) through the Accreditation Council for Continuing Medical Education (ACCME) attempt to eliminate conflicts of interest with strict guidelines for commercial sponsorship of accredited continuing education. The guidelines emphasize independence of content, transparency through conflict of interest disclosures by content developers, separation of promotion from educational activity, and appropriate use of funds (ANCC, n.d.; ACCME, 2007). The AMA Council on Ethical and Judicial Affairs recommends that physicians, medical schools, and professional associations stop accepting industry funding of education, and the American Psychiatric Association announced its intention to phase out industry-funded education (Kuehn, 2009).

However, discerning when education is sponsored by a pharmaceutical manufacturer is difficult because the money is often passed through medical-education corporations or industry foundations. Other times the information is clearly from a drug company with little concern over any real or perceived conflict of interest. A downloadable 3-part CE series titled *Counseling Points* (n.d.), designed to resemble journal articles and distributed by the American Psychiatric Nurses Association (APNA) in 2009, provides clinical information clearly marked with drug-company sponsorship, without claim of authorship. When I asked about the appearance of bias created by the lack of scholarly attribution in a commercially sponsored product, the APNA expressed no concern. We do not know how much commercial money is directed for nursing education, but it appears to be increasing as more nurses prescribe medications.

Industry-sponsored education is a form of marketing. Drugs are so integral to modern health care that comprehensive education in almost all areas involves extensive discussion of medications, and even unbiased appraisals may favor one drug over another. But when commercial interests sponsor education, it cannot be discerned where unbiased evaluation ends and promotion begins. For example, if two experts have an honest disagreement about treatments, and the company sponsors the one that holds their drug superior to the lifestyle change favored by the other expert, then the discourse is biased by giving one side resources to magnify their opinion. Social justice is achieved through fair and equal access to all forms of discourse (Horster, 1992). Distortion of the discourse on health care in the public and professional community occurs through marketing techniques applied to products with the potential to generate revenue. And so, in market-driven public discourse, health practices with modest or little profit potential, such as exercise and moderate eating, are unlikely to receive the attention accorded to highly profitable pharmaceuticals.

GIFTS

The giving of explicit or disguised gifts also creates potential conflicts of interest in clinicians. After years of anecdotal denial by clinicians that gifts carry influence, data suggest that physicians' prescribing practices are influenced by drug company gifts (Sierles et al., 2005; Chew et al., 2000). So, voluntary guidance from the industry (PhRMA, 2008b), the government (Office of Inspector General, 2003), and the AMA (2005) limits the practice of giving gifts. PhRMA guidelines prohibit both the most egregious types of gifts given in the past by drug companies (including cash kickbacks, event tickets, and "fees" for bogus consultations) as well as those once considered benign, including mugs or pens. Voluntary PhRMA guidelines suggest gifts be limited to educational or clinically useful items of less than $100. Provision of meals is still allowed at clinical sites when in conjunction with educational presentations.

While the AMA has issued ethical guidance for physicians, guidance for nurses is notably absent. Major U.S. nursing organizations say little about relations with the pharmaceutical industry. The ANA has issued no guidance specific to relations with industry. Despite calls for ethical guidance on this topic for nurse practitioners (Crigger, 2005), the American College of Nurse Practitioners (ACNP) has only two related items on their website: (1) a position paper calling for DTC marketing to include referrals "to all qualified health care professionals" and not just physicians, and (2) a presentation provided by PhRMA reviewing its guidelines for clinician relations that are blatantly self-promoting (e.g., "Pharmaceutical company representatives help speed the dissemination of valuable improvements in medical care...") (Brigner, 2009). The American Academy of Nurse Practitioners (n.d.) website has a "Petition to End the Use of Physician-Biased Language in DTC Advertising" but no guidance on the ethics of relations with industry.

Nurses represent a relatively untapped and naïve resource for pharmaceutical marketing (Jutel & Menkes, 2008). Although only some nurses prescribe, nurses influence the use and purchase of drugs in other ways, including suggesting the use of particular medications, distributing medications, reporting adverse effects, conducting research, as well as managing many clinical trials. In a survey of more than 500 nurse practitioners, Blunt (2005) reported that 80% altered their prescribing practice after a drug company interaction.

SAMPLES

Providing free samples of drugs is another controversial form of gifts given to clinicians. The claim is often made that prescribers use these to benefit the economically disadvantaged. However, research shows that recipients of sample medications are more likely the wealthy rather than the poor or uninsured (Cutrona et al., 2008). The free samples are usually of new, expensive drugs that the patient may not be able to afford after the samples run out.

SUMMARY

The most pervasive effect of having a market-driven industry expected to deliver a public good may be the subtle shift in the nature of the public benefit expected. The sum effect of the vast amount of money spent to promote drug sales through education and advertising to clinicians and advertising directly to the public may be to alter the public's concept of life and health to conform with the interests of the pharmaceutical industry. This means a worldview where life's problems are medical conditions visited on us through no fault of our own and whose solutions require external interventions—most often a pill. In this view, personal responsibility means recognizing and admitting to having a disorder and then being compliant with treatment.

Medications are a miracle of modern health care. But the tradition will continue only if unbiased information on their benefits and uses is distributed in accordance with rational decisions about the public's health, rather than the effect on industry profits.

For a list of related websites, please refer to your Evolve Resources at http://evolve.elsevier.com/Mason/policypolitics/

REFERENCES

Accreditation Council for Continuing Medical Education. (2007). ACCME standards for commercial support: Standards to ensure the independence of CME activities. Retrieved from www.accme.org/dir_docs/doc_upload/68b2902a-fb73-44d1-8725-80a1504e520c_uploaddocument.pdf.

Aikin, K., Swasy, J., & Braman, A. (2004). Patient and physician attitudes and behaviors associated with DTC promotion of prescription drugs—Summary of FDA survey research results. U.S. Department of Health and Human Services, Food and Drug Administration, Center for Drug Evaluation and Research. Retrieved from www.fda.gov/downloads/Drugs/Science Research/ResearchAreas/DrugMarketingAdvertisingandCommunications Research/UCM152860.pdf.

American Academy of Nurse Practitioners. (n.d.). Petition to end the use of physician-biased language in DTC advertising. Retrieved from http://aanp.org/AANPCMS2/AboutAANP/Marketing+and+PR/DTC+Advertising+Petition.htm.

American Medical Association (AMA). (2005). Ethical guidelines for gifts to physicians from industry. The Association. www.ama-assn.org/ama/pub/category/5689.html.

American Nurses Credentialing Center (ANCC). (n.d.). Standards for disclosure and commercial support. Retrieved from www.nursecredentialing.org/ContinuingEducation/Accreditation/How-to-Apply/CommercialSupport/CommercialSupportStandards.aspx.

Angell, M. (2004). The truth about the drug companies: How they deceive us and what to do about it. New York: Random House.

Applbaum, K. (2006). Pharmaceutical marketing and the invention of the medical consumer. PLoS Med, 3, e189.

Association of American Medical Colleges. (2008). Industry funding of medical education: Report of an AAMC task force. Retrieved from www.aamc.org/publications.

Blunt, E. (2005). The influence of pharmaceutical-company-sponsored educational programs, promotions, and gifts on the self-reported prescribing beliefs and practices of certified nurse practitioners in three states. 16th International Nursing Research Congress, Sigma Theta Tau, Hawaii. Retrieved from http://stti.confex.com/stti/inrc16/techprogram/paper_23835.htm.

Bradford, W., Kleit, A., Nietert, P., & Ornstein, S. (2005). The effect of direct to consumer television advertising on the timing of treatment. Publication of the AIE-Brookings Joint Center for Regulatory Studies. Retrieved from http://reg-markets.org/admin/authorpdfs/redirect-safely.php?fname=../pdffiles/php2J.pdf.

Brigner, S. (2009). Demonstrating value and ethics in pharmaceutical marketing. ACNP Summit 2009. Retrieved from www.acnpweb.org/files/public/PhRMA_Demonstrating_Value_and_Ethics_in_Pharmaceutical_Marketing-Brigner.pdf.

Centers for Medicare & Medicaid Services. (2008). National health expenditure projections 2008-2018. Retrieved from www.cms.hhs.gov/NationalHealthExpendData/downloads/proj2008.pdf.

Cherry, D., Hing, E., Woodwell, D., & Rechtsteiner, E. (2008). National ambulatory medical care survey: 2006 summary national health statistics reports. Number 3. Hyattsville, MD: National Center for Health Statistics.

Chew, L. D., O'Young, T. S., Hazlet, T. K., Bradley, K. A., Maynard, C., et al. (2000). A physician survey of the effect of drug sample availability on physicians' behavior. Journal of General Internal Medicine, 15(7), 478-483.

Counseling points. (n.d.) Retrieved from www.apna.org/i4a/pages/index.cfm?pageid=3578.

Crigger, B. (2005). Pharmaceutical promotions and conflict of interest in nurse practitioner's decision making: The undiscovered country. Journal of the American Academy of Nurse Practitioners, 17(6), 207-212.

Cutrona, S. L., Woolhandler, S., Lasser, K. E., Bor, D. H., McCormick, D., et al. (2008). Characteristics of recipients of free prescription drug samples: A nationally representative analysis. American Journal of Public Health, 98(2), 284-289.

Donohue, J. M., Cevasco, M., & Rosenthal, M. B. (2007). A decade of direct-to-consumer advertising of prescription drugs. New England Journal of Medicine, 357(7), 673-681.

Ekelund, M. & Persson, B. (2003). Pharmaceutical pricing in a regulated market. The Review of Economics and Statistics, 85(2), 298-306.

Fortune 500. (April 17, 2003). Honey, I shrunk the profits. Fortune, 147(7), 199, F-26, F-59.

Fuchs, V. R. & Sox, H. C. (2001). Physicians' views of the relative importance of thirty medical innovations. Health Affairs, 20(5), 30-42.

Horster, D. (H. Thompson, trans.). (1992). Habermas: An introduction. Philadelphia: Pennbridge.

Jutel, A. & Menkes, D. (2008). Soft targets: Nurses and the pharmaceutical industry. PLoS Medicine, 5(2), 0193-0198. Retrieved from www.plosmedicine.org/article/info:doi%2F10.1371%2Fjournal.pmed.0050005.

Kuehn, B. (2009). Associations say no to industry funding. Journal of the American Medical Association, 301(18), 1865-1866.

National Center for Health Statistics. (2009). Health, United States, 2008. Hyattsville, MD. Retrieved from www.cdc.gov/nchs/data/hus/hus08.pdf.

Office of Inspector General, U.S. Department of Health and Human Services. (DHHS) (2003, May 5). OIG compliance program guidance for pharmaceutical manufacturers. Washington, D.C. Federal Register, 68, No. 86.

PhRMA. (2008a). 2008 Annual report. Retrieved from www.phrma.org/files/PhRMA_annualreportFianl.pdf.

PhRMA. (2008b). Code on interactions with healthcare professionals. Washington, D.C. Retrieved from www.phrma.org/files/PhRMA%20Marketing%20Code%202008.pdf.

PhRMA. (2008c). Pharmaceutical marketing in perspective: Its value and role as one of many factors informing prescribing. Retrieved from www.phrma.org/files/attachments/PhRMA%20Marketing%20Brochure%20Influences%20on%20Prescribing%20FINAL.pdf.

Public Citizen's Congress Watch. (2002). United Seniors Association: Hired guns for PhRMA and other corporate interests. Retrieved from www.citizen.org/documents/UnitedSeniorsAssociationreport.pdf.

Reinhardt, U. (2001). Perspectives on the pharmaceutical industry. Health Affairs, 20(5), 136-149.

Rosenthal, M. B., Berndt, E. R., Donohue, J. M., Epstein, A. M., & Frank, R. G. (2003). Demand effects of recent changes in prescription drug promotion. Menlo Park, CA: Kaiser Family Foundation.

Sierles, F. S., Brodkey A. C., Cleary, L. M., McCurdy F. A., Mintz, M., et al. (2005). Medical students' exposure to and attitudes about drug company interactions: A national survey. Journal of the American Medical Association, 294(9), 1034-1042.

Steinbrook, R. (2005). Commercial support and continuing medical education. New England Journal of Medicine, 352(6), 534-535.

Steinbrook, R. (2008). Financial support of continuing medical education. *Journal of the American Medical Association, 299*(9), 1060-1062.

Taylor, T. (2007). *Principles of economics: Economics and the economy.* St. Paul, MN: Freeload Press.

Weissman, J. S., Blumenthal, D., Silk, A. J., Zapert, K., Newman, M., & Leitman, R. (2003). Consumers' reports on the health effects of direct-to-consumer drug advertising. Health Affairs Web Exclusive. Retrieved from http://content.healthaffairs.org/cgi/reprint/hlthaff.w3.82v1.pdf.

Wilkes, M. S., Bell, R. A., & Kravitz, R. L. (2000). Direct-to-consumer prescription drug advertising: Trends, impact, and implications. *Health Affairs, 19*(2), 110-128.

Woloshin, S., Schwartz, L., & Welch, H. (2004). The value of benefit data in direct-to-consumer drug ads. Health Affairs Web Exclusive. Retrieved from http://content.healthaffairs.org/cgi/content/abstract/hlthaff.w4.234.

CHAPTER 91

Where Policy Hits the Pavement: Contemporary Issues in Communities

Katherine N. Bent

"I am of the opinion that my life belongs to the community, and as long as I live it is my privilege to do for it whatever I can."

—George Bernard Shaw

Most people experience the effects of public policy-making in their communities. In daily living, people feel the outcome of policy, and in communities, individuals learn how to step up and take part in the policymaking process. In communities, nurses and other health professionals have immediate opportunities to advocate for policies that promote and protect health in multiple ways. Indeed, the *Healthy People 2010* (United States Department of Health and Human Services [USDHHS], 2000) priorities for national health place nursing in a key position to affect future health-related policies.

This chapter explores the nature of communities, prospects for health in community, and the health-related conditions that shape and are shaped by policy. It suggests how nurses, as they increasingly move across institutional walls, can support improvements in policies affecting health.

WHAT IS A COMMUNITY?

Although community is a part of our daily experiences, the idea of community is elusive and can mean many things, particularly in a health care context (Bent, 2003). Attitudes about the role of community in health care and health policy differ when compared with attitudes about the role of community in other areas. For example, health care entrepreneurs view health care communities as a market where they are likely to find a concentration of persons to buy health care goods or services; however, public health professionals must be concerned about entire populations in a given area regardless of people's ability to buy, knowing that where economic market potential is lower, health risks and needs may actually be higher (Geronimus, 2000). Although the concept of community has broad appeal, in a politically charged environment, claims of community often become moral claims that may serve to divide people more than bring them together (Monroe, 1997). For example, differing neighborhoods within cities or towns may have competing interests for zoning regulations that affect traffic flow in and out of the community, local job opportunities, and health risks associated with production waste. This effect has serious consequences for questions of public health and the policies that support or define public health, such as policies that mandate reporting of or vaccination against communicable diseases or policies that exclude certain health care treatments from government health insurance programs.

Milio (2002) has noted that the basis for health lies in physical communities, where we find homes, schools, recreation and entertainment centers, faith centers, businesses, and governmental and voluntary organizations. These assets, along with means of communication and transportation, form a community's infrastructure (Box 91-1). The quality, availability, and accessibility of the infrastructure make a difference in health prospects of the people who live in those communities.

Communities must share both spirit and a sense of place in order to build, achieve, and sustain health and well-being. Through attachment to place, communities share attachment to social responsibility for creating healthy surroundings. This attachment does not exist among detached groups that may share other

---

BOX 91-1 Components of Community Infrastructure

Infrastructure includes such elements as clean and pure water, air, and food; adequate housing; employment; childcare; health; education; police and fire services; open media; civic opportunities and social life; strong neighborhood, community, and labor groups; and a strong health care service safety net. In communities that have the resources, a sense of cohesion can bring about distribution of these resources to achieve sustainable health for the people who are part of those communities.

BOX 91-2 Evaluating a Healthy Community

Most communities have some process in place for evaluating quality of health care at the community level, though the means by which they do so usually vary greatly. Variation in quality assessment strategies may capture issues of local importance (e.g., lead paint screening in communities with old housing stock, health career programs in schools, or enrollment assistance in public programs) but also complicates comparisons on issues of common concern across communities. For example, the specific question of how nonprofit health care providers should be expected to benefit the communities they serve has gained attention at multiple levels, particularly since these organizations are exempt from federal taxes. Federal rules that are scheduled to take effect in 2010 will require non-profit hospitals to report spending on charitable care in their communities. This increase in public reporting is important and may improve hospitals' responsiveness to community needs, but nurses and others who are concerned with a broad range of community health experiences need to make the case that charity care expenditures are an imperfect and incomplete measure of community benefit (Gray & Schlesinger, 2009). Nurses who are interested in disease prevention and community health promotion should advocate supplementing these data with information about how hospitals and other providers assess local needs, set priorities for addressing them, and evaluate the results of these efforts in and across specific communities.

---

interests (Milio, 1996). The importance of the physical and socio-economic environments in determining the health and needs of communities and individuals is well-recognized. As noted by the Institute of Medicine, "the health risk conferred by place is above and beyond the risk that individuals carry with them" (IOM, 2003, p. 68), and there is international interest in understanding the relationships among communities of place and health of the population (Diez Roux, 2001; Durie & Wyatt, 2007). Commitments to community-level responsibility for healthy populations pose challenges to most of our current and emerging health policies, which overwhelmingly target health care service delivery and health insurance. Can you think about what kinds of actions or policies within your community may be affecting health or quality of life? How would you work within a multidisciplinary context to promote health at the community level in these areas?

HEALTHY COMMUNITIES

In the late 1970s, the World Health Organization (WHO) embraced the principles of social justice and equity and challenged nations to provide a basic level of health for all citizens. They called the principal means to this end primary health care (PHC) (WHO, 1978). PHC is essential, practical, scientific, socially accepted, universally accessible to all members of a community, affordable, and geared toward self-reliance and self-determination, and it involves multiple agencies and sectors in health. This marked a shift away from dependence on health professionals and toward personal and community involvement, which WHO reaffirmed in the 1980s.

Today, growing social significance of health and health care and economic burden, plus a current awareness of lost opportunities and important health inequities has given rise to widespread interest in reforming health systems. Many of today's authorities and leaders no longer limit their responsibility for health to survival and disease control, but undertake building systems that support health as a key resource and strength that people and societies value (WHO, 2008).

The goals of health care service delivery and better health for all in a population are not mutually exclusive, but the degree of emphasis on one or the other is important since public policy is a highly influential force at all levels of health care in this country. Questions of emphasis remain relevant as national policies "decentralize," state policies "localize," and individuals and communities are told they hold more responsibility than ever for their own health (Box 91-2). This implies that the individual or the single community is responsible for the success (manifested through personal or population health measures) or failure (seen in ill health) of public health policy.

PARTNERSHIP AND PARTICIPATION FOR IMPROVING COMMUNITY HEALTH

Nurses have a tradition of actively creating and fostering partnerships for health promotion and community health, and their role remains vitally important today, for they are named by the WHO as the critical professional link to create communities that are healthier for both individuals and for the entire population (WHO, 2000).

Healthy communities may be achieved through truly active and collaborative partnerships among a broad representation of professional and lay community members, but it is important to examine all partnerships critically (Aronson, 1993). Partnerships may become a substitute for accountability in organizations or governments, as individuals and small organizations are expected to assume labor and costs associated with initiatives to improve health. A caring partnership between nurse and community is a collaboration that is an informed, flexible, and negotiated distribution and redistribution of power among the participants in the process of seeking change for improved community health status, process, and structure. Effective community collaborations are far more than nursing "interventions"; rather, they evolve through a dynamic process and with philosophic underpinnings called for by true partnership (Box 91-3).

Roles for nurses in healthy community initiatives focus on community action, developing personal skills in community members, eliciting and supporting existing strengths within communities, reorienting health care services, creating supportive environments, and participating actively in the creation of healthy public policy. Nurses also foster critical reflections among community members who are acting in partnerships. Nurses cannot ignore political, social, or cultural structures, material conditions, or the play of power in relationships between and among individuals and groups in communities. Nurses must continue to explore health policy in ways that make the relevance of community involvement in health

> ### BOX 91-3 Partnering with Veterans
>
> Nurses can highlight the need to better use talents and skills of veterans to both meet communities' most pressing needs and aid in community reintegration and transitions for veterans themselves. Veterans who have volunteered and contributed service since returning home have better transitions than those who have not, and an overwhelming majority (92%) of veterans from Iraq and Afghanistan want to serve again in their communities in a diverse range of issues (Yonkman & Bridgeland, 2009). However, while 7 of 10 report receiving offers of assistance from service organizations, only 2 of 10 have been asked to contribute; nurses can identify and highlight concrete opportunities and links between the military, nonprofits, veterans service organizations, faith-based groups, and elected officials that aim to ensure that veterans have meaningful opportunities to serve alongside fellow citizens and to be appreciated as a community asset and strength.

development clear. This supports not only health status of individuals, but also structures and processes that are the community-based determinants of health (Box 91-4).

DETERMINANTS OF HEALTH IN COMMUNITIES

Within public policy arenas, views differ about the proper primary focus of health policy: Is the primary purpose of health policy to deliver health services to or to improve the health and well-being of populations? Researchers have increasingly documented that the portion of population health status attributable to health care services is modest when compared to the contributions of other factors, including the sociopolitical determinants of health. Indeed, *Healthy People 2010*, a federal effort to outline national public health objectives, identified access to health care as only 1 of 10 leading indicators that, in addition to income and education, could serve as measures for the health of the population (USDHHS, 2000).

Determinants of health are factors in the sociocultural and political environments that contribute to or detract from the health of individuals and communities. These factors include, but are not limited to, income, education, occupation, transportation, sanitation, housing, access to services and resources

BOX 91-4 The Boston Women's Health Collective Model

The story of the Boston Women's Health Book Collective illustrates the power of communities working on their own behalf. Women who met at a 1969 conference in Boston shared personal stories about frustrations with health care; they later met to generate lists of "good" doctors for women. They then expanded their purpose in meeting to include learning basic information about their bodies, health, and sexuality, from which they developed course content that they later published. Known as *Our Bodies, Ourselves* (Boston Women's Health Book Collective, 2005), their work is now published in over 30 languages, and the collective collaborates with other institutions and individuals to advocate for changes in the norms, policies, and laws that influence women's health, economic status, and roles in society. They raise awareness about biotechnologies that pose ethical questions about women's health, direct-to-consumer advertising, and risks and benefits of new drugs and devices marketed to women (Stephenson & Zeldes, 2008).

There are policy implications to all dimensions and experiences of health in communities. Also, nurses may not be needed to identify gaps, problems, or issues for a community or to drive the agenda or manage the process of solving problems. Rather, as the work grew in scope and impact, a role evolved for nurses to be one among many true partners to achieve policy-driven outcomes.

BOX 91-5 How Can Policy Affect Health?

Nurses eager to support health-related policies can analyze the health impact of policies, environments, and ways of living that flow from them (Durie & Wyatt, 2007). For example, emerging technologies, such as stem cell technologies, raise ethical questions with ramifications in community health policy because scientific breakthroughs that may serve individuals suffering from illness may not equally serve diverse populations and economically fragile communities or health systems (Giacomini, Baylis, & Robert, 2007).

BOX 91-6 Defining the Policy Focus

There are many examples of healthy public policy decisions that highlight both relationships and tensions in aspects of health and life. Some communities struggle as they consider fast-food franchises in public school areas, where tensions exist between income for the school district and health-related questions for students. Can you think of other examples of where multiple areas of public policy converge, perhaps compete, and have health-related outcomes?

as how to advocate for policies to address forces associated with poor health and quality of life outcomes.

PUBLIC POLICY

Efforts at healthy public policymaking rest on the following two explicit assumptions:

- Most people, most of the time, will make decisions and choices based on the options that are available. The results are not exclusively personal, nor are they the result of totally free choices about lifestyle made in isolation from social, economic, cultural, and political contexts.
- The options that are available, and from which people make choices, do not "just happen," but rather are the result of prior policy choices that represent the scope of health-sustaining policy, including energy, technology, pollution, employment, income maintenance, taxation, prices, food, agriculture, transportation, housing, health care, child care, and other services.

Within a framework of healthy public policy, health-damaging environments and options are eliminated or made more expensive; new programs or resources that are easier to access in areas that may lack health-promoting or health-sustaining resources are also part of a healthy public policy framework (Milio, 1981, 1996) (Box 91-6).

One common example of healthy public policy is the body of laws and regulations that prohibit tobacco smoking in workspaces or other public space. Along with tax measures, cessation measures, and education, policy supporting smoking bans is an important element in reducing smoking and promoting public health (WHO, 2004). Although smoking laws vary widely in the United States, as of October 2009, only 13 states have no statewide bans on smoking in any non-government owned space; 24

linked to health, social support, and environmental hazards. Social forces that act at a collective level, such as a community decision to build sidewalks to promote safe walking opportunities, shape individual biology, individual risk behaviors, environmental exposures, and access to resources that promote health (Box 91-5).

It is critical that nurses understand how determinants of health contribute to health inequities as well states ban smoking in all enclosed public spaces, 13 more states ban smoking in some or most enclosed public places. When also considering local laws, 71% of the U.S. population lives under a smoking ban in workplaces and/or restaurants and/or bars (Americans for Nonsmokers' Rights, 2009). The rationale for smoke-free laws may include: to protect people from the effects of secondhand smoke, lower health care costs, improve work productivity, reduce risk of fire, increase cleanliness and reduce litter, and create incentives for smokers to quit.

The increasing interest in smoke-free measures raises important questions for policymakers, and offers opportunities for nurses to be active in providing accurate information that will have a meaningful effect on policy decisions. Will a smoking ban improve the public health? Will a smoking ban hurt business for restaurants, bars, and other segments of the hospitality industry? How will communities enforce a smoking ban? Should smoking be allowed if a bar or restaurant modifies its ventilation system to keep cigarette smoke confined to special smoking sections? Extensive research shows that smoking bans do reduce exposure to secondhand smoke, do improve health, and do not have an adverse effect on the hospitality economy (Hyland, 2009). Most businesses and individuals willingly comply with the new laws, and the smoothest transition occurs in communities that make a strong effort to educate the public and affected business about the benefits of smoke-free establishments (Hyland, 2009); nurses are ideal partners for these efforts (Box 91-7).

SOCIOECONOMIC STATUS, HEALTH DISPARITIES, AND INEQUITIES

The link between health status of a population and socioeconomic status is well established in both the U.S. and other countries; many diseases are more common, and life expectancy is shorter at the lower ends of the scale (WHO, 2003). Low-income populations may delay care or treatment due to issues of access or cost, and poverty weakens an individual or family's ability to cope with new stressors in addition to exposing individuals to more acute and ongoing stress (Kessler & Cleary, 1980). Beyond a threshold of about $5000 to $10,000 U.S. dollars per capita income, the gap between rich and poor, called *income inequality*, is a greater health hazard than absolute low income itself (Population Health Forum, 2009). This

---

> ### BOX 91-7 Ballot Initiative: Gift Horse or Trojan Horse?
>
> Some communities address healthy public policy decisions through a policy tool that is used with increasing frequency, the ballot initiative, in which a policy measure is put directly to a vote by a population after being submitted by a petition. In Colorado, a broad coalition of public health nurses, farmers, ranchers, environmentalists, and grassroots community groups brought to a statewide vote a law to regulate the state's increasing numbers of large hog factories, which were polluting groundwater with waste and nitrates (Colorado Revised Statutes, Amendment 14, 1998). Although the law was crafted specifically to address problems of contaminated wells and soil associated with certain large-scale operations in Colorado, seven other states rely on the Ogallala Aquifer, which lies directly below most of Colorado's hog farms, as their primary source for drinking water and other water needs (USGS, 1998). On the one hand, citizens were directly involved in achieving a regulatory outcome likely to support health in many rural western states. What disadvantages to policymaking by ballot initiative can you think of?

appears to be related to both access to resources for health and relative social position among people with different levels of education, income, and types of jobs and among people who live in communities characterized by different levels of community wealth and infrastructure (Massey & Durrheim, 2007; Wilkinson & Marmot, 2003).

For example, although the average life expectancy is improving in the U.S. (Heron, Hoyert, Murphy, et al., 2009), the picture is not uniform. From 1990 to 2000, life expectancy for people with at least some college education increased, while remaining unchanged for less-educated people. Increasing levels of educational success and improving housing standards are examples of how nurses might focus their attention to improve health through its socioeconomic determinants.

Other policy interventions for nurses to address inequities in community health include taking leadership in community-level emergency preparedness efforts to assure that all members of communities, particularly vulnerable populations, such as public housing residents, single parent families, persons with functional limitations or disabilities, and low-income families, are equally protected by community interventions for all kinds of emergency preparedness

---

BOX 91-8 **Collaborative Processes for Information**

Although constructing and maintaining a resource database can be expensive, nurses working with the Red Cross in several locations have demonstrated the acceptability and success of engaging members of a local community itself to maintain this kind of resource economically. These nurses found that collaborative processes of gathering information raises awareness of risk and vulnerability within the community, leads to an assessment of community strengths and resources, and mobilizes these resources and partnerships to assure the ability to receive accurate information about resources quickly to support rapid assessment and response (Troy, Carson, Vanderbeek, & Hutton, 2008).

---

planning (Hutchins, Truman, Merlin, & Redd, 2009). Federal, state, and local authorities have made emergency preparedness one of their highest priorities (Lurie, Wasserman, Nelson, 2006); nevertheless, significant gaps (e.g., infection control in mass casualties, public education, internal and external communication, mental health, provision of prescription medication, postdisaster disease surveillance, physical infrastructure, and partnerships among interested agencies and community members) have been shown to exist in public health emergency response, particularly for vulnerable and underrepresented populations (Rebmann, Carrico, & English, 2008; Jenkins, Hsu, Sauer, Hsieh, & Kirsch, 2009).

Some health departments are conducting interviews and gathering data from diverse communities in other structured ways to identify barriers to emergency communication, preferred preparedness content, communication strategies (who and how as well as strategies for both translating and culturally adapting appropriate content), and opportunities for collaboration among organizations and community members when needed (Andrulis, Siddiqui, & Gantner, 2007) (Box 91-8). Nurses should be leaders in assuring that all populations are integrated into efforts in their own communities to formulate effective strategies for reaching diverse or vulnerable populations (Andrulis et al., 2007; Bouye et al., 2009).

In the U.S., although people of color have disproportionately high rates of poverty, poverty and its associated factors alone are not sufficient to explain all of the health disparities among people of different races (USDHHS, 2004). Because the effect of race on

health is controversial, particularly for its relationship to issues of poverty, further investigation is warranted to tease out contributions of each, as well as contributions of social processes in neighborhoods. Systematic differences in health status between different socioeconomic groups are socially produced and modifiable (WHO, 2007). Eliminating health disparities and inequities is a foundation of public health nursing practice (Association of State and Territorial Directors of Nursing [ASTDN], 2009). Communities that enable all members to contribute fully and that build from assets in the community will be healthier than those where people are excluded or face deprivation.

ENVIRONMENTAL HEALTH

Environmental health is a rich public policy domain; there is considerable evidence that local environments are related to health outcomes (Hawe & Shiell, 2000). Nurses in environmental health partnerships may address a wide range of topics, such as safety of fish consumption or of drinking water, bioterrorism, questions of environmental justice, or long-term health outcomes of community-wide exposures.

For example, Libby, Montana is a rural community affected by generations of exposure to asbestos-contaminated mineral ores that were mined there for 78 years (Kuntz et al., 2009). Although mining operations provided jobs, roads, and economic development for the community, there were health consequences to residents; Libby was designated a federal Superfund site in 2002, after an analysis of mortality conducted by the Agency for Toxic Substances and Disease Registry (ATSDR) in cooperation with the Montana Department of Public Health and Human Services (MDPHHS) found asbestosis mortality that was 40 to 80 times higher than expected when compared with Montana and the U.S. and found lung cancer mortality that was 20% to 30% higher than expected (ATSDR, 2008, 2009).

There is a patchwork of federal agencies involved in public health management, policymaking, and regulation related to the health hazards associated with asbestos, but no single agency is responsible for coordination or oversight of efforts. In addition, Libby is a highly uninsured/underinsured population in a Health Care Professional Shortage Area, thus is without access to health care services. Because community residents may or may not yet have disease, or may be in varying stages of disease, and because there

---

BOX 91-9 **Healthy Eating**

Nurses and others have increasingly focused attention on the role of neighborhood and social context in efforts to improve healthy eating because policy elements (e.g., access to affordable, good food) make the greatest difference in what people eat (Cheadle et al., 1991; McKevith, Stanner, & Butriss, 2005).

People eat their meals away from home with much greater frequency than ever before, and consumers want nutritional information for foods and beverages purchased at restaurants. While proposed laws to require the disclosure of nutritional information on a menu or board have considerable support among health groups, they are opposed by the restaurant industry (Pomeranz & Brownell, 2008). Through letters to the editor, Op-Ed essays, and organizing constituent visits to policymakers, nurses can communicate the public health rationale for menu labeling laws at local, state, and federal levels. Nurses can also ensure that legal voices have been included in working coalitions so that community-driven proposals reflect current legal standards, thus making them less vulnerable to subsequent challenges.

---

is no umbrella agency taking leadership for comprehensive strategies and oversight to protect the health of residents, workers, and others affected by the contaminated ores, public health nurses and community members have been the most active partners in working collaboratively to identify specific activities, strategies, and roles needed to address multiple, ambiguous health and policy issues such as community-level conflict, individual or community stigma, and generational health consequences and long-term cleanup (Kuntz et al, 2009) (Box 91-9).

SUMMARY

Many dimensions of community health suggest that there are needs and opportunities for nurses to be involved in setting the policy agenda to promote and sustain health. Identifying communities, working to create and sustain partnerships with community members and organizations, and advocating health-promoting policies at all levels are all important features of the nursing role. The nurse who is concerned with policies that support health in communities finds that the role crosses areas of food and agricultural policy, housing policy, labor policy, aging policy, environmental policy, and social policy, among many others. Nurses today are better educated than ever before and well positioned to be involved in initiatives that extend the traditional boundaries of health policy to the creation of public policies that will truly support the health of communities.

For a list of related websites, please refer to your Evolve Resources at http://evolve.elsevier.com/Mason/policypolitics/

REFERENCES

Agency for Toxic Substances Disease Registry [ATSDR]. (2008). Summary report: Exposure to asbestos-containing vermiculite from Libby, Montana, at 28 processing sites in the United States. Retrieved from www.atsdr.cdc.gov/asbestos/sites/national_map/index.html.

Agency for Toxic Substances Disease Registry [ATSDR]. (2009). Mortality review: Mortality in Libby, Montana, 1979 to 1998. Retrieved from www.atsdr.cdc.gov/asbestos/sites/libby_montant/mortality_review.html.

Americans for Nonsmokers' Rights. (2009). Overview list: How many smoke free laws? Retrieved from www.no-smoke.org/goingsmokefree.php?id=519.

Andrulis, D. P., Siddiqui, N. J., & Gantner, J. L. (2007). Preparing racially and ethnically diverse communities for public health emergencies. *Health Affairs, 26*(5), 1269-1279.

Aronson, J. (1993). Giving consumers a say in policy development: Influencing policy or just being heard? *Canadian Public Policy, 19*(4), 367-378.

Association of State and Territorial Directors of Nursing (ASTDN). (2009). The public health nurse's role in achieving health equity: Eliminating inequalities in health. Retrieved from www.astdn.org/downloadablefiles/ASTDN-health-equity-11-08.pdf.

Bent, K. N. (2003). The people know what they want: An empowerment process of sustainable, ecological community health. *Advances in Nursing Science, 26*(3), 215-226.

Boston Women's Health Book Collective. (2005). *Our bodies, ourselves: A new edition for a new era.* New York: Simon & Schuster.

Bouye, K., Truman, B. I., Hutchins, S., Richard, R., Brown, C., Guillory, J. A. (2009). Pandemic influenza preparedness and response among public-housing residents, single-parent families, and low-income populations. *American Journal of Public Health, 99*(S2), S287-S293.

Cheadle, A., Psaty, B. M., Curry, S., Wagner, E., Diehr, P., Koepsell, T., et al. (1991). Community-level comparisons between the grocery store environment and individual dietary practices. *Preventive Medicine, 20*(2), 250-261.

Colorado Revised Statutes. (1998). (Section 25-8-501.1) Amendment 14, "Regulation of Commercial Hog Facilities," amending Part 5 of Article 8 of Title 25, Colorado Revised Statutes (Section 25-8-501.1) (passed November 4, 1998).

Diez Roux, A. V. (2001). Investigating neighborhood and area effects on health. *American Journal of Public Health, 91*(11), 1783-1789.

Durie, R. & Wyatt, K. (2007). New communities, new relations: The impact of community organization on health outcomes. *Social Science & Medicine, 65*(9), 1928-1941.

Geronimus, A. (2000). To mitigate, resist, or undo: Addressing structural influences on the health of urban populations. *American Journal of Public Health, 90*(5), 762-767.

Giacomini, M., Baylis, F., & Robert, J. (2007). Banking on it: Public policy and the ethics of stem cell research and development. *Social Science & Medicine, 65*(7), 1490-1500.

Gray, B. H. & Schlesinger, M. (2009). Charitable expectations of nonprofit hospitals: Lessons from Maryland. *Health Affairs, 28*(5), w809-w821.

Hawe, P. & Shiell, A. (2000). Social capital and health promotion: A review. *Social Science & Medicine, 51*(6), 871-875.

Heron, M. P., Hoyert, D. L., Murphy, S. L., Xu, J. Q., Kochanek, K.D., & Tejada-Vera, B. (2009). Deaths: Final data for 2006. *National Vital Statistics Reports, 57*(14). Hyattsville, MD. National Center for Health Statistics.

Hutchins, S. S., Truman, B. I., Merlin, T. L., & Redd, S. C. (2009). Protecting vulnerable populations from pandemic influenza in the United States: A strategic imperative. *American Journal of Public Health, 99*(S2), S243-S248.

Hyland, A. (2009). Clean Indoor Air Knowledge Asset. Robert Wood Johnson Foundation's Substance Abuse Policy Research Program. Retrieved from http://saprp.org/knowledgeassets/knowledge_detail.cfm?KAID=2.

Institute of Medicine (IOM). (2003). *The future of the public's health in the 21st century.* Washington, D.C.: The National Academies Press.

Jenkins, J. L., Hsu, E. B., Sauer, L. M., Hsieh, Y., & Kirsch, T. D. (2009). Prevalence of unmet health care needs and description of health care–seeking behavior among displaced people after the 2007 California wildfires. *Disaster Medicine and Public Health Preparedness, 3*(2 Suppl), S24-S28.

Kessler, R. C. & Cleary, P. D. (1980). Social class and poverty. *American Sociological Review, 45*(3), 463-478.

Kuntz, S. W., Winters, C. A., Hill, W. G., Weinert, C., Rowse, K., Hernandez, T., et al. (2009). Rural public health policy models to address an evolving environmental asbestos disaster. *Public Health Nursing, 26*(1), 70-78.

Lurie, N., Wasserman, J., & Nelson, C. D. (2006). Public health preparedness: Evolution or revolution. *Health Affairs, 25*(4), 935-945.

Massey, P. & Durrheim, D. (2007). Income inequality and health status: A nursing issue. *Australian Journal of Advanced Nursing, 25*(2), 84-88.

McKevith, B., Stanner, S., & Butriss, J. (2005). Food choices in primary care: A summary of the evidence. *Nursing Times, 101*(40), 38-42.

Milio, N. (1981). *Promoting health through public policy.* Philadelphia: F.A. Davis.

Milio, N. (1996). Linking health, communities, information technology and policy. In N. Milio (Ed.), *Engines of empowerment: Using information technology to create healthy communities and challenge public policy.* Chicago: Health Administration Press.

Milio, N. (2002). Where policy hits the pavement: Contemporary issues in communities. In D. J. Mason, J. K. Leavitt, & M. W. Chaffee (Eds.), *Policy and politics in nursing and health care* (4th ed., pp. 659-668). St. Louis: W.B. Saunders.

Monroe, J. A. (1997). Enemies of the people: The moral dimension to public health. *Journal of Health Politics, Policy and Law, 22*(4), 993-1020.

Pomeranz, J. L. & Brownell, K. D. (2008). Legal and public health considerations affecting the success, reach, and impact of menu-labeling laws. *American Journal of Public Health, 98*(9), 1578-1583.

Population Health Forum, University of Washington. (2009). Advocating for action toward a healthier society. Retrieved from http://depts.washington.edu/eqhlth/pages/issues.html.

Rebmann, T., Carrico, R., & English, J. F. (2008). Lessons public health professionals learned from past disasters. *Public Health Nursing, 25*(4), 344-352.

Stephenson, H. & Zeldes, K. (2008). Write a chapter and change the world: How the Boston Women's Health Book Collective transformed women's health then—and now. *American Journal of Public Health, 98*(10), 1741-1745.

Troy, D. A., Carson, A., Vanderbeek, J., & Hutton, A. (2008). Enhancing community-based disaster preparedness with information technology. *Disasters, 32*(1), 149-165.

U.S. Department of Health and Human Services (USDHHS). (2000). *Healthy People 2010.* Retrieved from www.healthypeople.gov.

U.S. Department of Health and Human Services (USDHHS). (2004). *The initiative to eliminate racial and ethnic disparities in health: HHS fact sheet.* Washington, D.C.: USDHHS Office of Minority Health. Retrieved from www.omhrc.gov/rah/index.htm.

U.S. Geological Survey (USGS). (2003). Principal aquifers of the 48 conterminous United States, Hawaii, Puerto Rico, and the U.S. Virgin Islands: U.S. geological survey. Madison, WI. Retrieved from http://nationalatlas.gov/atlasftp.html.

U.S. Geological Survey Map. (1998). Principal aquifers of the conterminous United States: U.S. Geological Survey, Madison, WI. National Atlas Series, compiled by James A. Miller.

Wilkinson, R., & Marmot, M. (Eds.). (2003). *Social determinants of health: The solid facts.* Copenhagen, Denmark: World Health Organization.

World Health Organization (WHO). (1978). *Report of the International Conference on Primary Health Care, (Alma Ata, USSR).* Geneva, Switzerland: World Health Organization.

World Health Organization (WHO). (2000). Munich Declaration. Nurses and midwives: A force for health, 2000. Retrieved from www.euro.who.int/aboutwho/policy/20010828_4.

World Health Organization. (2003). In R. Wilkinson & M. Marmot (Eds.). *Social determinants of health: The solid facts.* (2nd ed.). Retrieved from www.euro.who.int/document/e81384.pdf.

World Health Organization. (2004). WHO Framework Convention on Tobacco Control. Retrieved from www.who.int.fctc/en.

World Health Organization. (2007). In M. Whitehead & G. Dahlgren (Eds.), *Concepts and principles for tackling social inequities in health: Levelling up. Part 1.* Retrieved from www.euro.who.int/document/e89383.pdf.

World Health Organization. (2008). *World Health Report 2008: Primary health care now more than ever.* Geneva, Switzerland: World Health Organization.

Yonkman, M. M. & Bridgeland, J. M. (2009). All volunteer force: From military to civilian service. Civic Enterprises. Retrieved from www.civicenterprises.net/allvolunteerforce.

CHAPTER 92

An Introduction to Community Activism

DeAnne K. Hilfinger Messias

"Action indeed is the sole medium of expression for ethics."

—Jane Addams

Community activism is the means through which individuals, groups, and organizations work together to bring about specific, often radical, changes in social, economic, environmental, and cultural policies and practices. The broad goal of community activism is to enact social transformation that contributes directly to improving living conditions, enhancing community environments, and eliminating health and social disparities. Community activists engage in collaborative, sustained actions focused on changing underlying structures or removing barriers—be they political, social, economic, environmental, or cultural—with the ultimate aim of improving the lives of individuals or groups subjected to disparate, discriminatory, or oppressive conditions (Table 92-1). The primary focus on changing underlying or contributing structures, practices, or policies is what distinguishes community *activism* from community *service*, the provision of goods or services for underserved or underprivileged individuals or groups (Jennings, Parra-Medina, Messias, & McLoughlin, 2006; Jennings, Messias, & Hardee, 2010). It is further distinguished from community *development*, in which the primary focus is to enhance existing social and economic infrastructures through the creation of new service programs, leadership training, and innovative partnerships (Larsen, 2004). Another distinguishing characteristic of community activism is that the primary commitment and motivation for change are generated from within the community of interest. In contrast, the motivation, expertise, and resources for community service and development often originate outside the local community.

KEY CONCEPTS

The concepts of social justice, community, consciousness-raising, critical reflection, praxis, and empowerment are integral to community activism (Figure 92-1).

SOCIAL JUSTICE

Social justice is a philosophical, political, and public health concept rooted in the ideal of human rights and social equity (Reichert, 2007). The equitable distribution of resources and opportunities for a productive and fulfilling life is a human rights concern. Prerequisites for social justice include the establishment and assurance of equal treatment under the law, equal access opportunities, and fair and equitable distribution of resources. Yet in many communities around the globe, availability and access to basic resources and opportunities (i.e., clean air and water, adequate and nutritious food, appropriate housing, safe and secure neighborhoods, equitable educational opportunities, the means to a productive and fulfilling livelihood, affordable culturally appropriate health services, and fair and equal treatment under the law) are not equitably distributed among all individuals and groups. Rather, factors such as social privilege or market forces determine the distribution of these key resources and opportunities, resulting in social injustices and inequities. Overcoming social injustice requires collective action and solutions on multiple fronts. One of the ways the ideal of social justice is translated into practice is through community activism.

TABLE 92-1 **Types and Definitions of Community Actions**

Type of Community Action	Definition
Community activism	Collaborative, sustained actions focused on changing structures or removing barriers with the ultimate aim of improving the lives of individuals or groups subjected to disparate, discriminatory, or oppressive social, economic, political, cultural, or environmental conditions
Community development	The creation of new programs and services in order to improve and enhance local social and economic infrastructures
Community service	The provision of goods or services for underserved or underprivileged individuals or groups

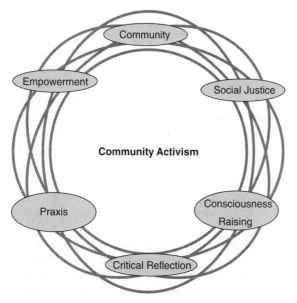

FIGURE 92-1 Key concepts of community activism.

COMMUNITY

Community is a dynamic and fluid concept, conceptualized and practiced in diverse ways. In relation to activism, community implies the actual involvement of individuals and groups directly impacted by the specific issues or conditions that are the focus of change. In a more traditional sense, community—or grassroots—activism is considered to be locally generated and locally focused. Many community activists are located within and focused on creating change in a specific geographic location, such as the neighborhood, school district, or city where they live, study, or work. Neighborhood activists frequently mobilize around issues related to public safety, environmental health, education, land use, zoning, and economic development. The focus may be location-specific (e.g., getting traffic signs installed at busy intersections, organizing a neighborhood watch or clean-up effort, eliminating the presence of alcohol and tobacco advertising in low-income and minority neighborhoods) or may address broader structural issues such as economic development or environmental pollution.

In the United States, education is a common focus of activism involving students, parents, teachers, and the broader community. For example, in 2002, Mayor Jerry Brown hired 100 police officers to patrol Oakland, California's underfunded public schools serving primarily African-American and Hispanic youth. This policy decision prompted the mobilization of the very youth intended as the target of armed police surveillance. In protest of the surveillance-based policy focus, Oakland students organized youth rallies and a march on City Hall, forcing the mayor to acknowledge other approaches to youth development and to allocate $7 million to Oakland youth programs (Ginwright & Cammarota, 2006). Similarly, the implementation of bilingual education programs in southwest Chicago public schools came about in response to Mexican-American community activism (Stovall, 2006).

Grassroots activists also mobilize across geographical and social communities. Historically, community activists have participated in broader social movements (e.g., the women's rights, civil rights, workers' rights, and environmental health movements). Much activism occurs within the context of communities formed through affiliation with a collective social identity (e.g., a cultural or ethnic group, race, or religion) or shared sense of political responsibility. Collective social identities related to specific health issues (e.g., HIV/AIDS, cancer, mental health, tuberculosis, women's reproductive health) have given rise to significant community activist movements. Over the past 25 years, what is now a global HIV/AIDS movement began as local activism within gay communities in the U.S., Canada, Western Europe, and Australia. These early activists mobilized to educate their own communities around HIV prevention and, at the same time, demand responsive public action from governments, medical researchers, health care providers, pharmaceutical companies, and legal systems (Piot, 2006). Subsequent HIV/AIDS grassroots mobilizations have involved diverse communities, including persons living with AIDS in Brazil, Uganda, and South Africa; sex-workers in Thailand; religious and community leaders in Senegal; and impoverished mothers of childhood AIDS victims in Romania. Through relentless advocacy and demands for changes in public policy as well as local health care systems, HIV/AIDS community activists have provoked governmental and industry responses, resulting in more effective prevention and access to treatment and significantly impacting the global HIV/AIDS epidemic (Marcolongo, 2002; Piot, 2006).

CONSCIOUSNESS RAISING, CRITICAL REFLECTION, AND PRAXIS

Consciousness raising, critical reflection, and *praxis* are three interrelated components of community activism. Underlying liberatory approaches to community activism is the premise that empowerment emerges from engagement in focused dialogue, listening, critical reflection, and reflective action (Freire, 1970, 1973). One of the first steps of engaging participants in activist endeavors is to increase public awareness of specific issues and the associated root causes.

CONSCIOUSNESS RAISING

Consciousness raising goes beyond simply presenting others with information to actually engaging with others in critical reflection. Popular educator and community activist Paulo Freire originally defined and applied the concept of *conscientização* (Portuguese for "conscientization") in his community-based work with illiterate Brazilian peasants. Conscientization is a reflective process in which individuals and

groups examine their own particular situations and contexts in order to identify social, economic, cultural, political, and environmental forces contributing to these situations. Critical awareness arises through the reflective processes of problem-posing and interpretive decoding of lived experiences.

CRITICAL REFLECTION

Critical reflection is integral to understanding the linkages and connections between a local community's issues and problems and those of other communities across the globe. By engaging in critical dialogue and reflection, community activists begin to envision possibilities for collective action leading to transformation (Jennings et al., 2010). Critical reflection also involves attention to the political processes and actions necessary to challenge inequalities and effect change. *Praxis* is purposeful, reflective action arising out of individual and collective conscientization and theorizing, grounded in a commitment to building a more just society, through diverse means, including culture circles, critical pedagogies, action research, and community activism (Freire, 1970, 1973; Hesse-Biber, 2007; Stovall, 2006). Community activism is a form of critical social praxis, an iterative cycle of conscientization-reflection-reflective action in which relations of power and inequality are identified, challenged, and changed.

EMPOWERMENT

Empowerment is a multilevel construct that incorporates processes and outcomes of social action through which individuals, families, organizations, and communities gain control and mastery within the social, economic, and political contexts of their lives in order to attain greater equity and improve the quality of life (Jennings et al., 2006). At the individual level, empowerment may result from the generation of new knowledge and understanding of issues and the development of new skills among community activists. This individual empowerment then can be linked to community organizing to support social action and political change, as well as to individual self-protective and other socially responsible behaviors (Wallerstein, Sanchez-Merki, & Velarde, 2005). Collective empowerment occurs within families, organizations, and communities. It involves processes and structures that enhance members' skills, provide them with mutual support necessary to effect change, improve their collective well-being, and strengthen intraorganizational and interorganizational networks and linkages to improve or maintain the quality of community life.

The process of making connections between personal experiences and broader social issues is integral to personal and community empowerment and to effective action. In describing a youth empowerment program at an alternative high school for youth unable to succeed within the traditional educational system, Mitra (2008) reported an adult advisor's observation that "The kids involved are changing [from] delinquent into activists. [They can see] how they got sucked into being delinquent and the criminal justice system through their upbringing—not just their family, but the community and the policies" (p. 210). The purpose of empowerment education is to develop the requisite knowledge and skills for community activism, particularly among youth. By participating in community action projects (e.g., peer teaching, the production of murals, cultural institutes, the creation of videos for use in educational efforts, or photo-voice projects), youth and other potential activists develop the requisite knowledge and skills for community activism as they engage in collective consciousness-raising, critical reflection, and reflective action (Messias, McLoughlin, Fore, Jennings, & Parra-Medina, 2008).

TAKING ACTION TO EFFECT CHANGE: CHARACTERISTICS OF COMMUNITY ACTIVISTS AND ACTIVISM

Activists not only recognize injustice but are willing to take action to correct it (Sherrod, 2006). Situated across the social, economic, and political spectrum, activists share a desire to contribute to the collective welfare and create a more just and equitable society. Motivation and commitment of personal time and energy to social involvement, a willingness to take risks, and the belief in power and efficacy of groups to effect change are common characteristics among community activists. The motivation may be rooted in personal or professional experience, empathy, or solidarity (Lewis-Charp, Yu, & Soukamneuth, 2006; Montlake, 2009). Due to the risks embedded in social justice work, activists must individually and collectively assess the potential harm that may come from

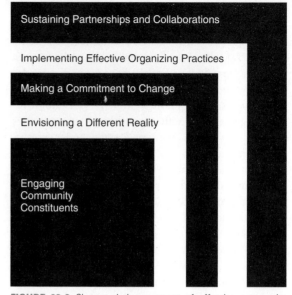

FIGURE 92-2 Characteristic processes of effective community activism.

actions, help each other prepare if they choose to take calculated risks, and take steps to protect themselves and others as best as possible when they do (Cohen, de la Vega, & Watson, 2001).

Community activism grows out of the desire to change existing social, political, or environmental conditions. In their commitment to change and transform the way power is distributed or controlled, activists draw on the power of the people and the community (power within) and exert pressure on those who hold institutional power (power over). Characteristics of successful community activism include the ability to *frame issues and envision a different reality*, a clear *commitment to change* at various levels, the implementation of *effective organizing practices and actions*, and the ability to develop and sustain *collaborative partnerships and relationships* (Figure 92-2).

ENVISIONING CHANGE AND POSSIBILITIES FOR DIFFERENT REALITIES

New ways of collective seeing, perceiving, and acting are essential for change (Jennings et al., 2010). To create the momentum and sustain process toward social change, activists may need to refocus issues around commonalities rather than fueling polarization around differences. When working toward the goal of a new and different reality, the processes of consciousness raising and critical reflection can result in collective redefinition and reframing of issues. For instance, in addressing problems such as educational inequality, activists may need to rethink commonly held wisdom and redirect the focus of their actions. Lightfoot (2008) provided an example of such rethinking and reframing, citing the case of local education activists changing the focus from replacing school segregation with integration to actively addressing the underlying racism that had fostered and perpetuated segregation in the first place. In the case of transnational activism to improve the lives of marginalized Filipino bar girls working in a country where prostitution is illegal, the commitment to change was informed by activists' understanding of the social and political context (Ralston & Keeble, 2009). Rather than framing the issue as eliminating prostitution, the activists focused on alleviating prostitutes' legal, financial, and social hardships, by changing the minds and practices of exploitative bar owners and clients, an unsympathetic community, and an insensitive court system.

TAKING ACTION

Beyond critical conceptualization and framing of issues, creating change requires action on multiple fronts and the participation of individuals with a wide range of skills, talents, and competencies. Activists work to create change in social norms, public policies, legislation, or environmental practices. Effecting change in policies, practices, and social structures entails integrated informational, mobilization, relationship-building, and communication work. This requires extensive research and analysis of complex issues; monitoring of local power dynamics; and ongoing planning, implementation, and evaluation of the effectiveness of organizing strategies and approaches.

Community activists organize and act to call attention to their issues, communicate and disseminate information, develop and maintain networks, and engage others in problem-solving and policy change strategies. Communication and information dissemination actions include door-to-door soliciting; writing letters to the editor; creating and distributing flyers, posters, and leaflets; and producing and disseminating print, radio, and television ads. Increasingly activists employ Internet formats (e.g., websites,

e-mail, blogs, social networking sites) to communicate within their existing networks and to reach new audiences. In tailoring their messages for specific audiences, community activists use a range of media, from art, storytelling, songs, theater, photography, videos, and multimedia presentations to expert panels, research reports, and policy briefs.

To engage community members and policymakers in problem solving and policy change, activists employ a variety of mobilization and organizing actions, such as conducting public meetings and forums; planning and carrying out mass demonstrations, rallies, and marches; supporting and participating in boycotts and strikes; collecting signatures on petitions and carrying out letter-writing campaigns; and conducting teach-ins, trainings, workshops, and community-based participatory research.

CREATING AND SUSTAINING COLLABORATIONS

Less visible, but clearly as important, is the behind-the-scenes work of networking, building relationships, and sustaining coalitions. Everyday social networks through home, school, and work provide potential connections and opportunities for activism (Martin, Hanson, & Fontaine, 2007). Collaboration is a key process within community activism and is necessary to develop and implement the policies and practices necessary to effect the desired changes. Similar to other organizing activities, collaboration requires considerable time, energy, skill, and the involvement of multiple stakeholders. But the power of collaboration is that by working together, concerned individuals and groups can create the synergy to produce a desired change that could not be generated by individual action alone.

Partnering with like-minded individuals and organizations strengthens activist movements, but to effect real change, activists often must build bridges and create collaborative relationships that cross differences in age, race, class, social position, location, or nationality and bring together groups on different sides of issues. Productive collaborations contribute to capacity-building among individuals, groups, and organizations, resulting in enhanced ability to achieve mutual goals. At its core, activism is relational work, as exemplified in the life and work of Ella Baker. Although not as well-known or recognized as Martin Luther King, Jr., Baker was an instrumental visionary and community organizer within the civil rights movement who dedicated her life to organizing with and mentoring students and community members. Born and educated in the Jim Crow South, in 1927 Baker moved to New York City, which became the base for her activist career over the next 50 years. Ella Baker worked on social justice issues ranging from child welfare, youth services, school reform, and consumer education to police brutality, desegregation, and voting rights. Through her collaborative associations with other activists, educators, and policymakers in various organizations (e.g., Parents in Action, National Association for the Advancement of Colored People, Southern Christian Leadership Conference, In Friendship, Student Nonviolent Coordinating Committee), Baker's activism was essential in developing the groundwork of legal and institutional changes of the civil rights movement and eventual de facto racial desegregation. Baker's approach to furthering human rights was to build "strong people" rather than to be or support a "strong leader" (Ransby, 2003).

CHALLENGES AND OPPORTUNITIES IN COMMUNITY ACTIVISM

Community activists in the twenty-first century face numerous challenges and opportunities, including making the choice between incremental or radical change; addressing local issues within the context of an increasingly globalized world; effectively harnessing the potential of new technologies; and encouraging and empowering new activists. A major strategic challenge is the decision to pursue incremental or radical change, concomitantly balancing the potential costs with prospective gains of either strategy. Ralston and Keeble (2009) provided an example of this challenge in their assessment of transnational collaborative efforts to improve the lives of Filipino prostitutes. Although some of the partner activist organizations were steadfast in their commitment to the eradication of prostitution and end to sexual exploitation, Ralston and Keeble recognized that to have begun with the explicit goal of "eliminating prostitution in such an exploitative context…would have prevented the germination of a project like ours, where the process of harm reduction to women in the sex trade began" (p. 161). Although making some headway in their collaborative effort to build the capacity of Filipino groups working directly with prostitutes, these activists also came to recognize the significance of actions

and change at the individual level, arguing that transcending differences to work for social justice involved both standing with others and changing minds.

The forces of globalization and its concomitant movement of people, goods, services, technology, information, and ideas across geographical and political borders have impacted the form and focus of community activism. Today's community activists address local issues within the context of an increasingly globalized world. There are enormous opportunities for ongoing activism and engagement to overcome environmental, economic, and social inequalities and injustice on many fronts, and the ability to transcend local boundaries and become part of global movements is both a challenge and an opportunity. The growth of the activist movement against gender-based violence is an example of the opportunities for local activism to translate into global action and policy change. In communities across the globe, activists have worked to raise awareness about gender-based violence and create and strengthen local resources to both support victims and prevent further violence against women and girls. The "16 Days of Activism" campaign against gender violence is an example of a global network of community activists. This campaign originated with local activists who came together at the 1991 Women's Global Leadership Institute. An outcome of this event was the creation of the 16 Days Campaign, anchored by November 25, International Day Against Violence Against Women, and December 10, International Human Rights Day, and symbolically linking gender-based violence and the violation of human rights. As part of the early 16 Days Campaigns, local activists circulated petitions and collected signatures that were instrumental in shaping the agenda of the 1993 World Conference on Human Rights in Vienna. In recent years, 16 Days Campaign activists have focused on the intersections of HIV/AIDS and gender-based violence (Center for Women's Global Leadership, n.d.; UNAIDS, 2006). Another example of transnational activism is the anti-sweatshop movement, linking students, community residents, workers, and labor activists, in the U.S. and other countries. These activists work concomitantly to change the working conditions of workers, most of whom are women, and the creation of "sweat-free" business policies and practices in cities and campuses (Student Labor Action Coalition, n.d.; United Students against Sweatshops, n.d.).

New technologies provide opportunities for activists to reach untapped audiences and disseminate interactive media. Media literacy can be both the means and an end in community activism. Duncan-Andrade (2006) described how engaging youth in critical production of media texts can serve as a site for critique and analysis of urban social inequalities as well as a site of production for social change. A new initiative of the Hesperian Foundation, the Community Action for Women's Health and Empowerment, combines the traditional print resource of a book with a Web-based tool that will include examples of action strategies and community-based organizational tools from groups around the world with expertise in particular areas of women's health (Hesperian Foundation, 2009). Beyond employing information technology as a tool, another challenge global health activists face is to create access to appropriate technology, such as renewable energy sources (e.g., solar, wind) for remote rural health care clinics in developing countries. Of course, technology does not come without costs and challenges such as investment costs, upkeep and maintenance, updates, as well as the costs of personnel and training. Ensuring intergenerational continuity of community work is another ongoing challenge among community activism movements (Naples, 1998). Thus, the work of successful community activists also includes encouraging, mentoring, and empowering new activists.

NURSES AS COMMUNITY ACTIVISTS

Nurses and other health professionals may be involved in activist endeavors as members of their local communities and in conjunction with their professional roles. The involvement of nurses in community activism is not surprising, given the shared ethics of care and social justice and the activism of early nursing leaders such as Florence Nightingale, Lillian Wald, and Lavinia Dock (Andrist, 2006; Drevdahl, 2006). Today's nurse activists work within a wide range of movements for social, environmental, cultural, and health systems change (Domrose, 2005). As environmental health activists, nurses have led efforts to implement smoke-free workplace policies, create physical-activity–friendly neighborhood environments, establish and monitor standards for clean air and water, and mobilize communities impacted by environmental toxins and pollutants. Within the women's health arena, examples of nurse-led activism

include the establishment of community-based maternity care for underserved populations, implementation of hospital breastfeeding policies and practices, and advocacy and policy work in the areas of reproductive health and human trafficking. Nurse activists can be an important force for change within the health care system, as evidenced by recent efforts to implement policy and practice changes in the areas of patient safety, workplace injury prevention, and health care reform. The professional expectation that advanced practice nurses be involved in policy development, implementation, and evaluation will require more nurses to develop an activist skill set in the future. As each new generation of nurses comes into practice, they must balance the need to sustain existing activist endeavors while addressing new challenges as they arise.

Opportunities for community activism and social justice work exist in every community, however defined. Every community faces the ongoing challenge of renewing the call to action, encouraging and empowering members to actively participate in the processes and institutions that shape their social and economic lives and their health and well-being.

For a list of related websites, please refer to your Evolve Resources at http://evolve.elsevier.com/Mason/policypolitics/

REFERENCES

Andrist, L. C. (2006). The history of the relationship between feminism and nursing. In L. C. Andrist, P. K. Nicholas, & K. A. Wolf (Eds.), *A history of nursing ideas* (pp. 5-22). Sudbury, MA: Jones & Bartlett.

Center for Women's Global Leadership. (n.d.). About the 16 Days: What is the 16 Days of Activism against Gender Violence Campaign? Retrieved from www.cwgl.rutgers.edu/16days/about.html.

Cohen, D., de la Vega, R., & Watson, G. (2001). *Advocacy for social justice: A global action and reflection guide.* Bloomfield, CT: Kumarian Press.

Domrose, C. (2005). Nurse activists strive for change: Four nurses make activism a part of their nursing practice. Retrieved from www.nurseweek.com/news/Features/05-04/NurseActivists_print.html.

Drevdahl, D. J. (2006). The concept of community in nursing history: Its narrative stream. In L. C. Andrist, P. K. Nicholas, & K. A. Wolf (Eds.), *A history of nursing ideas* (pp. 83-96). Sudbury, MA: Jones & Bartlett.

Duncan-Andrade, J. (2006). Urban youth, media literacy, and increased critical civic participation. In S. Ginwright, P. Noguera, & J. Cammarota (Eds.), *Beyond resistance! Youth activism and community change: New democratic possibilities for practice and policy for America's youth* (pp. 149-169). New York: Routledge.

Freire, P. (1970/1997). *Pedagogy of the oppressed: 20th-Anniversary edition.* (Trans.) Myra Bergman Ramos. New York: Continuum.

Freire, P. (1973/1993). *Education for critical consciousness.* (Trans.) Myra Bergman Ramos. New York: Continuum.

Ginwright, S., & Cammarota, J. (2006). Introduction. In S. Ginwright, P. Noguera, & J. Cammarota (Eds.), *Beyond resistance! Youth activism and* community change: New democratic possibilities for practice and policy for America's youth (pp. xiii-xxii). New York: Routledge.

Hesperian Foundation. (2009). Community action for women's health and empowerment. Retrieved from www.hesperian.org/projects_inProgress_womensactionguide.php.

Hesse-Biber, S. N. (2007). Feminist research: Exploring the interconnections of epistemology, methodology, and method. In S. N. Hesse-Biber (Ed.), Handbook of feminist research: Theory and praxis (pp. 1-26). Thousand Oaks: Sage.

Jennings, L., Messias, D. K. H, & Hardee, S. (2010). Addressing oppressive discourses and images of youth: Sites of possibility. In L. B. Jennings, P. C. Jewett, T. T. Laman, M. V. Souto-Manning, & J. L. Wilson (Eds.), Sites of possibility: Critical dialogue across educational contexts (pp. 39-67). Cresskill, NJ: Hampton Press.

Jennings, L. B., Parra-Medina, D., Messias, D. K. H., & McLoughlin, K. (2006). Toward a theory of critical social youth empowerment. Journal of Community Practice, 14(1/2), 29-54.

Larsen, S. C. (2004). Place, activism, and development politics in the Southwest Georgia United Empowerment Zone. Journal of Cultural Geography, 22(1), 27-49.

Lewis-Charp, H., Yu, H. C., & Soukamneuth, S. (2006). Civic activist approaches for engaging youth in social justice. In S. Ginwright, P. Noguera, & J. Cammarota (Eds.), Beyond resistance! Youth activism and community change: New democratic possibilities for practice and policy for America's youth (pp. 21–35). New York: Routledge.

Lightfoot, J. D. (2008). Separate is inherently unequal: Rethinking commonly held wisdom. In A. H. Normore (Ed.), Leadership for social justice: Promoting equity and excellence through inquiry and reflective practice (pp. 37-59). Charlotte, NC: Information Age Publishing.

Marcolongo, M. (2002). The good mothers: Romania's HIV/AIDS activists are mostly poor mothers of thousands of children who contracted the disease due to poor medical practices under the Ceausescu regime. Alternatives Journal, 28(2), 23-25.

Martin, D. G., Hanson, S., & Fontaine, D. (2007). What counts as activism? The role of individuals in creating change. Women's Studies Quarterly, 35(3/4), 78-94.

Messias, D. K. H., McLoughlin, K., Fore, E., Jennings, L., & Parra-Medina, D. (2008). Images of youth: Representations and interpretations by youth actively engaged in their communities. International Journal of Qualitative Issues in Education, 21(2), 159-178.

Mitra, D. L. (2008). Student voice or empowerment? Examining the role of school-based youth-adult partnerships as an avenue toward focusing on social justice. In A. H. Normore (Ed.), Leadership for social justice: Promoting equity and excellence through inquiry and reflective practice (pp. 195-214). Charlotte, NC: Information Age Publishing.

Montlake, S. (2009). People making a difference: After her husband disappeared, housewife Angkhana Neelepaichit became a human rights activist. Christian Science Monitor, 101(86), 47.

Naples, N. A. (1998). Grassroots warriors: Activist mothering, community work, and the war on poverty. New York: Routledge.

Piot, P. (2006, March 7). Diverse voices, common ground: Uniting the world against AIDS. Speech at Georgetown University, Washington D.C. Retrieved from www.unaids.org/en/AboutUNAIDS/Leadership/EXD/EXDHighSpeeches.asp.

Ralston, M., & Keeble, E. (2009). Reluctant bedfellows: Feminism, activism, and prostitution in the Philippines. Sterling, VA: Kumarian Press.

Ransby, B. (2003). Ella Baker and the Black freedom movement: A radical democratic vision. Chapel Hill: University of North Carolina Press.

Reichert, E. (2007). Challenges in human rights: A social work perspective. New York: Columbia University.

Sherrod, L. R. (2006). Promoting citizenship and activism in today's youth. In S. Ginwright, P. Noguera, & J. Cammarota (Eds.), Beyond resistance! Youth activism and community change: New democratic possibilities for practice and policy for America's youth (pp. 287-299). New York: Routledge.

Stovall, D. (2006). From hunger strike to high school: Youth development, social justice, and school formation. In S. Ginwright, P. Noguera, & J. Cammarota (Eds.), Beyond resistance! Youth activism and community change: New democratic possibilities for practice and policy for America's youth (pp. 97-109). New York: Routledge.

Student Labor Action Coalition. (n.d.). Retrieved from http://slac.rso.wisc.edu.

UNAIDS. (2006). Stop violence against women; stop HIV. Retrieved from www.unaids.org/en/KnowledgeCentre/Resources/FeatureStories/archive/2006/20061127_Women_violence_en.asp.

United Students against Sweatshops. (n.d.). Retrieved from www.studentsagainstsweatshops.org/index.php.

Wallerstein, N., Sanchez-Merki, V., & Velarde, L. (2005). Freirian praxis in health education and community organizing: A case study of an adolescent prevention program. In M. Minkler (Ed.), Community organizing and community building for health (2nd ed., pp. 218-239). New Brunswick, NJ: Rutgers University Press.

CHAPTER 93

TAKING ACTION
From Sewage Problems to the Statehouse: My Life as an Elected Official

Mary L. Behrens

"All politics is local."
—Thomas P. "Tip" O'Neill, former Speaker
of the United States House of Representatives

I have practiced as a family nurse practitioner, pediatric clinical specialist, and nurse educator. Running for political office was not one of my career goals. However, my father was a good role model; he served on our local school board for 12 years. I attended college in the 1960s during a period of student activism and protests; that experience influenced me also. But it was a problem in my town that sparked my work in politics.

SEWAGE CHANGED MY LIFE

My leap into the political arena came because of a call from an upset friend who lived on property along the river that ran through our community. She told me there was raw sewage on her lawn that was washing up from the river. She had called the health department. They told her to call the state Department of Environmental Quality. That state department referred her to the health department. Out of frustration, she called me.

SEEING IS BELIEVING

I drove to my friend's neighborhood and saw the raw sewage on people's lawns. My friend told me that it appeared like clockwork when everyone flushed their toilets and used their dishwashers in the morning and evening. I decided to take action. I contacted local daycare centers and learned that they had noticed an increase in diarrhea in the children. I then called the two local TV stations and three radio stations. I informed them of a serious problem on the river, and I gave them the time and location of a press conference I was planning.

At the press conference, I stated that I was a nurse and was concerned about the sewage being a serious health threat to citizens in our town. I discussed the increased diarrhea in children reported by local daycare centers. The news media representatives who attended my press conference could see the raw sewage and captured images with their cameras. The train was moving down the track! The city, the health department, and the state Department of Environmental Quality had to deal with the calls from the press and the citizens. Our local city government and the state had to provide funds to connect this housing development to city water and sewer in order to stop the pollution.

MY CAMPAIGNS

As I took action on the sewage problem, I attended several city council meetings. When I observed the city council in action, I thought to myself, "I can do this and bring a perspective to the council as a nurse, mother, and concerned citizen." At the next election, I ran for city council in my ward along with 13 other candidates. I won, and since then, I have held three elected offices: city councilor and mayor, chair of the

667

county commission, and representative in the state legislature.

I recognized the importance of being involved in my professional associations. I have served as president of the Wyoming Nurses Association, and as second vice president and first vice president of the American Nurses Association. Currently, I serve on the American Nurses Association (ANA) Congress on Nursing Practice and Economics and as chair of the ANA Political Action Committee.

THE VALUE OF POLITICAL ACTIVITY IN YOUR COMMUNITY

At the local level, you have the opportunity to help address problems that affect people's lives. For example, a citizen came to a city council meeting one evening and said he wanted passing lanes on a street in the community. He had a persuasive personality and a reputation for getting what he wanted. His initial presentation was very convincing to other council members. But I lived in this neighborhood and was concerned about the safety implications of this proposal. Part of this street abutted a park where children played. Parents parked along the street to watch or pick up their children. If passing lanes were established in this area, speeds would increase, and the potential risk of a serious accident would rise. I asked every councilperson to visit the area, particularly in the late afternoon. All of the members voted against establishing passing lanes on the street.

AN OPPORTUNITY TO LEARN THE ROPES

The local community is an excellent starting place if you want to run for higher office. You can gain experience, confidence, name recognition, and respect. I had the chance to testify before the Federal Energy Regulatory Commission in Washington, D.C. about the high natural gas prices we were paying in our community. Because I was the only mayor to testify (the others providing testimony were senators, representatives, or governors), I was quoted and praised for bringing a refreshing perspective to the Commission.

NETWORKING

As mayor, I worked with citizens, state legislators, and our state's congressional delegation in Washington, D.C. Richard B. (Dick) Cheney was our only representative in Congress when I served as mayor of

Casper, Wyoming. I formed an important connection with him because of my service. This type of connection was an important part of my network when I decided to run for the state legislature and international nursing endeavor.

Some of my work bridged both local and state-level work. I had joined the "Seatbelt Coalition" in Wyoming before running for the legislature. The coalition's mission was to educate Wyoming citizens about the need for seatbelt legislation and develop a model law for the Wyoming legislature to enact. As a freshman legislator, I co-sponsored the first seatbelt legislation aimed at reducing fatalities on Wyoming highways. I also sponsored several pieces of legislation to help assist communities with high natural gas prices. My experience on the city council prepared me to hit the ground running with issues like this when I arrived at the Wyoming state house.

LEADERSHIP IN THE INTERNATIONAL COMMUNITY

I had traveled five times to do humanitarian work in Vietnam and had attended International Council of Nursing conferences. I was concerned about the nursing shortage—not just in the U.S. but in the developing world. In 2006, I sent a one-page note to then–Vice President Cheney discussing how I might contribute to the World Health Assembly that meets annually in Geneva, Switzerland. I did not specify a year but rather how my experiences at the ANA and in Vietnam could add to the discussion for a future appointment.

I was invited to meet with the vice president but had health issues that caused me to cancel (I couldn't believe I had to do that!). I was so disappointed to have missed out on this opportunity but was surprised a few weeks later when I answered the phone.

Someone said, "This is the White House." I grabbed my chair. My mind raced—"am I dreaming this?" The vice president had recommended that I be part of the U.S. delegation to the World Health Assembly—in 3 weeks. I notified the ANA and planned to work with Barbara Blakeney, then–ANA president, who would be attending also.

Soon I was involved in phone calls with staff on logistics and schedule. Before I knew it, I arrived in Geneva for the first meeting with Health and Human Services Secretary Michael Leavitt. I told staff I wanted

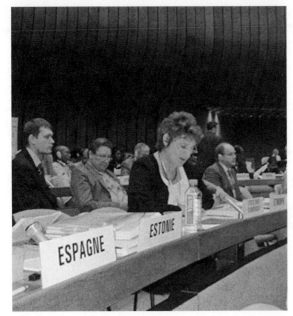

FIGURE 93-1 Mary Behrens testifying at the World Health Assembly in Geneva, Switzerland.

to testify on behalf of the international nursing shortage (Figure 93-1).

Representatives of several countries had testified before me and had discussed their struggle to find nurses to provide basic services. When it was my turn, I shared my concern about the lack of nurses worldwide, especially in countries in Africa. Several nurses came up to me afterward to thank me for my remarks.

RECOMMENDATIONS FOR BECOMING INVOLVED IN POLITICS

JOIN A POLITICAL PARTY

You don't have to agree with every part of a party's political platform, but joining a political party is an important step in learning the ropes. Organized political parties provide support and guidance on how to get started with a political campaign. They can provide you with the opportunity to gain experience by working on someone's campaign before actually running yourself. You can learn the steps for running a grassroots campaign, for example, how much money you need to raise, what forms are required, how to organize a campaign committee, and how to access mailing lists, voter registration, and past precinct results. The parties also raise money, which is used to support the total slate of offices in that particular

party. The party can help you get your message out and reach all voters, especially those who might "cross party lines."

CONNECT WITH OTHER NURSES

Nursing colleagues and associations can be extremely helpful in a political campaign. A group of nurses can send a powerful message of support when they back a candidate. Many state nurses associations have political action committees to assist with endorsements and financial assistance.

LEARN FROM OTHERS IN YOUR COMMUNITY

Another helpful activity is to join the League of Woman Voters. The name is derived from the woman's suffrage movement, but today membership is open to women and men. Local leagues will often hold public forums on various issues such as health care. It is a wonderful opportunity to contribute to the dialogue and make connections. The League of Women Voters is also concerned about getting the vote out and what motivates people to go to the polls.

DEVELOP COST-EFFECTIVE CAMPAIGN STRATEGIES

When you are a candidate, you cannot be afraid to ask for money, and you need to take advantage of free and low-cost opportunities to get your message out. Flyers, mailing labels (usually the party you have joined will provide this at a bulk price), newspaper and radio ads, yard signs, and billboards all cost money. Press releases, letters to the editor, speaking at meetings and forums, neighborhood cafes, and news coverage are free. My least expensive campaign was my first race for city council. We produced a one-page flyer and distributed it door to door. Whenever you choose a strategy like this, it is important to be aware of laws and regulations so you and your campaign staff don't run into problems. For example, you cannot leave flyers in a mailbox because it is a federal offense. If no one is at home, leaving a personal note stating "Sorry I missed you" can be an effective alternative. My husband made the political signs in our garage. It took a table saw, some nails, and stiff cardboard with name and logo on it.

GET THE MESSAGE OUT

Getting out your message is critical to success. You must reach the voters. It does help to get some media training to help frame your messages. The press wants a good story and good "sound bites," so your words should be carefully selected. Don't say anything you would not want to see in print or on TV. The press may not fully understand an issue, and you can help frame the story with your nursing knowledge. If you provide accurate information, members of the media will look forward to contacting you again. I've learned from my experience. Don't be afraid to tell the TV crew that you want a "head and chest only" shot of you because you did not have time to change your clothes.

Serving as an elected official can be a very rewarding experience and a great opportunity for advocating for community health improvements. We need nurses serving at all levels of government. We need nurses working for safe schools and safe drinking water at the local level, working for safe highways and seatbelt usage at the state level, and working for health care reform and funding for nursing education at the federal level.

For a list of related websites, please refer to your Evolve Resources at http://evolve.elsevier.com/Mason/policypolitics/

CHAPTER 94

TAKING ACTION
Community Advocacy in Pennsylvania: How I Worked to Make my Community Healthier

Patricia E. Tobal

"In every community, there is work to be done … In every heart, there is the power to do it."

—Marianne Williamson

MY PATH TO BECOMING A COMMUNITY ADVOCATE

Nursing has been my vocation for over 40 years. My roles in nursing have changed over time, from beginning as a staff nurse caring for hospitalized individuals to concluding as a manager of a community-based, prevention-focused program for 125 first-time, low-income mothers. Along the way, I continued my education, obtaining bachelor's and master's degrees in nursing, which expanded my professional opportunities. It is these experiences that have led me to my avocation: community advocacy and volunteerism.

After receiving a diploma in 1967 from the Uniontown Hospital School of Nursing, I practiced in the community in Pennsylvania where I grew up, married, raised my family, and retired. Over the course of my career, I saw many changes in the health care system. Yet one thing remains the same. Chronic health problems such as diabetes, chronic obstructive pulmonary disease, and coronary artery disease continue to plague our population, and individuals with these conditions consume tremendous portions of our health care resources. Current data indicates that obesity, smoking, and other unhealthy lifestyle choices are at all-time highs and do not bode well for our population.

I began my nursing career in a hospital and transitioned into oncology nursing. It was my experience at an outpatient radiation oncology center that would raise my awareness of the research being done, not only to find a cure for cancer but also to identify factors that contribute to the development of the disease and efforts being made to educate the public about ways to reduce individual risk and ultimately prevent its occurrence. While at the center, I became co-facilitator of a support group for individuals and their families who were receiving treatment or who were cancer survivors. The stories they shared gave me a greater understanding of the challenges faced by individuals in the community who were dealing with a serious illness.

After leaving the cancer center and completing my master's degree in 1998 at Duquesne University, I was approached to teach a community health nursing course for RN to BSN students at Penn State's Fayette campus. This reaffirmed my commitment to prevention. It also led to a career transition with the Nurse-Family Partnership (NFP). The NFP is a prevention-focused, home visitation program for low-income, at-risk pregnant women expecting their first child. NFP home visitors are registered nurses who have received additional education preparing them to deliver the program with fidelity to the evidence-based model that evolved from findings gathered from three separate randomized, controlled trials. After beginning in 1996, the NFP has expanded through a national initiative to over 25 states. The Fayette County, Pennsylvania site was established in

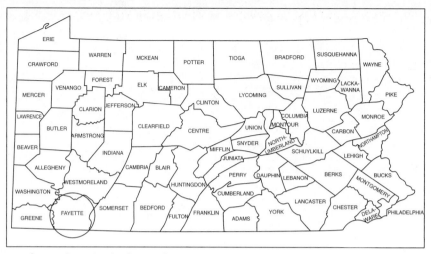

FIGURE 94-1 Fayette County, Pennsylvania. Source: State of Pennsylvania. (Retrieved from *www.dot.state.pa.us/Internet/Bureaus/pdPlanRes.nsf/infoBPRCartoCountyType3.*)

2001 under the auspices of the Fayette County Community Action Agency (FCCAA). Fayette County is located in southwestern Pennsylvania (Figure 94-1). The coal mining industry was the most significant employer until that industry's decline in the late twentieth century. This has resulted in a high rate of unemployment and dependence on government and social services. The FCCAA is an organization that assists individuals to work toward self-sufficiency through a myriad of services that include educational programming; a food bank; the Women, Infants and Children (WIC) program; nutrition education; senior centers; and medical and dental offices located at a central location to ease access. Thus began my "up close and personal" exposure to the unmet needs in my community.

THE HOPWOOD VILLAGE PROJECT—AN EXAMPLE OF COMMUNITY COLLABORATION

At the same time that I became involved with the NFP, my husband, Jim Tobal, and I joined the Hopwood Village Project, a group composed of people from the small community in which we live at the foot of the western slope of the Appalachian Mountains along the National Road (U.S. Route 40). The organization's dream was to install sidewalks, erect period streetlights, and landscape the streetscape along the historic Road. We envisioned an environment in which people could safely walk and enjoy the natural beauty and history of our area. However, there were barriers to accomplishing this, and many thought it impossible. We knew that we had an achievable plan that could only be accomplished with the cooperation of our elected officials. Our village is unincorporated, and the National Road divides two neighboring municipalities: the North Union and South Union Townships. If we were to be successful, we would need to get the two groups of township supervisors to work together in collaboration with us. We began by sponsoring a community "Light-Up Night" event to bring residents together. The supervisors of each township were asked to support the event by providing traffic control. The event was a success, the supervisors were recognized for their help, and the Hopwood Village Project demonstrated credibility. As a result, each township's board of supervisors began to send representatives to village project planning meetings.

We started work on a 7-year project that involved writing grant proposals that were completed with the assistance of the Fayette County Planning Office. We also reached out to local, state, and national elected officials. Township officials, county commissioners, state senators and representatives, and members of Congress representing our area received invitations to participate in each of our activities and often were in attendance. This provided an opportunity for them to see the progress that was being made in Hopwood as well as to interact with their constituents. They were included in our annual parade celebrating the National Road Festival, quoted in newspaper articles, and interviewed for television coverage. Hopwood was the site of community meetings with our U.S. representative, enabling us to keep him informed of our progress. These relationships proved invaluable as we continued to move forward. Communication with shopowners in the village was also critical. Information about every event was shared with them during the planning phase, and their input and involvement was sought.

The Hopwood Village Project was completed in stages and included the following:

- Erecting two stone welcome signs that were designed by a local resident and built and installed by vocational-technical school masonry students
- Installing streetlights and benches that were donated by families, organizations, and businesses
- Installing continuous stamped concrete sidewalks along the corridor, curbs, and landscaping

All of this was accomplished at a cost of over $1 million. The funding was secured from a variety of sources including federal and state grants, fundraising, and donations. We learned many lessons from this experience including the importance of a good plan, communication, teamwork, patience, perseverance, and flexibility.

ANOTHER OPPORTUNITY PRESENTS ITSELF

As progress was being made on the Hopwood Village Project, an opportunity presented itself that would build on the work we had done to create a safe place to walk in the village. Fayette County, Pennsylvania, has extremely high rates of chronic disease and unhealthy lifestyle behaviors. For this reason, the Pennsylvania Department of Health selected Fayette County to receive funding through the Centers for Disease Control and Prevention (CDC) as an initiative of the U.S. Department of Health and Human Services (DHHS) to establish the Steps to a Healthier PA-Fayette County program. (The Steps program has since been renamed CDC's Healthy Communities Program.) (Box 94-1).

Fayette was one of three Pennsylvania counties to implement community-appropriate programs. The programs were designed to encourage behavioral changes that would reduce the burden of diabetes,

---

> **BOX 94-1 The CDC's Healthy Communities Program**
>
> CDC's Healthy Communities program (formerly known as the Steps program) engages communities and mobilizes national networks to prevent chronic disease. Through the program, communities work to change the places and organizations that touch people's lives every day including schools, worksites, health care sites, and other community settings. The actions are focused on reversing the national epidemic of chronic diseases.
>
> Source: www.cdc.gov/healthycommunitiesprogram.

---

obesity, and asthma as well as impact the risk behaviors of physical inactivity, poor nutrition, and tobacco use. One of the programs offered by the Steps program in Fayette County was the Neighborhood Health Leadership program. The Hopwood Village Project chose to participate. I chaired a committee that was trained in a series of workshops that covered communications; data; statistics; and available resources, board management, and neighborhood assessment. We selected "Healthier Hopwood" as our goal and set out to plan a strategy.

WALKING TOWARD BETTER HEALTH

The committee decided to address the problem of physical inactivity by encouraging people to use the new sidewalks. With the guidance of Steps staff, a grant application for "Healthier Hopwood" was completed. Funding was received in 2008 to implement the program, which included creating and printing maps highlighting three walking routes in the village (including descriptions of points of interest on each); erecting custom signs at each end of the village to keep the maps accessible to walkers; and purchasing t-shirts imprinted with the Hopwood Village logo. The t-shirts were awarded to people who walked a total of 100 miles on the sidewalks. "Healthier Hopwood" was introduced at the dedication ceremony held to celebrate completion of the Hopwood Village streetscape project on May 24, 2008. The initiative was well received as measured by the positive feedback received, increased pedestrian traffic visible in the village, and the number of t-shirts being worn.

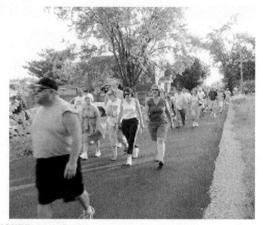

FIGURE 94-2 Participants enjoying the Wednesday Evening Walk in Hopwood, Pennsylvania.

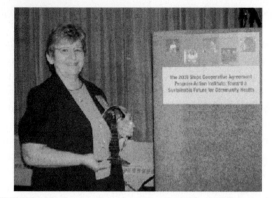

FIGURE 94-3 Patricia Tobal receiving the CDCs 2008 Community Hero Award for her community advocacy.

Shortly after the sidewalk dedication, Hopwood hosted the first of a series of Wednesday evening walks sponsored by the Steps program in various Fayette County communities (Figure 94-2). Led by my husband, a group of over 100 people traveled the walking route, stopping at points of interest to learn interesting facts about the history of the village. When planning community events, it can be difficult to predict the response. We were pleasantly surprised at the size of the turnout in Hopwood.

A SPIRITUAL ASPECT OF COMMUNITY SERVICE

Steps offered health ministry training by the Mercy Parish Nurse and Health Ministry Program sponsored by the Sisters of Mercy in Pittsburgh to our local community and provided resource materials and support to interested church groups. We began the health ministry at my church by assessing the congregation to determine health-related needs and wants. Blood pressure measurement, weight loss, and physical activity were identified as the top three areas of interest. We responded by offering blood pressure screenings, which included body mass index (BMI) measurement, education, and referral. We sponsored a "Big Losers" contest during the summer months to support those wanting to lose weight. The goal of the program was to lose an amount of weight equivalent to that of an average adult male by combining the amount of weight lost by all participants. Weekly

updates were published in the church bulletin accompanied by healthy recipes that used fresh fruits and vegetables available at the time. While we were successful in losing only "half a person," we did keep health on people's minds in a fun way. During the fall, we led the congregation on a virtual "Walk to Bethlehem" (the one in the West Bank). This activity drew parishioners of all ages. Participants submitted weekly walking totals that were combined and tracked on a map of the area from Pennsylvania to the Middle East. The total distance was 5975 miles, and, frankly, we weren't convinced that we would make it. Walking groups were organized for those interested, and we mapped out a route inside the church building, marking it with vinyl clings. By the end of the 12-week program, we had totaled over 8000 miles, equivalent to walking the entire way to Bethlehem and flying over the Atlantic on our return. We celebrated our achievement with an after-church social and served food typical of that eaten in the Middle East. It was a well-received, healthy change from the coffee and donuts typically seen at coffee hours.

AN UNEXPECTED RECOGNITION

I received an unexpected recognition for my community advocacy. For my work as the chair of Healthier Hopwood, I received an award from the CDC. At a ceremony in Washington, D.C., I and seven others from the 40 CDC-funded Steps communities received 2008 Steps Community Hero awards (Figure 94-3). Seven individuals were selected from the 40 CDC-funded Steps communities. Each honoree accepted the award not just for himself or herself, but on behalf of everyone in his or her community who is committed to the vision of creating a healthier America.

COMMUNITY ADVOCACY AND "GIVING BACK"

I encourage health care professionals to get involved in their communities. Community advocacy is one way of "giving back." It provides great opportunities for personal growth and satisfaction. However, community advocacy is not without challenges. I have been fortunate to work with others who share a passion and commitment for the projects. We've found it important to have a plan, but also to be willing to be able to make adjustments when necessary. Timelines may need to be extended when seeking funding sources. Relationships are critical, particularly with those outside the group who can help "make things happen." Local media are invaluable in raising awareness of a project and activities. It helps to provide prepared press releases for distribution. Elected officials at every level have a vested interest in supporting local communities. Opening lines of communication with officials assures that voices in the community are heard. Informing them of activities and thanking them for any assistance that they provide helps to maintain their awareness and support of projects. Volunteering with others to make a difference in the community is a meaningful experience. You get so much more than you give.

For a list of related websites, please refer to your Evolve Resources at http://evolve.elsevier.com/Mason/policypolitics/

CHAPTER 95

TAKING ACTION
A Nurse Practitioner's Advocacy Efforts in Nevada

Elena Lopez-Bowlan

"Service is the rent we pay for being. It is the very purpose of life, and not something you do in your spare time."

—Marian Wright Edelman

I remember the first time I was called an "activist." I was not sure if I was being criticized or complimented. A friend said, "How dare they call you an activist— you are much more than that." I had to think about this label. I came to realize I was being considered an "advocate," a label I embraced as part of my nursing heritage. When I was a student, I had been impressed when I learned that Florence Nightingale advocated for the improvement of sanitary conditions for the soldiers during the Crimean war. This type of patient advocacy has been a principle role of nurses, and I was proud that it was part of my work.

WANTING TO BE A NURSE

From the earliest time I can remember, I wanted to be a nurse and I wanted to help others. When I was a child, my idol was a nurse who was a neighbor of ours in South Texas. I loved watching her leave for work in her crisp, white uniform. I noticed the compassion she showed the worried mothers in the neighborhood. She would support and guide them when their children were sick. I remember the way she flicked the glass thermometer with confidence and authority. I wanted to be like her.

When I was about 4 years old, my older brother suffered with tonsillitis, and I volunteered to take him his medicine, juice, and food. At age 10, I bottle-fed some kittens we had found, and I made sure they were comfortable before I went to school. The start of my nursing career was delayed by some of my choices. I got married as a young woman and moved from Texas to New York.

At the age of 30, I found myself divorced and living on Long Island without a solid career. After trying many jobs, such as sales, secretarial work, and modeling, I moved to upstate New York, where Corning Community College offered a 2-year registered nurse program. While the program was intense, I enjoyed every minute of it. Nothing was going to distract me again. I would graduate and become a nurse.

MY FIRST NURSING JOB

My first job as an RN was at a skilled nursing facility, Founder's Pavilion, in Corning, New York. While I had not anticipated working with older adults, it was the only job available at the time. For a year, I wrote nursing plans, passed medications, did postmortem care, and supervised other nurses. I took my job seriously and begged the administrators to let me learn management skills. One day, I was called to the assistant director of nursing's office. I was not sure if I had done something wrong, and I took a deep breath as I entered her room.

The assistant director of nursing asked, "How brave are you? We do not have a supervisor for the 11 to 7 shift, and we were wondering if you could do it." I remember feeling both excitement and fear. I accepted the challenge and learned as I went along. I became the night nursing supervisor and thought that I would never leave this job. I then met a man who encouraged me to move to the west coast, where he would be working in San Francisco, and he became my husband a year later. While in San Francisco, I worked in challenging positions until my husband's work took us to Reno, Nevada, in 1992. This is where my advocacy work was launched.

BACK TO SCHOOL

After moving to Reno, I decided to return to school to get a bachelors degree in nursing. I learned a great deal in class, but working in the community allowed me to see problems that needed attention. In a community nursing class, I learned of a social service organization called Nevada Hispanic Services. The organization had a small AIDS education program. The state of Nevada had little money to fund agencies like this, and I became an advocate for the Hispanic population (who were becoming infected with HIV/AIDS at an alarming rate). Another student and I embarked on developing better services for the Hispanic community. I requested meetings with state officials to discuss data that substantiated my requests. The program at Nevada Hispanic Services received funding, and in 1996 we received the National Latino Children's Agenda La Promesa Award for program development in the Hispanic community.

After completing my bachelors degree, I decided to continue my education again and entered a family nurse practitioner program at the University of Nevada, Reno. One of my instructors, Dr. Alice Running, asked me if I would join some medical students in the development of a clinic for the area's homeless. The students met on Saturday mornings at the local Salvation Army office, and we would see many people with desperate needs. We had one volunteer attending physician, and our clinical setting was very basic. We had fun as a team, and I learned about the needs of underserved populations. I felt that my volunteer work was an integral part of my life.

While I attended graduate school full time, I started to volunteer and to serve on some local and state boards. I participated as honorary co-chair for the Susan G. Koman Race for the Cure (to support breast cancer research), and I volunteered to do cancer screening for Hispanic and African-American women at churches and health fairs. I found that I could make a real difference in people's lives through these activities, and I gained important experience.

THE VALUE OF VOLUNTEERING

You may wonder why I devoted so much time to do volunteer work and participate in many organizations. My desire to make the world a better place may seem "Pollyanna-ish," but it is the primary reason for my participation. The more I volunteered and the more problems I tackled, the more I realized how important it was to use my skills to advocate for others.

I believe that my service and advocacy have made a difference, but it has not always been easy. The members of one of the boards I served on completed Myers-Briggs personality assessments to improve how we worked together. We learned how we could work better together—even though we worked in different ways (Figure 95-1).

CHALLENGES IN ADVOCACY AND SERVICE

One of the most difficult experiences I recall occurred when I was attending a Nevada AIDS/HIV conference. Many different groups throughout the state were asked to set up tables and displays about the work they were doing in their communities. Since our state programs were new, we at Nevada Hispanic Services decided to invite some individuals from San Antonio to assist us in this forum. They were known nationwide for their ability to reach the Hispanic community. We were overjoyed when they accepted our invitation, and we felt that they might help shed some light on the development of educational HIV/AIDS programs. Unfortunately, this offended the other Nevada groups. They chose to boycott our educational display. I was extremely disturbed by this response since I felt we were all working toward the same purpose. I learned some political realities in this experience.

Another difficult experience that provided a lesson for me occurred when I served on a state regulatory board. I noticed that the president of the board would hand-pick people she felt should run for board positions—and they appeared to be her close friends. I was concerned when I witnessed people less qualified than I and others being selected for a board position simply because of friendship. I challenged the process. While I prevailed in ending this method of doing board business, I was not seen as a "popular"

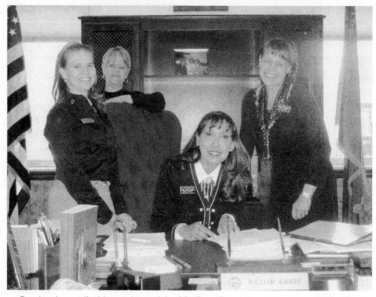

FIGURE 95-1 Elena Lopez-Bowlan *(seated)* with members of the Mt. Rose Republican Women at the legislature in Carson City, Nevada.

TABLE 95-1 **Examples of Elena Lopez-Bowlan's Community Advocacy Activities**

Agency or Appointment	Type of Volunteer Service or Activism
Truckee Meadows Fair Housing Advisory Board	Advocated for fair housing practices
HIV/AIDS Service Providers of Northern Nevada, State AIDS Task Force, and Nevada AIDS Foundation	Advocated for prevention education
Nevada Women's Fund	Raised money to help women return to school
The Angel Kiss Foundation	Raised money for families of children with cancer
Nevada Academy of Health Steering Committee	Advised legislators on health priorities
Governor's Maternal and Child Health Advisory Task Force	Advised the State Health Division
Latinos for Political Education	Encouraged Hispanics to vote and run for political office
Mt. Rose Republican Women	Promoted political awareness
Northern Nevada Breast and Cervical Cancer Coalition	Advocated for education about breast cancer awareness
Nevada State Board of Nursing	Appointed by governor to the state's nursing regulatory board
State Legislative Health Interim Advisory Committee	Advised Nevada state legislators
National American Latino Museum	Serving as member of a presidential commission planning a new museum

board member after that. Those were hard times, but I feel that I accomplished a lot. In addition to having the board abide by the open meeting laws, I led an effort to have our brochures translated into Spanish. It seemed an intelligent choice after learning that Hispanics were not calling this regulatory board.

WORKING IN THE MEDIA

I've had several opportunities to share my views and advocate for solutions in the media. Since 2006, I have been invited monthly to participate as a political pundit on a Reno television show entitled *Nevada*

Newsmakers. I have enjoyed writing an opinion column for our local newspaper, the *Reno Gazette Journal*. In this column, I write about diverse topics such as politics, nursing, health care, and culture. Through these activities, I am able to educate people, draw attention to problems, and use my background as a nurse to discuss solutions.

THE VALUE OF RECOGNITION

The work I've done has led to a number of awards and recognitions (Table 95-1). I was especially honored when I received the 2006 American Academy of Nurse Practitioners State Award for Excellence. My peers felt that I was deserving of this award for the advocacy work that I had done and for the newspaper articles that I have written about nursing. While I did not do this work expecting recognition, I have been honored to receive acknowledgement for it. Most importantly, the awards draw attention to the causes I believe in and to problems that still need solutions.

While much of my work has been at the local and state level, recently I was asked to serve on a presidential commission that will advise the president on the development of an American Latino museum of art in Washington, D.C. Writing this chapter has provided me with further insight as to why I believe in being a community activist. I recently made the decision to run for elective office, and I am campaigning for the Nevada state assembly. I feel that all of the advocacy experiences that I have had will make me an effective legislator. I clearly identify myself as a nurse in my campaign literature.

For a list of related websites, please refer to your Evolve Resources at http://evolve.elsevier.com/Mason/policypolitics/

CHAPTER 96

TAKING ACTION
One Nurse's Fight Against Gang Violence in California

Corazon Tomalinas

"We make a living by what we get, but we make a life by what we give."

—Winston Churchill

My husband and I were both nurses. We worked hard to have a good home to raise our children in. We love our children, and we were always involved in their lives and their education. We were close to our extended family, our church, and our community. Despite this, my beloved daughter got involved with "party crews" and drugs. That led our family on a painful journey filled with helplessness and guilt. At the end, though, the journey led me to a life in public service and to a world of people with great strength, hope, faith, and love.

MY CHILDHOOD IN THE PHILIPPINES

I was born in 1944 in a small barrio called San Jose, Agoo, La Union, in the Philippines. I was raised by my maternal grandparents, while my parents lived in neighboring Baguio City (a practice that was not common). My father was a taxicab driver. He was quick to help others—a poor man with a big heart. When I was 9 years old, while he was working late, he gave a ride home to a group of young men who didn't have money for the fare. He was murdered that night, leaving my mother with 6 children—the youngest barely 6 months old. With no means of support, the rest of the family moved in with my grandparents as well. My mother's brother, who had lived in the United States for many years, supported us. At age 9, I became a caregiver. I taught my siblings prayers, and I led the household chores. I graduated from Saint Mary's Academy High School in 1961 with no hope of pursuing my college education, even though I had graduated as the valedictorian.

Then a miracle occurred. My uncle invited me to the U.S. Against the odds, I was granted a student visa by a consul who heard about my mother's six children. That blessing meant that I had to leave my family and travel to a land and culture that was very alien to me. Upon reaching California, I lived with a family member who did not speak or understand my native language. I attended Jefferson High School in Daly City and found myself to be one of a handful of Filipino-Americans there. It was lonely and frightening, but it was also a challenge. Slowly, I traced my relatives and found a welcoming Filipino community in the San Francisco Bay Area. That "clan" became my family and support system in the U.S. The trauma of being a 16-year-old very far from home gradually eased.

BECOMING A NURSE, WIFE, MOTHER—AND U.S. CITIZEN

Two years after arriving in the U.S., I was admitted to San Francisco State College as a nursing student. It was not easy being a full-time student. I had no money for books. (I sent my uncle's allowance back to the Philippines to help support my family there.) Those were days of fear, as I had to have my student visa status changed to immigrant status. I approached a judge who was sensitive to my plight—and I had just passed by licensure exam! My request was approved, and I found my first job as a nurse.

I moved to San Jose and became a staff nurse at San Jose Medical Center in 1968. In this first nursing job, I met my husband Robert Tomalinas and became an American citizen. We were married in 1971, and I was able to continue to support my family in the Philippines with my salary. After 5 years at San Jose Medical Center, I moved to Santa Teresa Hospital while it was being built. I became the evening supervisor.

In my first nursing jobs, I learned to advocate for patients and their families. I learned to teach by example. I loved my patients and their families, and most of them loved me back. I made friends that have lasted for years. During this time, my daughter, Maria, was born in 1974 and then my son, Robert, in 1977. I remained at home until my son was almost 3 years old, and then worked as a float nurse for 2 days a week. My husband and I were very involved with our children. We volunteered on field trips, school plays, and the parent teacher association, where I served twice as president. Eventually, my mother finally joined us from the Philippines followed by my siblings. As an extended family, we took camping trips and went on retreats. Life was wonderful!

WHAT HAPPENED?

What happened next still haunts me, and I ask myself what I neglected to do or say. When my daughter turned 13, our family spiraled into a type of hell. My daughter became involved with "party crews." Party crews have been called the "junior varsity" of street gangs (Walbert, 2009). My daughter used drugs, ran away, and had crises at school—even failing physical education. My husband and I were caught off-guard, and we clung to each other and our son for strength and hope. My daughter said that she would attend classes stoned. She came home sober but kept to her room. Did her teachers notice? Did they care? She ran away for two days. She called home in the middle of the night to say she was okay but wouldn't reveal where she was. She was injured at a party and was arrested.

THE STRUGGLE TO FIND HELP

We were educated and articulate, but we struggled to find help for my daughter. We reached out to one organization that offered mental health services but no drug rehabilitation. Another organization provided rehabilitation but no mental health services. One organization would not admit patients on weekends, and another required that my daughter be arrested before they would help.

We sold our rental property (our only savings) to pay for my daughter to attend a 28-day program at a drug rehabilitation center; it cost us $18,000. We attended family therapy, and she had individual therapy at $97 per hour for 1 year. Most of this was not covered by insurance. Everything was hard. Her high school objected to her leaving school for therapy appointments, and the therapists had inflexible schedules. I maxed out credit cards for therapy and used them to keep my daughter busy shopping. I would do anything to keep her away from her "crew." I took on the school to create an Individual Education Plan (IEP) for her. My clergy became a critical source of support. And I prayed. One night we received a gift of grace—and my daughter's life changed dramatically. We got our daughter back, and her recovery since then has been a wonder. She caught up in school and graduated with her class (but at a different school in the district).

WE GOT HELP—BUT WHAT ABOUT OTHERS?

I believed I had been given a gift from God, but I was concerned about other families dealing with the same problems we had. I worried about other parents who did not have a house to sell to pay for care, who did not speak English, or who did not have the knowledge to seek help. The gift I received propelled me to help others.

I found a group called People Acting in Community Together (PACT), a faith-based community organization whose mission is to improve the quality of life in neighborhoods and families and to develop community leaders. In the 1980s, San Jose was besieged by drugs, gangs, and violence. The usual solutions (i.e., jails and police) were not effective. The youth involved in party crews and gangs were not receptive to professional psychologists deployed in the neighborhoods. PACT worked to get resources for a concentrated effort and a controversial solution: hiring ex-gang members who had turned their lives around to reach high-risk youth.

San Jose created the Mayor's Gang Prevention Task Force to convene all the service providers and to get the means to fund the work. County and city government, police, probation, schools, non-profit community organizations, faith organizations, and community representatives came to work together. The collaboration resulted in culturally-specific programs and an attempt at integrating services no one had ever done before. PACT supported citizens to empower themselves. A parents' safety council was organized to help and oversee the implementation of school safety plans and a new crisis response plan. The San Jose Mayor's Gang Prevention Task Force set out to save our youth and families—to heal a community one person at a time. Residents took up their responsibility and took action on behalf of others by the thousands.

I became one of the voices demanding accountability and compassion. These amazing events plunged me into the world of politics, committees, and commissions. I fought for tobacco settlement dollars to fund health insurance for children age 0 to 18 years. A partnership between county-city and private donations and foundations was formed to help families who were not eligible for medical care. I became a member of the First 5 Commission of Santa Clara County and helped shape the First 5 Santa Clara County Community Investment Plan. It funds neonatal intensive care units, Power of Preschool (an early care and education program that includes developmental assessment) and all other services First 5 offers, and advocates who steer families in court to appropriate services and bring dental care and medical referrals to the hearts of the neighborhood. I worked to encourage the stakeholders to integrate and align their services so they can be delivered in an appropriate and timely manner. I spoke to many people; the relationship of stakeholders must be strong and built on trust to foster such collaboration. I advocated for appreciation of our diversity, including the whole family in treatment and access to care without discrimination. I visited families, talked to groups, and cried with parents who are victims of violence. I also wept with many children who have lost hope because their parents find it difficult to forgive.

Presently I am working with the Mayor of San Jose's Gang Prevention Task Force to formalize a community-response protocol. This will bring help to the area of a violent incident— to both the victims and the perpetrators. We have a transition center that will reduce the amount of time an arrested youth is offered help and/or get them to court within 4 weeks instead of 12 weeks. Many people noticed my work and urged me to run for political office. I declined because I wish to advocate for any issue I wish. My loyalty is to my community and to God.

OPPORTUNITIES FOR ADVOCACY

A few years ago, we learned that my son is gay. Though often our culture is intolerant of homosexuality, our extended family rallied around us. They accepted and continue to love my son, and he and his sister remain very good friends. But I have concern for my son's welfare, and it presents another opportunity to advocate for a group of people who are often discriminated against. My husband passed away in 2001, and I lost my "bridge over troubled waters." For a short time, I wondered if I was strong enough to continue my mission. My faith became a beacon again as I picked up the pieces of my shattered heart and decided to be stronger. I accepted my vulnerability and leave myself as open as possible to share the pain of others—and then channel it to action.

My community efforts earned me many awards. They are all appreciated, but it often humbles me, for I do not act alone. The recognitions are valuable because they often lead to other opportunities to serve. My work with the schools brought me the Volunteer of the Year Award. I was awarded the Community Warrior from the Asian Pacific Democratic Club (although I am not a registered Democrat), the Community Star Award from Asian Americans for Community Involvement, the Martin Luther King Good Neighbor Award, an Outstanding Woman of Silicon Valley Award, California Assembly Woman of the Year, one for 100 Most Influential Women in the United States, the California Wellness Foundation's Peace Prize, and others (Figures 96-1 and 96-2).

I've made a difference in my community by participating on a number of boards that have brought about change in the community. These include the Board of Silicon Valley Education Foundation, the First 5 Santa Clara County Commission, the Mayor's Gang Prevention Task Force, the National League of Cities Crime and Gang Prevention Committee, and Sacred Heart Community Services. Today in San Jose,

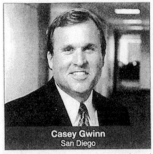

Casey Gwinn
San Diego

"We raise our criminals at home. Once we understand that, we need to focus on what we are doing with children early on and how we can break the generational cycle of violence. We have to start loving these children at five instead of locking them up at 17."

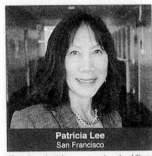

Patricia Lee
San Francisco

"If you have the right support services, the ability to work with the families, the ability to give a voice to and empower young people from within their own communities, the majority of youth will transition successfully out of the juvenile justice system."

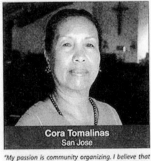

Cora Tomalinas
San Jose

"My passion is community organizing. I believe that you develop community one person at a time. I think that when people come together to look at a problem and really work together to do something about it, then we can prevent violence."

Violence Is Preventable!

◆

*The California Wellness Foundation
2007 Peace Prize*

◆

The California Wellness Foundation is proud to recognize its 2007 California Peace Prize awardees. In honor of their commitment to preventing violence and promoting peace in their communities, each will receive a $25,000 cash award.

These individuals are representative of thousands working throughout the state to prevent violence against youth. Each has offered practical, proven examples of how to build healthy communities and prevent violence.

The California Wellness Foundation recognizes these leaders for making California a healthier and safer place to live. To learn more about the Foundation and its 2007 California Peace Prize honorees, visit **www.tcwf.org**.

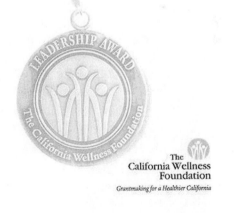

The
**California Wellness
Foundation**
Grantmaking for a Healthier California

FIGURE 96-1 California Wellness Foundation Peace Prize recognition of nurse activist Cora Tomalinas.

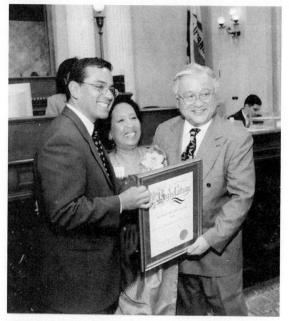

FIGURE 96-2 Cora Tomalinas receiving Woman of the Year recognition from the California legislature in 1996. Pictured: Antonio Villaraigosa, Cora Tomalinas, and Congressman Mike Honda.

California, a parent in need can call one number and get information from a live person (not a machine) on how to deal with problems from gang crime to food and shelter. Today in San Jose, children can get medical care from a clinic that asks only which insurance to use, not whether the child is insured. Today in San Jose, a child need not get arrested to be eligible for help. Today, one neighborhood has an alternative school directed by parents. Today, San Jose is one of the safest large cities in the U.S., but there is still much work to be done. The crumbling budget and economy threaten to close many vital services. I met Congressman Honda and his late wife while they were working at Franklin-McKinley School District where he was principal. He supports education not only in Washington, D.C., but also when he is at home in San Jose (Figure 96-3).

I retired from nursing in 2003 but continue to practice the vocation in a wider arena—caring as a volunteer in my community. When I was awarded the California Peace Prize, it came with $25,000. It sponsored two low-income families to visit Disneyland. It also funded an appreciation party for a gang task force

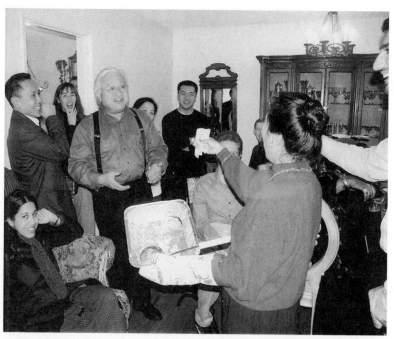

FIGURE 96-3 Cora Tomalinas shows fund-raising proceeds to Congressman Mike Honda during a Franklin-McKinley Education Foundation fund-raiser held annually at Tomalinas' home.

that was working very hard and for non-profit organizations to continue their work with high-risk youth. Every penny of that money touched a child's life.

I did not do it all myself. At times, I pushed others to the front, and at other times I pulled. Our children need resources, and the greatest of all is the gift of ourselves.

For a list of related websites, please refer to your Evolve Resources at http://evolve.elsevier.com/Mason/policypolitics/

REFERENCE

Walbert, M. (2009, March 10). Cracking down on party crews, "junior varsity" of street gangs. *The Arizona Republic*. Retrieved from www.azcentral.com/news/articles/2009/03/10/20090310partycrews0310.html.

CHAPTER 97

TAKING ACTION
The Canary Coalition for Clean Air in North Carolina's Smoky Mountains

Jonathan Bentley

"You cannot affirm the power plant and condemn the smokestack, or affirm the smoke and condemn the cough."

—Wendell Berry, *The Gift of the Good Land*, 1981

When I returned to the United States from living abroad, my goal was to settle down in a beautiful rural area and build a life there. I was impressed by Western North Carolina's richly forested mountains, kind people, plentiful rainfall, and huge tracts of protected land. But these blessings were marred by some of the worst air quality in the nation, due largely to pollution from motor vehicles and coal-fired power plants. My first impulse was to find another location with cleaner air, but I was reminded of Joe Louis' famous line, "You can run, but you can't hide." Air pollution in the Smoky Mountains is a symptom of a much more pervasive disorder. Human-derived environmental contamination can now be found from pole to pole, at the highest mountain peaks, and at the bottom of the deepest ocean trenches (WHO, 2007).

With this in mind, I decided to dig in and look for ways to directly address our local air quality problems. Fortunately, there were many other community members who valued clean air. In 2000, I met Avram Friedman, Executive Director of the Canary Coalition. This clean air advocacy organization had made significant progress with the people of the southern Appalachians and with state lawmakers in Raleigh. A prime example of this was North Carolina's Clean Smokestacks Act, one of the nation's strongest examples of clean air legislation. It promised to reduce emissions from the state's 14 coal-fired power plants by 70% to 80% by 2010.

With Avram's guidance, I joined eight other Canary Coalition members on a lobbying trip to Raleigh to meet with state legislators and highlight citizen support for this important clean air legislation. One representative showed us stacks of postcards and lists of e-mails and phone calls he had received on this issue, with an overwhelming majority supporting the Clean Smokestacks Act (Ross, 2009). Other lawmakers were less sympathetic, but there were already clear signs that our grassroots work was speaking more loudly than the deep pockets of the coal and electric industries. In 2002, the North Carolina General Assembly signed the Clean Smokestacks Act into law with an overwhelming majority (Figure 97-1).

THE CANARY COALITION AT WORK

The Canary Coalition's name and logo are derived from the old practice of taking caged canaries down into mines as an early warning device. The canaries were more sensitive to poor air quality than were the miners, who would take heed if their canary stopped singing. If deadly fumes or low oxygen levels killed the bird, the miners knew they could quickly be the next to perish. The Canary Coalition stresses that Fraser firs, trout, asthma patients, older adults, and human fetuses are the modern-day "canaries" in our current environment (Box 97-1). These sensitive harbingers suffer from excessive ground-level ozone as well as

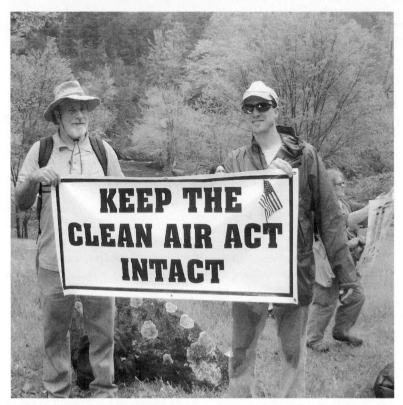

FIGURE 97-1 Jonathan Bentley (author) and David Wheeler protest legislative backsliding. Great Smoky Mountains National Park, Tennessee. (Reprinted with permission.)

dangerous levels of mercury, sulfuric acid, and nitrogen deposited on the earth by rain. Such toxins result from burning coal and other fossil fuels, and their health risks are well documented (NCDAQ, 2009a). Less understood are the extent and effects of global warming, which is related to the same outdated energy habits.

Drawing upon Avram Friedman's vision, dedication, and tireless leadership, the Canary Coalition pursues its goals through various methods, the most important of which is mobilizing public involvement. Education and public awareness are addressed at a personal grassroots level by talking with people at information booths and creating social events such as the 2005 Asheville Air Aid concert and the Blue Ridge Parkway Relay for Clean Air. The Canary Coalition also participates in high-profile protests in Raleigh and throughout Western North Carolina and amplifies the impact of these events by enlisting news media coverage. These events capture the attention of people who otherwise might not have even known that air

pollution is a problem. They also reach people who want to help but didn't know how. As a result, lawmakers hear more about the issues, and the Canary Coalition receives more support for its ongoing projects (Figure 97-2).

Passage of legislation requires relentless pressure from thousands of people, whose voices are organized by groups such as the Canary Coalition. We orchestrate petition drives, join well-publicized protests, and create public awareness events such as the Relay for Clean Air (Canary Coalition is leading in the right direction, 2006).

This annual 100-mile demonstration along the Blue Ridge Parkway covers a heavily polluted section of the southern Appalachians and highlights some of the devastation resulting from coal-fired power plants. Volunteers bike, run, and walk this epic course, joining the millions of tourists who become witness each year to dead and dying forests and thick haze.

Local residents endured especially bad air quality in 2002. As a teacher, I noticed a surge in students' use

BOX 97-1 Canary Coalition at a Glance

- Based primarily in North Carolina
- Membership as of January 15, 2010 was 2351
- Motto: "Clean air is a civil rights issue, and the Canary Coalition is building a movement."
- Mission Statement: "The Canary Coalition works to raise public awareness about the air quality crisis in the Smoky Mountains, the greater Appalachian region, and nationwide, generating a groundswell of public support to reduce or eliminate major sources of air pollution, thereby improving the health and quality of life enjoyed by all who breathe."

Organizational Goals

- Prevent construction of new coal-burning power plants.
- Expedite phase-out of existing coal-fired power plants.
- Assist in the enforcement of existing environmental regulations so that operational coal-fired power plants continuously employ the best available technology to reduce actual emissions of sulfur dioxides, nitrogen oxides, and mercury at each individual facility.
- Promote conservation, energy efficiency, and renewable energy technologies as the foundation of our regional, state, and national energy and transportation policies.

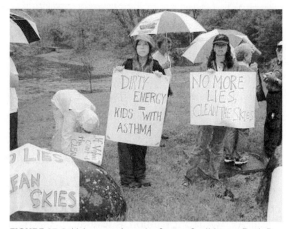

FIGURE 97-2 Volunteers from the Canary Coalition on Earth Day 2005 at the Great Smoky Mountains National Park.

of albuterol inhalers on the frequent "Ozone Action Days," when the ground-level pollutant reached unhealthy levels. I referred people on these same days to newspaper headlines that advised against outdoor activities because of increased risk of respiratory damage. I cited numerous studies that confirmed that repeated childhood exposure to ozone may lead not

only to immediate respiratory symptoms but also to reduced lung function in adulthood (NCDAQ, 2009b). Some people expressed concern, while others were not impressed. Why was an English teacher telling them about air pollution?

THE CONNECTIONS BETWEEN ENVIRONMENTAL ACTIVISM AND NURSING

In 2003, I decided to become a nurse, partly because I felt that the education and experience would help me work effectively in wellness promotion. When a reporter interviewed me at a protest in Great Smoky Mountains National Park, she seemed more interested when I told her I was a cardiac step-down nurse. Soon Canary Coalition members elected me to the governing board, allowing me to help guide the organization in strategic decisions and policy changes. Because of my work schedule, I was not always able to participate in organizational activities, but as a nurse, I could afford to contribute financially to help those who did. Nursing provided leverage to my environmental efforts and allowed me to become more effective, both as a citizen and as a Canary Coalition member.

Acute care nursing also provided direct observation of the relationship between air pollution and disease. In the past, I had felt my nasal passages burn from sharp-smelling ozone gas as it was emitted from fax machines and photocopiers, but I had not yet made the connection to similar symptoms experienced by patients living around hazy mountain ridges and valleys. I decided to shift my nursing career from cardiovascular progressive care to the emergency department in Bryson City, North Carolina. In this small town on the edge of Great Smoky Mountains National Park, I learned to recognize the transition from wheezing to respiratory failure. I also noticed certain COPD patients who would most often present on hazy days with high ground-level ozone levels. I clearly saw that bad air quality could be disastrous for high-risk patients.

My co-workers generally agreed that air pollution increased our workload, but they seemed puzzled about why I would ride my bicycle to work or participate in Canary Coalition protests to help our patients. It became clear to me that nursing education and practice had strayed from its core mission. In acute care settings, we were busy caring for sick patients and had little time to focus on prevention. Patient-based care pays the bills but neglects the root causes of disease in our society: lifestyle and environment. This lack of understanding among health care workers further underscores the need for public awareness groups such as the Canary Coalition.

POLITICAL STRATEGIES

TOGETHER WE STAND

Fortunately, the Canary Coalition is only one of many groups working toward sustainable environmental policies. Part of our work lies in coordinating with complementary organizations and individuals for maximum effect. For example, in 2007 Progress Energy was forced to abandon its plans to build an oil-fired power plant near Asheville, North Carolina. This victory was the result of a combined effort by several groups who organized public meetings, pooled resources for TV and newspaper ads, and waged an effective legal campaign against the plant. Once again, people were mobilized and empowered to protect the air they breathed.

With this broad-based foundation of support, the Canary Coalition can conduct lobbying efforts much more effectively. Avram Friedman writes, "Without public involvement, environmental lobbyists are viewed by most legislators as weak, inconsequential players. Legislators have bigger things to worry about than pleasing this thought-provoking but powerless small group" (Friedman, 2004). But when environmental lobbyists arrive on the coat-tails of several thousand letters, phone calls, and e-mails, our message has a much louder voice.

WALKING THE TALK

Ironically, once these voices are finally galvanized into law, the struggle has only just begun. Environmental legislation is only as good as its level of enforcement, and this keeps the Canary Coalition busy as a "watchdog" organization. Proactive surveillance is a continuous responsibility, as industry practices that pollute are often hidden from public scrutiny.

This was obvious in the recent licensing process for Duke Energy's proposed coal-fired power plant in Cliffside, North Carolina. Emissions from this huge 800-megawatt plant would directly affect millions of residents, including those in North Carolina's three largest urban population centers. As such, mandatory public hearings are required before construction licenses can be granted. Strangely, the sole public comment session for the new Cliffside plant was held in a rural location, hours from major population centers, at a time when many people would not be able to attend. In response to this, the Canary Coalition petitioned the Department of Air Quality to schedule additional public hearings. When this request was denied, the Canary Coalition and several other environmental groups held independent public hearings and submitted statements to the DAQ before the agency's deadline for written comments.

Construction of the Cliffside plant continues, despite growing public outcry and further revelations of procedural skullduggery. This has prompted the Canary Coalition to adapt its bylaws to embrace a new and controversial strategy: civil disobedience. At the "Call to Conscience" march, 44 people were arrested for peacefully trespassing on Duke Energy property in Charlotte, North Carolina. This presents a dilemma for many dedicated environmental activists, including nurses. What would be the long- and short-term consequences of being arrested for such a cause?

IS ENVIRONMENTAL STEWARDSHIP A LUXURY?

The Canary Coalition, like countless other grassroots movements, struggles not only with these personal challenges but also with those related to economic issues. For example, the recent "credit crunch" has affected cash flow for most organizations, especially those that rely on individuals and grant foundations for support. Faced with new financial constraints, many Canary Coalition supporters are unable to contribute as they have in the past. A downturn in the economy has also led to compromised environmental priorities for local governments and regulatory organizations.

A telling local example is the hasty modification of local zoning ordinances in 2009 to allow expansion of a paper plant in Sylva, North Carolina. Without providing the required opportunity for public input, the town council approved zoning changes to allow a second smokestack and accompanying facilities to be added to Jackson Paper's existing plant. This expansion promises 61 relatively high-paying jobs in a county hit hard by layoffs and other economic hardships. In this delicate environment, the Canary Coalition filed an appeal in the Superior Court to repeal the zoning modification, pending due process. Our hope was that in doing so, a stipulation would be added to prevent Jackson Paper from burning coal or rubber pellets as it had done in the past. Waste wood chips would remain as the primary fuel, with natural gas as a backup.

The Canary Coalition's appeal was denied. Without required input from informed members of the community, town council members inadvertently opened the door for an environmental Trojan Horse in exchange for the promise of financial betterment, and the courts supported their decision. The 61 jobs have yet to materialize, and the health-related costs will be difficult to quantify.

STEPPING UP

It is a nurse's duty not only to help those who suffer but to help those who might otherwise suffer. In 2009, air in our mountains was relatively clean, and the views occasionally rivaled the vistas that made the Smoky Mountains famous a century ago. Most of this can be attributed to fickle prevailing winds and plentiful rainfall, but to some degree it stems from Florence Nightingale and the people who continue to strive toward her fundamental provisions of fresh air, light, and cleanliness. As I join with others in clean air

marches and town hall meetings, I will also continue my work in the emergency department, where my patients and co-workers may not yet realize that we are all canaries.

Judith Hallock, MSN, CFNP, RN, has provided guidance and momentum in the writing of this chapter, both as a founding member of the Canary Coalition and through her ongoing example as an environmental activist.

For a list of related websites, please refer to your Evolve Resources at http://evolve.elsevier.com/Mason/policypolitics/

REFERENCES

Canary Coalition is leading in the right direction. (2006, August 30). *Smoky Mountain News*, p. 3.

Friedman, A. (2004, April). Creating a new political atmosphere in North Carolina and beyond. The Canary Coalition. Retrieved from www.canarycoalition.org/canary/create.htm.

North Carolina Division of Air Quality (NCDAQ). (2009a, November 6). Air quality, particle pollution, and ozone: Frequently asked questions: What's the problem? Retrieved from http://daq.state.nc.us/airaware/aqfaq.shtml#G1.

North Carolina Division of Air Quality (NCDAQ). (2009b, November 6). What are the health effects of ground-level ozone? Retrieved from http://daq.state.nc.us/airaware/aqfaq.shtml#O9.

Ross, W. G. Jr. (2009, May 13). North Carolina's Clean Smokestacks Act. North Carolina Division of Air Quality. Retrieved from http://daq.state.nc.us/news/leg/cleanstacks.shtml.

World Health Organization. (2007, November). Dioxins and their effects on human health. Retrieved from www.who.int/mediacentre/factsheets/fs225/en/index.html.

CHAPTER 98

TAKING ACTION
The Nightingales Take on Big Tobacco

Ruth E. Malone and Kelly Buettner-Schmidt

"Neglecting to discuss the industry's role as the disease vector in the tobacco epidemic is like refusing to discuss the role of mosquitoes in a malaria epidemic or rats in an outbreak of bubonic plague."

—Rob Cushman, MD, Medical Officer
of Health, Ottawa

RUTH'S STORY

"The latest news from me is that I died May 9, 1990, of lung cancer. Maybe my widower would like your free trip. Although I doubt it … You see, he has been mourning my death for 4 years. I was all he had left—me and my Benson & Hedges. Wish you were here" (Halpin, 1994). An elderly widower, perhaps sitting alone under the lamp at the kitchen table where he and his wife had eaten many meals together, wrote these words to the Philip Morris tobacco company in a trembling hand—on the back of a glossy Benson & Hedges cigarette brand mailer.

I found his letter online, one of perhaps thousands, written to tobacco companies by suffering customers and their families. Something about it caught me and wouldn't let me rest. In many ways, he and the many others whose letters I found were the founders of the Nightingales Nurses.

I smoked for years. I'd smoke feeling guilty as I cared for patients who were suffering from emphysema or lung cancer or heart disease. I tried to quit so many times, but I would slip back. I felt so alone. That was more than 20 years ago, but I vividly remember reading about new studies showing that smoking was not really so bad, comparing it with eating chocolate or having a glass of wine. I never dreamed, then, that

the tobacco industry was behind those phony "studies" (Smith, 2007).

What I didn't know then would fill a book. Mainly, I didn't realize that the tobacco industry (TI) had set up front groups, hired scientists, and organized massive campaigns to promote bogus ideas, had sponsored "distracting" scientific studies selected by industry lawyers to be sure they would result in findings favorable to the industry, and had promoted their intentionally deceptive ideas through an astonishingly large and varied assortment of paid "consultants" and front groups (Bero, 2003, 2005; Glantz, Slade, Bero, Hanauer, & Barnes, 1996). I had no idea that the tobacco companies had special marketing plans developed to reassure those, like me, who worried even as we lit up another cigarette (Brown and Williamson Tobacco Company, 1971; Cataldo & Malone, 2008) and that they were working on a global scale to fight tobacco control policies and ensure that smoking remained socially acceptable (Zeltner, Kessler, Martiny, & Randera, 2000; McDaniel, Intinarelli, & Malone, 2008).

THE PERSONAL BECOMES POLITICAL

I finally quit smoking for good, after struggling for years. Going back to school helped, building my confidence. In a postdoctoral study, I began working on tobacco-control policy research, and I learned more about tobacco than I ever had in nursing school.

I learned that until the advent of the machine-rolled cigarette in the late 1800s, almost nobody ever died from lung cancer. It was once such a rare disease that most physicians never saw a case in their lifetimes. Those same entrepreneurs who introduced machine-rolled cigarettes also introduced aggressive, innovative advertising techniques that linked cigarettes with glamour, freedom, sexuality, and status (Kluger, 1997). I realized that we were facing an industrially produced disease epidemic from tobacco.

More than 10 million internal tobacco company documents became publicly available as the result of multiple state attorney general lawsuits in the late 1990s and are accessible online *(http://legacy.library. ucsf.edu)*. They offer an amazing window into this incredibly destructive industry, including its business plans, budgets, scientific research, public relations and marketing plans, memos, letters, and much more. I developed a program of research drawing on them, and while doing this research, I stumbled on the letters.

COMPELLING VOICES

"My father died last October at the age of 50 due to lung cancer," one read. "He purchased many of your items in your *Marlboro Country Store Catalog* with his cigarette coupons…Now myself and my 16 year old sister are left fatherless…smoking does cause cancer, does kill and destroy families. You don't need to be a scientist or conduct a study to figure that out, just visit my Dad's grave if you want proof." The words were written in the fat, round script of a teenage girl, but the file I had found contained more such letters, written by every sort of human hand. Most were written on the backs of or in response to slick mailers from tobacco companies: catalogs, birthday cards, offers of coupons for cigarette discounts, surveys. There were letters from grieving mothers, widows, sons, and daughters; letters from friends and family; and letters from dying smokers and those struggling to escape tobacco addiction. They were testimony. "I know that we all have to work to put food on the table and pay bills," read one. "But are there no other choices?"

The letters weren't asking for money; they wanted their human pain and loss to be acknowledged by those who had furthered it through promoting tobacco use. A woman, grieving over her mother's death at 57 from lung cancer, wrote, "My mother wanted to quit so badly…When I close my eyes at night, all I can see is my mother's face as she lay dying,

and all the hell that she went through…that will haunt our family forever."

As a nurse I could easily fill in the terrible subtext accompanying every anguished word. Behind each letter were family members who had used every economic and emotional resource they had trying to cope with the suffering and loss of a loved one; orphaned children who would never have the guidance of a father or mother; and aging parents who helplessly watched their children die before them. I knew that the suffering from tobacco-related illnesses was often terrible to witness, much less to experience. And these stories were repeated more than 400,000 times every year, year after year, in the United States alone (Centers for Disease Control and Prevention [CDC], 2008).

I also knew that the products that had killed all these people had been engineered for addictiveness (Kessler, 2001). I knew that companies had targeted their aggressive marketing and outreach efforts to the most vulnerable groups: the poor, less educated, and minority groups (Apollonio & Malone, 2005; Balbach, Gasior, & Barbeau, 2003; Cook, Wayne, Keithly, & Connolly, 2004; Hackbarth, Silvestri, & Cosper, 1995; Landrine et al., 2005; Muggli, Pollay, Lew, & Joseph, 2002; Smith & Malone, 2003; Yerger & Malone, 2002).

I knew that tobacco companies had conspired to create "doubts" about the scientific evidence that cigarettes caused disease, and later, that secondhand smoke caused disease (U.S. Tobacco Companies, 1954), and that they had tried to undermine the work of the World Health Organization (WHO) and other public health bodies (Zeltner et al., 2000) and interfere with tobacco-control efforts (WHO, 2009a). I knew that the industry's political and philanthropic contributions bought silence from policymakers and groups that should have been protecting the public (Tesler & Malone, 2008; Yerger & Malone, 2002). But somehow, I had never once considered that these companies had been getting letters like these for decades and filing them away, year after deadly year. Although I tried to continue with my research projects, the letters would not let me rest. It simply wasn't right for them to remain forever hidden in the tobacco industry's files.

Inspired by youth activists who had attended the Altria/Philip Morris shareholders' meeting to speak out about the industry's targeting of youth, I decided to buy one share of stock and go to the shareholders'

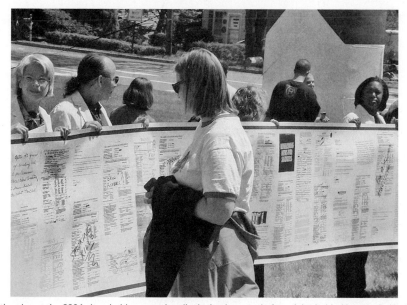

FIGURE 98-1 Nightingales at the 2004 shareholders meeting displaying banner. *Left to right, behind banner:* D. Hackbarth, Illinois; Terry Sayre, California; C. Southard, Illinois *(head turned);* P. Jones, California.

meeting as a nurse, taking some of the letters with me to read aloud in protest (Figures 98-1 and 98-2). Through networking, I recruited 11 other nurses from around the country who agreed to buy one share of Altria stock (only shareholders or their representatives could attend the meeting) and travel with me to the meeting in New Jersey. Other nurses paid for airfares for those who attended. We picked the Altria/Philip Morris meeting because Philip Morris is the largest U.S. tobacco company.

Our theme was "nurses bearing witness." We sought to point out the contradictions inherent in the company's claims to be "changed" and "socially responsible" while continuing the aggressive promotion of the most deadly consumer products ever made. Our key message: "A socially responsible company would not continue to promote products that it admits addict and kill." Initially, we focused on getting coverage in nursing media to help us spread the word about our group—the first nursing group to confront Big Tobacco on its own turf (Schwarz, 2004, 2005).

STRATEGIC PLANNING

A nurse in New Jersey who had been active with the American Lung Association scoped out the site for us.

Other activists working with youth invited us to be part of a postmeeting press conference. We assembled a selection of the letters into a 30-foot banner and made handouts about our efforts, including some of the letters and a press release (Box 98-1). We learned from other activists about the meeting format and how long we might have to speak. We would wear white lab coats and black armbands, indicating solidarity with those who suffered from tobacco. The next morning, and every year since, the Nightingales Nurses have borne witness at tobacco company shareholder meetings.

KELLY'S STORY: "THE NURSES ARE COMING..."

When I first heard about the Nightingales, I searched the Internet to learn more and immediately joined. I had never heard of shareholder advocacy, but I had a long history of activism and advocacy for tobacco control. My own journey in tobacco policy had begun with my first cigarette puff in junior high school. I was nauseated and then embarrassed. The next year, while playing basketball, I realized that smoking and playing ball was in conflict, and I quit. I was one of the lucky ones—I escaped addiction.

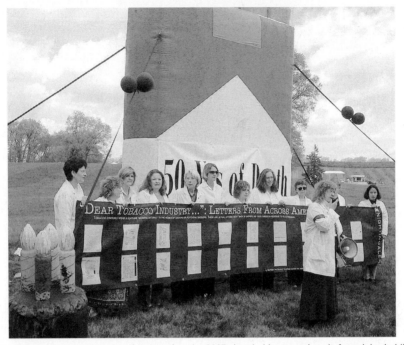

FIGURE 98-2 Nightingales conducting a press conference after the 2005 shareholders meeting. *Left to right, holding banner:* S. Toner, Missouri; D. Tasso, West Virginia; L. Greathouse, Kentucky; S. Brown, Pennsylvania; D. Hackbarth, Illinois; J. Buss, California; C. Southard, Illinois; M. Wertz, California; E. Wilson, New Jersey; M. J. Schymeinsky, California *(partially hidden);* A. Apacible, California; and Ruth Malone *(speaking),* California.

In my first nursing position, I saw so many who did not escape. I once shut off the oxygen in an elderly man's room in order to allow him to smoke. I did not tell him about the dangers of smoking, but I found it ironic that he needed oxygen because of his smoking and yet he still desired to smoke. I now recognize this was a testament to nicotine's addictiveness.

Teaching smoking cessation classes in the late 1980s was moving, frustrating, and unsettling. Unfortunately, at the time, tobacco was considered a "habit"; nicotine was not declared an addiction by the U.S. Surgeon General until 1988 (U.S. Department of Health and Human Services, 1988). Midway through the program was quit day, but often less than a quarter of the participants would remain quit for 48 hours; the disappointment and frustration showed clearly on their faces—if they came back to class at all. Seeing firsthand the power of addiction in people who strove so hard to quit was disturbing. Now, with advances in cessation practices, smoking cessation success rates have improved (Agency for Healthcare Research and Quality, 2008).

In 1992, I led a local public health tobacco prevention program in Minot, North Dakota. After developing a broad-based coalition, we successfully advocated for five local youth access laws. The policy and advocacy lessons learned through these efforts were invaluable for our later work on smoke-free environments that resulted in Minot being the first community in the state to pass a local smoke-free ordinance (Welle, Ibrahim, & Glantz, 2004; Buettner-Schmidt, Muhlbradt, & Brierley, 2003).

Our smoke-free environment efforts included public education events and billboard contests; collaborating with the American Cancer Society to encourage restaurants to be smoke-free the day of the Great American Smoke Out; and publicly recognizing restaurants that met public health standards and were smoke-free. In 2000, a new father and Minot city council member called me, asking if the coalition would assist him in having restaurants become smoke-free. With a newborn, he was concerned about the exposure of his child and others to secondhand smoke. A partnership began, and approximately 1

BOX 98-1 Nightingales' Press Release (Example)

PRESS RELEASE

NIGHTINGALES NURSES ACCUSE PHILIP MORRIS OF SOCIAL IRRESPONSIBILITY

DATE: Embargo release until 12:00 Noon Eastern Time Thursday April 29, 2010

CONTACT: Ruth Malone, RN, PhD, ruth.malone@ucsf.edu, (415) 123-4567

PRESS CONFERENCE: 12:00 Noon at Philip Morris entrance, 188 Rover Road, East Hanover, NJ

EAST HANOVER, NJ: Nurses from across America will attend the annual shareholders meeting of Philip Morris/Altria tomorrow to call on the company to demonstrate genuine corporate social responsibility by voluntarily ending all active promotion and marketing of tobacco products. A press conference will be held immediately after the meeting, with the Nightingale Nurses reading and sharing letters sent to the company by its dying customers and their families.

"We're here to say that this can't go on," said Nightingales organizer Ruth Malone, RN, Professor of Nursing at the University of California, San Francisco, School of Nursing. "The tobacco industry spends more than $1 million an hour, 24/7, on making their deadly, addictive products look fun, cool, and glamorous—but these letters show the terrifying, painful reality of what cigarettes do."

As the largest group of health care providers, the nation's 2.5 million nurses are in a unique position at the bedside and in the community to witness firsthand the deadly effects of tobacco products. "A socially responsible company would not continue to promote a product that they themselves admit addicts and kills," said Diana Hackbarth, RN, Professor of Nursing at Loyola University in Chicago and a Fellow of the American Academy of Nursing.

Wearing black armbands to honor the memories of their patients who have suffered and died from cigarette-caused diseases, nurses are attending the meeting to tell their patients' stories, giving voice to those who can no longer speak because tobacco addiction has robbed them of breath and life.

The Nightingales is a group of nurses who use advocacy, activism, and education to focus public attention on the role of the tobacco industry in creating the epidemic of tobacco-caused suffering, disease, and death.

For more information or to join, visit the Nightingales website at *www.nightingalesnurses.org.*

year later, after much political and media maneuvering, the city council passed the smoke-free ordinance. As we basked in our victory, however, opponents gathered enough signatures to put the new ordinance to a public vote. The battle-weary coalition began to meet weekly again to strategize how to defeat this referendum. Strategy for influencing city council members is vastly different from strategy to educate and influence an entire community. Thankfully, we did not have to fight alone. In conjunction with the Campaign for Tobacco Free Kids, Americans for Nonsmokers' Rights, the Robert Wood Johnson Foundation's Smokeless States grant program, the North Dakota Nurses Association, the North Dakota Medical Association, the American Lung Association, the American Cancer Society, the American Heart Association, and others, we defeated the referendum 55% to 45% on July 10, 2001. The new ordinance became effective January 1, 2002.

I later took a consulting position assisting other communities working on tobacco policy, helping pass several local ordinances and facilitating a statewide coalition that passed a bill banning tobacco use in public places and workplaces. I was involved in evaluating the effects of the local ordinance and the state law (Harstad Strategic Research Inc., 2003; Buettner-Schmidt, 2003, 2007; Buettner-Schmidt, Mangskau, & Boots, 2007; Buettner-Schmidt & Moseley, 2003). In a university faculty role, I developed a project within my Community Health Nursing course wherein senior nursing students conducted an assessment of college-age smoking and smoking policies on university campuses. The students developed a smoke-free campus recommendation and presented it to the university president. After going through many committees, our campus became smoke-free in June 2006. After all this, when I heard about the Nightingales' call for more nurse volunteers to speak out at the shareholder meeting, I could not resist. I had seen the industry in action before. Locally, lobbyists of organizations who collaborated with the tobacco industry attempted to derail our city-level policy efforts. Statewide, the tobacco industry lobbyists themselves would roam the halls of the legislature, something I never would have believed in my pre-tobacco activist years.

Now I was on my way into the belly of the beast. After a long flight and a meeting with other nurse activists the night before, feeling the solidarity among colleagues working on tobacco control in many different roles, I was excited as we drove through luxurious acreage leading to the corporate offices. As we parked and entered the building, there were "Men in Black" everywhere speaking into hidden microphones, and we could hear whispers: "The nurses are here...," "the nurses are coming..." It felt very James Bond–like, almost surreal.

Envision a cold-sounding CEO, a transfixing video presentation about cigarettes and other products, an opulent environment—these are my memories of the shareholder meeting. After the video, CEO Louis Camilleri highlighted how successful the company had been in increasing cigarette sales worldwide and how profitable an investment the stock was. Then it was time for the shareholder "question-and-answer" period. I told my family story and the stories of others who I knew. Other nurses spoke about the suffering they had witnessed: A nurse practitioner spoke about the harm tobacco does to pregnant women and children, and a burn nurse spoke about caring for burn victims from cigarette-caused fires. Each time, the room fell silent as we spoke; I felt the symbolic power of our white lab coats and our nursing presence. Some of the protesting youth stood boldly to interrupt the meeting; the CEO repeatedly told them to sit down. Then the Men in Black forced the youth to the back of the room and out the door. I remember wondering if we had made an impact.

In our debriefing later and in self-reflection, I realized that although we cannot know whether our words on that one day will create change, it is essential for nurses to continue to speak out *because we are nurses.* People who profit from selling death should not be able to do so without, at the very least, hearing about the suffering and devastation that their product causes. As nurses, we have a responsibility to "speak truth to power."

According to the WHO (2009b), tobacco caused 100 million deaths in the twentieth century and kills about 5.4 million people worldwide annually. Describing this in understandable numbers for laypeople should be among nurses' roles. This translates into 1 out of every 10 adult deaths or one person every 6 seconds. Meanwhile, in the U.S. alone, the tobacco industry spends more than $1 million an hour promoting its products (Federal Trade Commission, 2007). Globally, tobacco companies are now aggressively targeting low- and middle-income countries, seeking new generations of young people and women who will develop tobacco addiction.

EXTENDING THE MESSAGE

Currently, we have Nightingales in more than half the states and in Canada. We annually attend both the Altria and Reynolds American tobacco company shareholders' meetings. We've challenged the company's claims of "responsibility" at Philip Morris public relations events. Our website (*www.nightingalesnurses.org*) is a source for information about the industry. Our work has all been done with volunteer effort.

Of course, tobacco companies are still promoting tobacco products. We have a long way to go, and we will need to develop new and innovative strategies to get there. But our efforts have borne fruit in several respects. First, we have sent a strong message to the tobacco industry that nurses are their opponents. Nurses are trusted and respected by the public, and we owe it to our patients to speak out and tell the whole truth about Big Tobacco. Nurses need to promote public dialogue on an endgame for this industrially-produced tobacco disease epidemic— perhaps, as a recent article suggests, by phasing out cigarettes (Daynard, 2009) or by converting the tobacco market to a nonprofit entity with a public health mandate (Callard, Thompson, & Collishaw, 2005).

Whether our clients are starting to smoke or trying to quit, they receive constant messages from tobacco companies, straight into their homes, and increasingly through more subtle marketing methods, such as experiential programs, viral marketing, and music events. Philip Morris has a database of more than 20 million smokers, which it uses to establish personalized relationships and targeted communications (Philip Morris USA, 2003). We need to help clients understand how the industry has studied their every psychological weakness, segmenting the market to reach everyone from starter "replacement smokers," as the industry called youth, to worried older smokers whom they seek to reassure. We would not treat malaria victims without ever mentioning the mosquito that transmits the disease. As patient advocates, we must likewise name, discuss, and find ways to combat the industry vector of the tobacco disease epidemic.

Second, our efforts have inspired others. The youths we joined are still talking at meetings about "the nurses" and how we helped them feel part of something larger. Perhaps some of them will become nurses. We need their passion and political awareness in nursing. Finally, speaking out empowers us as nurses, as past shareholder meeting attendees have said: "This experience has changed the whole way I feel about being a nurse" and "Now I feel that I can say anything to anyone with confidence."

WHAT NURSES CAN DO

There is perhaps no other health issue on which nurses could have so much impact. Tobacco affects almost every body system and every demographic group across the lifespan. It affects individuals, families, and communities; there is no nurse for whom tobacco could not be relevant.

The tobacco industry has worried that nurses might take them on. Among the industry documents is a report on organizations the industry viewed as its opponents, with each one's strengths appraised, including the American Nurses Association, the American Public Health Association, the American Medical Association, and others. "Nurses, as a group, feel strongly and negatively about tobacco use," the report reads. "As they become more active in politics…at all levels, they could easily become formidable opponents for the tobacco industry" (Osmon, 1990). *Formidable opponents.* We aren't used to thinking of nurses in those terms. But when it comes to the tobacco industry, we need to be its "formidable opponents" in every possible way.

The Nightingales build on the great work of many nurses all over the country. Here are some other examples: Nightingale Jill A. Jarvie, RN, MSN, represented the San Francisco Department of Public Health on a workgroup that resulted in stronger restrictions on smoking in and around city-funded shelters for the homeless. Minnesota Nightingale Cheryl Bisping chairs two coalitions working on secondhand smoke, smoke-free restaurants, and tobacco-free youth recreation policies. Drs. Linda Sarna, Stella Bialous, and Erika Froelicher are continuing the Tobacco Free Nurses project *(www.tobaccofreenurses.org),* which is aimed at helping nurses quit smoking. At UCLA,

Professor Sarna helped pass a policy against accepting tobacco industry research funding.

In Kentucky, Nightingale Lisa Greathouse organized a World No-Tobacco Day display of our Nightingales banner showing the letters at the University of Kentucky (UK). Ellen J. Hahn, DNS, RN, and Carol A. Riker, MSN, RN, at the UK Tobacco Policy Research Program are actively involved in community engagement, smoke-free policy development, and research, helping 12 communities in Kentucky pass smoke-free policies since 2007.

Internationally, Nightingale and nursing professor Dr. Sophia Chan conducted the first Asia Pacific Workshop on Tobacco Control and Nurses inclusive of policy implications; developed the first smoking cessation counseling training program in Hong Kong; initiated a task force to help women smokers quit; launched the first youth quitline; and also influenced the government to fund 10 smoking cessation clinics.

Nightingales founding member Dr. Diana Hackbarth chairs the Illinois Coalition Against Tobacco, the oldest anti-tobacco coalition in the U.S., and for decades has worked on legislation, including clean indoor air legislation, outlawing bidis, banning tobacco billboards, and raising tobacco taxes. Nightingale Colleen Hughes of Nevada served as president of the Nevada Tobacco Prevention Coalition, working toward a smoke-free public places ballot initiative. Nightingale founding member Carol Southard, RN, MSN, was responsible for founding Chicago Second Wind, whose mission is to reduce tobacco use and increase quit attempts. In California, Gina Intinarelli worked to secure smoke-free campus policies for UCSF's medical center and to ensure that tobacco content (including content about the role of the tobacco industry) is incorporated into the curriculum of all health professions programs. In 2008, Nightingale Kelly Buettner-Schmidt worked on a statewide effort to mandate that certain tobacco settlement dollars be allocated to a fully funded, CDC Best Practices–based tobacco prevention program. North Dakota is the first tobacco prevention program in the country to be fully funded at the CDC recommended level.

Other nurses are organizing letter-writing campaigns, developing cessation services for special populations, conducting tobacco-related research, and working on a wide range of policy efforts to reduce tobacco's deadly toll. The Nightingales are always looking for more nurses to help—even writing a letter to the editor once a year can make a difference if enough letters appear at the right time.

NURSING IS POLITICAL

Some nurses are afraid of being "political." But let's face it: Health and disease are political; resources, education, and care are not distributed evenly in our society, and tobacco is a social justice issue. Just caring about those beyond ourselves and our immediate families is itself a deeply political act. Our most powerful nursing roots, after all, lie in our concern for those who feel voiceless and powerless, as exemplified by the early leaders in public health nursing.

As early as 1916, writings of Florence Nightingale referred to her knowledge of politics (Gourlay, 2004; Kopf, 1916; McDonald, 2006a, 2006b; Pfettscher, 2006). Nightingale emphasized having political will, using the media, and seeking the support of professionals and leaders (McDonald, 2006b). She encouraged others to lobby: "Agitate, agitate, agitate ..." (McDonald, 2006b). Ms. Nightingale would surely support the Nightingales' tobacco-control policy efforts (Nightingale, 1946).

LESSONS LEARNED

The first lesson is that it doesn't take a big organization and money to do something political. We started with a few committed nurses and a loosely organized network. If you have a good idea, the money often follows—if you're willing to ask for it. Second, try to get consensus on what goals and what kind of effort will be required, recognizing that this will need to be revisited as events change. For example, one of our group's aims was to get media coverage of our activism in order to change perspectives about the tobacco industry, and last year, for the first time, the *New York Times* covered the shareholder protests. However, initially we focused our efforts mostly on the nursing press, to build our network. Thirdly, coordinate efforts with other groups working on the same issues, recognizing that you may not always agree on everything. Build on common ground, and share resources. For example, we coordinated our press conference with Essential Action, a youth-focused tobacco-control group. Lastly, find ways to build on the strengths of all members. With activism, realize that not everyone is comfortable with public speaking or confrontation; however, they may contribute in other ways, such as preparing press releases, managing logistics, or working on a website.

For a list of related websites, please refer to your Evolve Resources at http://evolve.elsevier.com/Mason/policypolitics/

REFERENCES

Agency for Healthcare Research and Quality. (2008). Treating tobacco use and dependence: 2008 Update. Retrieved from www.ncbi.nlm.nih.gov/books/bv.fcgi?rid=hstat2.section.28165.

Apollonio, D., & Malone, R. E. (2005). Marketing to the marginalized: Tobacco industry targeting of the homeless and mentally ill. *Tobacco Control, 14*(6), 409-415.

Balbach, E. D., Gasior, R. J., & Barbeau, E. M. (2003). R.J. Reynolds' targeting of African Americans: 1988-2000. *American Journal of Public Health, 93*(5), 822-827.

Bero, L. (2003). Implications of the tobacco industry documents for public health and policy. *Annual Review of Public Health, 24,* 267-288.

Bero, L. A. (2005). Tobacco industry manipulation of research. *Public Health Reports, 120*(2), 200-208.

Brown and Williamson Tobacco Company. (1971). If you are worried about cigarettes—May we confuse you with some facts? (Advertisement). Retrieved from http://legacy.library.ucsf.edu/tid/mgw93f00.

Buettner-Schmidt, K. (2003). *Compliance of Minot restaurants with the Smoke-Free Restaurant Ordinance.* Minot, ND: Tobacco Education, Research and Policy Project, Minot State University, Department of Nursing.

Buettner-Schmidt, K. (2007). *The economic impact of North Dakota's smoke-free law on restaurant and bar taxable sales.* Minot, ND: Healthy Communities International, Minot State University, Department of Nursing. Retrieved from www.ndhealth.gov/tobacco/Reports/Impact_Report_2007.pdf.

Buettner-Schmidt, K., Mangskau, K., & Boots, C. (2007). *An observational assessment of compliance with North Dakota smoke-free Law.* Minot, ND: Healthy Communities International, Minot State University, Department of Nursing. Retrieved from www.ndhealth.gov/tobacco/Reports/Compliance_Report_2007.pdf.

Buettner-Schmidt, K., & Moseley, F. (2003, September). *An economic analysis of a smoke-free restaurant ordinance in a Midwestern frontier state.* Minot, ND: Minot State University, Department of Nursing, North Dakota Center for Persons with Disabilities, & College of Business.

Buettner-Schmidt, K., Muhlbradt, M., & Brierley, L. (2003). *Why not Minot: The battle over North Dakota's first smoke-free ordinance.* Minot, ND: Minot State University, Department of Nursing.

Callard, C., Thompson, D., & Collishaw, N. (2005). Transforming the tobacco market: Why the supply of cigarettes should be transferred from for-profit corporations to non-profit enterprises with a public health mandate. *Tobacco Control, 14*(4), 278-283.

Cataldo, J. K., & Malone, R. E. (2008). False promises: The tobacco industry, "low-tar" cigarettes, and older smokers. *Journal of the American Geriatrics Society, 56*(9), 1716-1723.

Centers for Disease Control and Prevention. (2008). Smoking-attributable mortality, years of potential life lost, and productivity losses—United States, 2000-2004. *Morbidity and Mortality Weekly Report, 57*(45), 1226-1228.

Cook, B. L., Wayne, G. F., Keithly, L., & Connolly, G. (2004). One size does not fit all: How the tobacco industry has altered cigarette design to target consumer groups with specific psychological and psychosocial needs. *Addiction, 98*(11), 1547-1561.

Daynard, R. A. (2009). Doing the unthinkable and saving millions of lives. *Tobacco Control*, *18*(1), 2-3.

Federal Trade Commission. (2007). Cigarette report for 2004 and 2005. Washington D.C. Retrieved from www.ftc.gov/reports/tobacco/2007cigarette 2004-2005.pdf.

Glantz, S., Slade, J., Bero, L., Hanauer, P., & Barnes, D. (1996). *The cigarette papers*. Berkeley: University of California Press.

Gourlay, J. (2004). Florence Nightingale: Still lighting the way for nurses. *Nurse Management*, *11*(2), 14-15.

Hackbarth, D. P., Silvestri, B., & Cosper, W. (1995). Tobacco and alcohol billboards in 50 Chicago neighborhoods: Market segmentation to sell dangerous products to the poor. *Journal of Public Health Policy*, *16*(2), 213-230.

Halpin, P. E. (1994). Letter to Benson and Hedges in response to mailed survey. In Legacy Tobacco Documents Library. Retrieved from http://legacy.library.ucsf.edu/tid/usc62e00.

Harstad Strategic Research Inc. (2003). *Poll shows Minot voters support the 2002 law prohibiting smoking in restaurants*. Boulder, CO: Author.

Kessler, D. (2001). *A question of intent: A great American battle with a deadly industry*. New York: Public Affairs.

Kluger, R. (1997). *Ashes to ashes: America's hundred-year cigarette war, the public health, and the unabashed triumph of Philip Morris*. New York: Vintage Books.

Kopf, E. W. (1916). Florence Nightingale as statistician. *Quarterly Publications of the American Statistical Association*, *15*(116), 388-405.

Landrine, H., Klonoff, E. A., Fernandez, S., Hickman, N., Kashima, K., Parekh, B., et al. (2005). Cigarette advertising in Black, Latino, and White magazines, 1998-2002: An exploratory investigation. *Ethnicity and Disease*, *15*(1), 63-67.

McDaniel, P. A., Intinarelli, G., & Malone, R. E. (2008, January 17). Tobacco industry issues management organizations: Creating a global corporate network to undermine public health. *Global Health*, *4*(2). Retrieved from www.globalizationandhealth.com/content/4/1/2.

McDonald, L. (2006a). Florence Nightingale and public health policy: Theory, activism and public administration: Paper for Origins of Public Health Policy, CSAA Meetings, York University, 2006. Retrieved from www.sociology.uoguelph.ca/fnightingale/Public%20Health%20Care/theory.htm.

McDonald, L. (2006b). Florence Nightingale as a social reformer. *History Today*, *56*(1), 9-15.

Muggli, M. E., Pollay, R. W., Lew, R., & Joseph, A. M. (2002). Targeting of Asian Americans and Pacific Islanders by the tobacco industry: Results from the Minnesota Tobacco Document Depository. *Tobacco Control*, *11*(3), 201-209.

Nightingale, F. (1946, p. 8). Notes on nursing: What it is, and what it is not. In *Notes on Nursing: What it is, and what it is not: Commemorative edition*. Philadelphia: Lippincott.

Osmon, H. E. (1990). Letter to T. C. Harris and others: Attached is the updated overview of anti-smoking organizations. In Legacy Tobacco Documents Library. Retrieved from http://legacy.library.ucsf.edu/tid/dkf24d00.

Pfettscher, S. A. (2006). Florence Nightingale, 1820-1910: Modern nursing. In A. M. Tomey & M. R. Alligood (Eds.), *Nursing theorists and their work*. (6th ed., pp. 71-90). St. Louis: Mosby-Elsevier.

Philip Morris USA. (2003). PM USA adult smoker database marketing past, present and future. In Legacy Tobacco Documents Library. Retrieved from http://legacy.library.ucsf.edu/tid/msh95a00.

Schwarz, T. (2004). Nightingales vs. Big Tobacco: Nurses confront the nation's biggest public health threat. *American Journal of Nursing*, *104*(6), 27.

Schwarz, T. (2005). Nightingales confront tobacco company, redux: Nurses from around the country gather to clear the smoke. *American Journal of Nursing*, *105*(6), 35.

Smith, E. A. (2007). "It's interesting how few people die from smoking": Tobacco industry efforts to minimize risk and discredit health promotion. *European Journal of Public Health*, *17*(2), 162-170.

Smith, E. A., & Malone, R. E. (2003). The outing of Philip Morris: Advertising tobacco to gay men. *American Journal of Public Health*, *93*(6), 988-993.

Tesler, L., & Malone, R. E. (2008, December). Corporate philanthropy, lobbying and public health policy. *American Journal of Public Health*, *98*(12), 2123-2133.

U.S. Department of Health and Human Services. (1988). The health consequences of smoking: Nicotine addiction. A report of the Surgeon General. Retrieved from http://profiles.nlm.nih.gov/NN/B/B/Z/D/_/nnbbzd.pdf.

U.S. Tobacco Companies. (1954). A frank statement (Advertisement). Retrieved from www.tobacco.neu.edu/litigation/cases/supportdocs/frank_ad.htm.

Welle, J. R., Ibrahim, J. K., & Glantz, S. A. (2004). *Tobacco control policy making in North Dakota: A tradition of activism*. San Francisco: University of California, Center for Tobacco Control Research and Education. Retrieved from http://repositories.cdlib.org/ctcre/tcpmus/ND2004.

World Health Organization. (2009a). Tobacco industry interference with tobacco control. Retrieved from www.who.int/tobacco/resources/publications/9789241597340.pdf.

World Health Organization. (2009b). Tobacco key facts. Retrieved from www.who.int/topics/tobacco/facts/en/index.html.

Yerger, V. B., & Malone, R. E. (2002). African American leadership groups: Smoking with the enemy. *Tobacco Control*, *11*(4), 336-345.

Zeltner, T., Kessler, D. A., Martiny, A., & Randera, F. (2000). Tobacco company strategies to undermine tobacco control activities at the World Health Organization. Geneva: World Health Organization. Retrieved from www.who.int/genevahearings/inquiry.html.

CHAPTER 99

Lactivism: Breastfeeding Advocacy in the United States

Diane L. Spatz

"Formula feeding is the longest lasting uncontrolled experiment lacking informed consent in the history of medicine."

—Frank Oski, MD

Lactivism is a term used to describe breastfeeding advocacy. *Lactivists* are those who support breastfeeding, advocate for the rights of breastfeeding mothers, ensure that breastfeeding mothers are not discriminated against, and aim to inform the general public regarding the health benefits of breastfeeding. Lactivism can occur in many ways, but the act that receives the most media attention is the "nurse-in." At a nurse-in, mothers gather in public places to breastfeed their children.

WHY ADVOCATE FOR BREASTFEEDING?

Breastfeeding is the preferred form of nutrition for all infants. The health benefits of breastfeeding are so significant that virtually every professional organization including the American Academy of Pediatrics and World Health Organization recommend exclusive breastfeeding for the first 6 months after birth followed by supplementary foods and continued breastfeeding for 1 to 2 years or more as mutually desirable by mother and child (Figure 99-1). The Agency for Health Care Quality and Research (AHRQ) (2007) conducted an extensive metaanalysis on the benefits of breastfeeding for both mother and child. Breastfed full-term infants receive the following health benefits: reduction in the risk of acute otitis media by 27% to 50%, a 42% reduction in the risk of atopic dermatitis, and a 27% reduction in the risk of asthma (Ip et al., 2007). Even more significant are the 64% risk

reduction for gastrointestinal infections and the 72% risk reduction for respiratory infections (Ip et al., 2007). Breastfeeding may also help protect the child from type I and type II diabetes (19% to 27%, and 39% risk reductions, respectively). Chen and Rogan (2004) report that infant mortality in the United States could be decreased by 21% if all infants received the recommended 6 months of human milk. The AHRQ also concluded that there is clear evidence to suggest an association between breastfeeding and a reduced maternal risk of breast cancer, ovarian cancer, and type II diabetes (Ip et al., 2007). Mothers who do not breastfeed or who have a short duration of breastfeeding are at higher risk for postpartum depression (Ip et al., 2007).

THE HISTORIC DECLINE IN BREASTFEEDING IN THE U.S.

What has led to the need for lactivism in the U.S.? Until the mid-1800s, almost all infants in the U.S. were breastfed. In the 1890s and early 1900s, a shift began that essentially transformed the culture to one in which bottle feeding became the cultural norm. Increasingly in the 1900s, baby formula manufacturers advertised their products in women's magazines and mothers had increasing doubts about being able to successfully breastfeed. As childbirth moved from the home into the hospital, medical practice began to interfere with successful establishment of lactation and breastfeeding. By 1948, only 38% of infants were receiving exclusively human milk feeds at 1 week of age, and by 1957, only 21% of infants were exclusively breastfed at the time of hospital discharge after birth (Apple, 1994).The culture of breastfeeding in the U.S. has eroded over the past 100 years, and, despite the

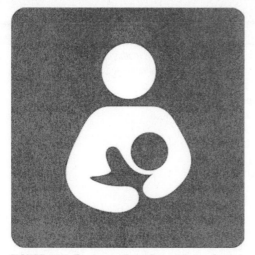

FIGURE 99-1 The International Breastfeeding Symbol.

fact that more women now "try" breastfeeding, preference for bottle feeding persists.

The federal government has tracked breastfeeding trends only since 1999. Prior to this, the earliest, and now the longest, ongoing survey of breastfeeding initiation rates in the U.S. was produced by the baby formula industry (the Ross Mothers Survey). According to the Centers for Disease Control and Prevention, breastfeeding initiation and duration rates have risen since 1999, however the increases have been modest at best. In 1999, approximately 68% of U.S. women initiated breastfeeding, and in 2006, 74% of women initiated breastfeeding—only a 6% increase. This includes mothers who may have only breastfed one time or just in the hospital before discharge. In 2006, only 13.6% of infants received human milk exclusively for 6 months, with any breastfeeding at 6 months increasing from 32.6% in 1999 to 43.4% in 2006 (Centers for Disease Control and Prevention [CDC], 2010).

A sociocultural issue that appears to underlie resistance to breastfeeding is the dual roles breasts have. Wolf (2008) wrote a commentary on why public breastfeeding remains so controversial in the U.S. Wolf asserted that American culture focuses on breasts for their sexual appeal—not for their primary function, which is to provide nourishment. The view that breastfeeding should be a private act, like sex, can make it challenging for some women to feel comfortable breastfeeding outside their homes (Wolf, 2008).

Because of these conflicting views, breastfeeding mothers have been met with discrimination in public areas, stores, and restaurants. At a Toys 'R Us at Times Square in New York, an employee asked a mother to move to a basement to breastfeed because there were children present. This resulted in a "nurse-in" at the Times Square location in 2006 (New York Civil Liberties Union, 2006). In 2004, Lori Charkoudian was asked by a Starbucks store employee in Silver Spring, Maryland, to cover up or use the women's restroom when she attempted to breastfeed her 15-month-old daughter. This led to a "nurse-in" involving 30 mothers and their babies as well as other family members and friends (Helderman, 2004). Similarly, a mother was ticketed for breastfeeding her son in Colorado at a beach, despite the fact that Colorado passed a law protecting breastfeeding in 2004 (The Denver Channel News, 2005). Table 99-1 provides a summary of breastfeeding incidents and lactivism events.

ACTION TO SUPPORT BREASTFEEDING

Efforts to improve breastfeeding rates have included federal and state legislation, changes in workplace policies, and individual activism to draw attention to discrimination against breastfeeding mothers.

FEDERAL EFFORTS

The federal government has attempted to address the need for changing breastfeeding outcomes in the U.S. The nation's national health goals, *Healthy People 2000* and *Healthy People 2010*, included the following objectives aimed at improving breastfeeding:

1. 75% breastfeeding initiation (28 states have met this objective)
2. 50% breastfeeding at 6 months (13 states have met this objective)
3. 25% breastfeeding at 12 months (20 states have met this objective) (CDC, 2009b).

Since none of the objectives have been met by the entire nation, *Healthy People 2020* also includes the previous objectives on breastfeeding rates in addition to three new objectives:

1. To increase the percentage of employers who have worksite lactation programs
2. To decrease the percentage of breastfed newborns who receive formula supplementation within the first two days of life

TABLE 99-1 Summary of U.S. Breastfeeding Incidents and Related Activities

Description of Breastfeeding Incident	Response	Source
Brooke Ryan was asked to cover the head of her infant while breastfeeding by a waitress and then the manager of an Applebee's restaurant in Lexington, Kentucky, in 2007. Both employees claimed that other customers were complaining about her breastfeeding in the restaurant.	A nurse-in was held on September 8, 2007. Jonathan R. Weatherby, Jr., Associate General Counsel for Applebee's attorney wrote "We regret that Ms. Ryan left without being served and would like the opportunity to personally invite her to return … we are also considering keeping blankets in the restaurants for use by breast-feeding mothers that may not have them readily available as a result of this incident."	*www.mothering.com/discussions/ showthread.php?t=739358*
Danielle Glanvill was harassed twice by a female security guard for breastfeeding in the children's section of a New York library in 2009.	A written apology was granted, and the security guard was transferred to another branch.	*www.nypost.com/seven/03242009/news/ regionalnews/mom_wins_booby_ prize_library_oks_breast__161094.htm*
A mother was asked to cover up while breastfeeding at a Denny's restaurant in North Carolina.	A nurse-in was held in protest on February 22, 2009.	*blogs.babiesonline.com/baby/ nationwide-dennys-nurse-in- february-22/*
Emily Gillette was asked to leave her Freedom Airlines flight if she would not cover her breasts while feeding her child.	News of the event spurred public "nurse-ins" at airports around the country, and Gillette filed a complaint with the Vermont Human Rights Commission.	*www.msnbc.msn.com/id/16773617/ wid/11915773/*
A lifeguard told Laurie Waldherr to leave a public pool in Washington state when she was breastfeeding at the pool's edge for risk of bodily fluids getting into the pool.	Waldherr sued the city and reached a settlement out of court.	*www.msnbc.msn.com/id/16773617/ wid/11915773/*
Julie Wheelan was asked to leave a shopping mall food court in Providence, Rhode Island, by a security guard when she was breastfeeding.	Wheelan suggested that the guard call the police, as she knew she was protected by law to breastfeed her child.	*www.msnbc.msn.com/id/16773617/ wid/11915773/*
Dorian Ryan was ticketed for indecent exposure on July 14, 2005, at the Carter Lake Swimming beach in Larimer County, Colorado.	Ryan requested an apology, and Colorado lawmakers agreed. A law passed that gives women the right to breastfeed anywhere she's allowed to be in public.	*www.thedenverchannel.com/ news/4785183/detail.html*
Lori Charkoudian was asked by a Silver Spring, Maryland, Starbucks store employee to cover up or use the women's restroom when she attempted to breastfeed her 15-month-old daughter in 2004.	A nurse-in was held in protest. A Starbucks spokesperson wrote "We will instruct our Maryland store partners to inform any concerned customer that by Maryland law, mothers have the right to breastfeed in public and to suggest to the customer that they either avert their eyes or move to a different location within the store."	*www.washingtonpost.com/wp-dyn/ articles/A50610-2004Aug8.html*

TABLE 99-1 Summary of U.S. Breastfeeding Incidents and Related Activities—cont'd

Description of Breastfeeding Incident	Response	Source
Chelsi Meyerson was harassed for breastfeeding her infant at the Times Square, New York, Toys "R" Us store. An employee asked her to move to the basement to breastfeed. Chelsi refused. Four other female employees also pressed her to move to the basement.	A nurse-in was held at Toys "R" Us Times Square on September 21, 2006. The New York Civil Liberties Union informed Toys "R" Us that it had violated civil rights law when employees told Meyerson she was not allowed to breastfeed in the store because her breastfeeding was inappropriate because there were children around. Toys "R" Us has apologized to Meyerson and informed stores of its nursing policy, which specifies that nursing women may breastfeed their children in the place "of their choice" at Toys "R" Us stores.	www.nyclu.org/news/ mothers-gather-toys-r-us-nurse-celebrating-right-breastfeed-public
Cheryl Cruz was asked to cover-up when breastfeeding at Universal Studios in Florida.	Cruz was permitted to breastfeed. A spokesman for the park said, "We're going to have the specific team members involved in this incident apologize to her, and we're going to make sure that our team members know how to proceed in these kinds of situations, moving forward."	www.cbc.ca/canada/newfoundland-labrador/story/2007/11/02/ breastfeeding-orlando.html
Lori Rueger asked if she could breastfeed her baby in a Victoria's Secret dressing room in Charleston, South Carolina. An employee told her no, it was against store policy, and suggested she go to the mall bathroom.	Anthony Hebron, spokesperson for The Limited Brands in Columbus, Ohio, said, "There was an unfortunate misunderstanding in the incident involving us, but you know what, if it's brought forth even greater things, that's fine."	abcnews.go.com/US/Health/ story?id=1378087
Heather Silvis was confronted in 2008 by a Walmart employee when she attempted to breastfeed. Her shopping cart and infant were taken from her and moved to a dressing room.	Two years earlier, Governor Mark Sanford signed an act protecting and promoting breastfeeding throughout the state. Walmart store management apologized to Silvis.	www.midlandsconnect.com/news/ news_story.aspx?id=221405

3. To increase the percentage of live births that occur in facilities that provide recommended care for lactating mothers and their babies (MICH HP 2020-18) (CDC, 2009b).

Workplace support for breastfeeding is critical. Breastfeeding mothers need support from supervisors and co-workers and need education regarding the benefits of continued breastfeeding. Co-workers can also benefit from education about the needs of breastfeeding employees. Mothers need time and a place to breastfeed or use a breast pump while at work. Unfortunately without regulations and policies, it is unlikely that most employers will adopt these practices. The Health Resources and Services Administration (HRSA) developed the Business Case for Breastfeeding program. It includes easy steps to support breastfeeding employees, an employee's guide to breastfeeding and working, an outreach marketing guide, and a tool kit. Representative Carolyn Maloney (D-NY) introduced the Breastfeeding Promotion Act of 2007 to amend the Civil Rights Act of 1964 to protect breastfeeding by new mothers, to provide performance standards for breast pumps, and to provide tax incentives for employers to encourage breastfeeding.

Language designed to protect the rights of working mothers was included in the historic passage of the Health Care Reform Act in 2010. The Affordable Care Act requires employers to provide reasonable unpaid break time and a non-bathroom location for an employee to express milk for her child for up to 1 year after the child's birth. Only employers with fewer than 50 employees are exempt if they claim undue hardship.

STATE EFFORTS

Forty nine states have enacted legislation to protect breastfeeding (CDC, 2009a). However, the legislation varies significantly from state to state. In some states, breastfeeding is merely exempted from public indecency laws, and in others, breastfeeding is protected by allowing a mother to breastfeed in any private or public location (Chang & Spatz, 2006). Unfortunately, many women are not aware of their individual state laws and rights. Chang and Spatz (2006) advocate that nurses inform childbearing women of their rights and provide them with patient family education sheets prior to discharge from the birth hospital.

BREASTFEEDING ADVOCACY ORGANIZATIONS

Much breastfeeding advocacy has occurred at the grassroots level led by organizations such as the La Leche League. The La Leche League was established in 1958 to provide mother-to-mother support and advocacy for breastfeeding. The National Alliance for Breastfeeding Advocacy was formed as the precursor to the U.S. Breastfeeding Committee (USBC). This committee is multidisciplinary and addresses the need for nationwide advocacy as it aims to move the breastfeeding agenda forward. The USBC was incorporated in Florida in 2000. Its mission is to improve the nation's health by working collaboratively to protect, promote, and support breastfeeding with a focus on collaboration, leadership, and advocacy (United States Breastfeeding Committee, 2008). USBC members consist of 34 non-profit organizations and 7 governmental agencies that all have vested interests in breastfeeding advocacy.

HOSPITAL POLICIES

Few U.S. hospitals provide evidence-based lactation care and support. To change infant feeding practices, the World Health Organization and UNICEF sponsored The Baby-Friendly Hospital Initiative (BFHI).

The BFHI is a global program designed to support and encourage hospitals to enact the most beneficial infant feeding practices. The BFHI recognizes hospitals that have achieved optimal infant feeding goals (BFHI USA, 2010). Only 86 U.S. hospitals are designated as "baby-friendly" facilities, though there are more than 19,000 worldwide. Fewer than 3% of all U.S. births occur in baby-friendly facilities. If hospital policies do not support, protect, and advocate for breastfeeding at all times, it is unlikely that women will be successful in their breastfeeding efforts. The BFHI is a designation available to birth hospitals only. Children and their mothers also may receive care at non–birth hospitals (for example, a children's hospital or an adult hospital where the mother is receiving care). These hospital personnel also need to be aware of the need for breastfeeding education and advocacy. Spatz (2005b) described the need for education of nurses and physicians, hospital-wide systems for managing breast milk, and the need for evidence-based standards of care.

THE NEED FOR BREASTFEEDING ADVOCACY EDUCATION

When the lack of hospital policies supporting breastfeeding and the lack of breastfeeding education received by health care providers is considered, the need for breastfeeding education becomes apparent. A model for integration of breastfeeding content into baccalaureate nursing curricula was developed that could be used for all health care disciplines (Spatz, Pugh, & American Academy of Nursing Expert Panel on Breastfeeding, 2007). A seminar course for undergraduate nursing students at the University of Pennsylvania serves as an example. Nursing students receive 28 hours of didactic and 14 hours of clinical experience related to current research topics in breastfeeding. A solid foundation in the science of breastfeeding makes nurses better prepared to serve as breastfeeding advocates in the community.

One nurse can make a big difference in breastfeeding outcomes. In a hospital, nurses can provide education and support for new mothers and can also be effective in community advocacy efforts (Spatz & Sternberg, 2005). Since 1995, over 200 students at the University of Pennsylvania have served as change agents in promoting breastfeeding. One student, who was motivated because her mother attempted breast-feeding her younger sibling born with spina bifida, wrote an article for the National Spina Bifida Association; this led to a second one published in a professional journal (Hurtekant & Spatz, 2007). A male Korean nursing student was alarmed by the lack of breastfeeding in the Korean immigrant community in the U.S. He contacted his church elders (in a church community of about 500 members) and developed educational sessions for the elders and families including written materials in Korean. Other students have targeted those not even planning to have children yet, such as presenting educational programs to their fraternity or sorority, athletic teams, and other organized groups (on and off campus). This type of advocacy work is vital because women make the decision on how they will feed their baby often before they are pregnant based on factors in their environment throughout their lifetime.

SUMMARY

Increased advocacy for breastfeeding in the U.S. is needed. Nurses are in ideal positions to influence breastfeeding in their clinical roles and as advocates in the workplace, community, and in legislatures. Nurses should be aware of the current state of breastfeeding as well as of forces that support and impede it. Armed with this information, nurses can advocate for breastfeeding and ultimately improve the health of the nation.

For a list of related websites, please refer to your Evolve Resources at http://evolve.elsevier.com/Mason/policypolitics/

REFERENCES

Agency for Health Care Research and Quality. (2007). Breastfeeding and maternal and infant health outcomes in developed countries. Retrieved from www.ahrq.gcv/downloads/pub/evidence/pdf/brfout/brfout.pdf.

Apple, R. (1994). The medicalization of infant feeding in the United States and New Zealand: Two countries, one experience. *Journal of Human Lactation*, *10*(1), 31-37.

The Baby-Friendly Hospital Initiative (BFHI) USA. (2010). Implementing the UNICEF/WHO Baby-Friendly Hospital Initiative in the U.S. Retrieved from www.babyfriendlyusa.org/eng/01.html.

Centers for Disease Control and Prevention. (2009a, October 20). Breastfeeding report card, United States: Process indicators. Retrieved from www.cdc.gov/breastfeeding/data/report_card3.htm.

Centers for Disease Control and Prevention. (2009b). *Healthy People 2020*. Retrieved from www.healthypeople.gov/hp2020/default.asp.

Centers for Disease Control and Prevention. (2010, March 16). Breastfeeding among U.S. children born 1999-2006, CDC National Immunization Survey. Retrieved from www.cdc.gov/breastfeeding/data/NIS_data/index.htm.

Chang, K., & Spatz, D. L. (2006). The family & breastfeeding laws: What nurses need to know. *American Journal of Maternal Child Nursing*, *31*(4), 224-230.

Chen, A., & Rogan, W. J. (2004). Breastfeeding and the risk of postneonatal death in the United States. *Pediatrics*, *113*(5), e435-e439.

The Denver Channel News. (2005). Mother ticketed for breast-feeding son in public wants apology. *The Denver Channel News*. Retrieved from www.thedenverchannel.com/news/4785183/detail.html.

Helderman, R.S. (2004, August 9). Md. mom says no to coverup at Starbucks. *The Washington Post*. Retrieved from www.washingtonpost.com/wp-dyn/articles/A50610-2004Aug8.html.

Hurtekant, K. M., & Spatz, D. L. (2007). Special considerations for breastfeeding the infant with spina bifida. *Journal of Perinatal and Neonatal Nursing*, *21*(1), 69-75. PMID: 17301670.

Ip, S., Chung, M., Raman, G., Chew, P., Magula, N., et al. (2007). *Breastfeeding and maternal and infant health outcomes in developed countries*. Evidence report/technology assessment No. 153 (Prepared by Tufts–New England Medical Center Evidence-based Practice Center, under Contract No. 290-02-0022). AHRQ Publication No. 07-E007. Rockville, MD: Agency for Healthcare Research and Quality.

New York Civil Liberties Union. (2006, September 20). Mother's gather at Toys-R-Us for "Nurse In" celebrating right to breastfeed in public. *The New York Civil Liberties Union*. Retrieved from www.nyclu.org/news/mothers-gather-toys-r-us-nurse-celebrating-right-breastfeed-public.

Spatz, D. L., Pugh, L. C., American Academy of Nursing Expert Panel on Breast-feeding. (2007). The integration of the use of human milk and breastfeeding in baccalaureate nursing curricula. *Nursing Outlook*, *55*(5), 257-263.

Spatz, D. L. (2005a). Breastfeeding education and training at a children's hospital. *Journal of Perinatal Education*, *14*(1), 30-38.

Spatz, D. L. (2005b). The breastfeeding case study: A model for educating nursing students. *Journal of Nursing Education*, *44*(9), 432-434.

Spatz, D. L., & Sternberg, A. (2005). Advocacy for breastfeeding: Making a difference one community at a time. *Journal of Human Lactation*, *21*(2), 186-190.

United States Breastfeeding Committee. (2003). *State breastfeeding legislation [issue paper]*. Raleigh NC: United States Breastfeeding Committee.

United States Breastfeeding Committee. (2005). *State legislation that protects, promotes, and supports breastfeeding: An inventory and analysis of state breastfeeding and maternity leave legislation*. Washington, D.C.: United States Breastfeeding Committee.

United States Breastfeeding Committee. (2008). Retrieved from www.usbreastfeeding.org.

Wolf, J. H. (2008). Got milk? Not in public! *International Breastfeeding Journal*, *3*(11), 1-3.

CHAPTER 100

TAKING ACTION
Postpartum Depression: The Convergence of Media Coverage and Community Activism to Influence Health Policy

Mary V. Muse, John T. Carlsen, and Vanessa D. Newsome

"The media's the most powerful entity on earth."

—Malcolm X

INTRODUCTION

The media can exert significant influence on social and public health issues, and it can reach the public through many means, such as print media like newspapers, billboards, and magazines, and electronic ones like television, radio, and the Internet. Through all of these, the media has the ability to encourage action, stimulate thinking, and propose solutions. This chapter examines a particular health problem—postpartum depression—and how, in one instance, the media played an influential role in addressing it. The chapter will present the story of Melanie Stokes, a young woman who suffered from postpartum depression and psychosis. She eventually committed suicide as a result of the disorder. The history of postpartum mood disorders, policy development, and the role that media played in focusing attention on the problem will be described.

In the past, the popular media's involvement in highlighting postpartum mood disorders has been limited. The focus has generally been on criminal events associated with the disorder, with less attention to the causes or management of the symptoms. Postpartum mood disorders can be debilitating if left untreated. When inadequately or not appropriately treated, they can lead to serious outcomes for the mother, child, and family. However, if these disorders are identified early and the mother receives appropriate treatment, postpartum depression and psychosis can have better outcomes. In the case of Melanie Stokes, the media played a valuable role in influencing policy change surrounding postpartum depression.

ONE MEDIA PORTRAYAL OF POSTPARTUM DEPRESSION

In 2009, the daytime television drama *General Hospital* featured a story line on postpartum depression. The character of Dr. Robin Scorpio (Robin) is portrayed as a married, respected physician. In this story line, Robin gives birth to her first child. Following the delivery, Robin becomes detached from her husband and her new baby. Her personality changes from focused, confident, and driven to withdrawn and disconnected from her family, child, and work. Robin does not bond with her baby and prefers that someone else care for her. She comments: "My baby doesn't like me." Robin is encouraged to get psychiatric help, but she is reluctant. She returns to her practice but refuses to take her medications and misrepresents her participation in therapy. After Robin's husband learns that she has not been seeing the psychiatrist, he arranges a family intervention. The intervention concludes with Robin and her husband in agreement to seek family therapy. The story line concludes with Robin's receiving treatment and, over time, she begins to engage with her husband and new baby. This media portrayal of postpartum mood disorder, although created as entertainment, provided an accurate glimpse into what can happen in a family's life when a postpartum mood disorder occurs.

BACKGROUND ON POSTPARTUM DEPRESSION

BABY BLUES

Current literature identifies three categories of postpartum mood disorders: "baby blues," postpartum depression, and postpartum psychosis (Harris, 1994). "Baby blues" is a time-limited experience that women might experience shortly after delivery of a baby. It can be a period of anxiety, and the new mother may experience a sense of feeling overwhelmed. It is considered normal because many women experience a period of anxiety and fatigue following delivery. This is usually associated with adjustments by the mother to the baby's feeding schedule and adjustments to the new baby. "Baby blues" usually peaks in 3 to 5 days and subsides within 2 weeks. For some mothers, anxiety and sleep disturbance extends beyond 2 weeks.

POSTPARTUM DEPRESSION

The symptoms of postpartum depression and postpartum psychosis are much more severe than those of baby blues. When depression lasts 2 weeks or longer, the symptoms are categorized as postpartum depression. Postpartum depression can affect new mothers within 2 weeks to 1 year after delivery. Women experiencing postpartum depression are frequently anxious and experience crying that lasts throughout the day. These women may develop feelings of inadequacy or detachment from their babies. Although these symptoms appear similar to those of "baby blues," the difference lies in their intensity, frequency, and duration. Women with postpartum depression worry that they cannot properly care for their babies or that they may hurt their children. The mothers may have appetite changes and sleep disturbances, difficulty concentrating and making decisions, fatigue, psychomotor agitation, and anxiety. Women displaying five of these symptoms should be considered to have postpartum depression (Gjerdingen & Yawn, 2007; WebMD, 2008). Women with postpartum depression may also have thoughts of suicide, death, feelings of worthlessness or

guilt, and a frequent focus on the child's health (WebMD, 2008). These symptoms may also be associated with postpartum psychosis.

POSTPARTUM PSYCHOSIS

Postpartum psychosis is the most severe form of postpartum disorders. While it usually develops around 3 weeks after delivery, it can occur earlier or up to 1 year after delivery (WebMD, 2007). Mothers with postpartum psychosis lose touch with reality; they become delusional and have distorted thinking. Hyperactivity, mania, hallucinations, disorganized speech, or disorganized behaviors are also features of the illness (WebMD, 2007).

MAGNITUDE OF THE PROBLEM

Postpartum mood disorders affect about 800,000 women annually (Menendez, 2010). A literature review found that 10% to 20% of women experience postpartum depression; the numbers most frequently reported are 15% to 20%. Postpartum psychosis is considered a medical emergency, affecting 0.1% and 0.2% of women (Joy, Contag, & Templeton, 2010; Gjerdingen & Yawn, 2007). The cause(s) of postpartum mood disorder and psychosis are not easily understood. There appears to be consensus among researchers that hormonal changes, stress, fatigue, anxiety, and sleep disturbance are factors that are likely to contribute to postpartum mood and psychotic disorders. A review of the literature finds research studies that have examined effects of hormones on mood, sleep disturbance, fatigue, mental illness, and prior history of depression. The findings from these various studies suggest that there is a sharp decrease in hormones following delivery, poor sleep is found to be associated with depression, and fatigue (not necessarily stress or depression) is a better indicator of postpartum mood disorders. Research also shows a link between a prior history of mental illness, depression, or anxiety and these disorders. The research also finds that women with a history of bipolar disorder are at risk for postpartum psychosis. Additional research shows that the risk of psychosis for mothers without a previous psychiatric illness (hospitalization) increases when the mother's age is at least 35 (Cassels & Murata, 2009). Despite the magnitude of this illness, its devastating effects on the mother, child, and society, and its recognition as a major public health issue, little attention has been paid to it by the general public. In 2001, an event raised awareness of the problem by capturing the attention of a local community and the nation. It was the death of Melanie Stokes.

MELANIE STOKES' STORY

On June 11, 2001, Melanie Stokes jumped to her death from a hotel in the Lincoln Park neighborhood of Chicago, Illinois. According to her mother, Carol Blocker, Melanie had every reason to live (personal communication, June 11, 2009). In 2001, Melanie was a successful pharmaceutical sales manager, was married to a physician, had a supportive family, and was expecting her first child (Figure 100-1). Mrs. Blocker, who was extremely close to her daughter, described Melanie as a beautiful and radiant woman who was excited about her new baby and looking forward to motherhood.

On February 23, 2001, Melanie had delivered her baby daughter, Sommer Skyy. After the delivery, there was a sudden change in Melanie. Her concerned family consulted Melanie's physician, who attributed Melanie's mood to "baby blues" and indicated that it would pass and she would bounce back. Despite this reassurance, Melanie's mother felt that things were

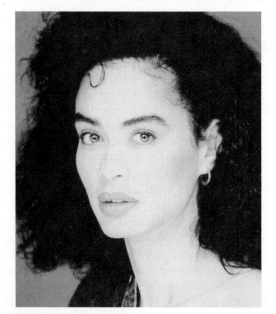

FIGURE 100-1 Melanie Blocker-Stokes. (Photo provided by Melanie Blocker-Stokes' family.)

not right. The family noticed that Melanie seemed to lose interest in the things she had previously viewed as important: her activities and friends. She had difficulty interacting and embracing her baby. Mrs. Blocker had difficulty getting the doctors to recognize that Melanie's depression was more than mild depression ("baby blues"). Carol reports telling the physician that "something is wrong."

Melanie stopped eating and drinking. Mrs. Blocker was shocked and scared, and she called her sisters for support. She called Melanie's physician, and, at one point, was told not to call the office again because of issues with patient privacy. Melanie's condition continued to deteriorate; she developed paranoid thoughts (she thought her neighbors closed their blinds because she was a bad mother). She thought her baby daughter did not like her and would be better off without her, and she began to contemplate suicide. At one point, she asked a family member for a gun. Mrs. Blocker states that her daughter told her: "Mommy, I am going to have to die. You are not going to be able to stop me." Melanie even picked out three outfits for her wake and funeral. With the persistence of her mother and the urging of her husband, Melanie was hospitalized. She was hospitalized 3 times in 7 weeks, received antipsychotic medication and antidepressants, and underwent electroconvulsive therapy. Unfortunately, this intervention had come too late. By this time, Melanie had developed serious depression and psychosis. She had concern for her baby, but she also felt that the baby rejected her and that she was unable to care for her. Despite the efforts of her husband and other family members, Melanie's condition worsened. On the morning of June 11, 2009, Melanie's husband went to work at Cook County Hospital, which was a short distance from their home. After he left, Melanie took a taxi to the North side and checked into a Chicago hotel. She wrote six letters and then jumped from a twelfth-floor window.

THE MEDIA'S ROLE IN CHANGING POLICY

The response to Melanie Stokes' death was immediate, drawing local and national attention. The newspapers, print, radio, television, and the Internet carried the story. The initial media response focused on "Why did it happen?" and "How did it happen?" How did a young woman from an upper middle-class family find so much despair that she would take her life? Why wasn't something done to help her? Questions were asked about the medical care she received and even about her family. The media scrutinized the events that had led to this tragedy. As more details emerged, the issues associated with postpartum mood disorder garnered increased media attention. Depression and psychosis became topics for mainstream media coverage. Eventually, experts were interviewed about postpartum disorders, and the media's focus became education rather than drama. The topic persisted in the media, both in print and on television, for years after Melanie's death. Tragically, several other cases of mothers' taking their own lives, or the lives of their children, followed Melanie's death (Jennifer Mudd-Houghtaling killed herself in Illinois, and Andrea Yates killed her children in Texas).

Why was the response to Melanie's story more than just one more sad story in the news? Public concern led to a call for appropriate diagnosis and treatment by clinical providers. Mothers like Carol Blocker, who lost a loved one, advocated for change. She was devastated by her daughter's death and became an advocate fighting for postpartum depression and psychosis awareness. She took her advocacy to the Internet, television, and public forums, forming coalitions with other mothers and organizations. Mrs. Blocker also created a website (Blocker, 2003), contacted her local and state representatives, called friends and former colleagues, contacted the media, and requested the opportunity to tell the story of her daughter's tragic death. The *Oprah Winfrey Show* featured a program on postpartum depression with Mrs. Blocker as a guest.

Mrs. Blocker organized a march along Lake Michigan. The march drew mothers and victims' relatives from surrounding suburbs who had lost loved ones to the disorder. The march and the stories on postpartum depression were featured in both Chicago newspapers, *The Chicago Tribune* and *The Chicago Sun Times*.

ACTION IN RESPONSE TO MEDIA ATTENTION TO MELANIE'S DEATH

Some health care organizations revised policies in the wake of Melanie's death. The mayor of Chicago joined in support of postpartum awareness and proclaimed Postpartum Awareness Day in the city (Allen, 2009). The Illinois Alliance for Postpartum Mood Disorders launched a website and convened conferences to address the issue. At the state level in Illinois,

legislation was enacted to promote education of mothers and to encourage (although not require) pediatricians to discuss postpartum illness with new mothers (Illinois Public Acts, 2008).

U.S. HOUSE ACTION

Illinois Representative Congressman Bobby Rush (D-IL-1) asked Carol Blocker how he could help. Mrs. Blocker and experts on postpartum disorders provided the congressman with information and recommendations. Congressman Rush began working on a bill that addressed postpartum depression and psychosis. In June 2001, he introduced H.R. 2380, the Melanie Blocker-Stokes Postpartum Depression Research and Care Act, into Congress. It required the Secretary of Health and Human Services, acting through the Director of the National Institute of Mental Health, to "expand and intensify research and related activities of the Institute with respect to postpartum depression and postpartum psychosis [and] to make grants to provide for projects for the establishment, operation, and coordination of effective and cost-efficient systems for the delivery of essential services to individuals with postpartum depression or postpartum psychosis and their families" (Melanie Blocker-Stokes Postpartum Depression Research and Care Act, 2001). The bill was referred to the House Subcommittee on Health but never made it out of committee. In 2003 and 2005, Congressman Rush attempted several times to advance legislation to enhance research on postpartum disorders, but the initiatives did not move forward. In January 2009, Congressman Rush introduced H.R. 20, the Melanie Blocker Stokes Mom's Opportunity to Access Health, Education, Research, and Support for Postpartum Depression (MOTHERS) Act, and the bill was referred to committee.

U.S. SENATE ACTION AND LEGISLATIVE SUCCESS

In 2001 and 2003, after Melanie's death, Senator Richard Durbin (D-IL) called to amend the Public Service Act to provide research and services for women with postpartum depression and psychosis. His bills were referred to the Senate committee on Health, Education, Labor, and Pensions but stalled there. In 2006, Senator Durbin and Senator Robert Menendez (D-NJ) introduced Senate Bill 3529 (the MOTHERS Act). In May 2009 the House passed the Melanie Blocker-Stokes Postpartum Depression Research and Care Act, and the bill was sent to the Senate. Finally, in March 2010, as part of the landmark health insurance reform bill passed by Congress, the Melanie Blocker Stokes MOTHERS Act became law (Menendez, 2010).

ANALYZING THE MEDIA'S INFLUENCE

The media has substantial influence in driving public policy and promoting health education. It is important to understand the media's ability to influence public opinion and the policy landscape (Brookings, 2008; Lefebvres, 2008). The media's focus on Melanie's death drew attention and led to action. However, not all of the media attention was felt by the public to be of value. While some print media featured useful stories (e.g., those that appeared in *Ebony* and *Jet* magazines), others drew criticism. An article in *Time* magazine, "The Melancholy of Motherhood" by Catherine Elton, drew such criticism. Elton was perceived by some to have written a distorted article. The readers of Postpartum Progress, a widely read blog, wrote a letter in response because they believed the article contained misinformation and further contributed to confusion and stigmatization of women with postpartum depression. The letter stated that "*Time* has done a disservice to all mothers who are suffering and will suffer from postpartum depression" (Codey et al., 2009). Forty-eight individuals signed this letter including several nurses, Valerie Plame, and the first lady of New Jersey.

SUMMARY

Generating policy is often the result of a grassroots effort that captures the attention of the public, media, and legislators (Brookings, 2008). The death of Melanie Stokes was an event that focused the media's and the public's attention on a health problem. The tragic nature of Melanie's death was a powerful story. In this case, most of the media coverage was valuable in educating the public, clinicians, and policymakers about the potentially devastating consequences of undiagnosed and untreated postpartum depression and psychosis.

Melanie's mother, Carol Blocker, advocated for change through the media and worked with others, including a national alliance, to gain attention. In this case, media attention led to a number of policymakers taking action—locally in Melanie's home of Chicago and on Capitol Hill. It is not easy obtaining the attention of elected officials due to the number of problems competing for attention, and the media played a critical role in the efforts to encourage a different response to postpartum disorders.

For a list of related websites, please refer to your Evolve Resources at http://evolve.elsevier.com/Mason/policypolitics/

REFERENCES

Allen, S. (2009). Governor Quinn proclaims May 2009 Postpartum Mood Disorders Awareness Month in Illinois. Postpartum Depression Alliance of Illinois. Retrieved from www.ppdil.org/ppdmonth.htm.

BabyCenter.com. (2006). Postpartum depression. Retrieved from www.babycenter.com/0_postpartum-depression_227.bc.

Blocker, C. (2003). Melanie's battle: The hidden plague of postpartum psychosis and depression. Retrieved from www.melaniebattle.org/index.html.

Brookings. (2008). Democracy in the age of new media: A report on the media and the immigration debate. Retrieved from www.brookings.edu/reports/2008/0925_immigration_dionne.aspx.

Cassels, C., & Murata, P. (2009). Half of first-time moms with postnatal psychosis have no history of mental illness. Retrieved from http://cme.medscape.com/viewarticle/588298.

Codey, M. J., Blocker, C., Murdock, S., Beck, C., Gagliardi, A. D., et al. (2009). An open letter to *Time* magazine about postpartum depression. Postpartum Progress. Retrieved from http://postpartumprogress.typepad.com/weblog/2009/07/open-letter-to-time-magazine-about-postpartum-depression.html.

Gjerdingen, D. K., & Yawn, B. P. (2007). Postpartum depression screening: Importance, methods, barriers and recommendations for practice. *Journal of the American Board of Family Medicine, 20*(3), 280-288. Retrieved from www.medscape.com/viewarticle/558440.

Harris, B. (1994). Biological and hormonal aspects of postpartum depressed mood working towards strategies for prophylaxis and treatment. *Br J Psych, 164,* 288-292.

Illinois Public Acts. (2008). Perinatal Mental Health Disorders Prevention and Treatment Act. 095-0469. Illinois Public Acts. January 1, 2008.

Joy, S., Contag, S., & Templeton, H. (2010). Postpartum depression. Retrieved from http://emedicine.medscape.com/article/271662-overview.

Lefebvres, R. C. (2008). Effects of media on health behaviors: Evidence from tobacco control. Retrieved from http://socialmarketing.blogs.com/r_craiig_lefebvres_social/2008/09/the-effects-of-media-on-health-behaviors-evidence-from-tobacco-control.html.

Melanie Blocker Stokes Mom's Opportunity to Access Health, Education, Research, and Support for Postpartum Depression (MOTHERS) Act. (2009). H.R. 20. 111th Congress, 1st Session. Retrieved from http://thomas.loc.gov/home/bills_res.html.

Melanie Blocker-Stokes Postpartum Depression Research and Care Act. (2001). H.R. 2380. 107th Congress, 1st Session. Retrieved from http://thomas.loc.gov/cgi-bin/query/z?c107:H.R.2380.IH:.

Menendez, R. (2010). Major initiative to combat postpartum depression to be signed into law as part of health insurance reform. Retrieved from http://menendez.senate.gov/newsroom/press/index.cfm?PageNum_rs=2.

WebMD. (2007). Understanding postpartum depression—The basics. Retrieved from www.webMD.com/hw-popup/postpartum-psychosis.

WebMD. (2008). Understanding postpartum depression—Symptoms. Retrieved from www.webMD.com/depression/postpartum-depression/postpartum-depression-symptoms.

CHAPTER 101

Nursing in the International Community: A Broader View of Nursing Issues

Judith A. Oulton

"We cannot live for ourselves alone. Our lives are connected by a thousand invisible threads ... our actions run as causes and return to us as results."

—Herman Melville

In the late 1960s, Marshall McLuhan coined the term *global village.* McLuhan was referring to the fact that through advances in communications, time and space have vanished. Not only was there a new, multisensory view of the world in 1967, but people from around the world could communicate as if they lived in the same village. Yet when McLuhan outlined his vision over 40 years ago, the Internet did not exist, nor did the World Trade Organization (WTO) (Box 101-1) and its Global Agreement on Trade in Services (GATS). AIDS was a little-known wasting disease in Africa, and the world was celebrating its first heart transplant and bypass operations.

During the past 40-odd years, we have witnessed the increased globalization of commerce, travel, information, trade, and disease. In 1955, there were 51 million airline passengers (IATA, 2005). According to Airports Council International, by 2025 the number of air travelers worldwide will be more than 9 billion per year (Metrics 2.0, 2007). Today people, images, and messages move around the world with ease, and we truly have a sense of being a global village. As a result, we have a professional obligation to understand the village-world in its broader context and to base our decision-making on a broader understanding of ourselves, our patients, and our circumstances. By having a global view, we are capable of synthesizing a broad range of information to make informed decisions. It begins with understanding the policies and politics of globalization and of other key international health and nursing issues.

GLOBALIZATION

Globalization is the growing interdependence of the world's people with an integration of economy, culture, technology, and governance. Globalization changes the way nations and communities work, shrinking time, space, and borders. It means that national policy and action are increasingly shaped by international forces. Globalization brings new people to our countries and communities. The increase in international travel means the ready spread of disease and threat to security as people move freely across borders and continents. SARS and H1N1 are two examples of global health risks. Today, nations and health professionals must learn to care for new as well as reemerging illnesses, deal with the added risks of exposure, and handle acts of terrorism.

With GATS and the general globalization of trade, health services and the health professions are increasingly seen as commodities. Health tourism is gaining popularity as nations vie for patients interested in traveling to another country for health care. As well, many countries are expressing an interest in mutual recognition agreements that lower barriers for health professionals to practice in other nations. Increased communication, easier air travel, and the easing of trade restrictions have made mobility and migration easier.

BOX 101-1 **World Trade Organization**

Established in 1995, the World Trade Organization (WTO) is the successor to the General Agreement on Tariffs and Trade (GATT). Its mandate is to ensure that trade in goods and services flows as smoothly, predictably, and freely as possible. It does so by doing the following:

- Administering trade agreements
- Acting as a forum for trade negotiations
- Settling trade disputes, and reviewing national trade policies
- Assisting developing countries in trade policy issues through technical assistance and training programs
- Cooperating with other international organizations
  Multilateral trade agreements are the legal ground rules for international commerce that countries trade rights to and that bind governments to keep their trade policies within agreed limits. The General Agreement on Trade in Services (GATS) is a multilateral agreement to reduce barriers to international trade in services. It seeks to improve trade in services and investment conditions through a set of mutually agreed-on rules, including a dispute settlement system.

  Headquartered in Geneva, the WTO includes 153 countries, with another 30 negotiating membership. Member countries today account for over 97% of world trade (WTO, 2001; WTO, 2005).

MIGRATION: A CASE IN POINT

Migration is a key issue for nursing. According to the International Organization on Migration (IOM), there were 214 million international migrants in 2005, which represents 3.1% of the world's population. Of this number, 49% were women (IOM, 2010). People, including nurses, move around for many reasons: to work; to study; to have fun; to receive health care; or to escape violence, poverty, persecution, and famine in their native countries. This movement brings with it the problems of unemployment, discrimination, racial tension, and harmful cultural practices, such as female genital mutilation. Today's nurses must understand health, illness, and coping mechanisms from the perspectives of many cultures. Equally important is the need for the profession to be an advocate for sound health and nursing policy that considers the well-being of the patient along with that of the profession and its practitioners.

Governments—bilaterally, regionally, or through the WTO—negotiate terms for the movement of goods and people for economic gain. With the global shortage of health professionals, individuals and institutions at all levels (i.e., governments, employers, policymakers, the public, the professions, and professionals) are interested in the movement of nurses. It affects policy, planning, and delivery of nursing education and patient care. It brings to the fore such issues as use of fraudulent credentials, ethical recruitment, and discriminatory workplace policy and practice.

While nursing migration has slowed recently, nurses are still on the move. The nursing community has been vocal nationally and internationally in addressing migration and workforce policy and practice. The following are examples:

- In 2001, the International Council of Nurses (ICN) (Figure 101-1) issued its policy on Ethical Nurse Recruitment, which supports the right of nurses to migrate but denounces unethical recruitment and condemns the practice of recruiting nurses to countries where authorities have failed to implement sound human resource planning. The ICN has called for regulated recruitment and implementation of 13 principles to support recruitment and retention (ICN, 2001) (Box 101-2).
- In line with the ICN Position on Nurse Migration, and its Position on Ethical Recruitment, nurses' associations have condemned the practice of recruiting offshore rather than effectively addressing human resource planning, including the problems that cause nurses to leave the profession and discourage them from returning to nursing (ICN, 2007; ICN, 2001). As well, associations are monitoring employers to ensure that the rights of migrant nurses are upheld and that adequate support systems are in place.
- The nursing shortage and lack of focus on nursing prompted the ICN to undertake a global study in 2004. The papers are available online at *www.icn.ch*.
- The ICN has created two new centers addressing workforce issues. The International Centre on Nurse Migration (ICNM) was launched in 2005 in partnership with the Commission on Graduates of Foreign Schools of Nursing. It serves as a global resource for the development, promotion, and dissemination of research, policy, and information on nurse migration (ICNM, 2010). The second center,

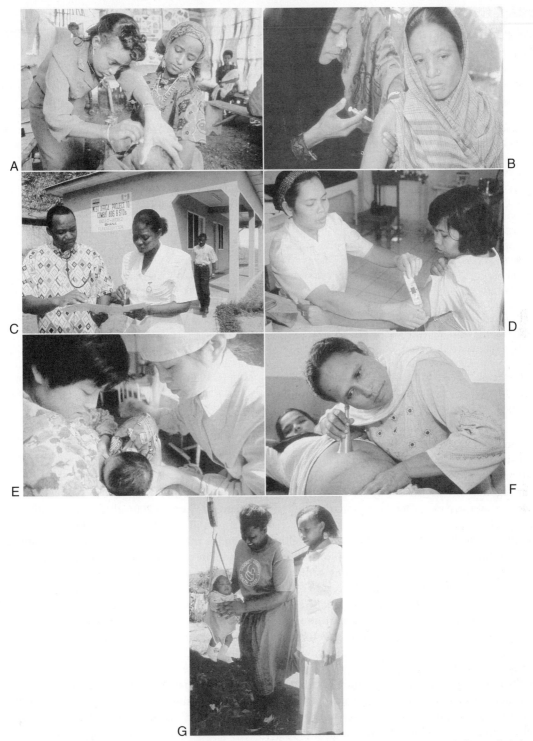

FIGURE 101-1 International Council of Nurses advocates: nurses and the world. **A,** Ethiopia; **B,** Bangladesh; **C,** Ghana; **D,** Indonesia; **E,** China; **F,** Pakistan; and **G,** Kenya. (Courtesy of David Barbour **[A]**, Nancy Durrell McKenna **[B, D,** and **F]**, Pierre St. Jacques **[C]**, Roger Lemoyne **[E]**, and Stephanie Colvey **[G]**, as well as ACDI/CIDA.)

BOX 101-2 International Council of Nurses

The International Council of Nurses is a federation of national nurses associations (NNAs) representing nurses in more than 130 countries. Founded in 1899, the ICN is the world's first and widest-reaching international organization for health professionals. Operated by nurses for nurses, the ICN works to ensure high-quality nursing care for all, sound health policies globally, the advancement of nursing knowledge, and the presence worldwide of a respected nursing profession and a competent and satisfied nursing workforce.

The ICN advances nursing, nurses, and health through its policies, partnerships, advocacy, leadership development, networks, congresses, and special projects and its work in the arenas of professional practice, regulation, and socioeconomic welfare. The ICN is particularly active in ethics, AIDS, advanced practice, research, leadership development, the international classification of nursing practice, women's health, regulation, human resources development, occupational health and safety, conditions of work, career development, and human rights.

The council works with agencies of the United Nations (UN) system, such as the WHO, UNAIDS, UNICEF, UNESCO, UNCTAD, and ILO; other intergovernmental organizations such as the World Bank, WTO, and the International Organization on Migration; and international, regional, and national nongovernmental organizations.

BOX 101-3 World Health Organization

The World Health Organization (WHO), established in 1948, is governed by 193 member countries through the World Health Assembly. It has a staff of more than 8000 people from over 150 countries who work in WHO's 147 country offices, 6 regional offices, and its Geneva-based headquarters. The Director General heads the staff and is appointed by the Assembly.

The WHO's objective is the attainment by all peoples of the highest possible level of health. It fulfills its mandate through its core functions as follows:

- Providing leadership on matters critical to health, and engaging in partnerships where joint action is needed
- Shaping the research agenda, and stimulating the generation, translation, and dissemination of valuable knowledge
- Setting norms and standards, and promoting and monitoring their implementation
- Articulating ethical and evidence-based policy options
- Providing technical support, catalyzing change, and building sustainable institutional capacity
- Monitoring the health situation, and assessing health trends

The WHO defines *health* as "a state of complete physical, mental and social well-being and not merely the absence of disease or infirmity." The definition, adopted in 1948, has not changed, though attempts have been made to persuade the WHO to add the concept of spiritual health to the definition (WHO, 2010b; WHO, 2010c).

---

the International Centre on Human Resources in Nursing (ICHRN), was established in 2006 as an online resource for information and tools on nursing human resources (ICHRN, 2010). The center produces papers, fact sheets, and case studies on a wide range of workforce issues.

- Beginning in 2006, the ICN, the World Health Organization (WHO), and the International Confederation of Midwives began hosting strategic biennial meetings in advance of the World Health Assembly, a body made up of representatives of ministries of health from 193 countries. Known as the Triad meetings and attended by government chief nursing officers, nursing and midwifery regulators, and leaders of national nursing and midwifery organizations, the group addresses key global issues, such as recruitment, retention, leadership, education, regulation, roles, and relationships. Triad statements are used in policy and advocacy at national and regional levels (Box 101-3).

- Migration has been on the WHO agenda for several years. In 2004, the World Health Assembly approved a resolution calling for a code of practice on the international recruitment of health personnel. The organization then spent 6 years discussing and drafting a code that, if approved, would be non-binding. It would, however, set out principles and guidelines for ethical recruitment (WHO, 2009). Several countries have developed guidelines for employers or introduced voluntary codes. In the United States, AcademyHealth, an organization that focuses on health services research and policy, and its partners created a voluntary code of conduct and a nonprofit organization—the Alliance for Ethical International Recruitment Practices—to increase transparency and accountability and monitor adherence to their Code (ICNM, 2009).

THE GLOBAL WORKFORCE CRISIS AND MILLENNIUM DEVELOPMENT GOALS

Migration and the shortage of health personnel have placed human resources for health care on the agenda as never before. In 2004, the Joint Learning Initiative (JLI) reported an estimated shortage of 4 million health workers globally. This figure is based on the density of 2.5 health workers (physician, nurse, midwife) per 1000 population that is required to achieve 80% coverage of measles immunization and skilled attendants at birth (JLI, 2004). It was supported in 2006 in the World Health Report, which identified 57 countries as falling below this threshold, 36 of them in sub-Saharan Africa (WHO, 2006). The crisis also saw the launch of the Global Health Workforce Alliance, a partnership with national governments, finance institutions, health workers, international agencies, professional associations, academic institutions and civil society, dedicated to identifying and facilitating solutions to the human resource crisis (GHWA, 2006). It champions universal access to health care and the message that a skilled, motivated, and supported health force is the cornerstone of a robust health system.

Attention to "health human resources" is part of the Millennium Development Goals (MDGs), launched in 2000. With a target date of 2015, the eight MDGs address poverty, education, women, child mortality, maternal health, HIV and malaria, the environment, and a global social compact (UN, 2005). Achieving the MDGs ultimately affects the health and well-being of the world's 6.8 billion people. Governments and others (e.g., the G8, made up of the heads of state of Canada, France, Germany, Italy, Japan, Russia, the United Kingdom, and the U.S.) who meet annually to deal with major national and international economic and political issues recognized that these ambitious goals could not be met unless two key issues were addressed: Africa and the global health human resource crisis, particularly the nursing shortage.

Today nearly all nations face a nursing shortage brought about by increasing demand and diminishing supply, an aging nursing workforce, a shortage of other professional and ancillary staff, increasing acuity of illness, a poor image of nursing, and continuing health sector reform. For Africa, HIV/AIDS further complicates the shortage. Shortages vary by field of nursing, geography, level of care, sector, and organization; but one commonality exists: there are two shortages—a real shortage and a pseudo-shortage.

Pseudo-shortages exist in both developed and developing countries and occur when there are enough nurses in the country but when posts are not funded and/or nurses are not willing to work under the conditions available. For example, South Africa is said to have 31,000 vacant public sector nursing posts and 35,000 unemployed nurses. The lack of a positive practice environment (low salaries, poor benefit packages, lack of supplies and equipment, inadequate nurse/patient ratios, unsatisfactory patient and staff safety, lack of access to professional development and promotions, lack of family-friendly policies, and lack of decision-making input) remains the most critical element everywhere and particularly in Africa.

Africa is in dire straits. As former Prime Minister Tony Blair noted, "Africa is the only continent which, without change, will not meet any of the Millennium Development Goals" (Blair, 2005). While mortality rates are improving, in 2008 the mortality rate among children under 5 years of age in sub-Saharan Africa was 144/1000 live births compared with 6/1000 in industrialized countries (UNICEF, 2009). This means that an Ethiopian child was 30 times more likely to die by age 5 than a child in Western Europe (UNICEF, 2010). In 2008, malaria killed approximately 850,000 people, 90% of which were in Africa, mostly among children under 5 years of age (UN, 2010). In 2008, over 30 million African children were not attending primary school (UN, 2010), and 14 million were AIDS orphans (UNAIDS, 2009b).

During this past decade, successive meetings of the G8 have focused on aid to Africa. In 2005, they agreed to increase annual aid to Africa by $25 billion per year and overall aid by an estimated $50 billion by 2010. They have since reaffirmed these commitments as well as specific commitments for health and the health workforce, especially in Africa (DFID, 2009; Guebert, 2009). It will be important that nurses and other stakeholders monitor and lobby national governments to keep these commitments. Ultimately, we need to decrease poverty and increase health for all nations.

BOX 101-4 World Bank Group

The World Bank, established in 1944, is composed of the International Bank for Reconstruction and Development, the International Development Association, the International Finance Corporation, the Multilateral Investment Guaranty Agency, and the International Centre for Settlement of Investment Disputes. The World Bank Group is owned by its member countries, whose numbers vary according to the agency. The International Bank for Reconstruction and Development (IBRD) is the largest, with 186 member countries. While governed by its members, day-to-day operations fall to the leadership of the president and the work of over 10,000 employees in more than 100 offices worldwide.

The Bank's mission is to fight poverty for lasting results and to help people help themselves and their environment by providing resources, sharing knowledge and building capacity, and forging partnerships in the public and private sectors. It is a development Bank that provides low-interest loans, interest-free credits, and grants to developing countries for a wide array of purposes that include investments in education, health, public administration, infrastructure, financial and private sector development, agriculture, and environmental and natural resource management. Also, it offers policy advice, technical assistance, and knowledge-sharing services to low- and middle-income countries to reduce poverty (WB, 2010).

POVERTY

Today, poverty is the world's most devastating scourge. The World Bank estimates that there are about 1.4 billion extremely poor people in the world, with women representing 70% of the absolute poor (World Bank, 2008). According to the UN Secretary General, the number of extreme poor in sub-Saharan Africa has risen by 92 million between 1990 and 2005, and by 8 million in West Asia. Children living in absolute poverty are 5 times more likely to die before the age of 5 than children who are not poor (WHO, 1999). Every day, almost 16,000 children die from hunger-related causes—1 child every 5 seconds; and 947 million people in developing countries are undernourished—a condition that affects one's health and well-being, hinders fetal development, and contributes to mental retardation (Bread for the World, 2009) (Box 101-4).

In 2009, over 1 billion people were hungry; this is the highest level ever due largely to high food prices, the global economic crises, and unemployment (UN,

2010). Unequal distribution of wealth and of health services has dire consequences for the poor, whether in developing countries or in the U.S. The poor and hungry have a greater burden of ill health and disability, attributable in large part to infectious diseases, malnutrition, and complications of childbirth.

Poor countries have few public services, and these are of poor quality. This means longer travel and waiting times for care, fewer drugs, shared beds, and more corruption and graft. Often it means user fees and out-of-pocket payments at a time when people are ill and most in need of care. Although user fees may bring in money to buy more supplies, they often create unanticipated problems. For example, they may keep the working poor from seeking care, leading to enhanced chronicity and disability. And in places where crime and hunger are rampant, user fees leave the nurse who handles the money vulnerable to attack. Today a number of African nations, such as Zambia, Liberia, Kenya, Senegal, Lesotho, and Ghana have abolished fees for key primary health care services (McCoy, 2009). Research shows that their removal has resulted in increased use of services by the poor.

Health care has deteriorated in many countries, and previous gains are being lost with the recent economic downturn and the 2008 energy and food crises, but we have also made considerable strides in demonstrating the economic advantage of good health. The WHO Report of the Commission on Macroeconomics and Health found that providing coverage of essential health services to the world's poor could save millions of lives each year, decrease poverty, stimulate economic development, and promote global security (WHO, 2001).

The G8 countries have committed billions of dollars to a massive effort to fight the diseases of poverty. These diseases—primarily tuberculosis, HIV and AIDS, malaria, childhood diseases (such as measles and diarrheal conditions), and the complications associated with pregnancy and delivery—inflict a terrible and disproportionate toll of death and disability on the world's poorest people. The Global Fund to Fight AIDS, Tuberculosis and Malaria (TGF) was created by the G8 in 2002 to scale up global effort and pool resources to fight these diseases. To date, it has committed $19.3 billion in 144 countries to support large-scale prevention, treatment, and care programs against the three diseases (TGF, 2010).

According to the ICN, nurses have a vital role in reducing poverty and its impact on health and well-being, including involving families and communities in defining their problems and seeking solutions; lobbying for antipoverty measures and for equity in health care and social services; supporting the shift to community-based care; working to initiate pro-poor social and health policy; and focusing attention on the impact of poverty on women and other vulnerable groups (ICN, 1999).

Education, particularly education of women, plays a key role in poverty reduction. It leads to lower fertility and infant mortality rates, better health and nutrition, higher productivity, better gender equity, and improved chances that the next generation will in turn be educated. However, because of poverty, illness, cultural practices, fear, and violence, girls are less likely than boys to be educated. According to the UN Secretary General, some 72 million children of primary school age around the world do not attend school. About half of them are in sub-Saharan Africa, where the percentage of enrollment of girls compared with boys continues to fall. In 2007, it stood at 79% (UN, 2010). Given the value of education to health and poverty reduction, in 2005 the ICN and its sister organization, the Florence Nightingale International Foundation (FNIF), launched the Girl Child Education Fund to support the primary and secondary schooling of orphaned daughters of nurses, beginning in sub-Saharan Africa, where there are an estimated 14 million AIDS orphans (Box 101-5).

HIV/AIDS

If poverty is the world's greatest scourge, then AIDS is surely second. AIDS is everywhere. In 2008, UNAIDS reported 33 million people living with HIV, and 2.7 million new infections, with 430,000 of these being newborns. Globally, 2 million people died of AIDS-related causes that year, and young people accounted for 40% of all new adult infections (UNAIDS, 2009a).

In the U.S., the Centers for Disease Control and Prevention (CDC) estimates that about 1 million people were living with HIV in 2007, around 470,000 had AIDS, and about 500,000 had died after developing AIDS. In 2006, 56,300 Americans became newly infected with HIV, with African Americans making up an estimated 45% of new infections, whites 35%, and Hispanic/Latinos 17% (Avert, 2010).

BOX 101-5 The Girl Child Education Fund: A Nursing Initiative for Orphaned Girls

The Need

Orphaned children, particularly girls, often have no access to schooling despite our understanding that educating girls and women plays a key role in poverty reduction, leading to lower fertility and infant mortality rates, better health and nutrition, higher productivity, better gender equity, and improved chances that the next generation will in turn be educated. Today, because of poverty, illness, cultural practices, fear, and violence, girls are less likely than boys to be educated, and they account for 60% of out-of-school children. Most out-of-school children (72 million) and most orphans (e.g., 14 million AIDS orphans) live in sub-Saharan Africa.

The Fund

The ICN and the FNIF are supporting the primary and secondary schooling of orphaned daughters of nurses in four sub-Saharan Africa countries: Kenya, Uganda, Swaziland, and Zambia. The fund provides for the cost of fees, uniforms, and books. An annual donation of $200 covers the costs of primary education, and $600 annually means an African colleague's orphaned daughter can attend secondary school.

For more information on this initiative, visit *www.fnif.org*.

While there are real concerns about rising rates of HIV infections in Central and Eastern Europe and in Asia, it is in Africa that the disease is devastating communities and nations and creating a generation of AIDS orphans. It is also taking its toll among the nurses who care for the ill, and who may be infected themselves. According to UNAIDS, sub-Saharan Africa, where 22.4 million people are infected, is home to over two-thirds of all people living with HIV and AIDS. In 2008, an estimated 1.9 million people became newly infected. Swaziland has the highest HIV prevalence rate (26%) with Lesotho second at 23.2%, while South Africa lays claim to the world's largest HIV population (2.7 million in 2007) (UNAIDS, 2009b).

Women account for 60% of HIV infections in the region, with young women and girls particularly vulnerable. In Kenya, young women are 3 times more likely to become infected than their male counterparts. The good news is that, as of 2008, 44% of infected adults and children in the region have access to ARV treatment, whereas in 2003 the rate was only 2% (UNAIDS, 2009b). As a result, people are living longer productive lives. However, 33% of people living with HIV are co-infected with tuberculosis, which is the leading cause of death among those living with HIV (UNAIDS, 2009a). In 2008, an estimated 1.3 million people died from tuberculosis according to the WHO. The highest incidence is found in Southeast Asia and sub-Saharan Africa. In the latter, the incidence rate is over 350 cases per 100,000 population, and it continues to rise (WHO, 2010a).

The severity of HIV and the workforce shortage have stretched resources, especially in sub-Saharan Africa, and limited access to care. As a result, the WHO, in collaboration with the Office of the U.S. Global AIDS Coordinator, came up with the idea of *task shifting*—the delegation of tasks to less specialized health workers (e.g., moving phlebotomy from nurses to community health workers in Ethiopia, or having nurses assume many tasks traditionally performed by physicians in Uganda, such as determining eligibility for anti-retroviral therapy [ART]) and managing those on ART who have minor side effects) (WHO, 2007). The World Health Professions Alliance (WHPA), concerned about the quality of care and the safety of task-shifting for patients and professionals, set out 12 principles for effective task shifting. These are available at *www.whpa.org*.

The impact of task shifting on nurses has yet to be determined. However, it is clear that nurses, if used to their full potential, could be the key to success. They form the core of care in most countries, particularly in the developing world, where money and drugs are scarce, beds are full, and myths flourish. The biggest problem for nurses in Africa is changing the social attitudes toward sex, including the myth that having intercourse with a virgin can rid a man of HIV.

AIDS increases nursing workloads and fuels burnout and frustration, thereby contributing to absenteeism, attrition, and migration. In addition to caring for HIV and AIDS patients at work, nurses often also care for family and friends after hours, and many are themselves ill. According to the WHO, anecdotal evidence and some recent African studies suggest that health systems may lose up to one-fifth of their employees to HIV/AIDS over the coming years (WHO, 2005). Fear of occupational exposure may be reducing entrants into the nursing workforce, as well as encouraging current members to leave. Few

sub-Saharan countries offer health workers counseling, support, or ART.

In 2004, the ICN began working with Zambia and Swaziland to develop proposals for providing ART and community-based care to health care workers and their families; this move resulted in the highly acclaimed Wellness Centres now in operation in Swaziland, Lesotho, Zambia, Uganda, and Malawi. The Centres offer HIV and tuberculosis care as well as stress management, lifestyle education, occupational health and safety services, a knowledge resource and training center for continuous professional development, and other services as needed. They have been singled out as a best practice example of the WHO strategy to treat, train, and retain the health care workforce. Sadly, nurses have yet to be used to their full potential within the UN system, where they play a minor role in health policy development.

NURSING, GOVERNMENTS, AND THE WORLD HEALTH ORGANIZATION

THE WORLD HEALTH ORGANIZATION

Today there are more dieticians and nutritionists than nurses on the WHO's staff. Needless to say, this handicaps nursing, which, at its height in 1968, had over 200 nursing posts at all levels within the WHO. In 2007, there were only 8, representing 1% of WHO professional posts in the category that includes dental, medical, nursing, and veterinary staff (Caughley, 2008). Not surprisingly, the majority of professionals are medical specialists and the Director General is a physician. The WHO has one nurse scientist within its Geneva-based secretariat, and, while all 6 regions have a nurse who oversees nursing issues, only 5 have designated Regional Nurse Advisors. The Pan-American Health Organization (PAHO), the regional office of the Americas, has none, although there is one nursing post within the human resources department. In the WHO, nurses do occupy non-nursing posts in program areas at headquarters, and at regional and country levels. Also, there are now two nurses who are WHO Country Representatives—the highest country-level WHO post.

Repeatedly, with senior staff changes at WHO, the question arises as to why the WHO needs a nurse scientist. The role has been further diluted recently as the Chief Nurse Scientist also assumed liaison responsibility for a number of other health professional groups, mostly paramedical. Several Regional Nurse Advisors are set to retire shortly, and it will be important for nursing to support continuation of these posts.

The global nursing shortage presents an opportunity to change the influence of nurses within the WHO and nationally. The World Health Assembly (WHA) has resolved to address nursing issues. In May 2006, it recognized the crucial contribution of nursing and midwifery to health systems, populations, and goals such as the MDGs; called for actions to recruit and retain nurses; and asked for progress reports in 2008 and 2010 (WHA, 2006). In preparation for the 2010 report, the WHO commissioned a survey of nursing in all regions.

NATIONAL GOVERNMENTS

Nurses hold staff, appointed, and elected posts in small numbers within national governments. Overall they are not making much headway with respect to government chief nurse posts, though the number is growing in Europe and in Central and Eastern Europe and the former Soviet Union. Lobbying for positions in South America continues, and the Caribbean and some African countries have lost posts as part of health care reform. There is little activity in the French-speaking states in Africa or Europe, where there is no history of the position and little call for it. The lack of a strong united nongovernmental nursing voice in many of these countries means that nursing continues to be disadvantaged in the policy arena.

NURSING'S POLICY VOICE

Achieving nursing's policy potential is perhaps the greatest challenge facing the profession in the twenty-first century. Nursing's success in shaping policy varies depending on the country, the issue, and the group under consideration. On the other hand, the limiting factors are fairly universal and include nursing's image, perceived value, and social status; educational requirements; gender issues; and numbers. The ratio of nurses to other health workers, the scope of practice, legislation, cultural norms, and the presence of strong national nursing associations affect the influence of nurses. Equally important is the extent to which nurses are perceived to be interested in

improving health for all, versus being interested in only personal and professional gains.

There is no doubt that policy influence is an uphill battle for many. In some newly independent countries, nurses are engaged in learning about nursing autonomy and lobbying for the right to chart their own actions. Nursing groups are lobbying in several countries to create a government Chief Nurse post, to maintain the position, or to reinstate it. Nursing too often lacks a single senior nurse let alone a cadre of influential nurses within the health department. Without nurses in key positions, there is little or no focus on nursing or the effects of decisions on nursing. This problem is compounded when there is no strong national nursing organization to monitor the quality of care or human resource issues.

Nursing's policy influence in this century will require more nurse politicians, more unity of voice, and more strategic alliances, along with leadership development and added political and policy skills for all new graduates. Currently, a real danger in many countries is the potential split in the nursing voice as more specialty organizations develop, particularly outside the umbrella of the national nurses association. The U.S. has felt the impact of divided nursing interests for many years and has developed mechanisms, such as forums and issue-specific lobbies, to bring the nursing voice together on key issues. Such strategic alliances are part of today's socioeconomic and political fabric. Touted first by management gurus and then applied to industry, strategic alliances have come to the fore in international health.

PARTNERSHIPS AND STRATEGIC ALLIANCES: A WAY FORWARD

There has been a long tradition of partnership between non-governmental organizations (NGOs) and United Nations agencies such as the WHO. The ICN was the first health professional group to attain official relations status with the WHO in 1948. More recently, the European Region of the WHO created the European Forum of National Nursing and Midwifery Associations and the WHO to exchange information and to formulate consensus and policy statements and recommendations on health-, nursing-, and midwifery-related issues. In 2005, the WHO South East Asia Regional Office (SEARO) created the South-East Asia Nursing and Midwifery

Educational Institutions Network as a forum for information and experience sharing, capacity building of educational institutions, and tackling common issues facing nursing and midwifery in the Region (WHO SEARO, 2008). WHO headquarters has had a Global Advisory Group on Nursing and Midwifery for nearly two decades. It meets annually and offers advice to the Director General. Unfortunately little action arises from this, and rarely is advice sought by the Director General's office.

The ICN is party to a number of strategic alliances. Some are joint ventures to deliver services such as the ICN Leadership for Change program. Others involve UN agencies, donor agencies, private sector companies, and NGOs in addressing common issues. For example, to strengthen collaboration among the professions and address key health issues, the World Health Professions Alliance brings together the ICN, the World Medical Association, the International Pharmaceutical Federation representing pharmacists, the World Confederation for Physical Therapy, and the World Dental Federation.

A new twist to strategic alliances within the UN system has been the addition of the corporate sector as partner. Recently, several new initiatives have involved key UN agencies, the World Bank, foundations, transnational corporations, and NGOs. The Global Alliance for Vaccines and Immunization (GAVI) is a case in point. Launched in 2000, the GAVI is a network of public and private-sector immunization stakeholders that includes the Gates Foundation, the financial community, vaccine manufacturers, governments, research and technical institutes, civil society organizations and multilateral organizations such as the World Health Organization (WHO), the United Nations Children's Fund (UNICEF), and the World Bank. Its mission is to save children's lives and protect poor people's health by increasing access to immunizations in poor countries. Since its launch in 2000, the Alliance has immunized more than 256 million children in poor countries and prevented the deaths of more than 4 million children. At the same time, nearly 24 million babies, mainly in the developing world, are not vaccinated against common illnesses (GAVI, 2009).

GETTING INVOLVED

Shared goals, vision, and values are key ingredients to policy and program initiatives such as the GAVI. The

---

> **BOX 101-6 How to Get Involved**
>
> - Begin at home—think globally, and act locally.
> - Cultivate a worldview; be sensitive to the cultural aspects of policy and practice.
> - Commit to learning more about trade agreements and how they affect your practice and your potential. Health services are now part of the WTO agenda.
> - Through the association or your workplace, help colleagues in other countries as they work to strengthen nursing and health care.
> - Undertake research to build evidence of nursing effectiveness.
> - Advocate, initiate, and document nursing's role in policy.
> - Know where your government stands on key international health and nursing matters, and lobby the government to support the initiative.
> - Join others in ensuring that national and local structures are in place so that nursing's voice is heard in policy and practice.
> - Ensure that new graduates know about policy and politics, how to analyze the environment, how to develop strategy, and how to work together.
> - Get involved in international issues, and team up with like-minded groups and individuals at home and internationally.
> - Know the stance taken by regional and international organizations, such as the ICN, on key nursing and health issues.
> - Share your ideas and achievements through publications and the Internet and papers presented at international conferences.

same is true for nursing. Any significant advancement toward realizing nursing's policy potential nationally, regionally, and internationally will require multiple strategies and joint efforts on many fronts. Ultimately, it means the commitment of individual nurses who share a vision and values and believe that nurses can make a difference for themselves and, most of all, for the people they serve. There are many ways to participate, as illustrated in Box 101-6.

If we are to achieve better health for all people, it will be through evidence that we are a strong profession that is committed to sound nursing and health policies and practices, and skilled in policy, politics, and care. One of the key tenets of primary health care is that communities should participate in decisions affecting them. It follows, then, that nursing, as a community and as part of the global society, needs to engage in all aspects of health policy.

For a list of related websites, please refer to your Evolve Resources at http://evolve.elsevier.com/Mason/policypolitics/

REFERENCES

Avert. (2010). United States statistical summary. Retrieved from www.avert.org/usa-statistics.htm.

Blair, T. (2005). Statement to Parliament on the G8 Summit. Retrieved from www.g8.gov.uk/servlet/Front?pagename=OpenMarket/Xcelerate/ShowPage&c=Page&cid=1078995903270&a=KArticle&aid=1119521193501.

Bread for the World. (2009). Hunger facts: International. World hunger and poverty: How they fit together. Retrieved from www.bread.org/learn/hunger-basics/hunger-facts-international.html.

Caughley, J. (2008). The International Council of Nurses and the World Health Organization: A growing and fruitful partnership. Sixty years of collaboration. Geneva: International Council of Nurses.

Department for International Development (DFID). (2009). About DFID: Who we work with: The G8. Retrieved from www.dfid.gov.uk/about-dfid/who-we-work-with1/the-g8.

Global Alliance for Vaccines and Immunization (GAVI). (2009). Facts and figures. Retrieved from www.gavialliance.org/media_centre/facts/index.php.

The Global Fund to Fight AIDS, Tuberculosis and Malaria (TGF) (2010). Home page. Retrieved from www.theglobalfund.org/en.

Global Health Workforce Alliance (GHWA). (2006). Global Health Workforce Alliance Strategic Plan 2006-2009. Geneva: World Health Organization.

Guebert, Jenilee (2009). G8 Commitments on Health, 1975-2009. G8 Research Group, December 16, 2009. G8 Information Centre, University of Toronto. Retrieved from www.g7.utoronto.ca/evaluations/g8-commitments-health-to-2009.html.

International Air Transport Association (IATA). (2005). Annual report 2005. Retrieved from www.iata.org/iata/Sites/agm/file/2005/file/Annual_report_2005.pdf.

International Centre on Human Resources in Nursing (ICHRN). (2010). ICHRN: About us. Retrieved from www.ichrn.org.

International Centre on Nurse Migration (ICNM). (2009). New Alliance for Ethical International Recruitment Practices created in the United States. ICNMeNews December 2009, Issue 9. Retrieved from www.intlnursemigration.org/assets/enews/ICNMeNews_2009_December.pdf.

International Centre on Nurse Migration (ICNM). (2010). International Centre on Nurse Migration: About us. Retrieved from www.intlnursemigration.org/sections/about/aboutus.shtml.

International Council of Nurses (ICN). (1999). ICN on poverty and health: Breaking the link. Nursing Matters fact sheet. Geneva: International Council of Nurses.

International Council of Nurses (ICN). (2001). Ethical nurse recruitment. ICN Position Statement. Geneva: International Council of Nurses.

International Council of Nurses (ICN). (2007). Nurse retention and migration. ICN Position Statement. Geneva: International Council of Nurses.

International Organization for Migration (IOM). (2010). About migration: Facts & figures. Retrieved from www.iom.int/jahia/Jahia/lang/en/pid/241.

Joint Learning Initiative (JLI) (2004). Human resources for health: Overcoming the crisis. Boston: The President and Fellows of Harvard College.

McCoy, D. (2009). The high level taskforce on innovative international financing for health systems. Health Policy and Planning, 24(5), 321-323.

Metrics 2.0. (2007). Air travelers worldwide to double to 9 billion a year by 2025: Report. Retrieved from www.metrics2.com/blog/2007/01/30/air_travelers_worldwide_to_double_to_9_billion_a_y.html.

UNAIDS/WHO Fact Sheet 09. (2009a). Global facts and figures. The global AIDS epidemic. Retrieved from http://data.unaids.org/pub/FactSheet/2009/20091124_FS_global_en.pdf.

UNAIDS/WHO Fact Sheet 09. (2009b). Sub-Saharan Africa. Latest epidemiological trends. Retrieved from http://data.unaids.org/pub/FactSheet/2009/20091124_FS_SSA_en.pdf.

United Nations (UN). (2005). The Millennium Development Goals report. New York: United Nations Department of Public Information.

United Nations (UN). (2010, February 12). Keeping the promise: A forward-looking review to promote an agreed action agenda to achieve the Millennium Development Goals by 2015. Report of the Secretary-General. 64th session of the General Assembly. New York: United Nations.

UNICEF. (2009). ChildInfo. Monitoring the situation of children and women. Overview. Retrieved from www.childinfo.org/mortality.html.

UNICEF. (2010). Millennium development goals. Goal: Reduce child mortality. Retrieved from www.unicef.org/mdg/childmortality.html.

World Bank (WB). (2008). Overview: Understanding, measuring and overcoming poverty. World Bank PovertyNet. Retrieved from http://web.worldbank.org/WBSITE/EXTERNAL/TOPICS/EXTPOVERTY/EXTPA/0,,contentMDK:20153855~menuPK:4350.

World Bank (WB). (2010). About us. Retrieved from http://web.worldbank.org/WBSITE/EXTERNAL/EXTABOUTUS/0,,pagePK:50004410~piPK:36602~theSitePK:29708,00.html.

World Health Assembly (WHA). (2006, May 27). Strengthening nursing and midwifery. Fifty Ninth World Health Assembly (WHA59.27). Agenda item 11.17. 27 May 2006.

World Health Organization (WHO). (1999). Making a difference. The World Health Report 1999. Geneva: World Health Organization.

World Health Organization (WHO). (2001). Macroeconomics and Health: Investing in Health for Economic Development. Report of the Commission on Macroeconomics and Health. Geneva: World Health Organization.

World Health Organization (WHO). (2005). The world health report 2005: Make every mother and child count. Geneva: World Health Organization.

World Health Organization (WHO). (2006). World Health Report 2006: Working together for health. Geneva: World Health Organization.

World Health Organization (WHO). (2007). Task shifting to tackle health worker shortages. Geneva: World Health Organization.

World Health Organization (WHO). (2009). A World Health Organization code of practice on the international recruitment of health personnel. Background paper. Geneva: World Health Organization.

World Health Organization (WHO). (2010a). Tuberculosis infection and transmission. Fact sheet No. 104. Retrieved from www.who.int/mediacentre/factsheets/fs104/en.

World Health Organization (WHO). (2010b). WHO: Its people and offices. Retrieved from www.who.int/about/structure/en/index.html.

World Health Organization (WHO). (2010c). WHO definition of health. Retrieved from www.who.int/about/definition/en/print.html.

WHO South-East Asia Regional Office (WHO SEARO). (2008). South-East Asia Nursing and Midwifery Educational Institutions Network. Report of the First Meeting, Chandigarh, India, 7-10 May 2007. New Delhi: World Health Organization.

World Trade Organization (WTO). (2001). The WTO. Retrieved from www.wto.org/english/thewto_e/thewto_e.htm.

World Trade Organization (WTO). (2005). The World Trade Organization in brief. Retrieved from www.wto.org/english/res_e/doload_e/inbr_e.pdf.

CHAPTER 102

TAKING ACTION
Ugandan Nurses Leading Health Policy Change

Stephanie L. Ferguson

"A policy is a temporary creed liable to be changed, but while it holds good it has got to be pursued with apostolic zeal."

—Mohandas Gandhi

Globally, the development of health care policy is often undertaken without the participation of health care professionals, particularly nurses. Poor communication and understanding between policy leaders and the professions most affected by health policy can result in initiatives that undermine the very health systems they purport to improve. This can occur through underinvestment, downgrading of work environments, undervaluing of health professionals' roles, and reductions in pay. In some cases, the very safety of health professionals has been put at risk.

These developments have contributed to an acute global shortage of nurses, exacerbating the challenges to all health systems and endangering the viability of some. In light of this, it is essential that nurses have tools, resources, and capabilities to communicate their interests to policymakers and drive health policy reform in strategic and beneficial directions. Individual nurses, the national nurses' associations (NNAs) to which they belong, and international non-governmental organizations (NGOs) such as the International Council of Nurses (ICN) have taken the lead in shaping policy solutions. The ICN and its member NNAs have made significant contributions to the personal and professional well-being of nurses, empowering them in the workplace through initiatives designed to improve practice environments, working conditions, and the quality of care.

This chapter presents my experience with assisting Ugandan nurses in taking hold of the reigns of policy reform and securing their interests. I conclude with a review of lessons learned with global relevance for the nursing profession.

THE CHALLENGE IN UGANDA

The world currently faces a drastic shortage of nurses. This shortage is the direct result of detrimental policies that have undermined the profession and health care environments, driving nurses to migrate out of intolerable work environments or leave the profession and deterring the next generation from joining the ranks. Around the world, nurses, NNAs and non-governmental organizations (NGOs) such as the ICN are working together to address these issues. They are training nurses for leadership roles to better influence public policy through the Leadership for Change program (Box 102-1). The ICN is also working on implementing the Positive Practice Environments campaign to improve the work environments and conditions of health care workers (Baumann, 2007; International Center for Human Resources in Nursing, 2010). The ICN Wellness Centres provide health care and counseling to health professionals and their families. The Girl Child Initiative supports the orphaned daughters of nurses through an education fund and other programs.

Uganda presents a salient example of health policymaking gone awry and the subsequent efforts of nurses from the Ugandan National Association for Nurses and Midwives (UNANM), with the support of ICN, to implement strategies in support of their

BOX 102-1 **International Council of Nurses and Major Initiatives**

The International Council of Nurses is a federation of NNAs representing nurses in more than 128 countries. It is the world's first and widest-reaching international organization for health professionals. The ICN works to ensure quality nursing care for all, sound health policies globally, the advancement of nursing knowledge, and the presence world-wide of a respected nursing profession and a competent and satisfied nursing workforce. The following are ICN initiatives to strengthen the nursing profession and health care systems globally. These initiatives are available online at *www.icn.ch.*

The ICN Leadership for Change™ (LFC) program aims to prepare nurses for leadership roles in nursing and the broader health sector. LFC focuses on health policymaking; leadership and management in health services; sustainable development; and creating networks nationally, regionally, and internationally. LFC has been deployed in over 70 countries. For more information, please refer to *www.icn.ch/ leadchange.htm.*

The ICN's Girl Child Initiative aims to influence and build sound national public policy, on a global scale, that supports the healthy development of girls. Within this framework, the Girl Child Education Fund was established in cooperation with the Florence Nightingale International Foundation (FNIF) to support schooling in developing countries of girls whose nurse parents have died. In Uganda, Kenya, Zambia, and Swaziland, 255 girls are currently receiving support through this initiative.

ICN Wellness Centres for health care professionals and their families provide health care and counseling to care-givers. The Centres, currently operated in Swaziland, Lesotho, Zambia, and Malawi (The Uganda Wellness Centre is currently under construction), have opened the door to improved retention practices, better health, and an increased sense of being valued for African health care workers, who work daily on the front lines of the battle against HIV/AIDS, tuberculosis, and other infectious diseases.

The Positive Practice Environments (PPE) for health care professionals was established to promote quality workplaces for quality care globally. Occupational health and safety, manageable workloads and work schedules, equal opportunity and treatment, fair pay, and access to required equipment and facilities are among the goals being pursued under the PPE campaign. For more information on PPE, download the information and action toolkit available at *www.icn.ch/ indkit2007.pdf;* for updates on PPE, visit *www.ichrn.org* or *www.whpa.org/ppe.htm.*

profession and the communities for whom they care. During my tenure as Director of the ICN Leadership for Change Program and Consultant for Nursing and Health Policy, I saw the devastating effects of nursing shortages, unhealthy practice environments, unfair nursing pay, and lack of incentives (Ferguson, 2008). While on an ICN field visit to meet with executives of the UNANM in 2003, I witnessed most of the critical nursing challenges facing nurses in Uganda. I saw the negative impact of having nurse-to-patient ratios averaging 1:100 at some health facilities. It was reported in 2004 that the nurse-to-population ratio in Uganda was approximately 6 nurses per 100,000, which is abhorrently low. In 2004, the United States had a ratio of 773 to 100,000 (Buchan & Calman, 2004).

Burdened with the impact of HIV/AIDS on the population and the health workforce, Uganda had tremendous hospital staffing problems. There was a geographic misdistribution of health workers from an urban-rural perspective, which saw rural areas facing an acute shortage of nurses. Health facilities had limited amounts of medicines and supplies, had unsafe water, and were overcrowded and plagued by lengthy waiting times for emergency care. Primary health care services were in short supply. National security was under threat from border conflict, pitting domestic tribes against Rwandan rebels. There was a lack of transparency in government affairs and a general distrust of political leaders by the citizenry.

At the time, more than 2000 non-governmental agencies and development organizations (including the U.S. government) were working to tackle the HIV/AIDS pandemic in Uganda. But the many organizations focusing on this challenge were delivering care that was fragmented and uncoordinated. Nursing was not involved.

The list of challenges in Uganda was daunting. Further compounding the disarray was the fact that nurses' roles were being undermined by new government policy seeking to establish a cadre of health workers with a less than sixth-grade education to replace some of the qualified registered nurses working in community health settings. Nurses' salaries had been cut from $80 per month to $30. At a time when Uganda needed its nurses more than ever, policymakers had chosen to demoralize and marginalize them, thus further eroding the health care system. Ugandan nurses realized it was time to take action.

THE STRATEGY

I worked with key nurse leaders and members of the UNANM to develop a strategic plan of action. We used the media to articulate a shared vision and message of change aimed at citizens, built an alliance with other health professionals and consumer groups, and renegotiated flawed policies through strategies such as policy assessment, data collection, and workforce planning. Among the most decisive factors in rallying popular support was UNANM's success in articulating the value of nursing and that nurses save lives precisely because of their professional skills and knowledge. They communicated that to replace them with lesser educated health workers would undermine the health care system and endanger the public. Both the Secretary General and President of UNANM were featured in local and national press reinforcing this messages. Ultimately, the image of nurses as skilled, essential care providers worthy of respect and decent wages was reinforced, and the Ugandan nursing workforce strengthened.

The UNANM developed strategies to implement workforce planning, including actions for recruitment and retention, performance management, and skill mix of nurses and other health professionals (Buchan & Calman, 2004). A strategic planning meeting was convened with all the nursing leaders in the nation (academia, regulation, government and non-governmental nursing and midwifery leaders, national nursing association) to determine the impact of the salary decrease, how to resolve the salary issue, and ensure that the policy to replace professional nurses was not implemented. During this critical meeting, key players participated in a situational analysis. An environmental scan determined strengths, weaknesses, opportunities, and threats (SWOT analysis), and a key stakeholders analysis revealed individuals, groups, or organizations who had an impact on or were impacted by nurses working in Uganda and the region. After completing the analysis phase, an action plan was developed, consisting of key results, goals, objectives, and indicators of progress in the context of workforce planning, strategies for recruiting and retaining nurses, performance management, and skill mix.

Another strategy was to meet with key stakeholders. During a meeting, the Minister of Health, the President of the UNANM, members of its executive

council, the country's Chief Nurse, and I were present. Accusations were made: Government officials said that nurses were not valued and respected by the citizens; and nurses did not fill out a survey sent from the government requesting that the nursing leadership articulate the value, roles, and responsibilities of all nursing positions in the nation. The Minister of Health noted that, since nurses did not complete the form, the government assigned salaries based on what they thought nurses "appeared to be doing" for the patients in various health facilities. The government viewed nursing care as "simple" daily care activities and duties. They assumed another health worker could do the job of the professional nurse at a lesser cost. After agreeing to disagree with the ministry officials, the nursing leadership present admitted they had not filled out the survey and asked for the opportunity to complete the salary survey. The request was denied. Government officials saw it in their best interest to maintain the salary decrease to lower the cost of health services. Important lessons were learned during the meeting: if the government calls on the nursing leadership of a nation to do a workforce planning survey, do it immediately and work with other government leaders to ensure that what you recommend is approved. If nurses do not take the lead in implementing such policy assessments, others who are not nurses will do it.

In spite of threats of a strike by the UNANM, government officials held firm in their refusal to reverse the salary decrease, further undermining the UNANM's negotiating position. The Ugandan government, specifically the Ministry of Health, had set a determined course of significant budget cuts in health care. All Ugandan health professionals had seen their salaries diminished.

The next steps included a media campaign and the formation of an alliance with other health professionals and hospital administrators. Building alliances with key stakeholders is invaluable in health policy development and advocacy. Networking and collaboration is crucial in forming partnerships and strategic alliances, and in carving out targeted media messages to reach citizens and officials.

The UNANM used the media to inform citizens of the challenges facing the nations' nurses. Their message justified a nursing strike in light of the governments undervaluing of nursing, emphasizing that salary cuts and the deployment of unqualified caregivers would be detrimental to the health and safety of the general population. In effect, the UNANM framed the value of nursing in the context of safe patient care. This message is appropriate worldwide.

Several articles and TV and radio stations carried the nurses' stories in Uganda. I was interviewed for a major newspaper story advocating for the rights of Ugandan nurses and patient safety. That article was seen by a Ugandan worker at the United Nations in Geneva, Switzerland, who also happened to be a member of my local church in Geneva. When I returned to Geneva, she called to thank me for the ICN's interventions on behalf of the nurses of Uganda and told me that the Ugandan government would be revising its policies related to nurses' salaries and roles.

Other steps in the plan included inviting the president of ICN, Christine Hancock, to meet with high-level officials including the Minister of Health, the International Red Cross, local World Health Organization officials, NGOs, foundations, and pharmaceutical companies with a vested interest in nurses and nursing care in Uganda. Getting a renowned leader or advocate to speak on your behalf can yield positive outcomes. ICN is respected by many international and national organizations and its positive reputation proved invaluable in Uganda.

Nurses' salaries were reinstated to their original levels. Additional gains included work incentives, such as an increase in uniform subsidy and allowances for housing and food. The Ugandan citizenry came out in support of their nurses, and government attitudes toward nursing were changed. The replacement of nurses by underqualified health workers was abandoned.

LESSONS LEARNED

The challenges faced and overcome by the UNANM in reversing negative health policy reform and securing influence over health policymaking holds the following valuable lessons for nurses and NNAs globally:

Be proactive and connected. Ugandan nurses were initially apathetic in responding to the government survey of nurses, which did them no good in the long run. Health care is a major concern for all governments, accounting for a significant share of national and regional budgets. It is essential for nurses to maintain a healthy connection to their government, particularly policymakers. This connection must be maintained by consistent engagement and exchange. Had this connection existed, government officials would have known all too well the challenges nurses face and the many roles they fulfill in their professional environments and in the society at large, and would not have questioned the value of nursing, attempted to decrease salaries, or sought to replace nurses with less-qualified health workers.

Be prepared and well trained. Nurses are an invaluable resource in all health care systems precisely because they are highly trained and provide indispensable care. Nurses' excellence in practice must be supplemented with training in policy making and politics, media relations, strategic timing, being articulate in presentations, forming partnerships with strategic alliances, and participating in debates in both health and social arenas (ICN, 2007).

Investigate, plan, communicate, lobby. Nurses must know the social and political environments in which they practice in order to fully understand their place and power within society. Nursing must have its finger on the popular pulse and that of their political leaders. Influencing or changing policy requires action plans, key performance measures, and targets. Nurses must develop strategies to effectively communicate their needs and aspirations as well as those of the communities they serve. Emphasizing the value of nursing to communities and societies as a whole is an essential part of any communication strategy, as is defining nursing positions on a range of issues of concern to their communities. ICN, the global federation of NNAs, regularly addresses issues of direct importance to nurses and the populations they care for, articulating position statements that help define the global voice of nursing. Continuous lobbying efforts by NNAs on behalf of their members, their colleagues in other health professions, and the public is an invaluable tool in keeping abreast of policy orientations and driving strategy, reform, and change in the right direction. Gaining a seat (or seats) at the policy table is the surest way to exert influence over health policy development, implementation, and evaluation.

Form alliances. Nurses represent the majority of health professionals but they are by no means alone in caring for populations. All health professionals share a stake in the quality of health systems, and this common interest makes them natural allies. No one group benefits from the exclusion of another group, and all benefit from mutual support. NNAs must endeavor to form global alliances linking them to sister organizations abroad as well as to international organizations, foundations, health industry interests, and national governments.

Rally your constituency. The communities nurses serve are their most natural constituency, as they are in constant contact with the public through the delivery of beneficial health care. Seeking out popular support in the face of challenges is an extremely effective way of influencing governments and policy leaders, who are almost inevitably responsive to public opinion.

Follow up and evaluate. Follow-up and evaluation of patients is an essential responsibility of nurses everywhere. This is just as true in the context of policymaking. Monitoring and evaluating the outcomes of policy initiatives is a must for nurses. This will allow for the recognition of positive and negative outcomes and for corrections and fine-tuning to be carried out in an informed and deliberate manner.

Nurses everywhere must secure their positions within the political landscape and insure their place at the policymaking table. Their professional well-being and the health and safety of those they care for demand this.

For a list of related websites, please refer to your Evolve Resources at http://evolve.elsevier.com/Mason/policypolitics/

REFERENCES

Baumann, A. (2007). *Positive practice environments: Quality workplaces = quality patient care.* Geneva, Switzerland: International Council of Nurses. Retrieved from www.icn.ch/indkit2007.pdf.

Buchan, J., & Calman, L. (2004). *The global shortage of registered nurses: An overview of issues and actions.* Geneva, Switzerland: International Council of Nurses.

Ferguson, S. (2008). Thriving while working on the edge: Nurses leading change worldwide. *International Nursing Review, 55*(4), 367-368.

International Center for Human Resources in Nursing. (2010). Positive Practice Environments Campaign. Retrieved from www.ichrn.org.

International Council of Nurses. (2010). ICN Leadership for Change™ Program Brochure. Retrieved from www.icn.ch/leadchange.htm.

International Council of Nurses (2007). *Health policy package: A guide for policy development.* Geneva, Switzerland: International Council of Nurses.

CHAPTER 103

Emerging and Reemerging Infectious Disease: A Global Challenge

James Mark Simmerman

"The deviation of man from the state in which he was originally placed by nature seems to have proven to him a prolific source of diseases."

—Edward Jenner

The relationship between infectious disease and human population growth, poverty, urbanization, climate change, industrialized food production, and rapid travel is increasingly well documented. The continual threat to public health from emerging and reemerging infectious diseases (EID) demands sustained attention, international cooperation, and resources. Innovative approaches are needed to improve the laboratory detection, surveillance systems, and control of EIDs in the context of rapidly changing human and pathogen ecology.

BACKGROUND

In 1962, immunologist and Nobel laureate Sir Mac-Farlane Burnet wrote that the middle of the twentieth century could be regarded as the end of one of the most important social revolutions in history, reflecting the virtual elimination of infectious disease as a significant factor in social life (Burnet, 1962). Indeed, the use of antibiotics, immunizations, and improved public health systems had significantly reduced deaths from infectious diseases in the United States. However, beginning in the early 1980s, human immunodeficiency virus infection and acquired immunodeficiency syndrome (HIV/AIDS) together with opportunistic infections such as multidrug-resistant tuberculosis, refocused global attention on the threat from emerging infectious diseases (Patton et al., 2009). Despite progress toward prevention and treatment, HIV/AIDS is still estimated to become the leading cause of disease burden in middle- and low-income countries by 2015 with 6.5 million deaths projected in 2030, even under the assumption that coverage with antiretroviral drugs reaches 80% (Mathers & Loncar, 2006). Outbreaks of other emerging pathogens have also occurred with increasing frequency. The majority (60%) of EID events are caused by zoonotic pathogens (a non-human animal source), and 72% of these events are caused by pathogens originating from wildlife (Jones et al., 2008). These pathogens can change hosts as a result of multiple complex factors that often work in combination (Cutler, Fooks, & Van Der Poel, 2010) (Figure 103-1).

DEFINING EMERGING AND REEMERGING INFECTIONS

In 1992, a report by the Institute of Medicine (IOM) called attention to the global problem of emerging infectious diseases (Lederberg, Shope, & Oaks, 1992). This was followed by two reports from the Centers for Disease Control and Prevention (CDC) that further characterized the issues (CDC, 1994, 1998). Emerging infectious diseases were defined as new, reemerging, or drug-resistant infections whose incidence in humans have increased within the past two decades or threatened to increase in the near future. Reemerging diseases refers to the reappearance of a known disease following a decline in incidence and (Lederberg et al., 1992) include newly recognized pathogens, new diseases caused by known organisms, and the extension of the geographic or host range of a pathogen (Lashley, 2003, 2004). The factors listed in Box 103-1 often operate in concert and have been associated with the emergence or reemergence of infectious diseases.

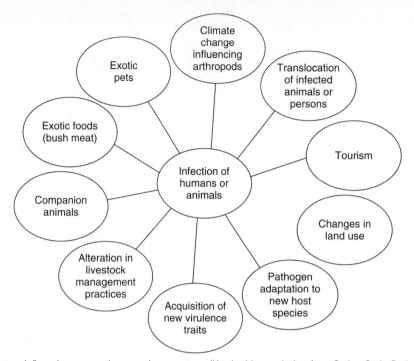

FIGURE 103-1 Factors influencing new and reemerging zoonoses. (Used with permission from Cutler, S. J., Fooks, A. R., & Van Der Poel, W.H. [2010]. Public health threat of new, reemerging, and neglected zoonoses in the industrialized world. *Emerging Infectious Diseases, 16*[1], 1-7. Retrieved from www.cdc.gov/EID/content/16/1/1.htm.)

A GLOBAL CONCERN

Since 1980, the emergence or reemergence of infectious diseases has had a significant impact on global health and economies (Binder, Levitt, Sacks, & Hughes, 1999; Morens et al., 2004). The speed and expansion of modern international air travel and global trade place every country at risk and require all to contribute to surveillance and control efforts. Recent examples of EID outbreaks include Avian Influenza A (H5N1), West Nile virus, SARS coronavirus, and Monkey pox.

AVIAN INFLUENZA A (H5N1)

The first confirmed case of avian influenza A (H5N1) infection identified in a human occurred in Hong Kong in May 1997. Six months later in November and December 1997 an additional 17 infections were detected (Chan 2002; Bridges et al., 2002). In 2001, the virus reappeared in humans in Hong Kong, and in late 2003 large-scale poultry die-offs and new human infections occurred in several countries in East and Southeast Asia (Uyeki, 2008). By 2006, the virus had

become endemic in most of East and Southeast Asian poultry, and human avian influenza infections had been documented in Eastern Europe and several African countries. While infections are often fatal, transmission from infected poultry to humans remains inefficient, and only limited human-to-human transmission has been observed (Ungchusak et al., 2005; Kandun et al., 2006). By October 2010, the World Health Organization (WHO) reported 507 confirmed cases with 302 deaths in 15 countries worldwide (WHO, 2010). Concern that the H5N1 virus could develop the ability to efficiently pass from person to person has led to the establishment of an aggressive global research and training agenda addressing surveillance, prevention, pandemic preparedness, epidemiological investigation, laboratory diagnostics, molecular virology, pathogenesis, and vaccine development (Oshitani, Kamigaki, & Suzuki, 2008; WHO, 2005a; Knobler, Mack, Mahmoud, & Lemon, 2005).

WEST NILE VIRUS

Emerging infectious diseases are increasingly due to the expanded geographic range of insect vectors.

BOX 103-1 Factors Associated with the Emergence or Reemergence of Infectious Diseases

- Increased use of antimicrobial and antiviral agents, including those used in animal feed
- Globalization of travel and trade; demands for imported food and exotic pets
- Industrialized food production and global distribution systems
- Widespread travel and recreational pursuits, bringing animals and people into closer contact
- Demographic factors such as population growth, migration, and aging societies
- Socioeconomic factors such as poverty and crowding
- Ecosystem changes such as dam projects, irrigation, and deforestation
- Anthropogenic climatic change resulting in increasingly severe and more frequent droughts, floods, and storms, as well as shifts in the distribution of humans, wildlife, and insect vectors
- Disasters and armed conflicts resulting in stress, crowding, and declines in health infrastructure
- Deterioration of public health infrastructure resulting in fewer and poorly trained health workers and decreased public health laboratory capacity
- Microbial evolution; mutation, new tissue specificities, and cross-species transmission
- Health care technology advances such as increases in organ transplantation and medical devices
- Human immune compromise from iatrogenic causes and malnutrition
- Lack of political will to address needed health measures
- Deliberate dissemination of microbial agents for political or military purposes

While vector-borne disease has long been a major cause of disability in poor, tropical countries, with the recent arrival of the West Nile virus it has become an important public health issue in temperate North America (Griffin, 2009). West Nile virus, a long-recognized cause of encephalitis in Africa and the Middle East, was first recognized in North America in 1999 (Hughes, 2001). Since that time, West Nile virus spread across the Western hemisphere and has become (Granwehr et al., 2004) the leading cause of arboviral disease in the U.S. While an estimated 80% of infections are asymptomatic, symptomatic

persons develop an acute febrile illness that includes headache, myalgia, arthralgia, rash, or gastrointestinal symptoms. Neuroinvasive disease typically presents as encephalitis, meningitis, or acute flaccid paralysis. Between 1999 and 2008, the U.S. CDC National Electronic Passive Surveillance System recorded a total of 28,961 confirmed and probable cases of West Nile virus disease, including 11,822 (41%) neuroinvasive cases from 47 states (Lindsey et al., 2009). In the absence of an effective human vaccine, West Nile virus prevention depends on community-level mosquito control and household and personal protection measures.

SARS CORONAVIRUS

The coronavirus associated with severe acute respiratory syndrome (SARS) first emerged in southern China in late 2002. A traveler who was incubating SARS traveled from Guangdong province to Hong Kong and subsequently infected other hotel guests. These individuals then traveled to other countries, seeding outbreaks in at least 26 countries (Christian, Poutanen, Loutfy, Muller, & Low, 2004; Skowronski et al., 2005). As the number of SARS cases increased in early 2003, the WHO and the CDC issued travel advisories (WHO, 2003). In just a few months, major economic losses resulted from curtailed business and tourist travel to various cities in East Asia as well as in Toronto, Canada. In all, 8096 cases were recorded with 774 deaths in 29 countries. For more information, visit *www.who.int/csr/sars/country/table 2004_04_21/en/index.html.*

The SARS outbreak was characterized by severe nosocomial outbreaks, often involving nurses, and the unprecedented and rapid international cooperation among the world's most sophisticated laboratories in order to identify the new viral pathogen (Simmerman 2003; Cheung et al. 2005). The SARS outbreak was contained in July 2003, but additional cases of infection have been reported in laboratory scientists studying the virus (Christian et al., 2004; Poon, Guan, Nicholls, Yuen, & Peiris, 2004).

MONKEY POX

Trade in domestic and exotic animals for food or pets has become an increasingly common source of infectious disease outbreaks. Monkey pox is an orthopox virus closely related to smallpox viruses. The virus was recognized in 1970 as a human pathogen in tropical Africa responsible for sporadic infections in rainforest hunters and rare outbreaks involving human-to-human transmission. Monkey pox was not considered to be a threat outside Africauntil 2003, when 82 children and adults in 11 Midwestern U.S. states contracted the infection. The outbreak resulted from contact with prairie dogs imported as exotic pets that had beeninfected during transport in cages with with Gambian giant rats (Reed et al., 2004; CDC, 2003b). An embargo on the import, sale, and transport of rodents from Africa and restrictions on the sale or movement of prairie dogs was announced in June 2003, and no cases have since been detected in North America (CDC, 2003a).

2009 PANDEMIC H1N1 INFLUENZA

Novel influenza A virus strains appear at unpredictable intervals and can cause outbreaks on a global scale (pandemics) with sharply increased morbidity and mortality, especially in children and young adults (Simonsen et al., 1998; Monto, 2009). Pigs are susceptible to infection from influenza viruses of both avian and human origins, efficiently transmit infection, and play an important role in the generation of novel influenza viruses (Ma et al., 2009). In early 2009, a multiple reassortant (with genes from swine, human, and avian viruses) influenza A/H1N1 virus emerged in southern Mexico (Brownstein, Freifeld, & Madoff, 2009). Beginning in late February 2009, national surveillance systems in Mexico detected an unusual increase in influenza-like illness (ILI) cases, and in March and April there were increasing reports of previously healthy young adults hospitalized with severe pneumonia. This led to active surveillance in 23 hospitals in Mexico City and the identification of non-subtypable influenza A viruses (Perez-Padilla et al., 2009). In March 2009, two epidemiologically unrelated children in southern California were detected that had been infected with the new reassortant virus, but neither had had contact with pigs. This set off national alerts and the establishment of syndromic surveillance systems in schools, cities, and states across the country. In New York, the first indication of an outbreak came from a telephone report from a school nurse reporting an increase in febrile illness after students returned from spring break vacation to Mexico. This novel virus rapidly spread around the world causing the WHO to declare a pandemic on June 11, 2009 (Novel Swine-Origin Influenza A

[H1N1] Virus Investigation Team et al., 2009; WHO, 2009). Fortunately, while the 2009 pandemic influenza A (H1N1) virus resulted in millions of illnesses, caused significant social disruption, and increased burden on health care systems, mortality rates from this virus were lower than that observed during previous pandemics.

Among the major policy domains associated with emerging and reemerging infectious disease outbreaks are surveillance and reporting, immunization, quarantine, travel and immigration restrictions, and restrictions related to the importation of food and animals.

GLOBAL SURVEILLANCE AND REPORTING

The International Health Regulations (IHRs) were adopted in 1969, amended in 1973 and 1981, and completely revised in 2005 at the 59th World Health Assembly to provide a legal framework for international cooperation. The main purpose of the IHRs is to prevent, control, and provide a public health response to the international spread of disease in ways that avoid unnecessary interference with international traffic and trade. The 2005 revision is legally binding on WHO member states and came into effect in 2007. This revision broadened the scope of the IHR from focusing on cholera, plague, and yellow fever to include any public health event of international concern (PHEIC). Under the IHRs, all WHO member states are required to develop, strengthen, and maintain core surveillance and response capacities, facilitate cross-border cooperation, and provide logistical and financial support to improve capacity to conduct surveillance and response activities (WHO, 2005b). The IHRs promote improved coordination with agricultural authorities such as the Food and Agriculture Organization (FAO) and the World Organization for Animal Health (OIE), to reduce the potential for EID outbreaks from food, livestock, and wild animal sources (Pavlin, Schloegel, & Daszak, 2009; Newell et al., 2010). The WHO also conducts a variety of global and regional surveillance activities under the umbrella of Communicable Disease Surveillance and Response (CSR), including the Global Outbreak Alert and Response Network (GOARN), which monitors communicable diseases as well as food and water safety.

SURVEILLANCE AND REPORTING SYSTEMS

Surveillance for infectious disease relies on formal and informal systems and may be syndromic or pathogen specific, depending on the objectives and available resources. Examples of these systems include the following:

- The U.S. CDC mandates reporting from the states for nationally notifiable diseases *(http://cdc.gov/mmwr/PDF/wk/mm5653.pdf)* through the National Notifiable Disease Surveillance System (NNDSS); reports are transmitted through the National Electronic Telecommunications System for Surveillance (NETSS).
- The CDC operates other syndromic and sentinel surveillance systems including the Global Disease Detection network; the domestic and international Emerging Infections Programs; the National Malaria Surveillance System; the Health Alert Network; the National Respiratory and Enteric Virus Surveillance System; the National West Nile Virus Surveillance System; and the National Tuberculosis Genotyping and Surveillance Network. Rapid electronic analysis of syndromic surveillance data for early detection of outbreaks is conducted through systems like the Early Aberration Reporting System (EARS).
- FoodNet (Foodborne Diseases Active Surveillance Network) is a collaborative project between the CDC Emerging Infections Program sites, the U.S. Department of Agriculture, and the U.S. Food and Drug Administration.
- GeoSentinel (Global Emerging Infections Sentinel Network) is funded through an agreement with CDC and consists of travel and tropical medicine clinics around the world that monitor trends in morbidity among travelers through the International Society of Travel Medicine.
- The National Healthcare Safety Network (NHSN) *(www.cdc.gov/nhsn)* is a voluntary, secure, Internet-based surveillance system that integrates health care personnel safety surveillance systems managed by the Division of Healthcare Quality Promotion (DHQP) at the CDC to provide data on emerging healthcare-associated infection and pathogens, assess the importance of potential risk factors, characterize their mechanisms of resistance, and evaluate alternative surveillance and prevention strategies in U.S. health care facilities. The Surveillance of Emerging Antimicrobial Resistance Connected to Healthcare (SEARCH) system is a network of hospitals and health departments that conducts surveillance on antibiotic-resistant *Staphylococcus aureus.*
- The Border Infectious Disease Surveillance (BIDS) project is an example of an interregional system that has been developed along the U.S.-Mexican border with the cooperation of the Mexican Secretariat of Health, the CDC, U.S. state and Mexican border health departments, and the Pan American Health Organization (PAHO). The BIDS project focuses on surveillance in border cities for hepatitis, dengue and West Nile virus.
- The Global Public Health Intelligence Network (GHPIN) *(www.phac-aspc.gc.ca/media/nr-rp/2004/2004_gphin-rmispbk-eng.php)* is a secure, Internet-based "early warning" system that gathers preliminary reports of public health significance in seven languages on a real-time, 24/7 basis. GHPIN is conducted by the Public Health Agency of Canada and focuses on chemical, biological, radiological, and nuclear public health threats throughout the world.

IMMUNIZATION POLICY

Most immunization laws concern children and immigrants. They specify the types of vaccinations that are required for school admission or entry into the U.S. as well as the information on the risks and benefits of vaccination that must be provided before vaccination. School immunization laws in the U.S. are state mandated, and exemptions, such as for religious reasons, are often permitted. Since July 1997, all individuals seeking permanent entry to the U.S. must prove that they have been inoculated against certain vaccine-preventable diseases (CDC, 2005). This includes infants or children entering as part of international adoption. Among the recommendations from an IOM report on immunization practices and policies were calls for strengthening federal and state immunization partnerships, developing a strategy for increasing financial support, and ensuring that immunization policy be national in scope (Guyer, Smith, & Chalk, 2000).

QUARANTINE POLICY

Quarantine is an important tool used to contain infectious diseases. The U.S. maintains a Division of

Global Migration and Quarantine (DGMQ) within the CDC's National Center for Emerging and Zoonotic Infectious Diseases. The DGMQ has statutory responsibility to make and enforce regulations necessary to prevent the introduction, transmission, or spread of communicable diseases from foreign countries into the U.S. The DGMQ achieves these objectives through its work in immigrant and refugee health, quarantine, animal importation, and traveler's health. U.S. Quarantine Stations are located at ports of entry and land-border crossings where international travelers arrive. DGMQ staff has authority to detain, medically examine, and conditionally release individuals and wildlife suspected of carrying a communicable disease. The DGMQ works in cooperation with other agencies, such as state and local health departments, the U.S. Customs Service, the Immigration and Naturalization Service (INS), the U.S. Fish and Wildlife Service, and the U.S. Department of Agriculture. Diseases that can result in quarantine include cholera, plague, infectious tuberculosis, yellow fever, and viral hemorrhagic fevers. In 2005, an executive order added "influenza caused by novel or reemergent influenza viruses that are causing, or have the potential to cause, a pandemic" (CDC, National Center for Infectious Diseases, Division of Global Migration and Quarantine, 2000; Bush, 2005).

TRAVEL AND IMMIGRATION POLICY

Throughout history, human travel and migration has introduced infectious diseases to vulnerable populations, often with devastating consequences. In the modern era of air travel and dramatically increased rates of migration, travel and immigration policy has become an important tool to slow the spread of EID (Arguin, Marano, & Freedman, 2009).

Several U.S. agencies are involved with processing immigration and implementing public health law, including the Public Health Service (PHS). In 1798, the U.S. Public Health Service was established following passage of an act that provided for the care and relief of sick and injured merchant seamen in a network of marine hospitals. Today the PHS is a cadre of more than 6000 commissioned nurses, physicians, dentists, engineers, and other professionals. The scope of activities of the PHS was expanded during the late nineteenth century to include the control of infectious disease and the enforcement of quarantine laws at sites such as Ellis Island in New York. PHS officers continue to play a major role in fulfilling the service's commitment to prevent infectious disease from entering the country.

Immigration laws in the U.S. have excluded aliens (defined as any person who is not a citizen or legal resident) for health-related reasons since 1879, when such legislation was first enacted. Distinction may be made among immigrants, long-term and short-term travelers, temporary residents, and refugees seeking political asylum. Among the criteria for exclusion of aliens is infection with any dangerous contagious disease (CDC, 2004b). For example, by the early 1990s, more than 50 countries had instituted mandatory HIV testing for visitors and immigrants despite the objections of various international organizations, including the WHO. In November 2009, HIV/AIDS was removed from the list of communicable disease of public health significance in the U.S. Prior to this final rule, aliens with HIV infection were inadmissible to the U.S. per the Immigration and Nationality Act (INA). Aliens are no longer barred from entry into the U.S. based solely on the grounds that they are infected with HIV, and they are not required to undergo HIV testing as part of the required medical examination for U.S. immigration.

RESTRICTIONS RELATED TO THE IMPORTATION OF FOOD AND ANIMALS

The importation of food and animals is another source of EID outbreaks, such as in England in February 2001, importation of infected animals resulted in a major foot-and-mouth disease outbreak (Haydon, Kao, & Kitching, 2004). Early responses were not well coordinated within the European Union. Responses included the banning of the importation of livestock, milk, and other bovine products first from Britain and then, as the disease spread, from other affected countries. Nearly 3 million farm animals in Great Britain were culled, mass immunization campaigns were conducted, compensation was made to farmers whose animals were destroyed, and increased restrictions were placed on travelers to agricultural areas in affected countries. Travelers returning from affected areas were questioned about whether they had visited farms and had their shoes and vehicles sprayed with disinfectants. The outbreak resulted in severe economic consequences, had an impact on tourism and other related industries, and demonstrated the need for rapid, global cooperation to more effectively respond and contain EIDs (Paton, Sumption, & Charleston, 2009).

SUMMARY

A renewed focus from governments, international organizations, and individual health professionals is needed to establish or improve public health policies to reduce the threat of emerging infectious diseases while respecting individual rights and protecting entire populations. Research, education, and sustainable program funding must be directed to shape and implement policies that will improve public health infrastructure in both mature and developing economies and ensure readiness to deal with future infectious disease emergencies. As population growth, urbanization, climate change, and the frequency of global travel accelerate, we can expect to encounter larger, more complex, and rapidly spreading outbreaks that will demand innovative approaches and increased global collaboration. As key actors in health care systems around the world, nurses will be expected to rise to meet these extraordinary challenges.

For a list of related websites, please refer to your Evolve Resources at http://evolve.elsevier.com/Mason/policypolitics/

REFERENCES

Arguin, P. M., Marano, N., & Freedman, D. O. (2009). Globally mobile populations and the spread of emerging pathogens. *Emerging Infectious Diseases*, *15*(11), 713-714.

Avian influenza—Eastern Asia (64): FAO/OIE/WHO. ProMed 2005 (No. 285), July 6, 2005, unpaginated.

Binder, S., Levitt, A. M., Sacks J. J., & Hughes J. M. (1999). Emerging infectious diseases: Public health issues for the 21st century. *Science*, *284*(5418), 1311-1313.

Bridges, C. B., Lim, W., Hu-Primmer, J., Sims, L., Fukuda, K., et al. (2002). Risk of influenza A (H5N1) infection among poultry workers, Hong Kong, 1997-1998. *Journal of Infectious Diseases*, *185*(8), 1005-1010.

Brownstein, J. S., Freifeld, C. C., & Madoff, L. C. (2009). Influenza A (H1N1) virus, 2009—online monitoring. *New England Journal of Medicine*, *360*(21), 2156.

Burnet, F. M. (1962). *Natural history of infectious disease* (3rd ed.). Cambridge, England: Cambridge University Press.

Bush, G. W. (2005). Executive order: Amendment to E. O. 13295 relating to certain influenza viruses and quarantinable communicable diseases. The White House, March 14, 2005. Retrieved from http://edocket.access.gpo. gov/cfr_2006/janqtr/pdf/3CFR13375.pdf

Centers for Disease Control and Prevention (CDC). (1994). *Addressing emerging infectious disease threats: A prevention strategy for the United States.* Atlanta: U.S. Department of Health and Human Services, Public Health Service.

Centers for Disease Control and Prevention (CDC). (1998). *Preventing emerging infectious diseases: A strategy for the 21st century.* Atlanta: U.S. Department of Health and Human Services.

Centers for Disease Control and Prevention (CDC). (2003a). Multistate outbreak of monkeypox—Illinois, Indiana, and Wisconsin, 2003. *Morbidity and Mortality Weekly Report*, *52*(23), 537-540.

Centers for Disease Control and Prevention (CDC). (2003b). Update: Multistate outbreak of monkeypox—Illinois, Indiana, Kansas, Missouri, Ohio, and Wisconsin, 2003. *Morbidity and Mortality Weekly Report*, *52*(24), 561-564.

Centers for Disease Control and Prevention (CDC). (2004b). History of quarantine. National Center for Infectious Diseases, Division of Global Migration and Quarantine. Retrieved from www.cdc.gov/ncidod/dq/history.htm.

Centers for Disease Control and Prevention (CDC). (2005). Immunization laws. National Vaccine Program Office. Retrieved from www.cdc.gov/od/nipo/law.htm.

Centers for Disease Control and Prevention (CDC), National Center for Infectious Diseases, Division of Global Migration and Quarantine. (2000, May). History of quarantine. Retrieved from www.cdc.gov/ncidod/dq/history.htm.

Chan, P. K. (2002). Outbreak of Avian Influenza A (H5N1) virus infection in Hong Kong in 1997. *Clinical Infectious Disease*, *34*(Suppl 2), S58-S64.

Cheung, T. K., Guan, Y., Ng, S. S., Chen, H., Wong, C. H., et al. (2005). Generation of recombinant influenza A virus without M2 ion-channel protein by introduction of a point mutation at the 5′ end of the viral intron. *Journal of Genetic Virology*, *86*(Pt 5), 1447-1454.

Christian, M. D., Poutanen, S. M., Loutfy, M. R., Muller, M. P. & Low, D. E. (2004). Severe acute respiratory syndrome. *Clinical Infectious Diseases*, *38*(10), 1420-1427.

Cutler, S. J., Fooks, A. R., & Van Der Poel, W. H. (2010). Public health threat of new, reemerging, and neglected zoonoses in the industrialized world. *Emerging Infectious Diseases*, *16*(1), 1-7.

Granwehr, B. P., Lillibridges, K. M., Higgs, S., Mason, P. W., Aronson, J. F., et al. (2004). West Nile virus: Where are we now? *The Lancet Infectious Diseases*, *4*(9), 547-556.

Griffin, D. E. (2009). Emergence and re-emergence of viral diseases of the central nervous system. *Progress in Neurobiology*, *91*(2), 95-101.

Guyer, B., Smith, D. R., & Chalk, R. (2000). Calling the shots: Immunization finance policies and practices. Executive summary of the report of the Institute of Medicine. *American Journal of Preventive Medicine*, *19*(3S), 4-12.

Haydon, D. T., Kao, R. R., & Kitching, R. P. (2004). The UK foot-and-mouth disease outbreak—The aftermath. *Nature Reviews, Microbiology*, *2*(8), 675-681.

Hughes, J. M. (2001). Emerging infectious diseases: A CDC perspective. *Emerging Infectious Diseases*, *7*(Suppl 3), 494-496.

Jones, K. E., Patel N. G., Levy M. A., Storeygard, A., Balk, D., et al. (2008). Global trends in emerging infectious diseases. *Nature*, *451*(7181), 990-993.

Kandun, I., Wibisono H., Sedyaningsih E. R., Yusharmen, Hadisoedarsuno, W., et al. (2006). Three Indonesian clusters of H5N1 Virus infection in 2005. *New England Journal of Medicine*, *355*(21), 2186-2194.

Knobler, S. L., Mack, A., Mahmoud, A., & Lemon, S. M. (Eds.). (2005). *The threat of pandemic influenza: Are we ready?* Washington, D.C.: National Academies Press.

Lashley, F. R. (2003). Factors contributing to the occurrence of emerging infectious diseases. *Biological Research for Nursing*, *4*(4), 258-267.

Lashley, F. R. (2004). Emerging infectious diseases: Vulnerabilities, contributing factors and approaches. *Expert Review of Anti-infective Therapy*, *2*(2), 299-316.

Lederberg, J., Shope, R. E., & Oaks, S. C., Jr. (Eds.). (1992). *Emerging infections: Microbial threats to health in the United States*. Washington, D.C.: National Academies Press.

Lindsey, N. P., Staples J. E., Lehman J. A., Fischer, M., & Centers for Disease Control and Prevention (CDC). (2009). Surveillance for human West Nile Virus disease—United States, 1999-2008. MMWR Surveillance Summaries. *Morbidity and Mortality Weekly Report. Surveillance Summaries/ CDC, 59*(2), 1-17.

Ma, W., Lager K. M., Vincent, A. L., Janke, B. H., Gramer, M. R., Richt, J. A. (2009). The role of swine in the generation of novel influenza viruses. *Zoonoses Public Health*, May 20. Epub ahead of print.

Mathers, C. D., & Loncar, D. (2006). Projections of global mortality and burden of disease from 2002 to 2030. *PLOS Medicine, 3*(11), E442.

Monto, A. S. (2009). The risk of seasonal and pandemic influenza: Prospects for control. *Clinical Infectious Diseases, 48*(Suppl 1), S20-S25.

Morens, D. M., Folkers, G. K., & Fauci, A. S. (2004). The challenge of emerging and re-emerging infectious diseases. *Nature, 430*(6996), 242-249.

Newell, D. G., Koopmans M., Verhoef, L., Duizer, E., Aidara-Kane, A., et al. (2010). Food-borne diseases—The challenges of 20 years ago still persist while new ones continue to emerge. *International Journal of Food Microbiology, 139*(Suppl 1), S3-S15.

Novel Swine-Origin Influenza A (H1N1) Virus Investigation Team, Dawood F. S., Jain, S., Finelli, L., Shaw, M. W., Lindstrom, S., et al. (2009). Emergence of a novel swine-origin Influenza A (H1N1) virus in humans. *New England Journal of Medicine, 360*(25), 2605-2615.

Oshitani, H., Kamigaki, T., & Suzuki, A. (2008). Major issues and challenges of influenza pandemic preparedness in developing countries. *Emerging Infectious Diseases, 14*(6), 875-880.

Paton, D. J., Sumption, K. J., & Charleston, B. (2009). Options for control of foot-and-mouth disease: Knowledge, capability and policy. Philosophical Transactions of the Royal Society of London, Series B, *Biological Sciences, 364*(1530), 2657-2667.

Patton, G. C., Coffey C., Sawyer S. M., Viner R. M., Haller D. M., et al. (2009). Global patterns of mortality in young people: A systematic analysis of population health data. *Lancet, 374*(9693), 881-892.

Pavlin, B. I., Schloegel, L. M., & Daszak, P. (2009). Risk of importing zoonotic diseases through wildlife trade, United States. *Emerging Infectious Diseases,15*(11), 1721-1726.

Perez-Padilla, R., de la Rosa-Zamboni, D., Ponce de Leon, S., Hernandez, M., Quiñones-Falconi, F., et al. (2009). Pneumonia and respiratory failure from swine-origin Influenza A (H1N1) in Mexico. *New England Journal of Medicine, 361*(7), 680-689.

Poon, L. L. M., Guan, Y., Nicholls, J. M., Yuen, K. Y., & Peiris, J. S. M. (2004). The aetiology, origins, and diagnosis of severe acute respiratory syndrome. *The Lancet Infectious Diseases, 4*(11), 663-671.

Reed, K. D., Melski, J. W., Graham, M. B., Regnery, R. L., Sotir, M. J., et al. (2004). The detection of monkeypox in humans in the Western Hemisphere. *New England Journal of Medicine, 350*(4), 342-350.

Simmerman, J. M. (2003). A close-up perspective on SARS. *Advances for Nurse Practitioners, 11*(11), 106.

Simonsen, L., Clarke, M. J., Schonberger, L. B., Arden, N. H., Cox, N. J., Fukuda, K. (1998). Pandemic versus epidemic influenza mortality: A pattern of changing age distribution. *Journal of Infectious Diseases, 178*(1), 53-60.

Skowronski, D. M., Astell, C., Brunham, R. C., Low, D. E., Petric, M., et al. (2005). Severe acute respiratory syndrome (SARS): A year in review. *Annual Review of Medicine, 56*, 357-381.

Swine-Origin Influenza A (H1N1) virus infections in a school—New York City, April 2009. *Morbidity and Mortality Weekly Report, 58*(17), 470-472.

Ungchusak, K., Auewarakul, P., Dowell, S. F., Kitphati R., Auwanit W., et al. (2005). Probable person-to-person transmission of Avian Influenza A (H5N1). *New England Journal of Medicine, 352*(4), 333-340.

Uyeki, T. M. (2008). Global epidemiology of human infections with highly pathogenic Avian Influenza A (H5N1) viruses. *Respirology,13*(Suppl 1), S2-S9.

World Health Organization (WHO). (2003). Acute respiratory syndrome, China. *Weekly Epidemiological Record, 78*, 41-48.

World Health Organization (WHO). (2005a). *Avian influenza: Assessing the pandemic threat.* Geneva, Switzerland: World Health Organization.

World Health Organization (WHO). (2005b). *Epidemic and Pandemic Alert and Response (EPR). Frequently asked questions about the international health regulations.* Geneva, Switzerland: World Health Organization. Retrieved from www.who.int/ihr/about/en.

World Health Organization (WHO). (2009). World now at the start of 2009 influenza pandemic. Retrieved from www.who.int/mediacentre/news/statements/2009/h1n1_pandemic_phase6_20090611/en/index.html.

World Health Organization (WHO). (2010). Cumulative number of confirmed human cases of avian influenza A/(H5N1) reported to WHO. Retrieved from www.who.int.esr.disease/avian_influenza/country/casestable_2006_04_12/en/index.html.

CHAPTER 104

Human Trafficking: The Need for Nursing Advocacy

Barbara Glickstein

"I freed a thousand slaves. I could have freed a thousand more if only they knew they were slaves."

—Harriet Ross Tubman, nurse abolitionist

Human trafficking is a serious crime of forced labor or enslavement. It is also a human rights tragedy. And it happens more often than we might think. The International Labour Organization (ILO) estimates that 12.3 million people are held as slaves around the world, representing a profit to the abusers of $32 billion and an additional loss to the victims of $20 billion (ILO, 2009). Many nurses have treated victims of human trafficking without realizing it. Encountering modern-day slavery can provoke a strong visceral response, often followed by the urge to distance ourselves from it. These feelings make it hard to imagine what you, one nurse, could possibly do to stop it. However, nurses are uniquely situated to make a difference.

When I speak about trafficking, nurses often approach me to discuss whether they may have cared for a person who was trafficked. One nurse told me she was a maternal child health nurse and worked at a community clinic. Once, a young woman presented in her final month of pregnancy but had no prenatal care, ID, or legal documents. She was accompanied by a man who was controlling and did most of the talking for the young woman, who introduced him as her "friend." The nurse who spoke with me had cared for domestic violence victims, but this felt different to her. Her skillful attempts to remove the male companion for part of the examination were met with resistance, but her persistence provided a few moments alone with the patient. However, the young woman repeated the same exact story, almost line by line, that she told in front of her male companion. The nurse knew that it would take time to learn the real story behind this patient and hoped there would be another chance on the next visit. There was no other encounter. Was she a victim of human trafficking? There is no way to know.

Nurses should ask themselves one question: "What role can nurses have in stopping human trafficking?" This question leads to the following important questions:
- What are the moments of intervention in the life of a woman/child/man who is a victim of trafficking when I can make a difference?
- What policies exist on a federal and state level?
- Does my place of employment or professional association have a policy or resolution on nursing's role in human trafficking?
- What is happening in the community where I live, and how can I stop human trafficking in my own neighborhood?

There are more than 13 million nurses worldwide providing up to 80% of the health services in most countries (International Council of Nurses, 2010). In every community where a nurse provides care, there are people who are vulnerable and could be targeted by traffickers. A trafficked person may be referred to a health care provider; a patient may disclose a trafficking experience; or a provider may detect signs that suggest an individual has been trafficked. To provide the best service to victims, it is imperative that nurses be aware of trafficking, be skilled in screening people who may be trafficked, and understand the needs of victims. Nurses can help to end trafficking by educating the public about this travesty and creating policies to protect those who are trafficked.

Nurses are also at risk for being trafficked. As poorer nations prepare nurses for export to other countries, questionable recruiting practices have led some migrating nurses to be threatened with criminal charges and deportation when they object to exploitative working conditions. Raising nurses' awareness about human trafficking can lower their own risk.

THE MYTHS

Anthropologist David Feingold says, "Trafficking is like a disease. If you don't change your response or if your response to the disease is 10 years out of date and made up of myths, the solution will not be effective, and may even be harmful" (Silverman, 2003). The following are four major myths about human trafficking:

1. Human trafficking is just an international problem.
2. Poverty and inequality are the causes of human trafficking.
3. Trafficking occurs only for the sex trade.
4. People who are traffickers have a common stereotypical profile.

The reality is that human trafficking occurs in almost every country including the United States—the second most frequent destination for trafficked persons. The U.S. State Department estimates that 15,000 victims enter the U.S. each year through trafficking rings, and that more victims are trafficked within our borders (U.S. Agency for International Development [USAID], 2004). These numbers are estimates because the trade is secretive, the victims are silenced, and the traffickers are dangerous. Although the majority of people trafficked are women and girls into sexual servitude, trafficking is not just forced prostitution. Victims of human trafficking may also be in forced labor situations as domestic servants (nannies, housekeepers, maids); sweatshop workers; janitors; restaurant workers; migrant farmworkers; fishery workers; hotel or tourist industry workers; or workers in nail salons.

Without recruiters and criminals, human trafficking would not exist. Poverty, unemployment, inflation, war, and the lack of a promising future are compelling factors that facilitate the ease with which traffickers recruit people, but they are not the cause of trafficking. Traffickers take advantage of poverty, unemployment, and the desire to emigrate to recruit people and traffic them into dangerous situations. Tragically, recruiters often know their victims. A common way that many victims are recruited is

through a friend or acquaintance (e.g., a cousin, neighbor, boyfriend, or fiancé) or by an individual recommended to them by someone they trusted.

Sometimes victims are recruited in groups. For example, an agency sets up a booth at a job fair in a high school gym. The legitimate-looking pamphlets, websites, and recruiters are quite professional looking. When victims arrive in a destination country, the methods used to control them include confiscation of travel documents, violence, threats to harm family members, and debt bondage. Whatever the recruitment method, the majority of people do not expect the exploitation and violence that awaits them. The ugly truth is that trafficking is big business. Traffickers make large profits due to high demand at low risk of prosecution.

Finally, traffickers can be anyone. Traffickers brazenly operate in our neighborhoods. They advertise in our newspapers and on Craigslist. They are men and women of all ages. They run legal employment agencies. They are diplomats who often get diplomatic immunity when caught, and they work in all kinds of professions (General Accounting Office, 2008). They act alone, or they may be members of international crime rings.

TRAFFICKING AS A GLOBAL PUBLIC HEALTH ISSUE

For nurses, trafficking in persons (TIP) can be best understood as a very serious health risk, because trafficking, like other forms of violence, is associated with physical and psychological harm (International Organization on Migration, 2009). It has serious public health implications related to the spread of infectious diseases such as tuberculosis, HIV, and other sexually transmitted diseases. Victims of trafficking are highly prone to social, economic, and legal issues that further put them at risk for a variety of mental health issues, including substance abuse, addiction, anxiety, depression, and even suicide (Hynes & Raymond, 2002). Common abuses experienced by trafficked persons include rape, torture, and other forms of physical, sexual, and psychological violence (Zimmerman, Hossain, Yun, Gajdadziev, & Guzun, 2008). Those who are sexually exploited may have multiple forced abortions, acquire sexually transmitted diseases, and experience other physical and psychological health problems (Moynihan, 2006). Paradoxically, these

---

BOX 104-1 What Can You Do about Human Trafficking?

1. Be well informed. Start with investigating what policy and protocols are in place at your health institution and if the issue of human trafficking is being addressed in the nursing curriculum in courses at your university or college.
2. If there are no policies in place, start an interdisciplinary task force to develop policies and pursue a plan to implement them.
3. Assess and educate community stakeholders, such as shelters, victim-assistance agencies, advocacy groups, and law enforcement agencies, and collaborate with them.
4. Become familiar with services and hotlines so that you can refer people who have been trafficked. Build a resource list, and keep it current.
5. Bring the issue of human trafficking to the public's attention in their local communities through public speaking in schools, places of worship, and social action groups. Use both traditional media and social media to launch campaigns and increase pressure on local authorities to act to stop human trafficking.

BOX 104-2 How Do You Know if Someone May Be a Victim of Human Trafficking?

The Signs
- Evidence of being controlled: watched, escorted.
- Traffickers may "coach" victims to answer questions with a cover story about being a wife, student, or tourist
- Bruises or other signs of battering
- Fear or depression
- Lack of passport, immigration, or identification documentation

Key Questions to Ask
- What type of work do you do? Are you being paid? Can you leave your job if you want to?
- Has your identification or documentation been taken from you?
- Have you or your family been threatened?
- What are your living conditions like?
- Where did you sleep last night? On a bed? On the floor?
- Do you have to ask permission to eat/sleep/go to the bathroom?
- Are there locks on your doors/windows so you cannot get out?

---

victims who desperately require health services are less likely to have access due to discrimination, social stigma, fear of law enforcement, and other factors. Nurses can contribute their expertise by conducting research on human trafficking as a global public health issue (Boxes 104-1 and 104-2).

INTERNATIONAL POLICY

The Universal Declaration of Human Rights (UDHR) was adopted by the United Nations General Assembly in Paris in 1948. The UDHR was the first international statement to use the term *human rights*. It states that human rights are rights inherent to all human beings, whatever our nationality, place of residence, sex, national or ethnic origin, color, religion, language, or any other status. Among several protections covered by the UDHR, Article 4 of the UDHR states: "No one shall be held in slavery or servitude: slavery and the slave trade shall be prohibited in all their forms." The UDHR made history and is used by human rights activists globally (General Assembly of the United Nations, 1948).

The first international legal instrument to address human trafficking as a crime and to define trafficking was passed in 2000, when The United Nations Office on Drugs and Crime passed the Protocol to Prevent, Suppress and Punish Trafficking in Persons. As of 2009, 136 Member States have signed the Protocol. It defines trafficking in persons as follows:

The recruitment, transportation, transfer, harbouring or receipt of persons, by means of the threat or use of force or other forms of coercion, of abduction, of fraud, of deception, of the abuse of power or of a position of vulnerability or of the giving or receiving of payments or benefits to achieve the consent of a person having control over another person, for the purpose of exploitation. Exploitation shall include, at a minimum, the exploitation of the prostitution of others or other forms of sexual exploitation, forced labour or services, slavery or practices similar to slavery, servitude or the removal of organs. (UN, 2000)

This international protocol established the standard approach for governments developing policies on trafficking: "The 3P Paradigm"—prevention, prosecution, protection of victims.

In 2007, The United Nations Global Initiative to Fight Human Trafficking (UN.GIFT) was established to coordinate global efforts to adopt the protocol. In addition to working with governments, the UN.GIFT works with business, academia, civil society, and the media to develop effective tools to fight human trafficking (United Nations Office on Drugs and Crime [UNODC], 2009).

The 2009 UN.GIFT Global Report on Trafficking of Persons challenged a widely held belief that sex slavery occurs more frequently than labor trafficking and suggested that this may be due to statistical bias resulting in more media attention to sex slavery. The report also identified that a growing number of women are traffickers due to a phenomenon called "the second wave" in which trafficked victims return home to recruit others. One of the few means of escaping the brutality of being a victim is to move from victim to perpetrator (UNODC, 2009).

U.S. RESPONSE TO HUMAN TRAFFICKING

The U.S. Department of State began monitoring trafficking in persons in 1994, when the issue began to be covered in the Department's Annual Country Reports on Human Rights Practices. Originally, coverage focused on trafficking of women and girls for sexual purposes. During the Clinton administration, the U.S. passed the Trafficking Victims Protection Act of 2000 (TVPA). This law defined human trafficking in persons as "sex trafficking in which a commercial sex act is induced by force, fraud, or coercion, or in which the person induced to perform such act has not attained 18 years of age" or "the recruitment, harboring, transportation, provision, or obtaining of a person for labor or services, through the use of force, fraud, or coercion for the purpose of subjection to involuntary servitude, peonage, debt bondage, or slavery " (TVPA, 2000). This act established the standard for federal policy on trafficking, and responses to act were all based on the 3P Paradigm. During the George W. Bush administration, there was a focus on the four Rs (Rescue, Rehabilitation, Restoration, and Reintegration) to describe the comprehensive sets of services for victims.

More recently, advocacy organizations globally are launching campaigns that focus on the demand side of slavery as a means of stopping this crime. These laws would take the focus off of the women and children in prostitution and put it on the end user or customer. Another demand-reduction strategy is an education and awareness campaign that is aimed at boys and young men and focuses on the negative consequences of purchasing sex—from public and private health problems like the spread of HIV and other STDs, to the grim facts about who runs the sex trade and how customers are helping traffickers flourish and hurting those who have been trafficked.

Ambassador Luis CdeBaca, the current Director of the Office to Monitor and Combat Trafficking in Persons, has called on every person to take personal responsibility for their contribution to this crime. He suggested that just as we evaluate and lesson our carbon footprint to protect the environment, we must assess our modern-day slavery footprint. He framed this self-assessment as "ask and act," where we ask questions such as, "Was the cotton that made my shirt picked by a trafficked woman?" or "Did my Valentines' Day chocolate come from children enslaved on cocoa farms?" (CdeBaca, 2010).

The ninth annual Trafficking in Persons Report (TIP) provides data from April 2008 to March 2009 (U.S. Department of State, 2009) and outlines major forms of human trafficking including forced labor, bonded labor, debt bondage among migrant laborers, involuntary domestic servitude, forced child labor, child soldiers, sex trafficking, and child sex trafficking and related abuses. The report notes that 5212 incidents of human trafficking were prosecuted globally in 2008—the lowest number since recording began in 2003. Of these cases, there were 2983 convictions. Some governments have yet to respond to the global call for victim protections or for effective law enforcement efforts against these crimes. As the UN Office on Drugs and Crime stated in its recent report on global human trafficking, two out of five countries have yet to achieve a single conviction of a human trafficker.

STATE LEGISLATION AND POLICY ON HUMAN TRAFFICKING

Criminalizing human trafficking in every state enables local and state law enforcement to investigate and prosecute these crimes and to work in partnership with federal law enforcement. The Center for Women

Policy Studies recommend that five key initiatives be included in every state law: making trafficking a state felony offense, providing victim-protection assistance programs, developing an interagency task force on human trafficking, regulating "bride trafficking" by international marriage brokers, and regulating travel service providers that facilitate sex tourism (U.S. Policy Advocacy to Combat Trafficking, 2010). Activists have been critical in moving this agenda forward.

Investigate and familiarize yourself with your state's legislation on human trafficking. If your state has legislation and an interagency anti-trafficking task force working on a comprehensive plan to provide services for persons who have been trafficked, ask if there is a nurse on the task force. Once identified, ask how you can help. If there is no nurse on the task force, work toward getting a nurse appointed, or nominate yourself. If your state is one of the remaining states without anti-trafficking laws, identify local and national advocacy organizations working toward this goal, and work with them to pass this legislation. Contact and engage your state nursing association to lobby to pass these comprehensive laws.

PROFESSIONAL NURSING ASSOCIATIONS

The International Council of Nurses (ICN) Code of Ethics for Nurses position statement, Nurses and Human Rights, requires nurses to safeguard and promote human rights (ICN, 2006a, 2006b). This statement, as well as other ICN advocacy and lobbying position statements, cover a wide range of health issues where nurses must act to enforce human rights and to promote and protect health as a fundamental human right and a social goal.

Success is attainable. In 2008, the New York State Nursing Association (NYSNA) invited me to deliver an address titled "Nurses Working to Stop Human Trafficking" at their annual convention. The NYSNA board's response was immediate. They drafted and submitted an action proposal on human trafficking to the American Nurses Association (ANA), which was passed by the ANA House of Delegates in 2008. The resolution states that it will advocate legislation to reduce the incidence of human trafficking and will work to ensure that nurses know how to identify and assist victims. This is a commendable action by the ANA to educate nurses nationally and support stronger enforcement of the federal laws (American Nurses Association, 2008).

SUMMARY

While there is much work that needs to be done to understand and end human trafficking, progress has been made since 2000. The international community has taken decisive action to end human trafficking. Greater research related to trafficking is a prerequisite to ending the abuse. Lack of data and failure to grasp the complexities that underlie human trafficking worldwide must be addressed. The media treatment of trafficking does not present the true dimensions of the problem and should work toward better reporting to help shatter the myths about human trafficking. Non-government agencies and advocacy groups dedicated to creating public awareness campaigns and developing victim services programs should be supported by volunteering your nursing expertise, time, and resources. Whether nurses are engaged in clinical care, advocacy, policy, or program activities, they can monitor human trafficking and have an impact on preventing it. One common agreement is that to stop human trafficking, global awareness of the problem must increase. Nurses can add their voices through advocacy and help build the global capacity needed to stop human trafficking.

For a list of related websites, please refer to your Evolve Resources at http://evolve.elsevier.com/Mason/policypolitics/

REFERENCES

American Nurses Association (ANA). (2008, July 1). RN delegates to ANA biennial meeting take action to work toward greater nurse retention, address public health issues. Press release.

CdeBaca, Luis. (2010). From bondage to freedom: The fight to abolish modern slavery. Retrieved from www.state.gov/g/tip/rls/rm/2010/136918.htm.

General Accounting Office (GAO). (2008, July). Human rights: U.S. government's efforts to address alleged abuse of household workers by foreign diplomats with immunity could be strengthened. Retrieved from www.gao.gov/new.items/d08892.pdf.

General Assembly of the United Nations. (1948). Universal declaration of human rights. Retrieved from www.un.org/en/documents/udhr.

Hynes, P., & Raymond, J. G. (2002). Put in harm's way: The neglected health consequences of sex trafficking in the United States. In J. Stillman & A. Bhattacharjee (Eds.), Policing the national body: Sex, race and criminalization (pp. 197-229). Cambridge: South End.

International Council of Nurses. (2006a). ICN code of ethics for nurses. Retrieved from www.icn.ch/images/stories/documents/about/icncode_english.pdf.

International Council of Nurses. (2006b). Nurses and human rights. Retrieved from www.icn.ch/images/stories/documents/publications/position_statements/C06_Nurse_Retention_Migration.pdf.

International Council of Nurses. (2010). About ICN. Retrieved from www.icn.ch/about-icn/about-icn.

International Labour Organization (ILO). (2009). *The cost of coercion.* Geneva, Switzerland: International Labour Organization. Retrieved from www.ilo.org/wcmsp5/groups/public/---ed_norm/---relconf/documents/meetingdocument/wcms_106230.pdf.

International Organization on Migration. (2009). *Caring for trafficked persons.* Geneva, Switzerland: International Organization for Migration. Retrieved from http://publications.iom.int/bookstore/free/CT_Handbook.pdf.

Moynihan, B. A. (2006). The high cost of human trafficking. *International Association of Forensic Nurses, 2*(2), 100-101.

Silverman, Vicki. (2003). "Trading Women" filmmaker shatters myths about human trafficking. Retrieved from www.america.gov/st/washfile-english/2003/September/20030911115501namrevlisv0.2781031.html.

United Nations (UN). (2000). Protocol to prevent, suppress, and punish trafficking in persons, especially women and children, supplementing the United Nations Convention Against Transnational Organized Crime. Retrieved from www.uncjin.org/Documents/Conventions/dcatoc/final_documents_2/convention_%20traff_eng.pdf.

United Nations Office on Drugs and Crime (UNODC). (2009). Global report on trafficking in persons. Retrieved from www.unodc.org/documents/human-trafficking/Global_Report_on_TIP.pdf.

U.S. Agency for International Development (USAID). (2004, March). Trafficking in persons: USAID's response. Retrieved from www.usaid.gov/our_work/crosscutting_programs/wid/pubs/trafficking_in_person_usaids_response_march2004.pdf.

U.S. Department of State. (2009). Trafficking in persons report. Washington, D.C.: Retrieved from www.state.gov/documents/organization/123357.pdf.

U.S. Policy Advocacy to Combat Trafficking. (2010). Fact sheet on state anti-trafficking laws. Washington, D.C.: Center for Women Policy Studies. Retrieved from www.centerwomenpolicy.org/news/newsletter/documents/FactSheetonStateAntiTraffickingLawsJanuary2010.pdf.

Victims of Trafficking and Violence Protection Act (TVPA) of 2000, 22 U.S.C. § 7102(8).

Zimmerman, C., Hossain, M., Yun, K., Gajdadziev, V., & Guzun N. (2008). The health of trafficked women: A survey of women entering posttrafficking services in Europe. *American Journal of Public Health, 98*(1), 55-59.

The Affordable Care Act: Historical Context and an Introduction to the State of Health Care in the United States

Andréa Sonenberg and Ellen S. Murray

Serious efforts to reform the U.S. health care system have been attempted since the 1930s. With increasing interest and petitioning from citizens groups and organized workers, Presidents Franklin D. Roosevelt, Harry S. Truman, and John F. Kennedy all attempted to implement National Health Insurance programs but ultimately failed due to opposition and pressure from Republicans, Southern Democrats, the American Medical Association, and the emerging private health insurance industry. In the 1960s, President Lyndon B. Johnson successfully passed the Social Security Act amendments of 1965 through Congress, establishing Medicaid and Medicare, but his success was followed by a string of failures during the administrations of Presidents Richard Nixon, Jimmy Carter, and Bill Clinton (Henry J. Kaiser Family Foundation [KFF], 2009).

Until recently, the lack of comprehensive health care reform in the United States had harmful effects on the health of the U.S. population and increased the cost of health care. While the United States has the most expensive health care system in the world, far exceeding expenditures in other Organization for Economic Co-operation and Development (OECD) countries, the U.S. ranks last among industrialized nations in preventable mortality (Gable, 2011) and ranks surprisingly low in other important health quality measures, such as maternal and child mortality. Even more astonishing, a 2009 study published in the *American Journal of Public Health* estimated that 45,000 people died each year due to a lack of health insurance (Wilper et al., 2009). The U.S. Census reported an increase in the number of uninsured people in the United States, reaching 49.9 million in 2010, and a decline in employer-based health insurance coverage for the eleventh year in a row (Physicians for a National Health Program [PHNP], 2011), Without government action, these problems would only increase in severity.

On March 23, 2010, President Barack Obama signed the Patient Protection and Affordable Care Act (PPACA) into law. A few days later, the U.S. Senate and House of Representatives negotiated and passed the Health Care and Education Reconciliation Act (HCERA), a piece of legislation that made significant amendments to the PPACA. President Obama signed HCERA into law on March 30, 2010, and the final, revised law—the PPACA as amended by HCERA—is commonly referred to as the Affordable Care Act (ACA). The ACA is a landmark piece of legislation that aims to transform the U.S. health care system by expanding health insurance coverage, controlling costs, and improving quality, delivery, and access to care (McDonough, 2011).

The ACA's ten titles tackle and reform specific elements of the current health care system. While implementation of the law began immediately after its signing, the biggest reforms are set to roll out in January of 2014, with full implementation of the law expected by 2019 (American Academy of Family Physicians [AAFP], n.d.). Table A-1 provides an overview of the law by title.

TABLE A-1 **The Affordable Care Act**

Title	Provisions
Title I (Quality, Affordable Health Care for All Americans)	• Immediate improvements are made to the health insurance system: eliminates lifetime and unreasonable annual limits on benefits, with annual limits prohibited in 2014; prohibits rescissions of health insurance policies; prohibits preexisting condition exclusions for children; extends dependent coverage to age 26; requires coverage of preventive services. • A minimum essential coverage provision (commonly referred to as the individual mandate) is established, requiring most individuals to obtain health care coverage for themselves and their dependents or face a shared responsibility payment (tax penalty) of either $95 or 1% of household income, starting in 2014 and increasing thereafter. • Coverage can be obtained through employer-sponsored health insurance, new state health exchanges, government programs (Medicaid/Medicare), or a grandfathered health plan. • State health exchanges will be established and implemented in January 2014 to help individuals and small employers obtain coverage. Plans participating in the exchanges will be rated (bronze through platinum options) based on their benefits. • Premium tax credits will be made available to households and individuals with incomes between 100% and 400% of the FPL to offset the cost of purchasing insurance through state health exchanges. Cost-sharing assistance will be made available for those at 250% FPL and under. • Employers with more than 200 employees must automatically enroll new full-time employees in coverage. Establishes penalties ($750 per full-time employee, capped) for employers with more than 50 full-time employees that do not offer coverage or offer coverage deemed unaffordable or below the minimum essential coverage standard.
Title II (Medicaid, CHIP, and the Governors)	• Starting in January 2014, states will be required to provide health coverage for all children, parents and childless adults who are not entitled to Medicare and are at or below 133 percent of the FPL. The federal government will initially cover 100% of the cost of the expansion, with federal aid dropping slightly starting in 2017. (Note: Per the Supreme Court's Decision, states may decide to "opt-out" of the ACA's Medicaid expansion. The HHS Secretary may withhold the funds noncompliant states would get if they chose to expand coverage, but the HHS Secretary may NOT withhold existing federal Medicaid funds from noncompliant states.) • States will be required to maintain income eligibility levels for the Children's Health Insurance Program (CHIP) through September 30, 2019, and will receive additional federal funding. • Federal Coordinated Health Care is established to integrate care under Medicare and Medicaid and improve coordination among both programs (dual eligibles). • Medicaid and Medicare reimbursement policies for hospitals are reformed, and additional funding is shifted to community-based care centers.
Title III (Improving the Quality and Efficiency of Health Care)	• Establishes a new Center for Medicare & Medicaid Innovation to research, develop, and test effective payment and delivery models. • Sets up incentives and guidelines for hospitals and ACOs to take responsibility for quality and cost of care and encourages the development of community health teams that emphasize coordinated care and prevention. • Adjusts Medicare reimbursement values based on preventable patient readmissions and increases Medicare fee schedules from providers in rural areas.
Title IV (Prevention of Chronic Disease and Improving Public Health)	• Creates a new Prevention and Public Health Investment Fund to support community and public health initiatives that aim to prevent injury and disease and eliminate access barriers to community health centers and clinical preventive services.

TABLE A-1 The Affordable Care Act—cont'd

Title	Provisions
Title V (Health Care Workforce)	• Enhances health care workforce education and training, particularly for primary care and mental and behavioral health education. • Provides training grants to schools for the development, expansion, and enhancement of training programs in social work, graduate psychology, professional training in child and adolescent mental health, and pre-service or in-service training to paraprofessionals in child and adolescent mental health. • Provides competitive grants for workforce planning and workforce development strategies on the state level, as well as competitive grants for coordinated and integrated care in mental and behavioral health.
Title VI (Transparency and Program Integrity)	• Requires greater transparency and reporting dealing with conflicts of interest between medical professionals and drug, device, and medical supply manufacturers and distributors. It also requires hospitals and health industry organizations to disclose greater financial information to the public and establishes a demonstration project to test and implement a national independent monitoring program to oversee interstate and large intrastate chains. Title VI also contains the Elder Justice Act, which help to prevent and eliminate elder abuse, neglect, and exploitation.
Title VII (Improving Access to Innovative Medical Therapies)	• Gives the FDA authority to license the production and sale of biosimilars and also extends drug discounts to certain children's hospitals, critical access and sole community hospitals, and rural medical centers treating high-need and low-income populations.
Title VIII (Community Living Assistance Services and Supports—CLASS Act)	• Establishes a national voluntary insurance program for purchasing community living assistance services and support (CLASS program). The HHS Secretary will develop a sound benefit plan that ensures solvency for 75 years. Allows for a 5-year vesting period for benefit eligibility. No taxpayer funds will be used to pay benefits under this provision.
Title IX (Revenue Provisions)	• Establishes and reforms taxes on medical-related expenses, introduces certain fees for hospitals and the pharmaceutical industry, and closes a number of tax deduction loopholes. The cost savings introduced through this title will pay for approximately half the cost of expanded coverage in Titles I and II.
Title X (Strengthening Quality, Affordable Health Care for All Americans)	• Makes a series of amendments to titles I through IX. Key provisions include adjusting the implementation and structure of the ban on lifetime and annual insurance caps, excluding the coverage of abortion services using federal funds, and reauthorizing the Indian Health Care Improvement Act.

SOURCE: McDonough, J.E. (2011). *Inside national health reform.* Los Angeles: University of California Press.

In the days after President Obama signed it into law, lawsuits were filed by various groups challenging the constitutionality of the ACA, focusing specifically on the law's two major provisions: the minimum essential coverage provision, known as the individual mandate (Title I), and Medicaid expansion (Title II). On November 14, 2011, after contentious judgments in the Eleventh Circuit Court and pressure from the Obama Administration, the U.S. Supreme Court agreed to consider two cases: one case brought by the state of Florida and joined by 25 additional U.S. states (*Florida v. U.S. Dept. of Health and Human Svcs.*), and one brought by a group of plaintiffs that included the National Federation of Independent Businesses (*National Federation of Independent Business v. Sebelius,* 2012).

Between Monday, March 26, and Wednesday, March 28, 2012, the court heard over 6 hours of oral arguments. They justices were to vote on whether the Anti-Injunction Act prevented the court from deciding the case until after taxpayers incurred the individual mandate penalty; the constitutionality of the individual mandate; the severability of the individual mandate from the rest of the law, allowing the Affordable Care Act to stand without the mandate;

and the constitutionality of the Medicaid expansion (KFF, 2012).

All nine justices agreed that the Supreme Court had jurisdiction to decide the case and that the Anti-Injunction Act did not apply. In a 5-4 vote, the majority of the court, including Chief Justice Roberts, held that the individual mandate is a constitutional exercise of Congress' power to tax and is therefore constitutional. The court also ruled in a 7-2 vote that Medicaid expansion under the ACA was unconstitutionally coercive to states because it lacked adequate notice to voluntarily consent and because the Secretary of Health and Human Services (HHS) held the power to withhold all existing Medicaid Funds from noncompliant states. To remedy this, the court ruled in a 5-4 vote that the HHS Secretary should be restrained from withholding existing Medicaid funds from noncompliant states. The majority ruled that the Secretary should still have authority to withhold the increased Medicaid expansion funds that the state would receive under the ACA, as well as that all other Medicaid reforms under the ACA would remain intact and on schedule (KFF, 2012).

While the Supreme Court voted largely in favor of the ACA, its decision to circumscribe the Secretary's power to withhold existing Medicaid funds renders the Medicaid expansion an "optional" element of the ACA, and analysts estimate that approximately 3 million fewer people will receive coverage due to states that opt-out of the Medicaid expansion funds (Pear, 2012); 25 states, including Florida, Texas, Georgia, Alabama, Louisiana and Mississippi, have indicated that they will not expand Medicaid in January 2014 together with the rest of the country, leaving their neediest populations without government-sponsored health care aid (Pear, 2013).

An estimated 32 million uninsured Americans will be covered as a result of the ACA (Title I and Title II), with half of them covered through the private insurance markets and half covered through the expansion of Medicaid. With the country and health care system poised for this influx of newly insured to come on to the Medicaid rosters in 2014, there is a growing concern regarding the existing capacity of primary care providers to meet the substantial and increasing demand for access to care that is emerging (Institute of Medicine [IOM], 2010). One answer that has been put forth to assist in meeting this growing demand for primary care is to optimize utilization of advanced

practice registered nurses (APRNs), specifically nurse practitioners (NPs) (Fairman, Rowe, Hassmiller, & Shalala, 2011; IOM, 2010). Evidence supports that APRNs and NPs deliver high quality health care and improved health outcomes at a lower cost than the traditional medical model (Newhouse et al., 2011).

The implications of the ACA for nursing fall into two categories: those that are related to the provisions directed specifically to nursing and those that are related to the provisions that will either indirectly affect nursing or invite and demand nursing's involvement by affording new opportunities. Through the creation of a National Health Care Workforce Commission established in Title V (Health Care Workforce) of the ACA, the law aims to monitor and influence national health workforce policy to further explore the health workforce needs of the nation (American Association of Colleges of Nursing [AACN], 2012 White House, n.d.), although this Commission remained unfunded as of 2013. Through a combination of training programs, loans, loan repayment programs, and scholarships (Commonwealth Fund, 2011), the ACA will fulfill one of its other more direct roles, that of capacity building of the primary care workforce. Title V also eases criteria and expands the federal student loan program for schools and students focusing on primary care and increases funding to community health centers and the National Health Service Corps. In striving to expand workforce resources, a substantial portion of the ACA plan addresses both the supply and regulation of practice of APRNs.

DIRECT IMPACTS ON NURSING AS A HEALTH WORKFORCE

Through a variety of funding and regulatory provisions, the ACA is directly focused on nursing by addressing (1) demand for a larger primary care workforce to improve patient access to care and (2) regulation of practice.

FUNDING

Expanded funding and payments will impact nursing in several ways, including through effects on patient census; nursing education funding; nursing services and roles; and regulation of nursing practice (American Academy of Nursing [AAN], 2010; American Nurses Association [ANA], 2010a, 2010b).

PATIENTS

Expanded funding for patient services will increase access to care. There will be (1) expanded Medicaid eligibility through state health insurance exchanges, a kind of marketplace for purchasing insurance with subsidies in some cases, and (2) expanded coverage of dependent children up to the age of 26 years old. Both of these measures will amplify the patient rosters and the demand for access to care (and therefore, for APRNs).

NURSING

To meet those growing demands for primary care, the legislation addresses the health care workforce shortage through provisions that expand funding in several areas, including nursing education and loan repayment and nursing services in a variety of models. These provisions are included in:

Education and Loan Repayment. Provisions for expanded funding for nursing education include:
1. Increased federal loan limits for nursing students
2. Expansion of the National Health Service Corps Loan repayment Program, which will repay 60% of a nursing student loan in exchange for a commitment of 2 years of service in a critical health workforce shortage area
3. Establishing a Medicare graduate nurse education demonstration program in up to five hospitals (already in progress)
4. Expanding the Public Health Service Act to provide demonstration grants for family NP training programs, offering 1-year residencies for NPs in federally qualified health centers (FQHCs) and nurse-managed health centers (AAN, 2010; American Association of Nurse Practitioners [AANP], 2013a; ANA, 2013).

Nursing Services. Provisions that increase funding for nursing services include:
1. Expansion of the National Health Service Corp (Title V)
2. An enhanced Medicare reimbursement rate for certified nurse-midwives (CNMs) to 100% of the physician schedule; this had been 65% since CNMs were first designated primary care providers with the Omnibus Reconciliation Act of 1987 (Centers for Medicare and Medicaid [CMS], 2011)
3. Home visits to low-income mothers, providing education during pregnancy and the early childhood years

4. Home care and education to chronically ill older adults, facilitating their ability to remain homebound
5. Nurse-managed health clinics to serve low-income community residents, including federally funded community health clinics and maternity care homes
6. A Medicare "readmission penalty" (AAN, 2012; AANP, 2013b; American College of Nurse-Midwives [ACNM], 2013; ANA, 2013a).

REGULATION OF PRACTICE

With its focus on expansion of the primary care NP workforce, the ACA only addresses two areas of regulatory policy, which historically have been barriers to NP practice. First, and as previously mentioned, in January 2011, the ACA expanded Medicare reimbursement for certified nurse-midwife services to 100% of the Medicare fee schedule from 65% (Title III, Section 3114) (ACA, 2010). The second reform in regulation, which directly improves access to NP services, is that, effective in 2014, the ACA will amend the Public Health Service Act entitled *Non-Discrimination in Health Care*. This Act mandates that neither group nor individual health plans shall discriminate against any health care provider's participation under the plan or coverage for their chosen provider, given that the health care provider is practicing within the scope of her or his applicable state license or certification (AAN, 2010). Once licensed, however, NP reimbursement under Medicaid continues to be determined by individual state regulations. Despite the disparity between the focus on expansion of an NP workforce and the regulatory barriers it faces in practice, both of these issues are significant concerns.

INDIRECT IMPACTS ON NURSING

In addition to the provisions that directly address and affect nursing, several of the other provisions of the ACA will have a profound impact on nursing by providing opportunities through expanded roles in leadership, practice, quality practice improvement, research, technology, and innovation. It is not within the scope of this discussion to elaborate upon the indirect implications of each and every provision or regulation; however, it is clear that there are numerous prospects for nurses in relation to the evolving ACA regulations on quality standards, state exchanges and the individual mandate, care coordination, increased primary care workforce needs, outcomes data gathering and reporting, communication with beneficiaries, health promotion and illness prevention, and patient-centeredness. How nurses avail themselves of these opportunities will depend greatly on their proactive actions and those of professional nursing organizations. The implementation of the ACA also requires monitoring of the progress and success of the legislation.

With its expertise in care coordination, health care informatics, and quality and practice performance improvement, nursing is keenly positioned to take a leadership role in this implementation. Indeed, doing so is a key recommendation of the IOM (2010) report on *The Future of Nursing* (AANP, 2013; ANA, 2010; Correia, 2011; Fairman, Rowe, Hassmiller, & Shalala, 2011; Flinter, 2012; IOM, 2010). Nurses have already begun to take leadership roles that have usually been held by those in other disciplines. For example:

- In May 2013, Congress confirmed Marilyn Tavenner as administrator of the Centers for Medicare & Medicaid Services (CMS). Tavenner began her career as a staff nurse, working her way up to chief executive officer (CEO) of two hospitals in Virginia, and later served as Virginia's Secretary of HHS. In 2010, President Obama appointed Tavenner as Deputy Administrator of CMS due to her experience working with a broad range of advocacy, health profession, and political organizations and networks.
- Mary Wakefield is administrator for the Human Resources and Services Administration (HRSA). Prior to the HRSA, Wakefield gained crucial experience on Capitol Hill as chief of staff to two North Dakota Senators and served on a number of commissions and committees, including the IOM, the Medicare Payment Advisory Commission, and President Clinton's Advisory Commission on Consumer Protection and Quality in the Health Care Industry. Wakefield earned a doctoral degree in nursing and served as associate dean for rural health at the School of Medicine and Health Sciences at the University of North Dakota, as well as director of the Center for Health Policy, Research and Ethics at George Mason University.
- Janet Heinrich heads the HHS Bureau of Health Professions. Heinrich has held numerous executive and policy analyst positions, including serving as the CEO of the American Academy of Nursing.

Heinrich, Wakefield, and Tavenner will prove critical to nurse leadership and hold a voice with a new perspective as new regulations are implemented. A summary of the indirect implications of the ACA for nursing can be reviewed in Table A-2, which is a table adapted with the permission of the ANA (2010).

REGULATIONS

The underpinnings of any health policy reform include access, cost, and quality. Much of the aforementioned discussion has been around cost and access to care. Reforms addressing these elements are largely achieved through the federal regulations instituted by the ACA. These regulations are assigned in a variety of categories along with those that also address quality. There are mandates to the federal level for oversight; to the states with relation to funding and quality monitoring; to insurance companies for nondiscrimination, rating, and coverage; to employers regarding employee health benefits; to various health care delivery models and to the providers delivering care through those models, primarily to ensure quality; and to individual citizens for securing individual coverage.

FEDERAL OVERSIGHT

A variety of additional departments and programs were created in the Centers for Medicare and Medicaid, including:

1. Centers for Medicare and Medicaid Innovation to generate and evaluate innovative service and payment programs
2. A hospital value-based purchasing program (Medicare) to incentivize hospitals meeting defined performance standards
3. Modification of provider reimbursement rates to a "composite measure of quality of care furnished compared to cost" (ANA, 2010, p. 3)
4. Mandates for more comprehensive monitoring for disparities, including data collection related to a variety of demographics, including geographic monitoring of rural residents and data analysis "to monitor trends in disparities" (p. 3)
5. A 10% Medicare bonus to all primary care providers, including NPs but excluding nurse-midwives

TABLE A-2 Provisions in the Affordable Care Act and the Implications for Nursing

Category	Provisions	Nursing Implications (Direct and Indirect)
Quality	• Quality reporting to HHS by group health insurers with respect to plan or coverage benefits and health care provider reimbursement structures that implement activities to improve patient safety and reduce medical errors through the appropriate use of best clinical practices, evidence-based medicine, chronic disease management, and health information technology (Title I, Section 1001). • Establishes the Center for Quality Improvement and Patient Safety (in AHRQ) to conduct and gather research on changes in processes of care that will reliably result in improved patient safety and reduced medical errors (Title III, Section 3501). • Establishes the Patient-Centered Outcomes Research Institute for comparative effectiveness research (Title 6, Section 6301), and the Center for Medicare and Medicaid Innovation within CMS to test innovative payment and service delivery models (Title III, Section 3021). • Establishes the Federal Coordinated Health Care office within CMS to improve care continuity and ensure safe and effective transitions for dual eligible individuals (Title II, Section 2602). • Establishes a hospital value-based purchasing program under which value-based incentive payments are made to hospitals that meet certain performance standards (Title III, Section 3001). • Establishes a payment modifier for physicians under the Medicare fee schedule based upon performance measures reflecting health outcomes. In 2017, this becomes applicable to all eligible health professionals, including APRNs (Title III, Section 3007). • Requires increased collection and reporting of demographic data to monitor trends in disparities (Title III, Section 3121). • Establishes the community-based Collaborative Care Network Program to support consortiums of health care providers for low-income, uninsured, and underinsured populations (Title X, Section 10333). • Awards grants for quality measure development, with priority given to measures that allow the assessment of, among other things, the safety, effectiveness, patient-centeredness, appropriateness, and timeliness of care; the efficiency of care; the equity of health services and health disparities; and the continuity of care (Title III, Section 3013). • Requires qualified plans to provide a floor of preventive services with no cost sharing, as recommended by the U. S. Preventive Service Task Force. The plans must also include recommended immunizations; preventive care for infants, children, adolescents; and certain screenings for women. The plans will also cover and eliminate cost-sharing for these services for Medicare and Medicaid.	• The provisions related to ensuring quality provide nurses with vast opportunities in the areas of research, evidence-based practice, health information technology, leadership, and innovation. • In May 2013, Congress confirmed Marilyn Tavenner as administrator of the CMS. She is a former Secretary of HHS for Virginia, hospital administrator, and intensive care nurse, and will prove critical to nursing leadership as new regulations are implemented. • Nurses should avail themselves of the opportunities to seek funding to support their efforts in quality improvement, including roles in research, leadership, and direct quality practice improvement initiatives. • Prevention has always been a keystone of the nursing philosophy. The opportunity to develop qualified plans in the area of preventive services affords nurses chances to embrace new roles in leadership, innovation, practice, and quality practice improvement.

Continued

TABLE A-2 Provisions in the Affordable Care Act and the Implications for Nursing—cont'd

Category	Provisions	Nursing Implications (Direct and Indirect)
Access	• Requires HHS Secretary to develop national quality improvement strategy, including priorities of improving delivery, outcomes, and population health. HHS Secretary will also consult with National Quality Forum, states, and other stakeholders and convene an Interagency Workgroup on Health Care Quality for federal departments to collaborate (Title III, Sections 3011 and 3012). • Workforce provisions promote cultural competence training of health care professionals and also promote training of a diverse workforce (Title V). • Funds $11 billion for Community health Centers and National Health Service Corp over 5 years (Title V). • Establishes new programs to support school-based health centers and nurse-managed health centers (Title IV, Section 4101).	• ANA holds representation on the National Quality Forum. • Cultural competence has always been one of the foundations of nursing. School-based clinics have often been one of the unique settings in which nursing has played a great role. The initiatives to expand access to care provide unique opportunities for APRNs as well as for nurse researchers and nurse leaders (coordinators)
Cost	• While all U.S and legal residents are covered under the ACA, undocumented immigrants are not included • Workforce provision supports development of interdisciplinary mental and behavioral health training programs and supports the development of training programs that focus on primary care models that integrate physical and mental health services • The ACA calls for individuals to obtain minimum essential coverage (individual mandate) for themselves and their dependents, effective 2014. Exemptions will be permitted on hardship or religious grounds (Title I). • States are required to establish health exchanges to facilitate individuals' and small business' purchase of coverage. States can join to form regional exchanges and can also opt out if they can create coverage systems that meet or exceed the federal requirements; HHS will help states with funding exchanges' set-up and will create exchange in states that do not comply (Title I). • 10% bonus Medicare payment to primary care providers, including nurse practitioners in 2011-2015. • Increase in Medicaid payments for primary care physicians to 100% Medicare rates for 2013 and 2014. • Increase in grant funding for programs and service that increase the primary care workforce. • The Center for Quality Improvement and Patient Safety (in AHRQ) is to conduct research that identifies best practices that are adaptable, scalable to diverse health care settings, or effective in improving care across diverse settings (Title III, Section 3501).	• Health care for all is part of ANA/ICN Code of Ethics and Mission. • The focus on primary health care and mental health provide numerous opportunities for APRNs to practice collaboratively in both areas. • With the expansion of Medicaid recipient base under the ACA and health exchanges, the extent of implications for nursing are related to the need to ensure Medicaid reimbursement for NP services. Without parity in provider reimbursement, the potential to expand access to care to this growing population of insured will not be realized fully. • The focus on corralling costs in the health care system while improving access to care provides opportunities for nurses in leadership and practice, including innovation in practice models. These opportunities are further enhanced by the the Center for Quality Improvement and Patient Safety (in AHRQ) research focus, affording nurses opportunities in leadership, research, quality practice improvement, and innovation.

Adapted with permission from the American Nurses Association. (2010). *ANA policy & provisions of health reform law April 27, 2010*. Retrieved from http://nursingworld.org/MainMenuCategories/Policy-%09Advocacy/HealthSystemReform/Policy-and-Health-Reform-Law.pdf.

6. Enhanced Medicaid payments to primary care physicians to 100% Medicare rate; however, this excludes primary care APRNs

7. Mental Health Parity, with a variety of Medicaid payment and program innovations to promote it

8. Requirement for Medicaid to cover tobacco cessation programs for pregnant women

Other federal oversight regulations include establishment of the Federal Coordinated Health Care Office; the Patient Centered Outcomes Research Institute; Centers for Quality Improvement and Patient Safety (in AHRQ) to monitor quality and safety from a variety of vantage points; and a few federal offices to stimulate a focus on health promotion and illness prevention (the National Prevention, Health Promotion, and Public Health Council; Prevention and Public Health Fund; and task forces on Preventive Services and Community and Preventive Services). Additionally, the Secretary of HHS was delegated to establish a national quality improvement strategy through a variety of measures and coalitions, of which ANA is often a member (ANA, 2010). Included in these is updating of provider-level national quality measures, which could ultimately lead to implementation of National Database of Nursing Quality Indicators (ANA, 2010). Finally, there are several regulations related to increased federal funding and loan repayment options, primarily through Title V, to promote growth in the primary care workforce, most of which have been summarized in previous sections of this appendix. The National Health Care Workforce Commission was also established to monitor the adequacy of the workforce to meet the growing needs of the expanding roster of insured.

STATE EXCHANGES

State-based health insurance exchanges are a major component of Title I of the ACA. They will enable individuals, families, and small employers to shop for coverage in a competitive marketplace. States are required to begin enrollment through exchanges by October 1, 2013 and have fully operational exchanges by January 1, 2014. States can either partner with the federal government to operate the exchange, default to a federally-facilitated exchange, or create their own exchange, provided it meets or exceeds the federal government's minimum coverage standards.

As of May 2013, 16 states along with the District of Columbia have received conditional permission from the HHS to establish a state-based marketplace, and 7 states are planning to implement a state-federal partnership exchange. Another 26 states have decided not to pursue a state-based marketplace and will likely default to a federally facilitated exchange (KFF, 2013a).

All exchanges must be accessible to potential enrollees via telephone, in person, and online. Nurses can play a key role in educating the public about the exchanges because informing the public about this opportunity for insurance coverage is a major challenge for the states and the federal government.

THIRD-PARTY PAYERS

Regulations imposed on third-party payers include:

1. No discrimination based on an employee's wages, health status, medical condition or history, claims experience, genetic information, disability, or evidence of insurability, as well as other factors HHS deems

2. Insurance rating variability only on age, family composition, geographic location, and tobacco use, with no rating based on health or gender

3. Medicaid expanded to all individuals under age 65 at 133% of the federal poverty level (FPL)

4. Third-party payers being required to cover dependents up until the age of 26 years

5. Full coverage, without co-pay, extended to preventive services, including most screening tests and contraceptive methods, with a waiver of that last aspect for payers furnishing coverage to religiously observant organizations and employers

6. Quality reporting to HHS being required in relation to coverage benefits and health care provider reimbursement structures that carry out patient safety initiatives through utilization of best clinical practices, evidence-based medicine, and health information technologies (ANA, 2010)

EMPLOYERS

Employers with more than 50 employees are mandated to provide "minimal essential benefits" (ANA, 2010, p. 6) to its employees, and employers with more than 200 employees are mandated to automatically enroll new employees into third-party plans. There are penalties for noncompliance with these regulations. Employers are also permitted to award participation in wellness programs (ANA, 2010; McDonough, 2011).

HEALTH CARE DELIVERY MODELS: AFFORDABLE CARE ORGANIZATIONS

There are several regulations that pertain to the eligibility, implementation, and quality monitoring of affordable care organizations (ACOs). The rule links the percentage of shared savings an ACO is eligible to receive to its quality standards performance. The quality measures on which the ACO is graded are in five key areas that impact the beneficiary's care:

1. Patient/caregiver experience of care
2. Care coordination
3. Patient safety
4. Preventive health
5. At-risk population/frail elderly health

There is a defined set of performance standards and a scoring procedure in the regulation, including a methodology to account for more complex patients (U.S. Department of Health and Human Services [USDHHS], 2012). Eligibility to be a member ACO that participates in the Shared Savings Program is dependent on the ACO's agreement to the following conditions:

1. Accountability to quality, cost, and complete care of its assigned Medicare beneficiaries
2. A 3-year commitment to participate in the program
3. Development of a legal structure to manage shared savings receipt and distribution
4. An adequate primary care workforce to care for the assigned number of beneficiaries
5. Submission of all required data and documentation to HHS
6. A management structure encompassing both clinical and administrative structures
7. Policies and procedures to implement evidence-based and coordinated care
8. Meeting of all patient-centered care standards
9. Requirements to provide certain notices to beneficiaries (Correia, 2011; USDHHS, 2012)

Although there are no rules directly assigned to them, federally qualified health centers are strongly impacted by many of the ACA regulations (National Association of Community Health Centers, 2012).

INDIVIDUAL MANDATE

Come January of 2014, individuals (and their dependents) will be required to be protected by "essential coverage" (ANA, 2010, p. 6). The only allowable exemptions will be for hardship and religious reasons.

The state exchanges are meant to provide competition among third-party plans to promote affordability (ANA, 2010).

OVERALL COST OF THE ACA

At the time the ACA was signed into law, scorekeepers estimated the net cost of the ACA to equal $940 billion. The Congressional Budget Office estimated that Title I and Title II, if fully implemented, would have a total gross cost of $974 billion ($540 and $434 billion, respectively). However, Titles III and IX were projected to bring over $800 billion in savings and revenues to offset this cost (McDonough, 2011). The final cost of the ACA will largely depend on the final implementation of the law and how closely it follows and resembles the original legislation.

COST FOR INDIVIDUALS AND HOUSEHOLDS

For individuals and families who do not fall under the Medicaid expansion (133% of the FPL and below), there are both premium tax credits and cost-sharing assistance available to lower the financial burden of purchasing health insurance. Subsidies for purchasing health insurance go into effect in January 2014 alongside the roll out of state health exchanges. Premium tax credits are available to all individuals and families with incomes between 100% and 400% of the FPL. In 2013, 100% FPL was $23,000 for a family of four, and 400% FPL was $94,000 for a family of four. Additionally, the ACA provides cost-sharing assistance for individuals and households with incomes under 250% FPL ($59,000 and under for a family of four in 2013). Families and individuals have the option to purchase four types of plans—bronze, silver, gold, and platinum—on the state exchange market. Coverage and benefits in these plans vary, with bronze plans beings the least comprehensive, and platinum plans being the most comprehensive. All premium credits are tax credits and will be delivered in advance directly to the insurers that a family or individual chooses in the health exchange. The remaining balance will be the responsibility of the family or individual. As an example, a family of four with an income of $47,000 that purchases a silver plan will end up paying approximately $247 a month to cover the entire family after factoring in premium credits and cost-sharing assistance (Angeles, 2013).

POLITICAL AND IMPLEMENTATION CHALLENGES

As stated above, the ACA provides subsidies to individuals and households with incomes between 100% and 400% FPL to purchase health insurance under the state exchanges. Those below 100% FPL do not receive subsidies for health insurance under the law because this population would be covered through Medicaid expansion. The Supreme Court's decision has given states the option to opt-out of the ACA Medicaid expansion and, as of June 2013, 20 states have confirmed that they will not be participating in Medicaid expansion; 8 states continue to debate the expansion (KFF, 2013). As a result, the very poorest populations living in noncompliant states will be left without support and without affordable health insurance options (Pear, 2013). As an example, Texas, a state that has refused to expand Medicaid, will leave 1.3 million uninsured people without viable health insurance options. In Florida, another nonparticipating state, 1 million people will be left without support (Kenney, Dubay, Zuckerman, & Huntress, 2012). Furthermore, the lack of Medicaid expansion in noncompliant states will have an even greater impact on rural communities where people are more likely to live in poverty and less likely to have employer-sponsored health coverage (Mueller, Coburn, Lundblad, MacKinney, McBride, & Watson, 2012). While many noncompliant states suggest that Medicaid expansion would overwhelm state budgets, independent and nonpartisan analysis has shown that states would have an incremental cost of only 0.3% ($8 billion) more between 2013 and 2022 if they implement the ACA's Medicaid expansion than they would without it (Holahan, Buettgens, Carroll, & Dorn, 2012).

In addition, polling suggests that the general public has a distinct lack of awareness and understanding of the ACA. According to a recent KFF (2013b) poll, 57% of individuals stated that they did not feel they had enough information about the ACA to understand how it will impact them personally. When filtered by income, this percentage increased to 68% for those with household incomes less than $40,000 (KFF, 2013b). Public awareness and understanding has been a challenge since the onset of the ACA's passage through Congress (McDonough, 2011). Increasing public awareness and decreasing the amount of misinformation regarding the ACA through mainstream media will be critical to the ACA's long-term success.

CONCLUSION

After a lengthy historical build-up and a few unsuccessful attempts at health care reform in the United States, the socio-political landscape was finally receptive and conducive to significant transformation. In 2010, President Obama successfully passed the ACA through Congress, and the ACA subsequently survived legal threats in the Supreme Court. Although there may be revisions throughout the period of implementation of this landmark legislation, the ACA holds promise to increase access to care; change the culture of health care from one of cure to one of health promotion and illness prevention; mitigate barriers to practice for primary care providers of all disciplines; capitalize on the skill and expertise of nursing in areas of leadership, practice, research, and innovation; and, through these mechanisms, improve population health outcomes. The challenge for nursing is to rise to the call and seize this moment of opportunity in becoming the leaders in health care that so many already recognize they should be. Understanding the reforms and realizing the potential implications to nursing are the first steps in achieving these roles.

REFERENCES

American Academy of Family Physicians. (n.d.). *The Patient Protection and Affordable Care Act implementation timeline.* Retrieved from http://www.aafp.org/online/etc/medialib/aafp_org/documents/policy/fed/hcr-timeline.Par.0001.File.dat/timeline.pdf.

American Academy of Nursing. (2010). *Implementing health care reform: Issues for nursing.* Washington, DC. Retrieved from http://http://www.aannet.org/assets/docs/implementinghealthcarereform.pdf.

American Association of Colleges of Nursing. (2012). *New AACN data show an enrollment surge in baccalaureate and graduate programs amid calls for more highly educated nurses.* Retrieved from: http://www.aacn.nche.edu/news/articles/2012/enrollment-data.

American Association of Nurse Practitioners. (2013a). *Provide sufficient funding for nurse practitioner education programs.* Retrieved from http://www.aanp.org/images/documents/federal-legislation/issuebriefs/Issue%20Brief%20-%20Provide%20Sufficient%20Funding.pdf.

American Association of Nurse Practitioners. (2013b). *Recognize NP practices as medicare shared savings accountable care organizations.* Retrieved from http://www.aanp.org/images/documents/federal-legislation/issuebriefs/Issue%20Brief%20-%20Recognize%20NP%20Practices.pdf.

American Nurses Association. (2010a). *ANA policy & provisions of health reform law April 27, 2010.* Retrieved from http://nursingworld.org/MainMenuCategories/Policy-%09Advocacy/HealthSystemReform/Policy-and-Health-Reform-Law.pdf.

American Nurses Association. (2010b). *Health care transformation: The Affordable Care Act and more—Nursing education and workforce.* Retrieved from http://www.nursingworld.org/MainMenuCategories/Policy-Advocacy/HealthSystemReform/AffordableCareAct.pdf.

American Nurses Association. (2013). *ANA working to ensure full contributions of RNs on 2nd anniversary of Affordable Care Act.* Retrieved from http://nursingworld.org/MainMenuCategories/Policy-Advocacy/HealthSystemReform/ANA-on-2nd-Anniversary-of-Affordable-Care-Act.html.

Angeles, J. (2013). Making health care more affordable: The New Premium and Cost-Sharing Assistance. Center on Budget and Policy Priorities. Retrieved from http://www.cbpp.org/cms/?fa=view&id=3190.

Centers for Medicare and Medicaid. (2011). Payment for certified nurse-midwife services. *MLN Matters.* Retrieved from http://www.cms.gov/Outreach-and-Education/Medicare-Learning-Network-MLN/MLNMattersArticles/downloads/mm7005.pdf.

Commonwealth Fund. (2011). *Realizing health reform's potential: How the affordable care act will strengthen primary care and benefit patients, providers, and payers.* Retrieved from http://www.commonwealthfund.org/~/media/Files/Publications/Issue%20Brief/2011/Jan/1466_Abrams_howACA_will_strengthen_primary_care_reform_brief_v3.pdf.

Correia, E. W. (2011). Accountable care organizations: The proposed regulations and the prospects for success. *American Journal of Managed Care, 17*(8), 560–568.

Fairman, U., Rowe, J. W., Hassmiller, S. & Shalala, D. E. (2011). Broadening the scope of nursing practice. *New England Journal of Medicine, 364,* 193–196.

Flinter, M. (2012). From new nurse practitioner to primary care provider: Bridging the transition through FQHC-based residency training. *Online Journal of Issues In Nursing, 17*(1), 1. doi:10.3912/OJIN.Vol17No01PPT04.

Gable, L. (2011). The Patient Protection and Affordable Care Act, public health, and the elusive target of human rights. *Journal of Law, Medicine, and Ethics, 39*(3), 340–354.

Henry, J., Kaiser Family Foundation. (2009). *National health insurance—A brief history of reform efforts in the U. S.* Retrieved from http://kaiserfamilyfoundation.files.wordpress.com/2013/01/7871.pdf.

Henry, J., Kaiser Family Foundation. (2013a) *Establishing health insurance marketplaces: An overview of state efforts.* Retrieved from http://kff.org/health-reform/issue-brief/establishing-health-insurance-exchanges-an-overview-of/.

Henry, J., Kaiser Family Foundation. (2013b). *Majority say they don't understand how ACA will impact them, including two-thirds of uninsured and low-income.* Retrieved from http://kff.org/health-reform/slide/majority-say-they-dont-understand-how-aca-will-impact-them-including-two-thirds-of-uninsured-and-low-income-2/.

Holahan, J., Buettgens, M., Carroll, C., & Dorn, S. (2012, November). *The cost and coverage implications of the ACA Medicaid expansion: National and state-by-state analysis.* The Kaiser Commission on Medicaid and the Uninsured &The Urban Institute. Retrieved from http://kaiserfamilyfoundation.files.wordpress.com/2013/01/8384.pdf.

Institute of Medicine. (2010). *Future of nursing: Leading change, advancing health.* Washington, DC: The National Academies Press.

Kenny, G., Dubay, L., Zuckerman, S., & Huntress, M. (2012, July) *Opting out of the Medicaid Expansion under the ACA: How many uninsured adults would not be eligible for Medicaid?* The Kaiser Commission on Medicaid and the Uninsured & The Urban Institute. Retrieved from http://www.urban.org/UploadedPDF/412607-Opting-Out-of-the-Medicaid-Expansion-Under-the-ACA.pdf.

McDonough, J. E. (2011). *Inside national health reform.* Los Angeles: University of California Press.

Mueller K., Coburn, A., Lundblad, J., MacKinney, A., McBride, T., & Watson, S. (2012, September). *The current and future role and impact of Medicaid in rural health.* Rural Policy Research Institute. Retrieved from http://www.rupri.org/Forms/HealthPanel_Medicaid_Sept2012.pdf.

National Association of Community Health Centers. (2012). *Final Medicaid and exchange regulations: Implications for federally qualified health centers.* Retrieved from http://www.nachc.org/client/documents/4.12%20IB%20-%20MCD%20and%20Exchange%20Final%20Rules%20-%20FINAL.pdf.

National Federation of Independent Business et al. v. Sebelius, Secretary of Health and Human Services, et al., 567 U.S. __ (2012).

Newhouse, R. P., Stanik-Hutt, J., White, K. M., Johantgen, M., Bass, E. B., Zangara, G., ... Weiner, J. P. (2011). Advanced practice nurse outcomes 1990-2008: A systematic review. *Nursing Economics 29*(5),1-21.

Pear, R. (2012). Court's ruling may blunt reach of the health law. *New York Times.* Retrieved from http://www.nytimes.com/2012/07/25/health/policy/3-million-more-may-lack-insurance-due-to-ruling-study-says.html.

Pear, R. (2013). States' policies on health care exclude some of the poorest. *New York Times.* Retrieved from http://www.nytimes.com/2013/05/25/us/states-policies-on-health-care-exclude-poorest.html.

Physicians for a National Health Program. (2011). *Number of uninsured climbs to highest figure since passage of Medicare, Medicaid.* Retrieved from http://www.pnhp.org/news/2011/september/number-of-uninsured-climbs-to-highest-figure-since-passage-of-medicare-medicaid.

U. S. Department of Health and Human Services. (2012). *Accountable care organizations: Improving care coordination for people with Medicare.* Retrieved from http://www.healthcare.gov/news/factsheets/2011/03/accountablecare03312011a.html.

White House. (n.d.) *Affordable Care Act: The new health care law at two years.* Retrieved from http://www.whitehouse.gov/sites/default/files/uploads/careact.pdf.

Wilper, A., Woolhandler, S., Lasser, K. E., McCormick, D., Bor, D. H., & Himmelstein, D. U. (2009). Health insurance and mortality in U.S. adults. *American Journal of Public Health, 99*(12), 2289–2295.

Health Policy Internships and Fellowships

Johnnie Sue Cooper

Name of Program	Type	Qualifications	Financial Data	Location/Duration	Application Requests
AARP/AAN Joint Fellowship	Prepares nurse leaders to play a more prominent role in national health policy development.	Must be a Fellow of the American Academy of Nursing and must demonstrate interest/experience in the area of aging.	$75,000 stipend (as well as in-kind support of office space at AARP, computer, phone, and so on).	AARP offices in Washington, DC. Duration is 1 year.	Manager, Policy & Development American Academy of Nursing 888 17th Street NW, Suite 800 Washington, DC 20006 Phone: 202-777-1178 Main Phone: 202-777-1170 Website: www.aannet.org
AcademyHealth	For health services research that has made a positive impact on health policy and/or practice.	Graduate students, postdoctoral students, and professionals.	$2000 award.	No specific location.	AcademyHealth 1150 17th Street NW, Suite 600 Washington, DC 20036 E-mail: awards@academyhealth.org Website: www.academyhealth.org/files/awards/NominationPacket.pdf
Albert Schweitzer Fellowship	For graduate students in health-related professional fields dedicated to addressing unmet health needs.	Graduate students in health-related professional fields who are dedicated to addressing unmet health needs in their local areas.	Stipends range from $2000 to $3000 depending on region.	Baltimore, San Francisco Bay area, Boston, Chicago, greater Philadelphia, Los Angeles, New Hampshire, Vermont, North Carolina, New Orleans, and Pittsburgh.	National Program Director Albert Schweitzer Fellowship 330 Brookline Avenue (BR) Boston, MA 02215 Phone: 617-667-3115 Website: www.schweitzerfellowship.org
Alliance Health Reform Internship	Focuses on health policy research and media relations.	Undergraduate and graduate students with solid academic records; strong writing, research, and communication skills; and an interest in public policy.	A small stipend may be available, and academic credit can be arranged.	Washington, DC. Duration is negotiable, but for best experience, interns should stay for a minimum of 1 quarter. Academic credit can be arranged.	Alliance for Health Reform Director of Operations 1444 Eye Street NW, Suite 910 Washington, DC 20005 Website: www.allhealth.org/aboutus_internships.asp

Name of Program	Type	Qualifications	Financial Data	Location/Duration	Application Requests
American Public Health Association International Health Internship	Provides an opportunity to gain hands-on experience and insight into the dynamic role of science in public health.	Undergraduate students, graduate students, postgraduate students, and fellows.	Unpaid, but interns are provided with administrative support.	Several terms; see website for more information.	APHA Fellowship Program American Public Health Association 800 I Street NW Washington, DC 20001-3710 Website: www.apha.org/ advocacy/fellowship
ASPIRA Public Policy Internship	Provides an opportunity for interns to work with public and health policy issues that affect and are important to the Hispanic community and to gain experience in a national nonprofit setting.	Undergraduate students and graduate students.	Spring and fall internships are unpaid; academic credit is available.	Interns are accepted throughout the year.	ASPIRA Association 1444 Eye Street NW, 8th Floor Washington, DC 20005 Website: www.aspira.org/ manuals/internships-fellowships
Australian-American Health Policy Fellowship, Packer Policy Fellowships	For outstanding, mid-career U.S. policy researchers and practitioners to conduct original research and work with policy experts in Australia.	Mid-career health policy researchers and practitioners.	Provides up to $55,000 (AUD).	Australia. Duration is 6 to 10 months; a minimum stay of 6 months is required. Application deadline is August 15.	Robin Osborn Vice President and Director International Program in Health Policy and Practice The Commonwealth Fund 1 East 75th Street New York, NY 10021-2692 Website: www. commonwealthfund.org/ fellowships
Barbara Jordan Health Policy Scholars Program	Allows scholars to gain knowledge about federal legislative procedure and health policy issues and to develop critical-thinking and leadership skills.	Undergraduate students or recent graduates. Professional school or graduate students are not eligible.	Scholars receive approximately $7500 in support, which includes a stipend of $2000. Academic credit is available for students of Howard University.	Washington, DC. Annual 9-week program from late May to late July. Applications are accepted in the fall before the summer program.	Barbara Jordan Health Policy Scholars Program, Kaiser Family Foundation 2400 Sand Hill Road Menlo Park, CA 94025 E-mail: bjscholars@howard.edu Website: www.kff.org/ minorityhealth/bjscholars/ index.cfm
Bazelon Mental Health Law Policy and Research Internship	Provides an opportunity to work with leading national legal-advocacy organization representing people with mental disabilities.	Individuals with strong analytic, research, and computer skills. The ideal candidate thrives on independence with an interest in health policy research.	Interns will be paid $12 per hour. This is not a legal research position.	Varying times throughout the year.	Bazelon Center for Mental Health Law Policy and Research Internships 1101 15th Street NW, Suite 1212 Washington, DC 20005-5002 Website: www.bazelon.org/ about/intern/policy.htm

Name of Program	Type	Qualifications	Financial Data	Location/Duration	Application Requests
Cecil G. Sheps Postdoctoral and Predoctoral Fellowship Program in Health Services Research and Policy Analysis	University of North Carolina at Chapel Hill offers predoctoral- and postdoctoral-level training in health care research and policy analysis for qualified candidates.	Individuals who have completed the requirements for all relevant doctoral degrees for postdoctoral fellowship. Must be considered in final year of graduate study to begin predoctoral fellowship.	Annual stipend set by the AHRQ is based on the number of years of relevant experience beyond the doctoral degree.	Chapel Hill, North Carolina. Duration is 1 to 2 years. Deadline for receipt of application is February 15 of each year.	Cecil G. Sheps Center for Health Services and Research, UNC 725 Airport Road, Campus Box 7590 Chapel Hill, NC 27599-7590 Website: *www.shepscenter.unc. edu/training_programs/ nrsaprepost.html* Other current information can be found at *www.ahrq.gov*
Center for Medicare Advocacy (CMA) Health Policy Internship	Provides an opportunity for law students and health policy students to engage in activities such as research, writing, and attending hearings and briefings on Capitol Hill.	Individuals who have completed at least 1 year of law school or an equivalent graduate program.	Summer internships come with a small stipend; those during the school year are for academic credit only.	Washington, DC. Summer internship lasts 8 to 10 weeks, during which students are expected to commit to a 40-hour workweek. Academic internships are also available for academic credit during the school year.	Center for Medicare Advocacy 1025 Connecticut Avenue NW, Suite 709 Washington, DC 20036 Website: *www. medicareadvocacy.org/ AboutUs/CareerOpps_Intern. htm* Summer applications are accepted on a rolling basis.
Center on Budget and Policy Priorities Health Policy Internship	Provides an opportunity to work with a leading national organization on public policy debates about Medicaid, child health insurance, and other health care issues that affect low- and moderate-income families.	Individuals with a demonstrated interest in health care policy and quantitative analytic skills. Must have an ability to work with spreadsheets. Knowledge of statistics is a plus.	Pay based on education.	Washington, DC. Duration is 1 semester.	Coordinator, Center on Budget and Policy Priorities 820 1st Street NE, Suite 510 Washington, DC 20002 E-mail: *internship@cbpp.org* Website: *www.cbpp.org/cms/ index.cfm?fa=view&id=2719*
Congressional Black Caucus Foundation's Louis Stokes Urban Health Policy Fellows Program	Provides a policy training and leadership development program that targets early to mid-level policy professionals who are committed to eliminating national and global health disparities.	Graduate or professional degree in a health-related field from an accredited institution completed prior to fellowship start date. Work experience may be substituted for educational requirements.	Compensation is $40,000 with benefits. Fellows are responsible for their own travel, housing, and other associated expenses.	Washington, DC. Duration is 12 months beginning in late August.	Congressional Black Caucus Foundation 1004 Pennsylvania Avenue SE Washington, DC 20003 Website: *www.cbcfinc.org/ images/pdf/Louis%20 Stokes%20Fellows%20 Program.%20Application.2009. pdf*

Continued

Name of Program	Type	Qualifications	Financial Data	Location/Duration	Application Requests
Congressional Budget Office Health Policy Intern	Health and Human Resources Division provides Congress with analyses in the areas of health, income security, education, and employment.	Ideal candidates are pursuing a graduate degree in economics, public health, health policy, or related discipline and desire to work in the analysis of the economic and budgetary impact of health-related issues.	Salary range based on education level and includes transportation.	Washington, DC. Fall semester.	Human Resources Congressional Budget Office Ford House Office Building, Room 410 Second and D Streets SW Washington, DC 20515 E-mail: *jobs@cbo.gov* Website: *www.cbo.gov/ employment/intern.cfm*
David A. Winston Fellowship	Provides a unique opportunity to learn about the political system through direct exposure to public and private sector roles in health policy development.	Graduate students from any program, department, or university that is a member of the Association of University Programs in Health Administration (AUPHA).	Monthly stipend and related expense provided for 12-month period of July through June.	Washington, DC. Duration is 1 year, beginning in July.	Dennis Morgan, AUPHA 2000 14th Street N, Suite 780 Arlington, VA 22201 E-mail: *winston@aupha.org* Website: *www. winstonfellowship.org*
Deland Fellowship in Health Care and Society, Brigham and Women's Hospital	Annual fellowship awarded to accomplished individuals who aspire to shape the future of health care delivery.	Candidates come from business, law, economics, public policy, and medicine. Must have an advanced degree.	Salary and benefits package, commensurate with experience. Reimbursement is provided for one health care conference of choice during the 12-month program.	Boston, Massachusetts. Based at Brigham and Women's Hospital; 1-year graduate fellowship.	Deland Fellowship Program Brigham and Women's Hospital 75 Francis Street Boston, MA 02115 Website: *www. brighamandwomens.org/ DelandFellowship/application. aspx*
Families USA: Health Policy Department Internship	Interns participate in regular internal seminars on key health policy issues and attend congressional hearings and policy briefings outside the office.	Strong research, writing, and computer skills are essential. Health care policy knowledge is a plus. Preference is given to law, MPH, and MPP students, although undergraduates may apply.	Interns are paid $7 per hour and normally work 40 hours per week.	Washington, DC. Duration is 1 semester.	Internship and Fellowship Program Director Families USA Foundation 1201 New York Avenue NW, Suite 1100 Washington, DC 20005. E-mail: *internship@familiesusa. org* Website (for application details): *www.familiesusa.org/about/ about-internship-opportunities. html*

Name of Program	Type	Qualifications	Financial Data	Location/Duration	Application Requests
Families USA: Villers Fellowship for Health Care Justice	Inspires and develops the next generation of health care justice leaders.	Demonstrated commitment to social and health care justice advocacy following their year of hands-on experience as a fellow. Fellows must also commit to mentoring at least one person.	Annual salary of approximately $35,000 and excellent health care benefits. One Villers Fellow is selected each year.	Washington, DC. Duration is 1 year from August through July of the following year. Application deadline is early February.	Families USA Villers Fellowship 1201 New York Avenue NW, Suite 1100 Washington, DC 20005 Website: *www.familiesusa.org/ fellowships/the-villers-fellowship.html*
Families USA: Wellstone Fellowship for Social Justice	Fosters the advancement of social justice through participation in health care advocacy work that focuses on the challenges facing many communities of color.	Interest in health care policy as a tool for reducing racial and ethnic health disparities and a commitment to contributing to social justice work after fellowship completion.	Annual salary of approximately $35,000 and excellent health care benefits. One Wellstone Fellow is selected each year.	Washington, DC. Duration is 1 year from August through July of the following year. Application deadline is early February.	Families USA Wellstone Fellowship 1201 New York Avenue NW, Suite 1100 Washington, DC 20005 Website: *www.familiesusa.org/ fellowships/wellstone-fellowship.html*
Greenwall Fellowship Program in Bioethics and Health Policy	Interdisciplinary fellowship program provides fellowship and faculty development and training in bioethics and health policy.	Doctoral degree in medicine (MD), philosophy (PhD), or law (JD or LLB). Fellows with doctoral degrees in public health, biomedical sciences, religious studies, social sciences, and nursing have also been accepted.	Two-year financial package of $122,003 includes health insurance for both years.	Washington, DC. Three 2-year postdoctoral fellowship positions beginning in September annually. Application deadline is December 1.	Greenwall Fellowship Program in Bioethics and Health Policy The Johns Hopkins Berman Bioethics Institute Johns Hopkins University 624 North Broadway Hampton House 352 Baltimore, MD 21205 Website: *www.bioethicsinstitute. org/web/page/408/ sectionid/378/interior.asp*
Harkness Fellowships in Health Care Policy and Practice	Fellows work with leading U.S. experts to conduct a research study that addresses a critical issue on the health policy agenda in both the U.S. and New Zealand.	Must be a citizen of NZ, AU, DE, NL, NO, SE, or UK. Master's or doctorate is required in health care services, health policy research, or a related discipline.	Up to $107,000 for airfare, U.S. living expenses, setup and shipping allowances, and support toward the portion of the project conducted in home country.	United States. Duration minimum is 7 months, with a maximum of 12 months, beginning in August-September of the year after applicant applies.	The Commonwealth Fund 1 East 75th Street New York, NY 10021 E-mail: *grants@cmwf.org* Website: *www. commonwealthfund.org/ Fellowships/Harkness-Fellowships/Harkness-Application.aspx*

Continued

Name of Program	Type	Qualifications	Financial Data	Location/Duration	Application Requests
Health and Human Services Emerging Leaders Program	Intended for the best of those eager to make contributions to HHS.	Must be a U.S. citizen. Must have a bachelor's degree, master's degree, JD, or PhD with one or more majors in scientific, public health, administrative, social sciences, or information technology studies.	Those selected are hired at the GS-9 level. At the end of the program, graduates are advanced to a GS12 level. (See the federal salary pay scale on the HHS website.)	Two-year program structure with devoted work in chosen career path on a full-time basis for the selecting operating division. Interviews held in April; selections made in May; and program begins in July.	ELP Program Coordinator 6010 Executive Boulevard, Suite 400 Rockville, MD 20852 E-mail: *ELP@hhs.gov* Website: *http://hhsu.learning.hhs.gov/elp/*
Helen Rodriguez-Trias Women's Health Leadership Program	Offers a unique 10- to 12-week experience that allows the intern to develop health research skills while exploring the worlds of public policy, health education, and feminist organizing.	Undergraduate and graduate students. Students of color and those with disabilities are encouraged to apply. Must submit 3- to 5-page writing sample.	Internships are full-time, and interns work 32 hours per week between 9:00 AM and 5:30 PM.	Washington, DC. Internships are available year-round and typically last 10 to 12 weeks.	Internship Coordinator National Women's Health Network 514 10th Street NW, Suite 400 Washington, DC 20004 E-mail: *nwhn@nwhn.org* Website: *http://nwhn.org/about*
Institute of Medicine (IOM), American Nurses Foundation (ANF), American Academy of Nursing (AAN) Scholar in Residence Program	Designed as an immersion experience to facilitate nurse leaders playing a more prominent role in health policy development at the national level.	Must have membership in the AAN and/or the IOM and have a congruent health policy interest with the priorities of the IOM and the AAN.	This carries an annual stipend of $50,000. An office at IOM with appropriate supports. A 2-month orientation in federal health policy formation.	Washington, DC. One year, annually beginning the day after Labor Day. Application deadline is April 30.	Contact: Beach Lagassa Phone: 202-777-1176 E-mail: *blagassa@aannet.org* Website: *www.aannet.org/i4a/headlines/headlinedetails.cfm?id=129&archive=1*
Joseph P. Kennedy Foundation Professional Public Policy Program	Fellows spend 1 year in Washington, DC, learning about the policymaking process that affects the rights of intellectually disabled people on a national level.	Mid-career professionals with significant disability policy experience.	Stipend and modest relocation expenses.	Washington, DC. One year. Start date is August of each year.	Professional Public Policy Fellowship Program The Joseph P. Kennedy, Jr. Foundation, 1010 Wayne Avenue, Suite 650 Silver Spring, MD 20910 Website: *www.jpkf.org/Fellowship_guidelines/Professional_Fellow_app.html*

Name of Program	Type	Qualifications	Financial Data	Location/Duration	Application Requests
Kellogg Health Scholars Program	Develops new leadership in the effort to reduce and eliminate health disparities and to secure equal access to the conditions and services essential for achieving healthy communities.	Doctoral-level degree from one of a variety of disciplines. Need not have engaged in previous work in health disparities, or produced a health-oriented dissertation.	Annual stipend of $63,000 in the first year and $64,000 in the second year, including fringe benefits and an annual research fund of $10,000.	Consists of two tracks (Community Track and Multidisciplinary Track). Offers 2-year postdoctoral fellowships at four training sites.	Kellogg Health Scholars Program Center for Advancing Health 2000 Florida Avenue NW, Suite 210 Washington, DC 20009-1231 E-mail: *healthscholars@cfah.org* Community Track Program Office Kellogg Health Scholars Program University of Michigan School of Public Health 109 Observatory Street Ann Arbor, MI 48109-2029 Website: *www.kellogghealthscholars.org*
National Center for Health Statistics (NCHS)/Academy Health Policy Fellowship	On-site fellowship at NCHS.	Applicants must demonstrate training or experience in health services research and may be at any stage in their career from doctoral students to senior investigators. Doctoral students must be in dissertation phase of study.	Salaries are commensurate with qualifications and experience and range from $43,365 to $135,136.	Hyattsville, Maryland. Duration for full-time fellowship is 13 to 24 months. Fellowship begins each September.	NCHS/Academy Health Fellowship Academy Health 1150 17th Street NW, Suite 600 Washington, DC 20036 Website: *www.academyhealth.org/nchs/program.htm*
National Consumer League Health Policy Intern	Provides an opportunity to gain knowledge about current health policy issues within the setting of a national nonprofit advocacy group.	Requires a high level of oral and written communication skills. Interns are frequently called on to write brief reports for NCL staff.	The League is able to offer a stipend when grant funding allows.	Washington, DC. Minimum commitment is 8 weeks, spending at least 20 hours per week working at the League. Longer commitments are welcome.	Health Policy Intern National Consumer League 1701 K Street NW, Suite 1200 Washington, DC 20006 Fax: 202-835-0747 E-mail: *intern@nclnet.org* Website: *www.nclnet.org/employment/108-health-policy-intern-part-time*
Nurse in Washington Internship (NIWI)	Three-day intensive learning experience that culminates in a trip to Capitol Hill for visits with senators and representatives.	Open to registered nurses and student nurses interested in better understanding health policy and the legislative and regulatory process.	A full scholarship for the internship is offered by Elsevier/Saunders, publishers and editors of this book. Some specialty nursing organizations fund attendance for their officers and boards.	Washington, DC. Three days in early spring.	Alliance Headquarters Offices Phone: 859-514-9157 E-mail: *alliance@AMRms.com* Website: *www.nursing-alliance.org/content.cfm/id/niwi?CFID=491612878&CFTOKEN=63400945#info*

Continued

Name of Program	Type	Qualifications	Financial Data	Location/Duration	Application Requests
Robert Wood Johnson Executive Nurse Fellowship	An advanced leadership program for nurses in senior executive roles in health services, public health, and nursing education who aspire to help lead and shape the U.S. health care system.	Open to senior-level nurses who hold executive positions in health services organizations, public health organizations and systems, and nursing education.	Fellowship resources of $35,000 over 3 years.	The 3-year fellowships allow participating nurses to remain in their current positions while they gain the experiences, insights, competencies, and skills necessary to advance in executive leadership positions in a health care system that is undergoing unprecedented change.	The Center for the Health Professions, Program Assistant University of California, San Francisco Website: *www.enfp-info.org*
Robert Wood Johnson Health Policy Fellows	Provides the nation's most comprehensive experience at the nexus of health science, policy, and politics in Washington, DC.	Exceptional candidates from academic faculties and nonprofit health care organizations are encouraged to apply. Applicants may have backgrounds in allied health professions, health services organization/ administration, medicine, nursing, public health, or social/ behavioral health.	Each fellow will receive up to $94,000 for the Washington stay (September 1 through August 31 of the following year) in salary plus fringe benefits or fellowship stipend.	A 12-month residential experience in Washington, DC, with continued health policy leadership development activities. Applications posted in mid-September.	The Robert Wood Johnson Health Policy Fellows Institute of Medicine The National Academies 500 5th Street NW Washington, DC 20001 Website: *www. healthpolicyfellows.org*

Name of Program	Type	Qualifications	Financial Data	Location/Duration	Application Requests
Society for Medical Decision Making (SMDM) and the Agency for Healthcare Research and Quality (AHRQ) Health Policy Fellowship	Provides hands-on comparative effectiveness program development and research experience working on intramural and extramural projects within the Effective Healthcare Program at the AHRQ (www.effectivehealthcare.ahrq.gov).	Must be a current member of the SMDM and demonstrate training or experience in medical decision-making, health policy, or health services research.	Salaries commensurate with qualifications and experience and will include salary and benefits.	Residential program in Rockville, Maryland. Duration of the full-time fellowship is 12 months.	Executive Director Society for Medical Decision Making Website: www.smdm.org/documents/2010-2011 SMDMAHRQFellowCallfor Applications_000.pdf Submit electronic application package per website specifications.
Washington Health Policy Institute	Provides an opportunity for individuals from a variety of disciplines to study the current issues confronting health care consumers, providers, and policymakers.	Health care professionals, health organization and association staff, health and policy scholars and educators, and others involved in health policy activities.	The institute fee is $1200 for three graduate credits or four CEUs. Housing is not included.	Washington, DC. Four and one-half day program.	George Mason University The Center for Health Policy and Research Ethics Website: www.gmu.edu/centers/chpre/policyinstitute/instituteinfo.html
White House Fellows Program	One of America's most prestigious programs for leadership and public service. Offers exceptional young men and women first-hand experience working at the highest levels of federal government. The program's mission is to encourage active citizenship and service to the nation.	Must be a U.S. citizen. Must have completed undergraduate education and be working in his or her chosen profession.	Fellows are considered federal employees, with the rank of GS-14 step 3. Salary of approximately $100,000 per year. Military personnel maintain their current salary and benefits.	Washington, DC. Duration runs from August 31 to September 1 of the following year.	Website (for additional application information): www.whitehouse.gov/fellows

Index